S0-BIM-233

TEXTBOOK OF

DIAGNOSTIC ULTRASONOGRAPHY

VOLUME ONE

TEXTBOOK OF

DIAGNOSTIC ULTRASONOGRAPHY

VOLUME ONE

SANDRA L. HAGEN-ANSERT
B.A., RDMS, RDCS

Program Director of Diagnostic Ultrasound, Department of Radiology;

Former Clinical and Research Echocardiographic Sonographer, Pediatric Cardiology Division;

Clinical Neonatal Echoencephalographic Sonographer, Neonatal Support Center,

University of California, San Diego Medical Center, San Diego, California

FOURTH EDITION

with 3,138 illustrations

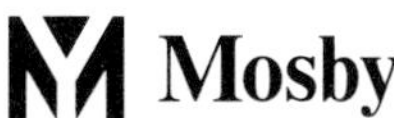

St. Louis Baltimore Boston Chicago London Madrid Philadelphia Sydney Toronto

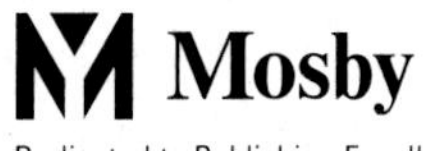

Dedicated to Publishing Excellence

Editor: Jeanne Rowland
Developmental Editor: Lisa Potts
Project Manager: Carol Sullivan Weis
Production Editors: Jennifer J. Byington, Diana Lyn Laulainen
Designer: Betty Schulz

FOURTH EDITION

Printed in the United States of America
Composition by Clarinda Company
Printing/binding by Maple-Vail Book Mfg. Group

Mosby–Year Book, Inc.
11830 Westline Industrial Drive
St. Louis, Missouri 63146

Library of Congress Cataloging in Publication Data
Hagen-Ansert, Sandra L.
Textbook of diagnostic ultrasonography / Sandra L. Hagen-Ansert.—4th ed.
p. cm.
Includes bibliographical references and index.
ISBN 0-8016-7948-6 (set)
1. Diagnosis, Ultrasonic. 2. Echocardiology. I. Title.
II. Title: Diagnostic ultrasonography.
[DNLM: 1. Ultrasonography. WB 289 H143t 1995]
RC78.7.U4H33 1995
616.07′543--dc20
DNLM/DLC 94-22472
for Library of Congress CIP

94 95 96 97 1 9 8 7 6 5 4 3 2 1

Contributors

KARA MAYDEN ARGO, B.S., RDMS, RDCS, RTR
Obstetric Ultrasound Specialist
The West Michigan Perinatal and Genetic Diagnostic Center
Grand Rapids, Michigan;
Assistant Adjunct Professor
Department of Obstetrics and Gynecology and Reproductive Biology
College of Human Medicine
Michigan State University
East Lansing, Michigan

KATHLEEN BAUMAN, RDMS
Department of Radiology/Ultrasound
University of California, San Diego Medical Center
San Diego, California

RAUL BEJAR, M.D.
Division of Neonatal Perinatal Medicine
Department of Pediatrics
University of California, San Diego Medical Center
San Diego, California

FRANK CHERVENAK, M.D.
Professor of Obstetrics and Gynecology
Director of Obstetrics;
Director, Maternal-Fetal Medicine
New York Hospital, Cornell Medical Center
New York, New York

DALE CYR, B.S., RDMS
Chief Sonographer
Diagnostic Ultrasound
Department of Radiology
University of Washington Medical Center;
Clinical Instructor
Department of Diagnostic Ultrasound
Seattle University
Seattle, Washington

SUZANNE DEVINE, RT, RDMS
Chief Sonographer
Division of Ultrasound
Department of Radiology
The Children's Memorial Medical Center
Chicago, Illinois

KATE A. FEINSTEIN, M.D.
Assistant Professor of Radiology
Northwestern University Medical School
Department of Radiology;
The Children's Memorial Medical Center
Department of Radiology
Northwestern Memorial Hospital
Chicago, Illinois

CRIS D. GRESSER, R.N., RDMS
Technical Director, Cardiology
Toronto Hospitals
Toronto, Ontario

SANDRA L. HAGEN-ANSERT, B.A., RDMS, RDCS
Program Director of Diagnostic Ultrasound
Department of Radiology;
Former Clinical and Research Echocardiographic Sonographer
Pediatric Cardiology Division, Neonatal Support Center;
Clinical Neonatal Echoencephalographic Sonographer
University of California, San Diego Medical Center
San Diego, California

OI LING KWAN, B.S., RDCS
Technical Director, Cardiology
Division of Cardiology
University of California, San Diego Medical Center
San Diego, California

DEBORAH LEVINE, M.D.
Imaging Fellow
Department of Radiology/Ultrasound
University of California, San Diego Medical Center
San Diego, California

HOLLY D. LLOYD, B.S., RDMS
Department of Radiology/Ultrasound
University of California, San Diego Medical Center
San Diego, California

LAURENCE A. MACK, M.D.
Professor of Radiology and Obstetrics and Gynecology;
Director, Diagnostic Ultrasound
Department of Radiology
University of Washington Medical Center
Seattle, Washington

HANH VU NGHIEM, M.D.
Assistant Professor
Department of Radiology
University of Washington Medical Center
Seattle, Washington

TRACI PARKER, RDMS
Department of Radiology/Ultrasound
University of California, San Diego Medical Center
San Diego, California

RICHARD E. RAE, RT(R), RDMS, RVT
Technical Director
Vascular Laboratory
Schumacker, Isch, Jolly, Fitzgerald, Fess, Glasser MD's, Inc.
Indianapolis, Indiana

JOANNE C. ROSENBERG, B.S., RDMS
Perinatal Ultrasound Manager
University of Medicine and Dentistry of New Jersey;
Robert Wood Johnson Medical School
St. Peter's Medical School
New Brunswick, New Jersey

ARNOLD SHKOLNIK, M.D.
Professor of Radiology
Northwestern University Medical School;
Head, Division of Ultrasound
Department of Radiology
The Children's Memorial Medical Center
Chicago, Illinois

LAURA J. ZUIDEMA, M.D.
Director, Maternal-Fetal Medicine
The West Michigan Perinatal and Genetic Diagnostic Center
Butterworth Hospital
Grand Rapids, Michigan

WILLIAM J. ZWIEBEL, M.D.
Professor of Radiology
University of Utah School of Medicine;
Chief of Radiology
VA Medical Center
Salt Lake City, Utah

To our own little sonic boomers,
Rebecca, Alyssa, and Katrina.

Foreword

I am once again pleased to offer a foreword for this prestigious text of ultrasonography. It has been several years since the previous edition, and growth in the field is certainly sufficient to warrant a revisit. It is noteworthy that the work now occupies two volumes, attesting to both thoroughness and an expanded knowledge base.

Sandra Hagen-Ansert and her colleagues have proved more than equal to the task. New in this edition are chapters on the gastrointestinal tract, peritoneal cavity, thyroid/parathyroid, and scrotum, complimenting existing chapters on general sonography. Special attention to neonates has resulted in new chapters on cranial, abdominal, and renal sonography. Obstetrical and gynecological sonography has also been enhanced by new offerings in normal anatomy and physiology, as well as embryosonology, congenital anomalies, and fetal echocardiography. The cardiology section offers new material on transesophageal, stress echocardiography, exercise treadmill echocardiography, right heart disease, and ischemia. As with previous editions the quality of the text and illustrations remains very high. The authors are to be commended for their efforts in making a very readable textbook.

The focus of this text has always been on the sonographer actually performing studies. Those who assume this role have an unique relationship with physicians responsible for interpreting sonographical studies. Real-time sonography provides the sonographer with vast amounts of information, most of which is discarded. Final images reaching the physician are a distillation of this information. In a very real sense the sonographer performs diagnosis during the study. Nowhere else in medicine does this relationship exist. Perhaps the closest analogy is in gastrointestinal fluoroscopy, where spot films are made of real-time images, often sacrificing functional information. Technologists perform these studies in virtually *no* institutions. Yet curiously, in these same institutions, sonographers daily churn out complex studies of the heart, abdomen, and pelvis—in my view a far more complex task.

This unique role as a physician's assistant clearly deserves recognition. It requires high-quality instruction, of which this book is an excellent example. It also requires outstanding and dedicated individuals, of which the book's principal author is an excellent example. She and her coauthors are to be congratulated on their success in advancing our knowledge in this discipline.

It is hard to overestimate the number of individuals who have benefited from previous editions of this text. While initially conceived for sonographers, I frequently see it used by sonologists as well. It is my belief that this usage typifies the close relationship between these groups, which is essential for top quality sonography. In this edition, Sandra Hagen-Ansert and her colleagues have once again shown us that through prodigious effort it is still possible to produce a text benefiting all who labor in this vineyard.

GEORGE R. LEOPOLD, M.D.

Preface

A Look Back.

Medicine has always been a fascinating field. I was introduced to it by Dr. Charles Henkelmann, who provided me with the opportunity to learn radiography. Although x-ray technology was interesting, it did not provide the opportunity to evaluate patient history or to follow through interesting cases, which seemed to be the most intriguing aspect of medicine and my primary concern.

Shortly after I finished my training, I was assigned to the radiation therapy department, where I was introduced to a very quiet and young, dedicated radiologist, whom I would later grow to admire and respect as one of the foremost authorities in diagnostic ultrasound. Convincing George Leopold that he needed another hand to assist him was difficult in the beginning, and it was through the efforts of his resident, Dan MacDonald, that I was able to learn what has eventually developed into a most challenging and exciting new medical modality.

Utilizing high-frequency sound waves, diagnostic ultrasound provides a unique method for visualization of soft tissue anatomic structures. The challenge of identifying such structures and correlating the results with clinical symptoms and patient data offers an ongoing challenge to the sonographer. The state of the art demands expertise in scanning techniques and maneuvers to demonstrate the internal structures; without quality scans, no diagnostic information can be rendered to the physician.

Our initial experience in ultrasound took us through the era of A-mode techniques, identifying aortic aneurysms through pulsatile reflections, trying to separate splenic reflections from upper-pole left renal masses, and, in general, trying to echo every patient with a probable abdominal or pelvic mass. Of course, the one-dimensional A-mode techniques were difficult for me to conceptualize, let alone believe in. However, with repeated successes and experience gained from mistakes, I began to believe in this method. The conviction that Dr. Leopold had about this technique was a strong indicator of its success in our laboratory.

It was when Picker brought our first two-dimensional ultrasound unit to the laboratory that the "skeptics" started to believe a little more in this modality. I must admit that those early images were weather maps to me for a number of months. The repeated times I asked, "What is that?" were enough to try anyone's patience.

I can recall when Siemens installed our real-time unit and we saw our first obstetrical case. Such a thrill for us to see the fetus move, wave his hand, and show us fetal heart pulsations.

By this time we were scouting the clinics and various departments in the hospital for interesting cases to scan. With our success rate surpassing our failures, the case load increased so that, soon, we were involved in all aspects of ultrasound. There was not enough material or reprints for us to read to see the new developments. It was for this reason that excitement in clinical research soared, attracting young physicians throughout the country to develop techniques in diagnostic ultrasound.

Because Dr. Leopold was so intensely interested in ultrasound, it became the diagnostic method of choice for our patients. It was not long before conferences were incomplete without the mention of the technique. Later, local medical meetings and eventually national meetings grew to include discussion of this new modality. A number of visitors were attracted to our laboratory to learn the technique, and thus we became swamped with a continual flow of new physicians, some eager to work with ultrasound and others skeptical at first but believers in the end.

In the beginning, education progressed slowly with many laboratories offering a one-to-one teaching experience. Commercial companies thought the only way to push the field was to develop their own national training programs, and thus several of the leading manufacturers were the first to put a dedicated effort into the development of ultrasound.

It was through the combined efforts of our laboratory and commercial interests that I became interested in furthering ultrasound education. Seminars, weekly sessions, local and national meetings, and consultations became a vital part of the growth of ultrasound.

Thus, as ultrasound grew in popularity, more intensified training was desperately needed to maintain the initial quality that the pioneers strived for. Through working with one of the commercial ultrasound companies conducting national short-term training programs, I became acquainted with Barry Goldberg and his enthusiasm for quality education in ultrasound. His organizational efforts and pioneer spirit led me to the east coast to further develop more intensive educational programs in ultrasound.

Introducing the New Fourth Edition.

The fourth edition of the *Textbook of Diagnostic Ultrasonography* has been vastly updated and reorganized from the first edition in 1975. The field of diagnostic ultrasound has changed so dramatically in the past 35 years that the approach to many procedures has been altered significantly.

The primary goal in preparing such a textbook was and continues to be to provide a complete resource for students studying sonography, as well as practitioners in hospitals, clinics, and private radiology, cardiology, and obstetrical settings. This new, fourth edition strives to keep up with this fast-moving field, giving students and practitioners not only complete, but also up-to-date information in sonography.

The first new distinguishing feature that readers will probably notice is that the *Textbook of Diagnostic Sonography* has been divided into two volumes. This was done for two reasons: to compensate for its expanded coverage and to make it more convenient and easier to use. The content has been completely reorganized to provide better flow for the reader. The first volume covers abdominal and retroperitoneal cavities, superficial structures, pediatric applications, and cerebrovascular and peripheral vascular Doppler. The second volume presents complete discussions on gynecology, obstetrics, and cardiology.

The physics section will now be available in a separate text by James B. Zagzebski. A separate text permits a complete presentation of ultrasound physics. In addition, this new and separate practical resource is an excellent tool for preparation to take the physics portion of the American Registry of Diagnostic Medical Sonographers certification examination.

This fourth edition has been completely revised and expanded to offer approximately 400 more pages than before, making this new edition more comprehensive than ever. About half of the book consists of entirely new or completely rewritten chapters. These chapters encompass everything from the gastrointestinal tract in Chapter 8 to cerebrovascular sonography, Doppler, and noninvasive examinations in Chapter 22 to prenatal diagnosis of congenital anomalies in Chapter 30.

Particularly noteworthy is the section on obstetrics and gynecology, which has been completely rewritten and updated by Kara Mayden Argo and several excellent, new contributors. The pediatric ultrasound section has been added by Suzanne Devine and her colleagues from Children's Hospital in Chicago. The cerebrovascular and peripheral vascular chapters have been extensively rewritten and updated by Richard E. Rae. And once again, many of the echocardiology chapters have been completely revised to include the latest in Doppler and color flow discussions.

Notable topics include peripheral vascular Doppler; obstetrics, including coverage of high-risk patients, along with transvaginal procedures; fetal echocardiography, with all new images demonstrating state-of-the-art resolution; and cardiology, with coverage of stress echocardiography and myocardial contrast agents.

As in all editions, concepts continue to be presented in a logical and consistent manner in each chapter. In an effort to help the student and the sonographer understand the total clinical picture that the patient presents before the sonographic examination, discussions on anatomy, physiology, laboratory data, clinical signs and symptoms, pathology, and sonographic findings are found in each specific chapter.

To keep up with the continually changing field of ultrasound, hundreds of new images have been incorporated. Out of more than 3000 images, approximately 70% are new. In addition, a multitude of anatomical illustrations cite many of the relevant landmarks the sonographer should look for when performing an ultrasound examination. A particularly nice assortment of new, anatomical line drawings can be found in Chapter 43, demonstrating important features of the heart.

To help the reader stay current with the latest technology, we have added a color insert, including approximately 380 color Doppler scans. These same images are also presented in black and white next to the corresponding text so that comprehension is not sacrificed. Each image included in the color insert has the notation "See color insert" after the figure mention in the text.

A glossary of useful terms and definitions has been included to assist the reader. References cited in the text are listed at the end of each chapter. In addition, review questions are a new feature of this edition and have been added so that readers can measure their comprehension.

It is my hope that this textbook will not only introduce the reader to the field of ultrasound, but also go a step beyond to what I have found to be a very stimulating and challenging experience in diagnostic patient care.

SANDRA L. HAGEN-ANSERT

Acknowledgments

I would like to acknowledge the individual who contributed most to my early interest in diagnostic ultrasound, Dr. George R. Leopold, for his personal perseverance and instruction, as well as for his outstanding clinical research. My thanks also go to the following:

Dr. Sam Halpern who encouraged me to publish;

Dr. Barry Goldberg for the opportunity to develop training programs in an independent fashion and for his encouragement to stay with it;

Drs. Barbara Gosink, Dolores Pretorius, Nancy Budorick, Wanda Miller-Hance, and David Sahn for their encouragement throughout the years at the UCSD Medical Center;

Dr. Daniel Yellon for his early hour anatomy dissection and instruction in clinical cardiology;

Dr. Carson Schneck for his excellent instruction in gross anatomy and sections of "Geraldine";

Dr. Jacob Zatuchni for the interest, enthusiasm, and understanding he showed me while at Episcopal Hospital;

Dr. Fred Sample whose quest for the anatomical ultrasound demonstration of the abdomen and pelvis was an inspiration to us all;

Drs. Howard Dittrich and Paul Walinsky for their enthusiastic support in echocardiology;

Dr. William Zwiebel for his contribution on the liver physiology and laboratory data for the liver chapter;

Becky Levzow and Kim Skerritt for their contributions in the Renal Transplant section of the Urinary System chapter;

Kim Warner for her contribution of the appendix for the GI chapter;

Tina Platon Siemba for her contribution of Budd Chiari syndrome;

Drs. Harry Rakowski and Bob Howard for their tremendous support and contributions to the chapters on adult and congenital heart disease;

Cris Gresser for her contribution of images throughout the cardiac chapters and for her chapter on cardiomyopathy;

The wonderful department of Diagnostic Ultrasound at the UCSD Medical Center, which includes John Forsythe, Holly Lloyd, Tracy Parker, Andrea Yerevanian, Kathleen Bauman, Jim Warner, and Chris Sahn, who have been helpful in retrieving interesting abdominal and pelvic cases;

The students I have taught in Diagnostic Ultrasound from the various medical institutions I have been involved with—Episcopal Hospital, Thomas Jefferson University Medical Center, University of Wisconsin, Madison Medical Center, and the UCSD Medical Center—who continually work toward the development of finer ultrasound techniques and instruction, and for their support I would like to thank them.

Special recognition goes to my recent graduates—Tracy Johnson, Candace Goldstein, Kim Warner, Mary Gregor-Nuxoll, Shelby Smith, Joanne Wong, Tami Worley, and Barbara Jimenez—for their critique, input, and patience during this revision.

I would also like to acknowledge the excellent staff at Mosby, especially Jeanne Rowland, Lisa Potts, Jennifer Byington, and Don Ladig, all of whom were most patient and enduring for the entire preparation of the manuscript.

Very special recognition goes to my patient and understanding family, Arthur, Rebecca, Alyssa, and Katrina, who were very tolerant of the hours upon hours of preparation and writing this edition bestowed upon all of our lives. The girls have grown up with these four editions and have volunteered their tiny hearts, and now abdominal vessels, for various illustrations throughout the book. They have vowed never to volunteer again.

Contents

Detailed Contents

PART 4 CEREBROVASCULAR AND PERIPHERAL VASCULAR NON-INVASIVE EVALUATIONS

TEXTBOOK OF

DIAGNOSTIC ULTRASONOGRAPHY

VOLUME ONE

• PART ONE •

Abdominal and Retroperitoneal Cavities

CHAPTER 1

Anatomic and Physiologic Relationships Within the Abdominal Cavity

Sandra L. Hagen-Ansert

The ability of the sonographer to understand anatomy as it relates to the cross-sectional, coronal, oblique, and sagittal projections is critical in performing a quality sonogram. Normal anatomy has many variations in size and position, and it is the responsibility of the sonographer to be able to demonstrate these findings on the sonogram. To complete this task the sonographer must have a thorough understanding of anatomy as it relates to the anteroposterior relationships, as well as the variations in sectional anatomy. This chapter provides a background for these anatomic relationships.

ANATOMIC TERMS

Several anatomic terms that relate to the human body are described below:

anatomic position (Figs. 1-1 and 1-2) The individual is standing erect, the arms are by the sides with the palms facing forward, the face and eyes are directed forward, and the heels are together, with the feet pointed forward.
median plane A vertical plane that bisects the body into right and left halves.
sagittal plane Any plane parallel to the median plane.
coronal plane Any vertical plane at right angles to the median plane.
transverse plane Any plane at right angles to both the median and coronal planes.
supine Lying face up.
prone Lying face down.
anterior (ventral) Toward the front of the body.
posterior (dorsal) The back of the body or in back of another structure.
medial Nearer to or toward the midline.
lateral Farther from the midline or to the side of the body.
proximal Closer to the point of origin or closer to the body.
distal Away from the point of origin or away from the body.
internal Inside.
external Outside.
superior Above.
inferior Below.
cranial Toward the head.
caudal Toward the feet.

ABDOMEN

The abdominal cavity, excluding the retroperitoneum and the pelvis, is bounded superiorly by the diaphragm, anteriorly by the abdominal wall muscles, posteriorly by the vertebral column, ribs, and iliac fossa, and inferiorly by the pelvis.

Abdominal Regions

The abdomen is commonly divided into nine regions by two vertical and two horizontal lines. Each vertical line passes through the midinguinal point, the point that lies on the inguinal ligament halfway between the pubic symphysis and anterior superior iliac spine. The upper horizontal line, referred to as the *subcostal plane,* joins the lowest point of the costal margin on each side of the body. The lowest horizontal line, the intertubercular plane, joins the tubercles on the iliac crests.

The nine abdominal regions include the following: (1) upper abdomen—right hypochondrium, epigastrium, and left hypochondrium; (2) middle abdomen—right lumbar, umbilical, and left lumbar; and (3) lower abdomen—right iliac fossa, hypogastrium, and left iliac fossa (Fig. 1-3).

Transpyloric Plane

The transpyloric plane is a horizontal plane that passes through the pylorus, the duodenal junction, the neck of the pancreas, and the hilum of the kidneys (Fig. 1-4).

Abdominal Viscera

Variations in abdominal viscera occur from patient to patient, with change in position, and with change in respiration.

Liver. The liver lies under the lower ribs with most of its structure in the right hypochrondrium and epigastrium.

Gallbladder. The fundus of the gallbladder lies opposite the tip of the right ninth costal cartilage.

Spleen. The spleen lies in the left hypochondrium under

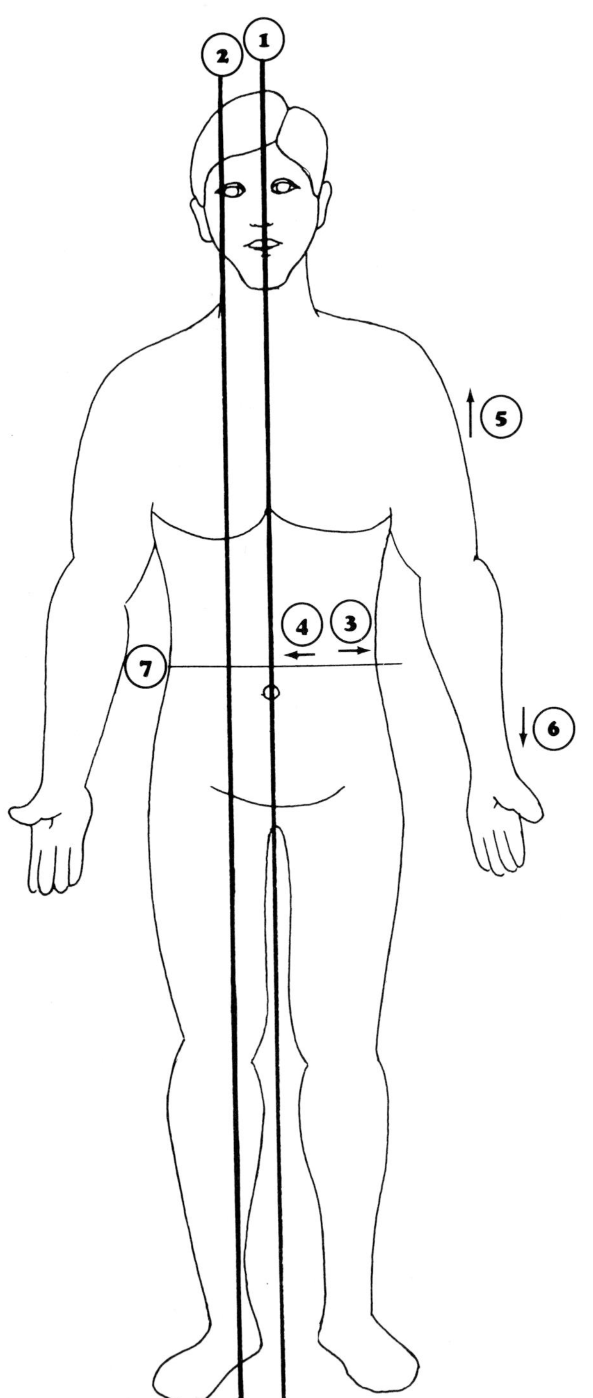

FIG. 1-1 Anterior view of the body in the anatomic position. Median sagittal plane, *1;* paramedian plane, *2;* lateral, *3;* medial, *4;* proximal, *5;* distal, *6;* and transverse plane, *7.* (From Hagen-Ansert SL: The anatomy workbook. Philadelphia, JB Lippincott, 1986.)

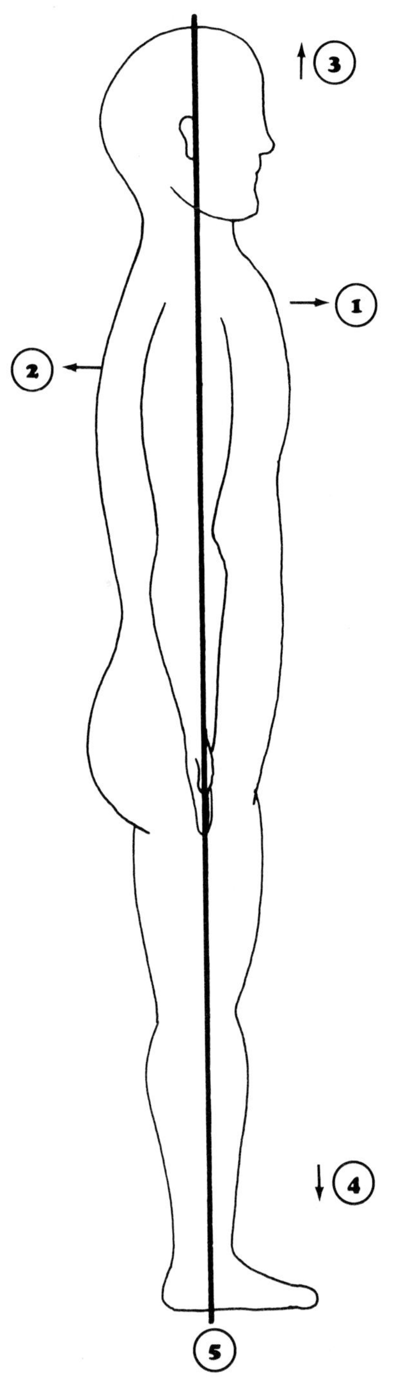

FIG. 1-2 Lateral view of the body. Anterior, *1;* posterior, *2;* superior, *3;* inferior, *4;* coronal plane, *5.* (From Hagen-Ansert SL: The anatomy workbook. Philadelphia, JB Lippincott, 1986.)

cover of the ninth, tenth, and eleventh ribs. Its long axis corresponds to the tenth rib, and in adults, it usually doesn't project forward of the midaxillary line.

Pancreas. The pancreas lies across the transpyloric plane. The head lies below and to the right, the neck lies on the plane, and the body and tail lie above and to the left.

Kidneys. The right kidney lies slightly lower than the left. Each kidney moves about 1 inch in a vertical direction during full respiratory movement of the diaphragm. The hilus of the kidney lies on the transpyloric plane, about three fingers from the midline.

Aorta and Inferior Vena Cava. The aorta lies in the midline, slightly to the left of the abdomen, and bifurcates into

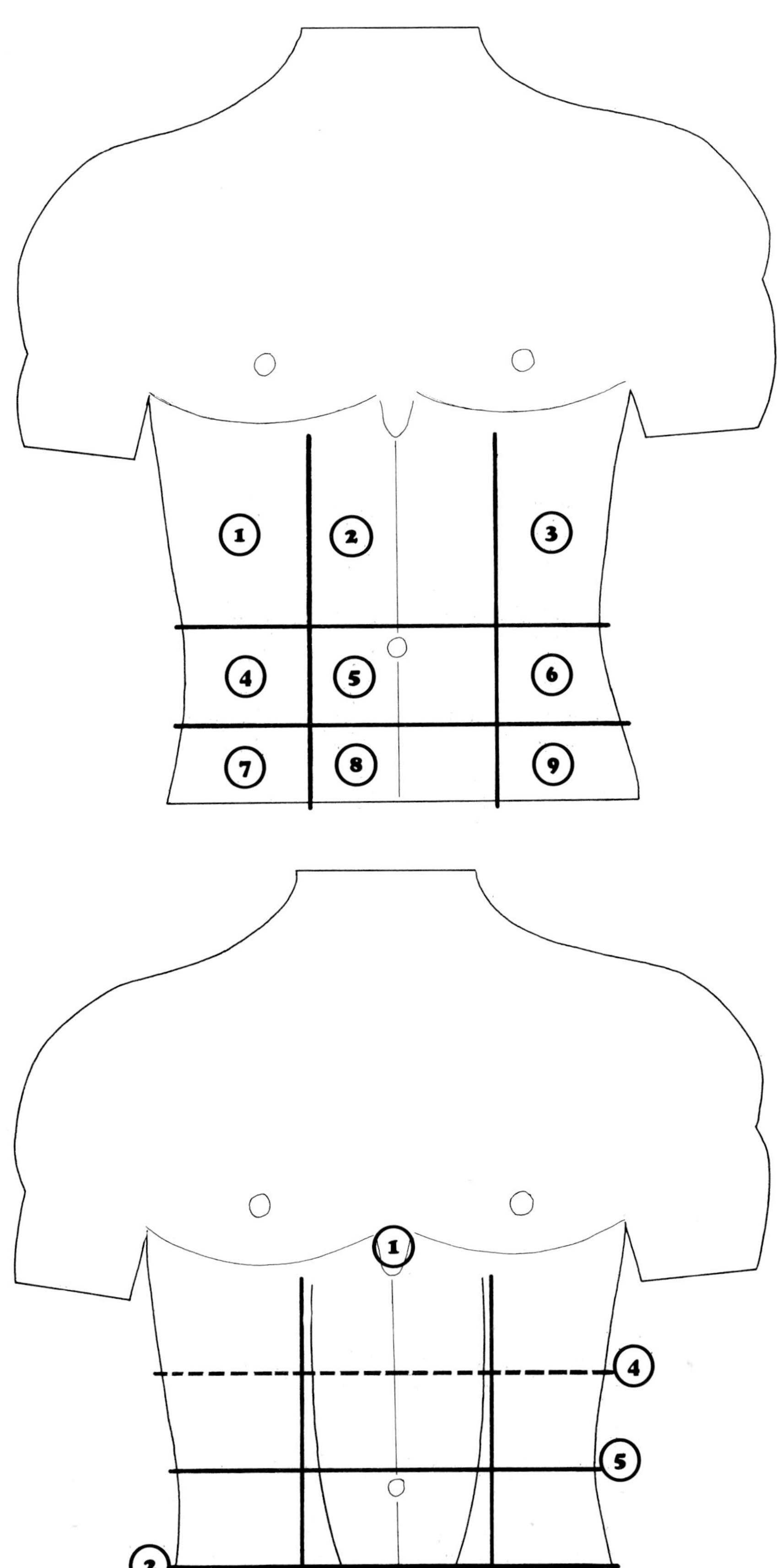

FIG. 1-3 Regions of the anterior abdominal wall are the right hypochondrium, *1;* epigastrium, *2;* left hypochondrium, *3;* right lumbar region, *4;* umbilical region, *5;* left lumbar region, *6;* right iliac fossa, *7;* hypogastrium, *8;* left iliac fossa, *9*. (From Hagen-Ansert SL: The anatomy workbook. Philadelphia, JB Lippincott, 1986.)

FIG. 1-4 Surface landmarks of the anterior abdominal wall are the xyphoid process, *1;* tubercle of crest, *2;* right lateral plane, *3;* transpyloric plane, *4;* subcostal plane, *5;* linea semilunaris, *6*. (From Hagen-Ansert SL: The anatomy workbook. Philadelphia, JB Lippincott, 1986.)

the right and left common iliac arteries opposite the fourth lumbar vertebra on the intercristal plane. The inferior vena cava lies in the midline, slightly to the right of the abdomen, and bifurcates into the right and left common iliac veins.

Bladder and Uterus. The bladder and uterus lie in the lower pelvis in the hypogastric plane.

The Abdominal Wall

Superiorly the abdominal wall is formed by the diaphragm. Inferiorly it is continuous with the pelvic cavity through the pelvic inlet. Anteriorly the wall is formed above by the lower part of the thoracic cage and below by several layers of muscles: the rectus abdominis, the external oblique, internal oblique, and the transversus abdominis. The linea alba is a fibrous band that stretches from the xyphoid to the symphysis pubis. It is wider at its superior end and forms a central anterior attachment for the muscle layers of the abdomen. It is formed by the interlacing of fibers of the aponeuroses of the right and left oblique and transversus abdominis muscles.

Posteriorly the abdominal wall is formed in the midline by five lumbar vertebrae and their disks. Laterally it is formed by the twelfth ribs, upper part of the bony pelvis, psoas muscles, quadratus lumborum muscles, and the aponeuroses of origin of the transversus abdominis muscles.

Laterally the wall is formed above by the lower part of the thoracic wall, including the lungs and pleura, and below by the external and internal oblique muscles and the transversus abdominis muscles.

Fascia. The fasciae of the abdominal wall are divided into superficial and deep fasciae (Fig. 1-5). The superficial fascia may be further divided into two layers. The superficial layer contains fatty tissue (Camper's fascia), whereas the deep layer is mostly membranous with little fat (Scarpa's fascia).

PERITONEUM

The peritoneum is a serous membrane lining the walls of the abdominal cavity and clothing the abdominal viscera. The peritoneum (Figs. 1-6 to 1-8) is formed by a single layer of cells called the *mesothelium,* which rests on a thin layer of connective tissue. If the mesothelium is damaged or removed in any area (as from surgery), there is danger that two layers of peritoneum may adhere to each other and form an adhesion. This adhesion may interfere with the normal movements of the abdominal viscera.

The peritoneum is divided into two layers. The parietal

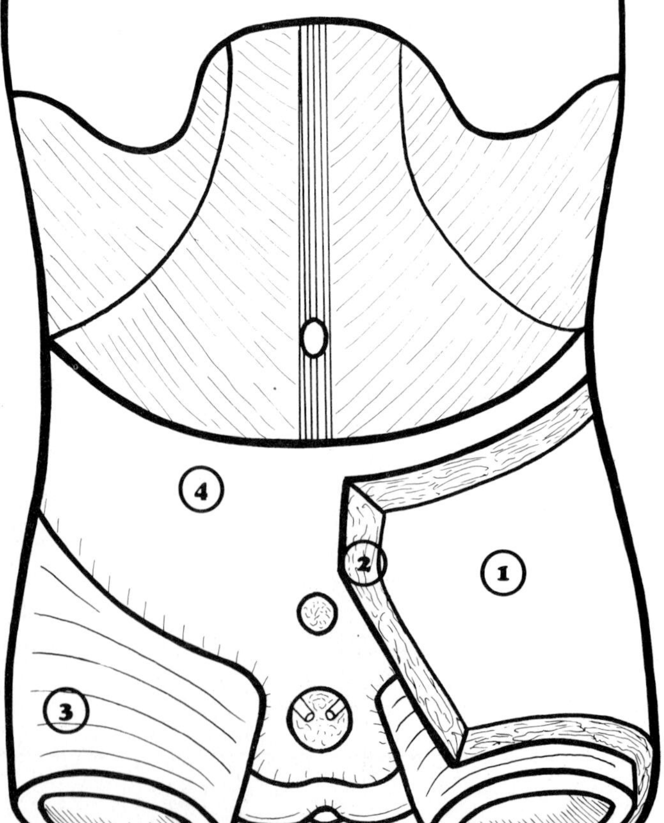

FIG. 1-5 Superficial fascia of the lower anterior abdominal wall include the superficial fascia, *1;* fatty layer (Camper's fascia), *2;* fascia lata, *3;* membranous layer (Scarpa's fascia), *4.* (From Hagen-Ansert SL: The anatomy workbook. Philadelphia, JB Lippincott, 1986.)

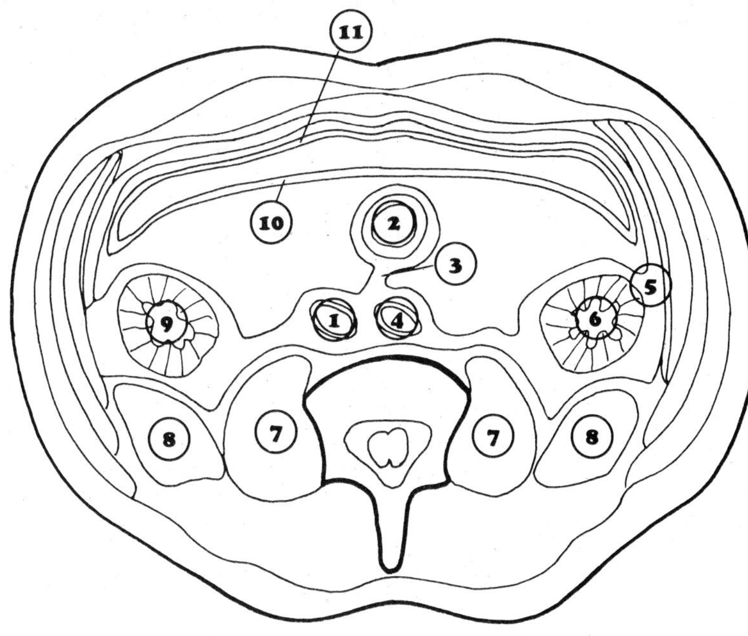

FIG. 1-6 Transverse section of the abdominal cavity showing the reflections of the peritoneum. Inferior vena cava, *1;* small intestine, *2;* mesentery of the small intestine, *3;* aorta, *4;* peritoneum, *5;* descending colon, *6;* psoas major muscle, *7;* quadratus lumborum muscle, *8;* ascending colon, *9;* posterior layers of the greater omentum, *10;* and anterior layers of the greater omentum, *11.* (From Hagen-Ansert SL: The anatomy workbook. Philadelphia, JB Lippincott, 1986.)

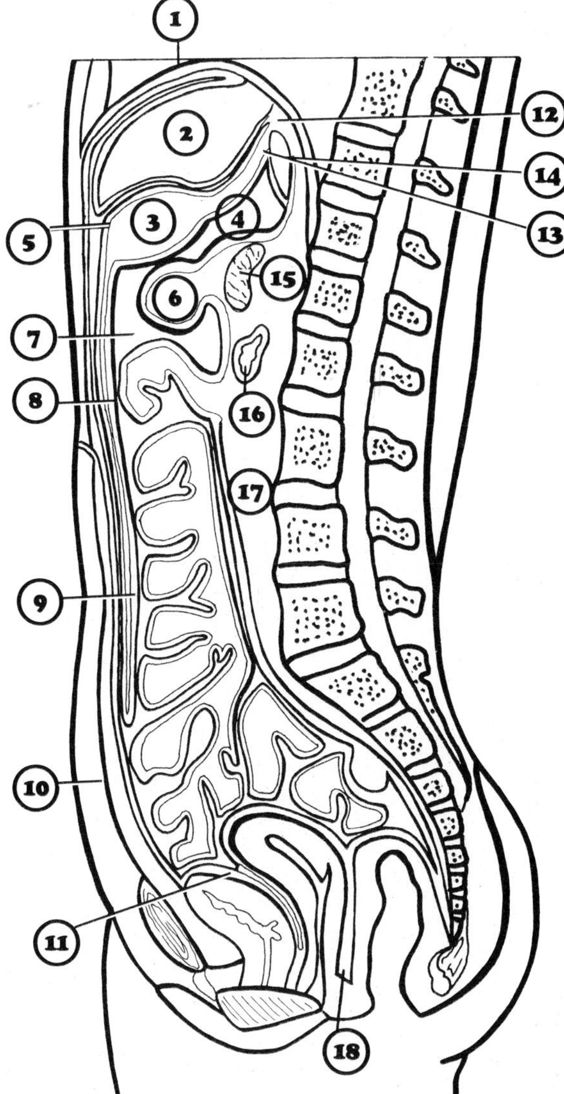

FIG. 1-7 Sagittal section through the abdomen and pelvis: Diaphragm, *1;* liver, *2;* stomach, *3;* omental bursa, *4;* gastric ligament, *5;* transverse colon, *6;* peritoneal cavity, *7;* greater omentum, *8;* parietal peritoneum, *9;* linea alba, *10;* vesicouterine pouch, *11;* subphrenic space, *12;* lesser omentum, *13;* caudate lobe of the liver, *14;* pancreas, *15;* duodenum, *16;* retroperitoneum, *17;* rectouterine pouch, *18.* (From Hagen-Ansert SL: The anatomy workbook. Philadelphia, JB Lippincott, 1986.)

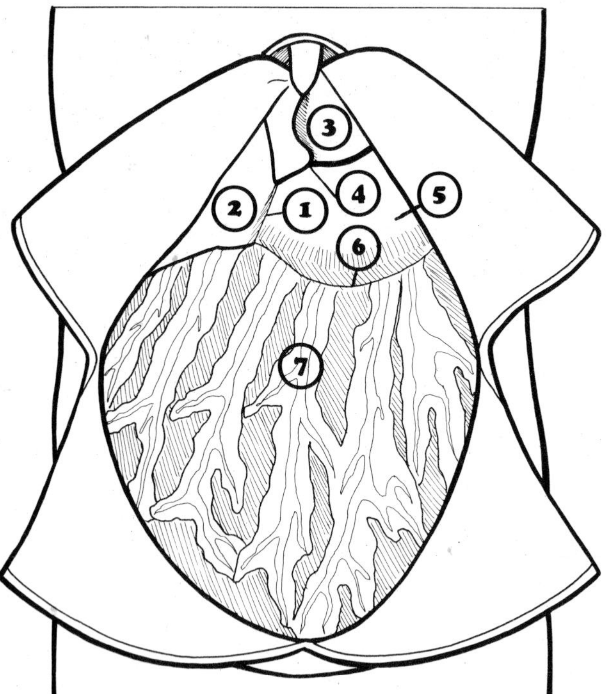

FIG. 1-8 The greater omentum is often referred to as an apron hanging between the small intestine and the anterior abdominal wall. Falciform ligament, *1;* right lobe of the liver, *2;* left lobe of the liver, *3;* ligamentum teres, *4;* stomach, *5;* greater curvature of the stomach, *6;* greater omentum, *7.* (From Hagen-Ansert SL: The anatomy workbook. Philadelphia, JB Lippincott, 1986.)

peritoneum is the portion that lines the abdominal wall but does not cover a viscus; the visceral peritoneum is the portion that covers an organ. The peritoneal cavity is the potential space between the parietal and visceral peritoneum. This cavity contains a small amount of lubricating serous fluid to help the abdominal organs move on one another without friction. Under certain pathologic conditions, the potential space of the peritoneal cavity may be distended into an actual space containing several liters of fluid. This accumulation of fluid is known as *ascites*. Other fluid substances, such as blood from a ruptured organ, bile from a ruptured duct, or fecal matter from a ruptured intestine, also may accumulate in this cavity.

The peritoneal cavity forms a completely closed sac in the male; in the female there is a communication with the exterior through the uterine tubes, uterus, and vagina. Retroperitoneal organs and vascular structures remain posterior to the cavity and are covered anteriorly with peritoneum. These include the urinary system, aorta, inferior vena cava, colon, pancreas, uterus, and bladder. The other abdominal organs are located within the peritoneal cavity.

The peritoneal cavity may be divided into two parts—the greater and lesser sacs. The greater sac is the primary compartment of the peritoneal cavity and extends across the anterior abdomen and from the diaphragm to the pelvis. The lesser sac is the smaller compartment and lies posterior to the stomach. The lesser sac is a diverticulum from the greater sac as it opens through a small opening, the epiploic foramen.

Mesentery

A mesentery is a two-layered fold of peritoneum that attaches part of the intestines to the posterior abdominal wall and includes the mesentery of the small intestine, the transverse mesocolon, and the sigmoid mesocolon.

Omentum

The omentum is a two-layered fold of peritoneum that attaches the stomach to another viscus organ. The greater omentum is attached to the greater curvature of the stomach and hangs down like an apron in the space between the small intestine and anterior abdominal wall. The greater omentum is folded back on itself and is attached to the inferior border of the transverse colon. The lesser omentum slings the lesser curvature of the stomach to the undersurface of the liver. The gastrosplenic omentum ligament connects the stomach to the spleen (Fig. 1-9).

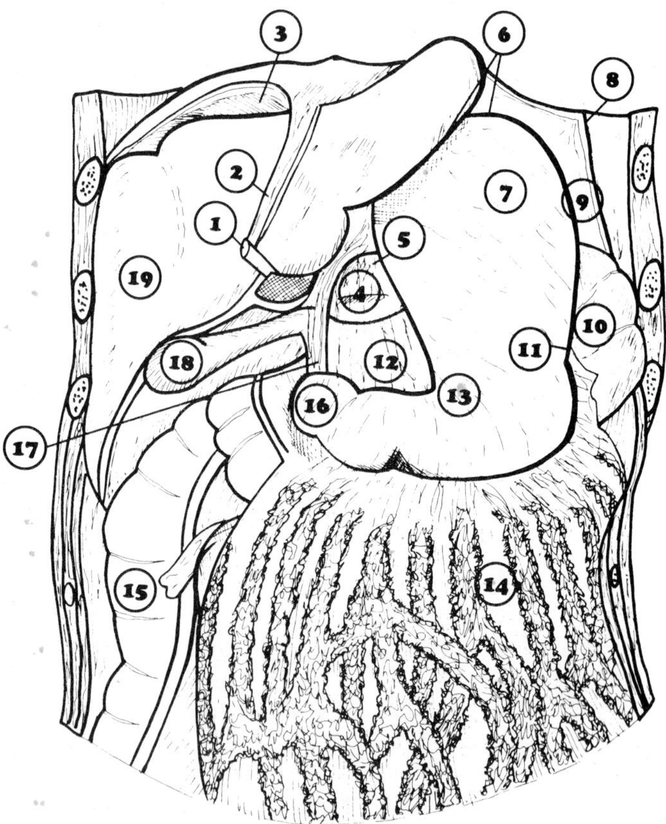

FIG. 1-9 Anterior view of the abdominal viscera with the liver pulled upward. Ligamentum teres, *1;* falciform ligament, *2;* hepatic coronary ligament, *3;* caudate lobe of the liver, *4;* hepatogastric ligament, *5;* cardiac ligament, *6;* fundus of the stomach, *7;* diaphragm, *8;* parietal peritoneum, *9;* spleen, *10;* gastrosplenic ligament, *11;* lesser omentum, *12;* lesser curvature of stomach, *13;* greater omentum, *14;* ascending colon, *15;* pylorus, *16;* epiploic foramen, *17;* gallbladder, *18;* liver, *19.* (From Hagen-Ansert SL: The anatomy workbook. Philadelphia, JB Lippincott, 1986.)

Ligament

The peritoneal ligaments are two-layered folds of peritoneum that attach the lesser mobile solid viscera to the abdominal walls. For example, the liver is attached by the falciform ligament to the anterior abdominal wall and to the undersurface of the diaphragm. The ligamentum teres lies in the free borders of this ligament. The peritoneum leaves the kidney and passes to the hilus of the spleen as the posterior layer of the lienorenal ligament. The visceral peritoneum covers the spleen and is reflected onto the greater curvature of the stomach as the anterior layer of the gastrosplenic ligament.

Peritoneal Fossae

Lesser Sac. The lesser sac is an extensive peritoneal pouch located behind the lesser omentum and stomach. It extends upward to the diaphragm and inferior between the layers of the greater omentum. The left margin is formed by the spleen and the gastrosplenic and lienorenal ligaments. The right margin of the lesser sac opens into the greater sac through the epiploic foramen (Fig. 1-10).

The epiploic foramen has the following boundaries: anteriorly, the free border of the lesser omentum containing the common bile duct, hepatic artery, and portal vein; posteriorly, the inferior vena cava; superiorly, the caudate process of the caudate lobe of the liver; and inferiorly, the first part of the duodenum.

Subphrenic Spaces. The subphrenic spaces are the result of the complicated arrangement of the peritoneum in the region of the liver. The right and left anterior subphrenic spaces lie between the diaphragm and the liver, one on each side of the falciform ligament. The right posterior subphrenic space lies between the right lobe of the liver, the right kidney, and the right colic flexure. This is also called *Morison's pouch*.

Peritoneal Recesses

The omental bursa normally has some empty places. Parts of the peritoneal cavity near the liver are so slitlike that they are also isolated. These areas are known as *peritoneal recesses* and are clinically important because infections may collect in them. Two common sites occur where the duodenum becomes the jejunum and where the ileum joins the cecum.

Paracolic Gutters. The arrangement of the ascending and descending colon, the attachments of the transverse mesocolon, and the mesentery of the small intestine to the posterior abdominal wall result in the formation of four paracolic gutters. The clinical significance of these gutters is their ability to conduct fluid materials from one part of the body to another. Materials such as abscess, ascites, blood, pus, bile, or metastases may be spread through this network.

The gutters are on the lateral and medial sides of the ascending and descending colon. The right medial paracolic gutter is closed off from the pelvic cavity inferiorly by the mesentery of the small intestine. The other gutters are in free communication with the pelvic cavity. The right lateral paracolic gutter communicates with the right posterior subphrenic space. The left lateral gutter is separated from the area around the spleen by the phrenicocolic ligament.

Inguinal Canal

The inguinal canal is an oblique passage through the lower part of the anterior abdominal wall. In the male, it allows structures to pass to and from the testes to the abdomen. In the female, it permits the passage of the round ligament of the uterus from the uterus to the labium majus.

Abdominal Hernias. A hernia is the protrusion of part of the abdominal contents beyond the normal confines of the abdominal wall. It has the following three parts: the sac, the contents of the sac, and the coverings of the sac. The hernial sac is a diverticulum of the peritoneum and has a neck and a body. The hernial contents may consist of any structure found within the abdominal cavity and may vary from a small piece of omentum to a large viscus organ. The hernial coverings are formed from the layers of the abdominal wall through which the hernial sac passes. Abdominal hernias are one of the following types: inguinal, femoral, umbilical, epigastric, or abdominis rectus.

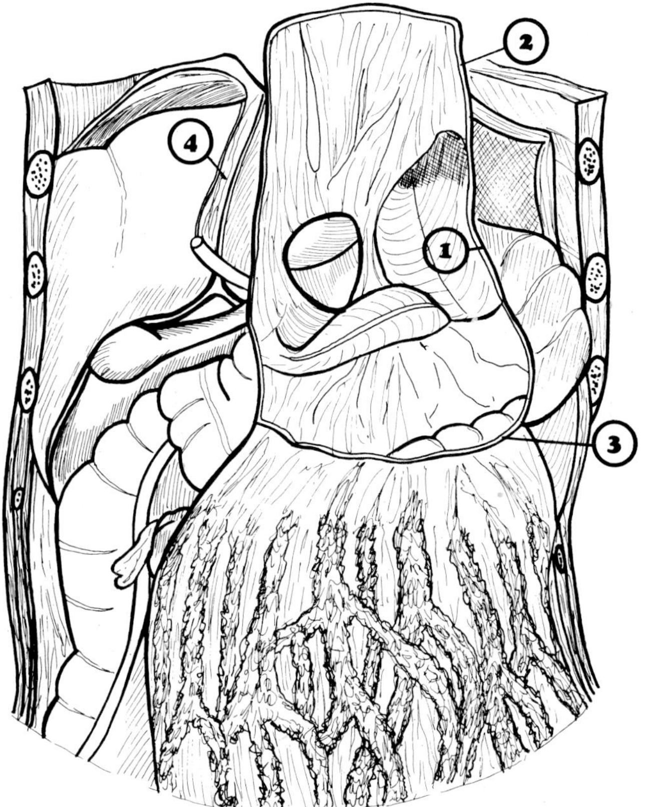

FIG. 1-10 Upper abdomen with the greater curvature of the stomach lifted. Gastrosplenic ligament, *1;* phrenic gastric ligament, *2;* gastrocolic ligament, *3;* falciform ligament, *4*. (From Hagen-Ansert SL: The anatomy workbook. Philadelphia, JB Lippincott, 1986.)

THE PELVIS

The pelvis is divided into the major and minor parts. The major or false pelvis is that portion of the pelvis found above the brim of the pelvis; its cavity is that portion of the abdominal cavity cradled by the iliac fossae. The minor or true pelvis is found below the brim of the pelvis. The cavity of the pelvis minor is continuous at the pelvic brim with the cavity of the pelvis major.

False Pelvis

The false pelvis is bounded posteriorly by the lumbar vertebrae, laterally by the iliac fossae and iliacus muscles, and anteriorly by the lower anterior abdominal wall.

True Pelvis

The true pelvis protects and contains the lower parts of the intestinal and urinary tracts and the reproductive organs. The true pelvis has an inlet, outlet, and cavity.

The walls of the pelvis are formed by bones and ligaments, which are partly lined with muscles covered with fascia and parietal peritoneum. It has anterior, posterior, and lateral walls and an inferior floor.

The piriformis muscles form the posterior pelvic wall. The obturator internus muscle lines the lateral pelvic wall. The pelvic floor stretches across the pelvis and divides it into the main pelvic cavity, which contains the pelvic viscera, and the perineum below. The pelvic diaphragm is formed by the levatores ani muscles and coccygeus muscles.

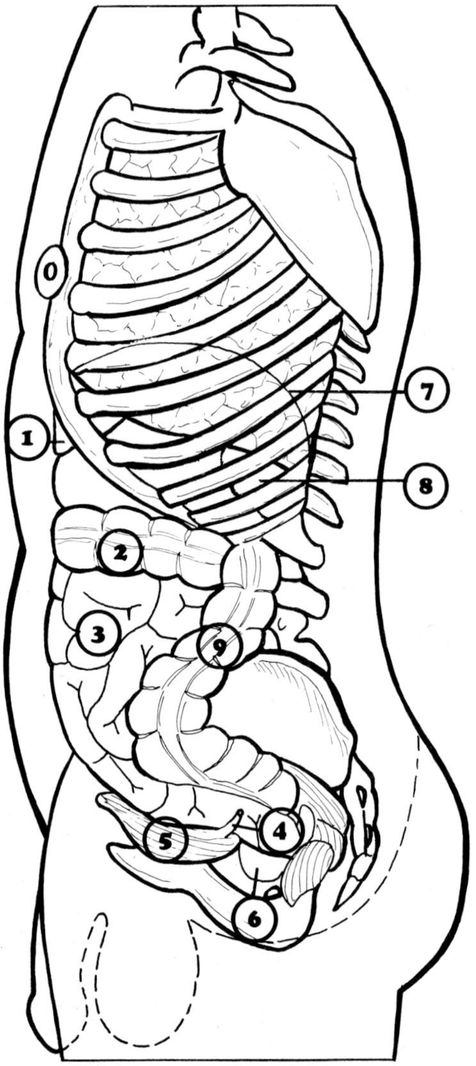

FIG. 1-11 Sagittal view of the abdomen and pelvis in the male. Liver, *1;* transverse colon, *2;* intestine, *3;* ureter, *4;* bladder, *5;* prostate, *6;* diaphragm, *7;* spleen, *8;* descending colon, *9*. (From Hagen-Ansert SL: The anatomy workbook. Philadelphia, JB Lippincott, 1986.)

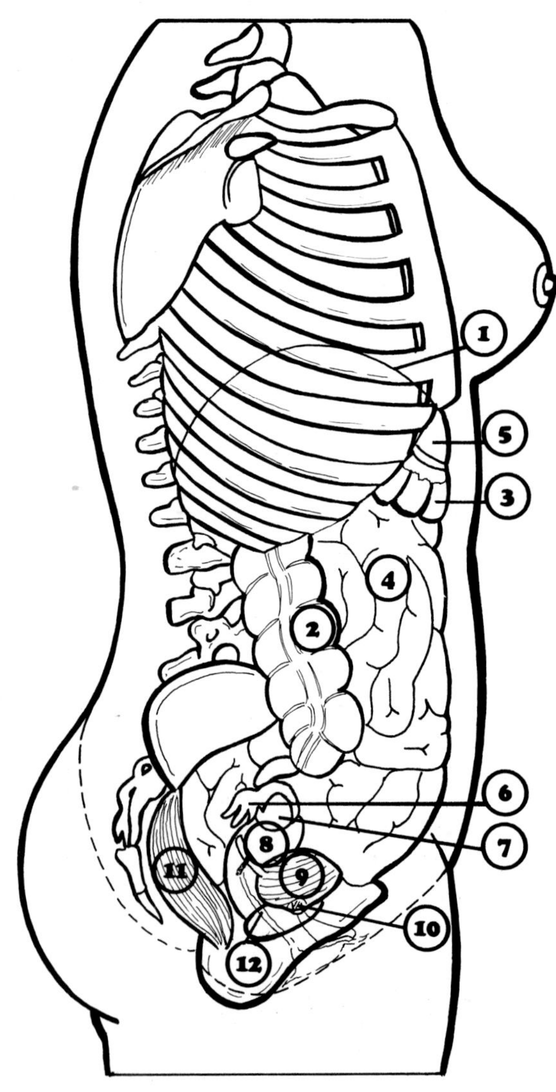

FIG. 1-12 Sagittal view of the abdomen and pelvis in the female. Diaphragm, *1;* ascending colon, *2;* transverse colon, *3;* intestine, *4;* stomach, *5;* fallopian tube, *6;* ovary, *7;* uterus, *8;* bladder, *9;* urethra, *10;* rectum, *11;* vagina, *12*. (From Hagen-Ansert SL: The anatomy workbook. Philadelphia, JB Lippincott, 1986.)

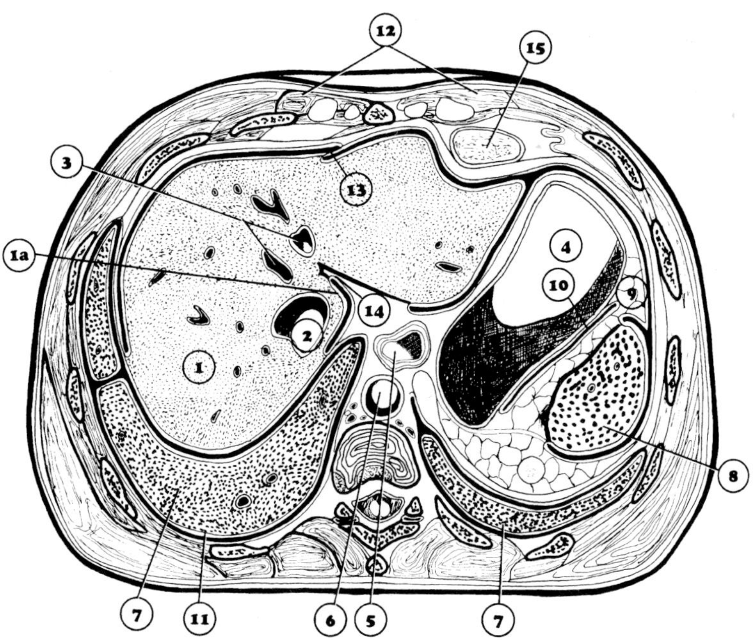

FIG. 1-13 Cross-section of the abdomen at the level of the tenth intervertebral disc. Right lobe of the liver, *1;* caudate lobe, *1a;* inferior vena cava, *2;* hepatic veins, *3;* stomach, *4;* esophagus, *5;* abdominal aorta, *6;* pleural cavity, *7;* spleen, *8;* gastrosplenic ligament, *9;* omental bursa, *10;* pleural sac, *11;* rectus abdominis muscle, *12;* falciform ligament, *13;* ligamentum venosum, *14;* pericardial sac, *15*. The lower portion of the pericardial sac is seen. The splenic artery enters the spleen, and the splenic vein emerges from the splenic hilum. The abdominal portion of the esophagus lies to the left of the midline and opens into the stomach through the cardiac orifice. The liver extends to the left mammillary line. The falciform ligament extends into the section above this. The upper border of the tail of the pancreas is seen. The spleen is shown to lie alongside the ninth rib. (From Hagen-Ansert SL: The anatomy workbook. Philadelphia, JB Lippincott, 1986.)

The peritoneal cavity invests several pelvic organs: the rectum, bladder, and uterus (Fig. 1-11 and 1-12). In the female the peritoneum descends from the anterior abdominal wall to the level of the pubic bone onto the superior surface of the bladder. It passes from the bladder to the uterus to form the vesicouterine pouch. The peritoneum covers the fundus and body of the uterus and extends over the posterior fornix and the wall of the vagina. Between the uterus and the rectum the peritoneum forms the deep rectouterine pouch.

INTRODUCTION TO CROSS-SECTIONAL AND SAGITTAL ANATOMY

The sonographer must have a solid knowledge of gross anatomy, sectional anatomy, sagittal anatomy, and the various obliquities of anatomic sections. Although "normal" anatomy is often shown in numerous line drawings and anatomic sections, the sonographer must keep in mind the normal variations that can occur in the anatomic structure. Thus the sonographer should carefully evaluate organ and vascular relationships to neighboring structures rather than memorizing where in the abdomen a particular structure ought to be. For example, it is better to recall the location of the gallbladder as anterior to the right kidney and medial to the liver than to remember that it is usually found 6 to 8 cm above the umbilicus.

Figs. 1-13 to 1-41 represent a combination of cross-sectional and sagittal anatomic sections of the abdominal and pelvic cavity. These are presented in descending order from the diaphragm to the symphysis pubis to help the sonographer understand the relationships between vascular structures and organs as one proceeds by 10-mm increments through the abdominal and pelvic cavity.

Text continued on p. 26.

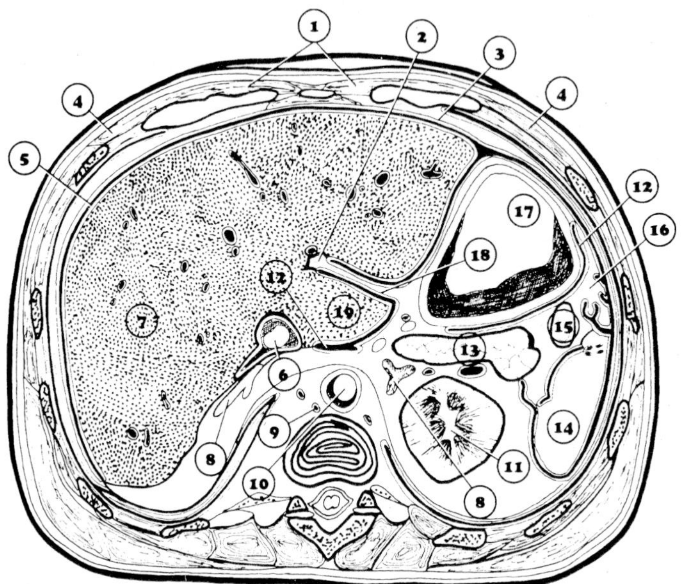

FIG. 1-14 Cross section of the abdomen at the level of the eleventh thoracic disc. Rectus abdominis muscle, *1;* ligamentum venosum, *2;* diaphragm, *3;* external oblique muscle, *4;* peritoneal cavity, *5;* inferior vena cava, *6;* right lobe of the liver, *7;* suprarenal glands, *8;* azygos vein, *9;* aorta, *10;* kidney, *11;* omental bursa, *12;* pancreas, *13;* spleen, *14;* colic flexure, *15;* gastric ligament, *16;* stomach, *17;* hepatogastric ligament, *18;* caudate lobe, *19*. The hepatic vein is shown to enter the inferior vena cava. The renal artery and vein of the left kidney are shown. The left branch of the portal vein is seen to arch upward to enter the left lobe of the liver. The upper part of the stomach is shown with the hepatogastric and gastrocolic ligaments. The lesser omental cavity is posterior to the stomach. The upper border of the splenic flexure of the colon is seen. The caudate lobe of the liver is in this section. The tail and body of the pancreas are shown anterior to the left kidney. The spleen is shown to lie along the left lateral border. The adrenal glands are lateral to the crus of the diaphragm. (From Hagen-Ansert SL: The anatomy workbook. Philadelphia, JB Lippincott, 1986.)

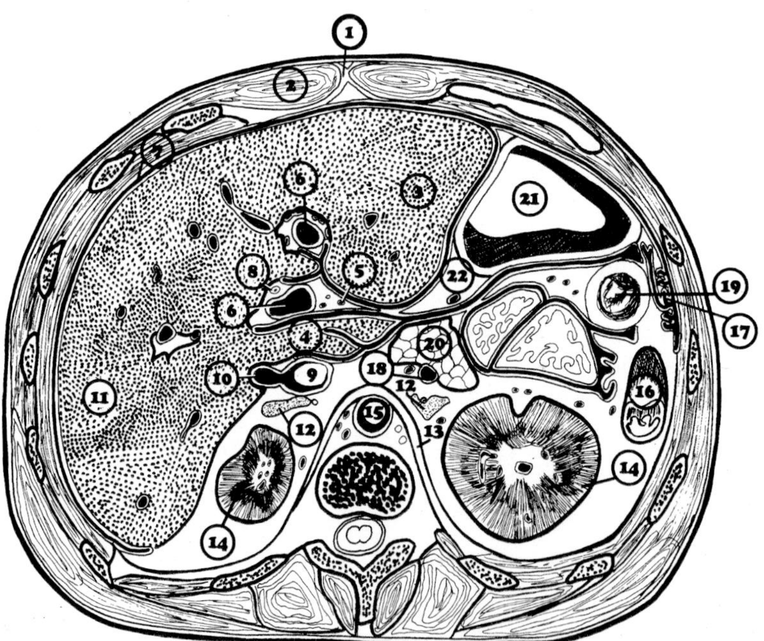

FIG. 1-15 Cross section of the abdomen at the level of the twelfth thoracic vertebra. Linea alba, *1;* rectus abdominis muscle, *2;* left lobe of the liver, *3;* caudate lobe, *4;* hepatic artery, *5;* portal vein, *6;* diaphragm, *7;* hepatic duct, *8;* inferior vena cava, *9;* hepatic vein, *10;* right lobe of the liver, *11;* suprarenal gland, *12;* crus of the diaphragm, *13;* kidney, *14;* aorta, *15;* descending colon, *16;* peritoneal cavity, *17;* splenic vein, *18;* transverse colon, *19;* pancreas, *20;* stomach, *21;* omental bursa, *22*. The celiac axis arises in the middle of this section from the anterior abdominal aorta. The right renal artery originates at this level. The hepatic vein isshown to enter the inferior vena cava. The greater curvature of the stomach and the pylorus are shown. The transverse and descending colon are shown inferior to the splenic flexure. The caudate lobe of the liver is well seen. The body of the pancreas, both kidneys, and the lower portions of the adrenal glands are shown.(From Hagen-Ansert SL: The anatomy workbook. Philadelphia, JB Lippincott, 1986.)

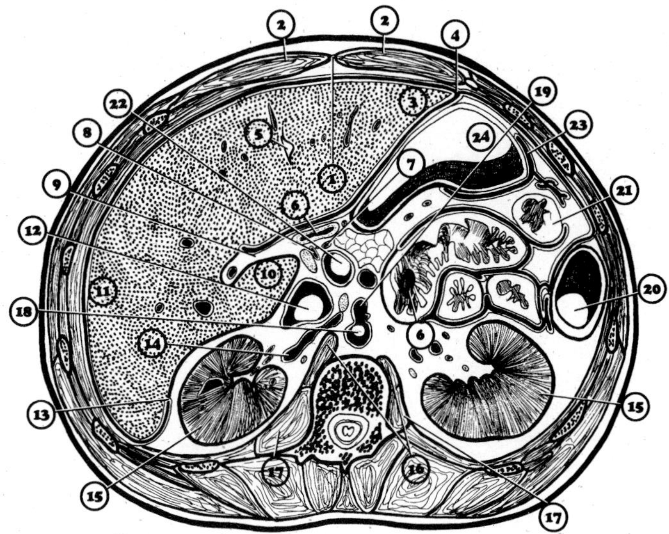

FIG. 1-16 Cross section of the abdomen at the first lumbar vertebra. Linea alba, *1;* rectus abdominis muscle, *2;* left lobe of the liver, *3;* peritoneal cavity, *4;* ligamentum teres, *5;* duodenum, *6;* gastroduodenal artery, *7;* hepatic duct, *8;* epiploic foramen, *9;* caudate lobe, *10;* right lobe of the liver, *11;* inferior vena cava, *12;* hepatorenal ligament, *13;* renal artery, *14;* kidney, *15;* crus of the diaphragm, *16;* psoas major muscle, *17;* aorta, *18;* superior mesenteric artery, *19;* descending colon, *20;* transverse colon, *21;* splenic vein, *22;* omental bursa, *23;* stomach, *24*. The psoas major muscle is seen. The crura of the diaphragm are shown on either side of the spine. The right renal artery is seen. The left renal artery arises from the lateral wall of the aorta. Both renal veins enter the inferior vena cava. The portal vein is seen to be formed by the union of the splenic vein and the superior mesenteric vein. The lower portions of the stomach and the pyloric orifice are seen, as is the superior portion of the duodenum. The duodenojejunal flexure and descending and transverse colon are shown. The greater omentum is very prominent. The small, nonperitoneal area of the liver is shown anterior to the right kidney. The round ligament of the liver and the umbilical fissure, which separates the right and left lobes of the liver, are seen. The neck of the gallbladder (not shown) is found just inferior to this section, between the quadrate and caudate lobes of the liver. The cystic duct is cut in two places. The hepatic duct lies just anterior to the cystic duct. The cystic and hepatic ducts unite in the lower part of the section to form the common bile duct. The pancreatic duct is found within the pancreas at this level. Both kidneys are seen just lateral to the psoas muscles. (From Hagen-Ansert SL: The anatomy workbook. Philadelphia, JB Lippincott, 1986.)

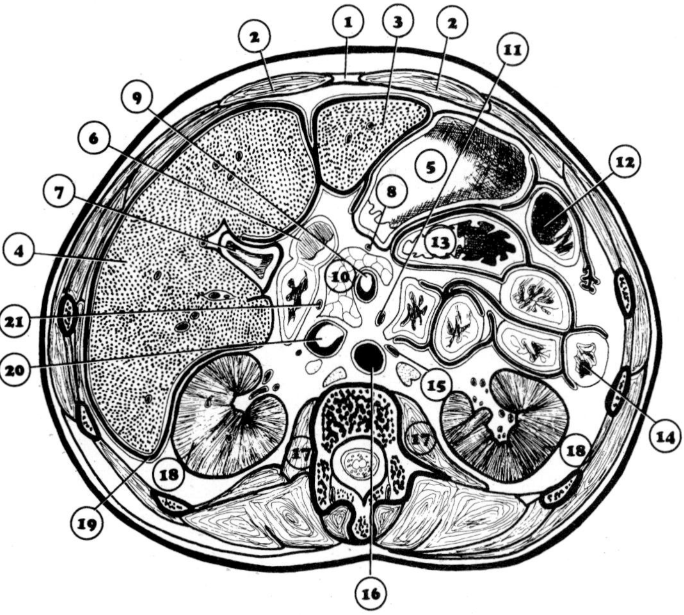

FIG. 1-17 Cross section of the abdomen at the level of the second lumbar vertebra. Linea alba, *1;* rectus abdominis muscle, *2;* left lobe of the liver, *3;* right lobe of the liver, *4;* stomach, *5;* duodenum, *6;* gallbladder, *7;* gastroduodenal artery, *8;* superior mesenteric vein, *9;* pancreas, *10;* superior mesenteric artery, *11;* transverse colon, *12;* jejunum, *13;* descending colon, *14;* left renal vein, *15;* aorta, *16;* psoas major muscle, *17;* kidney, *18;* peritoneal cavity, *19;* inferior vena cava, *20;* common bile duct, *21*. The superior pancreaticoduodenal artery originates in Fig. 1-16 and shows some of its branches in this section. The lower portion of the stomach is found in this section, and the hepatic flexure of the colon is seen. The lobes of the liver are separated by the round ligament. The left lobe of the liver ends at this level. The head and neck of the pancreas drape around the superior mesenteric vein. Both kidneys and the psoas muscles are shown. (From Hagen-Ansert SL: The anatomy workbook. Philadelphia, JB Lippincott, 1986.)

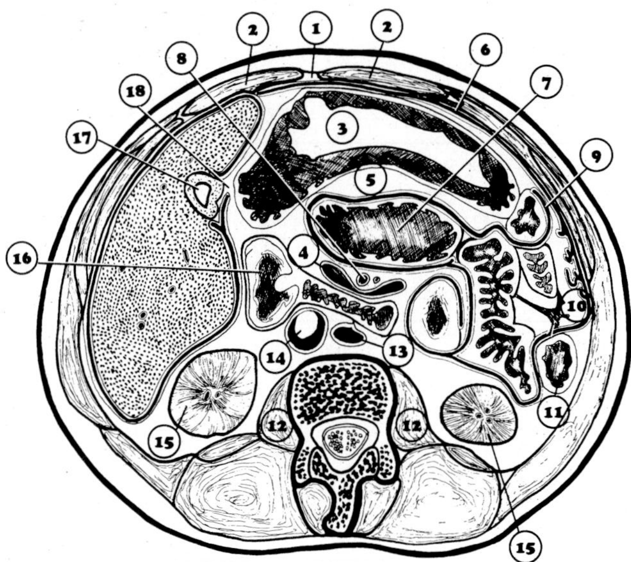

FIG. 1-18 Cross section of the abdomen at the level of the third lumbar vertebra. Linea alba, *1;* rectus abdominis muscle, *2;* transverse colon, *3;* superior mesenteric vein, *4;* transverse mesocolon, *5;* parietal peritoneum, *6;* jejunum, *7;* superior mesenteric artery, *8;* peritoneal cavity, *9;* greater omentum, *10;* descending colon, *11;* psoas major muscle, *12;* aorta, *13;* inferior vena cava, *14;* kidney, *15;* duodenum, *16;* gallbladder, *17;* hepatocolic ligament, *18*. The inferior mesenteric artery originates from the abdominal aorta at this level. The greater omentum is shown mostly on the left side of the abdomen. The descending and ascending portions of the duodenum lie between the aorta and the superior mesenteric artery and vein. The fundus of the gallbladder lies in the lower portion of this section. The lower poles of both kidneys lie lateral to the psoas muscles. (From Hagen-Ansert SL: The anatomy workbook. Philadelphia, JB Lippincott, 1986.)

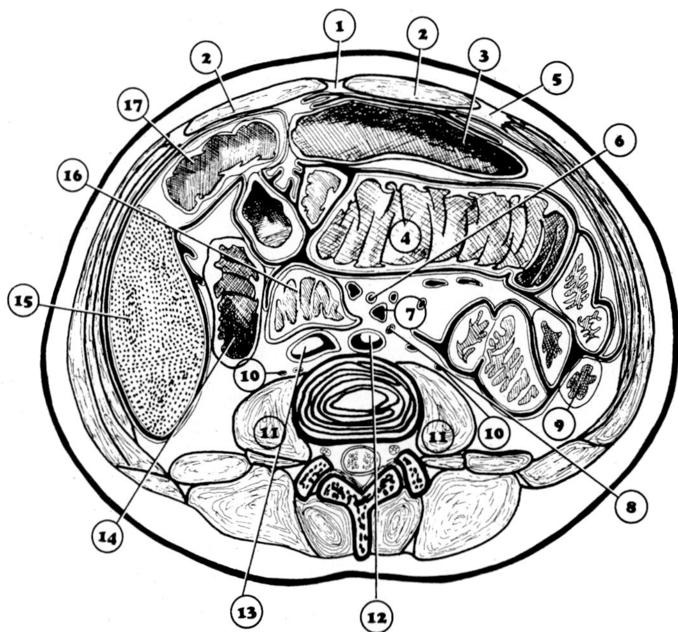

FIG. 1-19 Cross section of the abdomen at the level of the third lumbar disc. Linea alba, *1;* rectus abdominis muscle, *2;* transverse colon, *3;* jejunum, *4;* linea semilunaris, *5;* superior mesenteric artery, *6;* superior mesenteric vein, *7;* inferior mesenteric artery, *8;* descending colon, *9;* ureter, *10;* psoas major muscle, *11;* aorta, *12;* inferior vena cava, *13;* ascending colon, *14;* right lobe of the liver, *15;* duodenum, *16;* ileum, *17*. The lower portion of the duodenum is shown. The lower margin of the right lobe of the liver is seen along the right lateral border. (From Hagen-Ansert SL: The anatomy workbook. Philadelphia, JB Lippincott, 1986.)

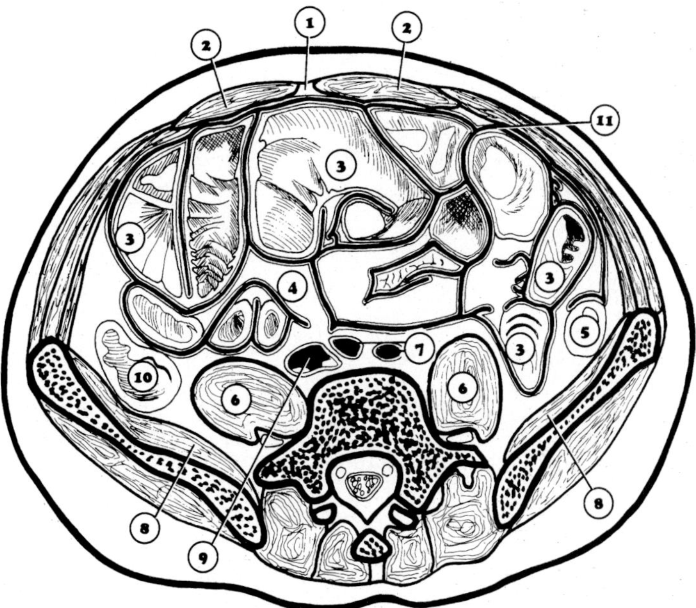

FIG. 1-20 Cross section of the abdomen at the level of the fifth lumbar vertebra. Linea alba, *1;* rectus abdominis muscle, *2;* ileum, *3;* mesentery, *4;* descending colon, *5;* psoas major muscle, *6;* iliac artery, *7;* iliacus muscle, *8;* inferior vena cava, *9;* ascending colon, *10;* peritoneal cavity, *11.* It cuts the ilium through the upper part of the iliac fossa and passes just above the wings of the sacrum. The gluteus medius and iliacus muscles are shown. The right common iliac artery bifurcates into the external and internal iliac arteries. The common iliac veins are shown to unite to form the inferior vena cava. The lower part of the greater omentum is shown in this section. (From Hagen-Ansert SL: The anatomy workbook. Philadelphia, JB Lippincott, 1986.)

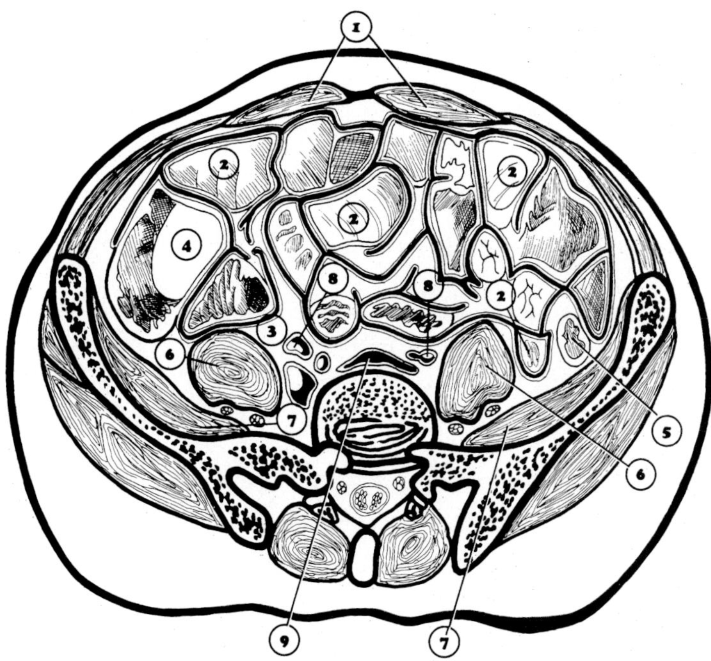

FIG. 1-21 Cross section of the pelvis taken at the lower margin of the fifth lumbar vertebra and disc. Rectus abdominis muscle, *1;* ileum, *2;* mesentery, *3;* ascending colon, *4;* descending colon, *5;* psoas major muscle, *6;* iliacus muscle, *7;* external iliac artery, *8;* iliac vein, *9.* The gluteus minimus muscle is shown on this section as are the right external and internal iliac arteries. The left common iliac artery branches into the external and internal arteries. The ileum is seen throughout this level, and the mesentery terminates at this level. (From Hagen-Ansert SL: The anatomy workbook. Philadelphia, JB Lippincott, 1986.)

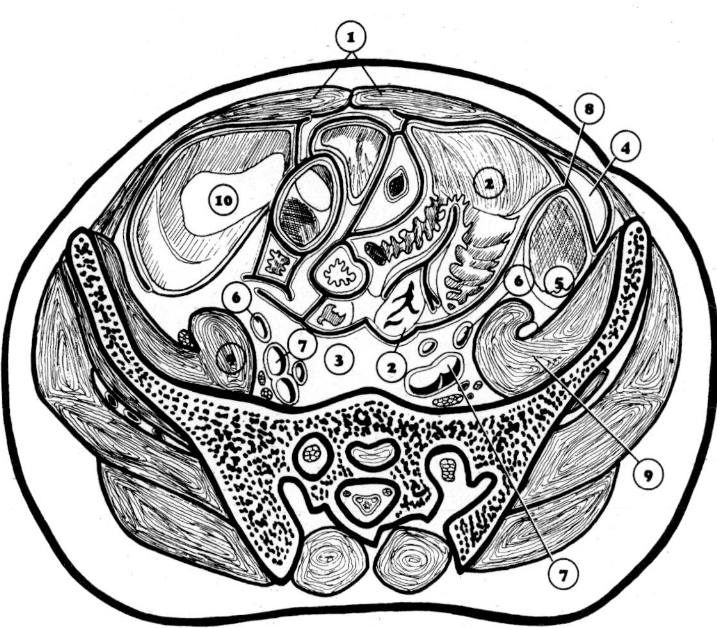

FIG. 1-22 Cross section of the pelvis taken at the level of the sacrum and the anterior superior spine of the ilium. Rectus abdominis muscle, *1;* ileum, *2;* mesentery, *3;* greater omentum, *4;* descending colon, *5;* external iliac artery, *6;* external iliac vein, *7;* peritoneal cavity, *8;* iliopsoas muscle, *9;* ascending colon, *10*. The gluteus maximus muscle appears on both sides. The internal and external iliac veins have united to form the common iliac vein. The ileum is seen throughout this section. (From Hagen-Ansert SL: The anatomy workbook. Philadelphia, JB Lippincott, 1986.)

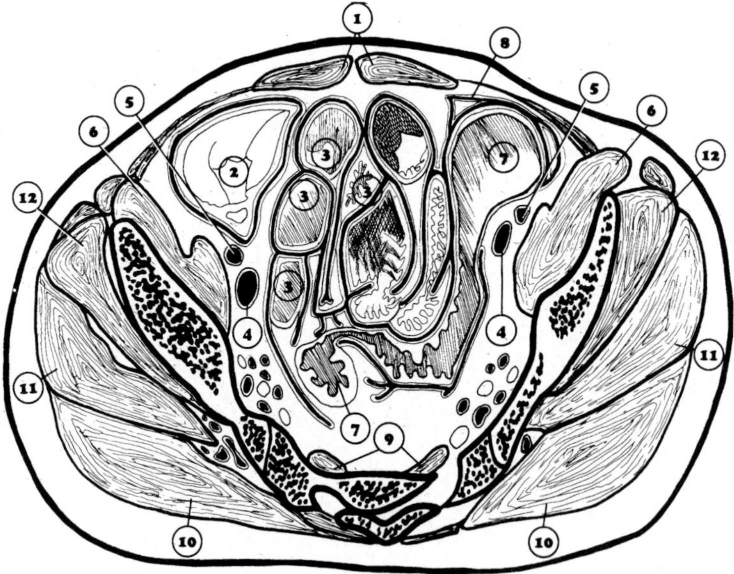

FIG. 1-23 Cross section of the pelvis taken through the third sacral vertebra near the upper margin of the third anterior sacral foramina. Rectus abdominis muscle, *1;* cecum, *2;* ileum, *3;* external iliac vein, *4;* external iliac artery, *5;* iliopsoas muscle, *6;* sigmoid colon, *7;* peritoneal cavity, *8;* piriformis muscle, *9;* gluteus maximus muscle, *10;* gluteus medius muscle, *11;* gluteus minimus muscle, *12*. The pyramidalis, obturator internus, and piriformis muscles are shown. The cecum is also seen in this section. The lower portion of the descending colon passes over the sigmoid colon, and the sigmoid colon passes over into the rectum. (From Hagen-Ansert SL: The anatomy workbook. Philadelphia, JB Lippincott, 1986.)

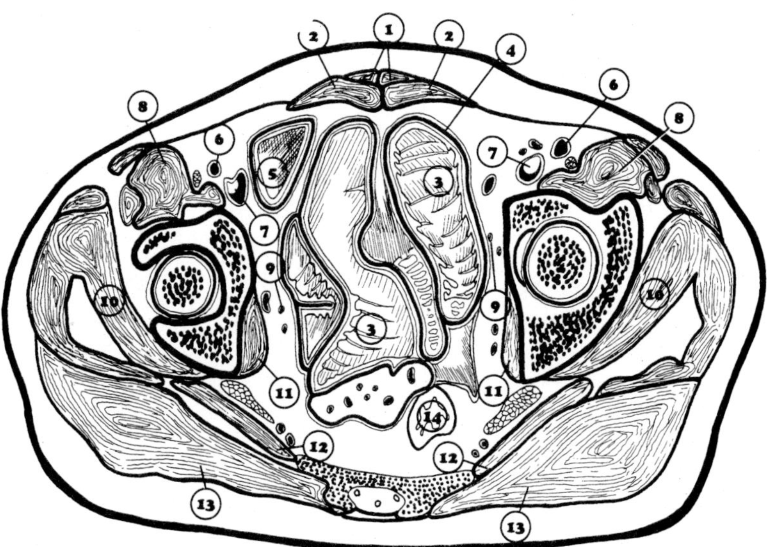

FIG. 1-24 Cross section of the pelvis taken above the margins of the fifth anterior pair of sacral foramina and head of the femur. Pyramidalis muscle, *1;* rectus abdominis muscle, *2;* ileum, *3;* peritoneal cavity, *4;* cecum, *5;* external iliac artery, *6;* external iliac vein, *7;* iliopsoas muscle, *8;* ductus deferens, *9;* gluteus minimus muscle, *10;* obturator internus muscle, *11;* piriformis muscle, *12;* gluteus maximus muscle, *13;* rectum, *14*. The external iliac arteries become the femoral arteries in this section. The femoral veins become the external iliac veins. The cecum and rectum are seen. (From Hagen-Ansert SL: The anatomy workbook. Philadelphia, JB Lippincott, 1986.)

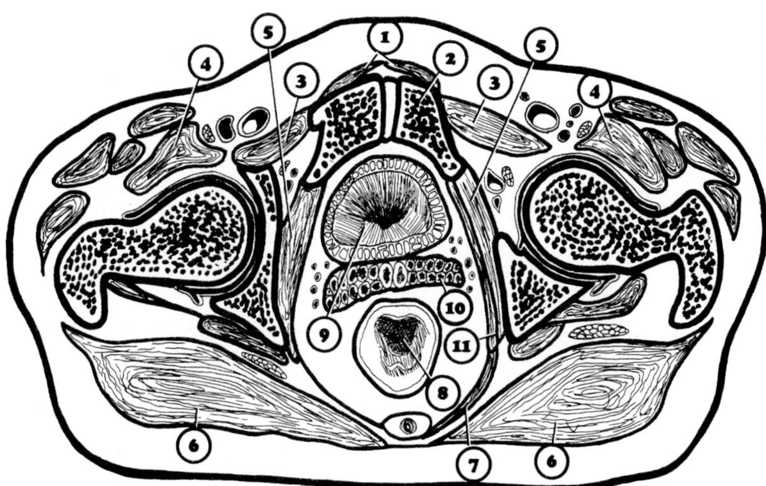

FIG. 1-25 Cross section of the pelvis at the level of the coccyx, the spine of the ischium, the femur, and greater trochanter. Pyramidalis muscle, *1;* pubic os, *2;* pectineus muscle, *3;* iliopsoas muscle, *4;* obturator internus muscle, *5;* gluteus maximus muscle, *6;* coccygeus muscle, *7;* rectum, *8;* bladder, *9;* seminal vesicles, *10;* levator ani muscle, *11*. This cross section passes through the coccyx, the spine of the ischium, the acetabulum, the head of the femur, the greater trochanter, the pubic symphysis, and the upper margins of the obturator foramen. The gemellus inferior and superior, coccygeus, and levator ani muscles are shown. The rectum is seen in the midline. The trigone of the bladder and the urethral orifice are well shown, and the seminal vesicles and the ampulla of the vasa deferentia can be identified. The ejaculatory ducts enter the urethra in the lower portion of this section. (From Hagen-Ansert SL: The anatomy workbook. Philadelphia, JB Lippincott, 1986.)

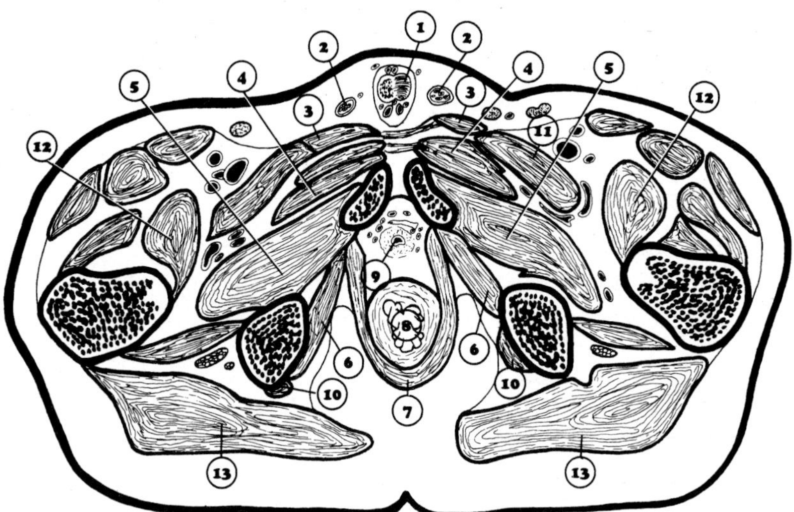

FIG. 1-26 Cross section of the pelvis at the tip of the coccyx, the inferior ramus of the pubis, and the neck of the femur. Penile fascia, *1;* ductus deferens, *2;* adductor longus muscle, *3;* adductor brevis muscle, *4;* obturator externus muscle, *5;* obturator internus muscle, *6;* levator ani muscle, *7;* anus, *8;* rectum, *9;* ischiocavernosus muscle, *10;* pectineus muscle, *11;* iliopsoas muscle, *12;* gluteus maximus muscle, *13*. This cross section passes below the tip of the coccyx, the upper portion of the tuberosity of the ischium and the inferior ramus of the pubis, the neck of the femur, and the lower portion of the greater trochanter. The rectum, prostate gland, penis, and corpus cavernosum are seen. (From Hagen-Ansert SL: The anatomy workbook. Philadelphia, JB Lippincott, 1986.)

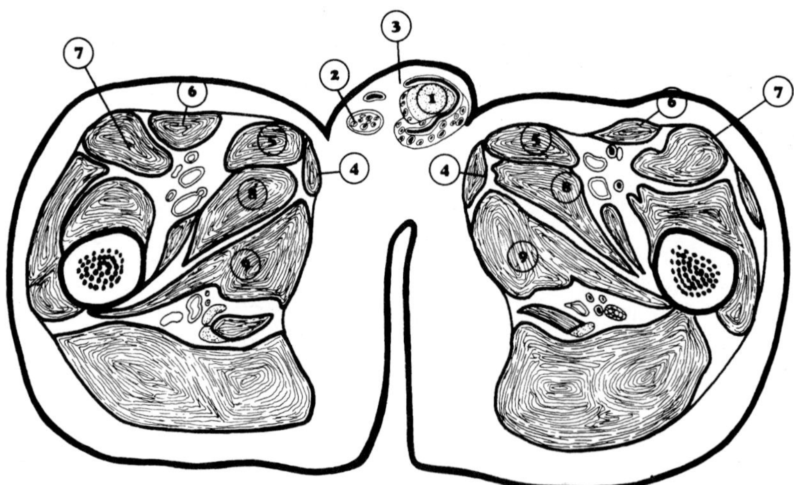

FIG. 1-27 Cross section of the pelvis at the femur, scrotum, testicle, and epididymis. Testis, *1;* plexus pampiniformis, *2;* scrotum, *3;* gracilis muscle, *4;* adductor longus muscle, *5;* sartorius muscle, *6;* rectus femoris muscle, *7;* adductor brevis muscle, *8;* adductor minimus muscle, *9*. This cross section passes through the femur, the scrotum, the upper portion of the left testicle, and the epididymis. The lining, membrane, and tunica vaginalis of the scrotal cavity are seen, as are the vas deferens and the vascular plexus. (From Hagen-Ansert SL: The anatomy workbook. Philadelphia, JB Lippincott, 1986.)

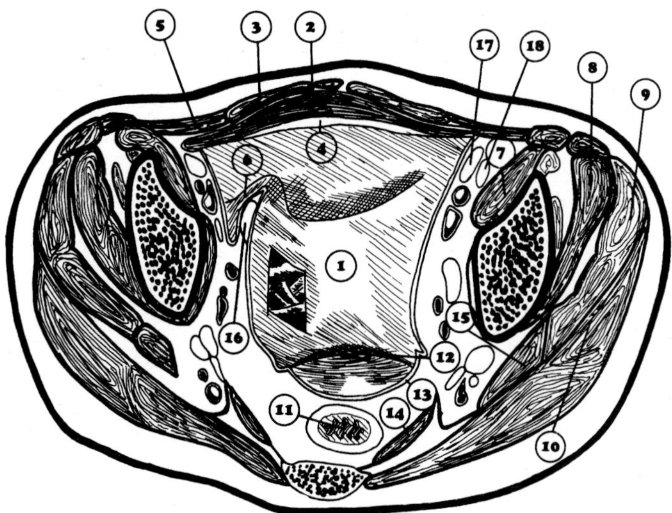

FIG. 1-28 Cross section of the female pelvis just below the junction of the sacrum and coccyx. Uterus, *1;* pyramidalis muscle, *2;* rectus abdominis muscle, *3;* peritoneal cavity, *4;* obturator internus muscle, *5;* fallopian tube, *6;* iliopsoas muscle, *7;* gluteus minimus muscle, *8;* gluteus medius muscle, *9;* gluteus maximus muscle, *10;* rectum, *11;* pouch of Douglas, *12;* peritoneum, *13;* coccygeus muscle, *14;* piriformis muscle, *15;* ovary, *16;* external iliac vein, *17;* external iliac artery, *18*. This cross section is a section through the female pelvis just below the junction of the sacrum and coccyx, through the anterior inferior spine of the ilium and the greater sciatic notch. The uterine artery and vein and the ureter are shown dissected beyond the uterine wall. The bladder is shown just anterior to the uterus, and the round ligament is shown. The ovaries are cut through their midsections on this level. (From Hagen-Ansert SL: The anatomy workbook. Philadelphia, JB Lippincott, 1986.)

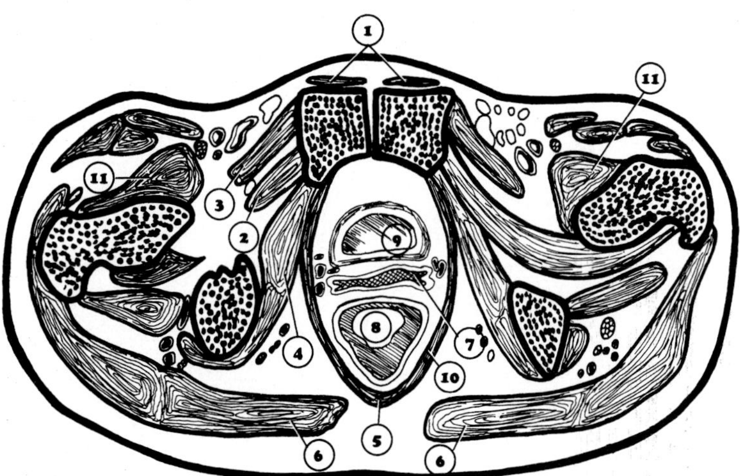

FIG. 1-29 Cross section of the female pelvis taken through the lower part of the coccyx and the spine of the ischium. Pyramidalis muscle, *1;* obturator externus muscle, *2;* pectineus muscle, *3;* obturator internus muscle, *4;* fascia of the pelvic diaphragm, *5;* gluteus maximus muscle, *6;* vagina, *7;* rectum, *8;* bladder, *9;* levator ani muscle, *10;* iliopsoas muscle, *11*. The superior gemellus muscles and the pectineus muscle appear in this section, and the coccygeus muscle terminates here. The gluteus maximus, gluteus minimus, and gluteus medius muscles all begin their insertions in the lower part of this section. The external os of the cervix is shown. The ureters empty into the bladder at the base. (From Hagen-Ansert SL: The anatomy workbook. Philadelphia, JB Lippincott, 1986.)

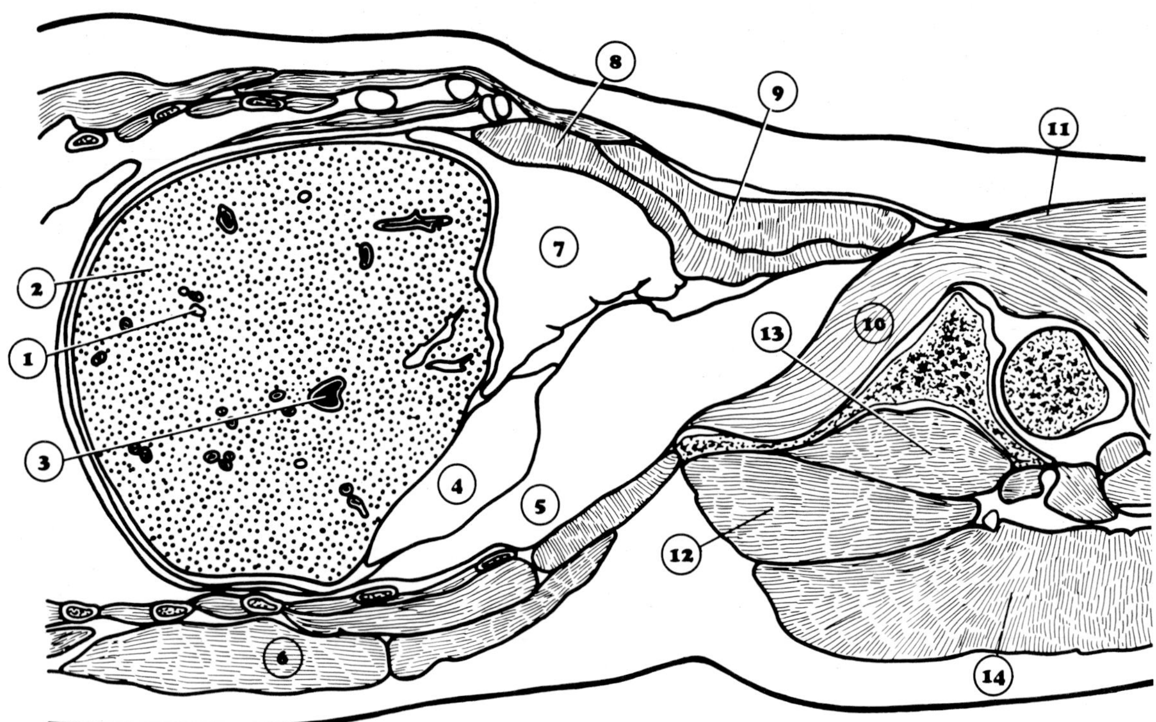

FIG. 1-30 Sagittal section of the abdomen taken along the right abdominal border. Portal vein, *1;* right lobe of the liver, *2;* hepatic vein, *3;* perirenal fat, *4;* retroperitoneal fat, *5;* latissimus dorsi muscle, *6;* omentum, *7;* internal oblique muscle, *8;* external oblique muscle, *9;* iliacus muscle, *10;* psoas major muscle, *11;* gluteus medius muscle, *12;* gluteus minimus muscle, *13;* gluteus maximus muscle, *14*. (From Hagen-Ansert SL: The anatomy workbook. Philadelphia, JB Lippincott, 1986.)

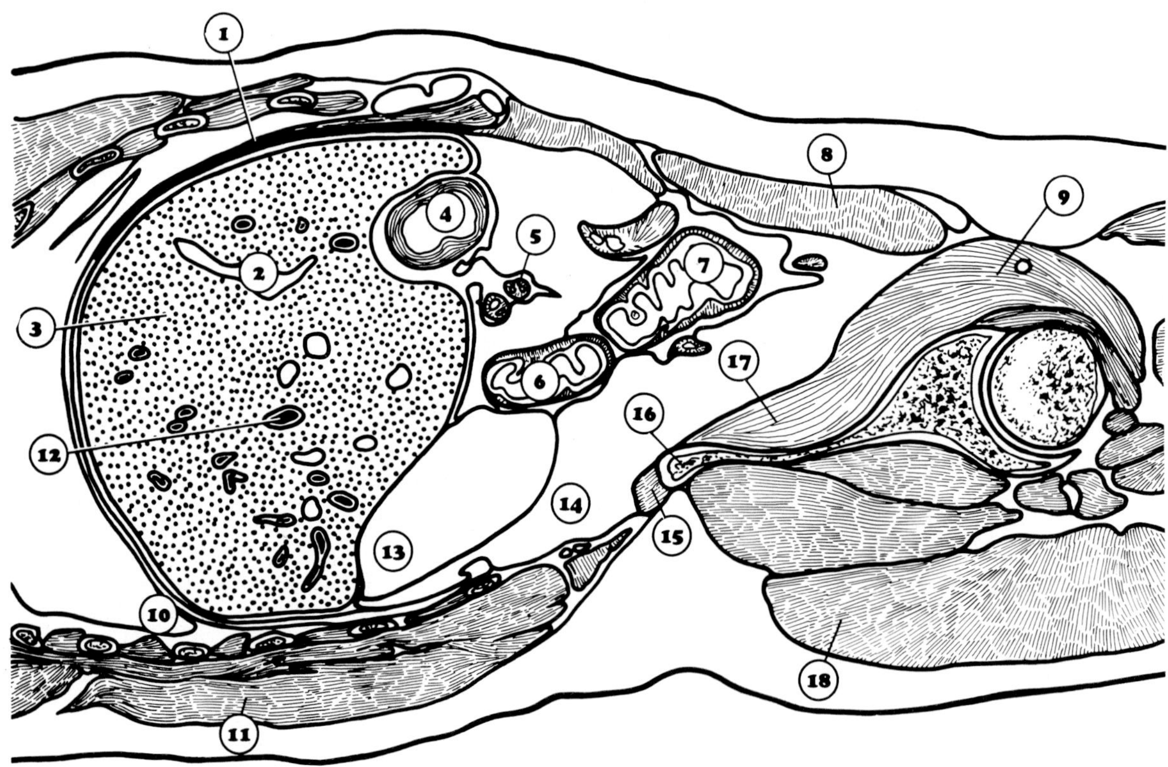

FIG. 1-31 Sagittal section of the abdomen 8 cm from the midline. Diaphragm, *1;* portal vein, *2;* liver, *3;* gallbladder, *4;* hepatic flexure, *5;* ascending colon, *6;* cecum, *7;* internal oblique muscle, *8;* psoas major muscle, *9;* costodiaphragmatic recess, *10;* latissimus dorsi muscle, *11;* hepatic vein, *12;* perirenal fat, *13;* retroperitoneal fat, *14;* quadratus lumborum muscle, *15;* ilium, *16;* iliacus muscle, *17;* gluteus maximus muscle, *18*. (From Hagen-Ansert SL: The anatomy workbook. Philadelphia, JB Lippincott, 1986.)

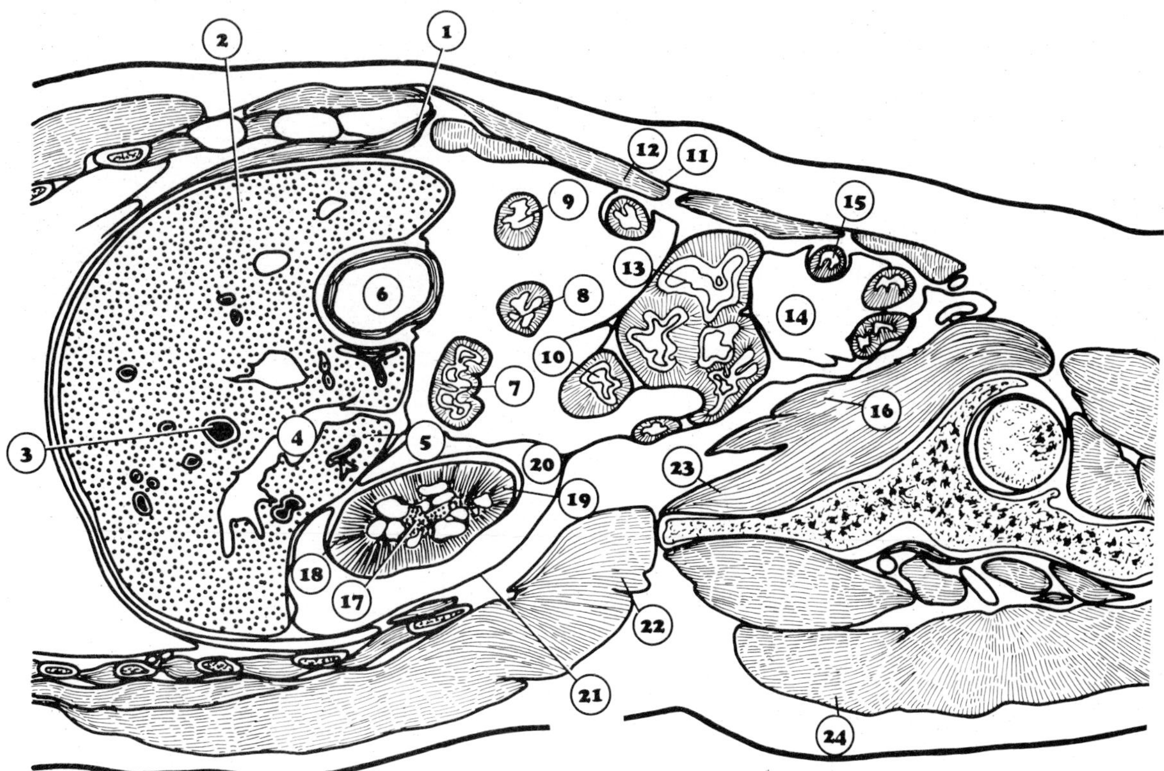

FIG. 1-32 Sagittal section of the abdomen 7 cm from the midline. Diaphragm, *1;* liver, *2;* hepatic vein, *3;* portal vein, *4;* caudate lobe of the liver, *5;* gallbladder, *6;* hepatic flexure, *7;* transverse colon, *8;* small bowel, *9;* ascending colon, *10;* rectus sheath, *11;* rectus abdominis muscle, *12;* cecum, *13;* mesentery, *14;* small bowel, *15;* psoas major muscle, *16;* renal medulla, *17;* right kidney, *18;* renal cortex, *19;* perirenal fat, *20;* perirenal fascia, *21;* quadratus lumborum muscle, *22;* iliacus muscle, *23;* gluteus maximus muscle, *24.* (From Hagen-Ansert SL: The anatomy workbook. Philadelphia, JB Lippincott, 1986.)

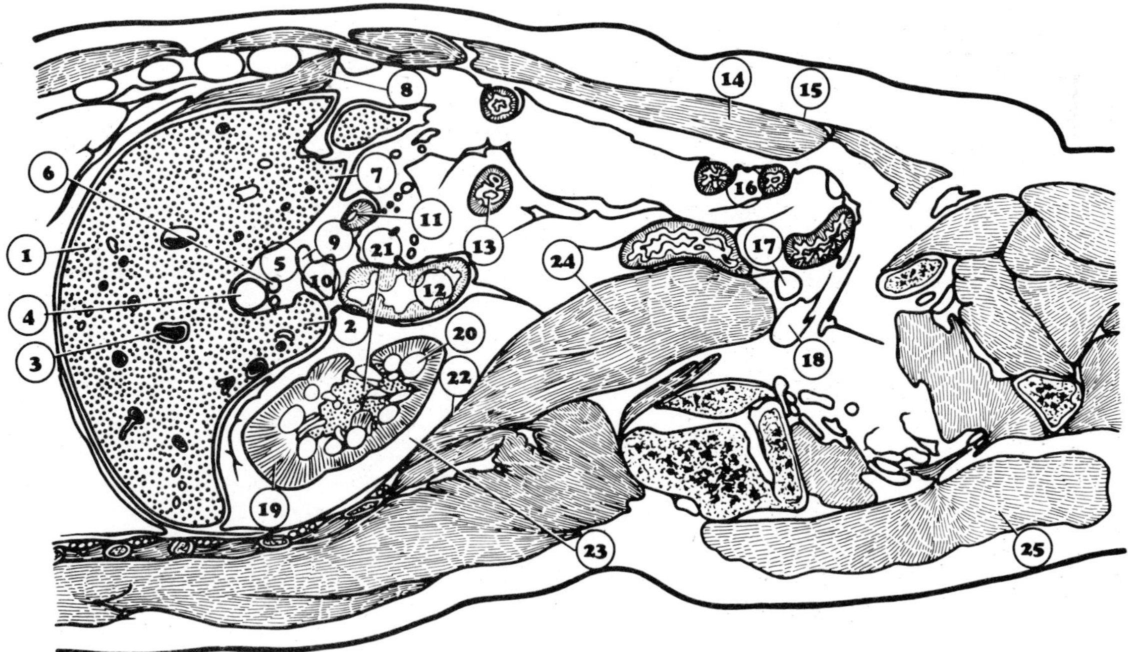

FIG. 1-33 Sagittal section of the abdomen 6 cm from the midline. Liver, *1;* caudate lobe, *2;* hepatic vein, *3;* portal vein, *4;* porta hepatis, *5;* hepatic artery, *6;* quadrate lobe of the liver, *7;* diaphragm, *8;* neck of the gallbladder, *9;* Hartmann's pouch, *10;* superior part of the duodenum, *11;* descending part of the duodenum, *12;* transverse colon, *13;* rectus abdominis muscle, *14;* anterior rectus sheath, *15;* mesentery, *16;* right external iliac artery, *17;* right external iliac vein, *18;* kidney, *19;* renal pyramid, *20;* renal sinus, *21;* perirenal fascia, *22;* perirenal fat, *23;* psoas major muscle, *24;* gluteus maximus muscle, *25.* (From Hagen-Ansert SL: The anatomy workbook. Philadelphia, JB Lippincott, 1986.)

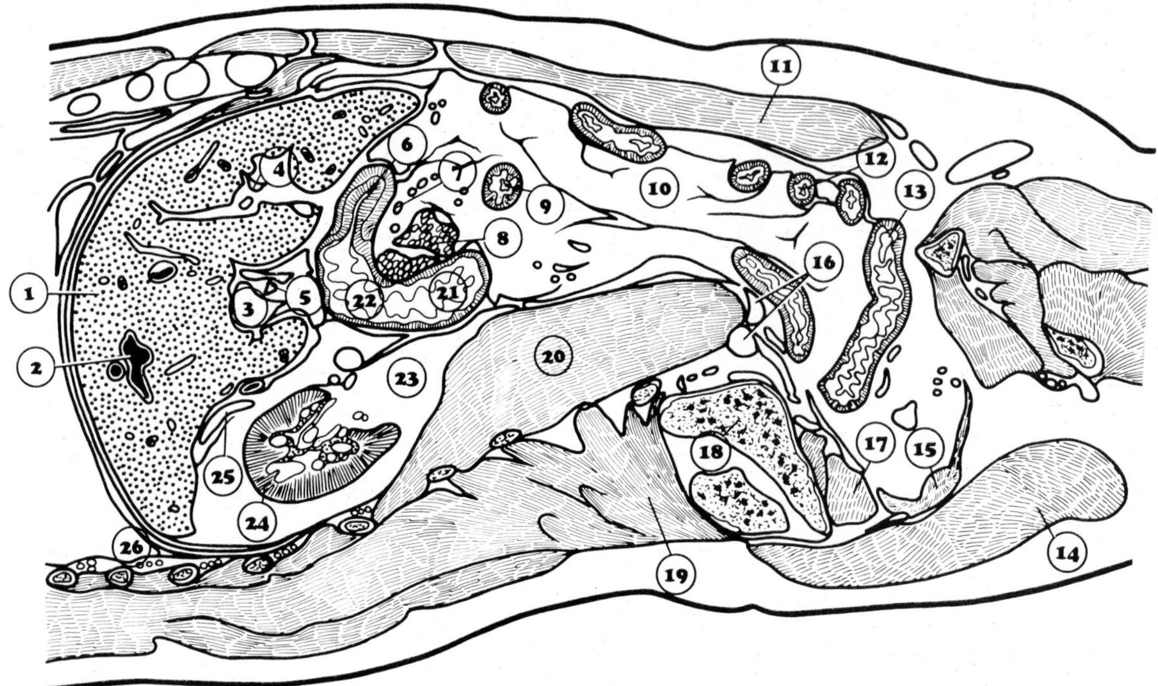

FIG. 1-34 Sagittal section of the abdomen 5 cm from the midline. Right lobe of the liver, *1;* hepatic vein, *2;* portal vein, *3;* left branch of the portal vein, *4;* cystic duct, *5;* pyloric sphincter, *6;* gastroduodenal artery, *7;* head of the pancreas, *8;* transverse colon, *9;* mesentery, *10;* rectus abdominis muscle, *11;* small bowel, *12;* ileum, *13;* gluteus maximus muscle, *14;* levator ani muscle, *15;* right external iliac artery, *16;* piriformis muscle, *17;* sacrum, *18;* erector spinae muscle, *19;* psoas major muscle, *20;* descending duodenum, *21;* superior duodenum, *22;* perirenal fat, *23;* right kidney, *24;* right suprarenal gland, *25;* costodiaphragmatic recess, *26.* (From Hagen-Ansert SL: The anatomy workbook. Philadelphia, JB Lippincott, 1986.)

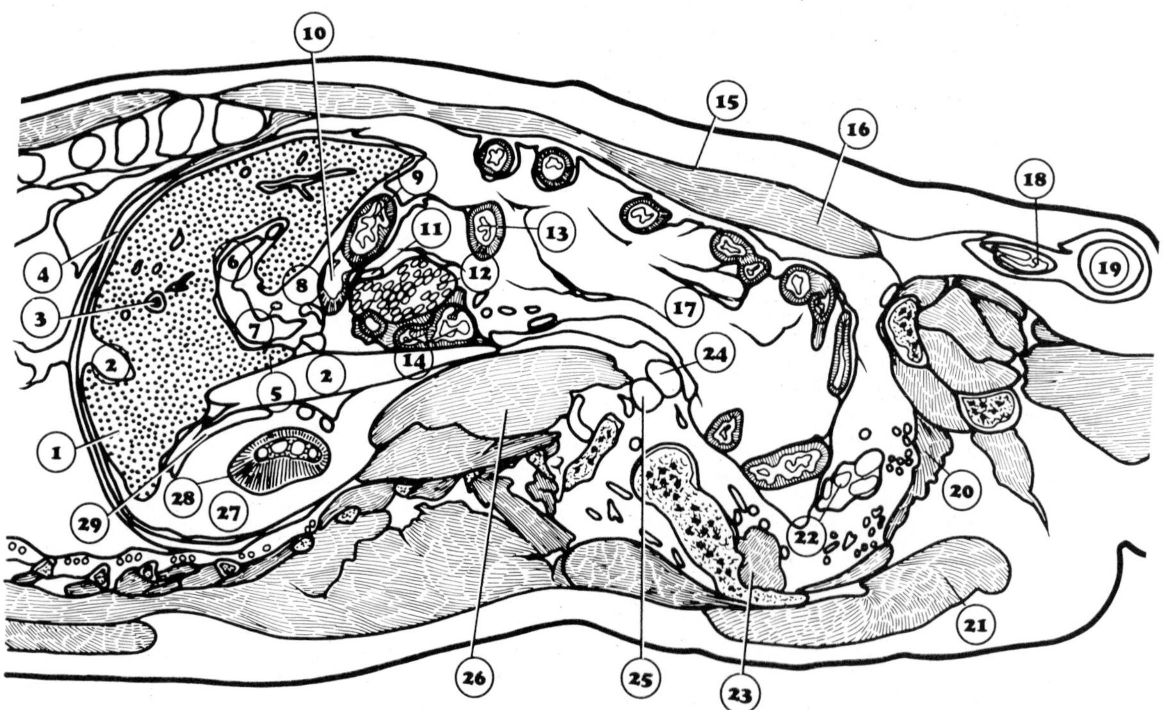

FIG. 1-35 Sagittal section of the abdomen 4 cm from the midline. Right lobe of the liver, *1;* inferior vena cava, *2;* hepatic vein, *3;* diaphragm, *4;* caudate lobe, *5;* left portal vein, *6;* hepatic artery, *7;* cystic duct, *8;* pylorus, *9;* descending part of the duodenum, *10;* gastroduodenal artery, *11;* head of pancreas, *12;* transverse colon, *13;* superior part of the duodenum, *14;* anterior rectus sheath, *15;* rectus abdominis muscle, *16;* mesenteric fat, *17;* spermatic cord, *18;* testis, *19;* levator ani muscle, *20;* gluteus maximus muscle, *21;* seminal vesicles, *22;* piriformis muscle, *23;* right common iliac artery, *24;* right common iliac vein, *25;* psoas major muscle, *26;* perirenal fat, *27;* right kidney, *28;* right suprarenal gland, *29.* (From Hagen-Ansert SL: The anatomy workbook. Philadelphia, JB Lippincott, 1986.)

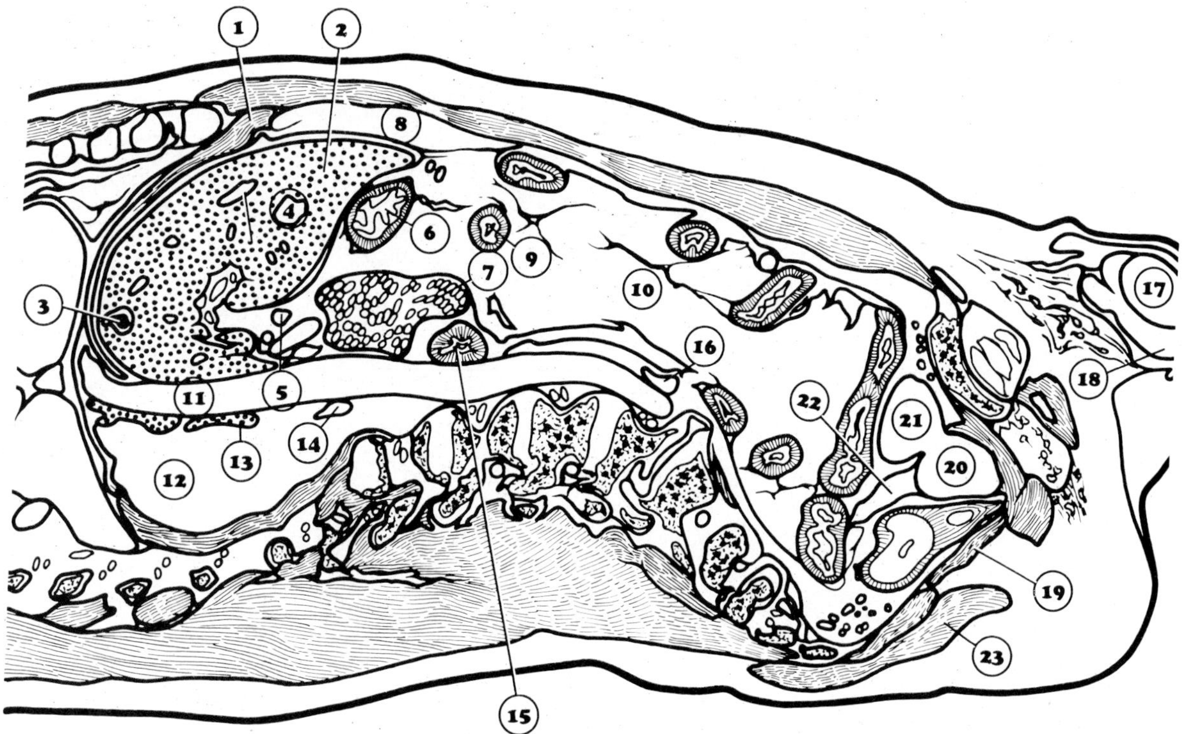

FIG. 1-36 Sagittal section of the abdomen 3 cm from the midline. Diaphragm, *1;* left lobe of the liver, *2;* hepatic vein, *3;* portal vein, *4;* hepatic artery, *5;* pyloric antrum, *6;* head of pancreas, *7;* falciform ligament, *8;* transverse colon, *9;* mesenteric fat, *10;* inferior vena cava, *11;* perirenal fat, *12;* right suprarenal gland, *13;* right renal artery, *14;* horizontal part of the duodenum, *15;* right common iliac artery, *16;* testis, *17;* scrotum, *18;* levator ani muscle, *19;* prostate, *20;* bladder, *21;* seminal vesicles, *22;* gluteus maximus muscle, *23.* (From Hagen-Ansert SL: The anatomy workbook. Philadelphia, JB Lippincott, 1986.)

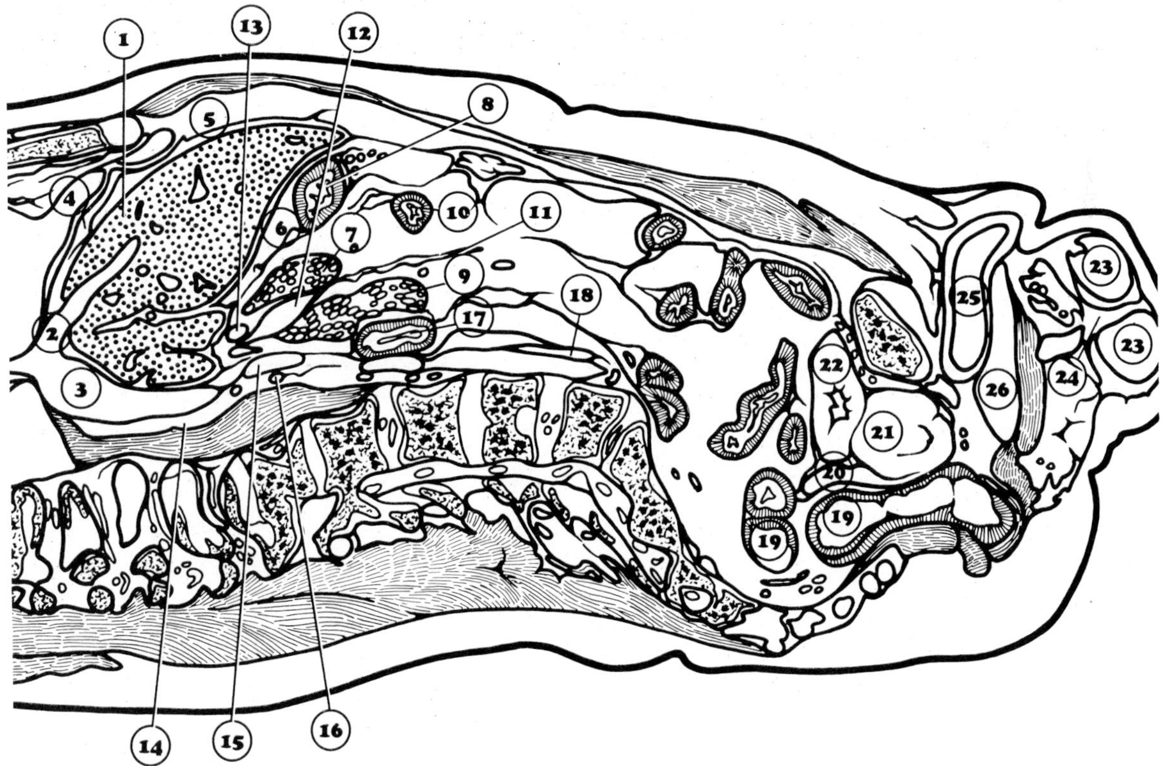

FIG. 1-37 Sagittal section of the abdomen 2 cm from the midline. Left lobe of the liver, *1;* hepatic vein, *2;* inferior vena cava, *3;* diaphragm, *4;* falciform ligament, *5;* lesser omentum, *6;* pancreas, *7;* pyloric antrum, *8;* uncinate process of pancreas, *9;* transverse colon, *10;* superior mesenteric vein, *11;* portal vein, *12;* hepatic artery, *13;* crus of diaphragm, *14;* left renal vein, *15;* right renal artery, *16;* horizontal part of the duodenum, *17;* right common iliac artery, *18;* rectum, *19;* seminal vesicles, *20;* prostate, *21;* bladder, *22;* testis, *23;* scrotum, *24;* corpus cavernosum penis, *25;* corpus spongiosum penis, *26.* (From Hagen-Ansert SL: The anatomy workbook. Philadelphia, JB Lippincott, 1986.)

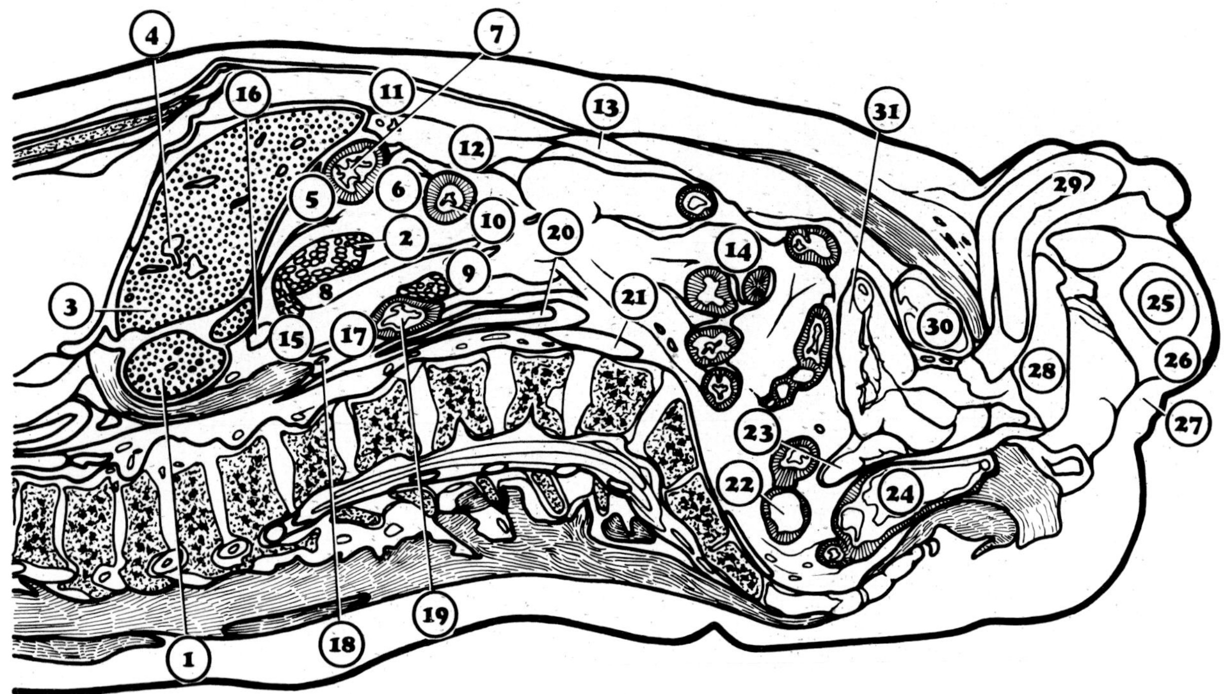

FIG. 1-38 Sagittal section of the abdomen 1 cm from the midline. Caudate lobe, *1;* body of pancreas, *2;* left lobe of liver, *3;* portal vein, *4;* lesser omentum, *5;* lesser sac, *6;* pyloric antrum, *7;* superior mesenteric vein, *8;* uncinate process of pancreas, *9;* transverse colon, *10;* falciform ligament, *11;* greater omentum, *12;* linea alba, *13;* mesenteric fat, *14;* crus of diaphragm, *15;* hepatic artery, *16;* left renal vein, *17;* right renal artery, *18;* horizontal part of the duodenum, *19;* aorta, *20;* left common iliac vein, *21;* rectum, *22;* seminal vesicles, *23;* rectum *24;* testis, *25;* epididymis, *26;* scrotum, *27;* corpus spongiosum penis, *28;* corpus cavernosum penis, *29;* symphysis pubis, *30;* bladder, *31*. (From Hagen-Ansert SL: The anatomy workbook. Philadelphia, JB Lippincott, 1986.)

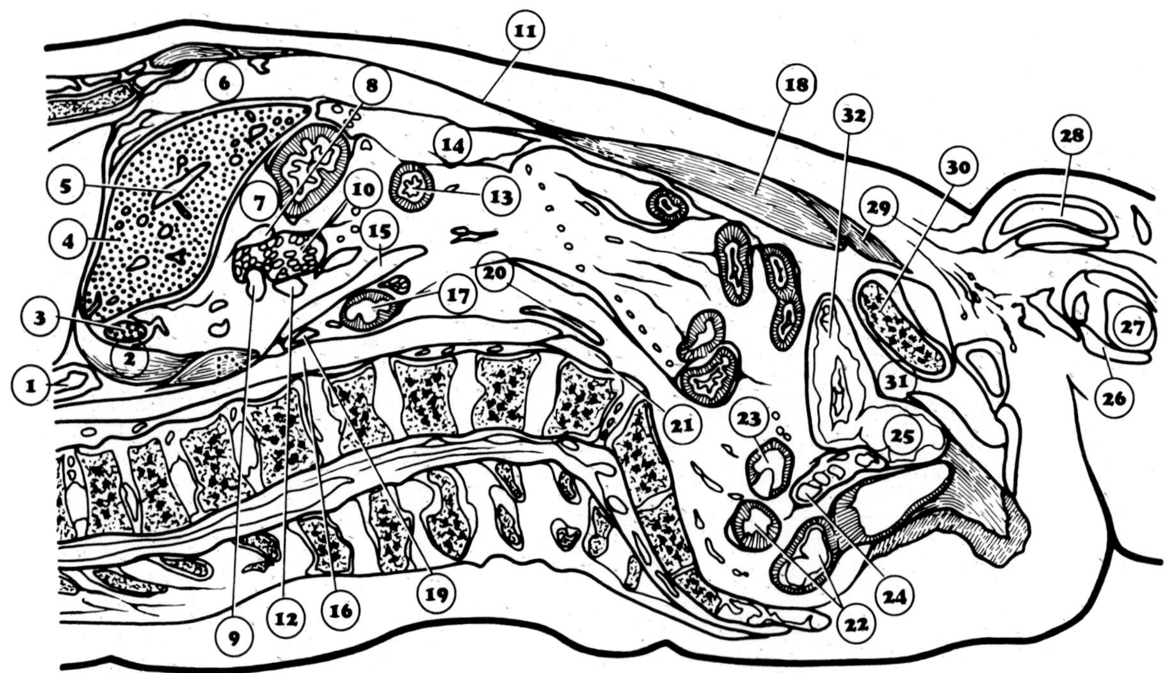

FIG. 1-39 Midline sagittal section of the abdomen. Esophagus, *1;* crus of the diaphragm, *2;* caudate lobe, *3;* left lobe of the liver, *4;* portal vein, *5;* falciform ligament, *6;* lesser omentum, *7;* lesser sac, *8;* splenic artery, *9;* pancreas, *10;* linea alba, *11;* splenic vein, *12;* transverse colon, *13;* greater omentum, *14;* superior mesenteric artery, *15;* aorta, *16;* horizontal part of duodenum, *17;* rectus abdominis muscle, *18;* left renal vein, *19;* inferior mesenteric artery, *20;* left common iliac vein, *21;* rectum, *22;* sigmoid colon, *23;* seminal vesicles, *24;* prostate, *25;* head of the epididymis, *26;* testis, *27;* corpus cavernosum penis, *28;* pyramidalis muscle, *29;* symphysis pubis, *30;* retropubic space, *31;* bladder, *32*. (From Hagen-Ansert SL: The anatomy workbook. Philadelphia, JB Lippincott, 1986.)

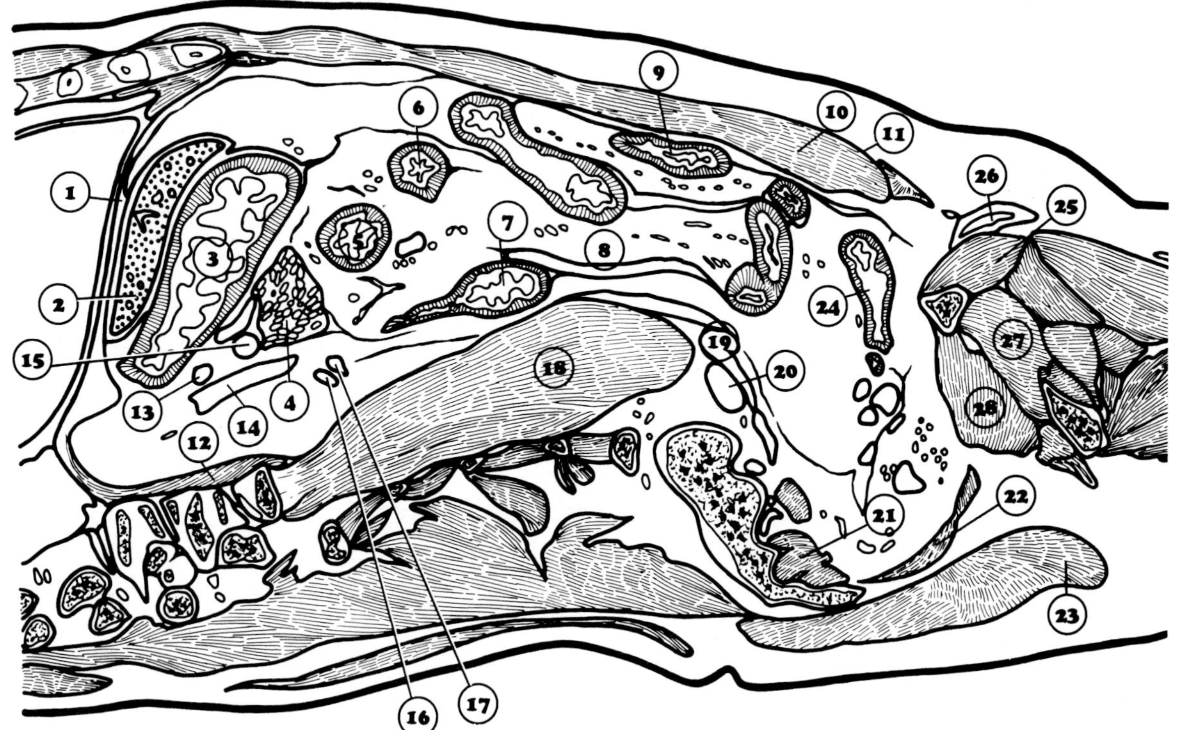

FIG. 1-40 Sagittal section of the abdomen 3 cm to the left of midline. Diaphragm, *1;* left lobe of the liver, *2;* body of the stomach, *3;* pancreas, *4;* ascending part of duodenum, *5;* transverse colon, *6;* jejunum, *7;* mesentery, *8;* small bowel, *9;* rectus abdominis muscle, *10;* rectus sheath, *11;* crus of the diaphragm, *12;* splenic artery, *13;* left suprarenal gland, *14;* splenic vein, *15;* left renal artery, *16;* left renal vein, *17;* psoas major muscle, *18;* left common iliac artery, *19;* left common iliac vein, *20;* piriformis muscle, *21;* levator ani muscle, *22;* gluteus maximus muscle, *23;* sigmoid colon, *24;* pectineus muscle, *25;* spermatic cord, *26;* obturator externus muscle, *27;* obturator internus muscle, *28.* (From Hagen-Ansert SL: The anatomy workbook. Philadelphia, JB Lippincott, 1986.)

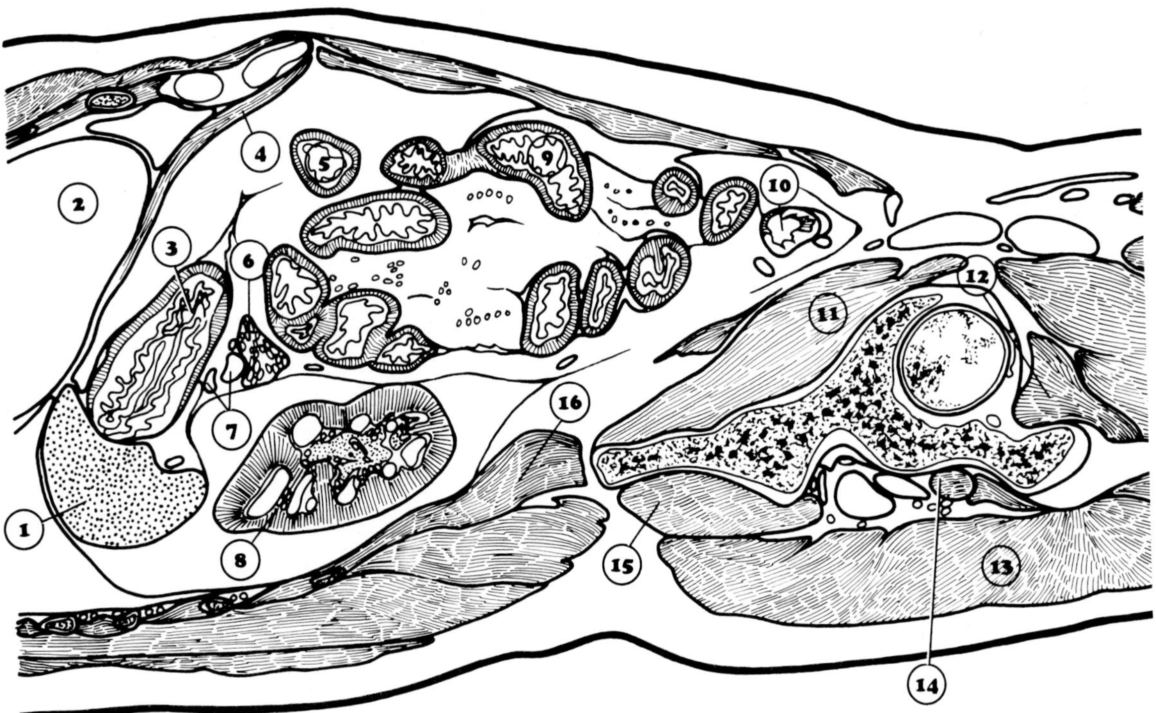

FIG. 1-41 Sagittal section of the abdomen along the left abdominal border. Spleen, *1;* heart, *2;* fundus of the stomach, *3;* diaphragm, *4;* transverse colon, *5;* pancreas, *6;* splenic artery and vein, *7;* left kidney, *8;* small bowel, *9;* sigmoid colon, *10;* iliacus muscle, *11;* obturator externus muscle, *12;* gluteus maximus muscle, *13;* obturator internus muscle, *14;* gluteus medius muscle, *15;* quadratus lumborum muscle, *16.* (From Hagen-Ansert SL: The anatomy workbook. Philadelphia, JB Lippincott, 1986.)

REVIEW QUESTIONS

1. Define the following anatomic terms: *median, sagittal, coronal,* and *transverse*.
2. Define anterior, posterior, medial, lateral, proximal, and distal as each relates to anatomic structures.
3. Name the nine regions of the abdomen.
4. What are the four quadrants of the abdomen?
5. What is the composition of the anterior abdominal wall?
6. Name and describe the two layers of the peritoneum.
7. What is the significance of the epiploic foramen?
8. What is the difference between the mesentery and the omentum?
9. Define the areas of the peritoneal fossae.
10. Name the muscles in the true pelvis that form the posterior pelvic wall and the muscle that lines the lateral pelvic wall.
11. Which muscles form the pelvic diaphragm?

BIBLIOGRAPHY

Crafts RC: A textbook of human anatomy, ed 2. New York, John Wiley & Sons, 1979.

Hagen-Ansert SL: The anatomy workbook. Philadelphia, JB Lippincott. 1986.

Healey JE: A synopsis of clinical anatomy. Philadelphia, WB Saunders, 1969.

Hollinshead WH: Textbook of anatomy, ed 3. New York, Harper & Row, 1974.

Kapit W and Elson LM: The anatomy coloring book. Philadelphia, Harper & Row, 1977.

Netter F: The CIBA collection, digestive system. West Caldwell, New Jersey, CIBA, 1989.

Snell RS: Clinical anatomy for medical students. Boston, Little, Brown & Company, 1992.

Swobodnik W, Herrmann M, Altwein JE, and Basting RF: Atlas of ultrasound anatomy. New York, George Thieme Verlag Stuttgart, 1991.

CHAPTER 2

Muscular System

Sandra L. Hagen-Ansert

Muscles comprise most of the superficial bulk of the human body, and it is useful for the sonographer to have a general understanding of the various muscle groups encountered during the sonographic examination. A brief description of the muscle groups is presented in this chapter.

An essential function of the human body is motion. This function is made possible by the development of the property of contractility in muscle tissue. Motion includes many movements, including body motion, breathing, heart contractility, gastrointestinal motility, as well as the rhythmic movement of the blood and lymph vessels.

TYPES OF MUSCLE

Three types of muscle can be identified by their function, structure, and location in the body—skeletal, smooth, and cardiac (Fig. 2-1).

Skeletal Muscle

Skeletal muscle produces movements of the skeleton and is sometimes called *voluntary muscle*. This muscle is composed of striped muscle fibers and has two or more attachments.

Tendons, ligaments, aponeuroses, and fasciae are the four basic forms of dense connective tissue. The tendons attach muscle to bone; the ligaments connect the bones that form joints; aponeuroses are thin, tendinous sheets attached to flat muscles; and the fasciae are thin sheets of tissue that cover muscles and hold them in their place.

The individual fibers of a muscle are arranged either parallel or oblique to the long axis of the muscle. With contraction, the muscle shortens to one half or one third its resting length. Examples of such muscles are the rectus abdominis and the sternocleidomastoid.

Pennate muscles have fibers that run oblique to the line of pull, resembling a feather. A unipennate muscle is one in which the tendon lies along one side of the muscle and the muscle fibers pass oblique to it. A bipennate muscle has a tendon in the center, and the muscle fibers pass to it from two sides. The pectus femoris is a bipennate muscle. A multipennate muscle may have a series of bipennate muscles lying alongside one another, such as the deltoid, or it may have the tendon lying within its center and the fibers converging into it from all sides.

Smooth Muscle

Smooth muscle is composed of long, spindle-shaped cells closely arranged in bundles or sheets. Its action is that of propelling material through vessels or the gastrointestinal tract and is known as *peristalsis*. In storage organs, such as the bladder and uterus, the fibers are arranged irregularly and are interlaced with one another. In these organs, contraction is slower and more sustained to expel its contents.

Cardiac Muscle

Cardiac muscle is only found in the myocardium of the heart and in the muscle layer of the base of the great blood vessels. These muscles consist of striated fibers that branch and unite with one another. The fibers tend to be arranged in spirals and have the ability to contract spontaneously and rhythmically. Specialized cardiac muscle fibers form the conducting system of the heart.

NECK

The larger muscle groups of the neck are presented in this section because they serve as landmarks for internal structures, such as the thyroid and vascular structures found within the neck. The neck is divided into two triangles, anterior and posterior, by the sternocleidomastoid muscle. (Fig. 2-2).

Anterior Triangle

The anterior triangle contains several important nerves and vessels and is bordered by the mandible above, the sternocleidomastoid muscle laterally, and the median plane of the neck. The infrahyoid muscle group consists of the sternohyoid, omohyoid, thyrohyoid, and sternothyroid muscles. These muscles arise from the sternum, the thyroid cartilage of the larynx, or the scapula and insert on the hyoid bone. Many vessels and nerves traverse this area.

Posterior Triangle

The posterior triangle is bounded anteriorly by the posterior border to the sternocleidomastoid, posteriorly by the

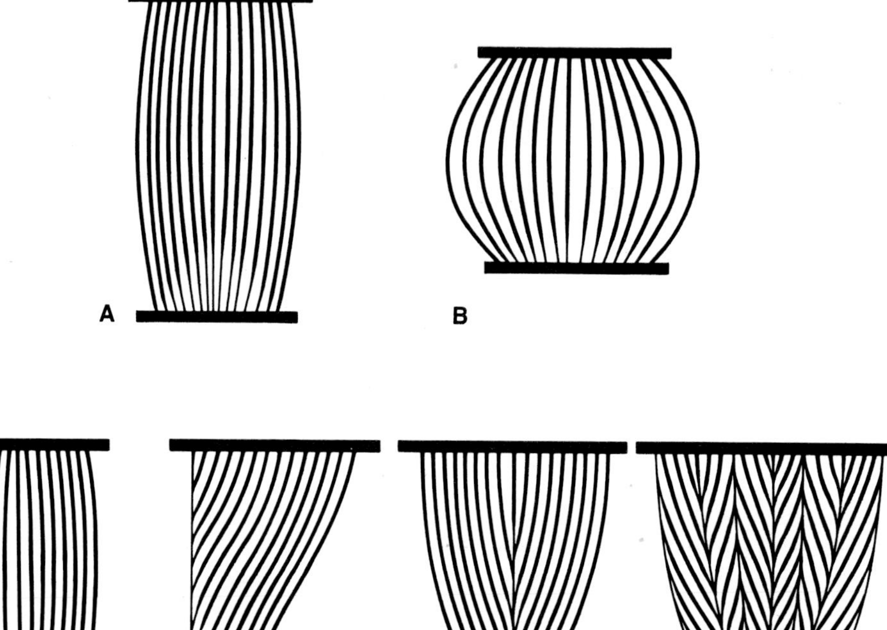

FIG. 2-1 Muscle groups. **A,** Resting muscle. **B,** Contracted muscle. **C** to **F,** Skeletal muscle. **C,** Parallel muscle. **D,** Unipennate muscle. **E,** Bipennate muscle. **F,** Multipennate muscle. (From Hagen-Ansert SL: The anatomy workbook. Philadelphia, JB Lippincott, 1986.)

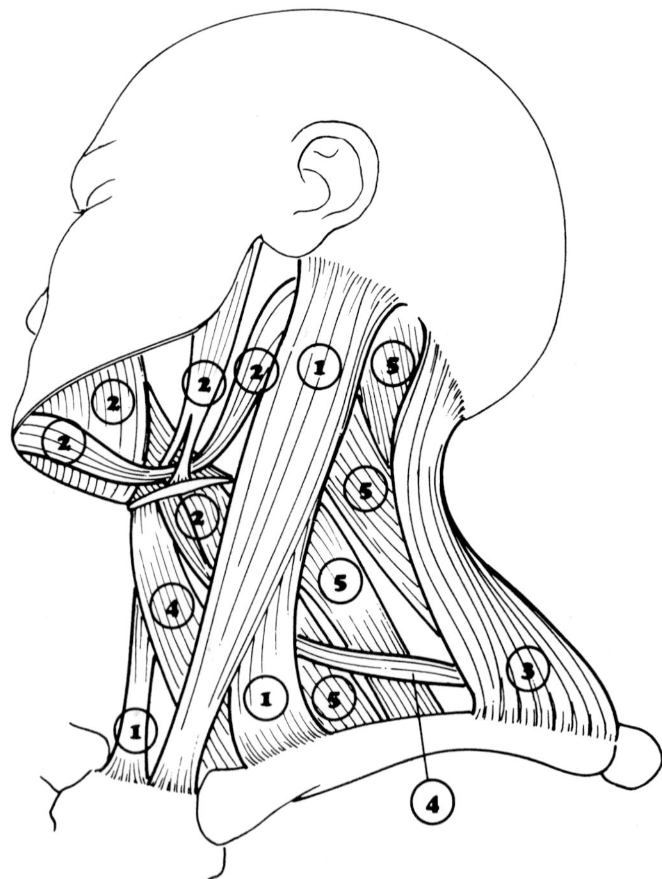

FIG. 2-2 Muscular system of the neck. *1,* Sternocleidomastoid muscles; *2,* suprahyoid muscles; *3,* trapezius muscles; *4,* infrahyoid muscles; *5,* posterior triangle of the neck. (From Hagen-Ansert SL: The anatomy workbook. Philadelphia, JB Lippincott, 1986.)

anterior border of the trapezius, and inferiorly by the middle third of the clavicle. The muscles of this area arise from the head, the cervical vertebrae, the head of the ribs, the scapula, and the cervical and thoracic vertebral spines.

ABDOMEN

Anterior Abdominal Wall

The anterior abdominal wall is a muscular wall; the muscles are attached to the thoracic cage, to the lumbar spine, to the ilium, and to the pubis (Fig. 2-3). In some cases, these attachments are indirect.

There are four muscles of the anterior abdominal wall. The central muscle is the rectus abdominis. The others are lateral to this muscle and are named, from the outside inwards, *external oblique, internal oblique,* and *transversus abdominis*.

Linea Alba

The linea alba is a fibrous band stretching from the xyphoid to the symphysis pubis. It is wider above than below and forms a central anterior attachment for the muscle layers of the abdomen. It is formed by the interlacing of the aponeuroses of the right and left oblique and transversus abdominis muscles.

Rectus Sheath

The sheath of the rectus abdominis muscle is a sheath formed by the aponeuroses of the muscles of the lateral group (Fig. 2-4). The rectus muscle arises from the front of the symphysis pubis and from the pubic crest. It inserts into the fifth, sixth, and seventh costal cartilages and the xyphoid process. On contraction, the lateral margin forms a palpable curved surface, termed the *linea semilunaris,*

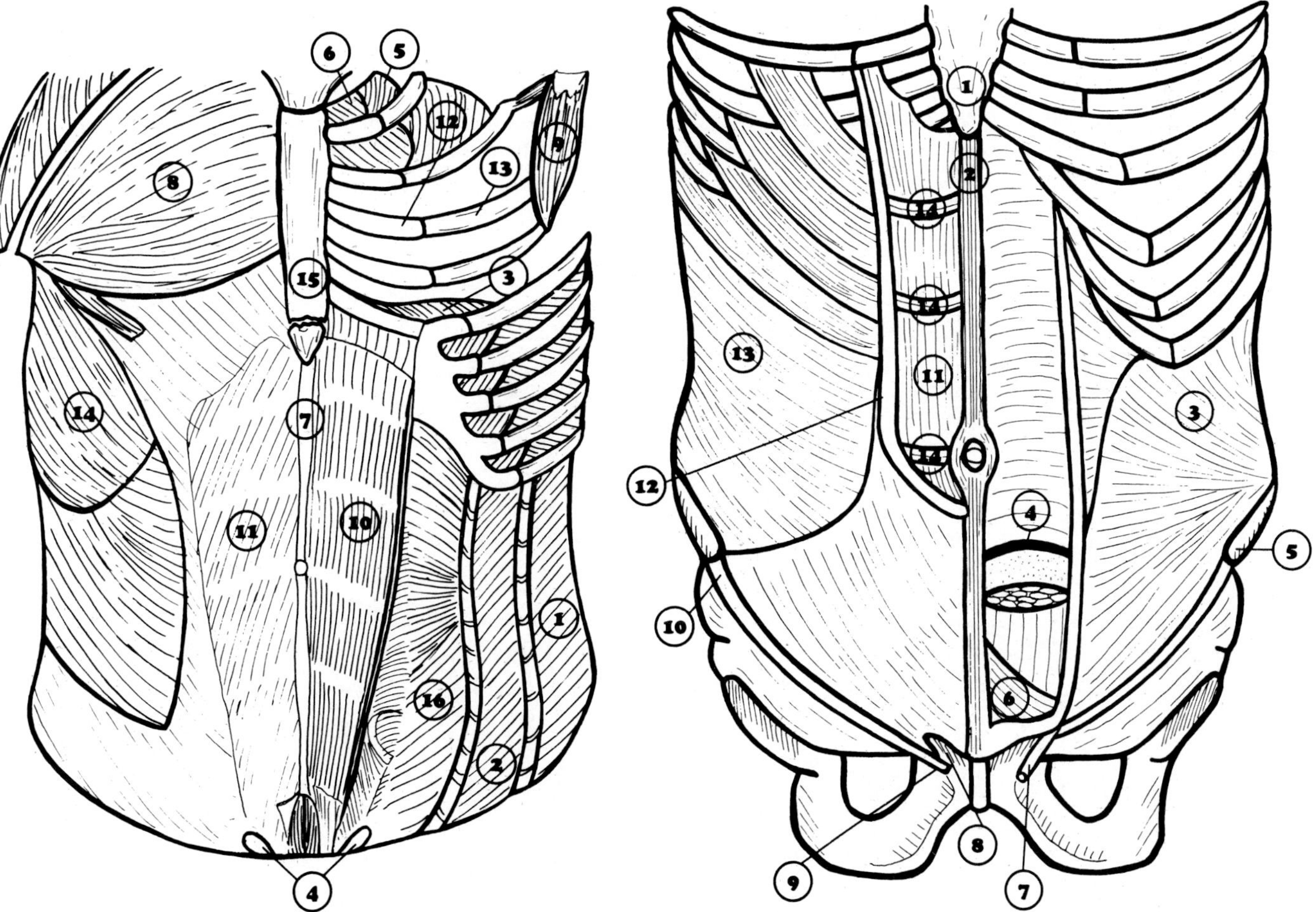

FIG. 2-3 Anterior view of the abdominal muscles. *1,* External oblique muscle; *2,* internal oblique muscle; *3,* diaphragm; *4,* external inguinal ring; *5,* external intercostal muscle; *6,* internal intercostal muscle; *7,* linea alba; *8,* pectoralis major muscle; *9,* pectoralis minor muscle; *10,* rectus abdominis muscle; *11,* rectus sheath; *12,* costal cartilage; *13,* rib; *14,* serratus anterior muscle; *15,* sternum; *16,* transversus abdominis muscle. (From Hagen-Ansert SL: The anatomy workbook. Philadelphia, JB Lippincott, 1986.)

FIG. 2-4 Anterior view of the rectus abdominis muscle and rectus sheath. *1,* Xyphoid process; *2,* linea alba; *3,* internal oblique muscle; *4,* arcuate line; *5,* anterior superior iliac spine; *6,* pyramidalis muscle; *7,* spermatic cord; *8,* superficial inguinal ring; *9,* pubic tubercle; *10,* inguinal ligament; *11,* rectus muscle; *12,* linea semilunaris; *13,* external oblique muscle; *14,* tendinous intersections. (From Hagen-Ansert SL: The anatomy workbook. Philadelphia, JB Lippincott, 1986.)

which extends from the ninth costal cartilage to the pubic tubercle. The anterior surface of the rectus muscle is crossed by three tendinous intersections and are firmly attached to the anterior wall of the rectus sheath.

External Oblique Muscle

The external oblique muscle arises from the lower eight ribs and fans out to be inserted into the xyphoid process, the linea alba, the pubic crest, the pubic tubercle, and the anterior half of the iliac crest (Fig. 2-5).

The superficial inguinal ring is a triangular opening in the external oblique aponeurosis and lies superior and medial to the pubic tubercle. (The spermatic cord or the round ligament of the uterus passes through this opening.)

The inguinal ligament is formed between the anterior superior iliac spine and the pubic tubercle, where the lower border of the aponeurosis is folded backward on itself.

The lateral part of the posterior edge of the inguinal ligament gives origin to part of the internal oblique and transverse abdominal muscles.

Internal Oblique Muscle

The internal oblique muscle lies very deep to the external oblique muscle (Fig. 2-6). The majority of its fibers are aligned at right angles to the external oblique muscle. It arises from the lumbar fascia, the anterior two thirds of the iliac crest, and the lateral two thirds of the inguinal ligament. It inserts into the lower borders of the ribs and their costal cartilages, the xyphoid process, the linea alba, and the pubic symphysis. The internal oblique has a lower free border that arches over the spermatic cord or the round ligament of the uterus and then descends behind it to be attached to the pubic crest and the pectineal line. The lowest tendinous fibers are joined by similar fibers from the transversus abdominis to form the conjoint tendon.

Transversus Muscle

The transversus muscle lies deep to the internal oblique muscle, and its fibers run horizontally forward (Fig. 2-7). It arises from the deep surface of the lower six costal cartilages (interlacing with the diaphragm), the lumbar fascia, the anterior two thirds of the iliac crest, and the lateral third of the inguinal ligament. It inserts into the xyphoid process, the linea alba, and the pubic symphysis.

Diaphragm

The diaphragm is a dome-shaped muscular and tendinous septum that separates the thorax from the abdominal cavity (Fig. 2-8). Its muscular part arises from the margins of the thoracic outlet. The right crus arises from the sides of the

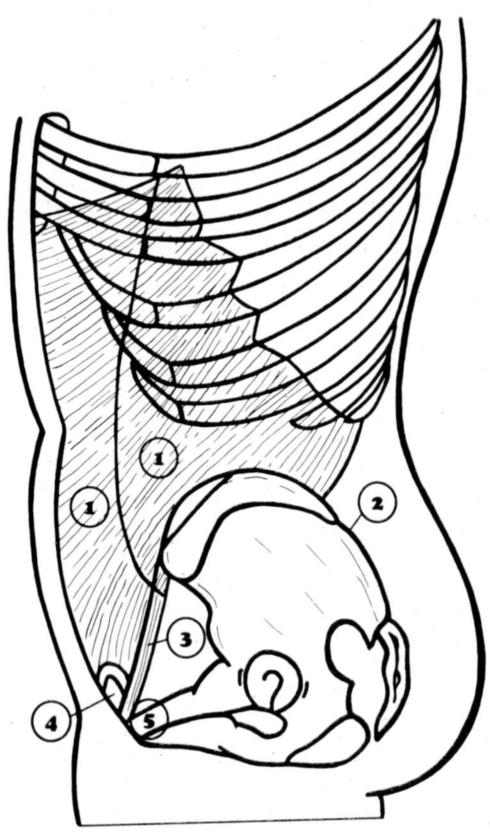

FIG. 2-5 External oblique muscle of the anterior and lateral abdominal wall. *1*, External oblique muscle; *2*, iliac crest; *3*, inguinal ligament; *4*, superficial inguinal ring; *5*, Pubic tubercle. (From Hagen-Ansert SL: The anatomy workbook. Philadelphia, JB Lippincott, 1986.)

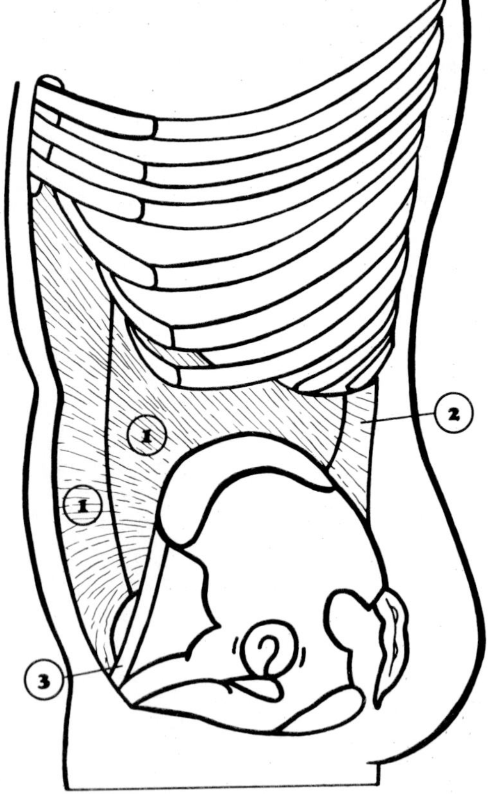

FIG. 2-6 Internal oblique muscle of the anterior and lateral abdominal wall. *1*, Internal oblique muscle; *2*, lumbar fascia; *3*, inguinal ligament. (From Hagen-Ansert SL: The anatomy workbook. Philadelphia, JB Lippincott, 1986.)

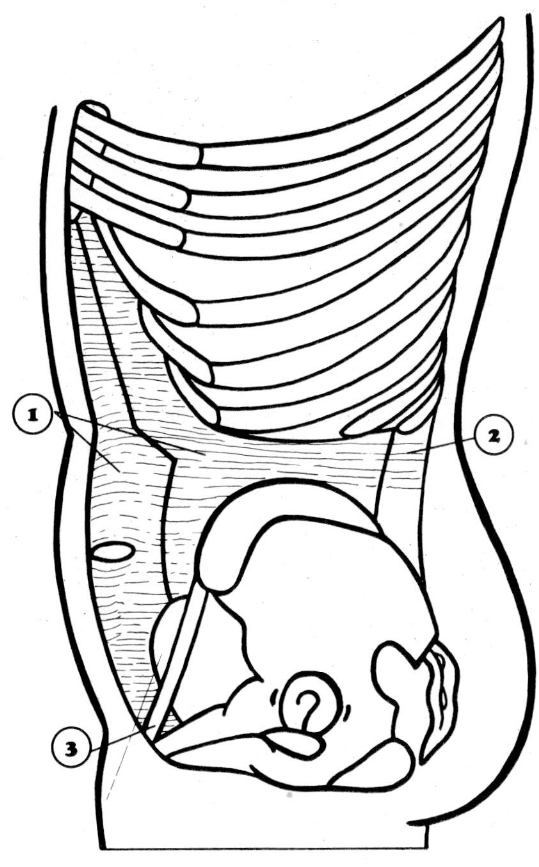

FIG. 2-7 Transversus muscle of the anterior and lateral abdominal wall. *1*, Transversus muscle; *2*, lumbar fascia; *3*, inguinal ligament. (From Hagen-Ansert SL: The anatomy workbook. Philadelphia, JB Lippincott, 1986.)

bodies of the first three lumbar vertebrae; the left crus arises from the sides of the bodies of the first two lumbar vertebrae.

Lateral to the crura, the diaphragm arises from the medial and lateral arcuate ligaments. The medial ligament is the thickened upper margin of the fascia covering the anterior surface of the psoas muscle. It extends from the side of the body or the second lumbar vertebra to the tip of the transverse process of the first lumbar vertebra. The lateral ligament is the thickened upper margin of the fascia covering the anterior surface of the quadratus lumborum muscle. It extends from the tip of the transverse process of the first lumbar vertebra to the lower border of the twelfth rib.

The median arcuate ligament connects the medial borders of the two crura as they cross anterior to the aorta.

The diaphragm inserts into a central tendon (Fig. 2-9). The superior surface of the tendon is partially fused with the inferior surface of the fibrous pericardium. Fibers of the right crus surround the esophagus to act as a sphincter to prevent regurgitation of the gastric contents into the thoracic part of the esophagus.

Back Muscles

The deep muscles of the back help to stabilize the vertebral column (Fig. 2-10). They also influence the posture and curvature of the spine. The muscles have the ability to extend, flex laterally, and rotate all or part of the vertebral column.

PELVIS

The pelvis is divided into two sections; the inferiormost section is called the *minor* or *true pelvis*. The superior section is named the *major* or *false pelvis*.

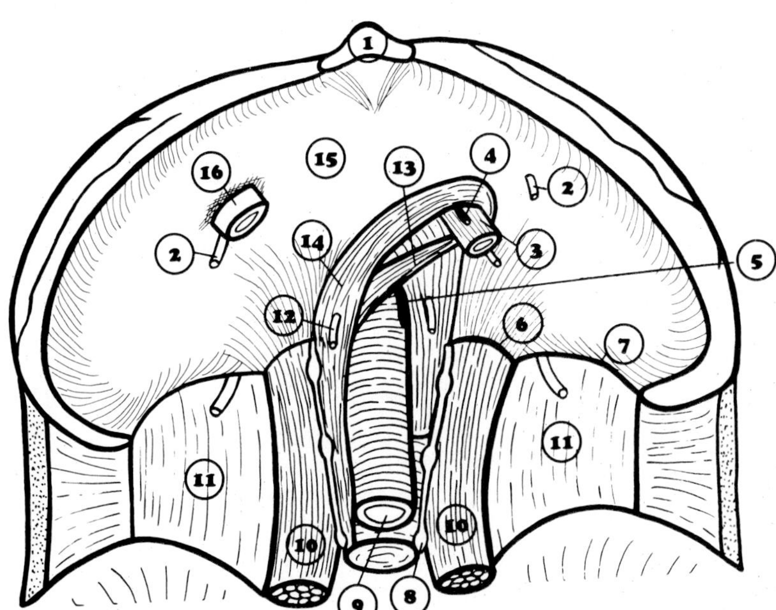

FIG. 2-8 Inferior view of the diaphragm. *1*, Xyphoid process; *2*, right and left phrenic nerves; *3*, esophagus; *4*, vagi; *5*, median arcuate ligament; *6*, medial arcuate ligament; *7*, lateral arcuate ligament; *8*, sympathetic trunk; *9*, aorta; *10*, psoas muscle; *11*, quadratus lumborum muscle; *12*, splanchnic nerves; *13*, left crus; *14*, right crus; *15*, central tendon; *16*, inferior vena cava. (From Hagen-Ansert SL: The anatomy workbook. Philadelphia, JB Lippincott, 1986.)

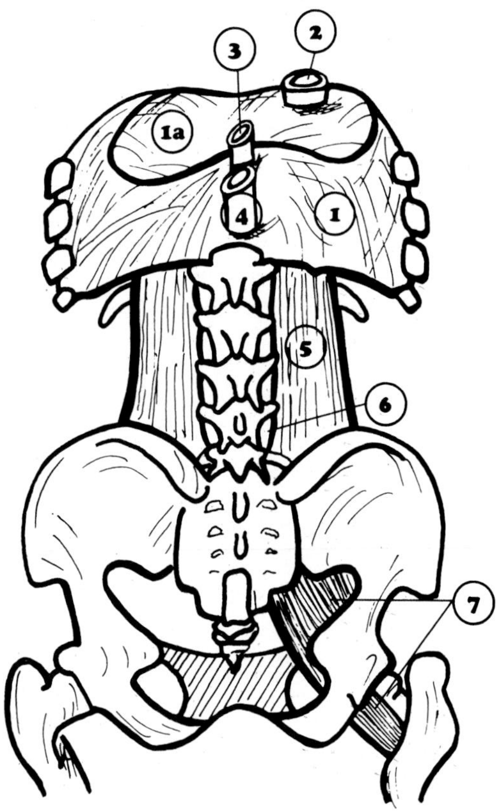

FIG. 2-9 Posterior view of the diaphragm. *1*, Diaphragm; *1a*, central tendon; *2*, inferior vena cava; *3*, esophagus; *4*, aorta; *5*, quadratus lumborum muscle; *6*, psoas major muscle; *7*, iliopsoas muscle. (From Hagen-Ansert SL: The anatomy workbook. Philadelphia, JB Lippincott, 1986.)

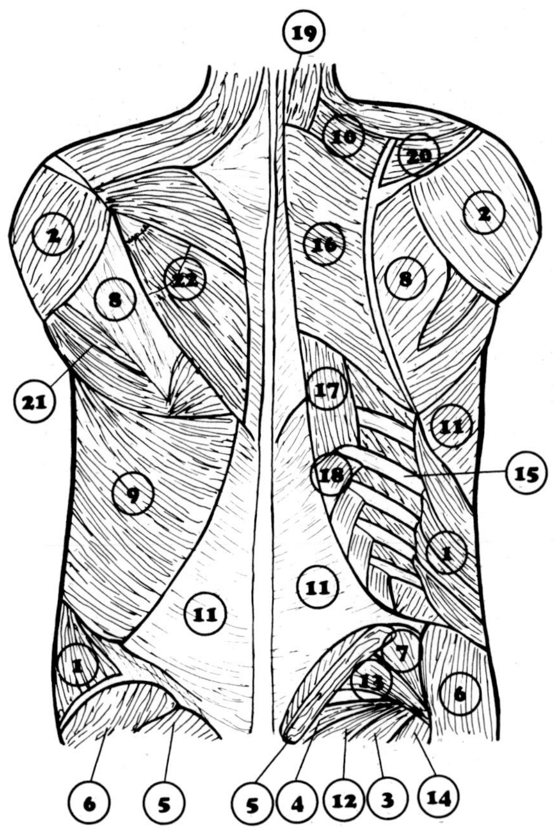

FIG. 2-10 Posterior view of the torso. *1*, External oblique muscle; *2*, deltoid muscle; *3*, gemellus inferior muscle; *4*, gemellus superior muscle; *5*, gluteus maximus muscle; *6*, gluteus medius muscle; *7*, gluteus minimus muscle; *8*, infraspinatus muscle; *9*, latissimus dorsi muscle; *10*, levator scapulae muscle; *11*, lumbodorsal fascia; *12*, obturator internus muscle; *13*, piriformis muscle; *14*, quadratus femoris muscle; *15*, ribs (7-12); *16*, rhomboid muscle; *17*, erector spinae muscle; *18*, serratus posterior inferior muscle; *19*, splenius capitis muscle; *20*, supraspinatus muscle; *21*, teres major muscle; *22*, trapezius muscle. (From Hagen-Ansert SL: The anatomy workbook. Philadelphia, JB Lippincott, 1986.)

True Pelvis

The true pelvis is bounded posteriorly by the sacrum and coccyx (Fig. 2-11). The anterior and lateral margins are formed by the pubis, the ischium, and a small portion of the ilium. A muscular "sling" composed of the coccygeus and levator ani muscles forms the inferior boundary of the true pelvis and separates it from the perineum.

The true pelvis is divided into anterior and posterior compartments. The anterior compartment contains the bladder and reproductive organs. The posterior compartment contains the posterior cul de sac, the rectosigmoid muscle, perirectal fat, and the presacral space.

False Pelvis

The false pelvis is defined by the iliac crests, the iliacus muscles, and the upper crest of the sacrum and is actually considered part of the abdominal cavity. The sacral promontory and the iliopectineal line form the boundary between the false pelvis and the true pelvis and delineate the boundary of the abdominal and pelvic cavities.

The uterus lies anterior to the rectum and posterior to the bladder and divides the pelvic peritoneal space into anterior and posterior pouches. The anterior pouch is termed the *uterovesical space*, and the posterior pouch is called the *rectouterine space* or *pouch of Douglas*. The latter is a common location for accumulation of fluids such as pus or blood.

The fallopian tubes extend laterally from the fundus of the uterus and are enveloped by a fold of peritoneum known as the *broad ligament*. This ligament arises from the floor of the pelvis and contributes to the division of the peritoneal space into anterior and posterior pouches.

Pelvic Muscles

The posterolateral surfaces of the true pelvis are lined by the obturator internus and pubococcygeus muscles (Fig. 2-12). The obturator internus muscles are symmetrically aligned along the lateral border of the pelvis with a concave medial border.

The pubococcygeus muscles are rounded, concave muscles that lie more posterior than the obturator internus muscles (Fig. 2-13). The psoas and iliopsoas muscles lie along

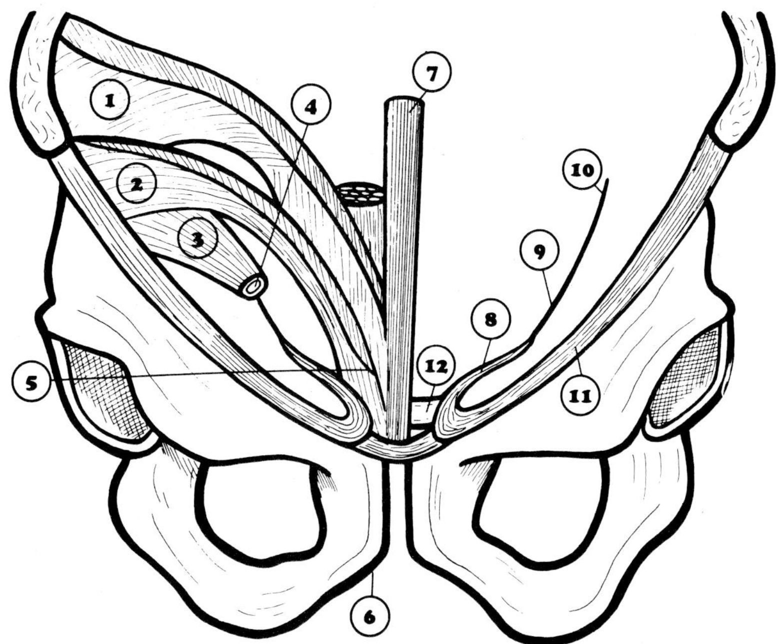

FIG. 2-11 Anterior view of the pelvis. *1,* Transversus muscle; *2,* internal oblique muscle; *3,* cremaster muscle; *4,* spermatic cord; *5,* conjoint tendon; *6,* aponeurosis of the external oblique muscle; *7,* linea alba; *8,* pectineal ligament; *9,* pectineal line; *10,* iliopectineal line; *11,* inguinal ligament; *12,* pubic crest. (From Hagen-Ansert SL: The anatomy workbook. Philadelphia, JB Lippincott, 1986.)

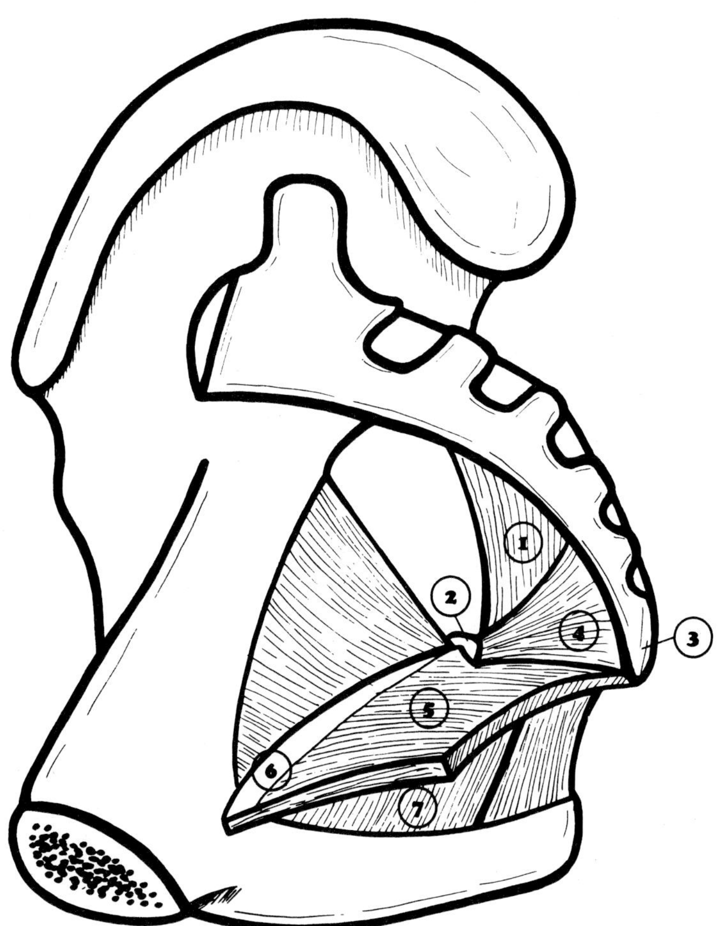

FIG. 2-12 Inferior wall of the pelvis. *1,* Sacrotuberous ligament; *2,* ischial spine; *3,* coccyx; *4,* coccygeus muscle; *5,* levator ani muscle; *6,* linear thickening of fascia covering the obturator internus muscle; *7,* obturator internus muscle. (From Hagen-Ansert SL: The anatomy workbook. Philadelphia, JB Lippincott, 1986.)

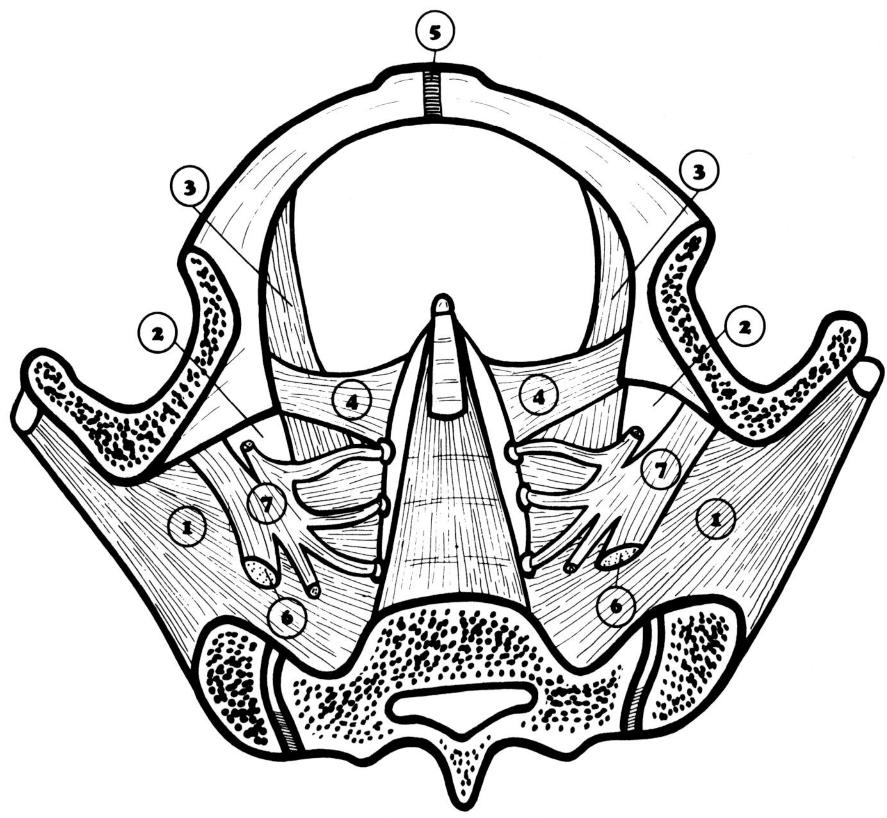

FIG. 2-13 Posterior wall of the pelvis. *1,* Piriformis muscle; *2,* greater sciatic foramen; *3,* sacrotuberous ligament; *4,* sacrospinous ligament; *5,* pubic symphysis; *6,* lumbosacral trunk; *7,* sciatic nerve. (From Hagen-Ansert SL: The anatomy workbook. Philadelphia, JB Lippincott, 1986.)

FIG. 2-14 Inferior view of the female pelvis. *1,* Urethra; *2,* ischiocavernosus muscle; *3,* urogenital diaphragm; *4,* bulbospongiosus muscle; *5,* vagina; *6,* transverse perineal muscle; *7,* ischial tuberosity; *8,* sphincter ani externus muscle; *9,* anus; *10,* levator ani muscle; *11,* anococcygeal ligament; *12,* coccyx. (From Hagen-Ansert SL: The anatomy workbook. Philadelphia, JB Lippincott, 1986.)

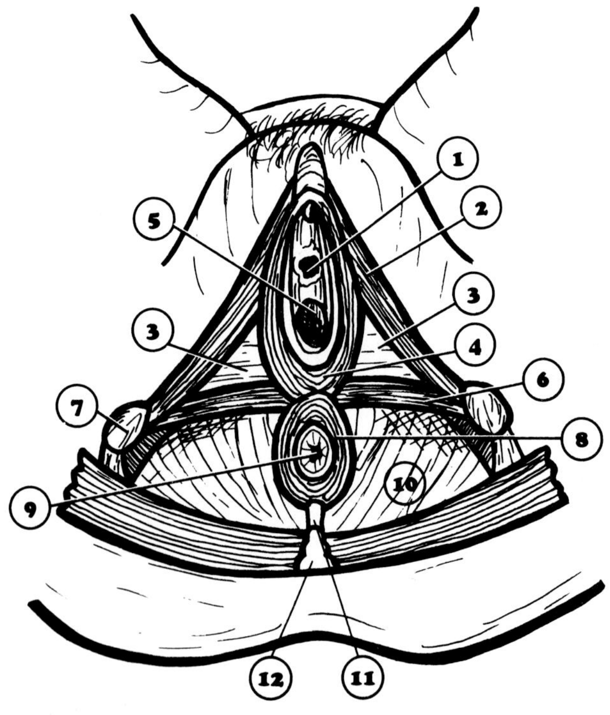

the posterior and lateral margins of the pelvis major. The fan-shaped iliacus muscles line the iliac fossae in the false pelvis. The psoas and iliacus muscles merge in their inferior portions to form the iliopsoas complex. The posterior border of the iliopsoas lies along the iliopectineal line and may be used as a separation landmark of the true pelvis from the false pelvis.

Perineum

The true pelvis is subdivided by the pelvic diaphragm into the main pelvic cavity and the perineum (Fig. 2-14). The perineum has these surface relationships—anterior is the pubic symphysis; posterior is the tip of the coccyx; and lateral are the ischial tuberosities. The region is divided into two triangles by joining the ischial tuberosities by an imaginary line. The posterior triangle is the anal triangle, and the anterior triangle is the urogenital triangle.

The anal triangle has a posterior border of the coccyx, the ischial tuberosities, the sacrotuberous ligament, and the gluteus maximus muscle. The anus lies in the midline, with the ischiorectal fossa on each side.

The urogenital triangle is bounded anteriorly by the pubic arch and laterally by the ischial tuberosities. The superficial fascia is divided into the fatty layer, fascia of Camper, and the membranous layer, Colles' fascia.

REVIEW QUESTIONS

1. What are the three basic muscle types?
2. Name the four basic forms of dense connective tissue.
3. The neck is divided into two triangles—name them.
4. What muscle group divides the neck into the two triangles?
5. Name the four muscle groups of the anterior abdominal wall.
6. What structure separates the thoracic cavity from the abdominal cavity?
7. What is the purpose of the back muscles?
8. What is the difference between the true and the false pelvis?
9. What muscles comprise the muscular "sling" in the inferior boundary of the true pelvis?
10. What is the pouch of Douglas? Where is it located and what is its significance?

BIBLIOGRAPHY

Crafts RC: A textbook of human anatomy, ed 2. New York: John Wiley & Sons, 1979.

Hagen-Ansert SL: The anatomy workbook. Philadelphia: J.B. Lippincott, 1986.

Healey JE: A synopsis of clinical anatomy. Philadelphia: WB Saunders, 1969.

Hollinshead WH: Textbook of anatomy, ed 3. New York, Harper and Row, 1974.

Kapit W and Elson LM: The anatomy coloring book. Philadelphia: Harper & Row, 1977.

Netter F: The CIBA collection III, digestive system, West Caldwell, New Jersey: CIBA, 1964.

Snell RS: Clinical anatomy for medical students, Boston: Little, Brown & Company, 1992.

CHAPTER

3

Introduction to Abdominal Scanning Techniques and Protocols

Sandra L. Hagen-Ansert

The state of the art of ultrasound demands a high degree of manual dexterity and hand-eye coordination, as well as a thorough understanding of anatomy, physiology, pathology, patient contours, equipment capabilities and limitations, and transducer characteristics. Ultrasound equipment today is so sophisticated that it demands a much greater understanding of the physical principles of sonography to produce quality images. The addition of Doppler techniques and color-flow mapping has enhanced the understanding of physiology as it relates to blood-flow dynamics.

Even though it is somewhat difficult to appreciate the actual scanning technique from a textbook, individual hands-on training in ultrasound is part of the sonographer's experience in producing high-quality scans. The sonographer must be aware of the special scanning techniques, artifacts encountered, and equipment malfunctions to be able to produce consistently high-quality scans. The specific applications of abdominal scanning are discussed in this chapter.

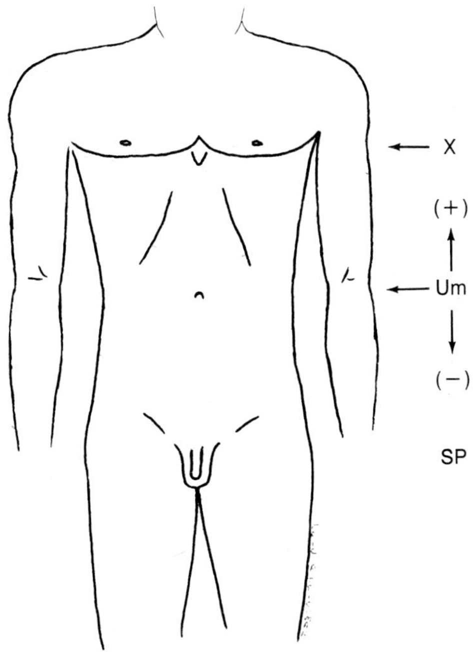

FIG. 3-1 Orientation for transverse labeling. *Um,* umbilicus; *SP,* symphysis pubis; *X,* xyphoid.

SCANNING TECHNIQUES

Ultrasound can distinguish interfaces among soft tissue structures of different acoustic densities. The strength of the echoes reflected depends on the acoustic interface and the angle at which the sound beam strikes the interface. The sonographer must determine which "window" on the patient is the best to record optimal ultrasound images. The small-diameter real time transducer allows the sonographer to go in between intercostal spaces from a supine, coronal, decubitus, or upright position.

ORIENTATION TO LABELING AND PATIENT POSITION

Labeling

An orderly procedure should be used to identify the anatomic position where the transverse and longitudinal scans have been taken. The illustrations in this book use the umbilicus or the symphysis pubis in the transverse supine position (Fig. 3-1); in the sagittal supine position the xyphoid and umbilicus are used (Fig. 3-2); for the prone position the iliac crest is used as a landmark.

All transverse supine scans are oriented with the liver on the left of the scan. Prone transverse scans orient the liver to the right. Longitudinal scans present the patient's head to the left and feet to the right of the scan. Longitudinal scans use the xyphoid, umbilicus, or symphysis to denote the midline of the scan plane. The longitudinal scans are labeled as midline, right, or left.

Real time scans are labeled as transverse or longitudinal for a specific organ, such as the liver, gallbladder, pancreas, spleen, or uterus. The smaller organs that can be imaged on a single plane, such as the kidney, are labeled as long-midline, long-lateral, or long-medial; whereas the transverse scans are labeled as low, middle, and high.

All scans should be appropriately labeled for future reference. This includes the patient's name, date, and anatomic position.

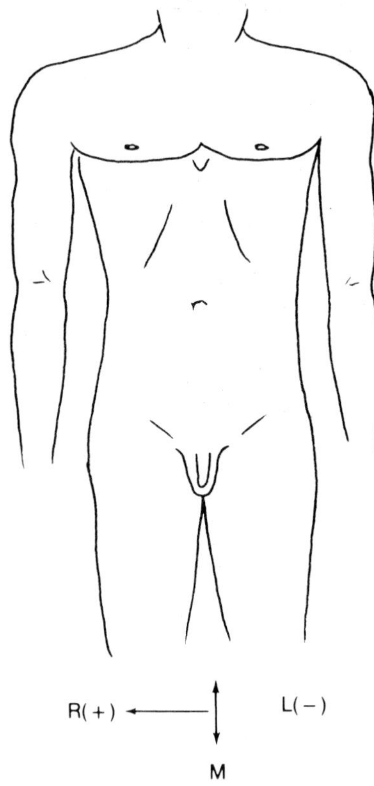

FIG. 3-2 Orientation for sagittal labeling. *M,* midline; *R,* right of midline; *L,* left of midline.

Patient Position

The position of the patient should be described in relation to the scanning table (i.e., a right decubitus would mean the right side down, a left decubitus would indicate the left side down). If the scanning plane is oblique, merely state that it is an oblique view without specifying the exact degree of obliquity.

CRITERIA FOR AN ADEQUATE SCAN

With the use of real time ultrasound, it is sometimes difficult to become oriented to all of the anatomic structures

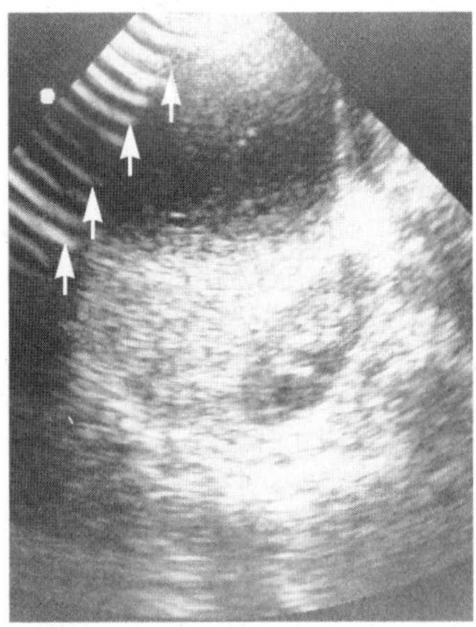

FIG. 3-4 A ring-down artifact is seen *(arrows)* whenever the sound beam strikes a bony interface, such as a rib. This artifact is equally spaced between each reflection as the beam strikes the rib and keeps sending and receiving the signal.

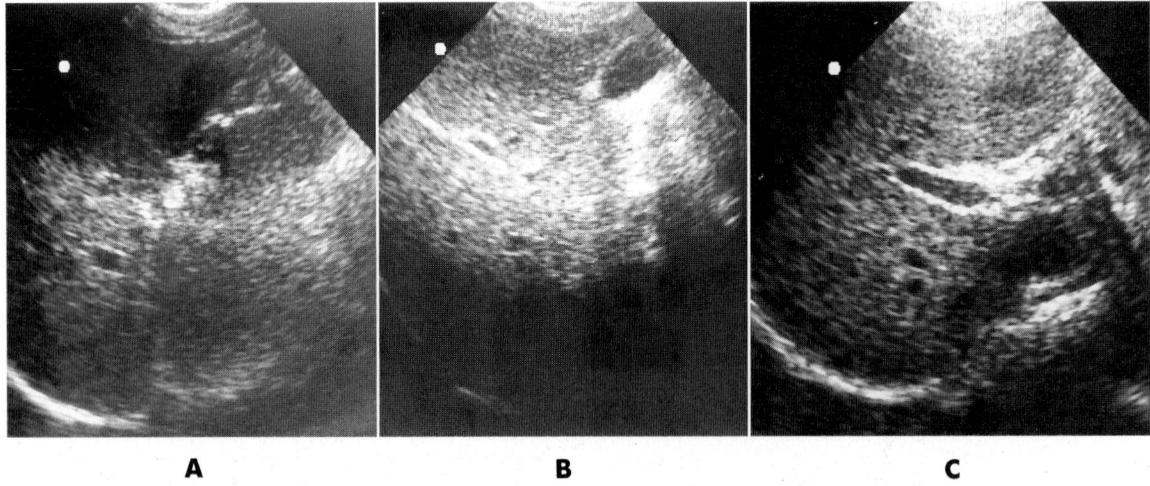

FIG. 3-3 A, Transverse scans of the right upper quadrant show the near-field gain decreased too much compared with the far field. The liver parenchyma should be homogeneous throughout. **B,** Adjustments in the near-field gain are now overcompensated, with a bright band of echoes across the liver parenchyma. The far-field gain has been decreased to the point that only the diaphragm reflection is seen. **C,** A balanced near and far field (time gain compensation) is now set correctly with uniform echoes throughout the liver parenchyma.

on a single scan. Therefore it is critical to obtain as much anatomy as possible in a single image. With careful scanning technique and experience, the sonographer can decide to use the appropriate transducer, equipment, and gain settings to perform a high-quality ultrasound examination (Fig. 3-3).

Avoiding rib interference is important to eliminate artifact "ring-down" reverberation that may destroy information (Fig. 3-4). The small-diameter real time transducers allow the sonographer to scan in between the ribs. Variations in the patient's respiration may also help eliminate rib interference (Fig. 3-5). Patients generally prepare for an upper abdominal scan by not eating for 6 to 8 hours before the ultrasound procedure. This helps to distend the biliary system and to avoid unnecessary bowel gas that may interfere with the visualization of the smaller abdominal and vascular structures (Fig. 3-6).

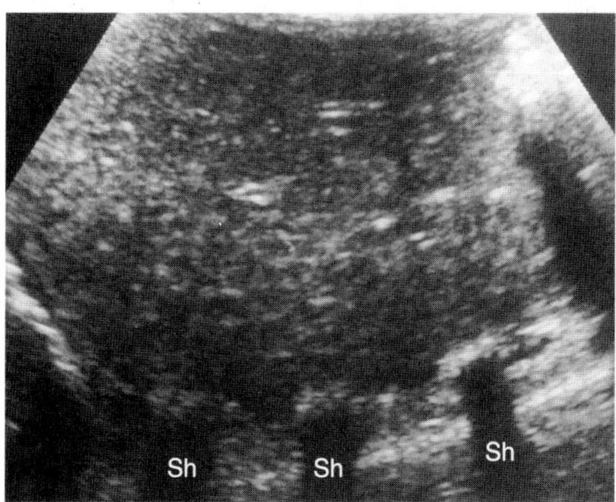

FIG. 3-5 Another artifact seen in the upper abdomen is complete shadowing, *sh*, from the ribs.

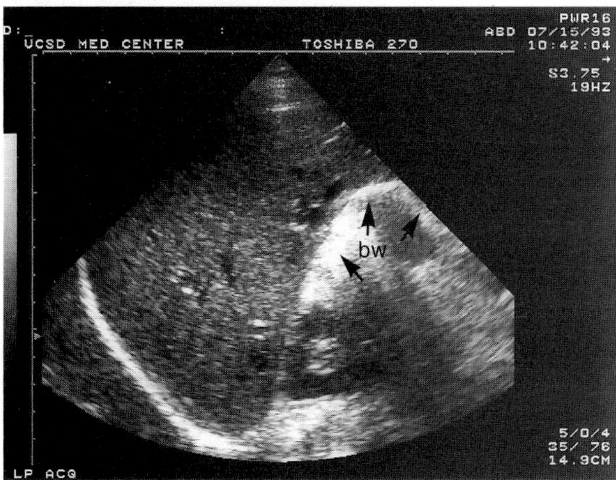

FIG. 3-6 The stomach or transverse colon may cause the gas- or air-filled material to completely reflect the sound beam. The transducer must be moved to avoid the air interference, or the liver may be used as an acoustic window to image the abdominal structures.

Transverse Scans (Fig. 3-7)

1. The horseshoe-shaped contour of the vertebral column should be well delineated to ensure sound penetration

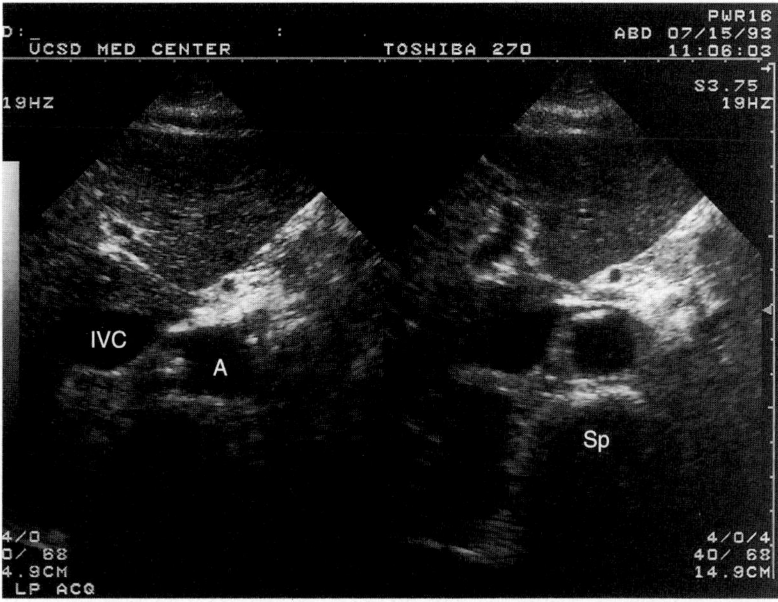

FIG. 3-7 Criteria for a transverse upper abdominal scan mean that the spine, *sp*, should be clearly delineated with the aorta, *A*, and inferior vena cava, *IVC*, directly anterior.

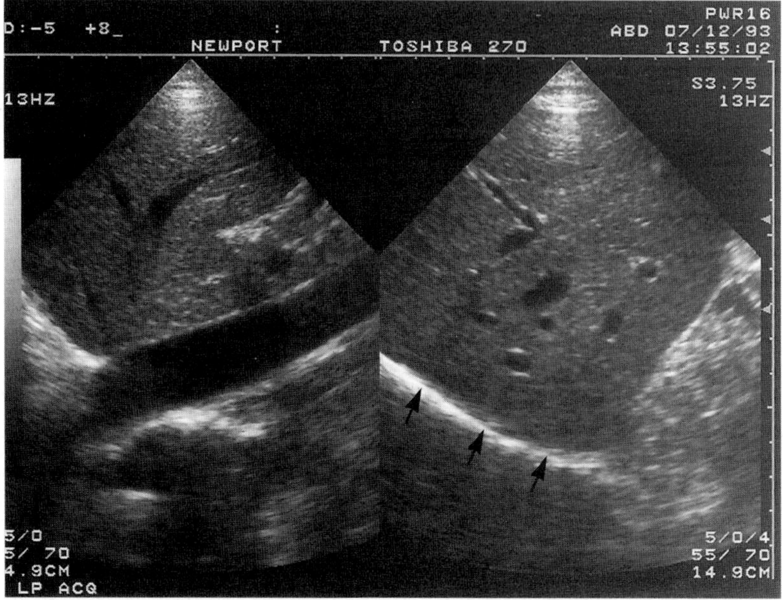

FIG. 3-8 Criteria for a longitudinal upper abdominal scan should show the vascular structures as echo-free. The liver should be homogeneous throughout with the bright reflection from the diaphragm along its posterior border *(arrows)*.

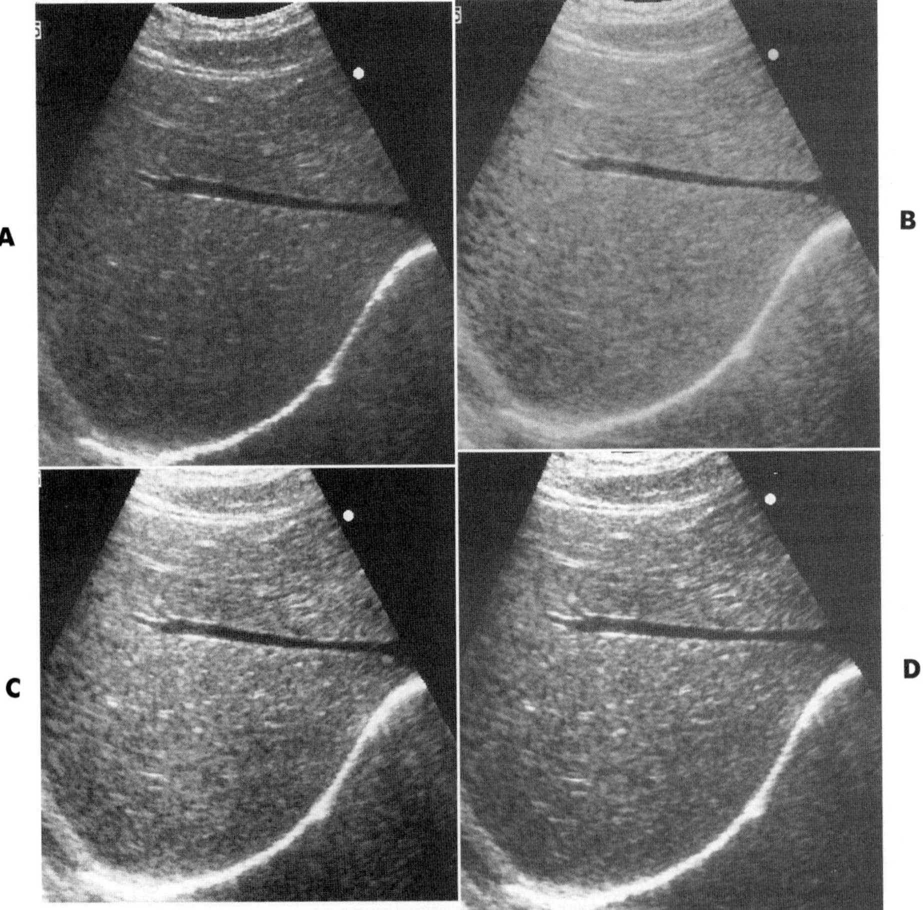

FIG. 3-9 A-D, Multiple scans over the right lobe of the liver with various photography or postprocessing curves allow the sonographer to reassign various gray levels within the liver parenchyma to produce a "softer" or more gray image, or to highlight the more reflective structures within the liver and thus produce a more contrasting type of image. Some structures stand out better when these processing levels are changed (i.e., some tumors, abscess collections, or hematomas may be more visible with this technique).

through the abdomen without obstruction from bowel gas interference.

2. The vascular structures, aorta and inferior vena cava, should be well seen anterior to the vertebral column as echo-free, or anechoic, structures.
3. The posterior border of the liver should be imaged as the transducer is angled from the dome of the liver to its inferior edge. This ensures that time gain compensation (TGC) is set correctly (at the back edge of the liver). The overall gain should be adjusted to provide a smooth, homogeneous liver parenchyma throughout. If there are too many echoes outside the liver, the overall gain should be decreased. If the near gain is set too low, the anterior surface of the liver is not delineated.

Longitudinal Scans (Sagittal) (Fig. 3-8)

1. The transducer should be angled from the diaphragm to the inferior border of the right lobe of the liver. The diaphragm should be well defined as a linear bright line superior to the dome of the liver. The liver parenchyma should be homogeneous and uniform throughout. If gain is maximum without good uniform penetration, a lower-frequency transducer could be used to provide increased sensitivity.
2. Vascular structures should be outlined with the patient in deep inspiration.

PATIENT CARE PROTOCOLS

It is the responsibility of the sonographer to ensure that patients are afforded the highest quality care possible during their ultrasound procedure. This entails identifying the patient properly, ensuring confidentiality of information and patient privacy, providing proper nursing care, and maintaining clean and sanitary equipment and examination rooms.

General Abdominal Ultrasound Protocol

The upper abdomen is scanned with high-resolution real time equipment. The transducer may be a sector or curved linear array, or in many cases, a combination of the two. The frequency depends on the size and muscle and fat composition of the patient. Generally a 3-MHz transducer is used, with variations of 2.25 to 7.5 MHz, depending on resolution and beam penetration (Fig. 3-9).

The baseline upper abdominal ultrasound examination includes a survey of the liver and porta hepatis, vascular structures, biliary system, pancreas, kidneys, spleen, and paraaortic area. If variations in anatomy or pathology are seen, multiple views are obtained over the area of interest (Fig. 3-10).

Liver and Porta Hepatis

The liver is imaged in the longitudinal, transverse, and coronal planes (Figs. 3-11 and 3-12). The echogenicity of the liver parenchyma should be compared with that of the renal parenchyma. The hepatic venous, inferior vena cava, and right and left portal structures should be imaged. The ligamentum teres should be identified in the left lobe of the liver (Fig. 3-13). The dome of the right lobe of the liver should be surveyed with the patient in deep inspiration. The right hemidiaphragm and right pleural gutter should be evaluated. The main lobar fissure, as it projects from the right portal vein to the neck of the gallbladder, should be imaged (Fig. 3-14).

Biliary System

The gallbladder should be imaged in the longitudinal, transverse, and decubitus or upright positions (Fig. 3-15). The fundus, body, and neck should be surveyed. The common bile duct should be imaged in at least the oblique long axis plane as it lies anterior to the main portal vein before coursing posterior to the head of the pancreas (Fig. 3-16). The transverse scan of the porta-hepatis may help delineate the portal vein from the common duct (anterior and to the right) and hepatic artery (anterior and to the left) (Fig. 3-17). Visualization of the intrahepatic ducts is not possible unless dilation is present. Ductal dilation may be seen as one scans the liver, demonstrating right and left branches of the portal vein as the hepatic ducts follow a parallel course.

Pancreas

The pancreas should be surveyed in the transverse, longitudinal, and if necessary, upright positions. The head, body, and tail should be well delineated once the celiac axis, superior mesenteric artery and vein, aorta, and inferior vena cava are identified (Fig. 3-18). The small pancreatic duct may be seen on the transverse scan as it courses through the body of the gland (Fig. 3-19). The longitudinal view of the pancreatic head should be made as it lies anterior to the inferior vena cava and inferior to the portal vein (Fig. 3-20). The superior mesenteric vein may be seen to course anterior to the uncinate process of the head and posterior to the body (Fig. 3-21). The pancreatic tail may be seen as gentle, firm pressure is applied to the abdomen to display overlying gas in the antrum of the stomach or transverse colon (Fig. 3-22).

Spleen

The spleen is imaged with the patient in a right lateral decubitus. Oblique coronal and transverse scans are made to demonstrate the spleen, left hemidiaphragm, and upper pole of the kidney (Fig. 3-23).

Kidneys

The right kidney is demonstrated in a supine or slightly decubitus position (Fig. 3-24). The liver is used as the acoustic window. The left kidney is surveyed with the patient in a right lateral decubitus position. The spleen is used as the acoustic window. The renal cortex and medulla should be well delineated. Longitudinal scans

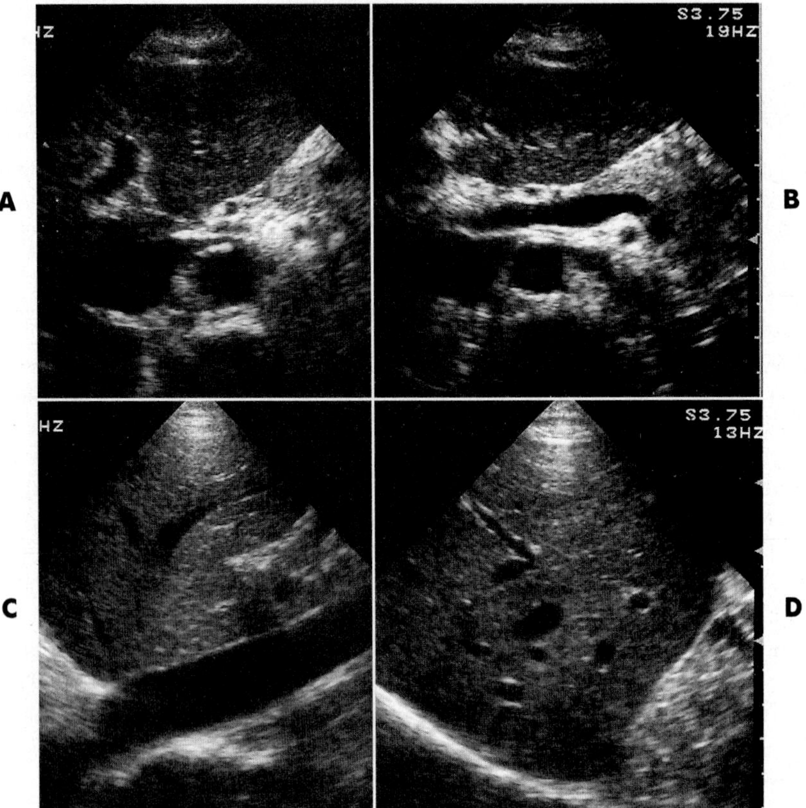

FIG. 3-10 **A** and **B,** Transverse, and **C** and **D,** longitudinal, scans of the upper abdomen show the proper gain settings (no low-level echoes seen within the vascular structures, a uniform liver parenchyma, and proper adjustment of the near and far gain settings).

are made through the midline and lateral and medial borders. Transverse scans are made through the upper pole, middle section at the level of the renal pelvis, and lower pole.

The bladder should be imaged in a longitudinal and transverse plane. The wall should be assessed for thickness or irregularities, and the presence of focal lesions documented. If the bladder is large, the evaluation of ureteral jets should be noted.

Aorta and Inferior Vena Cava

The aorta should be imaged in the longitudinal plane from the diaphragm to the bifurcation at the iliac junction (Fig. 3-25). Transverse scans should be made at the level of the diaphragm, superior to the renal arteries, inferior to the renal arteries, and at the bifurcation (Fig. 3-26). Lymph adenopathy should also be evaluated.

The inferior vena cava is best imaged on a longitudinal plane through the right lobe of the liver with the patient in full inspiration (Fig. 3-27).

An alternative imaging plane is the oblique-coronal window. The patient rolls onto his or her left side; the transducer is longitudinal and sharply angled from the right lobe of the liver to the left iliac wing. This allows the sonographer to image the inferior vena cava "anterior" to the aorta (Fig. 3-28). It usually allows one to follow the entrance and exit of the renal veins and arteries into the great vessels and provides an excellent window to perform color-flow or Doppler interrogation of the renal vessels.

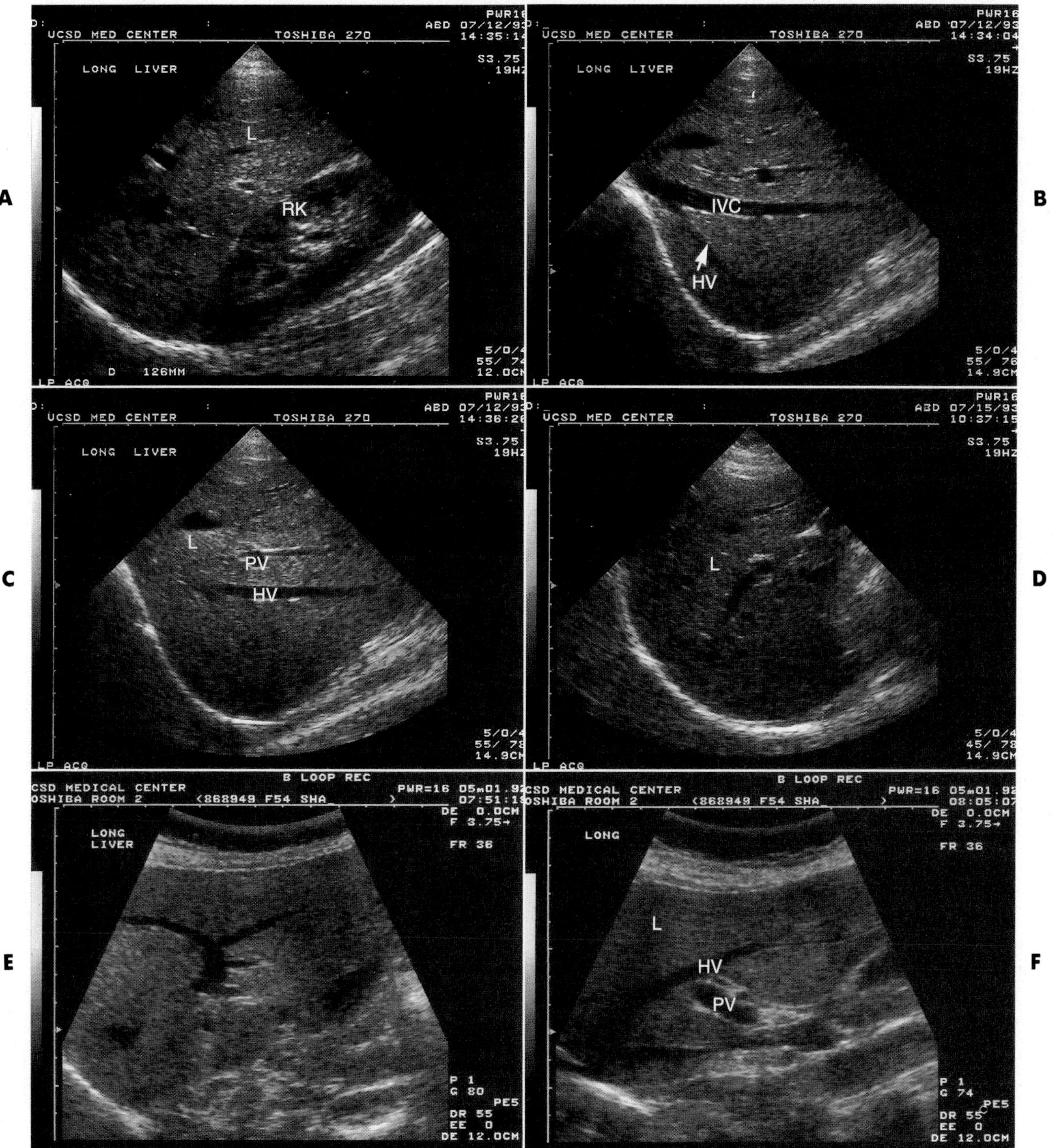

FIG. 3-11 Longitudinal views of the liver. **A,** Lateral border of the right lobe of the liver, *L,* and right kidney, *RK.* **B,** Right lobe of the liver with the inferior vena cava, *IVC,* and hepatic veins, *HV.* This view is made with the transducer angled medial from the lateral margin of the abdominal wall. **C,** Right lobe of the liver, *L,* hepatic veins, *HV,* and portal branches, *PV.* **D,** Right lobe of the liver, *L,* with portal and hepatic radicles throughout. **E,** Right lobe of the liver with the transducer approaching the midline of the abdomen. **F,** Left lobe of the liver, *L,* hepatic vein, *HV,* and portal vein, *PV.*

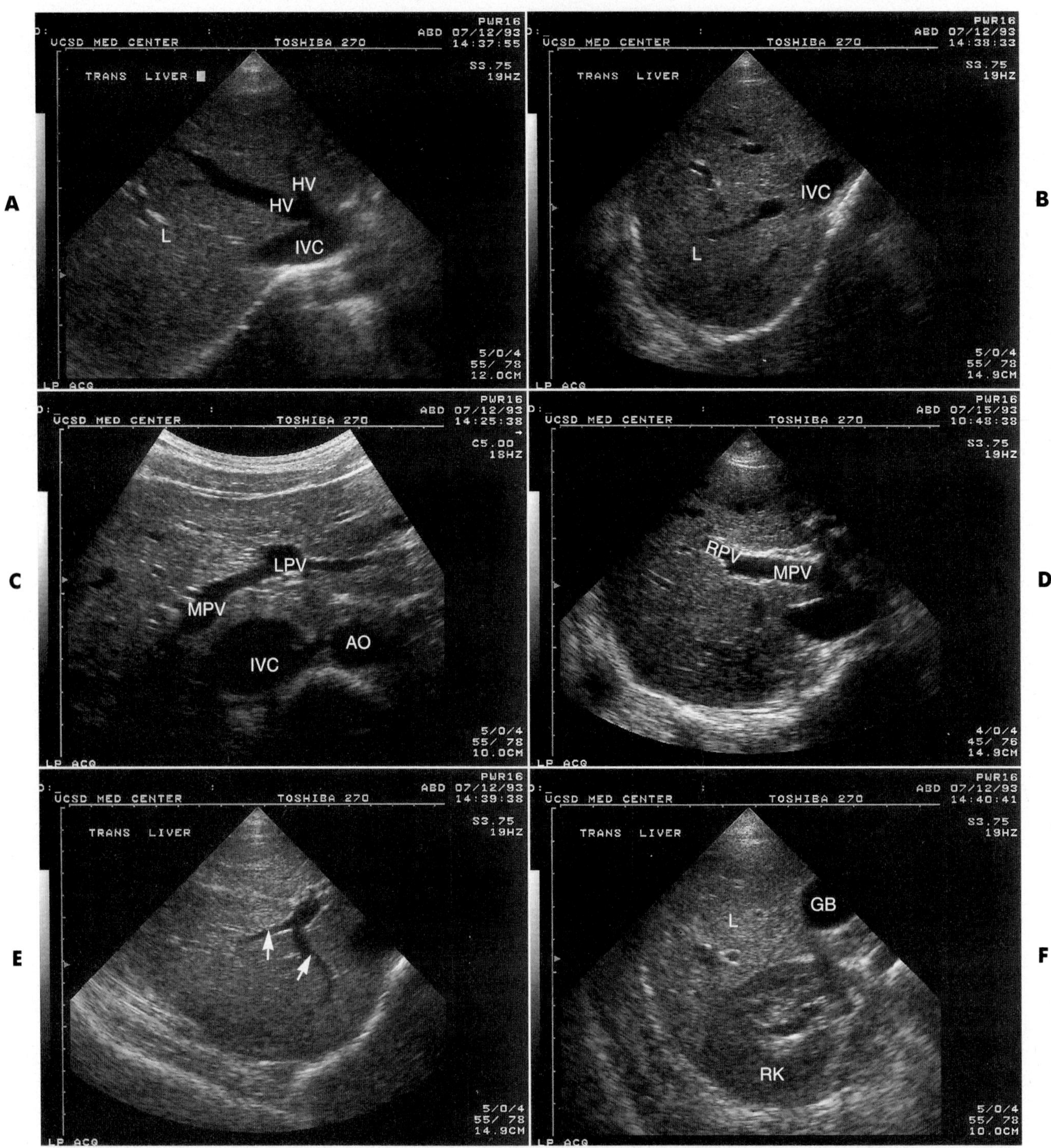

FIG. 3-12 Transverse scans of the liver. **A,** The patient is in full inspiration, and the transducer is sharply angled under the costal margin toward the diaphragm. The right and left lobes of the liver, *L,* are seen, with the hepatic veins, *HV,* draining into the inferior vena cava, *IVC.* **B,** The transducer is angled slightly inferior to record the right lobe of the liver, *L,* inferior vena cava, *IVC,* hepatic veins, and portal veins. **C,** The transducer is moved toward the midline to record the left lobe of the liver, main portal vein, *MPV,* left portal vein, *LPV,* inferior vena cava, *IVC,* and aorta, *AO.* **D,** The transducer is angled to the right and inferior to record the right lobe of the liver, main portal vein, *MPV,* and right portal vein, *RPV.* **E,** With various stages of inspiration, the sonographer may record the anterior and posterior branching of the right portal vein *(arrows).* **F,** The inferior part of the right lobe of the liver, *L,* gallbladder, *GB,* and upper pole of the right kidney, *RK,* are shown.

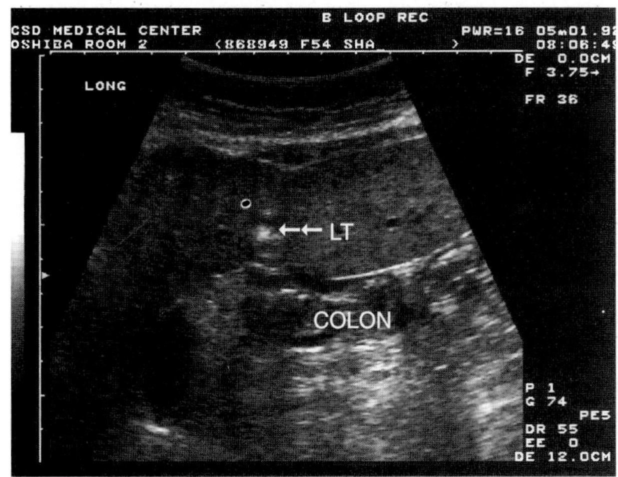

FIG. 3-13 The ligamentum teres, *LT*, is the bright echogenic focus seen in the left lobe of the liver on transverse scans.

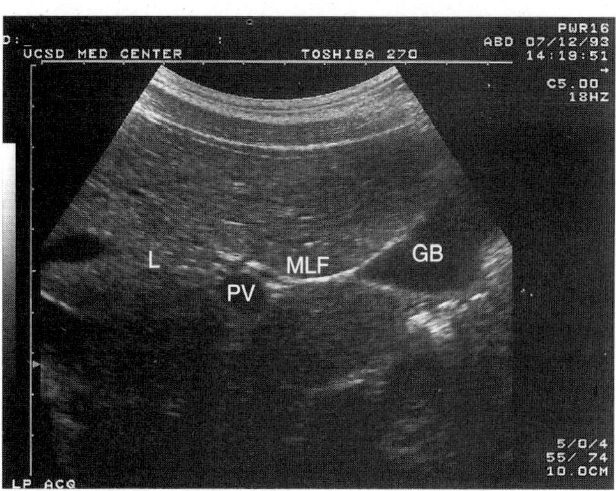

FIG. 3-14 The main lobar fissure, *MLF*, as it projects from the right portal vein to the neck of the gallbladder should be imaged.

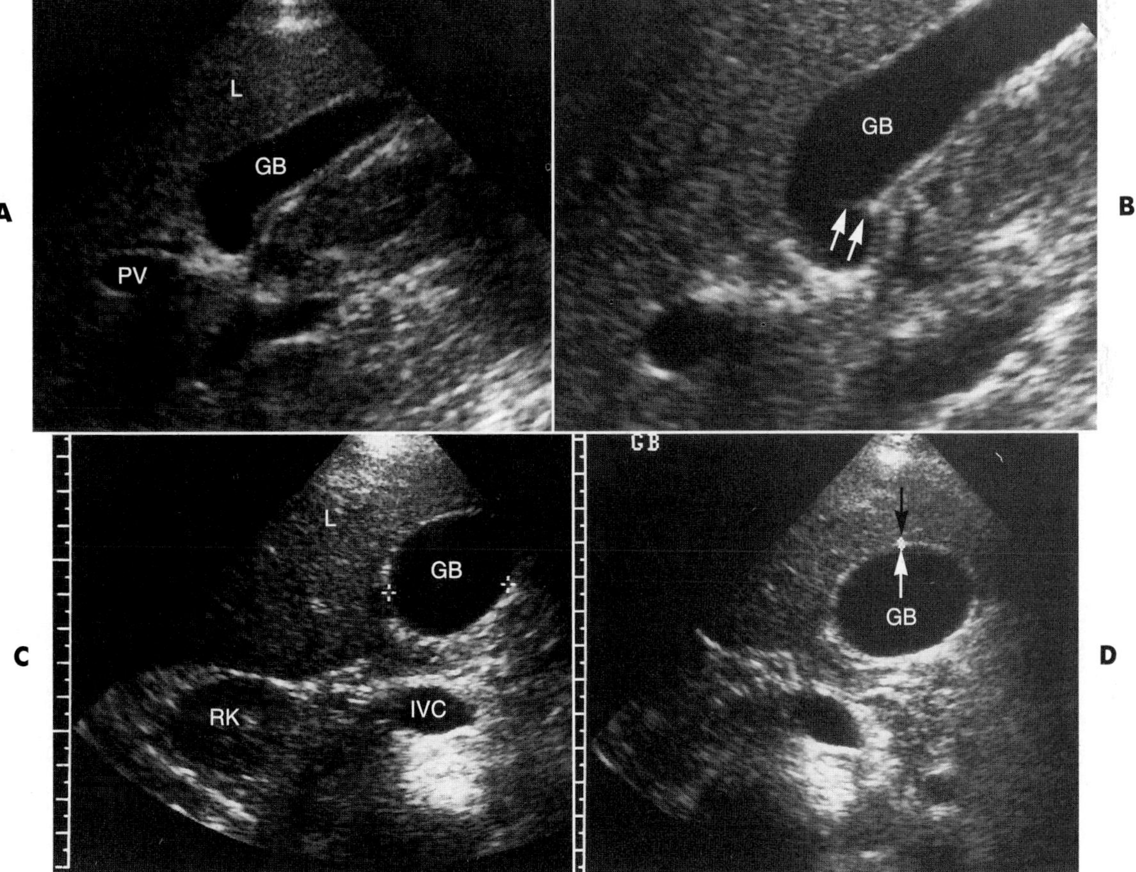

FIG. 3-15 Gallbladder images. **A,** The gallbladder is best imaged in the longitudinal plane under the right lobe of the liver. Gallbladder, *GB;* liver, *L;* portal vein, *PV.* **B,** Magnification of the gallbladder may help one see its internal structures—normal "folds" *(arrows)* are shown. **C,** The transverse scan is made to compare the size of the gallbladder with the right kidney—a normal gallbladder is usually smaller. Transverse measurements may be made to record the width of the gallbladder. **D,** Transverse scans are used to measure the wall of the gallbladder *(arrows).*

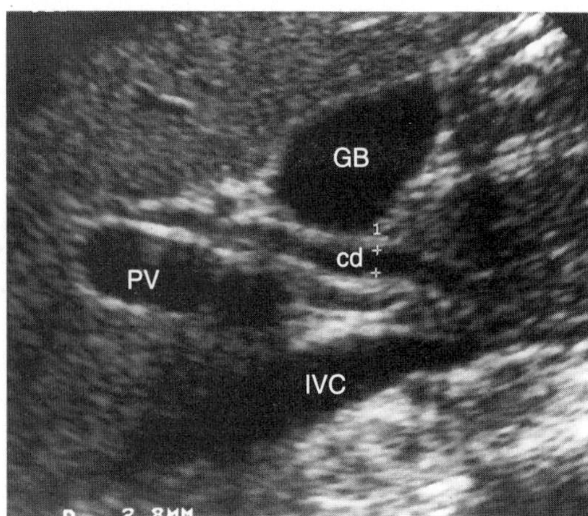

FIG. 3-16 A longitudinal oblique scan of the upper abdomen to show the common bile duct, *cd,* as it flows anterior to the portal vein, *PV,* and inferior vena cava, *IVC,* before it enters the head of the pancreas. Gallbladder, *GB.*

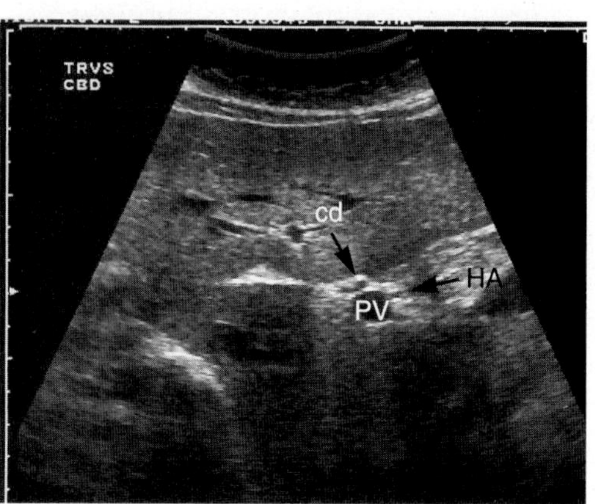

FIG. 3-17 A transverse oblique scan shows the "Mickey Mouse sign" with the portal vein, *PV,* as Mickey's face, the common duct, *cd,* as the right ear, and the hepatic artery, *HA,* as the left ear.

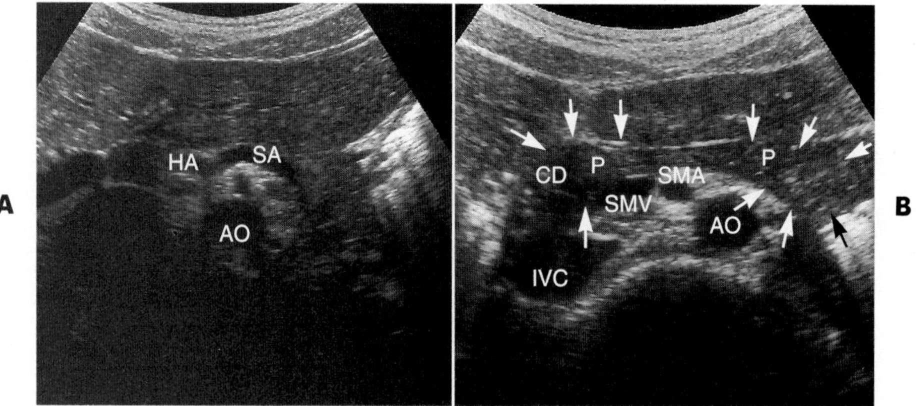

FIG. 3-18 **A,** The celiac axis is the superior transverse border of the pancreas. The sonographer should angle the transducer through as much of the left lobe of the liver as possible to provide a window to image the prevertebral vessels and pancreatic area. Aorta, *AO;* hepatic artery, *HA;* splenic artery, *SA.* **B,** The transducer should be angled slightly inferior from the celiac axis to record the pancreas *(arrows).* Inferior vena cava, *IVC;* aorta, *AO;* superior mesenteric vein, *SMV;* superior mesenteric artery, *SMA;* common duct, *cd;* pancreas, *P.*

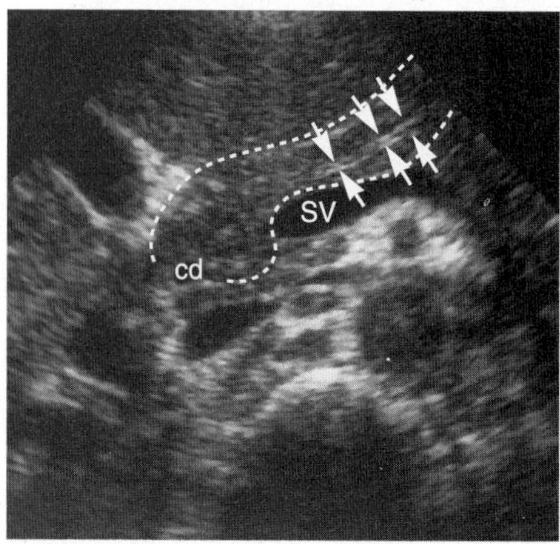

FIG. 3-19 The pancreatic duct *(arrows)* is usually seen best in the body of the gland. Common duct, *cd;* splenic vein, *SV.*

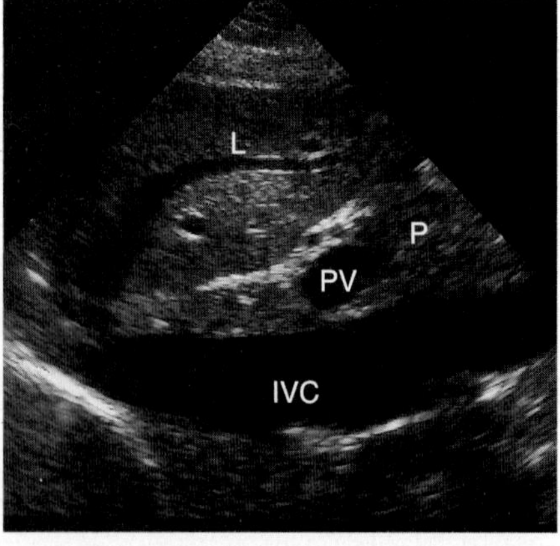

FIG. 3-20 The longitudinal view of the pancreatic head, *P,* should be made as it lies anterior to the inferior vena cava, *IVC,* and inferior to the portal vein, *PV.* Liver, *L.*

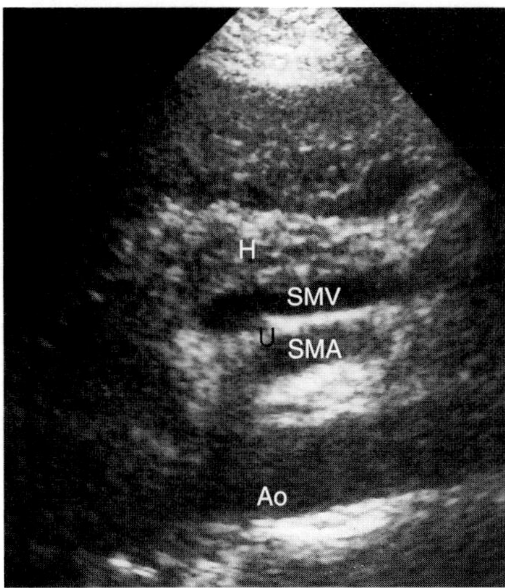

FIG. 3-21 Longitudinal scan. The superior mesenteric vein, *SMV*, may be seen to course anterior to the uncinate process of the head, *U*, and posterior to the head, *H*. Sometimes, with angulation, the superior mesenteric artery, *SMA*, may be seen posterior to the superior mesenteric vein and anterior to the aorta, *AO*.

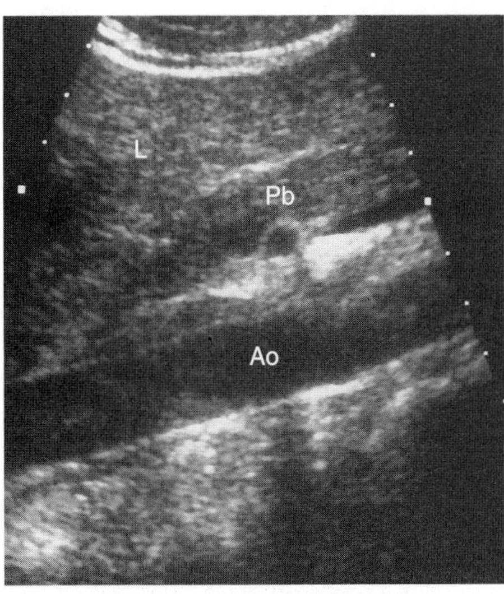

FIG. 3-22 The transducer is angled slightly to the left of midline to record the aorta, *AO*, and pancreatic body-tail, *Pb*, just inferior to the left lobe of the liver, *L*.

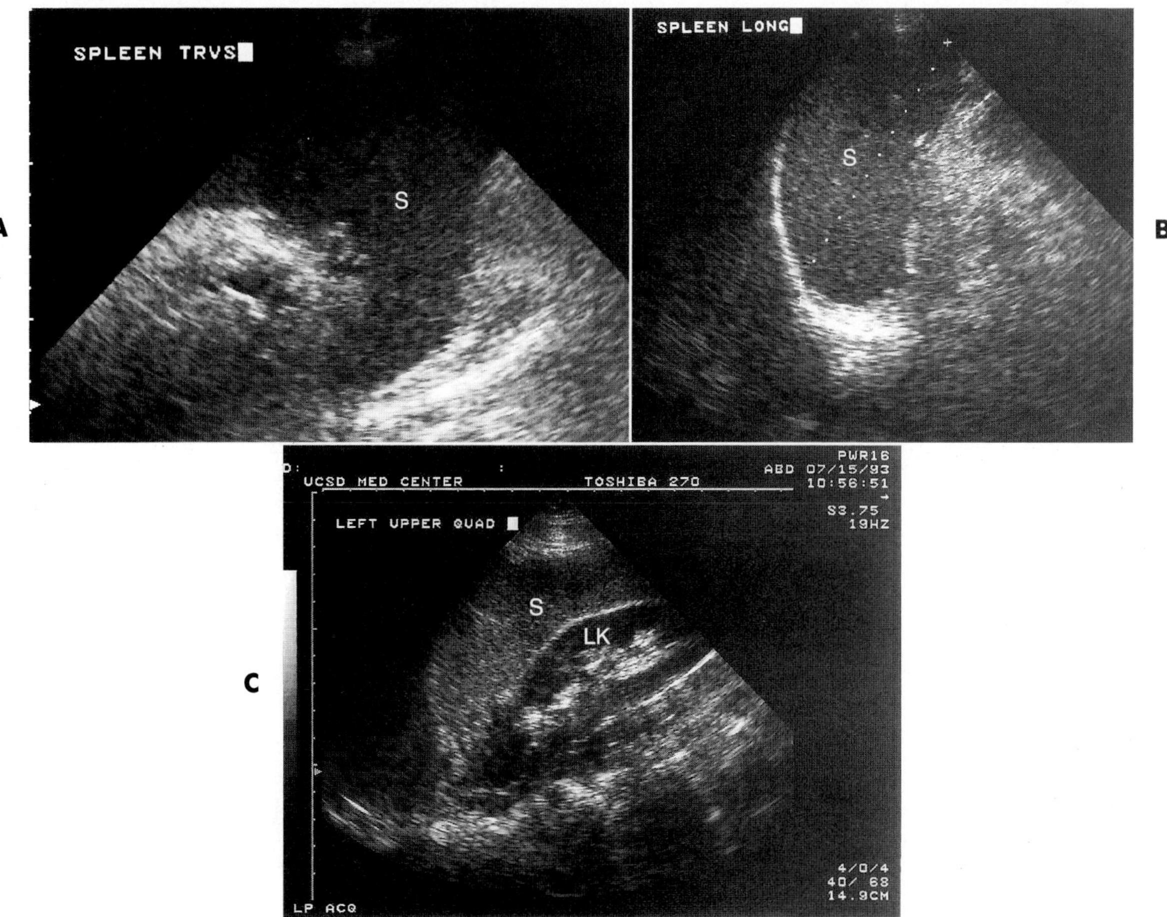

FIG. 3-23 The spleen, *S*, is seen in the transverse, **A**, and longitudinal, **B**, planes as a uniform, homogeneous organ in the left upper quadrant. The sonographer must be more creative with patient positioning and available windows to adequately record the splenic parenchyma. **C**, The longitudinal view of the spleen, *S*, may be used as a window to image the upper pole of the left kidney, *LK*.

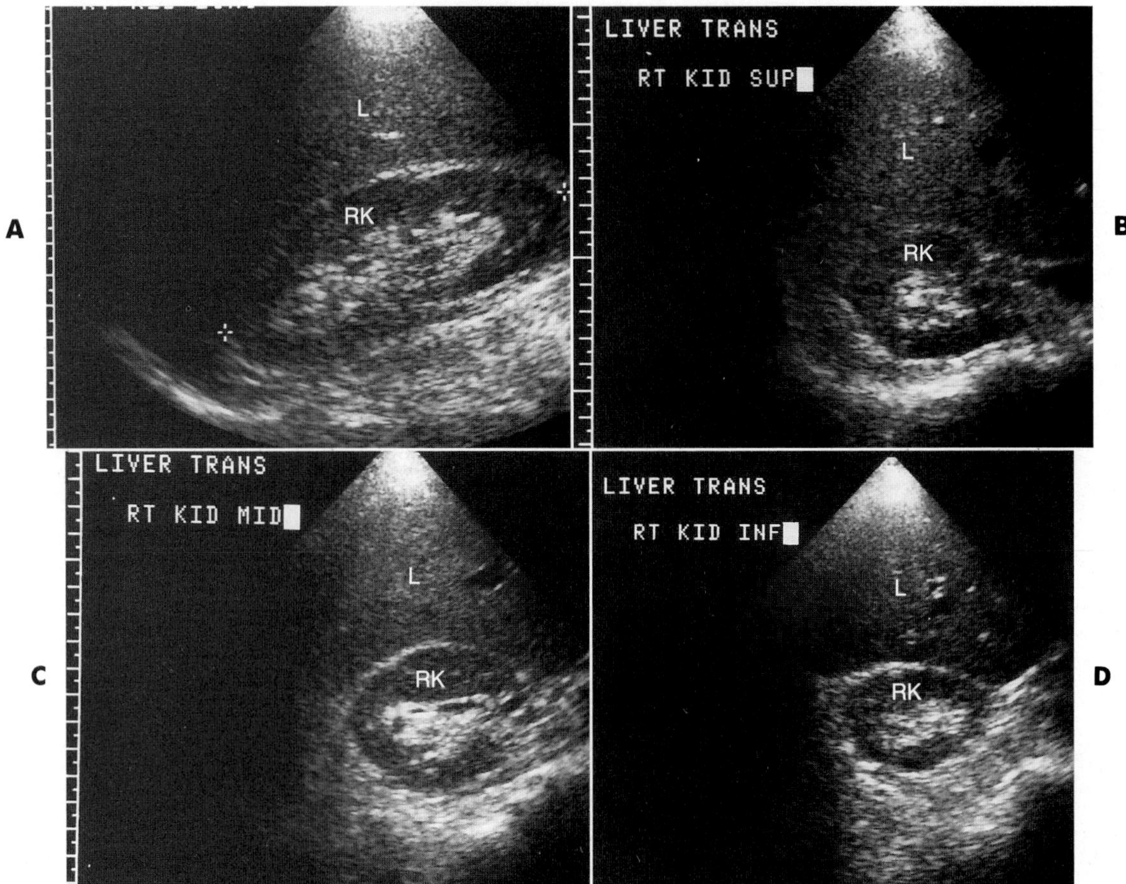

FIG. 3-24 Multiple views of the right kidney. **A,** A longitudinal scan of the right kidney, *RK,* is made with the patient supine. The transducer is angled through the right lobe of the liver, *L,* to provide an adequate window to image the renal parenchyma. The liver parenchyma should be more echo-producing than the cortex of the kidney. Subsequent scans are made through the lateral and medial borders of the kidney. Transverse scans of the right kidney are made in the, **B,** Superior pole, **C,** Midpole, and **D,** Inferior pole of the kidney.

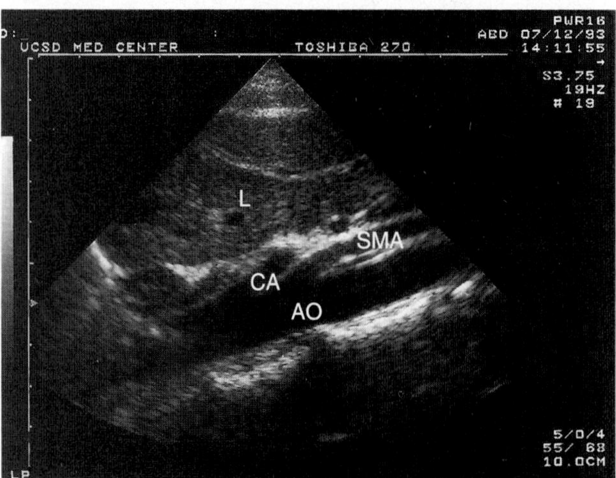

FIG. 3-25 The aorta should be imaged in the longitudinal plane from the diaphragm to the bifurcation. The celiac axis, *CA,* and superior mesenteric artery, *SMA,* arise from the anterior wall of the aorta, *AO*. Liver, *L*.

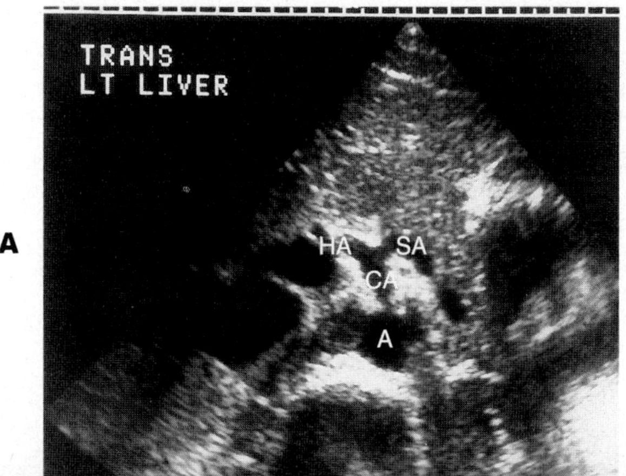

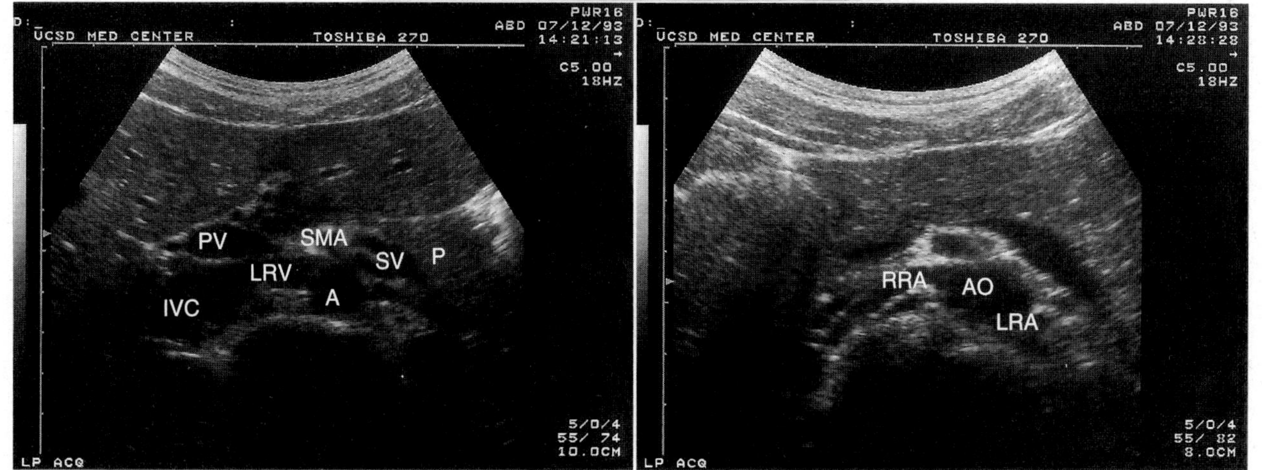

FIG. 3-26 A, Transverse scans of the aorta, should be made at the level of the celiac axis, *CA,* hepatic artery, *HA,* and splenic artery, *SA*. **B,** The transducer is angled inferior to record the aorta, *A,* at the level of the left renal vein, *LRV*. Other structures seen as the inferior vena cava, *IVC,* portal vein, *PV,* superior mesenteric artery, *SMA,* splenic vein, *SV,* and pancreas, *P*. **C,** The renal arteries, *RRA* and *LRA,* are seen just inferior to the above scan as they arise from the lateral borders of the aorta, *AO*.

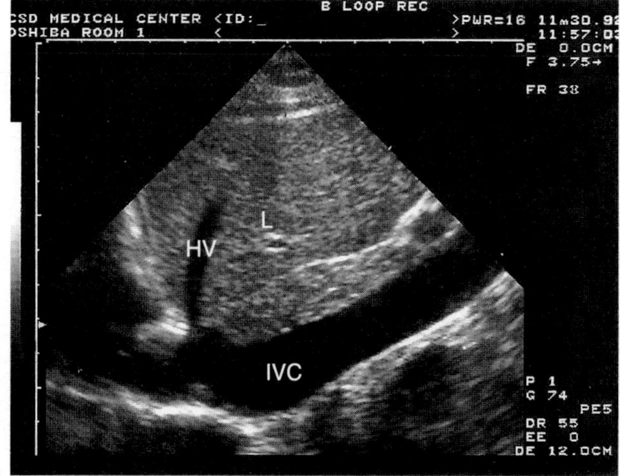

FIG. 3-27 The inferior vena cava, *IVC,* is best imaged when the patient is in full inspiration on a longitudinal plane through the right lobe of the liver, *L*. The hepatic vein, *HV,* is seen to enter the inferior vena cava at the level of the diaphragm.

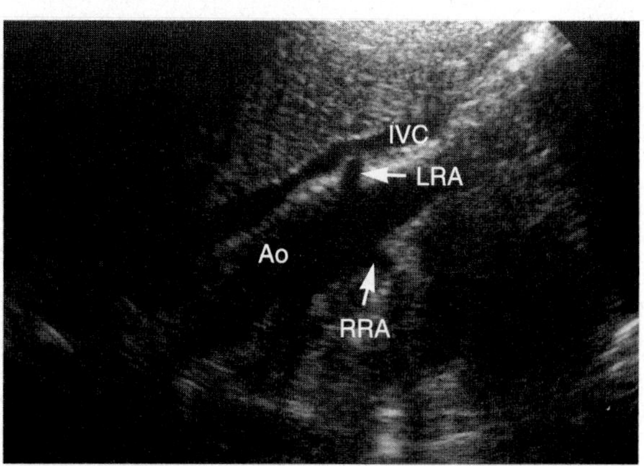

FIG. 3-28 The coronal "banana peel" oblique view of the great vessels is made with the patient rolled into a steep angle. The transducer is angled through the inferior vena cava, *IVC,* to record the aorta, *AO,* and renal arteries, *RRA* and *LRA*.

Liver Examination Protocol

General Considerations

The liver is examined as part of a comprehensive ultrasound evaluation of the abdomen. Abnormalities that can be evaluated include cirrhosis, fatty infiltration, hepatomegaly, portal hypertension, primary and metastatic tumors, abscess formation, and trauma. Pulsed and color flow Doppler are used to assess the hepatic vascular system.

Equipment Considerations

The liver is normally examined with a 3.5-MHz transducer. Lower-frequency transducers are often necessary in patients with fatty infiltration or cirrhosis.

Examination Protocol

Standard liver imaging protocol

1. Evaluation of the liver includes both longitudinal and transverse views. The echogenicity of the liver should be compared with that of the right kidney. The major vessels (aorta and inferior vena cava) in the region of the liver should be imaged, including the position of the inferior vena cava where it passes through the liver.
2. The regions of the ligamentum teres in the left lobe and the high dome of the right lobe (with the right hemidiaphragm and right pleural gutter) should be imaged. The main lobar fissure should be demonstrated.
3. Survey of the right and left lobes should include visualization of the hepatic veins. The right and left branches of the portal vein should be identified. This analysis can also serve to evaluate for possible intrahepatic bile duct dilation.
4. Document liver size in a parasagittal scan demonstrating the diaphragm and tip of the right lobe of the liver. Document the size of any demonstrated masses.
5. Evaluate and document the presence of ascites.

Doppler

1. Assess the patency and direction of flow of the main, right, and left portal veins.
2. Assess the patency of the right, middle, and left hepatic veins.
3. Assess the patency of the umbilical vein (recanalized umbilical vein).
4. Assess the patency of surgically or angiographically placed shunts.
5. Perform pulsed Doppler analysis of the hepatic artery with resistance measurements.

Disease-Specific Scanning Protocols

Abscess

1. Perform the standard liver imaging protocol.
2. Evaluate for hypoechoic or hyperechoic regions within the liver.
3. Evaluate extrahepatic spaces for the presence of fluid.

Cirrhosis

1. Perform the standard liver imaging protocol.
2. Evaluate and document liver echogenicity by comparing it with kidney texture.
3. Perform Doppler examination of the portal and hepatic venous systems.
4. Evaluate the size of the spleen and liver.
5. Evaluate associated findings and problems.
   a. Increased risk for hepatoma.
   b. Fatty infiltration.
   c. Pancreatitis.
   d. Ascites.
   e. Portal hypertension.

Budd-Chiari syndrome (thrombosis of the hepatic veins)

1. Perform the standard liver imaging protocol.
2. Document the patency of hepatic veins.
   a. Follow Doppler examination protocol.
3. Document the patency of the inferior vena cava.
4. Evaluate for abnormal collateral vessels draining the hepatic veins.
5. Assess for ascites.

Cysts

1. Perform the standard liver imaging protocol.
2. Evaluate the kidneys and pancreas for associated cysts.

Hematoma

1. Perform the standard liver imaging protocol.
2. Evaluate for free fluid.

Hepatitis

1. Perform the standard liver imaging protocol.
2. Evaluate associated findings and problems.
   a. Increased risk for hepatoma.
   b. Gallbladder wall thickening.

Hepatoma

1. Perform standard liver imaging protocol.
2. Evaluate for focal masses or diffuse involvement.
3. Evaluate the portal and hepatic venous system for tumor invasion.
4. Evaluate for isolated intrahepatic biliary obstruction.
5. Evaluate for local and distant metastases.
6. Evaluate for recanalization of the umbilical vein.
7. Follow the Doppler examination protocol.
8. Assess for ascites.

Metastatic work-up

1. Perform the standard liver imaging protocol.
2. Evaluate for focal masses or diffuse involvement.
3. Evaluate the portal and hepatic venous systems for tumor invasion.
4. Evaluate for isolated intrahepatic biliary obstruction.

Transplant

1. Perform the standard liver imaging protocol.
2. Follow the Doppler examination protocol.
3. Evaluate the hepatic artery for patency or stenosis,
4. Evaluate associated findings and problems.
   a. Rejection.
   b. Anastomotic stenosis.
   c. Abscess.
   d. Hematoma.
   e. Arteriovenous fistula.

Trauma

1. Perform the standard liver imaging protocol.
2. Evaluate for free fluid.

Gallbladder/Biliary Examination Protocol

General Considerations

Ultrasound examinations of the gallbladder and bile ducts are performed to document cholelithiasis, changes secondary to acute and chronic cholecystitis, obstruction, and primary or metastatic tumor involvement. The examination is performed as part of a comprehensive general abdominal evaluation.

Imaging Considerations

Scans are normally performed with a 3.5- to 5-MHz transducer. To evaluate stone disease, the focal point of the transducer is placed at the region of the posterior gallbladder wall and the gain reduced. This facilitates demonstration of acoustic shadowing. The bile ducts are evaluated using standard liver imaging protocols. Color Doppler helps distinguish between vascular structures and bile ducts.

Fasting Status

Ultrasound evaluation of the biliary system should be performed with the patient in a fasting state. Recommended periods of fasting are as follows:

- Infants and neonates—4-hour fast
- Pediatrics—6-hour fast
- Adults—8-hour fast

Examination Protocol

Gallbladder

1. Perform longitudinal and transverse scans with the patient in the supine and/or left posterior oblique position. The regions of the neck and fundus of the gallbladder must be demonstrated.
2. Observe and document gallbladder wall thickness (normal is less than 2 mm). If thickened, measure wall.
3. Evaluate for the presence of echogenic foci (e.g., stones or polyps) within the gallbladder lumen. If present, attempt to demonstrate acoustic shadowing and mobility. Remember that gallstones do not shadow if the diameter of the ultrasound beam is larger than the stone.
4. Acoustic shadowing can best be demonstrated by the following:
   a. Decreasing gain or power.
   b. Placing the focal point at the area of interest.
   c. Increasing the transducer frequency.
   d. Positioning the patient so that stones roll together, producing a larger reflective area.

Bile ducts

1. Measure the common hepatic duct. The normal duct measures less than 5 mm plus 1 mm per decade over 60 years of age. If the duct is enlarged it may be desirable to obtain a measurement 45 minutes after the patient has eaten or 5 to 10 minutes after injection of cholecystokinin. Consult with the radiologist before the patient leaves.
2. Observe for the presence of intrahepatic biliary dilation. It should be noted that isolated biliary obstruction can be seen in patients with tumor or inflammatory involvement of the bile ducts. Isolated biliary obstruction is most commonly seen involving the left hepatic ducts.
3. Attempt to demonstrate the common bile duct in the region of the pancreatic head.
4. If biliary obstruction is evident, attempt to demonstrate the cause (e.g., pancreatic carcinoma, stones, and nodes).

Disease-Specific Protocols

Acalculus cholecystitis

1. Take the standard gallbladder images.
2. Measure the wall thickness.
3. Measure gallbladder length and diameter.
4. Evaluate the pericholecystic area for fluid.
5. Evaluate the biliary ducts.

AIDS

1. Take the standard gallbladder images.
2. Evaluate the wall thickness.
3. Evaluate the biliary ducts.

Cholecystitis

1. Take the standard gallbladder images.
2. Evaluate for cholelithiasis.
3. Evaluate the biliary ducts.

Cholelithiasis

1. Take the standard gallbladder images.
2. If a filling defect is demonstrated,
   a. Demonstrate acoustic shadowing.
   b. Demonstrate mobility.
3. Document wall thickness.
4. Document biliary ducts.

Gallbladder carcinoma

1. Take the standard gallbladder images.
2. Evaluate wall thickness.
3. Evaluate for mass effect.
4. Evaluate the adjacent liver for extension.
5. Evaluate for other evidence of metastatic disease.
6. Evaluate for stones.

Bile duct carcinomas

1. Evaluate the intrahepatic ducts.
   a. Right and left hepatic.
   b. Observe for general or segmental dilation.
2. Evaluate and measure the common hepatic duct.
   a. Normal is less than 6 mm.
   b. If more than 5 mm, the patient may need a fatty meal.
3. Attempt to visualize the distal common bile duct.
   a. Longitudinal lateral aspect pancreatic head.
   b. Transverse pancreatic head.
4. If the patient is obstructed attempt to document the level of obstruction and cause.

Pancreatic Examination Protocol

General Considerations

The pancreas is examined as part of a comprehensive general abdominal study. Specific indications for pancreatic scanning include abdominal pain, clinically manifested acute or chronic pancreatitis, abnormal laboratory values, cholecystitis, and obstructive jaundice. The examination documents the presence of cystic and solid masses, biliary and ductal dilation, and the presence of extrapancreatic masses and fluid collections.

Examination Preparation

The pancreatic area is best examined with the patient fasting. The recommended periods of fasting are as follows:

1. Infants and neonates—2 to 4 hours
2. Pediatrics—4 to 6 hours
3. Adults—8 hours

Equipment Considerations

Examinations are normally performed with a 3.5-MHz transducer, but lower or higher frequencies may be desirable depending on the patient's body habitus.

Examination Protocol

1. Perform transverse scans along the region of the splenic vein to demonstrate the body and tail of the pancreas.
2. Perform transverse scans inferior to the splenic vein to demonstrate the pancreatic head.
3. Perform longitudinal scans along the region of the superior mesenteric vein to demonstrate the body and uncinate process portions of the pancreas.
4. Perform longitudinal scans along the region of the inferior vena cava to demonstrate the pancreatic head and pancreatic portion of the common bile duct.
5. Perform longitudinal scans left of the aorta and superior mesenteric vein to demonstrate the body and tail regions of the pancreas.
6. Assess for the presence of dilated pancreatic or biliary ducts and measure their size.
7. Assess for the presence of cystic or solid masses.
8. Assess for the presence of peripancreatic nodes.
9. Assess for the presence of peripancreatic fluid collections (e.g., pseudocysts).
10. Document the presence of any pancreatic calcifications detected.

Disease-Specific Protocols

Acute and chronic pancreatitis

1. Perform the standard pancreatic imaging protocol.
2. Assess for pseudocyst formation (pseudocysts may be distant from the pancreas).
3. Evaluate for biliary obstruction.
4. Evaluate for the presence of free fluid.
5. Evaluate for the following associated findings:
   a. Cholecystitis or cholelithiasis.
   b. Cirrhosis or fatty liver infiltration.

Pancreatic carcinoma

1. Perform the standard pancreatic imaging protocol.
2. Demonstrate and measure the pancreatic duct.
3. Evaluate the uncinate process.
4. Evaluate for pancreatic pseudocyst.
5. Assess for biliary obstruction.
6. Evaluate the following for metastases:
   a. Liver.
   b. Peripancreatic nodes.
7. Evaluate for superior mesenteric vein thrombosis or splenic vein thrombosis.

Spleen Examination Protocol

General Considerations

Ultrasound examinations are performed to assess overall splenic architecture, to evaluate or detect intrasplenic masses, to evaluate the splenic hilum and vasculature, and to determine splenic size.

Imaging Modality

Images are obtained with the patient in a right lateral decubitus position with a 3.5-MHz sector transducer. Color flow and pulsed Doppler tracings are performed to assess splenic vasculature or to determine increased tumor flow if pathology is present.

Examination Protocol

1. Perform coronal scans of the long axis of the spleen. Demonstrate the left hemidiaphragm, splenic hilus, and upper and lower borders of the spleen. Measure the splenic length.
2. Compare the texture of the spleen with that of the liver. The splenic parenchyma should be homogeneous with the liver.
3. Perform a transverse scan of the spleen at the level of the splenic hilus. Look for increased vascularity or splenic nodes.

Renal Examination Protocol

General Considerations

Ultrasound examinations are performed to assess overall renal architecture, evaluate or detect intrarenal and extrarenal masses, document hydronephrosis, detect calculi, evaluate renal vasculature, and determine renal size and echogenicity. The bladder and ureters are evaluated as part of the examination protocol.

Imaging Modalities

Images are obtained with a 3.5-MHz sector transducer. Lower or higher frequencies may be appropriate for patients with large or small body habitus. Curved linear array transducers may also be used, but they may be limited in scanning between the ribs. Flat linear array transducers may be used for pediatric patients.

Color flow and pulsed Doppler tracings are performed to assess renal vasculature.

Examination Protocol

Gray-scale images

1. Perform coronal or sagittal scans of the anterior, middle, and posterior aspects of the kidneys. Demonstrate the upper and lower poles. Obtain a measurement of the length of each kidney.
2. Perform transverse scans of the upper, middle, and lower segments of each kidney.
3. Perform transverse and longitudinal scans of the urinary bladder.
4. Perform general survey scans of the perirenal spaces to assess for extrarenal masses or fluid collections.

Doppler flow analysis

1. All Doppler studies of the kidneys include pulsed Doppler tracings with resistance measurements taken of the main, interlobar, and arcuate arteries. The patency of the main renal vein is documented.

Disease-Specific Protocols

Renal artery stenosis

1. Perform the normal gray-scale imaging protocol.
2. A measurement of the time from end-diastole to peak systole is obtained of the interlobar or segmental arteries of each kidney (normally less than 70 msec). The spectral sweep speed should be increased to the fastest setting for this measurement.
3. Angle-corrected flow-velocity measurements of the abdominal aorta at the level of the renal arteries and the main renal artery are obtained for suspected renal artery stenosis. A renal-artery-to-aorta ratio is calculated (normally less than 3.5 to 1).

Renal vein thrombosis

1. Perform standard gray-scale imaging protocol. Observe for increased kidney size and decreased echogenicity. Include images of the inferior vena cava and main renal vein.
2. Perform the standard renal Doppler protocol. Observe for significantly increased resistance or reversal of flow in diastole.
3. Perform pulsed Doppler tracing to document patency of the inferior vena cava.

Solid renal mass

1. Perform the standard gray-scale imaging protocol. Measure the size of the mass.
2. Assess for tumor invasion of the main renal vein and inferior vena cava. Document patency with pulsed or color Doppler.
3. Evaluate for metastatic involvement of other organs (e.g., contralateral kidney, liver, nodes).
4. Assess for tumor vascularity with pulsed and color Doppler. Obtain resistance measurements if possible.

Cystic renal mass

1. Perform the standard gray-scale imaging protocol. Observe and demonstrate smooth walls, acoustic enhancement, and the anechoic nature of the mass.

Polycystic disease

1. Perform the standard gray-scale imaging protocol. Curved-array transducers may be better for documenting kidney size.
2. Evaluate the liver and pancreas for associated cystic changes.

Hydronephrosis

1. Perform the standard gray-scale imaging protocol. Longitudinal scans should be performed in the coronal plane to better demonstrate the renal pelvis.
2. If there is mild hydronephrosis, empty the urinary bladder and rescan the kidneys.
3. Attempt to document the cause of obstruction (e.g., pelvic masses, renal calculi, and prostatic enlargement).
4. If hydronephrosis is demonstrated, perform color Doppler study of the bladder to observe the number of ureteral jets occurring in a 3- to 5-minute period.

Renal stones

1. Perform the standard gray-scale imaging protocol.
2. Observe for echogenic foci.
3. Attempt to demonstrate acoustic shadowing.
4. Assess for the presence of hydronephrosis.

Medical renal disease

1. Perform the standard gray-scale imaging protocol.
2. Observe and document the echogenicity of kidneys. Use adjacent organs for texture comparison (e.g., liver or spleen).
3. Perform the standard renal Doppler examination.

Renal abscess

1. Perform the standard gray-scale imaging protocol.
2. Evaluate for the presence of a hypoechoic or complex mass.
3. Evaluate for extrarenal fluid collections.

Aorta and Iliac Artery Examination Protocol

General Considerations

The aorta is examined primarily to document the presence of aneurysmal dilation. Aortic aneurysms are defined as those with vessel diameters greater than 3 cm or with focal dilation of the vessel. Iliac aneurysms are defined as vessels with diameters greater than 2 cm. Aneurysms above 5 cm or those with documented rapid rates of expansion have an increased risk of catastrophic rupture. The radiologist must be made aware of these patients before they leave the department.

Imaging Considerations

A 3.5-MHz transducer is normally used, although a lower frequency may be necessary in large patients. Scans are normally performed in an anteroposterior plane. Coronal scans may be helpful in patients with overlying bowel gas.

Examination Protocol

1. Perform longitudinal scans of the aorta from the level of the diaphragm to the bifurcation.
2. Perform transverse scans of the aorta at its proximal,

middle, and distal segments and at any area of dilation.
3. Take outer to inner measurements of the aorta in the longitudinal scan plane.
4. Take longitudinal scans of each iliac vessel from the bifurcation to the most distal segment.
5. Perform transverse scans of the iliacs below the bifurcation.

Thyroid Examination Protocol

General Considerations

The role of ultrasound in evaluating the thyroid is primarily limited to differentiating cystic from solid masses, documenting the number of masses, assessing overall echogenicity and homogeneity, and evaluating the size of the gland. It is normally performed as a result of an abnormal physical examination or to correlate with nuclear medicine scans. It is noteworthy that approximately 20% of thyroid nodules are cysts, 20% cancers, and the remaining 60% benign adenomas.

Imaging Modalities

Thyroid scans should routinely be performed with a 7-MHz transducer. Lower-frequency transducers may be necessary for patients with large necks or thyroid enlargement associated with multinodular goiters.

Examination Protocol

1. Perform and document longitudinal scans of each lobe. Landmarks include the carotid artery laterally and the trachea medially. Scans should be made along the lateral, middle, and medial portions of each lobe.
2. Make transverse scans of each lobe, including the most inferior, middle, and superior portions of the gland.
3. Perform transverse and longitudinal scans of the thyroid isthmus.
4. Obtain size measurements of the gland and any detected nodules.
5. If possible, make split-screen images of the right and left lobes for texture comparison.

Parathyroid Examination Protocol

General Considerations

The role of ultrasound in evaluating the parathyroid is primarily to detect adenomas. The examination is normally performed as a result of abnormal calcium levels or an abnormal physical examination. There are normally four parathyroid glands, two on each side at the upper and lower aspects of the thyroid gland. It should be noted, however, that parathyroid adenomas can be positioned distinctly separate from the thyroid gland.

Imaging Modalities

Parathyroid scans should routinely be performed with a 7-MHz transducer. Lower-frequency transducers may be necessary for patients with large necks.

Examination Protocol

1. Perform the standard thyroid imaging protocol.
2. Scan well below the inferior aspect of the thyroid gland.
3. Observe for discreet hypoechoic masses adjacent to or separate from the thyroid.
4. Measure the size of any detected nodules.

Breast Examination Protocol

General Considerations

The role of ultrasound in evaluating the breast is primarily to determine if a mass is a simple cyst from a complex or solid lesion. The patient generally has a palpable mass or an abnormal mammogram without a palpable mass, is pregnant, or has other complications that may prevent her from receiving a mammogram.

Imaging Modalities

Breast ultrasound should be performed with a 7-MHz transducer. The linear array transducer allows a bigger field of view. If the lesion is very superficial, an acoustically matched stand-off pad may be used with gel placed on the skin and the pad to afford adequate contact.

Examination Protocol

1. All scans should be labeled in relation to the clock. A lesion may be located at 3 o'clock or 11 o'clock, for example.
2. Scans should be made in the transverse and longitudinal planes over the area of interest.
3. Adjust the gain to note the borders, through-transmission, and internal echo pattern of the lesion.
4. Measure the size of the lesion.

Scrotal Examination Protocol

General Considerations

High-resolution ultrasound imaging is the primary screening modality for most testicular pathology. Applications include inflammatory processes of the testes and epididymus, tumor detection, trauma, torsion, hydroceles, varicocele, hernia, and undescended testis.

Imaging Modalities

The scrotum should normally be scanned with a minimum transducer frequency of 7 MHz. A lower-frequency transducer should only be used in cases of enlargement of the scrotum. Color flow and pulsed Doppler are used to evaluate vascular flow to the testicles.

Examination Protocol

Gray-scale imaging

1. Obtain longitudinal scans of each testis. Documented images should include scans from the lateral, middle, and medial segments of the testis.
2. Obtain transverse scans of each testis. Documented images should include the upper, middle, and lower poles.

3. Obtain longitudinal and transverse scans of the head and tail of the epididymus.
4. Document additional scans for any area of abnormality.
5. Measure each testis.
6. If possible, obtain a split-screen image to compare the echogenicity of each testis.
7. Obtain images of the extratesticular area to document the presence of hydrocele, hernia, or other conditions.

Doppler flow analysis

1. When indicated, obtain color and pulsed Doppler analysis of intratesticular flow with resistance measurements.
2. Optimize the scanning instrument for slow flow detection (e.g., decrease PRF/scale, lower filters, or increase gain or power).

Disease-Specific Protocols

Hernia detection

1. Perform the standard gray-scale imaging protocol.
2. Evaluate for the presence of bowel in the scrotal sac.
   a. Perform with the Valsalva maneuver.

Infertility work-up

1. Perform the standard gray-scale imaging protocol.
2. Assess for the presence of dilated veins.
   a. Perform color flow Doppler
   b. Evaluate with the Valsalva maneuver or with the patient standing erect.

Testicular torsion

1. Perform the standard gray-scale imaging protocol.
2. Document the presence or absence of intratesticular flow.
   a. Optimize the instrument for slow flow.
   b. Scan the normal side first. If unable to detect flow on the normal side, torsion of the affected side cannot be excluded.
3. Scans must be performed on an emergency basis. A testis in torsion has decreased chance of salvage beyond 6 hours of onset of pain.

Testicular trauma

1. Perform the standard gray-scale imaging protocol.
2. Assess for areas of decreased echogenicity.
3. Assess for interruption of the testicular capsule.
4. Evaluate for extratesticular fluid collections.

Undescended testis

1. Perform the standard gray-scale imaging protocol.
2. Evaluate the inguinal groove for the presence of an undescended testis.

Hydrocele

1. Perform the standard gray-scale imaging protocol.
2. Document the presence or absence of fluid.
3. Lower-frequency transducers may be necessary for patients with large hydroceles.
4. Evaluate for increased size of the epididymus secondary to associated inflammatory processes.

Orchitis and epididymitis

1. Perform the standard gray-scale imaging protocol.
2. Assess for the presence of extratesticular fluid.
3. Use color-flow Doppler to assess for increased vascularity.

Testicular carcinoma

1. Perform the standard gray-scale imaging protocol.
2. Assess for the echogenicity and homogeneity of the testis.
3. Use color-flow Doppler to assess for increased vascularity.
4. Pulsed Doppler tracings of intratesticular vessels for evaluation of resistance measurements.

Prostate Examination Protocol

General Considerations

High-resolution ultrasound imaging and the blood test for prostatic surface antigen are the current screening modalities for prostate pathology. The prostate, seminal vesicles, vas deferens, and perirectal space should be visualized. The prostate is divided into the central and peripheral zones. The central zone is distinct from and posterior to the central gland. The peripheral zone comprises 75% of the prostatic volume. Ten percent of prostatic cancer occurs in the central zone, 20% in the transitional zone, and 70% in the peripheral zone. Color flow should be used if an abnormal mass is seen, to determine the vascularity of the lesion.

The transrectal probes should be covered by a disposable sheath before insertion. The probe should be soaked in an antimicrobial solution after the procedure. Applications include the detection of hyperplasia, prostatitis, and prostatic intraepithelial neoplasia, as well as tumor localization and biopsy aspiration.

Imaging Modalities

Images are obtained with a transrectal high-frequency probe (5 to 7.5 MHz).

Examination Protocol

1. Image the prostate in the following two planes:
   a. Sagittal and axial.
   b. Sagittal and coronal.
2. Image from the apex to the base of the gland.
3. Thoroughly image the peripheral zone.
4. Evaluate the gland for size, echogenicity, symmetry, and continuity of margins.
5. Evaluate the periprostatic fat and vessels for asymmetry and disruption in echogenicity.
6. Examine the seminal vesicles in two planes from their insertion into the prostate via the ejaculatory ducts to their cranial and lateral extents.
7. Evaluate the seminal vesicles for size, shape, position, symmetry, and echogenicity.
8. Evaluate the vas deferens.
9. Survey the perirectal space with attention to the rectal wall and lumen.

ABDOMINAL DOPPLER

Doppler ultrasound has been used for many decades to evaluate cardiovascular flow patterns. As in other areas of ultrasound, there have been many improvements in the technology, such as the development of pulsed-wave Doppler, spectral analysis of the returning wave form, and color-flow mapping. These advances in Doppler instrumentation, combined with high-resolution real time imaging of the vessels, have led to duplex scanning equipment, which combines these modalities into a single probe.

Duplex scanning is used to ascertain the presence or absence of flow. It can be used to differentiate vessels from nonvascular structures with confusingly similar images (e.g., common duct from hepatic artery, arterial aneurysm from a cyst). The documentation and direction of flow may also be of diagnostic value. Once the presence and direction of flow have been documented, spectral analysis of the flow gives further information on flow velocity and turbulence. Increased velocity and poststenotic turbulence may be seen in vascular stenoses. In postoperative patients, increased turbulence alone may be present at the site of a graft anastomosis with the native vessel. The evaluation of the shape of the wave form, with comparison of the systolic and diastolic components, may give information on increased vascular impedance, such as is seen in renal transplant rejection.

The specific Doppler patterns of the vascular system are found in Chapter 4. Only brief comments are listed in this section.

Doppler Scanning Techniques

The normal, routine sagittal, transverse, coronal, and oblique scans of vascular structures are used to produce adequate images of vascular structures. Doppler techniques supplement the routine examination by permitting blood flow within those vessels to be detected and characterized. Flow toward the transducer is positive, or above the baseline, whereas flow away from the transducer is negative, or below the baseline. Arterial flow pulsates with the cardiac cycle and shows its maximal peak during the systolic part of the cycle. Venous flow shows no pulsatility and has lower flow than arterial structures.

As seen in echocardiology, many of the abdominal vessels have characteristic waveforms. If the sample volume can be directed parallel to the flow, quantification of peak gradients can be estimated. However, in the tortuous course of most vascular structures, this is very difficult.

Pulsed Doppler is the most common instrumentation used to evaluate abdominal flow patterns. This equipment uses a combined real time with pulsed or continuous-wave Doppler. The pulsed Doppler allows placement of the small sample volume within the vascular structure of interest by means of a trackball.

Aorta

The Doppler flow in the pulsatile aorta demonstrates arterial signals in the patent lumen. If the vessel were occluded, no arterial signals would be recorded.

Aortic dissection and pseudoaneurysms

Flow, often with two distinct patterns, can be seen in the true and false lumina by Doppler ultrasound.[1] The development of a pseudoaneurysm as a complication of an aortic graft procedure may be difficult to determine if pulsations are present or transmitted through the aortic wall. Doppler ultrasound may be useful to detect flow within the pseudoaneurysm.

Inferior Vena Cava

The Doppler waveform recorded in the inferior vena cava shows a lower flow than is found in arterial structures. The flow is increased in the presence of thrombus formation.

Portal Venous System

Doppler flow patterns can be used to diagnose varices or collaterals in the portal venous system. They can evaluate changes of flow patterns occurring in the course of portal hypertension. Bidirectional flow may also be seen. As liver function improves, normal hepatopetal flow is restored. If pressures worsen, there may be increased shunting away from the liver.

If a shunt is present in the porta hepatis, Doppler may be useful to determine the patency of the shunt.

Portal Hypertension Protocol

General Considerations

Portal hypertension is caused by increased resistance to venous flow through the liver. It is associated with cirrhosis, hepatic vein thrombosis, portal vein thrombosis, and thrombosis of the inferior vena cava. Ultrasound findings include dilation of the portal, splenic, and mesenteric veins, reversal of portal venous blood flow, and the development of collateral vessels (e.g., patent umbilical vein, gastric varices, or splenorenal shunting).

Equipment Considerations

A 2.25-MHz transducer frequency may be necessary because of decreased penetration into the liver as a result of fatty infiltration.

Examination Protocol

1. Perform the routine abdominal imaging protocol.
   a. Assess for the presence of ascites.
2. Obtain diameter measurements of the splenic and main portal veins on inspiration and expiration.
3. Assess for the presence of collateral blood vessels.
   a. Splenic hilum.
   b. Porta hepatis.
   c. Umbilical vein.
4. Document the flow direction of the portal veins. Include the main, left, and right portal veins.
5. Document the flow direction of the splenic and superior mesenteric veins.

6. Assess for the presence of splenorenal shunting.
   a. Collateral vessels along surface of kidney.
   b. Increased size and flow of the renal vein.
7. Assess for patency of the umbilical vein.
8. Document patency and direction of flow in the hepatic veins.
9. Document the patency of the hepatic artery.
10. Document the patency of the inferior vena cava.
11. Assess and document the patency of surgically placed shunts.

Transjugular Intrahepatic Portal Systemic Shunt (TIPS) Protocol

General Considerations

The Transjugular Intrahepatic Portal Systemic Shunt (TIPS) procedure is an angiographic placement of an indwelling stent to relieve portal hypertension. The stent is placed into the proximal segment of the right portal vein and across to the distal end of the right hepatic vein. The angiographer should, if possible, be present during the procedure. If this is not possible, the films should be shown to the angiography staff or fellow before the patient leaves the department.

Procedure Before TIPS

1. Document the patency of the portal venous system (main, left, and right portal veins).
2. Document the direction of flow in all portal branches.
3. Document the patency of the right, middle, and left hepatic veins.
4. Assess the relationship of hepatic and portal veins near the portal bifurcation.
5. Document the patency of the right jugular vein and optimal position (external landmarks) for puncture.
6. Assess the patency of the umbilical vein.
7. Assess for the presence of ascites.

Procedure After TIPS

1. Document the patency and diameter of the stent at all levels.
2. Obtain angle-corrected velocity measurements of flow in the stent. Samples should be taken at the proximal, middle, and distal segments of the stent, as well as at any area of narrowing. If stenosis is present, obtain samples proximal, at, and distal to the area of narrowing.
3. Document the caliber of hepatic veins above the stent and measure their flow velocities.
4. Document the patency and direction of flow in the right, middle, and left portal veins.
5. Document the distance between the distal end of the stent (hepatic vein end) and the inferior vena cava.
6. Determine umbilical vein patency and flow of patient on previous exam.
7. Assess for the presence of ascites.

Hepatic Artery

The hepatic artery from the common bile duct may be reliably identified by pulsed Doppler techniques. The sample volume may be placed directly in the pulsatile structure assumed to be the hepatic artery, and arterial flow may be recorded. If this were the common bile duct, no flow or color would be recorded.

Aneurysms of Gastrointestinal Tract

Real time imaging can detect small aneurysms of the hepatic, splenic, superior mesenteric, and gastroduodenal arteries. However, with perianeurysmal fibrosis, arterial pulsations may be reduced, and thus pulsed Doppler may help make a specific diagnosis. If color flow is available, the low-power mode may allow one to precisely outline the vascular structures, including the lumen and the aneurysm.

Renal Artery

The normal right renal artery arises anterolaterally from the aorta and passes anterior to the right crus of the diaphragm and posterior to the inferior vena cava. The left renal artery arises posterolaterally from the aorta. These points of origin are important in understanding the difficulties encountered when performing a Doppler study of the renal arteries. It may be difficult to accurately record Doppler tracings from this vessel because of the somewhat tortuous nature of the artery. This is one of the reasons it is difficult to evaluate renal artery stenosis, since the beam must be parallel to blood flow to accurately record maximum-velocity flow patterns.

The evaluation of renal artery occlusion is quite accurate with Doppler. The arterial waveforms should always be present from within the parenchyma of the kidneys. Their absence is diagnostic of arterial occlusion.[1]

Renal Vein

Doppler ultrasound of renal vein thrombosis has been well described. If the occlusion is complete, no Doppler flow is visualized. The entire vein should be evaluated so as not to miss a partial occlusion. The smaller veins within the kidney may also be evaluated. The absence of a flow signal from within the parenchyma may suggest venous thrombosis.

Liver and Pancreas Transplants

Not all patients with fatal liver disease are good candidates for transplant. It is important to identify patients whose vessels are anomalous, thrombosed, absent, or too small for satisfactory transplantation. In the pediatric patient, portal vein diameter must be at least 4 mm for the anastomosis to be surgically possible. Patency of the inferior vena cava is also an important finding in these children, since agenesis of the inferior vena cava is a known accompaniment of biliary atresia.

After liver transplantation, hepatic artery occlusion is one of the most feared complications, typically resulting in liver necrosis and death. Timely detection of such occlusion may allow revascularization of the transplant. Arterial stenosis at the anastomosis or in the donor hepatic artery may also be seen. Portal venous thrombosis and thrombosis of the inferior vena cava are also major complications.

Pancreatic transplantation is too new for much experience to have been collected. Doppler evaluation, however, may be used to evaluate the integrity of the vascular pedicle.

Renal Transplants

Visualization of vascular signals in a renal transplant is much easier than in the normotopic kidney, because of its superficial position. The renal artery normally shows some turbulence near the site of anastomosis. For this reason, it is important to have a baseline study to compare with subsequent examinations if stenosis of the transplanted artery is suspected. Up to 12% of patients with renal transplants develop this complication. It is important, when searching for renal artery stenosis, that the entire vessel be examined, because the high-velocity jet and distal turbulence are typically present only over a short section of the vessel.

Renal artery occlusion may occur immediately after transplant and is readily diagnosed with duplex scans. Generally this complication reflects technical problems during surgery.

The evaluation of graft rejection is another application of duplex scanning of the transplanted kidney. In patients with acute rejection, there is an increase in peripheral vascular resistance characterized by a loss or even reversal of diastolic flow and an eventual decrease in the amplitude of systolic flow. In contrast, with acute tubular necrosis, no abnormality in Doppler signals has been identified.

Acute rejection generally occurs within the first few weeks after transplant. It may be divided histologically into two forms—interstitial and vascular. In general, Doppler studies are more sensitive in detecting the more severe, vascular rejection. The diagnosis depends on identification of reduced blood flow during diastole. Normally, initial diastolic velocity is approximately 30% to 50% of peak systole throughout the renal arterial system, including the arcuate arteries. In patients with rejection, this ratio between peak systolic and peak diastolic velocity is increased, reflecting the decreased diastolic flow. Ideally, comparison with a baseline study obtained within 24 hours of surgery is necessary to identify milder forms of vascular rejection.

Other major complications of renal transplantation include renal artery stenosis (12%), renal artery occlusion (12%) (this generally occurs secondary to severe vascular rejection), renal vein stenosis (less common than arterial stenosis), arteriovenous fistula, and rejection.

Renal Transplant Protocol

General Considerations

Renal transplants are performed on patients with end-stage renal failure secondary to various types of medical renal disease or on children with congenital renal problems. The majority of renal transplants are positioned extraperitoneally in the right iliac fossa with anastomosis to the external iliac vasculature in an end-to-side fashion. The ureter is normally implanted directly into the bladder. The renal transplant can also be placed intraperitoneally or extraperitoneally within the right iliac fossa and anastomosed to the internal or external iliac vasculature. Ureteral anastomosis can be to the bladder or to a segment of bowel. All of these variations affect the sonographic appearance of the transplant and any complications that may occur.

The role of ultrasound is to evaluate the general anatomic appearance of the kidney, assess for hydronephrosis, document the presence of extrarenal masses, and provide a qualitative assessment of blood flow to the kidney.

Imaging Considerations

Because of the relatively superficial location of the transplanted kidney it is difficult to image it in its entirety with sector-type transducers. For this reason, it is best to image the transplant with a curved-array or long-flat-linear-array transducer. A 3.5- or 5-MHz transducer is ideal.

Examination Protocol

Gray-scale images

1. Obtain longitudinal scans of the lateral, middle, and medial segments of the kidney. Demonstrate the upper and lower poles. Measure the kidney length.
2. Perform transverse scans of the upper, middle, and lower segments of the kidney.
3. Perform transverse and longitudinal scans of the bladder.
4. Perform general survey scans of the pelvis to assess for the presence of extrarenal masses or fluid collections.

Doppler flow analysis

1. Take pulsed Doppler tracings with resistance measurements of the main, interlobar, and arcuate arteries.
2. Take a pulsed Doppler tracing of the main renal vein.

Neoplasms

Recent studies have shown Doppler imaging to be useful in evaluating abdominal neoplasms. Arteriovenous shunts occur in many tumors and are seen angiographically as early venous opacification. Such shunts cause high-velocity flow, frequently exceeding 100 cm per second and reaching as high as 700 cm per second. Typically, they are most obvious around the periphery of tumors. There is some evidence that Doppler ultrasound is more sensitive than angiography in identifying arteriovenous shunting. In some tumors, large thin-walled sinusoidal spaces are present, with dense parenchymal staining on angiography. The Doppler signal from such spaces is of relatively high velocity (100 to 200 cm per second) but not as high as in tumors with arteriovenous shunting. The signal characteristically shows very little systolic-diastolic variation (low pulsatility).

Both types of signals may coexist in a single tumor. Evaluation of these Doppler signals may sometimes give a clue as to the cell type of the tumor. Hepatocellular carcinomas tend to show the highest-velocity signals, usually exceeding 250 cm per second. In liver metastases the Doppler velocities are generally lower. Hemangiomas may show signals of less than 50 cm per second and often demonstrate no detectable signal at all. Spectral broadening is characteristic of tumor signals.

Much work remains to be done on the characterization of Doppler signals in neoplastic disease.

REVIEW QUESTIONS

1. How is ultrasound able to differentiate soft tissues within the abdomen?
2. Define the ring-down artifact seen in ultrasound. What causes this artifact?
3. What is the purpose of time gain compensation?
4. On a transverse scan, what structures should be identified to know that the correct transducer, gain setting, and time gain compensation have been selected?
5. What structures should be seen on a longitudinal scan to know that the proper settings have been used?
6. What organ is used to establish correct time gain compensation, gain settings, and transducer selection?
7. What is a baseline abdominal ultrasound? What organ structures are imaged?
8. How can one distinguish the right, caudate, and left lobes of the liver? What landmarks are used?
9. How would the sonographer separate the common bile duct from the hepatic artery?
10. What vascular landmarks are used to identify the pancreas?
11. In what patient position is the spleen best imaged?
12. What scans should be made to demonstrate the urinary system?
13. Define the "oblique-coronal" plane used to delineate the aorta and inferior vena cava. Why is this view useful?

BIBLIOGRAPHY

Hagen-Ansert SL: The anatomy workbook, Philadelphia, 1986, JB Lippincott.

Mittelstaedt CA: Abdominal ultrasound, New York, 1987, Churchill Livingstone.

Needdleman L and Rifkin M: Vascular ultrasonography: abdominal applications, Radiol Clin North Am 24:1986.

Sanders RC: Clinical sonography, Boston, 1991, Little, Brown and Co.

Swobodnik W, Herrmann M, Altwein JE, et al: Atlas of ultrasound anatomy, New York, 1991, Thieme Medical Publishers.

CHAPTER 4

The Vascular System

Sandra L. Hagen-Ansert

The sonographer's ability to recognize vascular structures within the abdomen, retroperitoneum, and pelvis is extremely useful in identifying specific organ structures. To understand the origin and anatomic variation of the major arterial and venous structures, the sonographer must be able to identify the anatomy correctly on the ultrasound image.

Function of the Circulatory System

The function of the circulatory system, along with the heart and lymphatics, is to transport gases, nutrient materials, and other essential substances to the tissues and subsequently transport waste products from the cells to the appropriate sites for excretion.

Anatomic Composition of Vascular Structures

Blood is carried away from the heart by the arteries and returned from the tissues to the heart by the veins. Arteries divide into smaller and smaller branches, the smallest of which are the arterioles. These lead into the capillaries, which are minute vessels that branch and form a network where the exchange of materials between blood and tissue fluid takes place. After the blood passes through the capillaries, it is collected in the small veins or venules. These small vessels unite to form larger vessels that eventually return the blood to the heart for recirculation.

A typical artery in cross-section consists of the following three layers (Fig. 4-1):

1. Tunica intima (inner layer), which itself consists of the following three layers: a layer of endothelial cells lining the arterial passage (lumen), a layer of delicate connective tissue, and an elastic layer made up of a network of elastic fibers.
2. Tunica media (middle layer), which consists of smooth muscle fibers with elastic and collagenous tissue.
3. Tunica adventitia (external layer), which is composed of loose connective tissue with bundles of smooth muscle fibers and elastic tissue.

Specific differences exist between the arteries and the veins. The arteries are hollow elastic tubes that carry blood away from the heart. They are enclosed within a sheath that includes a vein and nerve. The smaller arteries contain less elastic tissue and more smooth muscles than the larger arteries. The elasticity of the larger arteries is important in maintaining a steady blood flow.

The veins are hollow collapsible tubes with diminished tunica media that carry blood toward the heart. The veins appear collapsed because they have little elastic tissue or muscle within their walls. Veins have a larger total diameter than the arteries, and they move blood more slowly. The veins contain special valves that prevent backflow and permit blood to flow only in one direction—toward the heart. Numerous valves are found within the extremities, especially the lower extremities, because flow must work against gravity. Venous return is also aided by muscle contraction, overflow from capillary beds, gravity, and suction from negative thoracic pressure.

The capillaries are minute, hair-size vessels connecting the arterial and venous systems. Their walls have only one layer. The cells and tissues of the body receive their nutrients from the fluids passing through the capillary walls; at the same time, waste products from the cells pass into the capillaries. Arteries do not always end in capillary beds; some end in anastomoses, which are end-to-end grafts between different vessels that equalize pressure over vessel length and also provide alternate flow channels.

Major Vessels

AORTA

Anatomy

The aorta is the largest principal artery of the body. It may be divided into the following five sections: (1) root of the aorta, (2) ascending aorta, (3) descending aorta, (4) abdominal aorta, (5) and the bifurcation of the aorta into iliac arteries (Fig. 4-2).

Root of the Aorta. The systemic circulation leaves the left ventricle of the heart by way of the aorta. The root of the aorta arises from the left ventricular outflow tract in the heart. It is comprised of three semilunar cusps that prevent blood from flowing back into the left ventricle. The cusps

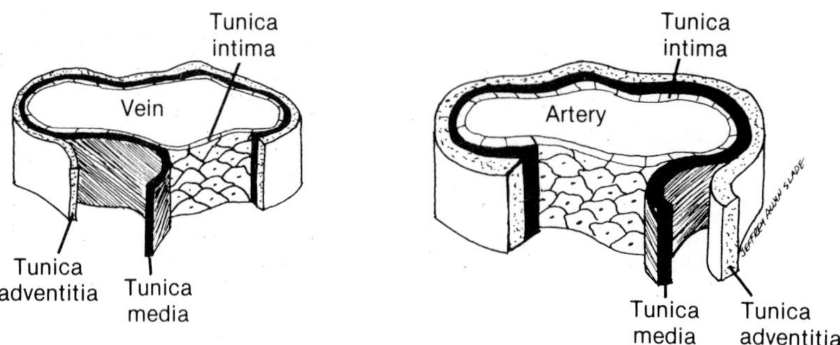

FIG. 4-1 Cross-section of an artery and vein showing the distinctions among the three layers of each vessel: tunica intima (inner layer), tunica media (middle layer), and tunica adventitia (external layer).

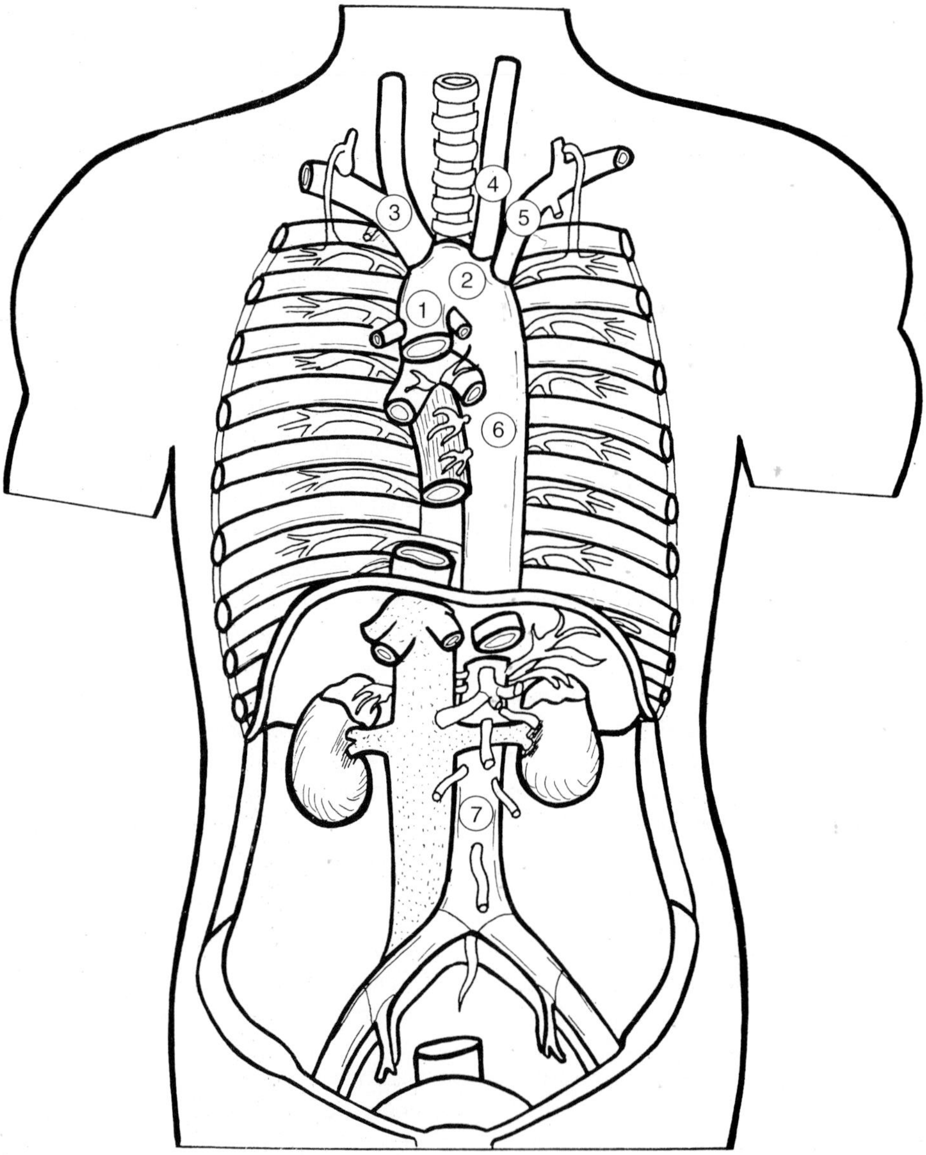

FIG. 4-2 The aorta is divided into seven sections. Ascending aorta, *1;* aortic arch, *2;* brachiocephalic artery, *3;* common carotid arteries, *4;* subclavian artery, *5;* thoracic (descending) aorta, *6;* abdominal aorta, *7;* (Modified from Hagen-Ansert SL: The anatomy workbook, Philadelphia, 1986, JB Lippincott.)

open with ventricular systole to allow blood to be ejected into the ascending aorta; the cusps are closed during ventricular diastole. The coronary arteries arise superiorly from the right and left coronary cusps to form the right and left coronary arteries, respectively. These coronary arteries further bifurcate to supply the vasculature of the cardiac structures. After the aorta arises from the left ventricle, it ascends posterior to the main pulmonary artery to form the ascending aorta.

Ascending Aorta. The ascending aorta arises a short distance from the ventricle and arches superior to form the aortic arch. Three arterial branches arise from the superior border of the aortic arch to supply the head, neck, and upper extremities: the right innominate, left common carotid, and left subclavian arteries.

Descending Aorta. From the aortic arch, the aorta descends posteriorly along the back wall of the heart through the thoracic cavity, where it pierces the diaphragm. The descending aorta enters the abdomen through the aortic opening of the diaphragm in front of the twelfth thoracic vertebra in the retroperitoneal space.

Abdominal Aorta. The aorta then continues to flow anterior to the vertebral column to the level of the fourth lumbar vertebra, where it bifurcates into the right and left common iliac arteries. At this point the aorta measures 2 to 3 cm in diameter. The aorta has four branches that supply other visceral organs and the mesentery: the celiac trunk, the superior and inferior mesenteric arteries, and the renal arteries.

Abdominal Aortic Branches. The celiac trunk is the first anterior branch of the aorta, arising 1 to 2 cm from the diaphragm. The celiac trunk gives rise to three smaller vessels: the splenic, hepatic, and left gastric arteries (Fig. 4-3). The superior mesenteric artery is the second anterior branch, arising approximately 2 cm from the celiac trunk. The right and left renal arteries are lateral branches arising just inferior to the superior mesenteric artery. The small inferior mesenteric artery arises anteriorly near the bifurcation. The distribution of these branch arteries is to the visceral organs and the mesentery.

Common Iliac Arteries. The common iliac arteries arise at the bifurcation of the abdominal aorta at the fourth lumbar vertebra. These vessels divide into the internal and external iliac arteries. The internal iliac artery enters the pelvis anterior to the sacroiliac joint, at which point it is crossed anteriorly by the ureter. It divides into anterior and posterior branches to supply the pelvic viscera, peritoneum, buttocks, and sacral canal. The external iliac artery runs along the medial border of the psoas muscle, following the pelvic brim. The inferior epigastric and deep circumflex iliac branches branch off before they pass under the inguinal ligament to become the femoral artery. The portion of the femoral artery posterior to the knee is the popliteal artery. This artery further divides into the anterior and posterior tibial arteries.

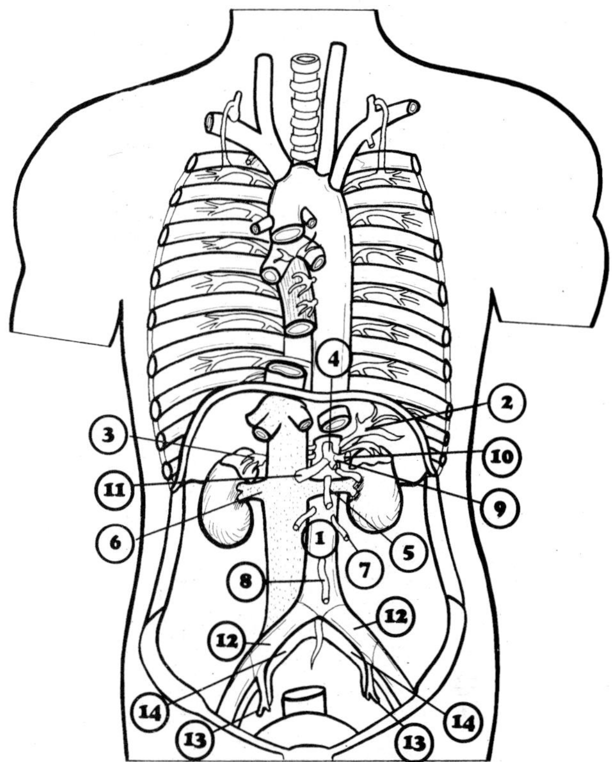

FIG. 4-3 The abdominal aorta and its tributaries. Abdominal aorta, *1;* inferior phrenic artery, *2;* suprarenal artery, *3;* celiac trunk, *4;* superior mesenteric artery, *5;* renal artery, *6;* testicular or ovarian artery, *7;* inferior mesenteric artery, *8;* left gastric artery, *9;* splenic artery, *10;* hepatic artery, *11;* common iliac arteries, *12;* internal iliac arteries, *13;* external iliac arteries, *14.* (From Hagen-Ansert SL: The anatomy workbook, Philadelphia, 1986, JB Lippincott.)

Ultrasound Findings. The abdominal aorta is usually one of the easiest abdominal structures to visualize by ultrasound because of the marked change in acoustic impedance between its elastic walls and its blood-filled lumen. Sonography provides the diagnostic information needed to provide an image of the entire abdominal aorta, to assess its diameter, and to visualize the presence of thrombus, calcification, or dissection within the walls.

The patient is routinely scanned in the supine position. Gas-filled or barium-filled loops of bowel may prevent adequate visualization of the aorta, but this can sometimes be overcome by applying gentle pressure with the transducer or by changing the angle of the transducer to move the gas out of the way.

Sagittal scans should be made beginning in the midline with a slight angulation of the transducer to the left, from the xyphoid to well below the level of bifurcation. In the normal individual the luminal dimension of the aorta gradually tapers as it proceeds distally in the abdomen (Fig. 4-4). A low to medium gain should be used to demonstrate the walls of the aorta without "noisy" artifactual internal echoes. These weak echoes may result from increased gain, reverberation from the anterior abdominal wall, or poor lateral resolution. These factors result in echoes being recorded at the same level as those from soft tissues that surround the vessel lumen, particularly if the vessels are smaller in diameter than the transducer.

Since the aorta follows the anterior course of the vertebral column, it is important that the transducer also follow a perpendicular path along the entire curvature of the spine. The anterior and posterior walls of the aorta should be easily seen as two thin lines. This facilitates measuring the anteroposterior diameter of the aorta, which in most institutions is done from the leading outer edge of the anterior wall to the leading inner edge of the posterior wall.

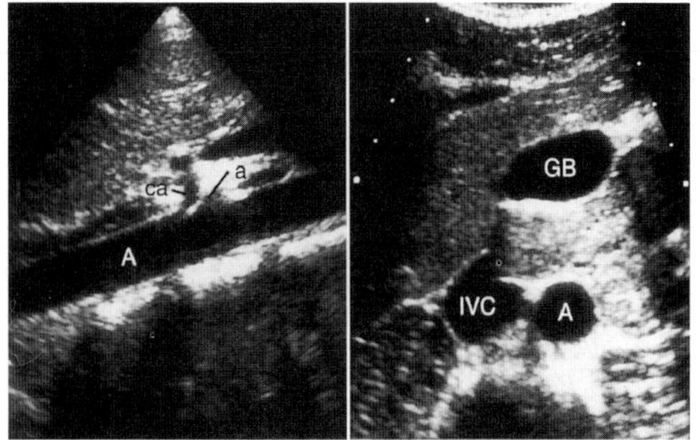

FIG. 4-4 A, The abdominal aorta is best visualized slightly to the left of the midline, from the level of the xyphoid to the bifurcation. The vessel follows the anterior surface of the vertebral bodies. The celiac axis *ca;* and superior mesenteric artery, *a;* arise from its anterior border. **B,** Transverse scans along the midabdomen show the aorta, *A,* and inferior vena cava, *IVC,* at the same horizontal level to the spine. As the transducer is angled in the cephalic direction, the inferior vena cava moves more medially and anterior to the spine. The gallbladder, *GB,* is seen anterior to the vascular structures.

In the transverse plane the aorta is imaged as a circular structure anterior to the spine and slightly to the left of the midline. In some cases the transverse diameter of the aorta differs from that found in longitudinal measurements; thus it is important to identify the vessel in two dimensions. Multiple scans should be made from the xyphoid to the bifurcation.

If the patient has a very tortuous aorta, scans may be difficult to obtain in a single plane. As one scans in the longitudinal plane, the upper portion of the abdominal aorta may be well visualized, but the lower portion may be out of the plane of view. In this case the sonographer should obtain a complete scan of the upper segment and then concentrate fully on the lower segment. In some patients, we have seen the aorta stretch from the far right of the abdomen to the far left.

To better visualize the aortic bifurcation, use the lateral decubitus position (Fig. 4-5). The patient should be examined in deep inspiration, which projects the liver and diaphragm into the abdominal cavity and provides an acoustic window to image the vascular structures. The patient should be rotated 5 to 10 degrees from the true lateral position. Slight medial to lateral angulation may be needed to image the bifurcation in the longitudinal plane. In this oblique plane the inferior vena cava is visualized anterior to the aorta.

INFERIOR VENA CAVA

The inferior vena cava is formed by the union of the common iliac veins posterior to the right common iliac artery (Fig. 4-6). The inferior vena cava ascends vertically through the retroperitoneal space on the right side of the aorta posterior to the liver, piercing the central tendon of the diaphragm at the level of the eighth thoracic vertebra to enter the right atrium of the heart. Its entrance into the lesser sac separates it from the portal vein. Caudal to the

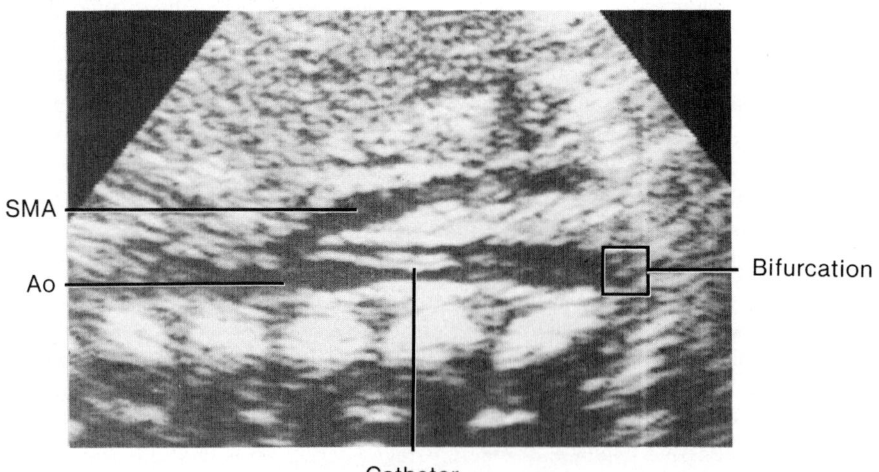

FIG. 4-5 Bifurcation of the abdominal aorta at the level of the umbilicus as seen in this neonatal abdomen. Superior mesenteric artery, *SMA;* Aorta, *Ao.*

renal vein entrance, the inferior vena cava shows posterior "hammocking" through the bare area of liver.

The tributaries of the inferior vena cava are the hepatic veins, the right adrenal vein, the renal veins, the right testicular or ovarian vein, the inferior phrenic vein, the four lumbar veins, the two common iliac veins, and the median sacral vein. The distribution of the venous system is such that blood drains from all organs and structures into the upper and lower abdomen through the system's major tributaries.

Ultrasound Findings. The inferior vena cava serves as a landmark for many other abdominal structures and should be routinely visualized on all examinations. On the sagittal image, the distended inferior vena cava can be seen with the patient in full inspiration from the diaphragm to its bifurcation (Fig. 4-7). The aorta is easily differentiated from the cava since the latter has a horizontal course, its proximal portion curving slightly anterior as it empties into the right atrial cavity; the aorta follows the curvature of the spine, its distal portion moving more posterior before bifurcating into the iliac vessels.

On transverse scans, the almond-shaped inferior vena cava serves as a landmark for localizing the superior mesenteric vein, which is generally found anterior and slightly to the right of or just medial to the cava (Fig. 4-8). On sagittal scans, it serves as a landmark for the portal vein, which is located just anterior to or midway down the anterior wall of the cava. It is also useful in identifying the pancreas and common bile duct (Fig. 4-9). The head of the pancreas is seen just inferior to the portal vein and anterior to the inferior vena cava as it makes a slight impression or indentation on the anterior wall of the cava. The common duct is seen anterior to the portal vein as it dips posterior to enter the head of the pancreas.

The inferior vena cava is first imaged on a sagittal scan beginning at the midline, the transducer being angled slightly to the right with a slight oblique tilt until the entire vessel is seen. The patient should be instructed to hold their breath; this causes the patient to perform a slight Valsalva

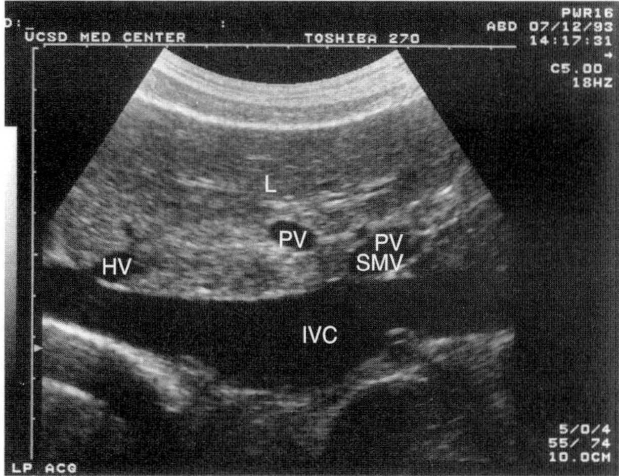

FIG. 4-7 On the sagittal image, the distended inferior vena cava, *IVC*, can be seen with the patient in full inspiration from the diaphragm to its bifurcation. Hepatic vein, HV; portal vein, *PV;* superior mesenteric vein, *SMV;* and liver, *L*.

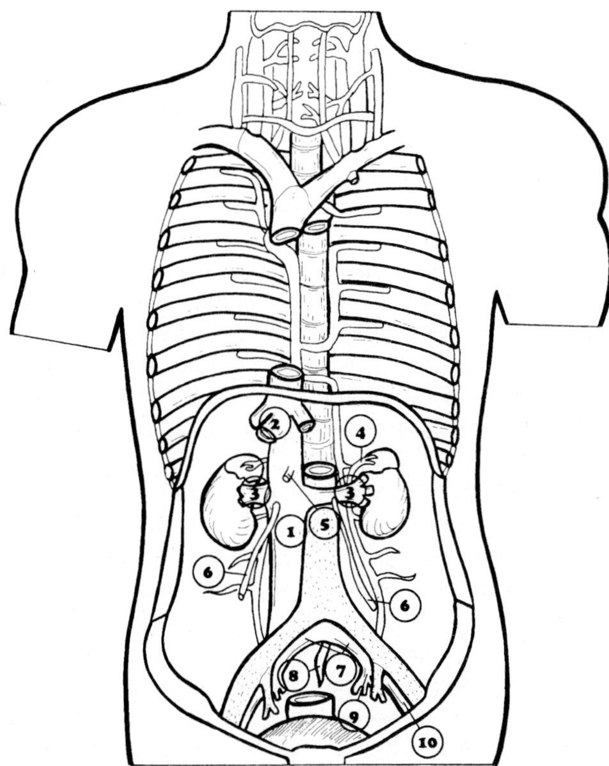

FIG. 4-6 The inferior vena cava and its tributaries. *1*, Inferior vena cava; *2*, hepatic vein; *3*, renal veins; *4*, suprarenal vein; *5*, phrenic vein; *6*, testicular or ovarian veins; *7*, right and left iliac veins; *8*, middle sacral vein; *9*, internal iliac vein; *10*, external iliac vein. (From Hagen-Ansert SL: The anatomy workbook, Philadelphia, 1986, JB Lippincott.)

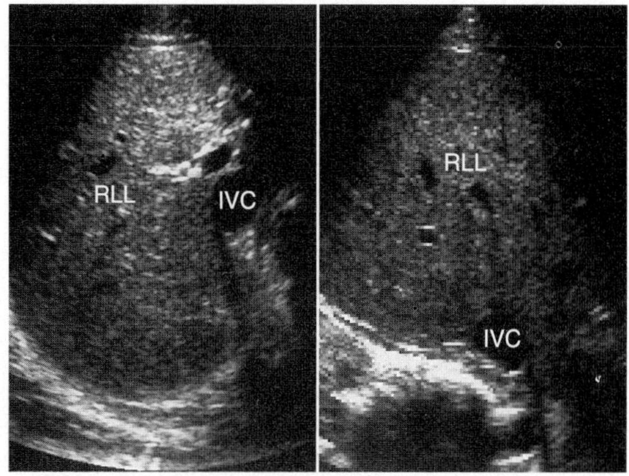

FIG. 4-8 Transverse scans show the inferior vena cava as an almond-shaped structure anterior to the spine. As the patient is rolled into a slight decubitus position, the inferior vena cava, *IVC*, is well seen through the window of the right lobe of the liver, *RLL*.

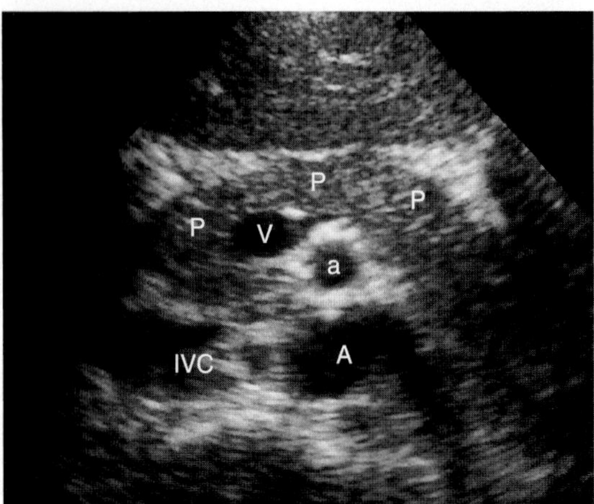

FIG. 4-9 Transverse scan of the vascular structures and the pancreas, *P*. The aorta, *A*, and inferior vena cava, *IVC*, lie anterior to the spine, and the superior mesenteric artery, *a*, is posterior to the body of the pancreas, whereas the superior mesenteric vein is posterior to the body and anterior to the uncinate process of the pancreas.

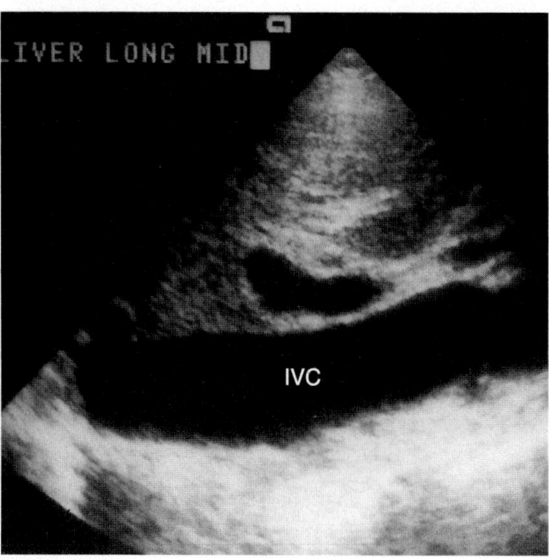

FIG. 4-10 Sagittal scan of the dilated inferior vena cava, *IVC*, as seen in this patient with right heart failure.

maneuver toward the end of inspiration, which dilates the inferior vena cava and other venous structures. The inferior vena cava may expand to as much as 3 to 4 cm in diameter with this maneuver.

Dilation of the inferior vena cava is noted in several pathologic conditions (Fig. 4-10), including right ventricular heart failure, congestive heart disease, constrictive pericarditis, tricuspid disease, and right heart obstructive tumors. In patients with hepatomegaly the hepatic veins are dilated and increased pressure is transmitted through the sinusoids, resulting in portal vein distention. If severe cirrhosis is present, the sinusoids may be unable to transmit pressure, and the portal veins will not distend. The presence of thrombus within the vessel should be evaluated, especially in patients with a known renal tumor. Other distortions of the inferior vena cava may be caused by an extrinsic retroperitoneal mass, hepatic neoplasm, or pancreatic mass.

Minor Arterial Vessels

ANTERIOR BRANCHES OF THE ABDOMINAL AORTA

Celiac Trunk

The celiac trunk originates within the first 2 cm from the diaphragm (Fig. 4-11). It is surrounded by the liver, spleen, inferior vena cava, and pancreas. After arising from the anterior wall it immediately branches into the following three vessels: the common hepatic, left gastric, and splenic arteries.

Common Hepatic Artery. The common hepatic artery arises from the celiac trunk and courses to the right of the abdomen at almost a 90-degree angle. It courses along the upper border of the head of the pancreas, behind the posterior layer of the peritoneal omental bursa, to the upper margin of the superior part of the duodenum, which forms the lower boundary of the epiploic foramen. The head of the pancreas, the duodenum, and parts of the stomach are supplied by the gastroduodenal artery and the right gastric artery. Along with the hepatic duct and the portal vein, the common hepatic then ascends into the liver, where it divides into two branches, the right and left hepatic arteries.

Left hepatic artery. The left hepatic artery is a small branch supplying the caudate and left lobes of the liver.

Right hepatic artery. The right hepatic artery supplies the gallbladder via the cystic artery.

Left Gastric Artery. The left gastric artery is a small branch of the celiac trunk, passing anterior, cephalic, and left to reach the esophagus and then descending along the lesser curvature of the stomach. It supplies the lower third of the esophagus and the upper right of the stomach.

Splenic Artery. The splenic artery is the largest of the three branches of the celiac trunk. From its origin, the artery takes a somewhat tortuous course horizontally to the left as it forms the superior border of the pancreas. At a variable distance from the spleen, it divides into two branches. One of these branches, the left gastroepiploic, runs caudally into the greater omentum toward the right gastroepiploic artery. The other courses in a cephalic direction and divides into the short gastric artery, which supplies the fundus of the stomach, and a number of splenic branches, which supply the spleen.

Several smaller arterial branches originate at the splenic artery as it courses through the upper border of the pancreas: the dorsal pancreatic, great pancreatic, and caudal pancreatic arteries. The dorsal or superior pancreatic artery originates from the beginning of the splenic artery or from

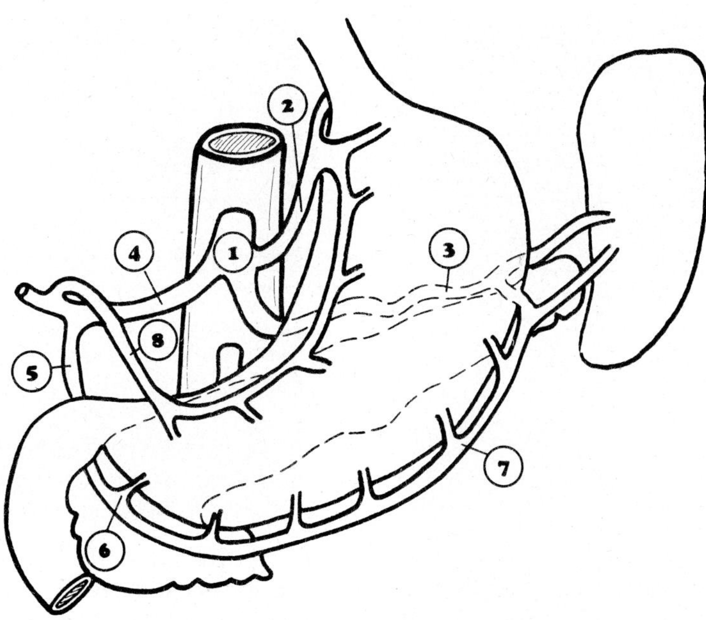

FIG. 4-11 Celiac artery and its branches. The celiac trunk originates within the first 2 cm of the abdominal aorta and immediately branches into the left gastric, splenic, and common hepatic arteries. Celiac artery, *1;* left gastric artery, *2;* splenic artery, *3;* common hepatic artery, *4;* gastroduodenal artery, *5;* right gastroepiploic artery, *6;* left gastroepiploic artery, *7;* right gastric artery, *8*. (From Hagen-Ansert SL: The anatomy workbook, Philadelphia, 1986, JB Lippincott.)

the hepatic artery, celiac trunk, or aorta. It runs behind and in the substance of the pancreas, dividing into right and left branches. The left branch is the transverse pancreatic artery. The right branch constitutes an anastomotic vessel to the anterior pancreatic arch and also a branch to the uncinate process. The great pancreatic artery originates from the splenic artery farther to the left and passes downward, dividing into branches that anastomose with the transverse or inferior pancreatic artery. The caudal pancreatic artery supplies the tail of the pancreas and divides into branches that anastomose with terminal branches of the transverse pancreatic artery. The transverse pancreatic artery courses behind the body and tail of the pancreas close to the lower pancreatic border. It may originate from or communicate with the superior mesenteric artery.

The distribution of the celiac trunk vessels is to the liver, spleen, stomach, pancreas, and duodenum.

Ultrasound Findings. The celiac trunk is best visualized sonographically on the longitudinal scan (Fig. 4-12). It is usually seen as a small vascular structure arising anteriorly from the abdominal aorta just below the diaphragm. Since it is only 1 to 2 cm long, it is sometimes difficult to record unless the area near the midline of the aorta is carefully evaluated. Sometimes the celiac trunk can be seen to extend in a cephalic rather than a caudal presentation. The superior mesenteric artery is usually just inferior to the origin of the celiac trunk and may be used as a landmark in locating the celiac trunk. Transversely, one can differentiate the celiac trunk as the "wings of a seagull" arising directly anterior from the abdominal aorta.

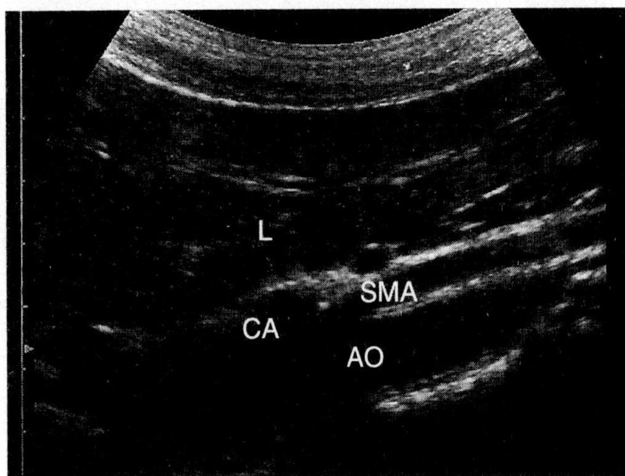

FIG. 4-12 Sagittal scan of the anterior branches of the abdominal aorta, *AO*, celiac axis, *CA*, and superior mesenteric artery, *SMA*, as imaged through the left lobe of the liver, *L*.

The splenic artery may be seen to flow from the celiac trunk toward the spleen (Fig. 4-13). Since it is so tortuous, it may be difficult to follow on the transverse scan. Generally small pieces of the splenic artery are visible as the artery weaves in and out of the left upper quadrant.

The hepatic artery can be seen to flow anterior and to the right of the celiac trunk, where it then divides into the right and left hepatic arteries (Figs. 4-14 to 4-18).

The left gastric artery is of very small diameter and often is difficult to visualize by ultrasound. It becomes difficult to separate from the splenic artery unless distinct structures are seen in the area of the celiac trunk branching to the left of the abdominal aorta.

A

B

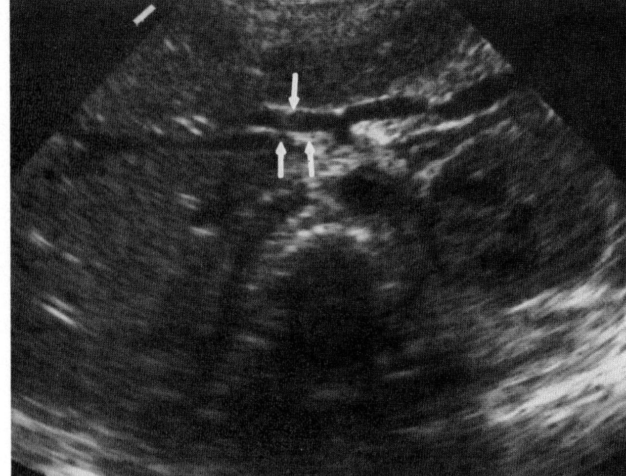

FIG. 4-13 A, Transverse scan of the splenic artery. This vessel may serve as the superior posterior border of the body and tail of the pancreas. **B,** The hepatic artery serves as the superior border of the head of the pancreas.

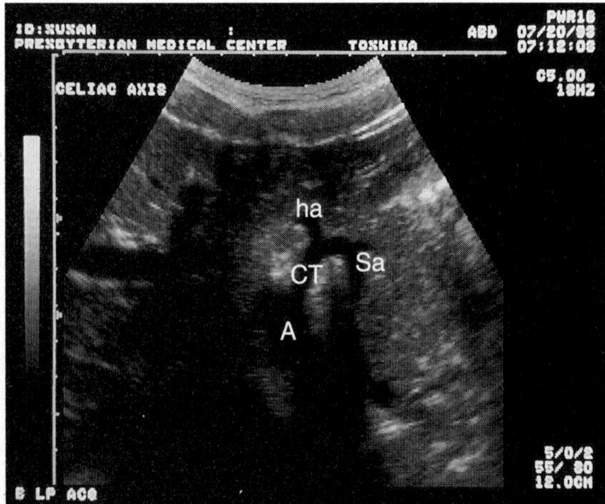

FIG. 4-14 Transverse scan of the upper abdomen shows the celiac trunk, *ct,* arising from the anterior wall of the aorta. The branches of the splenic artery, *sa,* and hepatic artery, *ha,* are seen.

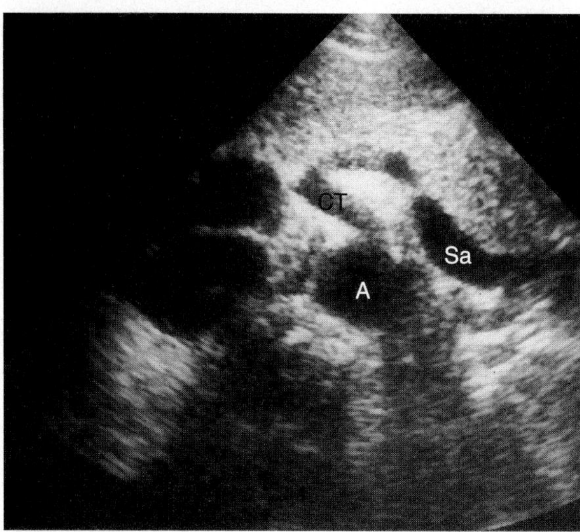

FIG. 4-15 The splenic artery, *sa,* takes a tortuous course from the celiac trunk, *ct,* to the splenic hilum on transverse scans.

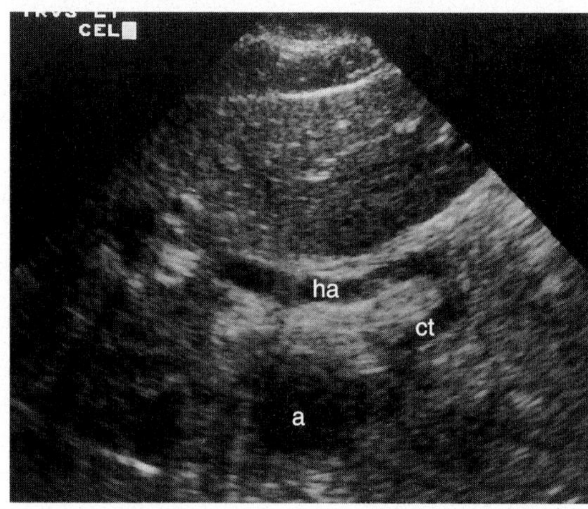

FIG. 4-16 The hepatic artery, *ha,* is well seen as it arises from the celiac trunk, *ct.*

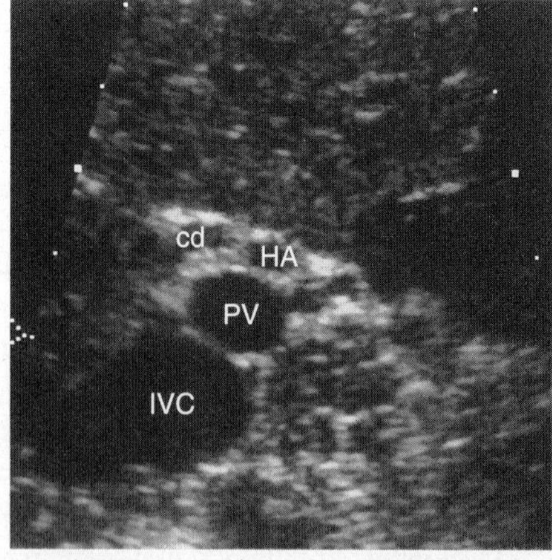

FIG. 4-17 Transverse scan of the upper abdomen shows the inferior vena cava, *IVC,* portal vein, *pv,* common bile duct, *cd,* and hepatic artery, *HA.*

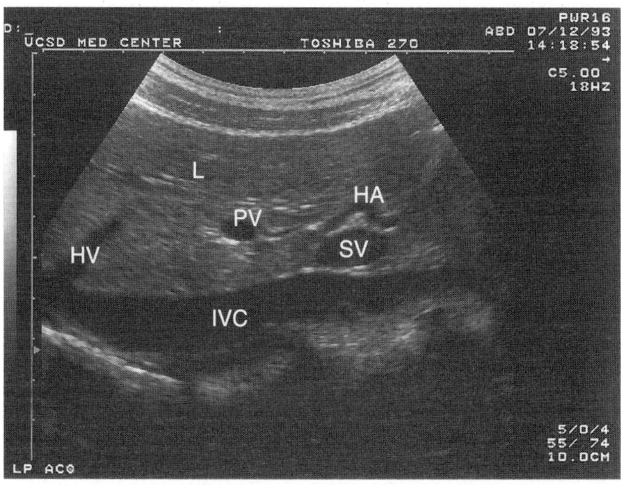

FIG. 4-18 Sagittal view of the hepatic artery, *HA,* as it courses anterior to the splenic vein and superior mesenteric vein, *SV,* and the pancreas. Hepatic vein, *HV,* portal vein, *PV,* liver, *L.*

Superior Mesenteric Artery

The superior mesenteric artery arises from the anterior abdominal aortic wall approximately 1 cm inferior to the celiac trunk (Fig. 4-19). It runs posterior to the neck of the pancreas and anterior to the uncinate process, which is anterior to the third part of the duodenum; it then branches into the mesentery and colon. The right hepatic artery is sometimes seen to arise from the superior mesenteric artery.

The superior mesenteric artery has the following five main branches (Fig. 4-20):

1. Inferior pancreatic artery
2. Duodenal artery
3. Colic artery
4. Iliocolic artery
5. Intestinal artery

These branch arteries supply the small bowel; each consists of 10 to 16 branches arising from the left side of the supe-

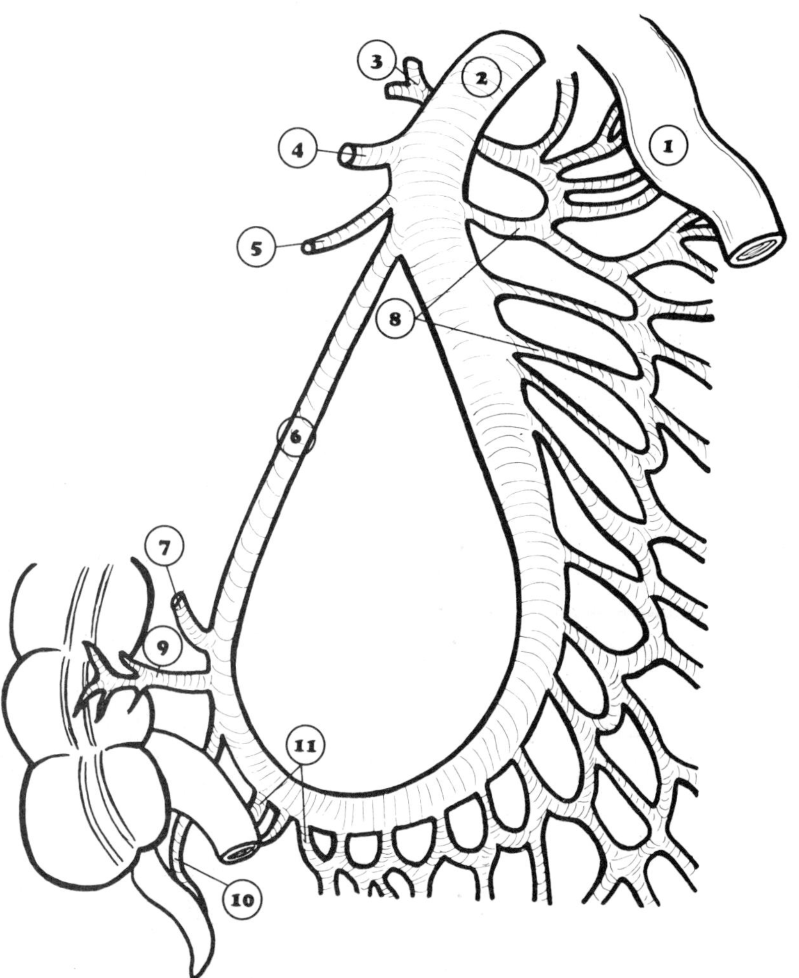

FIG. 4-19 The superior mesenteric artery arises anteriorly from the abdominal aorta approximately 1 cm below the celiac trunk. It supplies the proximal half of the colon and small intestine. Duodenojejunal flexure, *1;* superior mesenteric artery, *2;* inferior pancreaticoduodenal arteries, *3;* middle colic artery, *4;* right colic artery, *5;* ileocolic artery, *6;* ascending branch of ileocolic artery, *7;* intestinal arteries, *8;* cecal arteries, *9;* appendicular artery, *10;* ileal branches of the ileocolic artery, *11.* (From Hagen-Ansert SL: The anatomy workbook, Philadelphia, 1986, JB Lippincott.)

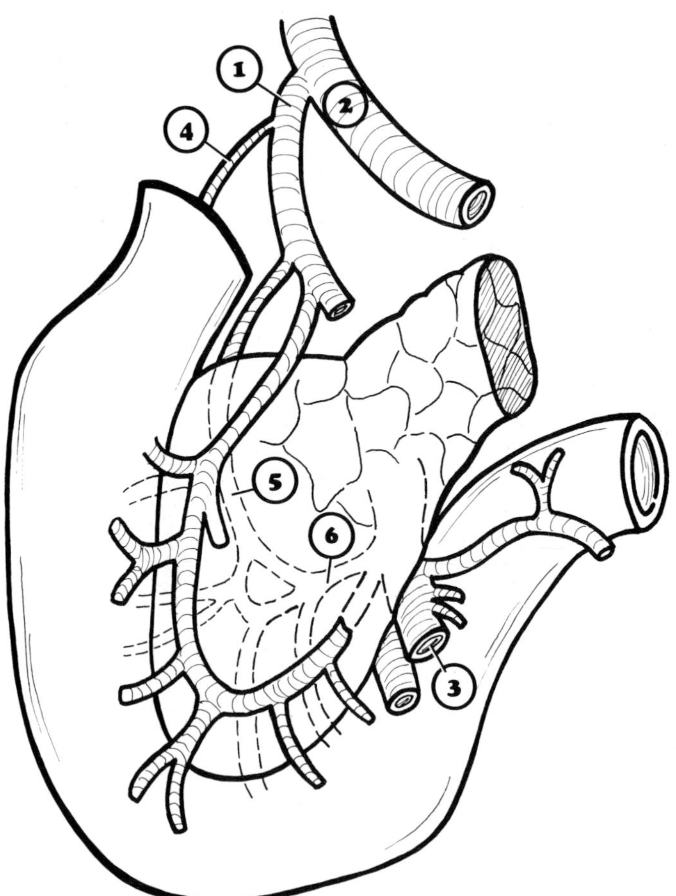

FIG. 4-20 The gastroduodenal artery is very useful in locating the head of the pancreas and serves as the lateral border of the gland. Gastroduodenal artery, *1;* hepatic artery, *2;* superior mesenteric artery, *3;* supraduodenal artery, *4;* anterior superior pancreaticoduodenal artery, *5;* posterior and anterior inferior pancreaticoduodenal artery, *6.* (From Hagen-Ansert SL: The anatomy workbook, Philadelphia, 1986, JB Lippincott.)

rior mesenteric trunk. They extend into the mesentery, where adjacent arteries unite with them to form loops or arcades. Their distribution is to the proximal half of the colon (cecum, ascending, and transverse) and the small intestine.

Ultrasound Findings. The superior mesenteric artery is well seen on both transverse and longitudinal scans. As it arises from the anterior aortic wall, it may follow a parallel course along the abdominal aorta or branch off at a slight angle to the anterior wall of the aorta and then follow a parallel course (Figs. 4-21 to 4-23; see color image). If the angle is severe (greater than 15 degrees), adenopathy should be considered.

Transversely the artery can be seen as a separate small circular structure anterior to the abdominal aorta and posterior to the pancreas. Characteristically it is surrounded by highly reflective echoes from the retroperitoneal fascia.

Inferior Mesenteric Artery

The inferior mesenteric artery arises from the anterior abdominal aorta approximately at the level of the third or

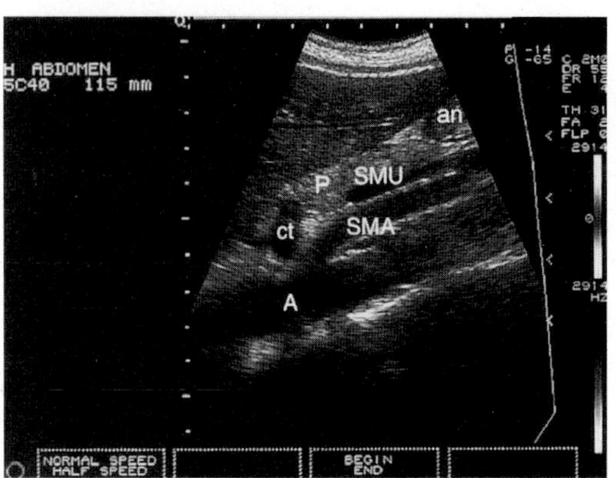

FIG. 4-21 Sagittal scan of the pancreas and mesenteric vessels. Aorta, *A;* celiac trunk, *ct;* superior mesenteric artery, *sma;* superior mesenteric vein, *v;* pancreas, *P;* antrum of stomach, *an.*

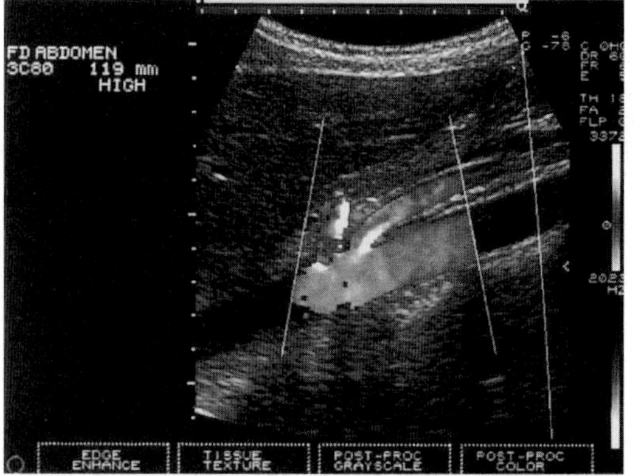

FIG. 4-22 Color flow of the image in Fig. 4-21 highlighting the arterial vessels (see color image).

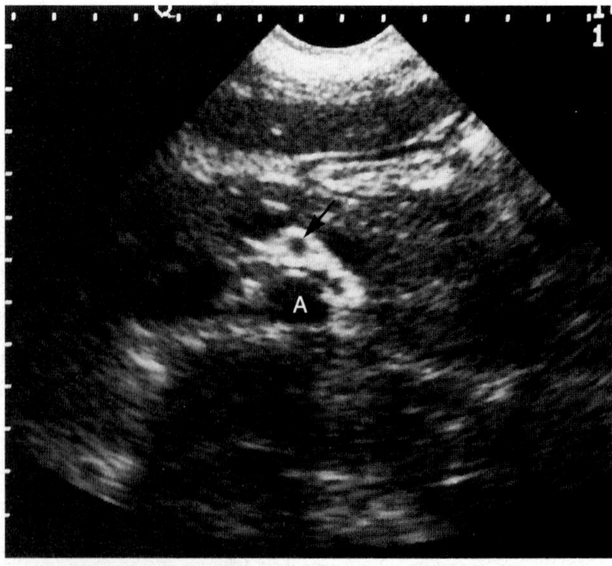

FIG. 4-23 Transverse scan of the superior mesenteric artery *(arrow)* with the highly reflective fatty tissue surrounding the vessel. The superior mesenteric artery lies anterior to the left renal vein and aorta, *A.*

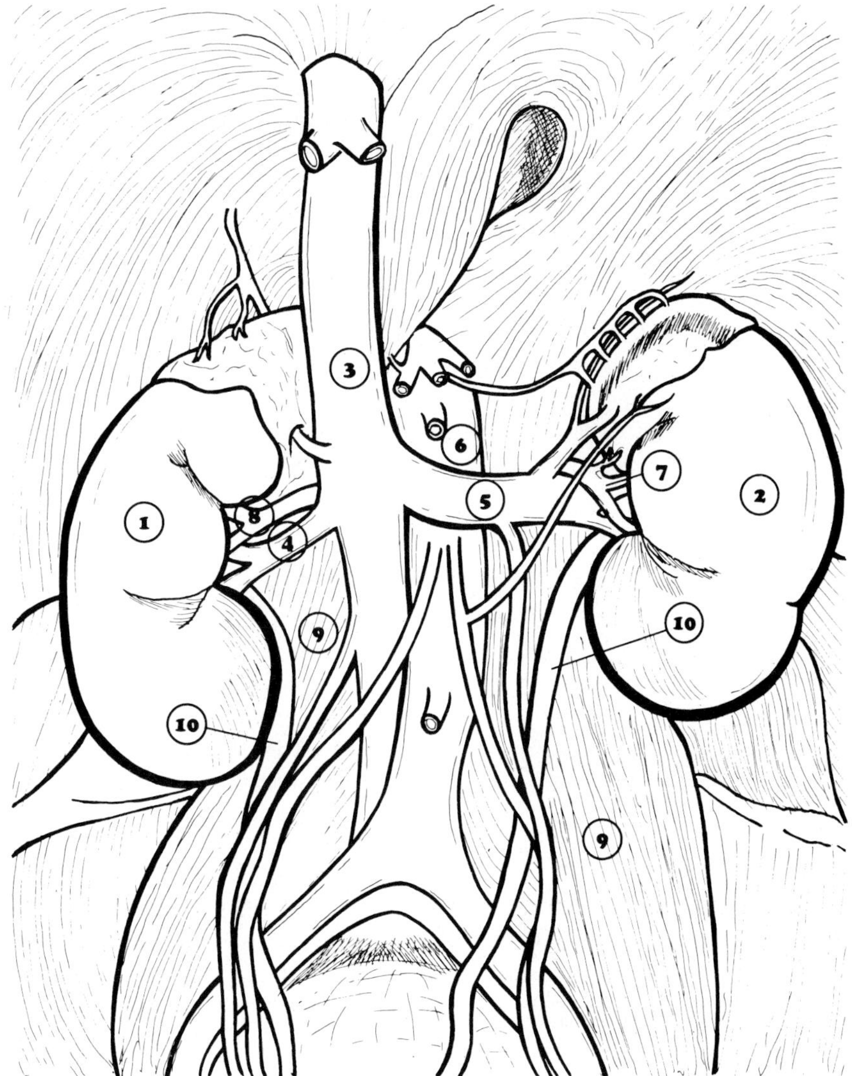

FIG. 4-24 The kidneys and their vascular relationships. Right kidney *1;* left kidney *2;* inferior vena cava, *3;* right renal vein, *4;* left renal vein, *5;* aorta, *6;* left renal artery, *7;* right renal artery, *8;* psoas muscle, *9;* ureter, *10.* (From Hagen-Ansert SL: The anatomy workbook, Philadelphia, 1986, JB Lippincott.)

fourth lumbar vertebra. It proceeds to the left to distribute arterial blood to the descending colon, sigmoid colon, and rectum. It has the following three main branches: the left colic, sigmoid, and superior rectal arteries. The distribution is to the left transverse colon, descending colon, sigmoid colon, and rectum.

Ultrasound Findings. The inferior mesenteric artery is more difficult to visualize by ultrasound; when it is seen, it is generally on a longitudinal scan. It is a small structure inferior to the superior mesenteric artery. On transverse scans it is difficult to separate from small loops of bowel within the abdomen.

LATERAL BRANCHES OF THE ABDOMINAL AORTA

Phrenic Artery

The phrenic artery is a small vessel that clings to the undersurface of the diaphragm which it supplies.

Renal Arteries

The renal arteries arise anterior to the first lumbar vertebra and inferior to the superior mesenteric artery (Fig. 4-24). Both vessels divide into the anterior and inferior suprarenal arteries.

Right Renal Artery. The right renal artery is a longer vessel than the left; it courses from the aorta posterior to the inferior vena cava and anterior to the vertebral column in a posterior and slightly caudal direction to enter the hilus of the right kidney. The renal artery passes posterior to the renal vein before entering the renal hilus.

Left Renal Artery. The left renal artery courses from the aorta directly into the hilus of the left kidney.

Ultrasound Findings. Both renal arteries are best seen on transverse sonograms (Fig. 4-25). The right renal artery passes posterior to the inferior vena cava and anterior to the vertebral column in a posterior and slightly caudal direction. Occasionally on longitudinal scans, a segment of

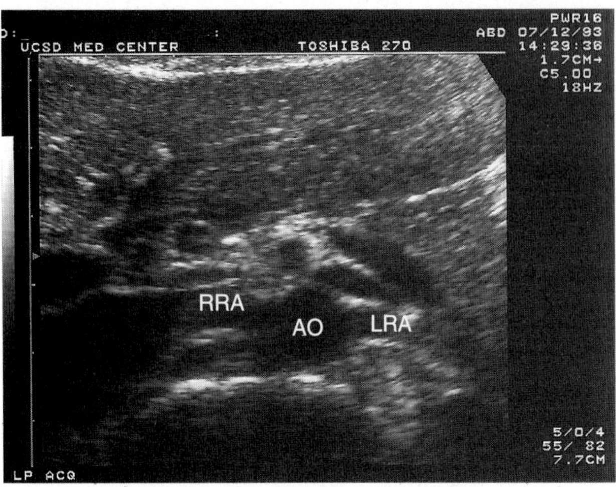

FIG. 4-25 Transverse scan of the aorta and both renal arteries.

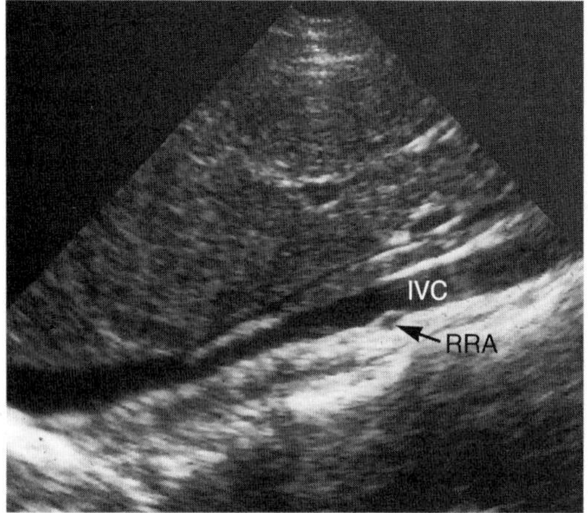

FIG. 4-26 Sagittal scan shows the inferior vena cava, *IVC*, anterior to the right renal artery, *RRA*.

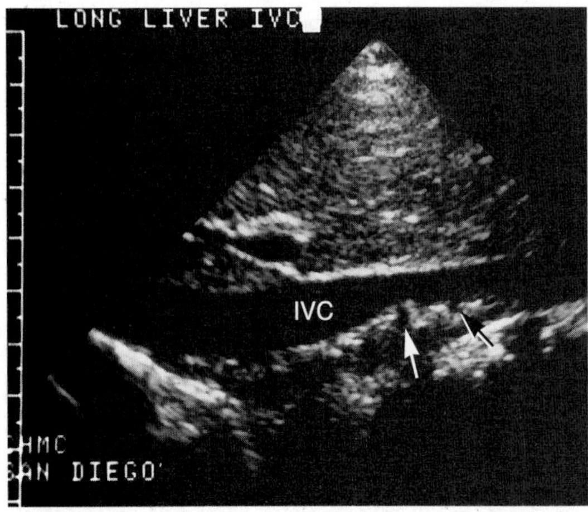

FIG. 4-27 Young patient with duplicated right renal arteries seen posterior to the inferior vena cava *(arrows)*.

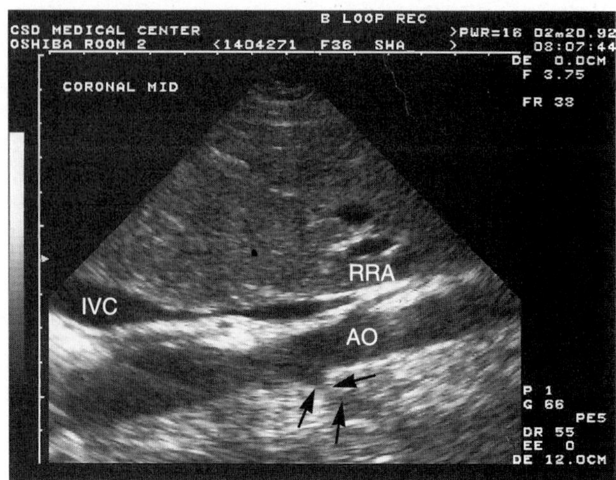

FIG. 4-28 The modified coronal oblique view shows the inferior vena cava anterior to the aorta. The right renal artery, *RRA*, and left renal artery *(arrow)* may be seen along the lateral margins of the abdominal aorta. This is an excellent view for Doppler analysis of the renal arteries.

the right renal artery is seen as a circular structure posterior to the inferior vena cava (Figs. 4-26 and 4-27). The left renal artery takes a direct course from the aorta anterior to the psoas muscle to enter the renal sinus.

The coronal oblique scan of the aorta and inferior vena cava is excellent for demonstrating the origin of the renal arteries and veins (Fig. 4-28). The patient is rolled into a steep decubitus position. The transducer is directed longitudinally with its axis across the inferior vena cava and aorta in efforts to see the origin of the renal vessels. The patient should be in full inspiration to dilate the venous structures for better visualization.

Gonadal Artery

The gonadal artery arises inferior to the renal arteries and courses along the psoas muscle to the respective gonadal area.

DORSAL AORTIC BRANCHES

Lumbar Artery

There are usually four lumbar arteries on each side of the aorta. The vessels travel lateral and posterior to supply muscle, skin, bone, and spinal cord. The midsacral artery supplies the sacrum and rectum.

Minor Venous Vessels

LATERAL TRIBUTARIES TO THE INFERIOR VENA CAVA

Renal Veins

Five or six branches of the renal vein unite to form the main renal vein. The vessels arise anterior to the renal ar-

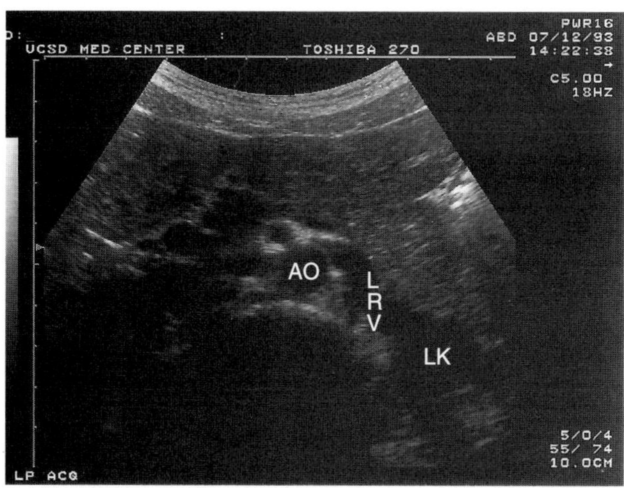

FIG. 4-29 Transverse scan of the left renal vein, *LRV*, as it exits the medial aspect of the kidney and flows anterior to the aorta and posterior to the superior mesenteric artery to enter the lateral wall of the inferior vena cava.

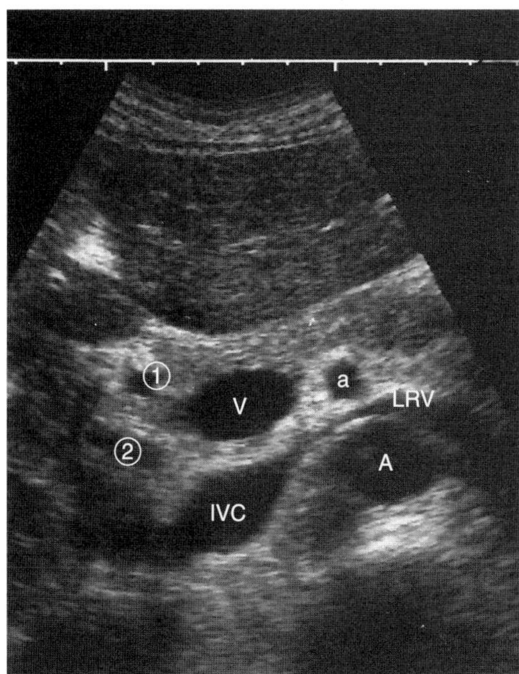

FIG. 4-30 Transverse scan of the left renal vein, *LRV*, aorta, *A*, inferior vena cava, *IVC*, superior mesenteric artery, *a*, and vein, *v*, gastroduodenal artery, *1*, and common bile duct, *2*.

teries at their respective sides of the inferior vena cava at the level of L2.

Left Renal Vein. The left renal vein arises medially to exit from the hilus of the kidney (Fig. 4-29). It flows from the left kidney posterior to the superior mesenteric artery and anterior to the aorta to enter the lateral wall of the inferior vena cava (Fig. 4-30). Above the entry of the renal veins, the inferior vena cava enlarges because of the increased volume of blood returning from the kidneys. The

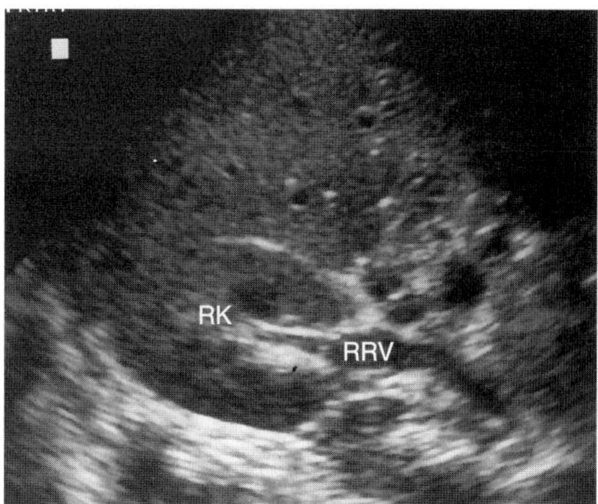

FIG. 4-31 Transverse scan of the right renal vein, *RRV*, as it leaves the hilus of the kidney to directly enter the inferior vena cava.

left vein is larger than the right renal vein. It accepts branches from the left adrenal, left gonadal, and lumbar veins.

Right Renal Vein. The right renal vein is seen best on transverse images as it flows directly from the right kidney into the posterolateral aspect of the inferior vena cava (Fig. 4-31). It seldom accepts tributaries—the right adrenal and right gonadal enter the cava directly.

Gonadal Veins

The gonadal veins (testicular and ovarian) course anterior to the external and internal iliac veins and continue cranially and retroperitoneally along the psoas muscle until their terminus. The left gonadal vein usually enters the left renal vein or the left adrenal vein, which empties into the inferior vena cava. The right gonadal vein enters the inferior vena cava on the anterolateral border above the entrance of the lumbar veins.

Suprarenal Veins

The right suprarenal vein arises from the suprarenal gland and usually drains directly into the inferior vena cava. The left arises from the suprarenal gland and drains into the left renal vein.

ANTERIOR TRIBUTARIES TO THE INFERIOR VENA CAVA

Hepatic Veins

The hepatic veins are the largest visceral tributaries of the inferior vena cava. They originate in the liver and drain into the inferior vena cava at the level of the diaphragm (Fig. 4-32). The hepatic veins return unoxygenated blood from the liver. The veins collect blood from the three minor tributaries within the liver: the right hepatic vein drains the right lobe of the liver, the middle hepatic drains the caudate lobe, and the left hepatic drains the left lobe of the liver.

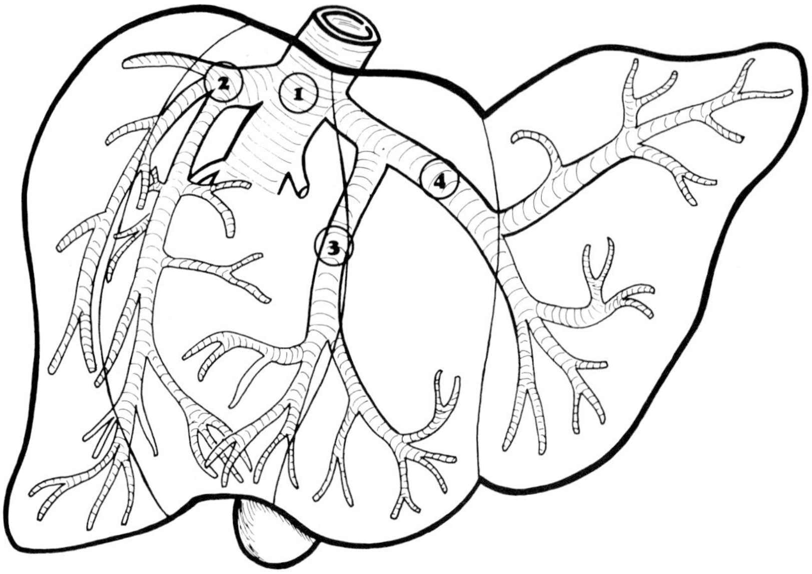

FIG. 4-32 The hepatic veins are divided into three components: right, middle, and left. They all drain into the inferior vena cava at the level of the diaphragm. Inferior vena cava, *1;* right hepatic vein, *2;* middle hepatic vein, *3;* left hepatic vein, *4.* (From Hagen-Ansert SL: The anatomy workbook, Philadelphia, 1986, JB Lippincott.)

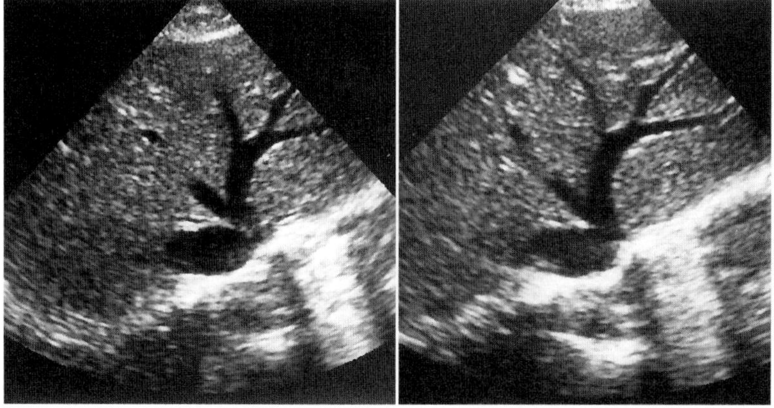

FIG. 4-33 Transverse view of the hepatic veins as they drain into the inferior vena cava at the level of the diaphragm.

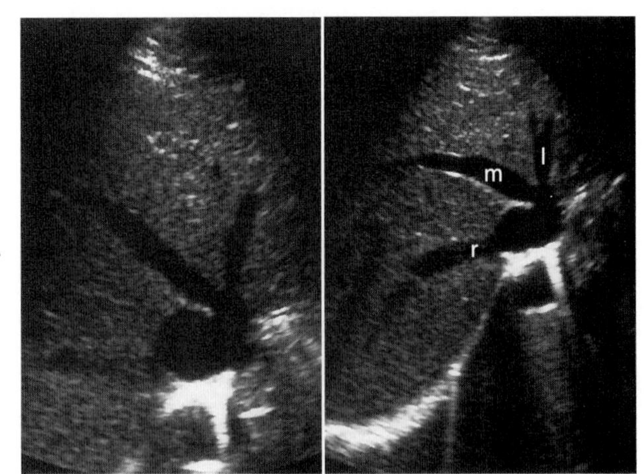

FIG. 4-34 A, The hepatic veins often look like "bunny ears" as they drain into the inferior vena cava. **B,** Transverse scan of the right, *r,* middle, *m,* and left, *l,* hepatic veins.

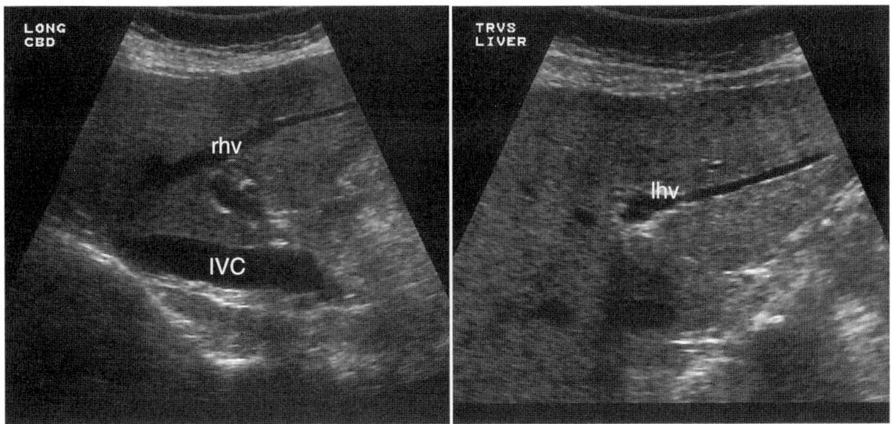

FIG. 4-35 Sagittal view of the middle hepatic vein, *mhv*, on the left, and left hepatic vein, *lhv*, on the right.

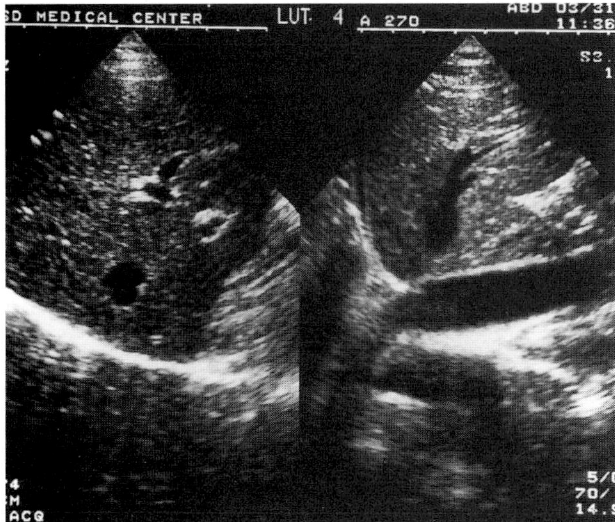

FIG. 4-36 Sagittal scan shows the hepatic veins with their thin walls, as compared with the portal veins, with bright acoustic reflections.

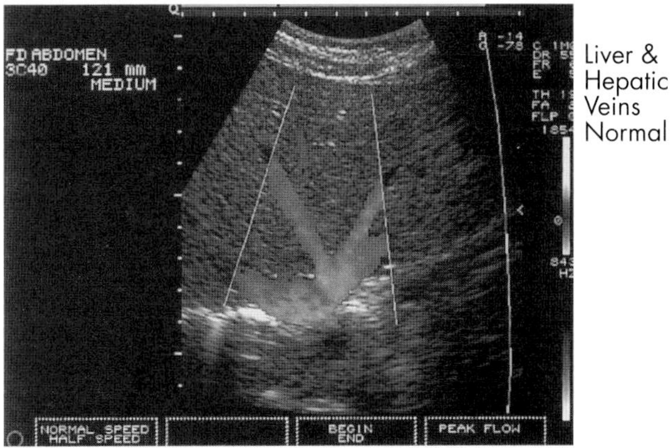

FIG. 4-37 Normal color flow showing the flow of the hepatic veins into the inferior vena cava (see color image).

Ultrasound Findings. The hepatic veins are best visualized on longitudinal scans of the liver as they drain into the inferior vena cava at the level of the diaphragm. Transverse scans obtained with a cephalic angle of the transducer at the level of the xyphoid often show at least two of the three veins draining into the inferior vena cava (Figs. 4-33 and 4-34). The hepatic veins resemble the "playboy" bunny or "reindeer" sign on the sonogram.

To distinguish hepatic veins from other vascular structures requires recognition of their anatomic patterns. Hepatic veins drain cephalad toward the diaphragm and then dorsomedially toward the inferior vena cava (Figs. 4-35 to 4-37; see color image of Fig. 4-37). Hepatic veins increase in caliber as they approach the diaphragm. Unlike portal veins, they are not surrounded by bright acoustic reflections, although a slight amount of acoustic enhancement may be seen along their posterior border.

Portal Vein

The portal vein is formed posterior to the pancreas by the union of the superior mesenteric and splenic veins at the level of L2. Its trunk is 5 to 7 cm in length (Fig. 4-38). The portal vein courses posterior to the first portion of the duodenum and then flows between the layers of the lesser omentum to the porta hepatis where it bifurcates into its hepatic branches. It carries blood from the intestinal tract to the liver by means of its two main branches, the right and left portal veins. It drains blood from the gastrointestinal tract from the lower end of the esophagus to the upper end of the anal canal, from the pancreas, gallbladder, bile ducts, and spleen. It has an important anastomosis with the esophageal veins, rectal venous plexus, and superficial abdominal veins. The portal venous blood traverses the

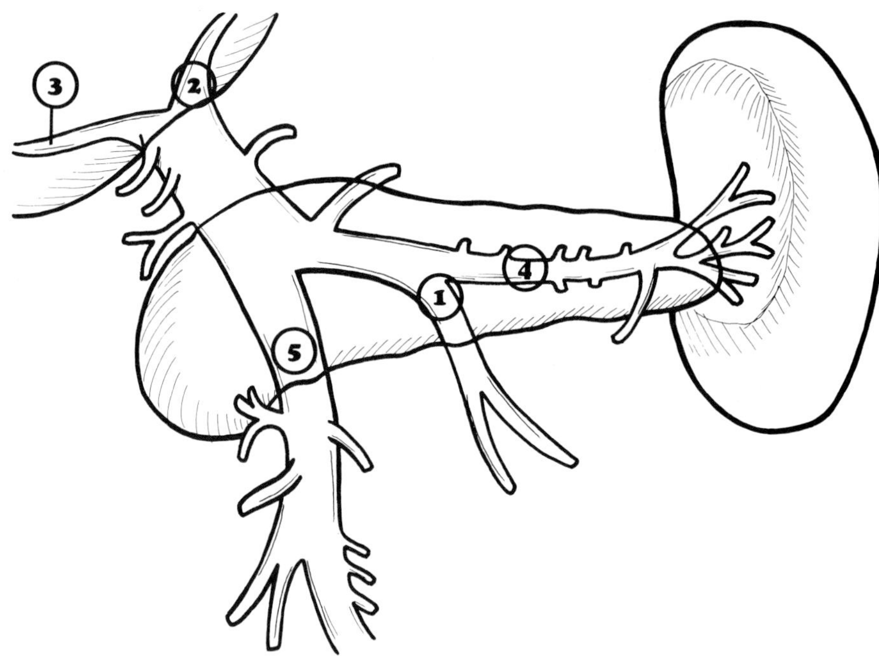

FIG. 4-38 The superior and inferior mesenteric veins join the splenic vein to form the portal vein. Inferior mesenteric vein, *1;* left branch of the portal vein, *2;* right branch of the portal vein, *3;* splenic vein, *4;* superior mesenteric vein, *5.* (From Hagen-Ansert SL: The anatomy workbook, Philadelphia, 1986, JB Lippincott.)

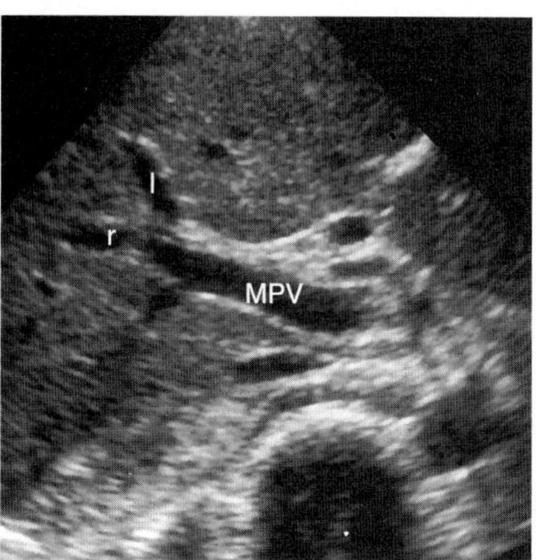

FIG. 4-39 Transverse scan of the main portal vein, *mpv,* and its right *r,* and left, *l,* branches in the liver.

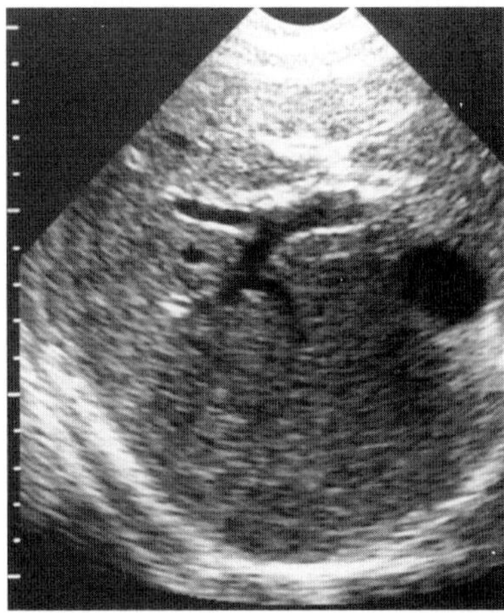

FIG. 4-40 Transverse scan of the right portal vein as it bifurcates into the posterior branch.

liver and drains into the inferior vena cava via the hepatic veins.

Ultrasound Findings. The portal vein is clearly seen on both transverse and sagittal scans. On transverse scans the main portal vein is a thin-walled circular structure, generally lateral and somewhat anterior to the inferior vena cava. It is often possible to record the splenic vein as it crosses the midline of the abdomen to join the superior mesenteric vein to form the main portal trunk. Thus a long section of the splenic vein can be visualized. Often the right or left portal vein can be seen branching from the portal trunk to enter the hilum of the liver.

Portal veins become smaller as they progress into the liver from the porta hepatis. Large radicles situated near or approaching the porta hepatis are portal veins, not hepatic veins. The portal veins are characterized by high-amplitude acoustic reflections that presumably arise from the fibrous tissues surrounding the portal triad as it courses through the liver substance (Figs. 4-39 to 4-42).

The right and left portal veins course transversely through

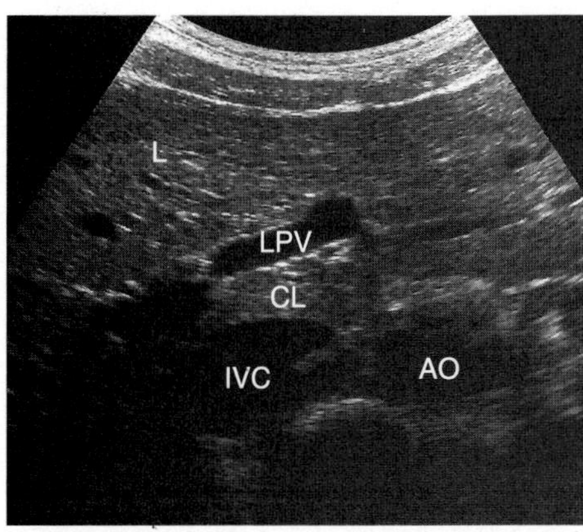

FIG. 4-41 The left portal vein, *LPV,* demarcates the caudate lobe, *CL,* of the liver.

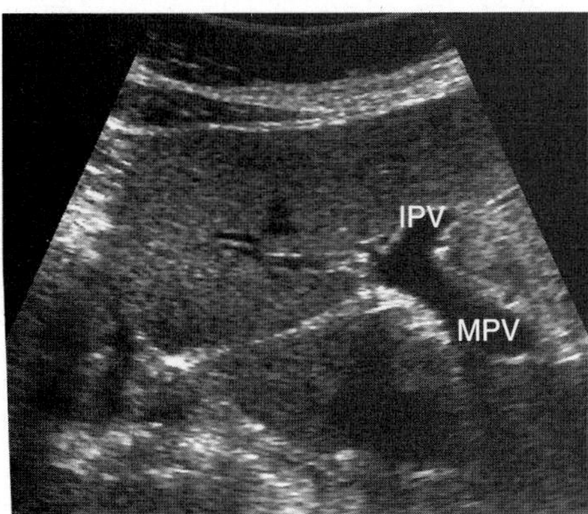

FIG. 4-42 Sagittal scan of the main portal vein, *mpv,* as it bifurcates into the left portal vein, *lpv.*

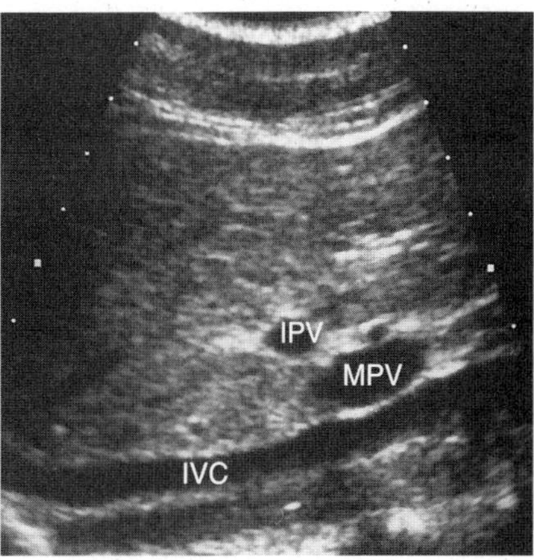

FIG. 4-43 Sagittal view of the inferior vena cava, *IVC,* main portal vein, *mpv,* and left portal vein, *lpv.*

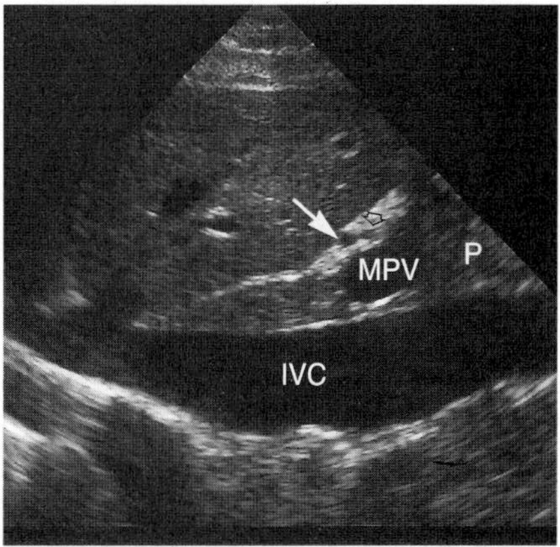

FIG. 4-44 Sagittal view of the inferior vena cava and main portal vein. The hepatic artery *(arrow)* and common bile duct *(open arrow)* are seen anterior to the main portal vein. The head of the pancreas is inferior to the main portal vein.

the liver. Thus transverse scans display their longest extent. The right portal vein is most consistently demonstrated on the sonogram. Anatomically any intraparenchymal segment of the portal venous system lying to the right of the lateral aspect of the inferior vena cava is a branch of the right portal system. The left portal vein has a narrow-caliber trunk and may be seen coursing transversely through the left hepatic lobe from a posterior to an anterior position (Figs. 4-43 and 4-44).

Since the portal radicle may have many different variations, it is important to become familiar with their patterns to be able to distinguish them from dilated biliary radicles.

Splenic Vein

The splenic vein is a tributary of the portal circulation. It begins at the hilum of the spleen, where it is formed by the union of several veins. It is subsequently joined by the short gastric and left gastroepiploic veins. The portal vein passes to the right within the ileorenal ligament and runs along the posteromedial border of the pancreas. It joins the superior mesenteric vein posterior to the neck of the pancreas to form the portal vein. Additional veins from the pancreas and inferior mesenteric vein join the splenic vein. It drains blood from the stomach, spleen, and pancreas.

Ultrasound Findings. The splenic vein is best visualized in the transverse plane as it crosses the upper abdomen from the hilum of the spleen to join the superior mesenteric to form the portal vein slightly to the right of midline (Figs. 4-45 and 4-46). The splenic vein crosses anteriorly to the aorta and the inferior vena cava and generally relates to the medial and posterior borders of the pancreatic body and tail. Its course is variable, so small degrees of obliquity may be necessary to image the vein entirely. It is usually smaller than the superior mesenteric vein and the main portal vein.

On sagittal scans the splenic vein can be visualized posterior to the left lobe of the liver and anterior to the major vascular structures. The pancreas may be seen inferior and slightly anterior to the vein. The larger diameter of the portal vein is the result of the influx of blood from the superior mesenteric vein. An obvious widening is demonstrated

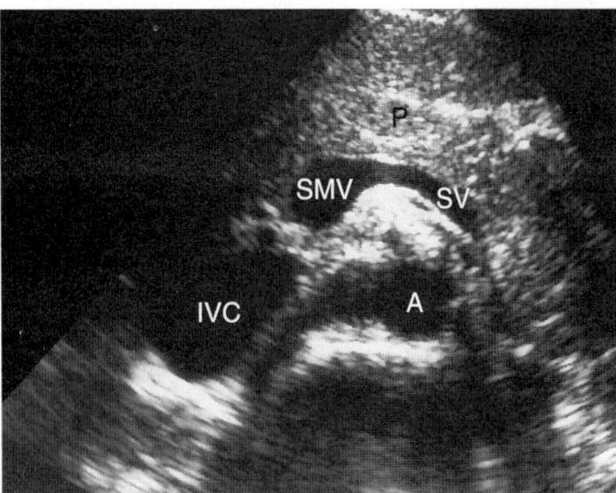

FIG. 4-45 The splenic vein is best visualized in the transverse plane as it crosses the upper abdomen from the hilum of the spleen to join the main portal vein. The prominent area above the inferior vena cava is the junction of the superior mesenteric vein.

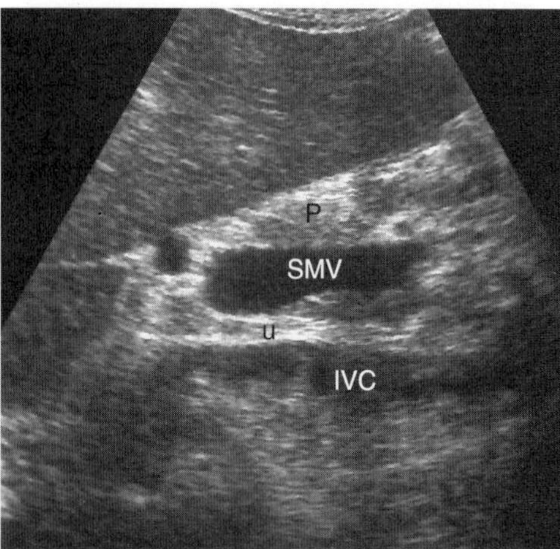

FIG. 4-46 Sagittal view of the superior mesenteric vein, *smv*. The body of the pancreas, *P*, is anterior, the uncinate process, *u*, is posterior.

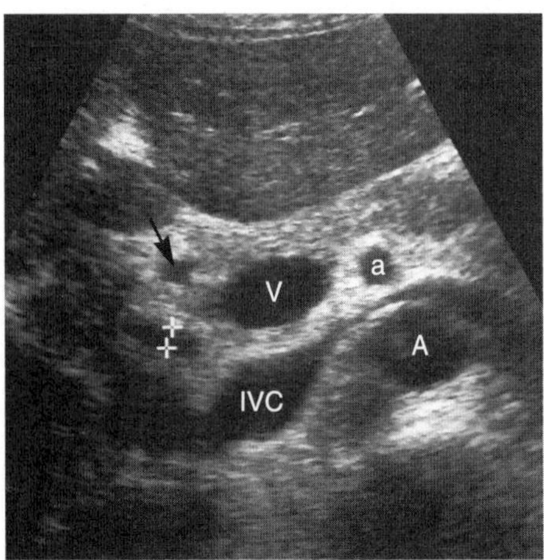

FIG. 4-47 Transverse view of the superior mesenteric vein, *v*, as it lies to the right of midline, anterior to the inferior vena cava, *IVC*. The gastroduodenal artery *(arrow)* marks the anterior lateral margin of the head of the pancreas; the common bile duct is denoted by crossbars.

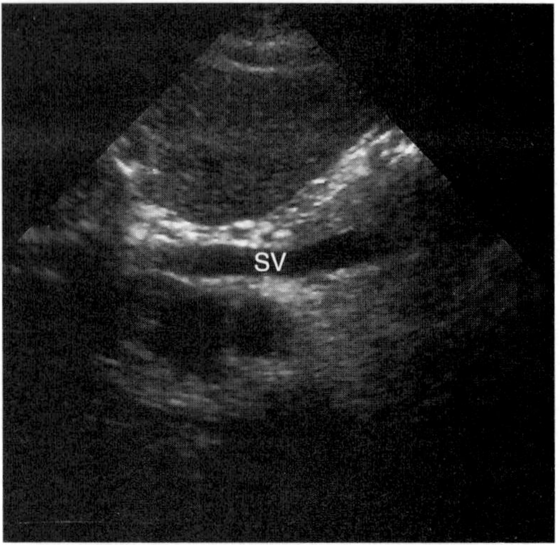

FIG. 4-48 Transverse scan of the splenic vein, *sv*.

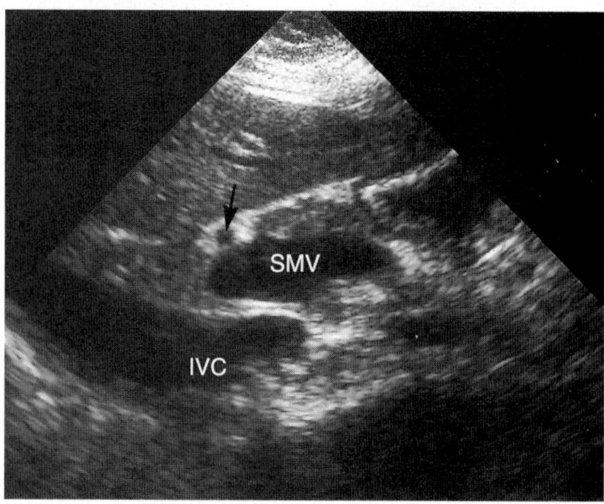

FIG. 4-49 Sagittal scan of the long tubular superior mesenteric vein, *smv*, as it lies anterior to the inferior vena cava, *IVC*. The small circle is the splenic artery *(arrow)*.

at the junction of the portal and splenic veins. When splenomegaly is present, it is often possible to identify the origin of the splenic vein at the splenic hilum.

Superior Mesenteric Vein

The superior mesenteric vein is also a tributary to the portal vein. It begins at the ileocolic junction and runs cephalad along the posterior abdominal wall within the root of the mesentery of the small intestine to the right of the superior mesenteric artery. The superior mesenteric vein passes anterior to the third part of the duodenum and posterior to the neck of the pancreas, where it joins the splenic vein to form the main portal vein. It also receives tributaries that correspond to the branches of the superior mesenteric artery, where it is joined by the inferior pancreaticoduodenal vein to the right gastroepiploic vein from the right aspect of the greater curvature of the stomach. The superior mesenteric vein drains blood from several smaller veins: the middle colic vein (transverse colon), right colic vein (ascending colon), and pancreatic duodenal vein.

Ultrasound Findings. The superior mesenteric vein is somewhat variable in its anatomic location. Generally it is anterior to the inferior vena cava and to the right of the superior mesenteric artery. The superior mesenteric vein drains into the main portal vein (with the splenic vein), therefore the sonographer should not be able to demonstrate these three structures together on a single transverse scan (Fig. 4-47). The superior mesenteric vein is the posterior border of the neck of the pancreas and the anterior border of the uncinate process of the pancreatic head.

On sagittal scans, the vein is seen as a long tubular structure anterior to the inferior vena cava (Figs. 4-48 and 4-49). With correct oblique angulation of the transducer, the path of the superior mesenteric vein can be followed as it enters the portal system.

The following points help to distinguish the superior mesenteric artery from the vein:

1. The superior mesenteric vein is of larger caliber than the artery.
2. Respiratory variations are seen in the vein.
3. On sagittal scans the superior mesenteric artery angles away from the aorta, whereas the vein tends to parallel the aorta or course anteriorly away from the aorta near the portal-splenic confluence.
4. Real time identification of the confluence of the superior mesenteric vein—portal vein or superior mesenteric artery is possible as the superior mesenteric artery originates from the aorta.

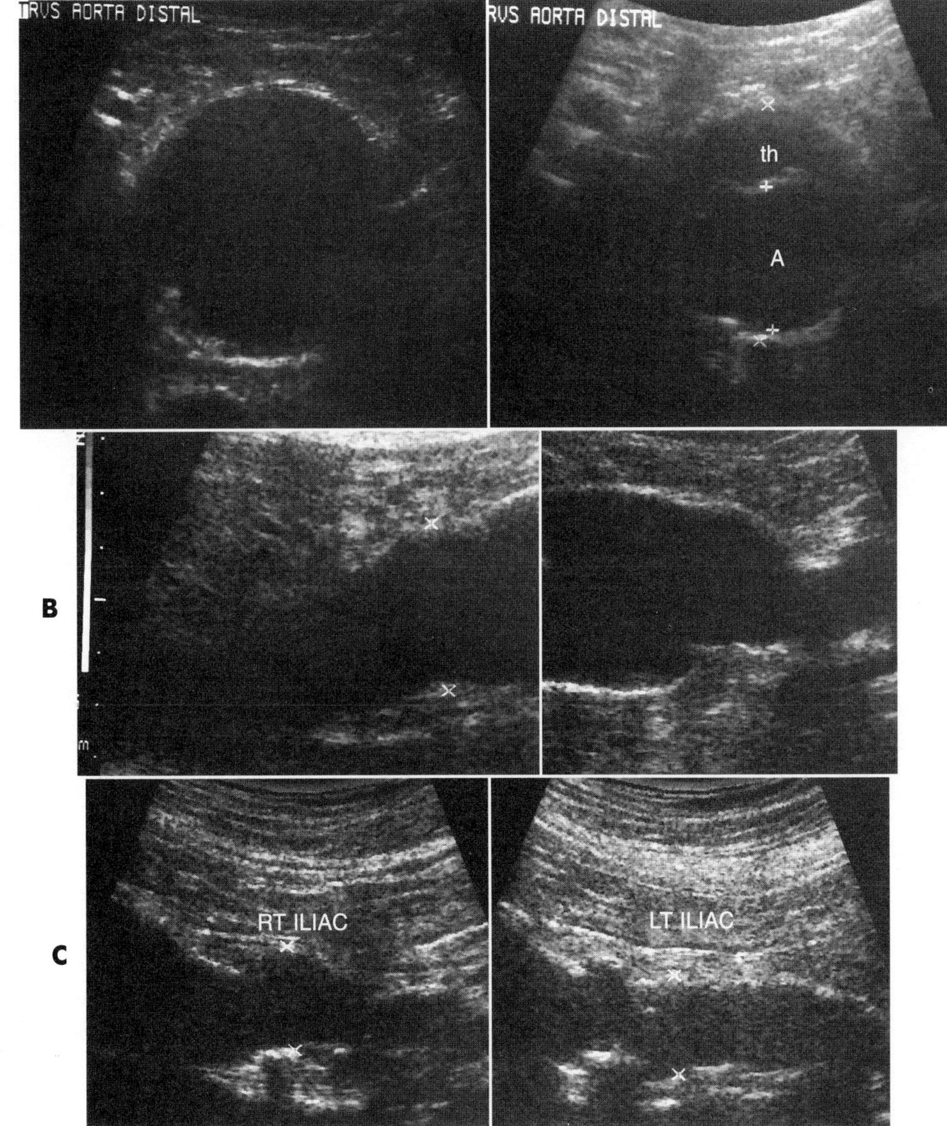

FIG. 4-50 The most common atherosclerotic aneurysm is a fusiform dilation of the distal aorta at the aortic bifurcation. The gain should be adjusted so the lumen may be separated from the thrombosis. **A,** Transverse views. Lumen, *L;* thrombus, *th.* **B,** Sagittal view of the fusiform dilation of the aorta as it extends into the iliac artery. **C,** Sagittal views of both distended iliac arteries.

Inferior Mesenteric Vein

The inferior mesenteric vein arises from the left third of colon and upper colon and ascends retroperitoneally along the left psoas muscle. It begins midway down the anal canal as the superior rectal vein. It runs cranial in the posterior abdominal wall on the left side of the inferior mesenteric artery and duodenojejunal junction to join the splenic vein posterior to the pancreas. It receives many tributaries along its way, including the left colic vein. The inferior mesenteric vein drains several tributaries: the left colic vein (descending colon), sigmoid vein (sigmoid colon), and superior rectal vein (upper rectum).

Ultrasound Findings. The inferior mesenteric vein is difficult to recognize on ultrasound because of its anatomic location and small diameter. It is generally covered by small bowel and has no major vascular structures posterior to it to aid in its recognition.

Pathophysiology of Vascular Disease

AORTIC ABNORMALITIES

Aortic Aneurysm

The visualization of the abdominal aorta has traditionally been an asset in diagnosing the clinical problem. Ultrasound is very capable of demonstrating abnormalities in the diameter, length, and extent of the abdominal aortic aneurysm. An aneurysm is defined as a localized abnormal dilation of any vessel. Three important factors predispose to aneurysm formation: arteriosclerosis, syphilis, and cystic medial necrosis.

Arteriosclerosis. Arteriosclerosis is the most common cause of aneurysms. It is found more often in middle-aged men than women, and involves the aorta, often with extension into the common iliac arteries. The disease sometimes involves the ascending and descending aorta. The aneurysm may be fusiform, cylindrical, or saccular in nature. It usually begins below the renal arteries (inferior to the superior mesenteric artery) and extends to the bifurcation.

Classifications of Aneurysms. The most common presentation of an atherosclerotic aneurysm is as a fusiform dilation of the distal aorta at the aortic bifurcation (Figs. 4-50). Atherosclerosis causes decreased pulsations of the aortic walls with bright echoes reflecting the degree of thickening and calcification (Fig. 4-51).

Saccular aneurysms are somewhat spherical and larger (5 to 10 cm) than the fusiform aneurysm. This type of aneurysm is connected to vascular lumen by a mouth that varies in size but may be as large as an aneurysm. It may be partially or completely filled with thrombus (Fig. 4-52).

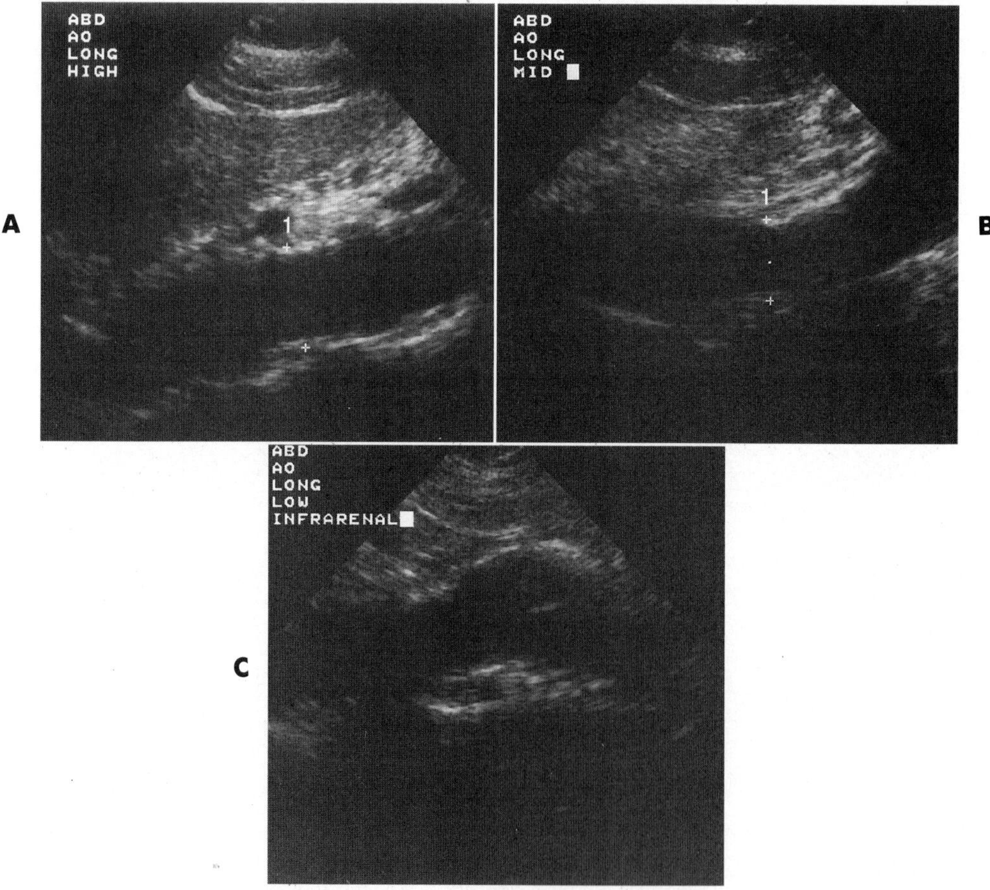

FIG. 4-51 Fusiform dilation of the aorta arising below the renal arteries. **A,** Sagittal view. **B,** Oblique sagittal view with iliac extension. **C,** Dilation of the aorta at the level of the umbilicus.

The sonographer must carefully follow the course of such an aneurysm to separate it from a retroperitoneal mass or lymphadenopathy. Pulsations are usually diminished secondary to clot formation.

The aneurysm may extend into the iliac arteries. The sonographer should examine both iliac arteries in at least two planes (Fig. 4-53). At the level of the bifurcation the iliac vessels may be seen as circular, pulsatile vessels just anterior to the spine. The oblique longitudinal scan is used to produce an image of the vessel in its entire length. Nor-

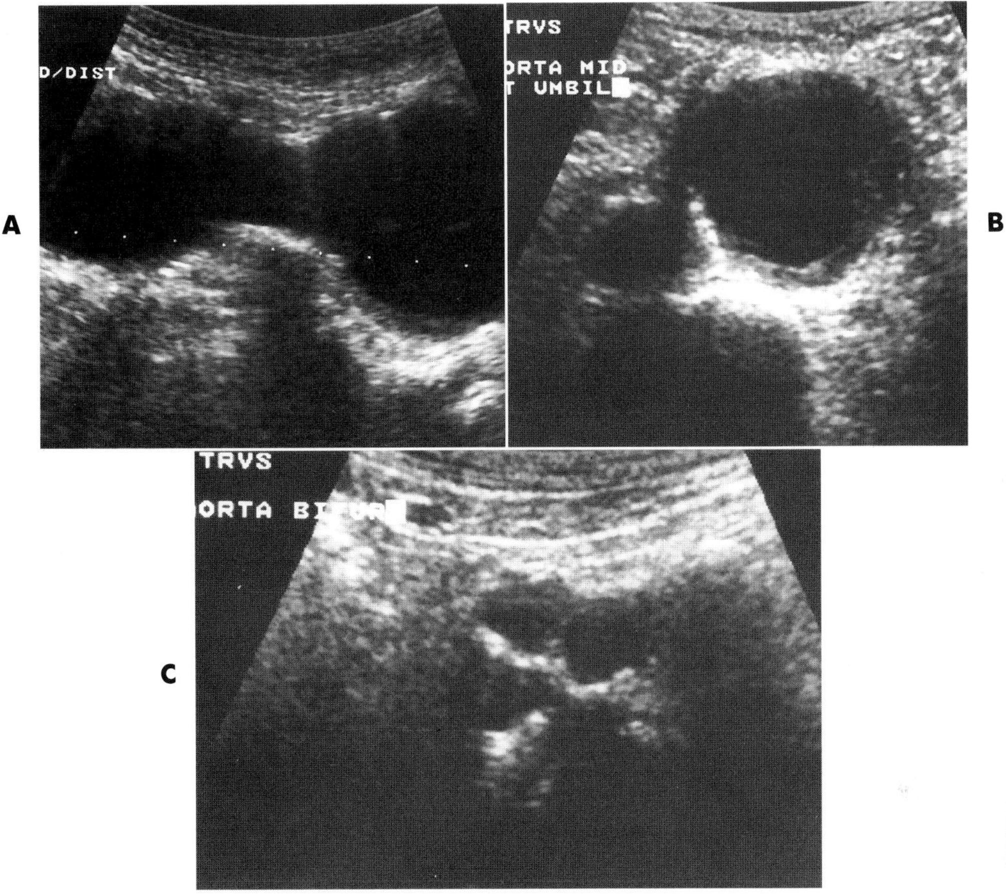

FIG. 4-52 Saccular aneurysms are spherical and larger than the fusiform aneurysm. This patient had a "dumbbell" type of aneurysm, more typically seen in a patient with cystic medial necrosis. **A,** Sagittal view. **B,** Transverse at the umbilicus. **C,** Transverse at the umbilicus with caudal angulation.

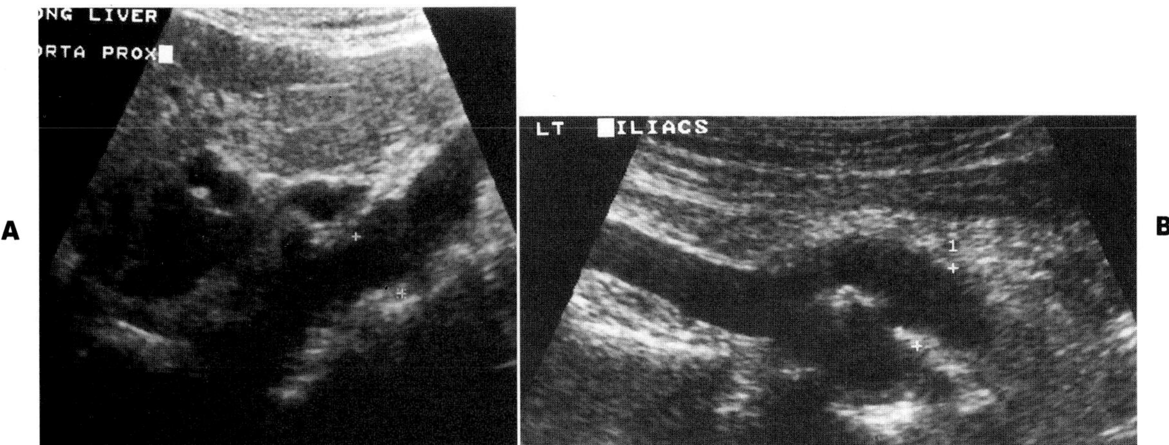

FIG. 4-53 This patient had fusiform dilation with irregular walls secondary to plaque formation. **A,** Sagittal view. **B,** Sagittal view with dilation of the iliac arteries.

mal iliac arteries do not measure over 1 cm in diameter. If the artery becomes so enlarged, it has an increased chance of rupture.

Clinical Symptoms. Symptoms may vary in the patient with an abdominal aneurysm. The enlarged vessel may produce symptoms by impinging on adjacent structures, or it may occlude a vessel by direct pressure or thrombus with resulting embolism. The large aneurysm may rupture into the peritoneal cavity or retroperitoneum, causing intense back pain and a drop in hematocrit.

Growth Patterns for Abdominal Aneurysm.* The normal aortic lumen diameter is under 3 cm. With careful sonographic technique, ultrasound has a 98.8% accuracy in detecting aneurysms. Aneurysms under 6 cm show a very slow growth pattern, so patients are followed at yearly intervals. The following information has been found on follow-up of aneurysms:

- Seventy-five percent of patients have 1-year survival if the aneurysm is under 6 cm.
- Fifty percent of patients have 1-year survival if the aneurysm is over 6 cm.
- Twenty-five percent of patients have 1-year survival if the aneurysm is over 7 cm.
- There is a 75% risk of fatal rupture if the aneurysm is over 7 cm.
- One percent of aneurysms under 5 cm rupture.
- Operative mortality before rupture is 5%, but with emergency surgery, mortality increases to 50%.

The patient who presents with an aneurysm probably has a number of other medical problems as well. It is important that the clinician be able to evaluate the size of the aneurysm noninvasively and follow it sequentially over a 3- to 6-month period by sonography (Fig. 4-54). It is also important in these cases to mark on the films the exact location of the aneurysm and measurements so follow-up information will be accurate.

Another important consideration is the relationship of the aneurysm to the renal arteries (Fig. 4-55). Thus not only should the diameter be measured, but also the longitudinal extent of the aneurysm as it relates to the origin of the renal vessels. Often bowel gas impairs adequate visualization of the renal arteries, and a more indirect method must be used to locate the origin of the superior mesenteric artery and renal arteries. Color Doppler may be useful to produce an image of arterial flow from the lateral margins of the abdominal aorta to the kidneys.

Ultrasound Findings. The aorta is thought to be aneurysmal when the diameter is increased to over 3 cm in an anteroposterior measurement. This measurement should be made from leading edge to leading edge. The sonographer should search for focal dilation of the abdominal aorta or lack of normal tapering distally. When an aneurysm is present, the presence of thrombus should be evaluated. Thrombus usually occurs along an anterior or anterolateral wall. Old clot is easier to see because of calcification that appears as thick, echogenic echoes, sometimes with posterior shadowing.

If an aneurysm extends beyond the diaphragm into the thoracic aorta, it may be difficult to trace with ultrasound because of lung interference in the beam. Several attempts may be necessary to demonstrate this thoracic aneurysm. The transducer can be sharply angled from the xyphoid toward the sternal notch to visualize the lower extent of the aorta. Another technique allows the sonographer to make a

*Mittelstaedt C: Abdominal ultrasound, 1987 Churchill Livingstone.

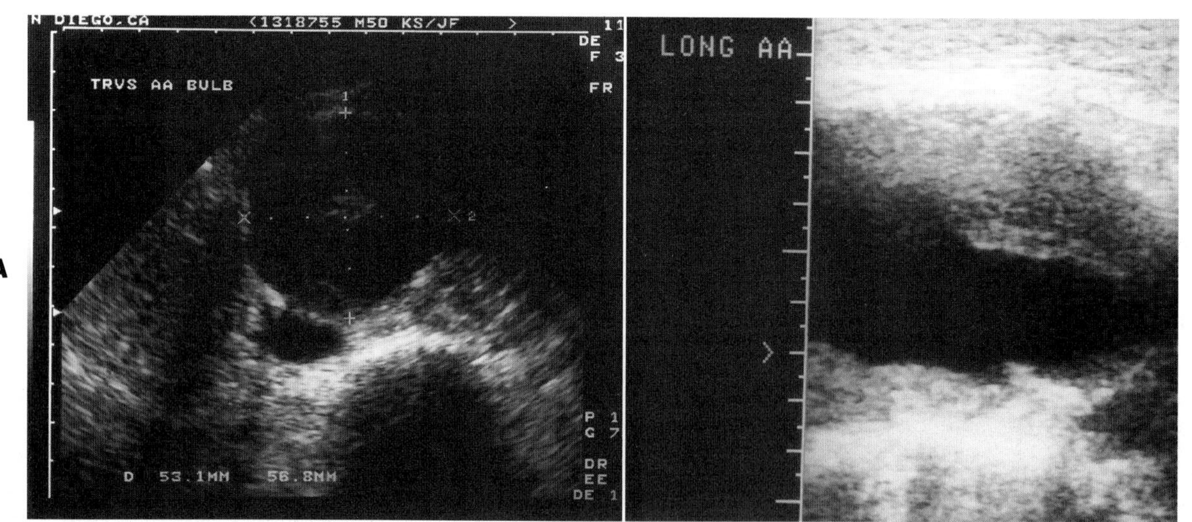

FIG. 4-54 The aorta's in its A-P, width, and length should be carefully measured. **A,** Transverse measurements. The shape of the aorta should be symmetric and rounded. **B,** In the sagittal scan, the A-P dimension and how far it extends into the upper abdomen or into the iliac arteries should be evaluated. If thrombus is present, the gain should be reduced to measure the wall from its leading edge to the outer edge.

longitudinal parasternal scan over the long axis of the heart. The thoracic aorta should be seen posterior to the cardiac structures. A third alternative is to scan along the patient's back with the patient sitting upright or prone. The transducer should be angled slightly medially and placed in a sagittal plane along the left intercostal space. This is very effective if the thoracic aorta is deviated slightly to the left of the spine. Scalloped reverberations from the ribs will be recorded, with the luminal echoes of the thoracic aorta directly posterior.

Thrombus within an aneurysm is shown ultrasonically as medium- to low-level echoes (Fig. 4-56). Generally increased sensitivity is likely to highlight the thrombus echoes. The echoes should be seen in both planes on more than one scan to be separated from low-level reverberation echoes. Thrombus formation is usually more frequent along the anterior and lateral walls than along the posterior wall of the aorta.

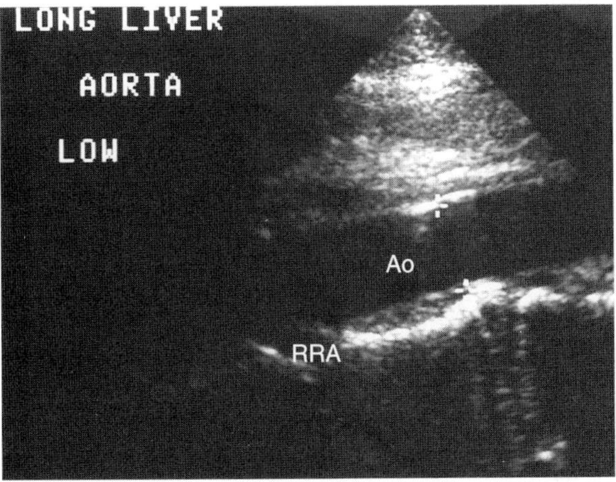

FIG. 4-55 Evaluation should be made with attention to the renal arteries. It is important to know if the aneurysm extends beyond the level of the renal arteries. Rotation of the patient with oblique scanning permits the sonographer to open the renal arteries for visualization.

Aortic Dissection

A dissecting aneurysm may be detected by ultrasound and usually displays one or more clinical signs and symptoms (Fig. 4-57). The patient is usually known to have an aneurysm, and sudden, excruciating chest pain radiating to the back may develop because of a dissection. The sonographer should look for a dissection "flap" or recent channel with or without frank aneurysmal dilation. The dissection of blood is along the laminar planes of the aortic media with formation of a blood-filled channel within the aortic wall. Most aneurysms enlarge fairly symmetrically in the anteroposterior and lateral dimensions; therefore an irregular enlargement with scattered internal echoes may represent an aneurysm with clot.

The typical patients are 40 to 60 years old and hypertensive; males predominate over females. When the dissection develops, hemorrhage occurs between the middle and outer thirds of the media. An intimal tear is considered if the tear is found in the ascending portion of the arch. This type of dissection extends proximally toward the heart, as well as distally, sometimes to the iliac and femoral arteries. A small portion of dissections do not have an obvious intimal tear. Extravasation may completely encircle the aorta or extend along one segment of its circumference, or it may rupture into any of the body cavities.

Types of Dissections. There are three classifications of aortic dissection. The first begins at the root of the aorta and may extend the entire length of the arch, descending

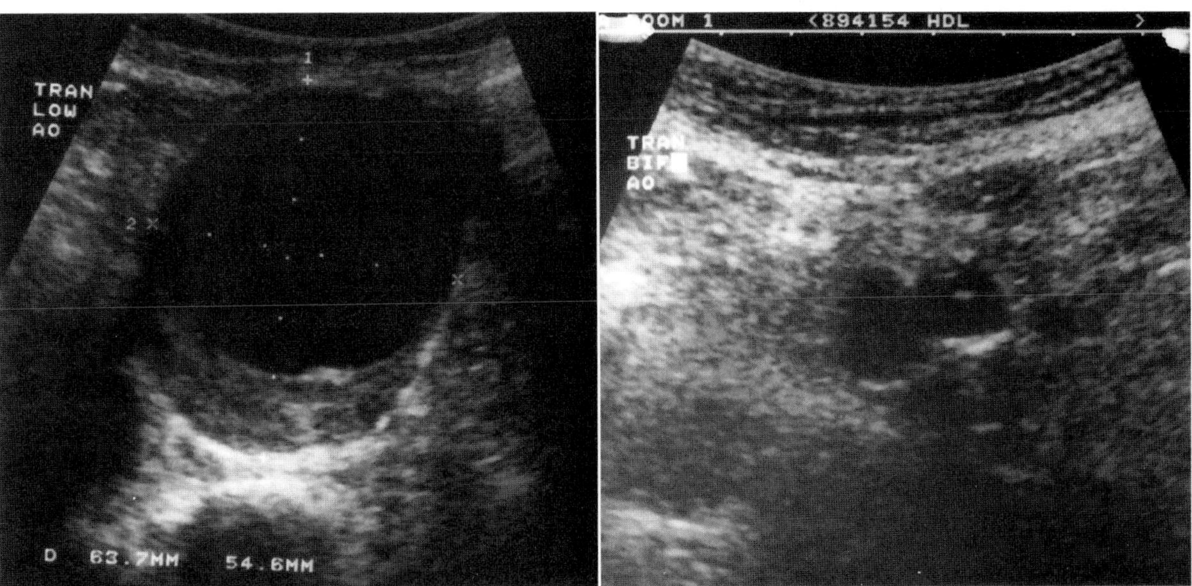

FIG. 4-56 Thrombus within an aneurysm is shown as medium- to low-level echoes with uniform consistency.

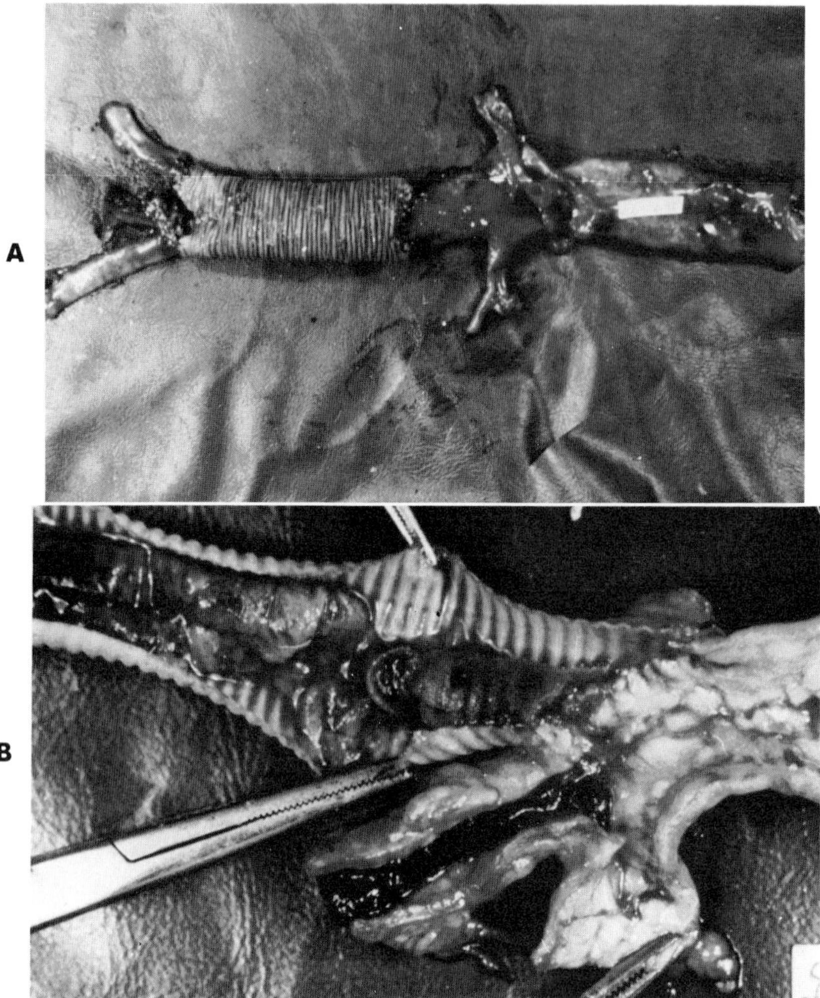

FIG. 4-57 **A,** Gross specimen of the abdominal aorta with a graft attached below the renal arteries and above the iliac arteries. **B,** Thrombus and clot within the vessel at dissection.

to the aorta and into the abdominal aorta. This is the most dangerous, especially if the dissection spirals around the aorta, cutting off the blood supply to the carotid, brachiocephalic, and subclavian vessels. The second type of dissection begins at or below the level of the left subclavian artery and extends down the descending aorta. It may or may not continue into the abdominal aorta. The third type of dissection begins at the lower end of the descending aorta and extends into the abdominal aorta. This may be critical if the dissection spirals around to impede the flow of blood into the renal vessels.

Dissection of the aorta may be secondary to cystic medial necrosis (weakening of the arterial wall), to the inherited disease of Marfan's syndrome (individuals with this disorder are extremely tall, lanky, and double-jointed; a progressive stretching disorder exists in all arterial vessels, especially in the aorta, causing abnormal dilation, weakened walls, and eventual dissection, rupture, or both), or hypertension.

Pulsatile Abdominal Masses

Masses other than an aortic aneurysm that can simulate a pulsatile abdominal mass are retroperitoneal tumor, fibroid uterus, or paraortic nodes. After aneurysm, the most common etiology for a pulsatile abdominal mass is nodes (Fig. 4-58; see color image). This mass is usually the result of lymphoma in the middle-aged patient. Symptoms include fever, weight loss, or malaise. On ultrasound the nodes are homogeneous masses surrounding the aorta. The aortic wall may be poorly defined because of the close acoustic impedance of the nodes and the aorta. The sonographer should also look for splenomegaly (Fig. 4-59).

Pancreatic carcinoma may appear as a hypoechoic mass and may displace the normal pancreas; biliary dilation with a enlarged gallbladder may be present.

A retroperitoneal sarcoma may present as a pulsatile mass; it may extend into the root of the mesentery and give rise to a larger intraperitoneal component. The echodensity

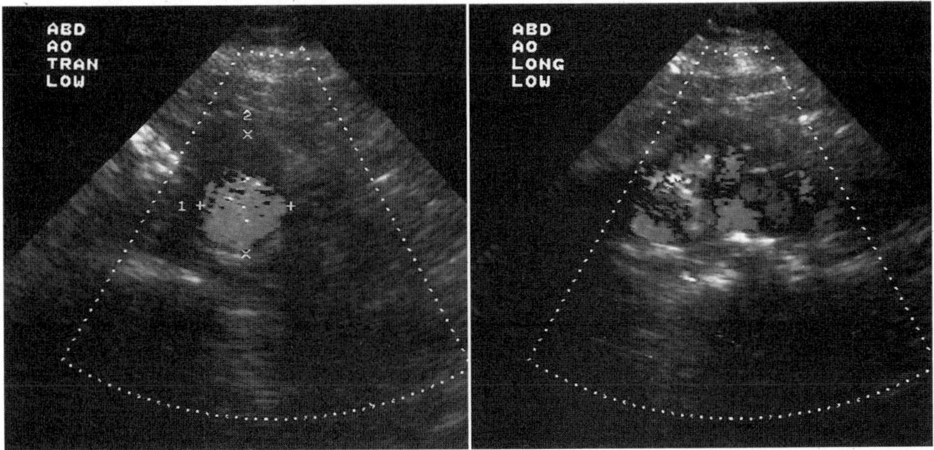

FIG. 4-58 Color flow helps the sonographer determine the direction of aortic flow, the presence of false channels (dissection), and the amount of lumen that remains open secondary to clot formation.

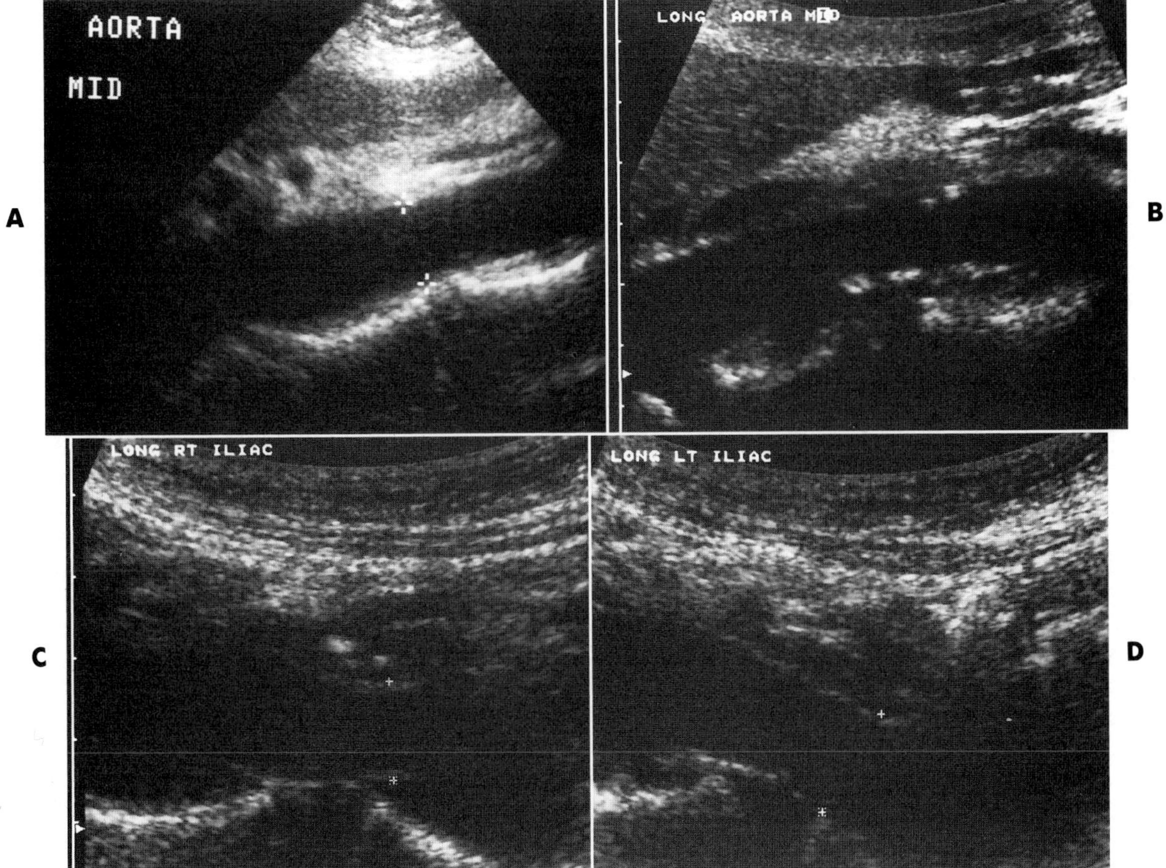

FIG. 4-59 A 64-year-old male presents with a pulsatile abdominal mass. The abdominal aorta is diffusely enlarged in **A. B,** The aorta is surrounded by low-level reflections. As one scans to the iliac vessels **(C** and **D),** the borders become aneurysmal, with continued low-level masses surrounding the aorta. Careful analysis should be made to ensure that retroperitoneal adenopathy is not present.

depends on the tissue type that predominates: fatty lesions are more echodense than fibrous or myomatous lesions.

Ruptured Aortic Aneurysms

The classic symptoms of ruptured aortic aneurysm are excruciating abdominal pain, shock, and an expanding abdominal mass. The operative mortality for such ruptures is 40% to 60%. The rupture may be into perirenal space with displacement of renal hilar vessels, effacement of the aortic border, and silhouetting of the lateral psoas border at the level of the kidney. The most common site is the lateral wall below the renal vessels. The hemorrhage into the posterior pararenal space accounts for a loss of lateral psoas muscle merging inferior to the kidney and may also displace the kidney.

Other Complications of Aortic Aneurysms. A large aneurysm may compress the neighboring structures (i.e., the common bile duct, causing obstruction, and the renal artery, causing hypertension and renal ischemia). Retroperitoneal fibrosis with aneurysm may involve the ureter.

Aortic Grafts

An abdominal aortic aneurysm may be surgically repaired with a flexible graft material attached to the end of the remaining aorta. The synthetic material used for a graft produces bright echo reflections compared to those from the normal aortic walls. After surgery, the attached walls may swell at the site of the attachment and form another aneurysm or pseudoaneurysm. Other complications of prosthetic grafts include hematoma, infection, and degeneration of graft material.

Arteriovenous Fistulas

The development of an arteriovenous fistula is not a common finding with ultrasound. The majority of fistulas are acquired secondary to trauma. Some may develop as a complication of arteriosclerotic aortic aneurysms.

Clinical Signs. The patient may develop low back and abdominal pain, progressive cardiac decompensation, a pulsatile abdominal mass associated with a bruit, and massive swelling of the lower trunk and lower extremities. Clinical signs are explained on the basis of the altered hemodynamics produced by a high-velocity shunt leading to increased blood volume, increased venous pressure, and cardiac output with cardiac failure and cardiomegaly.

If there is lower trunk and leg edema and a dilated inferior vena cava, an arteriovenous fistula should be suspected. If the fistula is large, the vein becomes very distended. A normal inferior vena cava is less than 2.5 cm wide. Right-sided heart disease or failure can also cause inferior vena cava distention.

Renal arteriovenous fistulas can be congenital or acquired. Congenital arteriovenous fistulas may be of the crisoid type or the aneurysmal type. Acquired fistulas are secondary to trauma, surgery, or inflammation or associated with a neoplasm such as renal cell carcinoma.

Ultrasound Findings. The sonographer finds multiple anechoic tubular structures feeding the malformation with an enlarged renal artery and vein, confirming increased blood flow to the kidney. It may look like hydronephrosis or a parapelvic cyst in association with a dilated inferior vena cava. The diagnosis is made by identifying one or more channels that enter the mass, suggesting that the lesion is related to the renal vasculature. The sonographer should look for pulsations. The crisoid type of fistula has a characteristic ultrasound appearance of a cluster of tubular anechoic structures within the kidney; it is supplied by an enlarged renal artery and drained by a dilated renal vein. In the aneurysmal type of fistula a vascular lesion should be suspected when the presence of thrombus is noted in the periphery of a mass with a tubular anechoic lumen with pulsations. Occasionally renal cell carcinoma is associated with arteriovenous shunting resulting from invasion of larger arteries and venous structures.

INFERIOR VENA CAVAL ABNORMALITIES

Congenital Abnormalities

The inferior vena cava is formed by three pairs of cardinal veins in the retroperitoneum; these veins undergo sequential development and regression. The posterior cardinal veins appear at 6 weeks and form no part of the cava but may be part of the anomalies. The subcardinal veins appear at 7 weeks to produce the prerenal segment of the inferior vena cava. The supracardinal system at 8 weeks produces the postrenal segment of the inferior vena cava. The supracardinals form the azygos and hemiazygos system above the diaphragm. The anastomosis between the subcardinal and supracardinal systems forms the renal veins. The normal left cardinal system involutes and the right is composed of the posterior infrarenal vein, supracardinal vein, renal segment, anterior suprarenal subcardinal vein, and the confluence of hepatic veins.

Double Inferior Vena Cava. This condition has an incidence of under 3%. The size of the two vessels can be the same or vary depending on the dominant side. The most common type is where the left inferior vena cava joins the left renal vein, which crosses the midline at its normal level to join the right inferior vena cava. There is no continuation of the left inferior vena cava above the left renal vein. Less commonly, the right inferior vena cava joins the left inferior vena cava to join the hemiazygos.

Infrahepatic Interruption of the Inferior Vena Cava. This condition is the failure of union of the hepatic veins and the right subcardinal vein; with it there can be azygos or, less commonly, hemiazygos continuation. It is associated with acyanotic and cyanotic congenital heart disease, abnormalities of cardiac position, and abdominal situs with asplenia and polysplenia.

Ultrasound Findings. In patients with an interruption of the inferior vena cava the azygos vein continuation is identical to or larger than the inferior vena cava that passes along the aorta medial to the right crus of the diaphragm. The hepatic veins drain into an independent confluence that passes through the diaphragm to enter the right atrium. A membranous obstruction of the inferior vena cava may simulate infrahepatic interruption of the cava with azygos continuation. A web or membrane obstructs the inferior vena cava at the level of the diaphragm and leads to chronic congestion of the liver with centrilobular and periportal fibrosis.

There are three types of obstruction:

1. A thin membrane at the level of the entrance to the right atrium
2. An absent segment of the inferior vena cava without characteristic conical narrowing
3. Complete obstruction secondary to thrombosis

Clinically patients present in their third to fourth decade of life with portal hypertension.

Ultrasound shows obstruction at the diaphragm and dilation of the azygos system. On longitudinal scans it is very difficult to identify the presence of the inferior vena cava. The azygos system is dilated on the right side of the midline, "acting" as the inferior vena cava.

Inferior Vena Caval Dilation

In patients with right ventricular failure the inferior vena cava does not collapse with expiration. This may be because of atherosclerosis, pulmonary hypertension, pericardial tamponade, constrictive pericarditis, or atrial tumor (Fig. 4-60).

Inferior Vena Caval Tumor

It is important for the sonographer to identify the entire inferior vena cava; bowel gas can make the distal cava difficult to identify.

Hepatic Portion of Inferior Vena Cava. Masses posterior to the hepatic portion of the inferior vena cava are the right adrenal, neurogenic, and hepatic. With enlargement of the liver, the cava is compressed rather than displaced. A localized liver mass would produce posterior, lateral, or medial displacement of the inferior vena cava, whereas a mass in the posterior caudate lobe and right lobe may elevate the cava.

Middle or Pancreatic Portion of the Inferior Vena Cava. The middle or pancreatic portion of the inferior vena cava may elevate the cava from abnormalities of the right renal artery, right kidney, lumbar spine, or lymph node masses.

Lower or Small Bowel Segment. Lumbar spine abnormalities or lymph nodes would elevate the inferior vena cava.

Ultrasound Findings. The inferior vena cava may become obstructed by tumor formation. The ultrasound appearance of tumor is of a single or multiple echogenic nodules along the wall. The cava may be distended and filled with tumor. The most common tumor is renal cell carcinoma, usually from the right kidney. Wilms' tumor is also seen to extend into the inferior vena cava and right atrium. Other less common tumors are retroperitoneal liposarcoma, leiomyosarcoma, pheochromocytoma, osteosarcoma, and rhabdomyosarcoma. Benign tumors, such as angiomyolipoma, can have venous involvement.

Inferior Vena Caval Thrombosis

Complete thrombosis of the inferior vena cava is life-threatening. Patients present with leg edema, low back pain, pelvic pain, gastrointestinal complaints, and renal and liver abnormalities (Figs. 4-61 to 4-63).

Ultrasound Findings. Thrombosis within the inferior vena cava appears as homogeneous echo-mass. Color Doppler is useful to determine if the vessel is occluded.

Inferior Vena Caval Filters

The most common origin of pulmonary emboli is venous thrombosis from the lower extremities. Surgical and angiographic placement of transvenous filters into the cava has been used to prevent recurrent embolization in patients who cannot tolerate anticoagulants. The preferred location of the filter is in the iliac bifurcation below the renal veins.

Some filters can migrate cranially or caudally and perfo-

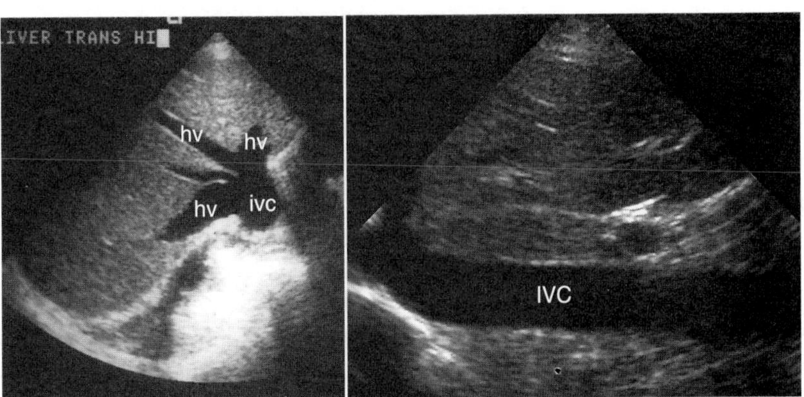

FIG. 4-60 Transverse and sagittal scans of a patient in right ventricular heart failure show a dilated inferior vena cava, *IVC*, and hepatic veins, *HV*.

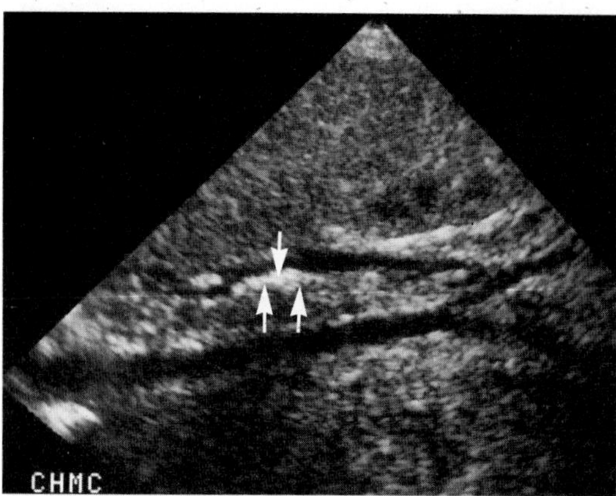

FIG. 4-61 A coronal oblique view in a neonate with inferior vena cava thrombosis *(arrows)*.

rate the cava, producing a retroperitoneal bleed. Filters can also perforate the duodenum, aorta, ureter, and hepatic vein.

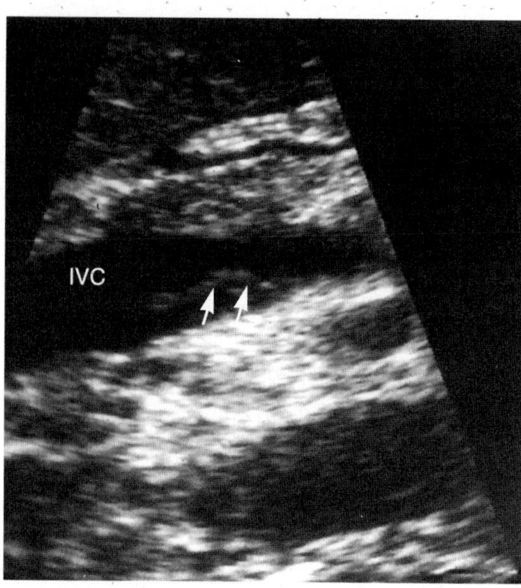

FIG. 4-62 A sagittal scan of the dilated inferior vena cava, *IVC*, with thrombus *(arrow)*. Real time showed that the thrombus moves with respiration.

RENAL VEIN OBSTRUCTION

Renal vein obstruction is seen in the dehydrated or septic infant. It may also be seen in adults with multiple renal abnormalities (nephrotic syndrome, shock, renal tumor, kidney transplant, or trauma).

Left renal vein obstruction may result from the spread of such nonrenal malignancies as carcinoma of the pancreas or lung or lymphoma. A retroperitoneal tumor can occlude the left renal vein by direct extension into the vein lumen or compression of the lumen by a contiguous mass.

Clinical Signs

The patient presents with flank pain, hematuria, flank mass, and proteinuria. The condition may be associated with maternal diabetes and transient high blood pressure.

Ultrasound Findings

Ultrasound can be used to confirm that a palpable mass is kidney and to exclude hydronephrosis and multicystic kidney as causes of a nonfunctioning kidney. In infants with renal vein obstruction, enlarged kidneys without cysts are seen. Medium echoes or "clumps" of echoes may be randomly scattered within the kidney with surrounding echo-free spaces. The parenchymal anechoic areas are the result of hemorrhage and infarcts. The renal pattern progresses to atrophy over 2 months. Late findings are increased parenchymal echoes, loss of corticomedullary junction, and decreased renal size.

RENAL VEIN THROMBOSIS

If the following are present on ultrasound, renal vein thrombosis can be diagnosed:

1. Direct visualization of thrombi in the renal vein and inferior vena cava
2. Demonstrated renal vein dilation proximal to the point of occlusion
3. Loss of normal renal structure
4. Increased renal size (acute phase)
5. Doppler shows decreased or no flow

Clinical Signs

The patient presents with pain, nephromegaly, hematuria, or thromboembolic phenomena elsewhere in the body. A variety of lesions may be associated with this abnormality.

Abdominal Doppler Techniques

APPLICATIONS

Doppler ultrasound has been a clinically useful tool in diagnosing many disease processes. Here we present an overview of abdominal applications that have been used with color-flow detection and pulsed Doppler techniques. Doppler has helped detect the presence or absence of blood flow, the direction of blood flow, and flow-disturbance patterns. It has also been used in tissue characterization and wave-form analysis.

Presence or Absence of Blood Flow

Doppler ultrasound frequently is used to differentiate vessels from nonvascular structures. For example, to distinguish the common bile duct from the hepatic artery, look for absence of flow in the common duct; to distinguish the

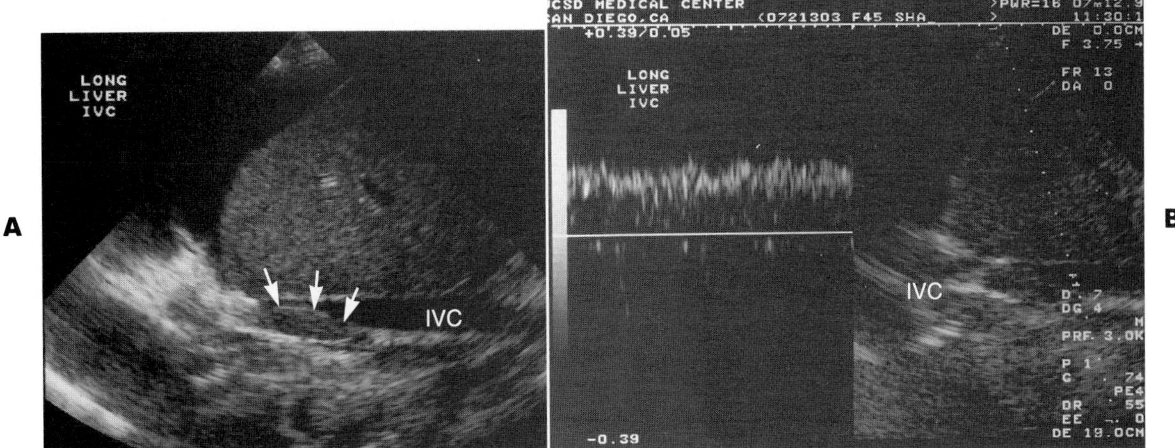

FIG. 4-63 Complete thrombosis of the inferior vena cava is life-threatening. Patients present with leg edema, ascites, and liver abnormalities. This patient had cirrhosis. The abdomen was tense, ascites was present. A large clot was seen in the inferior vena cava near the diaphragm *(arrow)*. **A,** Sagittal. **B,** Pulsed Doppler flow in the inferior vena cava shows turbulent flow just inferior to the clot.

hepatic artery from the splenic artery, look for direction of flow; to differentiate aneurysm from pancreatic pseudocyst, look for slow flow in the aneurysm; to differentiate dilated intrahepatic bile ducts and prominent hepatic artery, again look for absence of flow in the bile duct.

Direction of Blood Flow

In patients who develop portal venous hypertension, the portal blood flow becomes hepatofugal (away from the liver) instead of hepatopetal (toward the liver). This may be secondary to portal venous shunts or varices. The sonographer detects a high-velocity flow pattern at the site of the shunt with a turbulent flow pattern on color Doppler.

Flow Disturbance

A flow disturbance (increased velocity or obstruction of flow) may result from the formation of an atheroma or aneurysmal dilation.

Tissue Characterization

Research is currently under way in the area of tissue characterization. Doppler is thought to be capable of characterizing tissue because of the specific perfusion patterns characteristic of some tissues or states of tissue activity. Hepatocellular carcinomas of the liver appear to have a specific pattern. Pseudoaneurysms of peripancreatic arteries have turbulent flow patterns. Pancreatic tumors may have specific flow patterns.

Doppler Waveform Analysis

The shape of the waveform provides information on the vascular impedance of the organ the vessel supplies. Spectral analysis tells the velocity and turbulence of blood flow.

Nonresistive versus Resistive. Nonresistive vessels have a high diastolic component and supply organs that need constant perfusion, such as the internal carotid artery, the hepatic artery, and the renal artery.

Resistive vessels have very little or even reversed flow in diastole and supply organs that do not need a constant blood supply, such as the external carotid and the iliac and brachial arteries.

Compare peak systole with minimum diastole to quantify a vessel's impedance. This ratio is the resistive index.

$$\text{Resistive index} = \frac{A - B}{A}$$

$$\text{Pulsatility index} = \frac{A - B}{\text{Mean}}$$

(A = systole, B = Diastole)

Spectral display shows us the following:

x = Time is depicted on the horizontal axis.

y = Doppler shift frequency (velocity) is on the vertical axis (flow toward the transducer equals positive shift, above baseline; flow away from transducer equals negative shift or below baseline).

z = Gray scale is the quantity of blood flowing at a given velocity. More red blood cells produce a brighter gray-scale assignment.

Plug flow is a pattern of blood flow, typically seen in large arteries, in which most cells are moving at the same velocity across the entire diameter of the vessel. In other vessels the different velocities are the result of friction between the cells and arterial walls. A "clear window" under systole is typical of plug flow. When plug flow is present the volume of blood flow can be calculated.

DOPPLER TECHNIQUE

Unlike visualization of the heart, where high-velocity flows are present, visualization of abdominal vessels requires very sensitive Doppler instrumentation. Abdominal vessels generally have low velocity and flow.

Methods

Doppler is performed as part of the routine real-time examination. The patient should be fasting and suspend respirations for the best color and pulsed Doppler sample volume to be obtained. The Doppler sample volume (sometimes referred to as the *Doppler "gate"*) should be adjusted to encompass but not exceed the diameter of the vessel. If the sample volume exceeds the diameter, noise and ghost echoes may appear. This is because too wide a Doppler gate causes interference from the surrounding vessels and structures. The sonographer has the ability to control the velocity of the returning echoes to prevent the alias pattern. Another feature of Doppler is that the beam only records accurate velocity patterns when the beam is parallel to the flow (the angle of flow can be changed up to 60 degrees and still be accurate). The more perpendicular the beam is to the flow, the less signal is recorded; it falls to zero velocity when the beam is directly perpendicular to flow. Thus Doppler causes the sonographer to be creative in attempting to record accurate velocity flow patterns. The patient must be rolled into various obliquities with different angulations of the transducer to be parallel to many vascular structures.

Color Doppler is a relatively new and exciting modality that makes it easier to localize and identify smaller vessels from the biliary tree, lymphadenopathy, or other pathology (Fig. 4-64; see color images). The colors are arbitrarily assigned on all equipment and refer to the direction of flow. If red is assigned as a positive flow signal, all the flow toward the transducer is coded in various shades of red, depending on their returning velocity. If blue is assigned a negative flow signal, the flow away from the transducer is coded in various shades of blue. The sonographer may select the particular color scheme to be used; some labs choose to code all positive-flow patterns red and negative patterns blue. Other labs code all arterial flows red and venous flows blue.

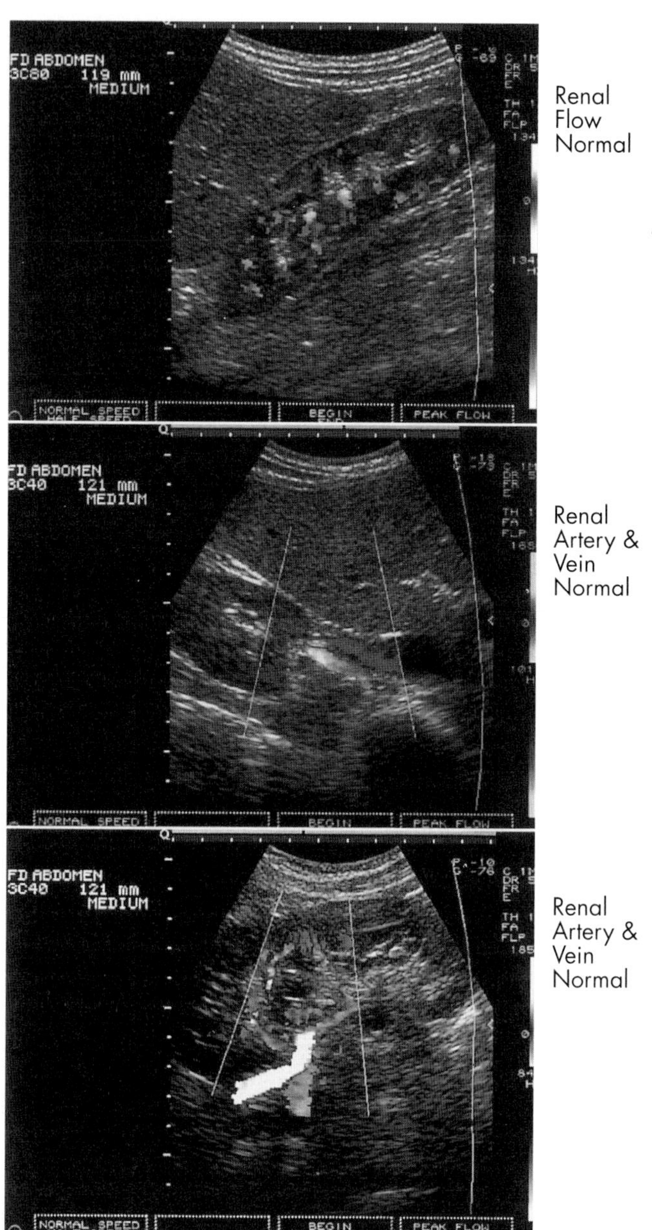

FIG. 4-64 Color Doppler makes it easier to localize and identify the smaller vessels in the renal parenchyma. **A,** Sagittal. **B,** Transverse of the right kidney, renal artery *(red)* and vein *(blue)*. **C,** Sagittal view of the main renal artery *(red)*, renal vein *(blue)* and interlobar and arcuate arteries and veins. (See color images.)

DOPPLER FLOW PATTERNS IN THE ABDOMINAL VESSELS

Aorta

The patient should be scanned in the longitudinal plane (Fig. 4-65). The pattern of blood flow in the abdominal aorta differs with the level at which the vessel is scanned. The flow pattern of the proximal abdominal aorta above the renal arteries shows a high systolic peak and a relatively low diastolic component. There is little spectral broadening. A clear window under systole means there is plug flow.

The distal abdominal aorta below the renal arteries shows flow with a small reversed component present during diastole. The closer one approaches the common iliac vessels, the greater the reverse component becomes. This is because of the high impedance of the peripheral circulation in the leg as it becomes triphasic, crossing the baseline three times.

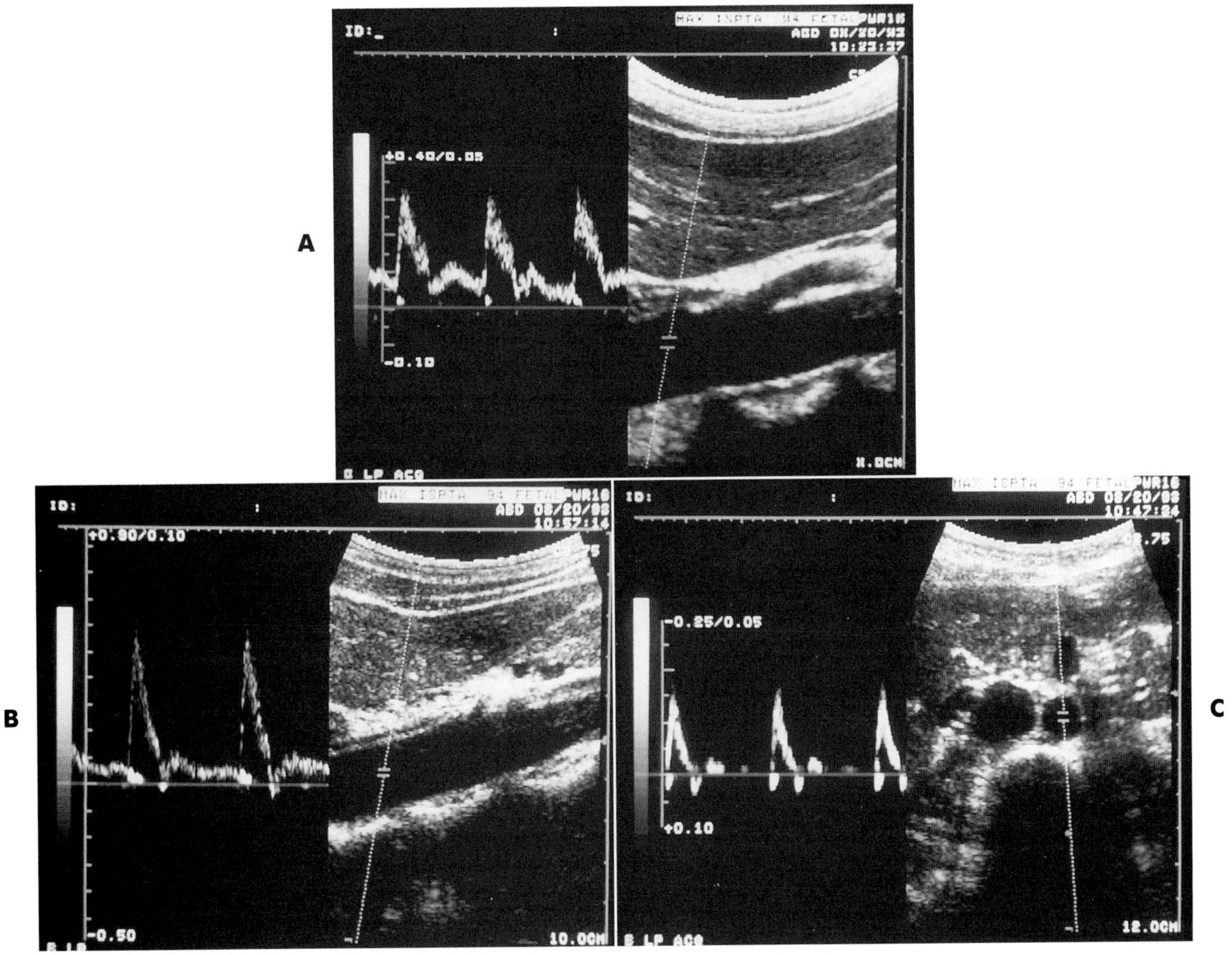

FIG. 4-65 **A** and **B,** Sagittal scans of the normal flow in the abdominal aorta. The flow pattern of the proximal aorta above the renal arteries shows a high systolic peak and a relatively low diastolic component. **C,** Transverse.

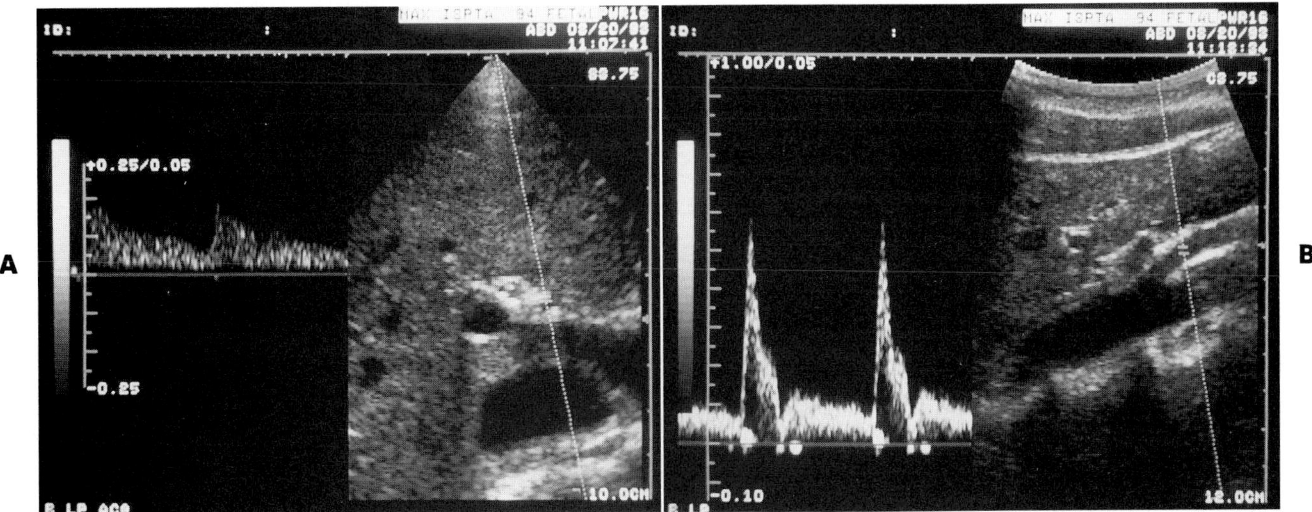

FIG. 4-66 **A,** Transverse view of the hepatic artery flow. More spectral broadening is seen during systole and diastole. **B,** Sagittal scan of the superior mesenteric artery flow. This vessel has high resistance in the fasting state with little flow in diastole.

Celiac Axis

The sonographer should scan transversely to search for the seagull sign, celiac trunk, hepatic artery, and splenic artery. If they can't be seen, scan longitudinally. Typically the spectral analysis of the celiac trunk shows some window under systole with spectral broadening (turbulence) in diastole. There is no change in the flow pattern after meals.

Hepatic Artery

It has been reported that 11% of the population has replaced hepatic arteries arising from the superior mesenteric artery (Fig. 4-66, *A*). Flow in diastole persists because of the low vascular impedance of the liver. Similar waveforms are seen in the main hepatic and intrahepatic arteries. Typically, there is more spectral broadening during both systole and diastole.

In a patient with a liver transplant, always document flow in the hepatic artery. Occlusion is one of the most dangerous complications, potentially resulting in death.

Splenic Artery

This vessel shows the most turbulence of all the celiac branches (probably because of its tortuosity). Aneurysms of the celiac branches have been described most commonly in the splenic branch. Patients with chronic pancreatitis are particularly prone to these. Always apply Doppler to pancreatic pseudocysts—their appearance is very similar to that of vascular aneurysms.

Superior Mesenteric Artery

Typically the superior mesenteric artery is a highly resistive vessel (with decreased diastolic flow) in the fasting state with little or no flow in diastole (Fig. 4-66, *B*). However, after a meal, the pattern of the superior mesenteric

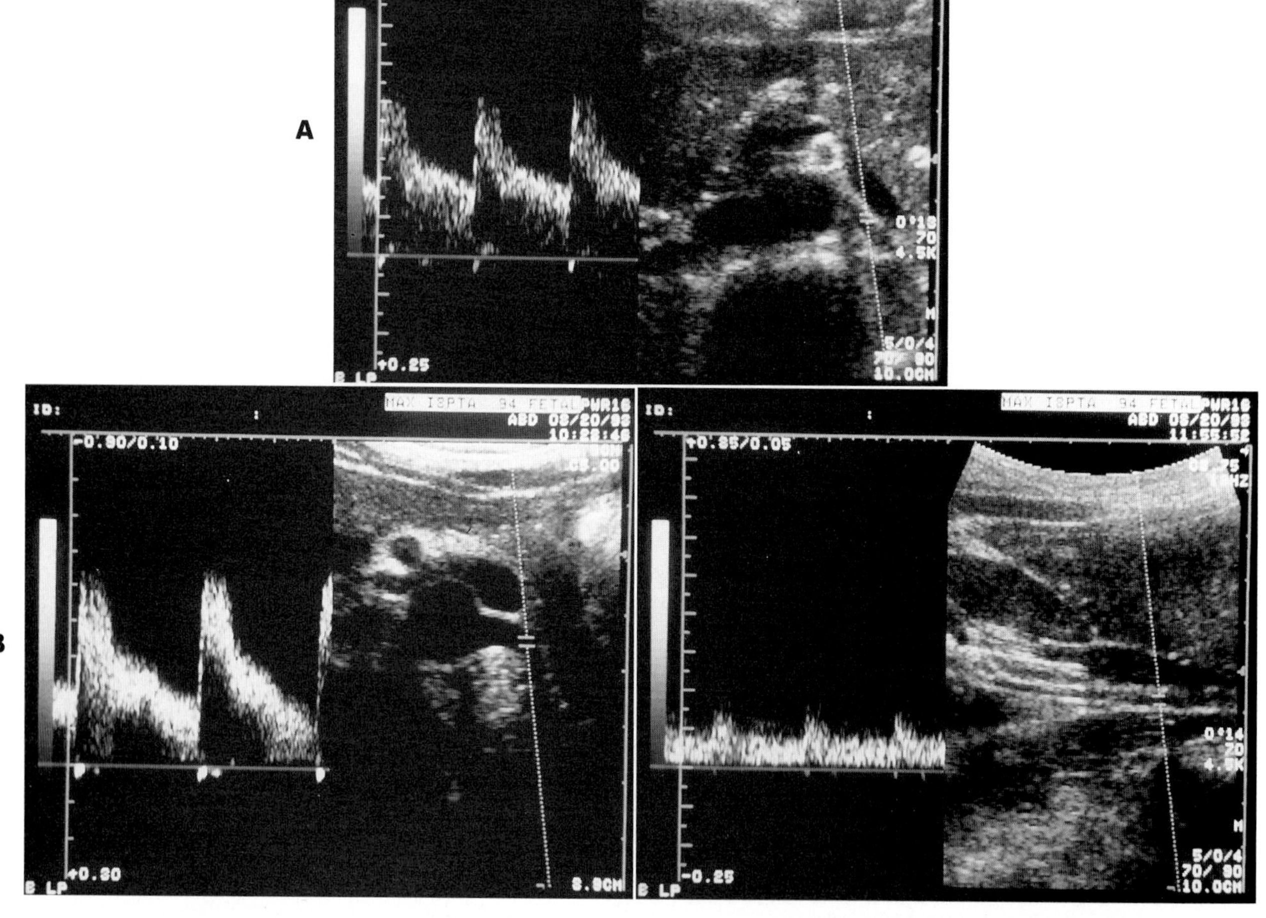

FIG. 4-67 A and **B,** Transverse scans of the left renal artery flow. The main renal artery has a low impedance (nonresistive) pattern with significant diastolic flow, usually 30% to 50% of peak systole. **C,** Transverse scans of the right renal artery. In this view it is much more difficult to obtain an adequate Doppler flow because the beam is perpendicular to the flow pattern. As a result, decreased velocities are obtained.

artery changes to a low-resistive waveform demonstrating enhanced diastolic flow. Doppler analysis of the superior mesenteric artery has the potential to diagnose mesenteric arterial occlusion and abdominal angina.

Renal Artery

The main renal artery has a low impedance (nonresistive) pattern with significant diastolic flow—usually 30% to 50% of peak systole (Fig. 4-67). The continuous diastolic flow gives us continuous perfusion of the kidneys. There is spectral broadening in systole and diastole. The segmental, interlobar, and arcuate arteries demonstrate a pattern similar to that of the main renal artery. However, the flow is progressively dampened in the periphery and shows reduced velocity patterns.

Renal Artery Stenosis

It is very hard to demonstrate renal artery stenosis in a native kidney because of the difficulty in seeing the vessel at its origin and in its entirety. Renal artery occlusion can only be declared when the artery is unquestionably imaged. The sonographer should be careful because with complete obstruction of the native artery, collaterals may be mistaken for a patent renal artery. At least 30% of the population has multiple renal arteries, which makes it more difficult to rule out obstruction.

Renal Hydronephrosis

When there is even minimal separation of the renal pelvis, the sonographer should Doppler the area. Surprisingly, no hydronephrosis may be found, just prominent renal vessels in the renal pelvis.

Renal Transplants

In the main renal artery, there is turbulence near the anastomosis. Only 12% of patients develop renal artery stenosis after transplantation; it is characterized by a high-velocity jet with distal turbulence. Renal artery occlusion is easier to diagnose in transplants than in native kidneys because there is no flow throughout the entire transplant.

Rejection

Normal transplants have a diastolic flow that is 30% to 50% of that of systole. During rejection, the vascular impedance increases, resulting in a decrease or even reversal of the diastolic flow. There are a few methods to quantify the Doppler signals.

$$\text{Pulsatility index} = \frac{A - B}{\text{Mean}}$$

$$\text{Resistive index} = A - B / A$$

A resistive index (RI) is the most popular method in use. An RI of 0.7 or less indicates good perfusion, whereas an RI of 0.7 to 0.9 indicates possible rejection and over 0.9 indicates probable rejection.

Renal Vein

The renal vein shows variable flow like the inferior vena cava. The sonographer should closely evaluate the renal veins in any patient with a suspected tumor or renal obstructive lesion because they may be invaded by tumor or clot (Fig. 4-68). In renal transplant patients, always look for a patent renal vein. An occlusion backs up the whole blood supply and the kidney acts like it is rejecting (with elevated blood, urea, nitrogen, creatinine, and proteinuria).

Inferior Vena Cava and Hepatic Veins

The inferior vena cava and hepatic veins present a complex waveform, which flows above and below the baseline,

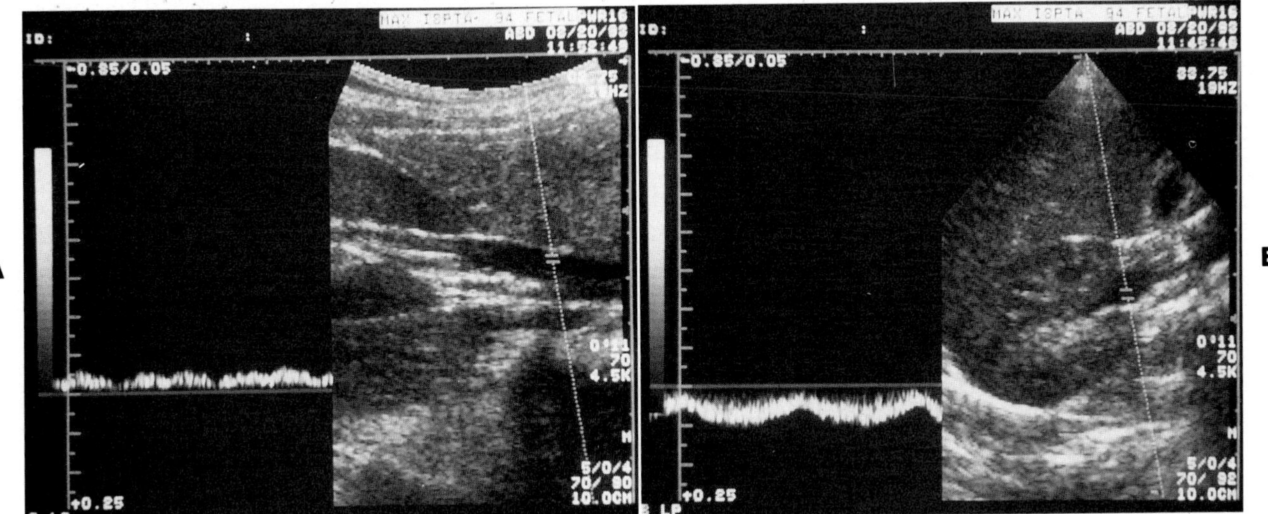

FIG. 4-68 **A** and **B**, Transverse scans of right renal vein flow show variable flow like the inferior vena cava pattern.

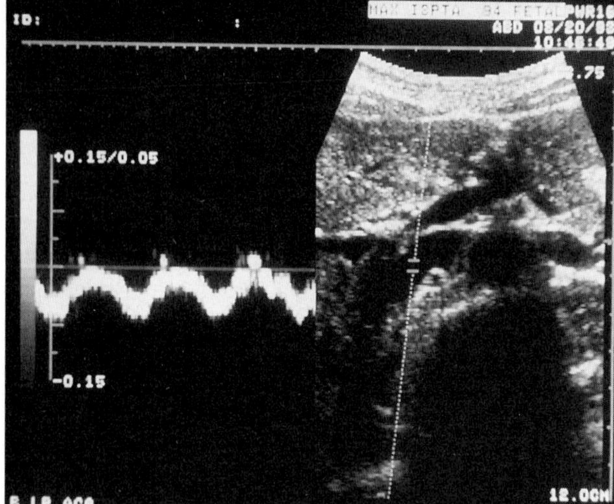

FIG. 4-69 The inferior vena cava and hepatic veins show a complex waveform flowing above and below the baseline. This reflects the reflux of blood from the right atrium during systole and variations with the respiratory cycle. **A**, Sagittal. **B**, Transverse.

reflecting the reflux of blood from the right atrium during systole and variations with the respiratory cycle (Figs. 4-69 and 4-70; see color image). Always look at the cava and renal veins for tumor invasion when you see a renal cell carcinoma.

Budd-Chiari Syndrome

Budd-Chiari Syndrome is thrombosis of hepatic veins. Duplex Doppler is an effective method for screening patients suspected of having Budd-Chiari Syndrome. Sonographically, hepatic veins appear reduced in size and may contain echogenic thrombotic material. The presence of "typical" blood flow in the hepatic veins permits the exclusion of Budd-Chiari Syndrome. Budd-Chiari Syndrome is a rare disease; 30% of cases are idiopathic. It is associated with hematologic disorders, oral contraceptives, collagen disease, echinococcus, and the periods before or after pregnancy.

Portal Vein

In the normal superior mesenteric vein and splenic vein, flow is hepatopetal (toward the liver) (Figs. 4-71 and 4-72). The portal vein shows a relatively continuous flow at low velocities, which may vary slightly with respirations. Portal vein thrombosis can be easily diagnosed with sonography. A direct sign is visualization of thrombus. Indirect signs are the loss of normal portal venous landmarks, dilation of the superior mesenteric artery and splenic vein, and venous collaterals in the porta hepatis (cavernous transformation of the portal vein).

Pulsed Doppler adds to these findings; lack of Doppler signals from the lumen indicates absence of blood flow. In cirrhotic patients, thrombosis is often suspected when ascites suddenly worsens. Consequently, in these patients, special attention must be paid to the portal vein to identify thrombus. It is often difficult to visualize the portal vein in such patients.

Cavernous Transformation of the Portal Vein

Cavernous transformation of the portal vein demonstrates periportal collateral channels in patients with chronic portal vein obstruction (Fig. 4-73). The Doppler analysis of the tubular structures is characteristic of portal venous flow—hepatopetal (toward the liver) with continuous low-velocity flow. Diagnosis can be made sonographically based on the following indications:

1. Extrahepatic portal vein is not visualized.
2. High-level echoes produced by fibrosis are present in the porta hepatis.
3. Multiple tubular structures are present in the porta hepatis, representing periportal collaterals.

Portal Venous Hypertension

The majority of portal venous hypertension is the result of intrinsic liver disease. Doppler techniques can determine whether portal flow is hepatopetal (toward) or hepatofugal (away). In portal venous hypertension, portal blood is diverted in a hepatofugal (away) direction via various collateral venous pathways with the formation of multiple portosystemic anastomoses. Doppler findings include the following:

- The portal vein shows low velocity.
- A patent paraumbilical vein is the definitive diagnosis.
- Typical portal hypertensive venous flow varies.
- The condition is most frequently caused by cirrhosis and obstruction of portal venous radicles by fibrosis and regenerating nodules.
- The condition is less frequently caused by portal venous thrombosis or other obstruction.
- Respiratory variation of vessels is usually lost in portal hypertension (there is no collapse of veins).

Spontaneous Shunting

Spontaneous shunting occurs at the following four main sites:

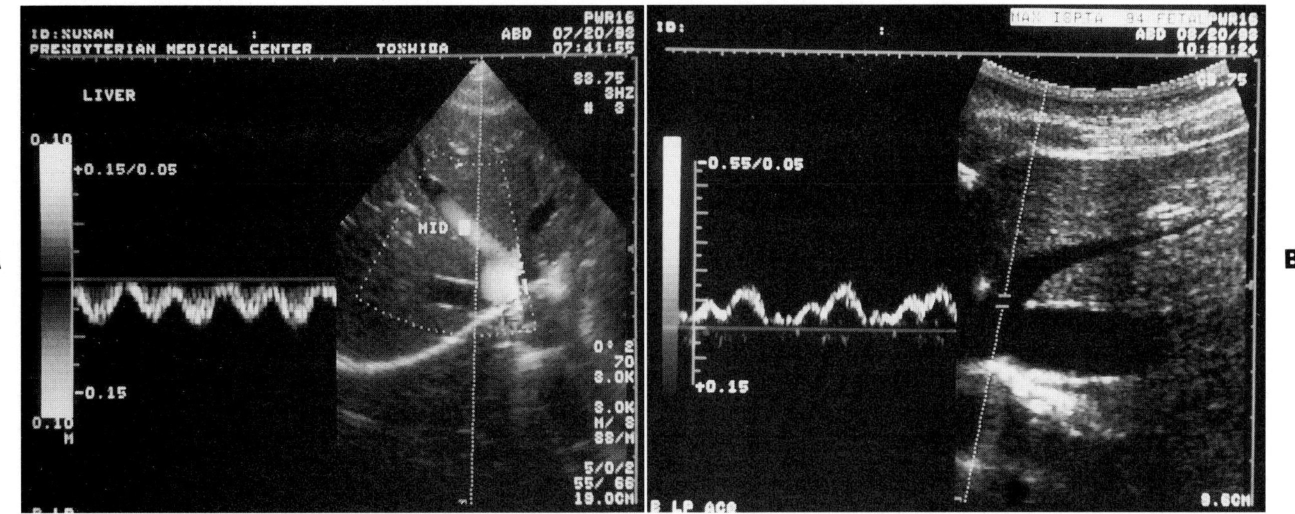

FIG. 4-70 **A,** Transverse scan of the middle hepatic vein flow shows normal flow patterns (see color image). **B,** Sagittal scan shows the complex waveform above and below the baseline.

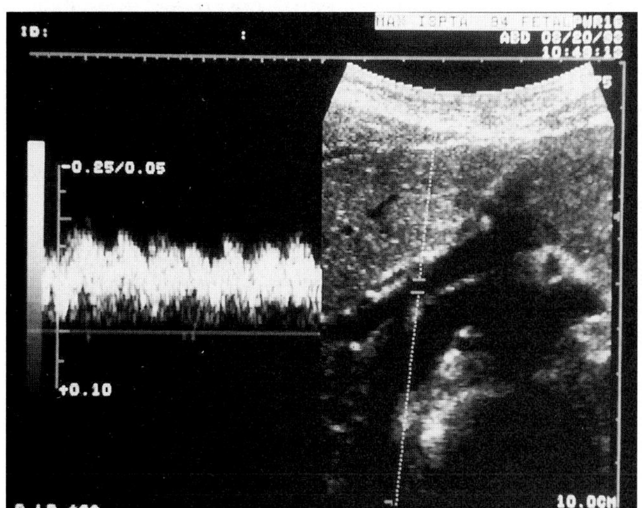

FIG. 4-71 Transverse scan of the main portal vein shows positive flow as it proceeds into the liver (hepatopetal).

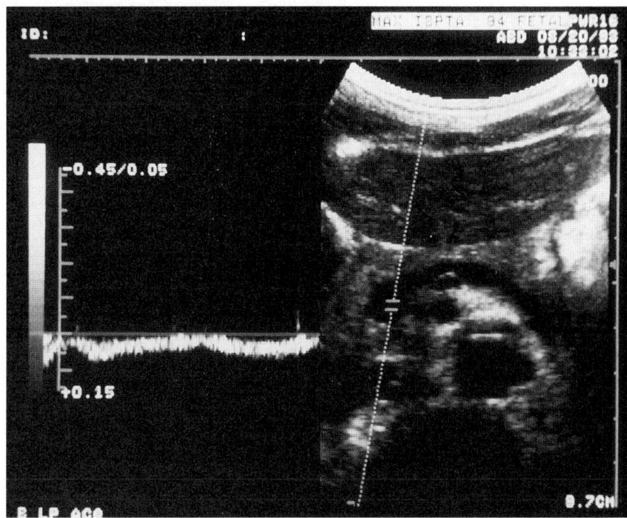

FIG. 4-72 Transverse scan of the superior mesenteric vein-portal vein flow.

1. Gastroesophageal—lower esophageal varices occur where esophageal branches of the left gastric vein form anastomoses with branches of the azygos and hemiazygos veins in the submucosa of the lower esophagus.
2. Paraumbilical vein—this appears as a continuation of the left portal vein and extends down the anterior abdominal wall to the umbilicus.
3. Hemorrhoidal anastomoses—these occur between the superior and middle hemorrhoidal veins.
4. Retroperitoneal anastomoses—vascular structures within the lesser omentum may cause thickening of the omentum (especially in children). Small vessels may be seen around the pancreas. Doppler is useful in distinguishing these vessels from nodes.

Ultrasound findings in portal hypertension:
Dilated portal vein
Dilated splenic and superior mesenteric vein (SMV)
Patent paraumbilical vein
Varices
Splenomegaly with dilated splenic radicles
Diminished response to respiration in splenic vein and SMV
Dilated hepatic and splenic arteries
Ascites
Small liver with irregular surface or large liver with abnormal texture

In patients with portal hypertension the blood flow may take one of several pathways—through splenic varices,

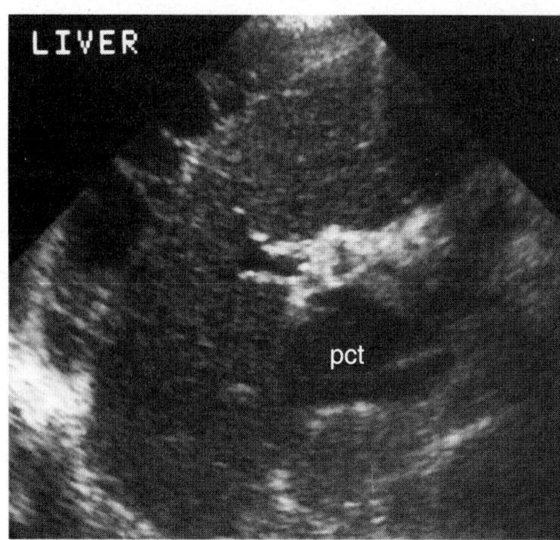

FIG. 4-73 Transverse scan over the area of the porta hepatis shows a complex mass medial to the right lobe of the liver. With color, the numerous collateral channels were seen within to represent cavernous transformation, *pct,* of the portal vein.

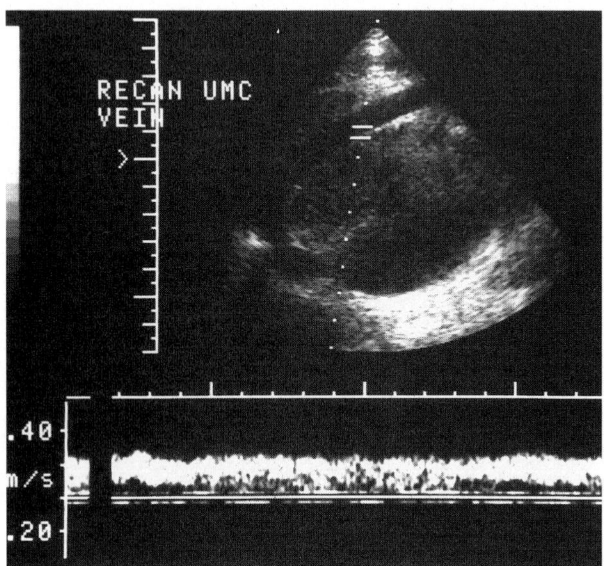

FIG. 4-74 In patients with portal hypertension the blood flow may take one of several pathways, through splenic varices, splenorenal shunts, recannalized umbilical vein, or surgical shunts.

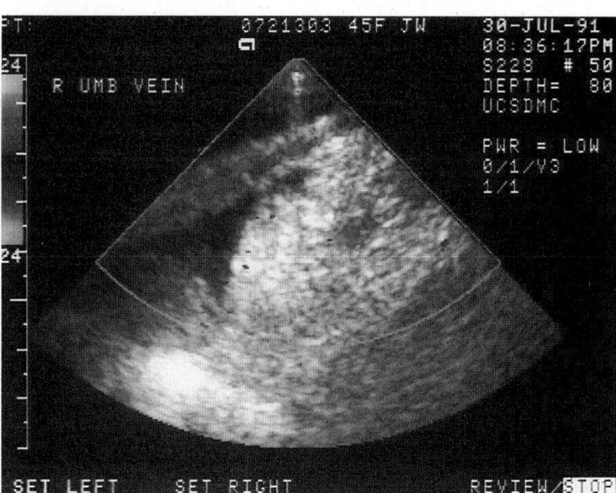

FIG. 4-75 Color-flow sagittal scans in a patient with a recannalized umbilical vein *(red)* (see color image).

splenorenal shunts, a recanalized umbilical vein, or surgical shunts.

With splenic varices, flow in the main, right, and left portal veins is reversed (hepatofugal), flow in the splenic vein is reversed, and flow in the superior mesenteric vein is normal.

With splenorenal shunts, all portal flows are reversed, as are flows in the splenic vein. The superior mesenteric vein is normal.

With a recanalized umbilical vein, the main portal vein and the left portal vein show normal flow, but the flow in the right portal vein is reversed (Figs. 4-74 and 4-75; see color image). The superior mesenteric vein and splenic veins are normal.

Once a portosystemic shunt has been performed, shunt patency can be directly identified with Doppler. This is usually easier with direct portacaval shunts (portal vein drains into inferior vena cava) than with mesocaval (superior mesenteric vein and inferior vena cava) shunts or splenorenal (splenic vein to renal vein) shunts.

If the PC shunt itself cannot be identified, the demonstration of hepatofugal (away) flow in the intrahepatic portal veins and hepatopetal flows in the superior mesenteric vein and splenic veins is a reliable indication of shunt patency.

REVIEW QUESTIONS

1. What are the three layers of the vascular wall structure? What is the difference between an artery and a vein?
2. What are the five divisions of the aorta?
3. Name the three head and neck vessels that arise from the aortic arch.
4. Describe the celiac trunk—where does it arise, into what branches does it ramify?
5. On ultrasound how can the sonographer distinguish between an artery and a vein? Between the aorta and the inferior vena cava?
6. Describe the path of the inferior vena cava and its tributaries.
7. Name the causes of dilation of the inferior vena cava.
8. What structures do the right and left hepatic artery supply?
9. What is the distribution of the celiac trunk vessels?
10. What is the echogenic "ring" surrounding the superior mesenteric artery on the transverse scan?
11. What is the relationship of the superior mesenteric artery to the pancreas, left renal vein, splenic artery, and left lobe of the liver?
12. What is the distribution of the superior mesenteric artery?

13. What is the significance of an abnormal angle of the superior mesenteric artery as it arises from the anterior wall of the aorta?
14. Describe the renal arteries and veins—their pathways from the aorta and inferior vena cava and their relationship with the other renal structures in the renal hilum.
15. Define the pathway of the renal artery as it enters the kidney.
16. Describe the portal vein and its tributaries.
17. What is the significance of the superior mesenteric vein, the gastroduodenal artery, and the common bile duct to the head of the pancreas?
18. Define the types of aortic aneurysms.
19. What is the most common cause of aortic aneurysms?
20. What are the growth patterns and mortality rates for aneurysms?
21. How does an aortic dissection present on ultrasound? What types of dissection can occur?
22. What are the causes of other abnormalities in the abdomen that may present as a pulsatile abdominal mass?
23. What is the ultrasound appearance of an aortic graft?
24. Describe an arteriovenous fistula and the signs associated with this abnormality.
25. Name the congenital anomalies in the development of the inferior vena cava.
26. What are the causes of tumor or thrombosis of the inferior vena cava or renal vein?
27. What are the applications of Doppler in abdominal vascular structures?
28. How can Doppler help diagnose a vascular problem?
29. Describe hepatofugal and hepatopetal flow patterns in the liver.
30. What is a flow disturbance?
31. What is the resistive index and what does it measure?
32. What is "plug flow"?
33. What is color-flow Doppler?
34. Describe the Doppler flow patterns in the following vascular structures: aorta, inferior vena cava, hepatic veins, portal venous system, superior mesenteric artery and vein, celiac axis, renal vessels.
35. How would arterial stenosis appear on pulsed or color-flow Doppler?
36. What Doppler measurement may be useful in evaluating a renal transplant?
37. What is the Budd-Chiari syndrome?
38. What are the causes of portal hypertension?
39. At what four sites does spontaneous shunting occur from portal hypertension?
40. What is a recanalized umbilical vein?
41. What is a portacaval shunt and when is it used?

BIBLIOGRAPHY

Abdomen and Pelvis

Abu-Yousef MM: Duplex Doppler sonography of the hepatic vein in tricuspid regurgitation, Am J Roentgenol 156:79, 1991.

Becker CD and Cooperberg PL: Sonography of the hepatic vascular system, Am J Roentgenol 150:999, 1988.

Bolondi L, Bassi SL, Gaiani S, et al: Liver cirrhosis: changes of Doppler waveform of hepatic veins, Radiology 178:513, 1991.

Fellmeth BD, Roberts AC, Bookstein JJ, et al: Postangiographic femoral artery injuries: nonsurgical repair with US-guided compression, Radiology 178:671, 1991.

Helvie MA, Rubin JM, Silver TM, and Kresowik TF: The distinction between femoral artery pseudoaneurysms and other causes of groin masses: value of duplex Doppler sonography, Am J Roentgenol 150:1177, 1988.

Moneta GL, Taylor DC, Helton WS, et al: Duplex ultrasound measurement of postprandial intestinal blood flow: effect of meal composition, Gastroenterology 95:1294, 1988.

Ohnishi K and Nomura F: Ultrasonic Doppler studies of hepatocellular carcinoma and comparison with other hepatic focal lesions, Gastroenterology 97:1489, 1989.

Sato S, Ohnishi K, Sugita S, and Kuda K: Splenic artery and superior mesenteric artery blood flow: nonsurgical Doppler US measurement in healthy subjects and patients with chronic liver disease, Radiology 164:347, 1987.

Taylor KJW and Burns PN: Duplex Doppler scanning in the pelvis and abdomen, Ultrasound Med Biol 11:643, 1985.

Taylor KJW, Burns P, Woodcock JP, and Wells PNT: Blood flow in deep abdominal and pelvic vessels: ultrasonic pulsed-Doppler analysis, Radiology 154:487, 1985.

Taylor KJW, Ramos I, Carter D, et al: Correlatin of Doppler US tumor signals with neovascular morphologic features, Radiology 166:57, 1988.

Taylor KJW, Ramos I, Morse SS, et al: Focal liver masses: differential diagnosis with pulsed Doppler US, Radiology 164:643, 1987.

Portal System

Abu-Yousef MM, Milam SG, and Farner RM: Pulsatile portal vein flow: a sign of tricuspid regurgitation on duplex Doppler sonography, Am J Roentgenol 155:785, 1990.

Alpern MB, Rubin JM, Williams DM, and Capek P: Porta hepatis: duplex Doppler US with angiographic correlation, Radiology 162:53, 1987.

Duerinckx AJ, Grant EG, Perrella RR, et al: The pulsatile portal vein in cases of congestive heart failure: correlatin of duplex Doppler findings with right atrial pressures, Radiology 176:655, 1990.

Goldberg REA, Rada C, Knelson M, et al: The response of the portal vein to an oral glucose load, J Clin Ultrasound 18:91, 1990.

Goyal AK, Pokharna DS, and Sharma SK: Ultrasonic measurements of portal vasculature in diagnosis of portal hypertension: a controversial subject reviewed, J Ultrasound Med 9:45, 1990.

Grant EG, Perella R, Tessler FN, Lois J, and Busuttil: Budd-Chiari syndrome: the results of duplex and color Doppler imaging, Am J Roentgenol 152:377, 1989.

Kawasaki T, Moriyasu F, Nishida O, et al: Analysis of hepatofugal flow in portal venous system using ultrasonic Doppler duplex system, Am J Gastroenterol 84:937, 1989.

Lafortune M, Patriquin H, Pomier G, et al: Hemodynamic changes in portal circulation after portosystemic shunts: use of duplex sonography in 43 patients, Am J Roentgenol 149:701, 1987.

Nelson RC, Lovett KE, Chezmar JL, et al: Comparison of pulsed Doppler sonography and angiography in patients with portal hypertension, Am J Roentgenol 149:77, 1987.

Patriquin H, Lafortune M, Burns PN, and Dauzat: Duplex Doppler examination in portal hypertension: technique and antomy, Am J Roentgenol 149:71, 1987.

Rice S, Lee KP, Johnson MB, et al: Portal venous system after portosystemic shunts or endoscopic sclerotherapy: evaluation with Doppler sonography, Am J Roentgenol 156:85, 1991.

Stanley P: Budd-Chiari syndrome, Radiology 170:625, 1989.

Kidney

Greene ER, Avasthi PS, and Hodges JW: Noninvasive Doppler assessment of renal artery stenosis and hemodynamics, J Clin Ultrasound 15:653, 1987.

Keller MS: Renal Doppler sonography in infants and children, Radiology 172:603, 1989.

Mostbeck GH, Kain R, Mallek R, et al: Duplex Doppler Sonography in renal parenchymal disease: histopathologic correlation, J Ultrasound Med 10:189, 1991.

Park CH, Gottlieb RP, Yoo Hs, and Pasto ME: Noninvasive diagnosis and follow-up of childhood renal vein thrombosis by ultrasound, Doppler, and renal scintiscan, Uremia Invest 9:305, 1985-1986.

Patriquin HB, O'Regan S, Robitaille P, and Paltiel H: Hemolytic-uremic syndrome: intrarenal arterial Doppler patterns as a useful guide to therapy, Radiology 172:625, 1989.

Platt JF, Rubin JM, and Ellis JH: Distinction between obstructive and nonobstructive pyelocaliectasis with duplex Doppler sonography, Am J Roentgenol 153:997, 1989.

Reuther G, Wanjura D, and Bauer H: Acute renal vein thrombosis in renal allografts: detection with duplex Doppler US, Radiology 170:557, 1989.

Scola FH, Cronan JJ, and Schepps B: Grade I hydronephrosis: pulsed Doppler US evaluation, Radiology 171:519, 1989.

Organ Transplantation

Liver and Pancreas Transplants

Dalen K, Day DL, Ascher NL, et al: Imaging of vascular complications after hepatic transplantation, Am J Roentgenol 150:1285, 1988.

Letourneau JG, Day DL, Ascher NL, et al: Abdominal sonography after hepatic transplantation: results in 36 patients, Am J Roentgenol 149:299, 1987.

Letourneau JG, Maile CW, Sutherland DER, and Feinberg SB: Ultrasound and computed tomography in the evaluation of pancreatic transplantation, Radiol Clin N Amercia 25:345, 1987.

Segel MC, Zajko AB, Bowen A, et al: Hepatic artery thrombosis after liver transplantation: radiologic evaluation, Am J Roentgenol 146:137, 1986.

Snider JF, Hunter DW, Kuni CC, et al: Pancreatic transplantation: radiologic evaluation of vascular complications, Radiology 178:749, 1991.

Wozney P, Zajko AB, Bron KM, et al: Vascular complications after liver transplantation: a 5-year experience, Am J Roentgenol 147:657, 1986.

Zonderland HM, Lameris JS, Terpstra OT, et al: Auxiliary partial liver transplantation: imaging evaluation in 10 patients, Am J Roentgenol 153:981, 1989.

Renal Transplants

Allen KS, Jorkasky DK, Arger PH, Velchik MG, et al: Renal allografts: prospective analysis of Doppler sonography, Radiology 169:371, 1988.

Buckley AR, Cooperberg PL, Reeve CE, and Magil AB: The distinction between acute renal transplant rejection and cyclosporine nephrotoxicity: value of duplex sonography, Am J Roentgenol 149:521, 1987.

Genkins SM, Segel MC, Sanfillippo FP, and Carroll BA: Duplex Doppler sonography of renal transplants: lack of sensitivity and specificity in establishing pathologic diagnosis, Am J Roentgenol 152:5335, 1989.

Grant EG and Perrella RR: Wishing won't make it so: duplex Doppler sonography in the evaluation of renal transplant dysfunction, Am J Roentgenol 155:538, 1990.

Grenier N, Douws C, Morel D, et al: Detection of vascular complications in renal allografts with color Doppler flow imaging, Radiology 178:217, 1991.

Kelcz F, Pozniak MA, Pirsch JD, and Oberly TD: Pyramidal appearance and resistive index: insensitive and nonspecific sonographic indicators of renal transplant rejection, Am J Roentgenol 155:531, 1990.

Platt JF, Ellis JH, and Rubin JM: Renal transplant pyelocaliectasis: role of duplex Doppler US in evaluation, Radiology 179:425, 1991.

Reuther G, Wanjura D, and Baver H: Acute renal vein thrombosis in renal allografts: detection with duplex Doppler US, Radiology 170:557, 1989.

Taylor KJW and Marks WH: Use of Doppler imaging for evaluation of dysfunction in renal allografts, Am J Roentgenol 155:536, 1990.

Townsend RR, Romlanovich SJ, Goldstein RB, and Filly RA: Combined Doppler and morphologic sonographic evaluation of renal transplant rejection, J Ultrasound Med 9:199, 1990.

CHAPTER 5

Liver

Sandra L. Hagen-Ansert • William J. Zwiebel

The liver is the largest organ in the body and is quite accessible to sonographic evaluation. The parenchyma of the normal liver is used to evaluate other organs and glands in the body (e.g., the kidneys are equally echogenic or less echogenic than the liver, the spleen is about the same echogenicity, and the pancreas is about as echogenic or slightly more echogenic than the liver). The size and shape of the liver determine the quality of the sonographic examination performed; that is, a prominent left lobe of the liver facilitates visualization of the pancreas, which is situated just inferior to the border of the left lobe, whereas if the right lobe extends just below the costal margin, it may facilitate visualization of the gallbladder and right kidney.

ANATOMY

The liver occupies almost all of the right hypochondrium, the greater part of the epigastrium, and the left hypochondrium as far as the mammillary line. The contour and shape of the liver vary according to patient habitus and lie. Its shape is also influenced by the lateral segment of the left lobe and the length of the right lobe. The liver lies close to the diaphragm. The ribs cover the greater part of the right lobe (usually a small part of the right lobe is in contact with the abdominal wall). In the epigastric region the liver extends several centimeters below the xyphoid process. Most of the left lobe is covered by the rib cage.

Projections of the liver may be altered by some disease states. Downward displacement is often caused by tumor infiltration, cirrhosis, or a subphrenic abscess, whereas ascites, excessive dilation of the colon, or abdominal tumors can elevate the liver. Retroperitoneal tumors may move the liver slightly forward.

Lobes of the Liver

Right Lobe

The right lobe is the largest of the four lobes of the liver (Fig. 5-1). It exceeds the left lobe by a ratio of 6:1. It occupies the right hypochondrium and is bordered on its upper surface by the falciform ligament, on its posterior surface by the left sagittal fossa, and in front by the umbilical notch. Its inferior and posterior surfaces are marked by three fossae: the porta hepatis, the gallbladder fossa, and the inferior vena cava fossa. A congenital variant, Riedel's lobe, can sometimes be seen as an anterior projection of the liver and may extend to the iliac crest.

Left Lobe

The left lobe lies in the epigastric and left hypochondriac regions (Fig. 5-2). Its upper surface is convex and molded onto the diaphragm. Its undersurface includes the gastric impression and omental tuberosity. The quadrate lobe (medial segment of the left lobe) is oblong and situated on the posteroinferior surface of the left lobe (Fig. 5-3). In front it is bounded by the anterior margin of the liver, behind by the porta hepatis, on the right by the fossa for the gallbladder, and on the left by the fossa for the umbilical vein.

Caudate Lobe

The caudate lobe is a small lobe situated on the posterosuperior surface of the left lobe opposite the tenth and eleventh thoracic vertebrae (Fig. 5-4). It is bounded below by the porta hepatis, on the right by the fossa for the inferior vena cava, and on the left by the fossa for the ductus venosus.

Portal and Hepatic Venous Anatomy

As described by Marks et al. the portal venous system is a reliable indicator of various ultrasonic tomographic planes throughout the liver (Fig. 5-5).

Main Portal Vein

The main portal vein approaches the porta hepatis in a rightward, cephalic, and slightly posterior direction within the hepatoduodenal ligament. It comes in contact with the anterior surface of the inferior vena cava near the porta hepatis and serves to locate the liver hilum (Figs. 5-6 and 5-7). It then divides into two branches, the right and left portal veins.

Right portal vein

The right portal vein is the larger of the two branches and requires a more posterior and more caudal transducer approach. It usually is possible to identify the anterior and posterior divisions of the right portal vein on sonography. The anterior division closely parallels the anterior abdominal wall.

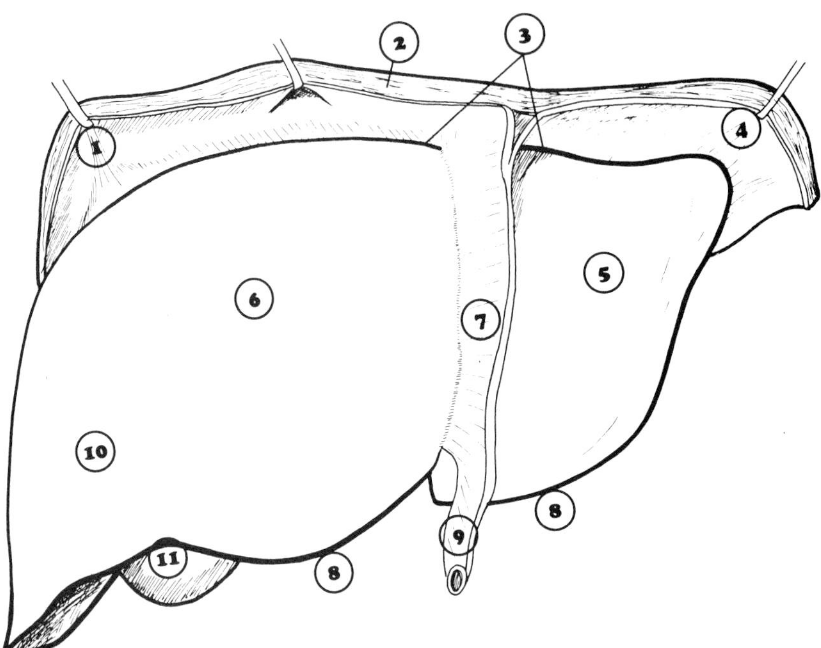

FIG. 5-1 A, Anterior view of the liver. The right lobe is the largest of the four lobes of the liver. Right triangular ligament, *1;* diaphragm, *2;* coronary ligament, *3;* left triangular ligament, *4;* left lobe, *5;* right lobe, *6;* falciform ligament, *7;* inferior margin, *8;* ligamentum teres; *9;* costal surface, *10;* gallbladder, *11.* (From Hagen-Ansert SL: The anatomy workbook, Philadelphia, 1986, JB Lippincott.)

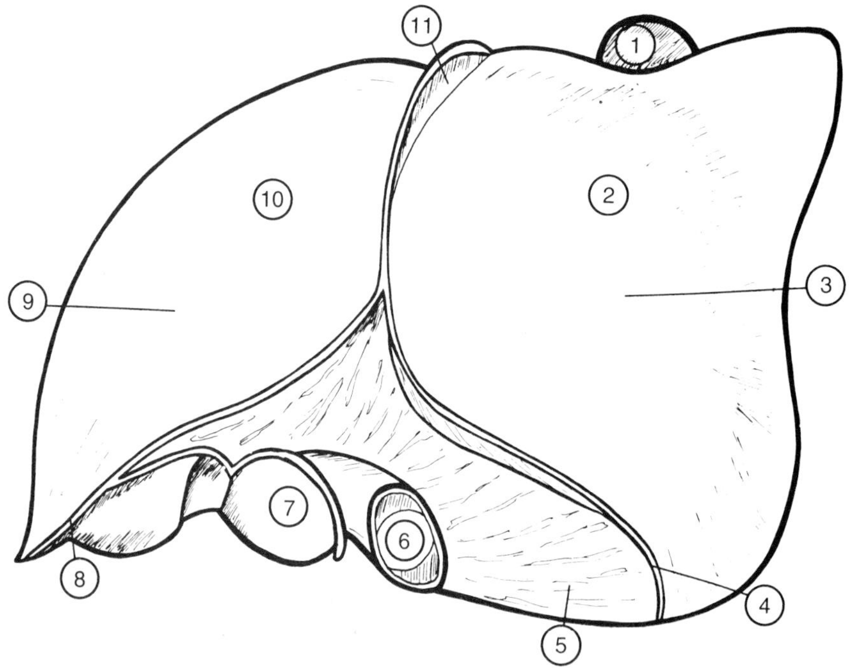

FIG. 5-2 Superior view of the liver. The left lobe of the liver lies in the epigastric and left hypochondriac regions. Fundus of the gallbladder, *1;* right lobe, *2;* diaphragmatic surface, *3;* coronary ligament, *4;* bare area, *5;* inferior vena cava, *6;* caudate lobe, *7;* left triangular ligament, *8;* diaphragmatic surface, *9;* left lobe, *10;* falciform ligament, *11.* (From Hagen-Ansert SL: The anatomy workbook, Philadelphia, 1986, JB Lippincott.)

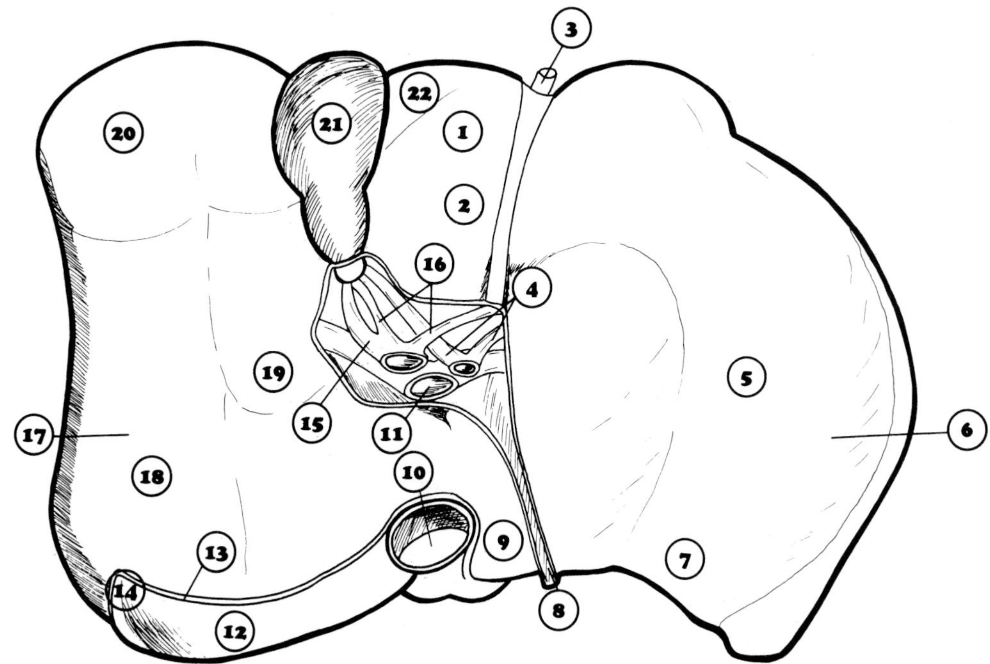

FIG. 5-3 Inferior view of the visceral surface of the liver. The quadrate lobe is located on the posteroinferior surface of the left lobe. Quadrate lobe, *1;* pyloric area, *2;* ligamentum teres, *3;* hepatic arteries, *4;* gastric impression, *5;* left lobe, *6;* esophageal impression, *7;* ligamentum venosum, *8;* caudate lobe, *9;* inferior vena cava, *10;* portal vein, *11;* bare area, *12;* coronary ligaments, *13;* right triangular ligament, *14;* cystic duct, *15;* hepatic duct, *16;* right lobe, *17;* renal impression, *18;* duodenal impression, *19;* colic impression, *20;* gallbladder. (From Hagen-Ansert SL: The Anatomy workbook, Philadelphia, 1986, JB Lippincott.)

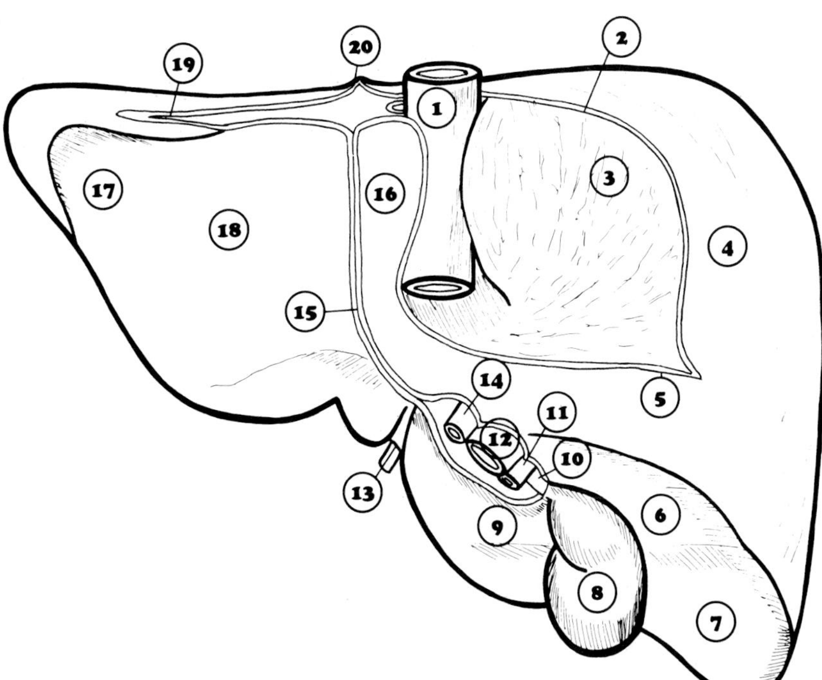

FIG. 5-4 Posterior view of the diaphragmatic surface of the liver. The caudate lobe is located on the posterosuperior surface of the right lobe, opposite the tenth and eleventh thoracic vertebrae. Inferior vena cava, *1;* coronary ligaments, *2;* bare area, *3;* right lobe, *4;* right triangular ligament, *5;* renal impression, *6;* colic impression, *7;* gallbladder, *8;* quadrate lobe, *9;* cystic duct, *10;* hepatic duct; *11;* portal vein, *12;* ligamentum teres, *13;* hepatic artery, *14;* attachment of the lesser omentum, *15;* caudate lobe, *16;* gastric impression, *17;* left lobe, *18;* left triangular ligament, *19;* falciform ligament, *20.* (From Hagen-Ansert SL: The anatomy workbook, Philadelphia, 1986, JB Lippincott.)

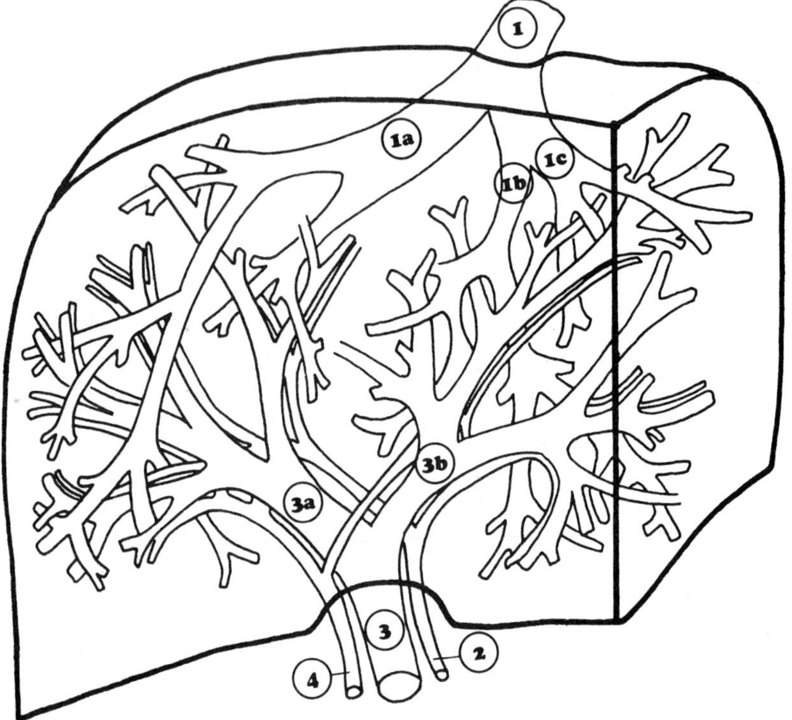

FIG. 5-5 Vascular system of the liver. Hepatic veins, *1* (right, *1a;* middle, *1b,* left, *1c*) hepatic artery, *2;* portal vein, *3* (right main, *3a;* left main, *3b*) bile duct, *4*. (From Hagen-Ansert SL: The anatomy workbook, Philadelphia, 1986, JB Lippincott.)

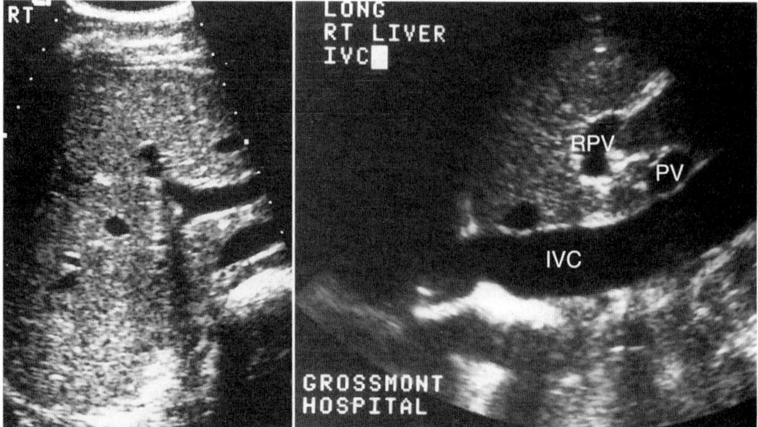

FIG. 5-6 Transverse and longitudinal scans of the main portal vein as it approaches the porta hepatis in a rightward, cephalic, and slightly posterior direction within the hepatoduodenal ligament.

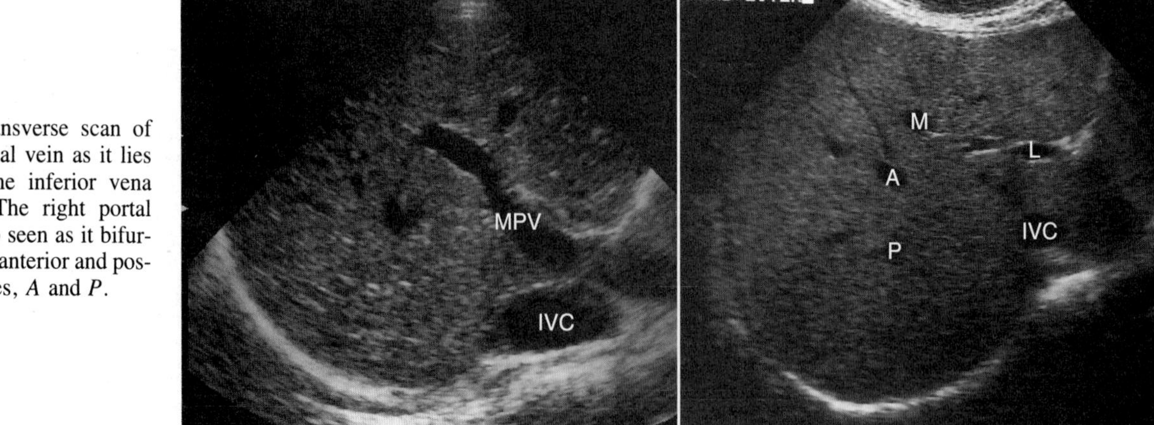

FIG. 5-7 Transverse scan of the main portal vein as it lies anterior to the inferior vena cava, *IVC*. The right portal branch is also seen as it bifurcates into the anterior and posterior branches, *A* and *P*.

Left portal vein

The left portal vein lies more anterior and cranial than the right portal vein. The main portal vein is seen to elongate at the origin of the left portal vein. The vessel lies within a canal containing large amounts of connective tissue, which results in the visualization of an echogenic linear band coursing through the central portion of the lateral segment of the left lobe.

Hepatic Veins

The hepatic veins are divided into three components: right, middle, and left (Figs. 5-8 to 5-10). The right hepatic vein is the largest and enters the right lateral aspect of the inferior vena cava. The middle hepatic vein enters the anterior or right anterior surface of the inferior vena cava. The left hepatic vein, which is the smallest, enters the left anterior surface of the inferior vena cava.

Often it is possible to identify a long horizontal branch of the right hepatic vein coursing between the anterior and posterior divisions of the right portal vein.

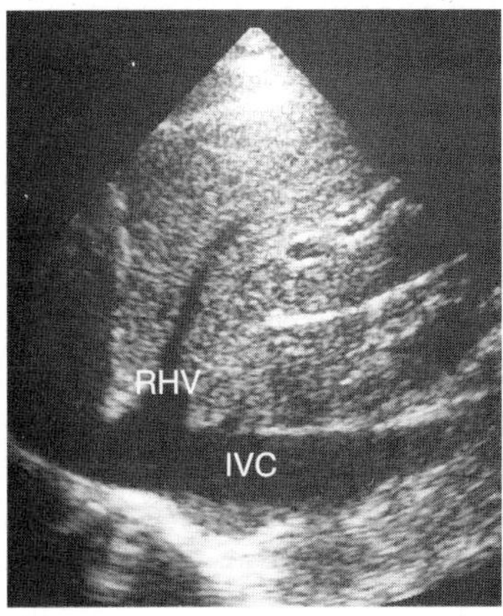

FIG. 5-8 Sagittal scan of the right hepatic vein, *RHV*, as it drains into the anterior wall of the inferior vena cava, *IVC*.

Distinguishing Characteristics of Hepatic and Portal Veins

The best way to distinguish the hepatic from the portal vessels is to trace their points of entry to the liver. The hepatic vessels flow into the inferior vena cava, whereas the portal system drains into the main portal vein. Real time sector allows the sonographer to make this assessment within a few seconds (Fig. 5-11).

Two other characteristics help distinguish the vessels:

1. Hepatic veins course between the hepatic lobes and segments; the major portal branches course within the lobar segments.
2. Hepatic veins drain toward the right atrium; the portal veins emanate from the porta hepatis (i.e., hepatic veins are larger near the diaphragm, whereas portal veins are larger nearer the porta hepatis).

Segmental Liver Anatomy

The liver is divided essentially into two lobes, each of which has two segments. The right lobe is divided into anterior and posterior segments, and the left lobe into medial and lateral segments. The quadrate lobe is a portion of the medial segment of the left lobe. The caudate lobe is the posterior portion of the liver lying between the fossa of the inferior vena cava and the fissure of the ligamentum venosum. The caudate lobe receives portal venous and hepatic arterial blood from both the right and the left systems. The anatomic features that assist in determining the positions of the various hepatic segments are listed in Table 5-1.

Functional Division of the Liver

The purpose of a functional division of the liver is to separate the liver into component parts according to the blood

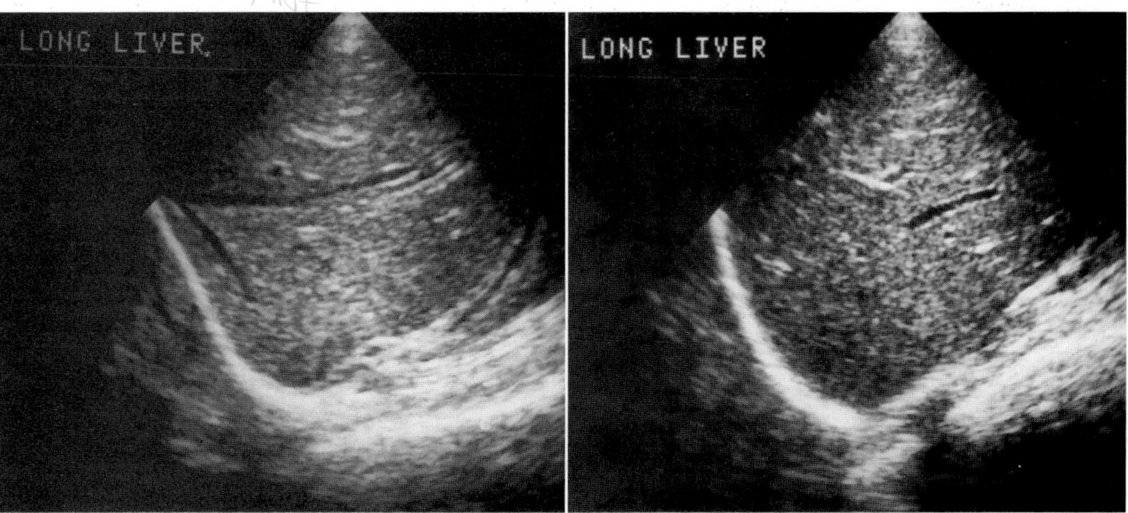

FIG. 5-9 The middle hepatic vein enters the anterior or right anterior surface of the inferior vena cava.

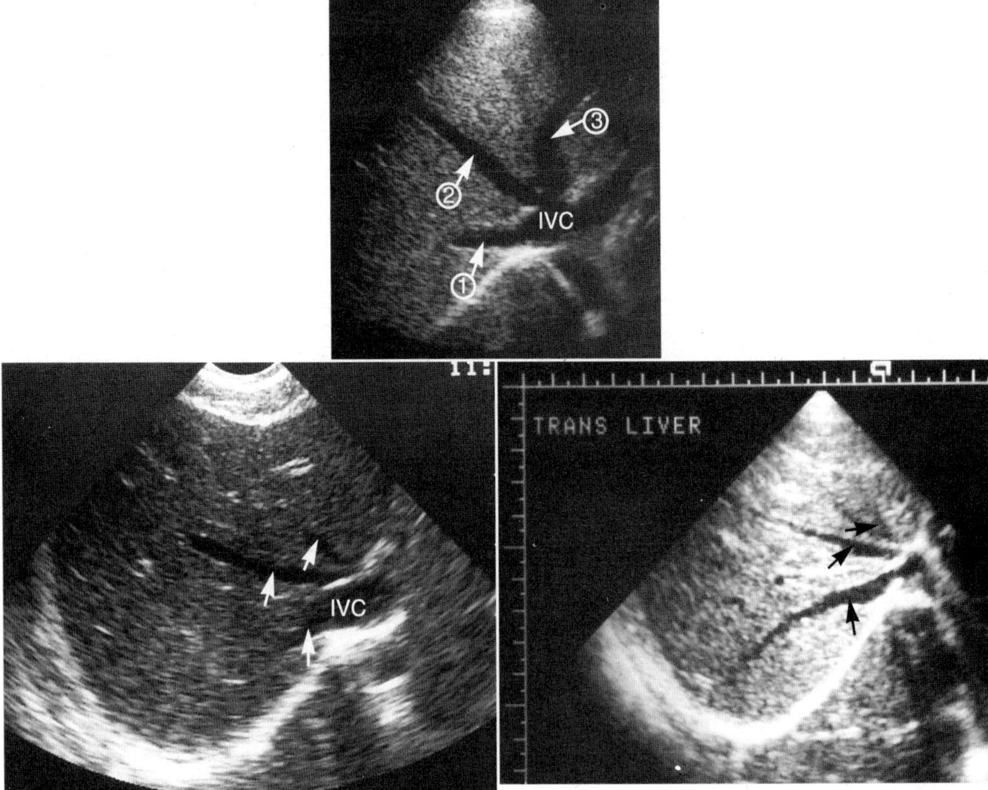

FIG. 5-10 Transverse view of the right, *1*, middle, *2*, and left, *3*, hepatic veins.

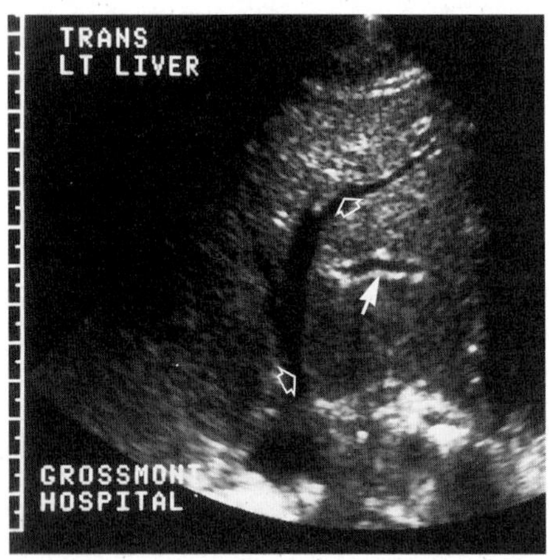

FIG. 5-11 Transverse scan of the portal vein *(small arrow)* and hepatic vein *(large arrow)*.

supply and biliary drainage so that one component can be removed in the event of tumor invasion or trauma. There are two functional divisions, a right and a left lobe. The right functional lobe includes everything to the right of a plane through the gallbladder fossa and inferior vena cava (which corresponds to the anatomic right lobe) (Fig. 5-12). The left functional lobe includes everything to the left of the above plane (which corresponds to the left lobe and caudate lobe).

Ligaments and Fissures

There are three important ligaments and fissures to remember in the liver. The falciform ligament extends from the umbilicus to the diaphragm in a parasagittal plane, containing the ligamentum teres (Fig. 5-13). In the anteroposterior axis the falciform ligament extends from the right rectus muscle to the bare area of the liver, where its reflections separate to contribute to the hepatic coronary ligament and attach to the undersurface of the diaphragm. The ligamentum teres appears as a bright echogenic focus on the sonogram and is seen as the rounded termination of the falciform ligament (Fig. 5-14). Both the falciform ligament and the ligamentum teres divide the medial and lateral segments of the left lobe of the liver. The fissure for the ligamentum venosum separates the left lobe from the caudate lobe (Figs. 5-15 and 5-16).

Relational Anatomy

The fundus of the stomach lies posterior and lateral to the left lobe of the liver and may frequently be seen on transverse sonograms (Fig. 5-17). The remainder of the stomach lies inferior to the liver and is best visualized on

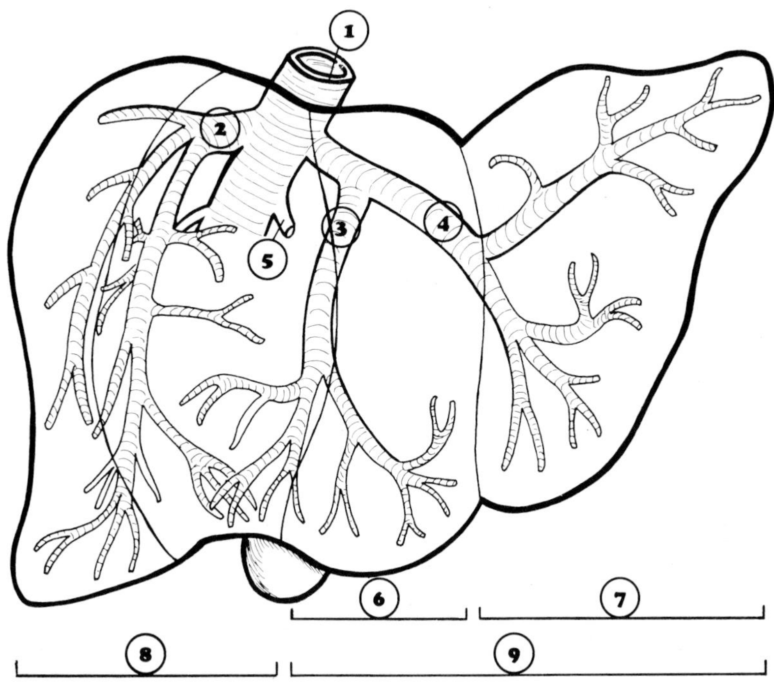

FIG. 5-12 Functional division of the liver. Inferior vena cava, *1;* right hepatic vein, *2;* middle hepatic vein, *3;* left hepatic vein, *4;* caudate lobe, *5;* medial segment, *6;* lateral segment, *7;* right lobe; *8;* left lobe, *9.*

TABLE 5-1 Anatomic Structures Useful for Dividing and Identifying the Hepatic Segments

Structure	Location	Usefulness
RHV	Right intersegmental fissure	Divides anterior and posterior segments of right hepatic lobe and courses between anterior and posterior branches of RPV
MHV	Main lobar fissure	Separates right and left lobes
LHV	Left intersegmental fissure	Divides medial and lateral segments of left lobe
RPV (anterior)	Intrasegmental in anterior segment of right hepatic lobe	Courses centrally in anterior segment of right hepatic lobe
RPV (posterior)	Intrasegmental in posterior segment of right hepatic lobe	Courses centrally in posterior segment of right hepatic lobe.
LPV (initial)	Courses anterior to caudate lobe	Separates caudate lobe posteriorly from medial segment of left lobe anteriorly
LPV (ascending)	Turns anteriorly in left intersegmental fissure	Divides medial and lateral segments of left lobe
IVC fossa	Posterior aspect of main lobar fissure	Separates right and left hepatic lobes
Gb fossa	Main lobar fissure	Separates right and left hepatic lobes
Ligamentum teres	Left intersegmental fissure	Divides caudal aspect of left hepatic lobe into medial and lateral segments
Fissure of ligamentum venosum	Left anterior margin of caudate lobe	Separates caudate lobe from medial and lateral segments of left lobe

From Callen PW: J Clin Ultrasound 7:81, 1979.

sagittal sonograms. The duodenum lies adjacent to the right lobe and medial segment of the left lobe of the liver. The pancreas is usually seen just inferior to the liver. The posterior border of the liver contacts the right kidney, inferior vena cava, and aorta. The diaphragm covers the superior border of the liver. The liver is suspended from the diaphragm and anterior abdominal wall by the falciform ligament and from the diaphragm by the reflections of the peritoneum. Most of the liver is covered by peritoneum, but a large area rests directly on the diaphragm; this is called the *bare area*. The subphrenic space between the liver (or spleen) and the diaphragm is a common site for abscess formation. The lesser sac is an enclosed portion of the peritoneal space posterior to the liver and the stomach. This sac

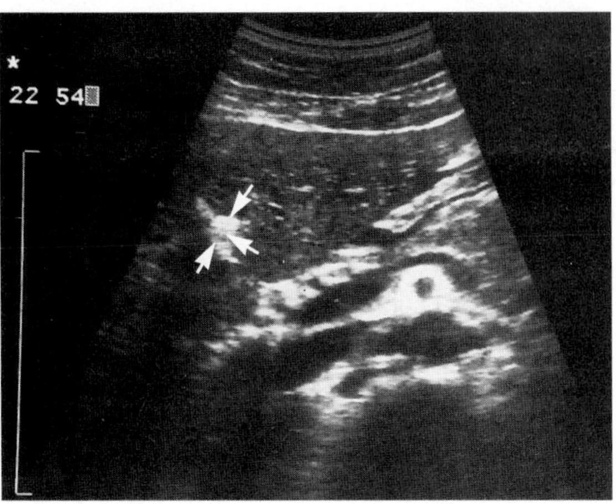

FIG. 5-13 The ligamentum teres appears as a bright echogenic focus on the ultrasound *(arrows)* and is seen as the rounded termination of the falciform ligament.

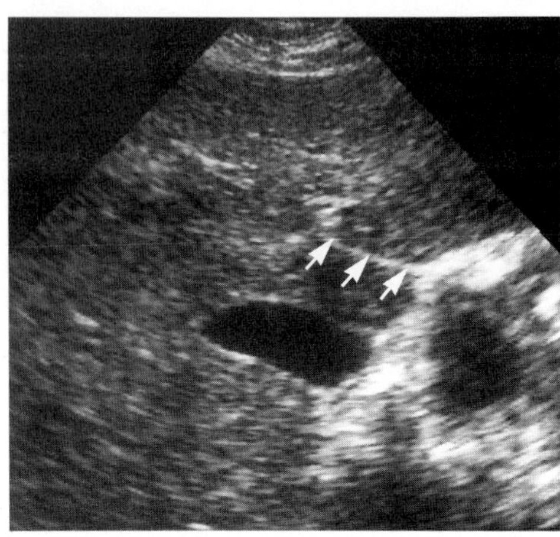

FIG. 5-15 The fissure for the ligamentum venosum *(arrows)* separates the left lobe from the caudate lobe of the liver.

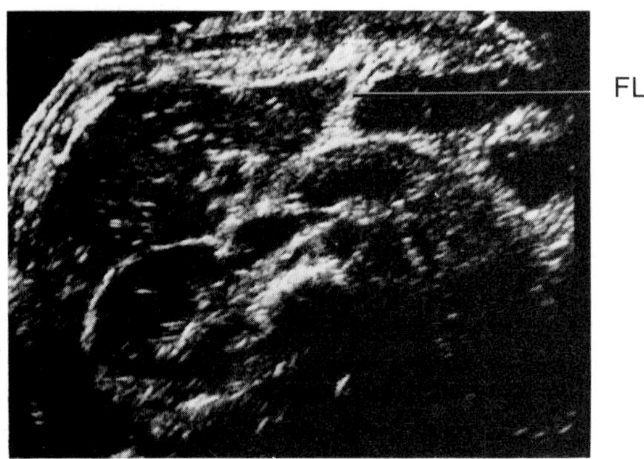

FIG. 5-14 The falciform ligament, *FL,* is shown in this transverse scan; it divides the left lobe from the quadrate lobe of the liver.

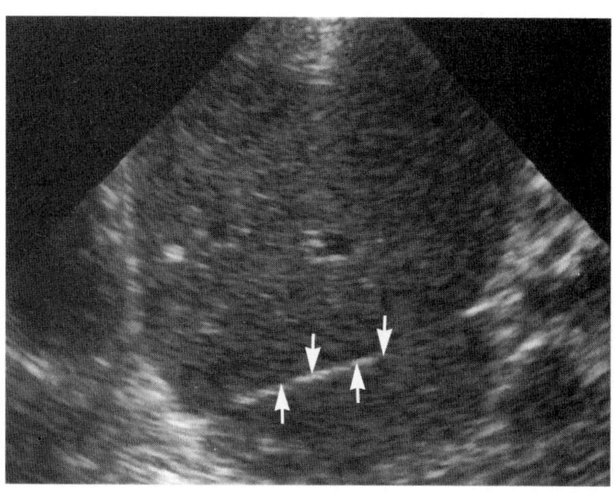

FIG. 5-16 Longitudinal view of the intersegmental fissure *(arrows)* in the posterior segment of the right hepatic lobe.

communicates with the rest of the peritoneal space at a point near the head of the pancreas. It also may be a site for abscess formation.

Intrahepatic Vessels and Ducts

The portal veins carry blood from the bowel to the liver, whereas the hepatic veins drain the blood from the liver into the inferior vena cava (see Fig. 5-5). The hepatic arteries carry oxygenated blood from the aorta to the liver. The bile ducts transport bile, manufactured in the liver, to the duodenum.

HEPATOBILIARY PHYSIOLOGY AND LABORATORY DATA

The liver, bile ducts, and gallbladder constitute the hepatobiliary system, which performs metabolic and excretory functions essential to physical well-being. Ultrasonography is an important method for detecting anatomic changes associated with hepatobiliary disease; but accurate ultrasound evaluation can be accomplished only when other diagnostic information, including signs, symptoms, and laboratory results, are considered with the ultrasound findings. The task of correlating these clinical and ultrasound data falls primarily to the sonologist. However, the sonographer must also understand the entire clinical picture to be able to plan and properly perform the ultrasound examination. It is necessary, therefore, that the sonographer be aware of the normal and abnormal physiology of the hepatobiliary system. This section is intended as a primer of hepatobiliary physiology with particular attention to physiologic alterations that commonly occur in hepatobiliary disease.

Liver

The liver is a major center of metabolism, which may be defined as the physical and chemical process whereby

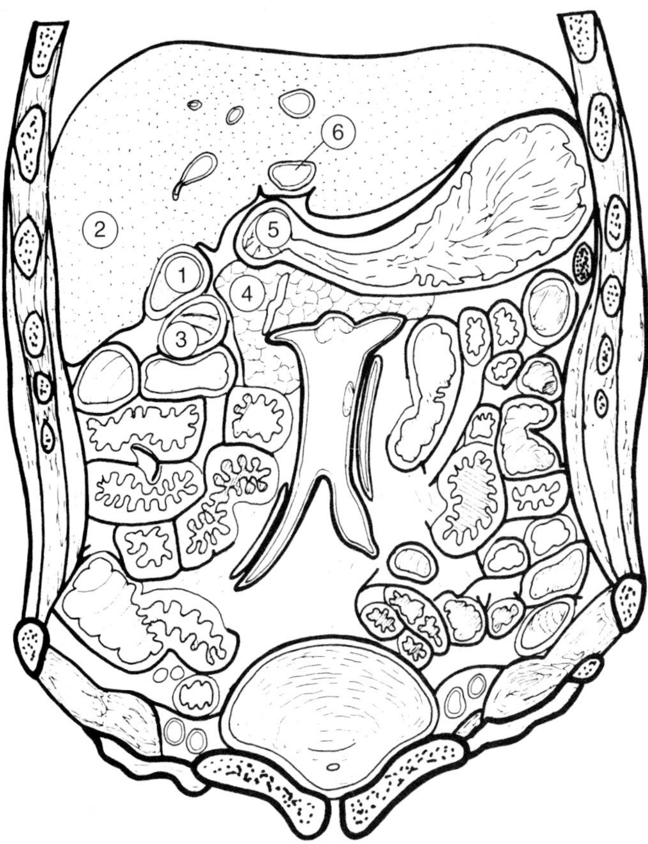

FIG. 5-17 Coronal view of the relational anatomy of the liver. The stomach lies posterior and lateral to the left lobe of the liver. The duodenum lies adjacent to the right lobe and medial segment of the left lobe. The pancreas is inferior to the liver. The posterior border of the liver contains the right kidney, inferior vena cava, and aorta. The diaphragm covers the superior border of the liver.

foodstuffs are synthesized into complex elements, complex substances are transformed into simple ones, and energy is made available for use by the organism. The liver is also a center for detoxification of the waste products of metabolism accumulated from other sources in the body and foreign chemicals (usually drugs) that enter the body. The liver expels these waste products from the body via its excretory product, bile, which also plays an important role in fat absorption. Finally, the liver is a storage site for several compounds used in a variety of physiologic activities throughout the body. In hepatobiliary disease, each of these functions may be altered, leading to abnormal physical, laboratory, and sonographic findings.

Hepatocellular Versus Obstructive Disease

Diseases affecting the liver may be classified as hepatocellular, when the liver cells or hepatocytes are the immediate problem; or obstructive when bile excretion is blocked.

Viral hepatitis is an example in which the virus attacks the liver cells and damages or destroys them, resulting in an alteration of liver function. In obstructive disorders the flow of bile from the liver is blocked at some point and secondarily results in liver malfunction.

The differentiation between hepatocellular and obstructive diseases is of considerable importance clinically. Hepatocellular diseases are treated medically with supportive measures and drugs; obstructive disorders are usually relieved by surgery. In some cases the distinction between hepatocellular and obstructive disease can be made through clinical laboratory tests, but often the laboratory findings are equivocal. Ultrasonography has been of great benefit, since it allows the physician to accurately separate hepatocellular and obstructive causes of liver disease.

Hepatic Metabolic Functions

Raw materials in the form of carbohydrates (sugars), fats, and amino acids (the basic components of proteins) are absorbed from the intestine and transported to the liver via the circulatory system. In the liver, these substances are converted chemically to other compounds or are processed for storage or energy production. The following is a brief discussion of the metabolic functions of the liver and basic disturbances in these functions that result from liver disease.

Carbohydrates

Sugars may be absorbed from the blood in several forms, but only glucose can be used by cells throughout the body as a source of energy.

The liver functions as a major site for conversion of dietary sugars into glucose, which is released into the blood stream for general use. The body requires only a certain amount of glucose at any one time, however, and excess sugar is converted by the liver to glycogen (a starch), which may be stored in the liver cells or transported in the blood to distant storage sites. When dietary sugar is unavailable, the liver converts glycogen released from stores into glucose; it can also manufacture glucose directly from other compounds, including proteins or fats, when other sources of glucose have been depleted. Thus the liver helps to maintain a steady state of glucose in the blood stream. In very severe liver disease, unless glucose is administered intravenously, the body may become glucose deficient (hypoglycemic) with profound effects on the function of the brain and other organs. Alternately, uncontrolled increases in blood glucose (hyperglycemia) may occur in severe liver disease if a large dose of glucose is administered, since the liver fails to convert the excess glucose to glycogen.

Fats

The liver is also a principal site for metabolism of fats, which are absorbed from the intestine in the form of monoglycerides and diglycerides.

Dietary fats are converted in the hepatocytes to lipoproteins, in which form fats are transported throughout the body to sites where they are used by other organs or stored. Conversely, stored fats may be transported to the liver and converted into energy, yielding glucose or other substances, such as cholesterol, that have important and widespread uses.

In severe liver disease, abnormally low blood levels of cholesterol may be noted because the liver is the principal site for cholesterol synthesis. Furthermore, failure of hepatic conversion of fat to glucose in liver disease may contribute to hypoglycemia. A striking histologic manifestation of many forms of hepatocellular disease is the so-called fatty liver. On gross pathologic examination the fatty liver has a yellow color and a greasy feel; on microscopic study globules of fat (primarily triglycerides) crowd the hepatocytes. The cause of fat accumulation in the liver cells is poorly understood, but it is believed to result from failure of the hepatocytes to manufacture special proteins, called *lipoproteins,* that coat small quantities of fat making the fat soluble in plasma and allowing for its release into the bloodstream. Fatty liver is a nonspecific finding that may be seen in a variety of illnesses including viral hepatitis, alcoholic liver disease, and exposure to toxic chemicals.

Proteins

The liver produces a wide variety of proteins, either indirectly from amino acids absorbed from the gut or directly from raw materials stored within the body.

Albumin, in particular, is produced in great quantities. In the bloodstream, it functions as a transport medium for a wide variety of molecules. Since it is nonionic, it also functions to draw water into the vascular system from tissue spaces; stated more technically, it helps to maintain oncotic pressure within the vascular system. When the liver is chronically diseased, clinical laboratory results may reveal a significant lowering of the serum albumin (hypoalbuminemia). The accompanying loss of oncotic pressure in the vascular system allows fluid to migrate into the interstitial space, resulting in edema (swelling) in dependent areas, such as the lower extremities. In patients with severe liver disease, especially advanced cirrhosis, ascites also develops. Hypoalbuminemia may account in part for the ascites, but the development of ascites is principally caused by portal hypertension.

In addition to being the primary source of albumin synthesis, the liver is the principal source of proteins necessary for blood coagulation, including fibrinogen (Factor I), prothrombin (Factor II), and Factors V, VII, IX, and X. In liver disease, decreased production of these proteins may lead to inadequate blood coagulation and uncontrollable hemorrhage. Commonly such hemorrhages occur into the bowel after rupture of a dilated vein or development of ulcer disease. These hemorrhages are often the immediate or contributing cause of death. Deficiencies of clotting Factors II, VII, IX, and X also may result from failure of intestinal absorption of vitamin K, which is a precursor (raw material) required for synthesis of these factors. Vitamin K is a fat-soluble vitamin (so are vitamins D, A, and E) and is absorbed only from the intestine in solution with fat. Fat absorption is severely limited in cases of bile duct obstruction because of the absence of bile salts (discussed later), and absorption of fat-soluble vitamins is therefore severely reduced. Ultimately the deficiency of vitamin K lowers the amount of the above-mentioned factors and coagulation is retarded. Deficiency of prothrombin and other vitamin K–dependent factors can be corrected in cases of obstruction through parenteral administration of vitamin K. In hepatocellular disease, administration of vitamin K may improve the coagulopathy but frequently does not restore normal clotting function, since the primary problem is hepatocyte dysfunction.

Clotting deficiencies related to liver disease may be detected with several laboratory tests. Of particular interest are the prothrombin time (pro time) and partial thromboplastin time (PTT). The results of these tests are presented as percentages of the time required for certain coagulation steps to occur in the patient's blood as compared with normal blood. Longer periods (lower percentages) indicate greater degrees of abnormality in each of these tests.

Hepatic enzymes

Enzymes are protein catalysts used throughout the body in all metabolic processes. Since the liver is a major center of metabolism, large quantities of enzymes are present in hepatocytes, and these leak into the bloodstream when the liver cells are damaged or destroyed by disease. The presence of increased quantities of enzymes in the blood is a very sensitive indicator of hepatocellular disorder. In hepatobiliary disease the enzymes AST (aspartase aminotransferase, ALT (alanine aminotransferase), and alkaline phosphatase are of particular interest. Serum levels of all three of these enzymes are increased in both hepatocellular dis-

FUNCTIONS OF THE LIVER

The numerous functions of the liver include the following:

1. Secretes bile, which is important in the digestion of fats. Bilirubin, a pigment released when red blood cells are broken down, is excreted in the bile.
2. Removes nutrients from the blood.
3. Converts glucose to glycogen and stores it—when glucose is needed, it breaks down the glycogen and releases glucose into the blood.
4. Stores iron and certain vitamins.
5. Converts excess amino acids to fatty acids and urea.
6. Performs many important functions in metabolism of proteins, fats, and carbohydrates.
7. Manufactures many of the plasma proteins found in the blood.
8. Detoxifies many drugs and poisons that enter the body.
9. Phagocytizes bacteria and worn-out red blood cells.

ease and biliary obstruction, but the patterns of elevation may help differentiate hepatocellular and obstructive causes (Table 5-2). In biliary obstruction, elevation of AST and ALT is usually mild (serum levels typically do not exceed 300 units). However, in severe hepatocellular destruction, such as acute viral or toxic hepatitis, striking elevation of AST and ALT may be seen (levels frequently exceed 1000 units). Marked elevation of alkaline phosphatase, on the other hand, is typically associated with biliary obstruction or the presence of mass lesions in the liver (e.g., metastatic disease or abscesses). Low levels of alkaline phosphatase are very unusual in obstruction, and high levels (greater than 15 Bodansky units) are uncommon in hepatocellular disorders. Alkaline phosphatase is such a sensitive indicator of obstruction that it may become elevated before the serum bilirubin in cases of acute obstruction. Hence a disproportional increase of alkaline phosphatase relative to bilirubin always suggests obstruction. Elevation of serum alkaline phosphatase may be the only abnormal laboratory finding in metastatic disease.

Whereas the pattern of enzyme abnormality may strongly suggest hepatocellular disease or obstruction in some cases, it may not allow this distinction to be made in others because obstruction may be superimposed on preexisting hepatocellular disease or unrelieved obstruction may cause hepatocellular damage. Confusion in interpretation of serum enzyme abnormalities may also occur when AST, ALT, or alkaline phosphatase is released from diseased tissues other than the liver. For instance, AST and ALT are increased with damage to heart and skeletal muscle, and alkaline phosphatase is elevated in bone disease and in normal pregnancies. Since ALT is somewhat more specific for liver disease than AST, elevation of ALT above AST suggests a hepatic cause.

Hepatic detoxification functions

The liver is a major location for detoxification of waste products of energy production and other metabolic activities occurring throughout the body. It is also the principal site of breakdown of foreign chemicals, such as drugs. Although these functions fall under the general definition of metabolism and could therefore be grouped in the preceding section, it is useful for instructional purposes to think of these functions as separate categories of hepatic activity.

Ammonium, a toxic product of nitrogen metabolism, is converted to nontoxic urea in the liver, which is practically the only site where this conversion occurs. Urea is subsequently eliminated from the body by the kidneys. The level of urea in the blood is measured as the blood urea nitrogen (BUN), and in severe liver disease (acute or chronic) the BUN may be abnormally low because of fall-off of urea production. The exhaled breath of patients with severe liver disease may have a fruity or pungent odor (known as fetor hepaticus) because of ammonium (NH_4) accumulation. More important, the concentration of NH_4 in the blood may rise to toxic levels and cause brain dysfunction (including confusion, coordination disturbances, tremor, and coma). Gastrointestinal hemorrhage frequently leads to the accumulation of toxic levels of NH_4 in the blood. Blood lost into the intestine is broken down by bacteria into nitrogen-containing substances, which are absorbed into the bloodstream. The failing liver may therefore be presented with a large amount of NH_4 that it cannot detoxify; coma may result and is frequently a precursor to death if the patient does not succumb to the direct effects of blood loss. Thus failure of ammonium detoxification is a serious consequence of liver failure.

Bilirubin detoxification

Bilirubin, the breakdown product of hemoglobin, is also an important substance detoxified in the liver. Besides detoxification, the liver also excretes bilirubin into the gut via the biliary tree.

Red blood cells survive an average of 120 days in the circulatory system; they are then trapped and broken down by reticuloendothelial (RE) cells, primarily within the spleen. Hemoglobin released from the red cells is converted to bilirubin within the RE system and is then released into the bloodstream. The bilirubin molecules become attached to albumin in the blood and are transported to the liver, where the following metabolic steps take place in the hepatocytes:

1. Uptake. The bilirubin is separated from albumin, probably at the cell membrane, and is taken within the hepatocytes.
2. Conjugation. The bilirubin molecule is combined with two glucuronide molecules, forming bilirubin diglucuronide.
3. Excretion. The bilirubin molecule is actively transported across the cell membrane into the bile canaliculi, which are the microscopic "headwaters of" the biliary system. Bilirubin released from the hepatocytes passes through the bile ducts with other components of bile and is de-

TABLE 5-2 Comparison of Laboratory Abnormalities in Hepatocellular Disease and Biliary Obstruction

	Bilirubin	Serum albumin	AST	ALT	Alkaline phosphatase
Hepatocellular disease	↑ ↑↑ ↑↑↑	↓ ↓↓		↑↑ ↑↑↑	↑ ↑↑
Obstruction	↑ ↑↑	→	↑ ↑↑	↑ ↑↑	↑↑↑

↑ Minimal; ↑ ↑ moderate; ↑ ↑ ↑ severe increase; → normal.

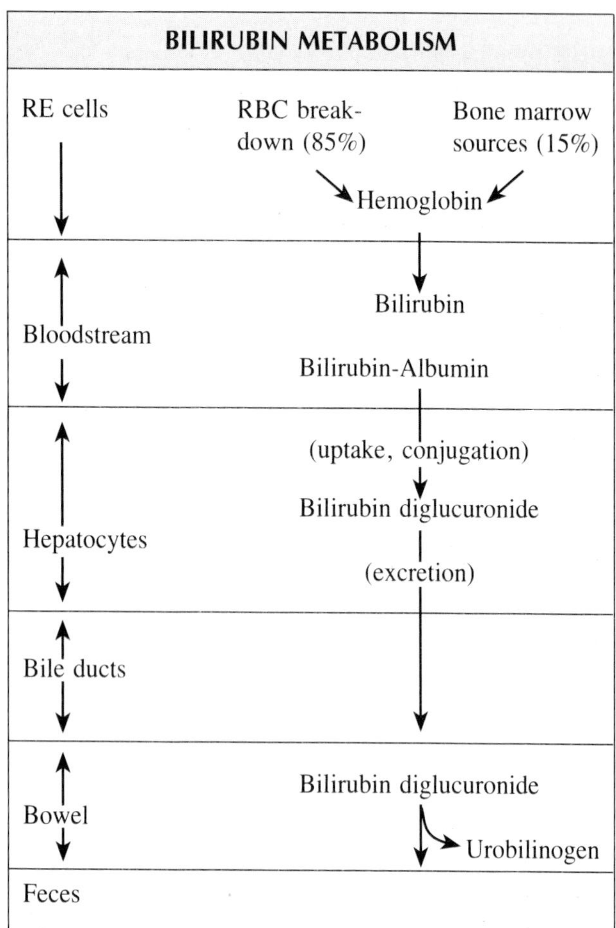

livered to the bowel, where most bilirubin diglucuronide is excreted into the feces (a small portion is broken down into urobilinogen by intestinal bacteria, absorbed into the portal system, and reexcreted by the liver).

Measurement of the concentration of bilirubin in the blood is a standard laboratory test for hepatocellular disease. The following two fractions of bilirubin are measured: the direct-acting fraction, which reacts chemically in an aqueous medium and consists of conjugated bilirubin, and the indirect-acting fraction, which consists of unconjugated bilirubin released from the RE system. Indirect bilirubin reacts only in a nonaqueous (alcohol) medium. The total bilirubin is the sum of the direct-acting and the indirect-acting fractions and normally does not exceed 1 mg/100 ml of serum. In hematologic diseases associated with abrupt breakdown of large numbers of red blood cells (hemolytic anemias, transfusion reactions), the liver may receive more bilirubin from the RE system than it can detoxify. The level of indirect or unconjugated bilirubin therefore is elevated.

In biliary obstruction the hepatocytes pick up bilirubin and conjugate it with glucuronide molecules but cannot dispose of it. The conjugated form is then regurgitated into the bloodstream, with resultant elevation of the direct-acting bilirubin fraction. The indirect-acting bilirubin may also rise slightly in biliary obstruction, but the direct bilirubin predominates.

The direct or conjugated form also predominates in hepatocellular disease. Excretion of bilirubin is the step most readily affected when the hepatocytes are damaged; therefore the diseased hepatocytes continue to take in and conjugate bilirubin but are unable to excrete it. As in biliary obstruction, the accumulated conjugated bilirubin is regurgitated into the blood.

The direct/indirect patterns may be summarized as follows:

	Direct bilirubin predominates	**Indirect bilirubin predominates**
Hemolysis		X
Hepatocellular disease	X	
Biliary obstruction	X	

Elevation of serum bilirubin results in jaundice, which is a yellow coloration of the skin, sclerae, and body secretions. Jaundice is a nonspecific finding seen in massive blood breakdown, hepatocellular disease, or biliary obstruction. Chemical separation of bilirubin into direct and indirect fractions helps to specify a hepatocellular or hematologic cause for jaundice. Furthermore, if jaundice results from liver disease, the level of bilirubin may help to separate hepatocellular disease from obstruction since it is uncommon for the total bilirubin to rise above 35 mg/100 ml of serum with obstruction.

Hormone and drug detoxification

The liver breaks down several hormones that otherwise would accumulate in the body. For example, failure to metabolize estrogen in men with chronic hepatocellular disease, such as cirrhosis, causes gynecomastia (breast enlargement), testicular atrophy, and changes in body-hair patterns. Reduced detoxification of the hormone glucagon, which is an insulin antagonist, occurs in liver disease and may contribute to the fluctuations in blood-sugar levels seen in severe hepatic disorders. The liver is also the primary location for breakdown of medications and other foreign chemicals administered orally or parenterally. It is of particular concern that doses of medications be reduced to compensate for the loss of this function in patients with severe liver disease; otherwise accumulation of drugs may lead to overdosage.

Bile

Bile is the excretory product of the liver. It is formed continuously by the hepatocytes, collects in the bile canaliculi adjacent to these cells, and is transported to the gut via the bile ducts. The principal components of bile are water, bile salts, and bile pigments (primarily bilirubin diglucuronide). Other components include cholesterol, lecithin, and protein. The primary functions of bile are the emulsification of intestinal fat and the removal of waste products excreted by the liver.

Fats are absorbed into the portal blood and intestinal lymphatics in the form of monoglycerides and triglycerides by the action of the intestinal mucosa, but efficient absorption occurs only when the fat molecules are suspended in solution through the emulsifying action of bile salts. As emulsifiers, bile salts act like nonionic detergents to suspend fats in solution within the watery medium of the intestinal contents. Both hepatocellular disease and biliary obstruction affect the amount of bile salts available for fat absorption, but obstruction generally has the more profound effect. Absence of bile salts may lead to steatorrhea (fatty stools), but a more important effect is failure of absorption of the fat-soluble vitamins (D, A, K, and E). As previously noted, vitamin K is an essential precursor for hepatic production of several clotting factors; the absence of this vitamin leads to bleeding tendencies in patients with hepatobiliary disease.

Bile Pigments

According to Filly et al., bile pigments are the principal cause of ultrasonic scattering in echogenic bile, although cholesterol crystals may also contribute to this finding. The presence of echogenic bile indicates stasis, but this stasis is not always pathologic and may simply result from prolonged fasting.

Portal Hypertension

The majority of blood passing through the small and large bowel is collected in the portal venous system and transported to the liver. In the liver, it passes through an intricate system of vascular channels, which allows maximum contact of the blood with hepatocytes. Many hepatocellular diseases, particularly those associated with chronic inflammation (i.e., cirrhosis), result in scarring of the hepatic parenchyma and distortion of the hepatic architecture. The narrow passageways through which the portal blood travels are obstructed by the scarring process, which interferes with the flow of portal blood through the hepatic parenchyma. When flow restriction is advanced, portal hypertension (increased venous pressure) occurs and portal blood is forced to bypass the liver via collateral channels. Many of these collateral pathways include small veins in submucosal locations in the stomach and esophagus. These vessels are not equipped to accept the pressure and flow associated with portal hypertension and they are therefore subject to rupture. Major blood loss into the gastrointestinal tract may ensue, especially in the presence of coagulation disorders, which are commonly associated with severe liver disease. The combination of anatomic and metabolic abnormalities produces a dangerous situation that, as noted previously, is often the direct or indirect cause of death.

Liver Function Tests

The term *liver function tests* refers to a group of laboratory tests established to analyze how the liver is performing under normal and diseased conditions.

In patients with known liver disease a number of laboratory tests are used to help in the diagnosis, including the following:

1. Aspartate aminotransferase (AST, formerly SGOT)
2. Alanine aminotransferase (ALT, formerly SGPT)
3. Lactic acid dehydrogenase (LDH)
4. Alkaline phosphatase (Alk Phos)
5. Bilirubin (indirect, direct, and total)
6. Prothrombin time
7. Albumin and globulins

Aspartate Aminotransferase (AST or SGOT)

Aspartate aminotransferase is an enzyme present is tissues that have a high rate of metabolic activity, one of which is the liver. As a result of death or injury to the producing cells, the enzyme is released into the bloodstream in abnormally high levels. Any disease that injures the cells causes an elevation in AST levels. This enzyme is also produced in other high-metabolic tissues, so an elevation does not always mean liver disease is present. Significant elevations are characteristic of acute hepatitis and cirrhosis. The level is also elevated in patients with hepatic necrosis, acute hepatitis, and infectious mononucleosis.

Alanine Aminotransferase (ALT or SGPT)

Alanine aminotransferase is more specific than AST for evaluating liver function. This enzyme is slightly elevated in acute cirrhosis, hepatic metastasis, and pancreatitis. There is a mild to moderate increase in obstructive jaundice. Hepatocellular disease and infectious or toxic hepatitis produce moderate to highly increased levels. (In alcoholic hepatitis, AST is higher.)

Lactic Acid Dehydrogenase

Lactic acid dehydrogenase is found in the tissues of several systems including the kidneys, heart, skeletal muscle, brain, liver, and lungs. Cellular injury and death cause this enzyme to increase. This test is moderately increased in infectious mononucleosis and mildly elevated in hepatitis, cirrhosis, and obstructive jaundice. Its primary use is in detection of myocardial or pulmonary infarction.

Alkaline Phosphatase

Alkaline phosphatase is produced by the liver, bone, intestines, and placenta. It may be a good indicator of intrahepatic or extrahepatic obstruction, hepatic carcinoma, abscess, or cirrhosis. In hepatitis and cirrhosis the enzyme is moderately elevated.

Bilirubin

Bilirubin is a product of the breakdown of hemoglobin in tired red blood cells. The liver converts these byproducts into bile pigments, which, along with other factors, are secreted as bile by the liver cells into the bile ducts.

The following are three ways this cycle can be disturbed:

1. With an excessive amount of red blood cell destruction
2. With malfunction of liver cells
3. With blockage of ducts leading from cells

These disturbances cause a rise in serum bilirubin, which leaks into the tissues and thus gives the skin a jaundice, or yellow coloration.

Indirect bilirubin is unconjugated bilirubin. Elevation of this test is seen with increased red blood cell destruction (anemias, trauma from a hematoma, or hemorrhagic pulmonary infarct).

Direct bilirubin is conjugated bilirubin. This product circulates in the blood and is excreted into the bile after it reaches the liver and is conjugated with glucuronide. Elevation of direct bilirubin is usually related to obstructive jaundice (From stones or neoplasm).

Specific liver diseases may cause an elevation of both direct and indirect bilirubin levels, but the increase in the direct level is more marked. These diseases are hepatic metastasis, hepatitis, lymphoma, cholestasis secondary to drugs, and cirrhosis.

Prothrombin Time

Prothrombin is a liver enzyme that is part of the blood-clotting mechanism. The production of prothrombin depends on adequate intake and use of vitamin K. The prothrombin time is increased in the presence of liver disease with cellular damage. Cirrhosis and metastatic disease are examples of disorders that cause prolonged prothrombin time.

Albumin and Globulins

Assessment of depressed synthesis or proteins, especially serum albumin and the plasma coagulation factors, is a sensitive test for metabolic derangement of the liver. In patients with hepatocellular damage a low serum albumin suggests decreased protein synthesis. A prolonged prothrombin time indicates a poor prognosis. Chronic liver diseases commonly show an elevation of gamma globulins.

SONOGRAPHIC EVALUATION OF HEPATIC STRUCTURES

Evaluation of the hepatic structures is one of the most important procedures in sonography for many reasons. The normal, basically homogeneous parenchyma of the liver allows one to image the neighboring anatomic structures in the upper abdomen. Echo amplitude, attenuation, transmission, and parenchymal textures may be physically assessed with proper evaluation of the hepatic structures.

Within the homogeneous parenchyma lie the thin-walled hepatic veins, the brightly reflective portal veins, the hepatic arteries, and the hepatic duct. Color flow is useful in determining the direction of flow of the portal and hepatic veins. The portal flow is shown to be hepatopedal (toward the liver), whereas the hepatic venous flow is hepatofugal (away from the liver) (Figs. 5-18 and 5-19; see color image). The portal vein serves as the landmark to locate the smaller hepatic duct and artery. Near the porta hepatis, the hepatic duct can be seen along the anterior lateral border of the portal vein, whereas the hepatic artery can be seen along the anterior medial border. With color Doppler, the hepatic artery would show flow toward the liver, whereas the ductal system would show no flow (Fig. 5-20; see color image).

The system gain should be adjusted to adequately penetrate the entire right lobe of the liver as a smooth, homogeneous echo-texture pattern (Fig. 5-21). Enough sensitivity must be present to image the normal smooth liver parenchyma. If too much gain is used, the electronic "noise" or "snow" produced as low-level echoes appears in the background of the image (outside the liver parenchyma—above the diaphragm or within the vascular structures). The ultrasound manufacturers have made it possible to preselect various preprocessing and postprocessing controls to allow the sonographer to emphasize or highlight various aspects of the liver parenchyma.

The time-gain compensation should be adjusted to balance the far-gain and the near-gain echo signals. The easiest way to do this is to hold the transducer over a large

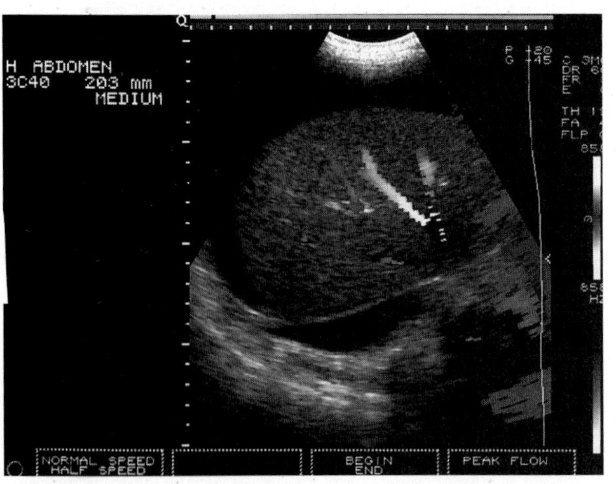

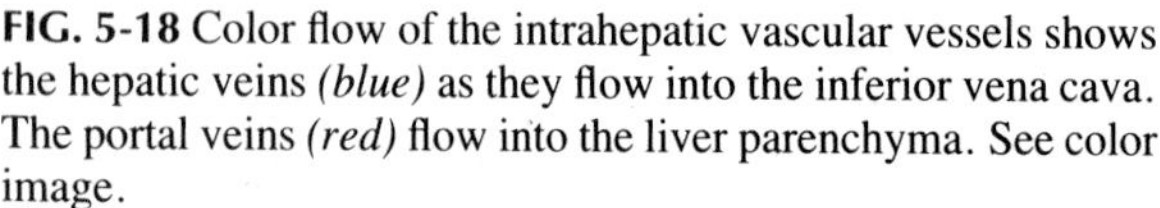

FIG. 5-18 Color flow of the intrahepatic vascular vessels shows the hepatic veins *(blue)* as they flow into the inferior vena cava. The portal veins *(red)* flow into the liver parenchyma. See color image.

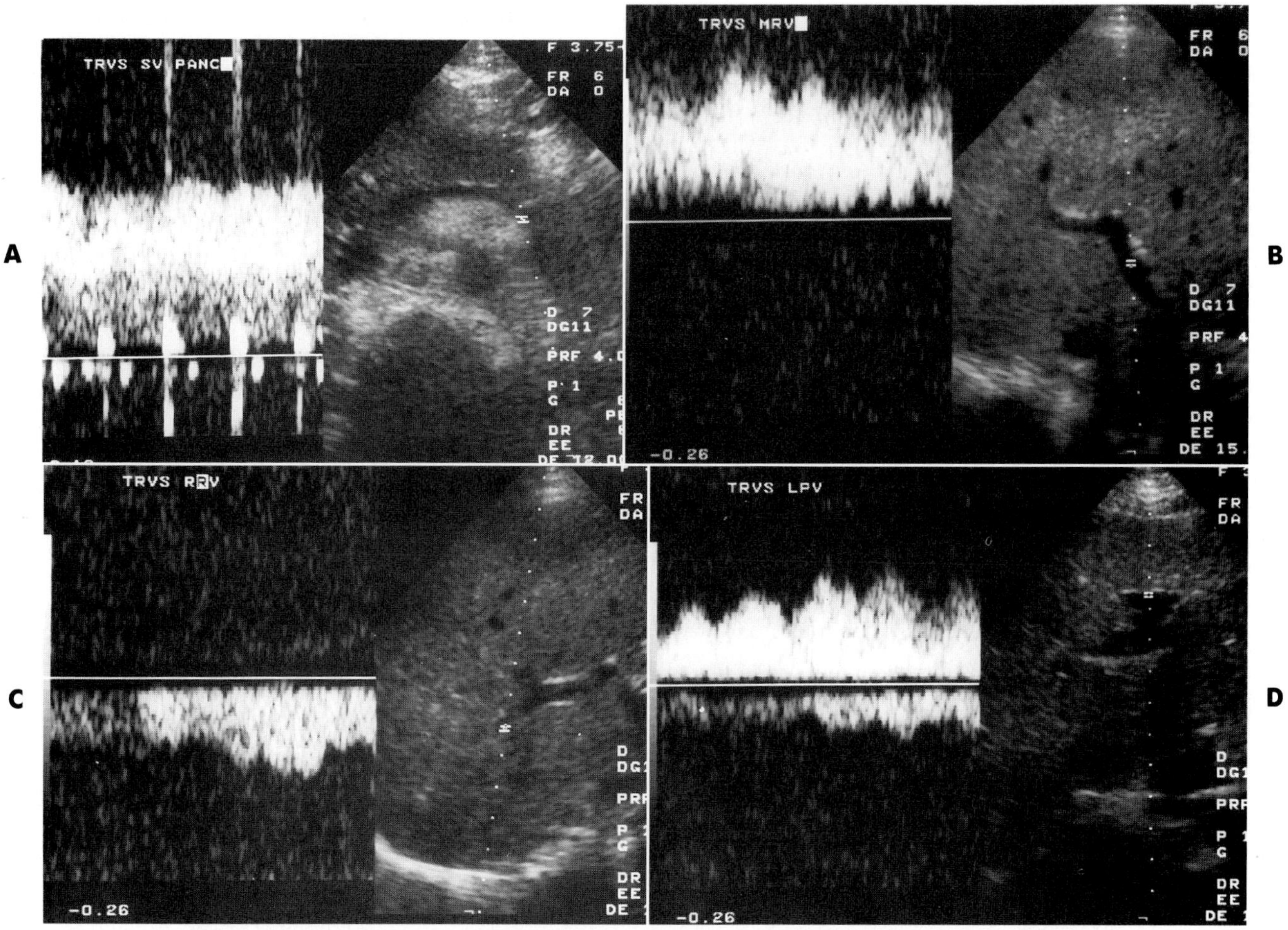

FIG. 5-19 Normal Doppler flow patterns of the splenic vein, **A;** main portal vein, **B;** posterior right portal vein, **C;** and left portal vein, **D.**

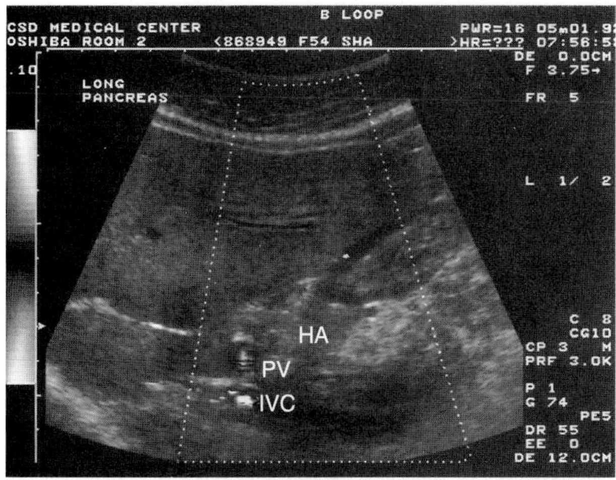

FIG. 5-20 Color Doppler in the longitudinal plane shows the hepatic arterial flow, *HA*, anterior to the portal vein, *PV*, and inferior vena cava, *IVC*. See color image.

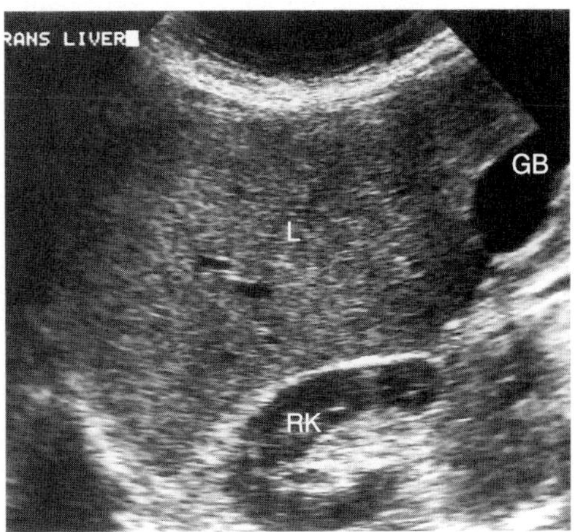

FIG. 5-21 The liver parenchyma should be smooth, uniform, and homogeneous throughout. The right kidney should be well-defined and the gallbladder should be echo-free.

segment of the right lobe of the liver. The far–time–gain control pods should gradually be increased until the posterior aspect of the liver is well seen. The near-field time-gain controls should be adjusted to image the anterior wall and musculature, the anterior hepatic capsule, and the near field of the hepatic parenchyma. The depth should be adjusted so the posterior right lobe is positioned at the lower border of the screen. The electronic focus on the equipment is positioned near the posterior border of the liver, or the multiple focus points may be positioned equidistant throughout the liver to further enhance the hepatic parenchyma. The multiple-focus technique causes the frame rate to decrease and causes a "slower sweep" of the real time picture. If the patient cannot take a deep breath, the sonographer may chose not to use the multiple-frequency focus with decreased frame rate. In most patients who can suspend their respiration for a variable amount of time, this multifocal technique works very well, since the liver is a nondynamic organ and does not need a high frame rate for a quality image to be obtained.

The appropriate transducer would depend on the patient's body habitus and the clinical request for the ultrasound examination. The transducer frequency depends on the body habitus and size. The average adult abdomen usually requires a 3.5-MHz frequency, whereas the more obese adult may require a 2.25-MHz. Slender adults and young children may require a 5-MHz frequency, and the neonate may need a high-frequency 7.5-MHz transducer.

Generally, a wider "pie" sector or curved linear array transducer is the most appropriate to optimally image the near field of the abdomen. This transducer is especially useful in detecting liver abscesses or metastases. To image the far field better, a sector or annular array transducer with a longer focal zone is used. Often the transducers are interchanged throughout the examination to obtain the ideal image pattern.

Adequate scanning technique demands that each patient be examined with the following criteria (Figs. 5-22 and 5-23):

1. The sonographer needs to assess:
   a. The size of the liver in the longitudinal plane
   b. The attenuation of the liver parenchyma
   c. Liver texture
   d. The presence of hepatic vascular structures

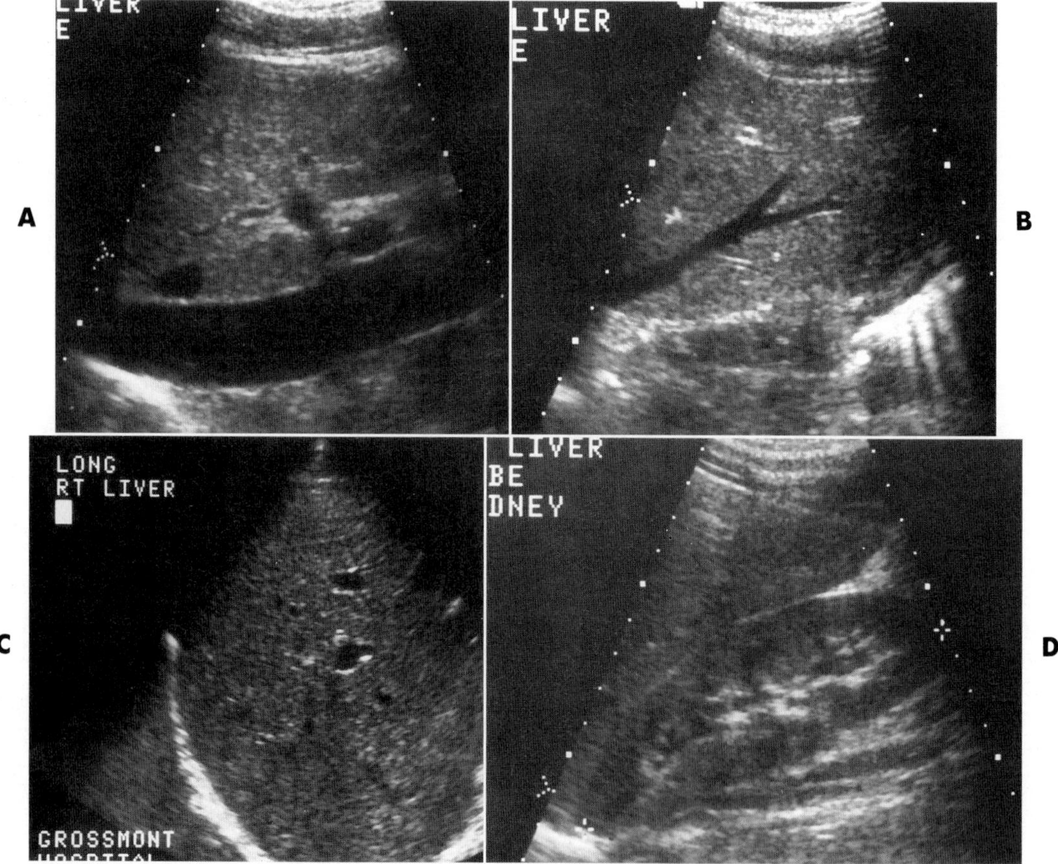

FIG. 5-22 A normal liver examination includes evaluation of the left lobe, caudate lobe, right lobe, and vascular structures. The following scans are longitudinal examples of the liver: **A,** Inferior vena cava and left lobe of the liver with portal and hepatic vascular structures. **B,** Right lobe with right hepatic vein. **C,** Right lobe of the liver with the echogenic diaphragm. **D,** Lateral edge of the right lobe of the liver and long axis of the right kidney.

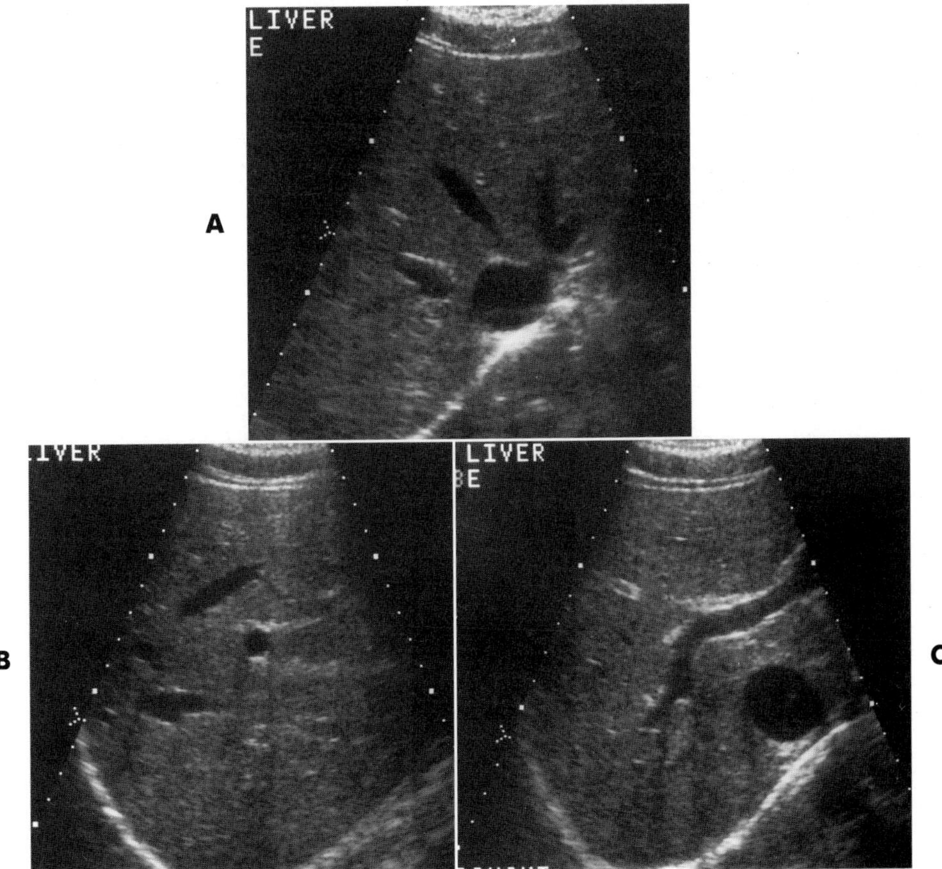

FIG. 5-23 Transverse scans of the normal liver include: **A,** Cephalic angulation to image the hepatic veins as they drain into the inferior vena cava at the level of the diaphragm. **B,** Right lobe of the liver with portal and hepatic branches. **C,** Right lobe of the liver with the main portal vein and posterior branch of the right portal vein.

2. The basic instrumentation should be adjusted in the following parameters:
   a. Time gain compensation
   b. Overall gain
   c. Transducer frequency
   d. Depth

Ultrasound Examination Technique

Supine Longitudinal Scan Plane

The longitudinal or sagittal scan offers an excellent window to visualize the hepatic structures. With the patient in full inspiration, the transducer may be swept under the costal margin (with slight to medium pressure) to record the liver parenchyma from the anterior abdominal wall to the diaphragm.

Scan I. The initial scan should be made slightly to the left of the midline to record the left lobe of the liver and the abdominal aorta. The left hepatic and portal veins may be seen as small circular structures in this view (Fig. 5-24).

Scan II. As one moves midline or slightly to the right of midline, a larger segment of the left lobe and the inferior vena cava may be seen posteriorly. In this view, it is useful to record the inferior vena cava as it is dilated near the end of inspiration. The left or middle hepatic vein may be imaged as it drains into the inferior vena cava near the level of the diaphragm. The area of the porta hepatis is shown anterior to the inferior vena cava as the superior mesenteric vein and splenic vein converge to form the main portal vein. The common bile duct may be seen just anterior to the main portal vein. The head of the pancreas may be seen just inferior to the right lobe of the liver and main portal vein and anterior to the inferior vena cava (Figs. 5-25 to 5-27).

Scan III. The next image should be made slightly lateral to this sagittal plane to record part of the right portal vein and right lobe of liver. The caudate lobe is often seen in this view (Fig. 5-28).

Scans IV, V, and VI. The next three scans should be made in small increments through the right lobe of the liver (Figs. 5-29 to 5-31). The last scan is usually made to show the right kidney and lateral segment of the right lobe of the liver. The liver texture is compared to the renal parenchyma. The normal liver parenchyma should have a softer, more homogeneous texture than the dense medulla and hypoechoic renal cortex. Liver size may be measured from

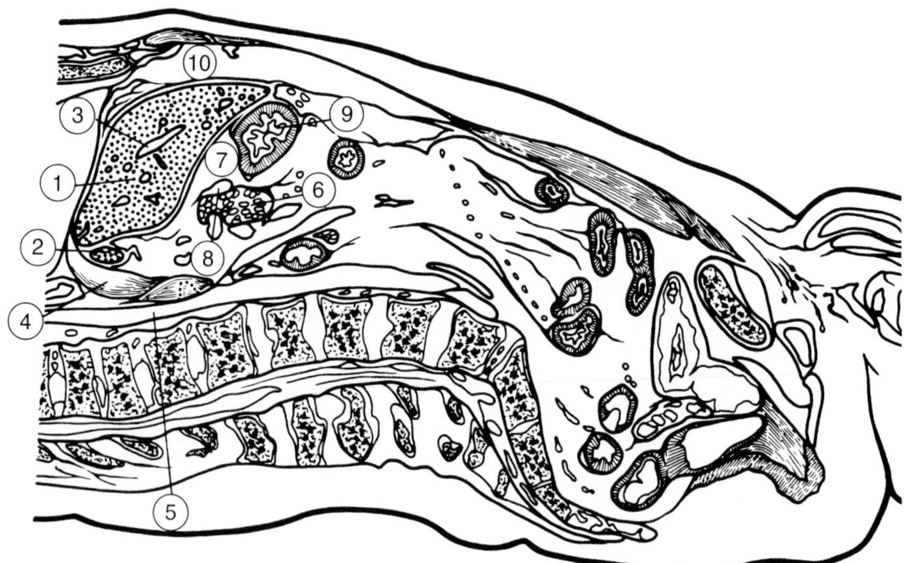

FIG. 5-24 Scan I, see text. Left lobe, *1;* caudate lobe, *2;* portal vein, *3;* crus of the diaphragm, *4;* arota, *5;* pancreas, *6;* lesser omentum, *7;* lesser sac, *8;* stomach, *9;* falciform ligament, *10*. (From Hagen-Ansert SL: The anatomy workbook. Philadelphia, 1986, JB Lippincott.)

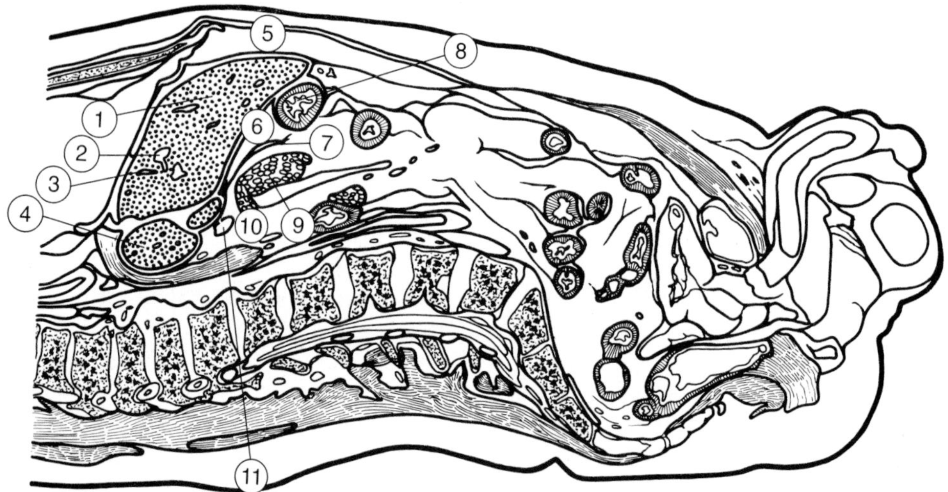

FIG. 5-25 Scan II, see text. Left lobe, *1;* portal vein, *2;* hepatic vein, *3;* caudate lobe, *4;* falciform ligament, *5;* lesser omentum, *6;* lesser sac, *7;* pyloric antrum, *8;* pancreas, *9;* crus of the diaphragm, *10;* hepatic artery, *11*. (From Hagen-Ansert SL: The anatomy workbook. Philadelphia: 1986, JB Lippincott.)

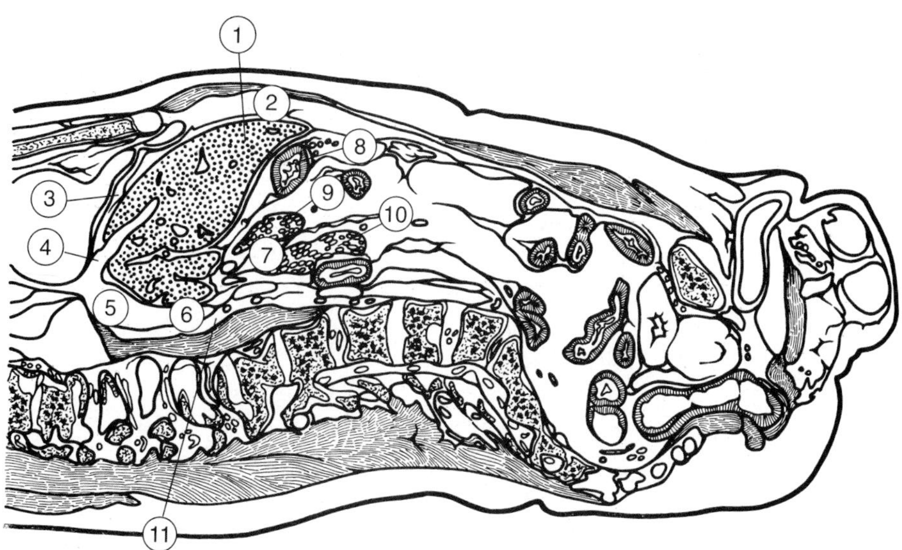

FIG. 5-26 Scan II, see text. Left lobe, *1;* falciform ligament, *2;* diaphragm, *3;* hepatic vein, *4;* inferior vena cava, *5;* hepatic artery, *6;* portal vein, *7;* pyloric antrum, *8;* pancreatic head, *9;* uncinate process, *10;* crus of the diaphragm, *11*. (From Hagen-Ansert SL: The anatomy workbook. Philadelphia: 1986, JB Lippincott.)

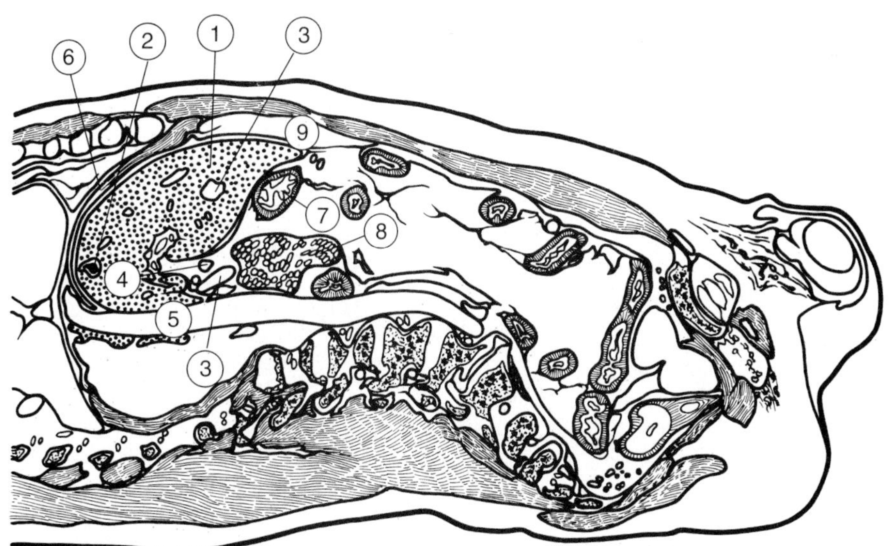

FIG. 5-27 Scan II, see text. Left lobe, *1;* hepatic vein, *2;* portal vein, *3;* hepatic artery, *4;* inferior vena cava, *5;* diaphragm, *6;* pyloric antrum, *7;* pancreas, *8;* falciform ligament, *9*. (From Hagen-Ansert SL: The anatomy workbook. Philadelphia, 1986, JB Lippincott.)

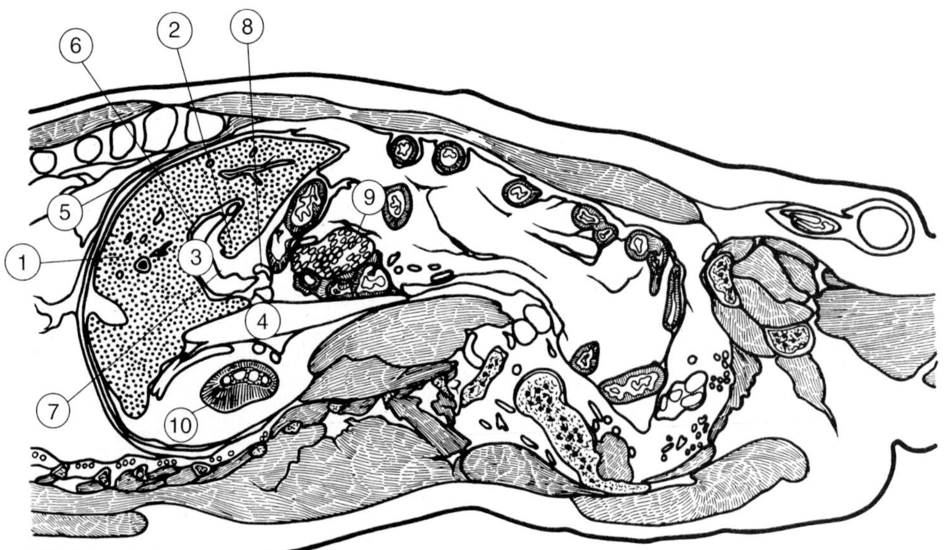

FIG. 5-28 Scan III, see text. Right lobe, *1;* caudate lobe, *2;* left portal vein, *3;* inferior vena cava, *4;* diaphragm, *5;* fissure of the ligamentum teres, *6;* hepatic artery, *7;* common bile duct, *8;* head of the pancreas, *9;* right kidney, *10*. (From Hagen-Ansert SL: The anatomy workbook. Philadelphia, 1986, JB Lippincott.)

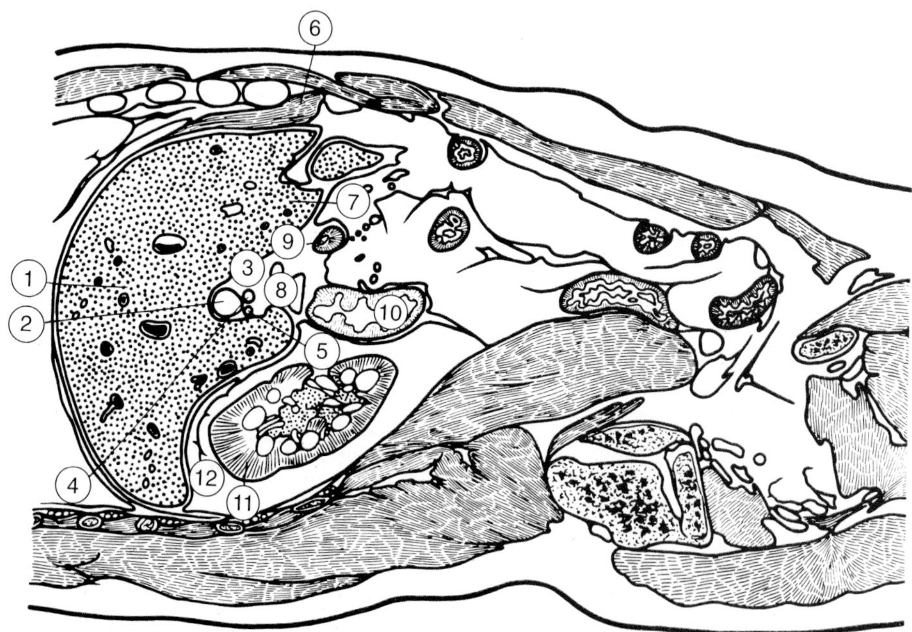

FIG. 5-29 Scan IV, see text. Right lobe, *1;* right portal vein, *2;* port hepatis, *3;* hepatic artery, *4;* common bile duct, *5;* diaphragm, *6;* quadrate lobe, *7;* neck of gallbladder, *8;* superior part of the duodenum, *9;* descending part of the duodenum, *10;* right kidney, *11;* perirenal fat, *12*. (From Hagen-Ansert SL: The anatomy workbook. Philadephia, 1986, JB Lippincott.)

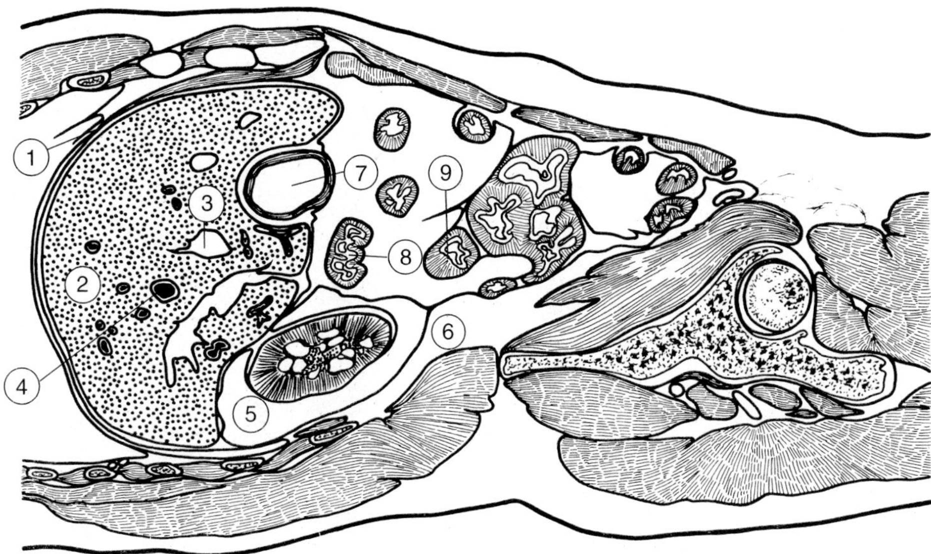

FIG. 5-30 Scan V, see text. Diaphragm, *1;* right lobe, *2;* portal vein, *3;* hepatic vein, *4;* perirenal fat, *5;* retroperitoneal fat, *6;* gallbladder, *7;* hepatic flexure, *8;* ascending colon, *9.* (From Hagen-Ansert SL: The anatomy workbook. Philadelphia, 1986, JB Lippincott.)

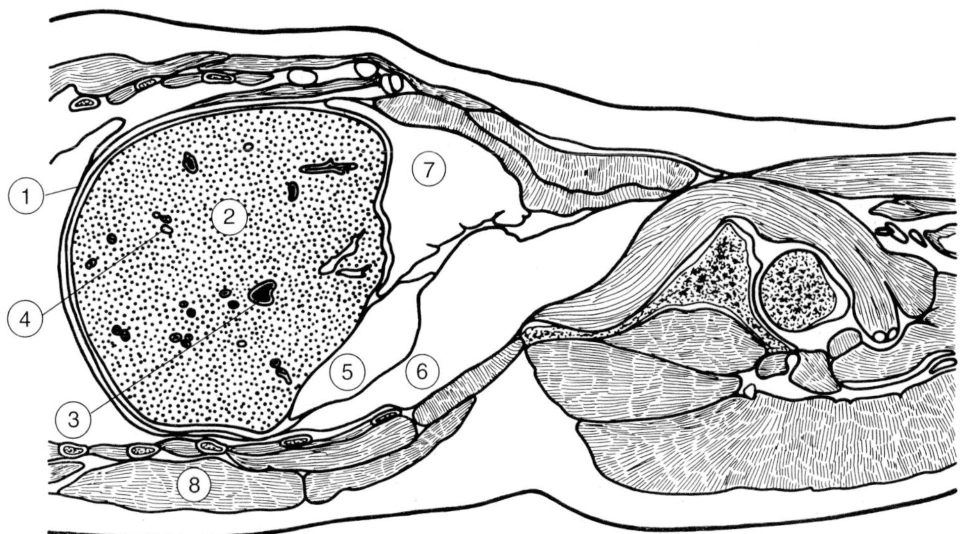

FIG. 5-31 Scan VI, see text. Diaphragm, *1;* right lobe, *2;* hepatic vein, *3;* protal vein, *4;* perirenal fat, *5;* retroperitoneal fat, *6;* omentum, *7;* latissimus dorsal muscle, *8.* (From Hagen-Ansert SL: The anatomy workbook. Philadelphia, 1986, JB Lippincott.)

the tip of the liver to the diaphragm. Generally this measurement is less than 15 cm, with 15 to 20 cm representing the upper limits of normal. Hepatomegaly is present when the liver measurement exceeds 20 cm.

Supine Transverse Scan Plane

Multiple transverse scans are made across the upper abdomen to record specific areas of the liver. The transducer should be angled in a steep cephalic direction to be as parallel to the diaphragm as possible. The patient should be in full inspiration to maintain detail of the liver parenchyma, vascular architecture, and ductal structures.

Scan I. The initial transverse scan is made with the transducer under the costal margin at a steep angle perpendicular to the diaphragm (Fig. 5-32). The patient should be in deep inspiration to adequately record the dome of the liver. One should identify the inferior vena cava and three hepatic veins as they drain into the cava. This pattern has

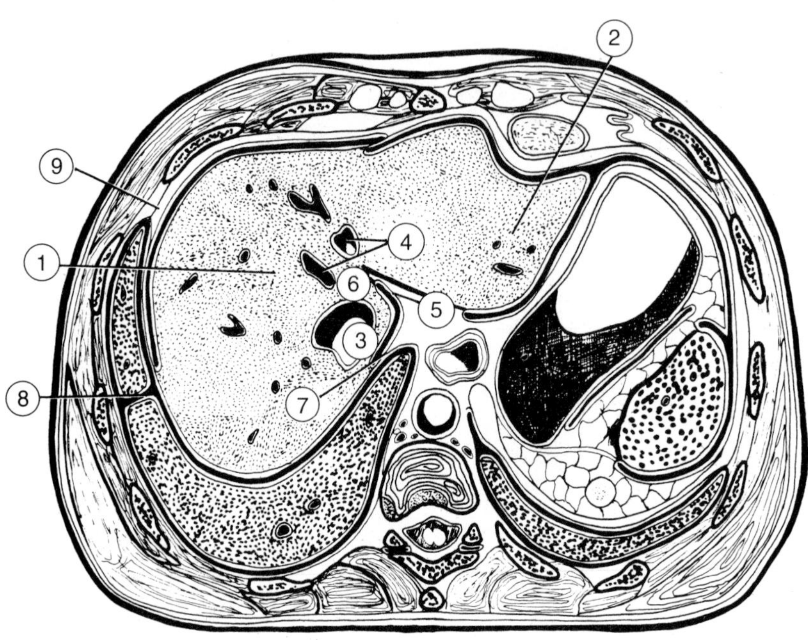

FIG. 5-32 Scan I, see text. Right lobe, *1;* left lobe, *2;* inferior vena cava, *3;* hepatic vein, *4;* ligamentum venosum, *5;* caudate lobe, *6;* coronary hepatic ligament, *7;* pleural cavity, *8;* diaphragm, *9.* (From Hagen-Ansert SL: The anatomy workbook. Philadelphia, 1986, JB Lippincott.)

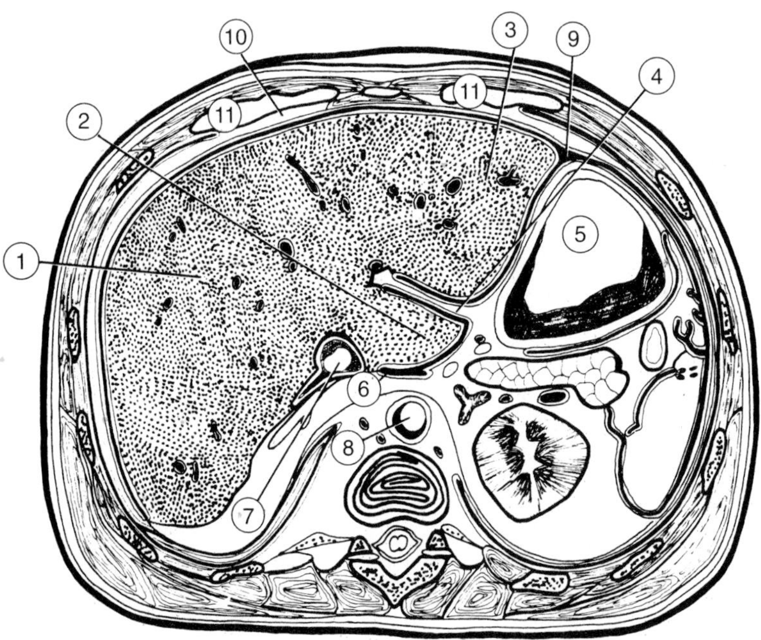

FIG. 5-33 Scan III, see text. Right lobe, *1;* caudate lobe, *2;* left lobe, *3;* hepatogastric ligament, *4;* stomach, *5;* omental bursa, *6;* inferior vena cava, *7;* aorta, *8;* peritoneal cavity, *9;* diaphragm, *10;* rectus abdominis muscle, *11.* (From Hagen-Ansert SL: The anatomy workbook. Philadelphia, 1986, JB Lippincott.)

sometimes been referred to as the *reindeer sign* or *playboy bunny sign*.

Scan II. The transducer is then directed slightly inferior to this point to record the left portal vein as it flows into the left lobe of the liver.

Scan III. The porta hepatis is seen as a tubular structure within the central part of the liver. Sometimes the left or right portal vein can be identified. The caudate lobe may be seen just superior to the porta hepatis; thus, depending on the angle, either the caudate lobe is shown anterior to

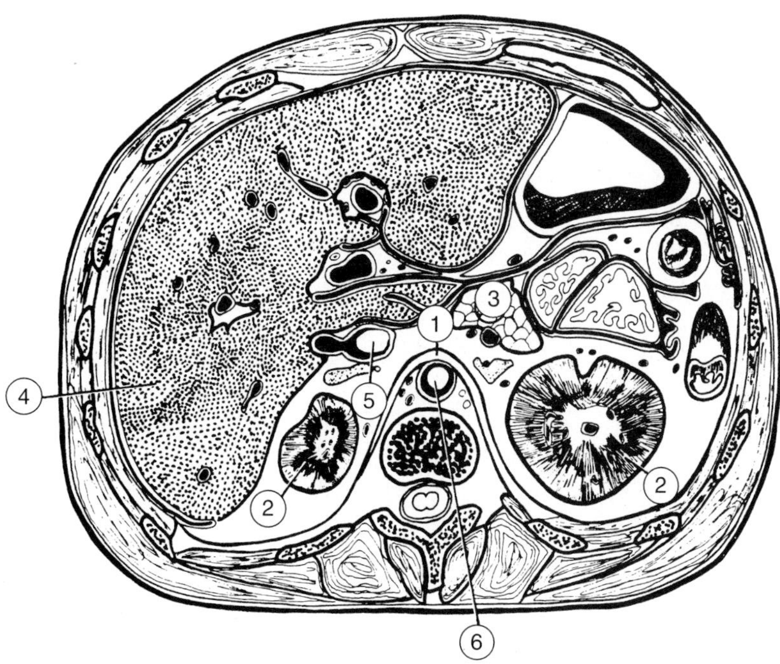

FIG. 5-34 Scan IV, see text. Crus, *1;* kidneys, *2;* pancreas, *3;* right lobe of the liver, *4;* inferior vena cava, *5;* aorta, *6.* (From Hagen-Ansert SL: The anatomy workbook. Philadelphia, 1986, JB Lippincott.)

the inferior vena cava, or as you move inferior, the porta hepatis is identified anterior to the inferior vena cava (Fig. 5-33).

Scan IV. The fourth scan should show the right portal vein as it divides into the anterior and posterior segments of the right lobe of the liver. The gallbladder may be seen in this scan as an anechoic structure medial to the right lobe and anterior to the right kidney (Fig. 5-34).

Scans V and VI. These two scans are made through the lower segment of the right lobe of the liver. The right kidney is the posterior border (Fig. 5-35). Usually intrahepatic vascular structures are not identified in these views (Fig. 5-36).

Left Anterior Oblique Scans

The left anterior oblique scan requires that the patient roll slightly to the left. A 45-degree sponge or pillow may be placed under the right hip to support the patient. This view allows better visualization of the lower right lobe of the liver, usually displacing the duodenum and transverse colon to the midline of the abdomen, out of the field of view. Transverse, oblique, or longitudinal scans may be made in this position.

Left Lateral Decubitus Scans

If the previously described scans do not allow adequate visualization of the liver and vascular structures, the lateral decubitus position may be used. If the body habitus allows the transducer to image in between the intercostal spaces, additional views may be obtained of the dome of the liver and medial segment of the the left lobe of the liver.

PATHOLOGY OF THE LIVER

The evaluation of the liver parenchyma includes the assessment of its size, configuration, homogeneity, and contour. Liver volume can be determined from serial scans in an effort to detect subtle increases in size or hepatomegaly. The development and clinical utility of three-dimensional ultrasound in determining organ volumes is currently under clinical investigation in many academic institutions.

As in other organ systems, the hepatic parenchyma pattern changes with disease processes. Hepatocellular disease affects the hepatocytes and interferes with liver function enzymes. Cirrhosis, ascites, or fatty liver patterns may be detected with the ultrasound examination. In an effort to provide a differential diagnosis for the clinician, intrahepatic, extrahepatic, subhepatic, and subdiaphragmatic masses may be outlined and their internal composition recognized as specific echo patterns.

In subsequent pages we discuss the pathology of liver disease in the following categories: diffuse disease, functional disease, abscess formation, hepatic trauma and transplantation, benign disease, malignant disease, and vascular problems.

Diffuse Disease

Diffuse hepatocellular disease both affects the hepatocytes and interferes with liver function. The hepatocyte is a parenchymal liver cell that performs all the functions ascribed to the liver. This abnormality is measured through the series of liver function tests. The hepatic enzyme levels are elevated with cell necrosis. With cholestasis (i.e.,

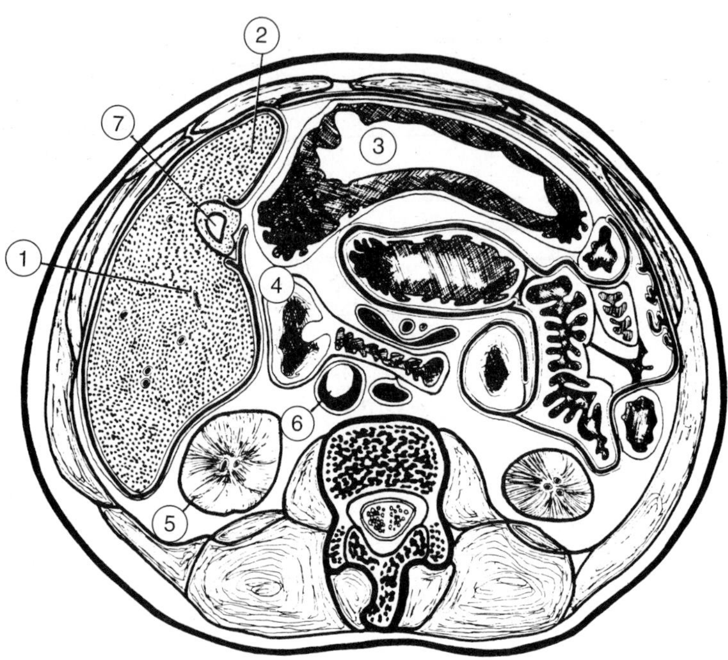

FIG. 5-35 Scan V, see text. Right lobe, *1;* quadrate lobe, *2;* stomach, *3;* duodenum, *4;* right kidney, *5;* inferior vena cava, *6;* gallbladder, *7.* (From Hagen-Ansert SL: The anatomy workbook. Philadelphia, 1986, JB Lippincott.)

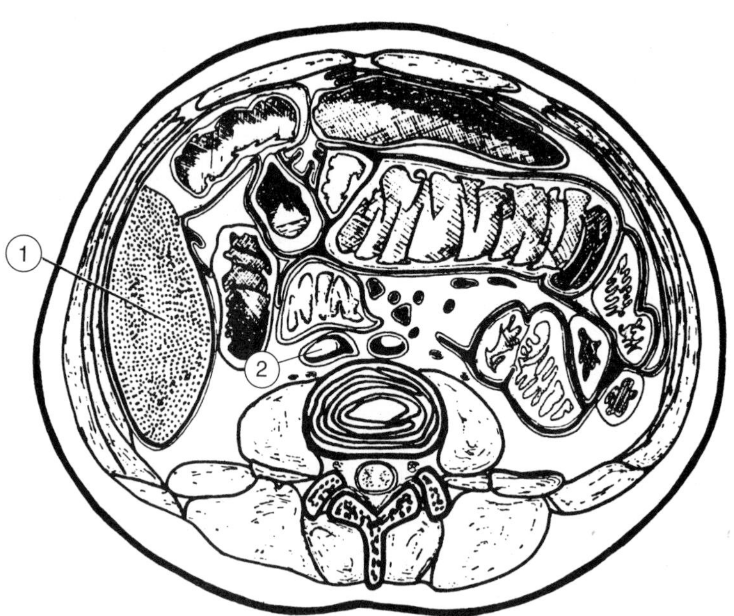

FIG. 5-36 Scan VI, see text. Right lobe, *1;* inferior vena cava, *2.* (From Hagen-Ansert SL: The anatomy workbook. Philadelphia, 1986, JB Lippincott.)

interruption in the flow of bile through any part of the biliary system, from the liver to the duodenum) the alkaline phosphatase and direct bilirubin levels increase. Likewise, when there are defects in protein synthesis, there may be elevated serum bilirubin levels and decreased serum albumin and clotting factor levels.

There are many subcategories of diffuse parenchymal disease, including fatty infiltration, acute and chronic hepatitis, early alcoholic liver disease, and acute and chronic cirrhosis.

Fatty Infiltration

Fatty infiltration implies increased lipid accumulation in the hepatocytes and results from significant injury to the

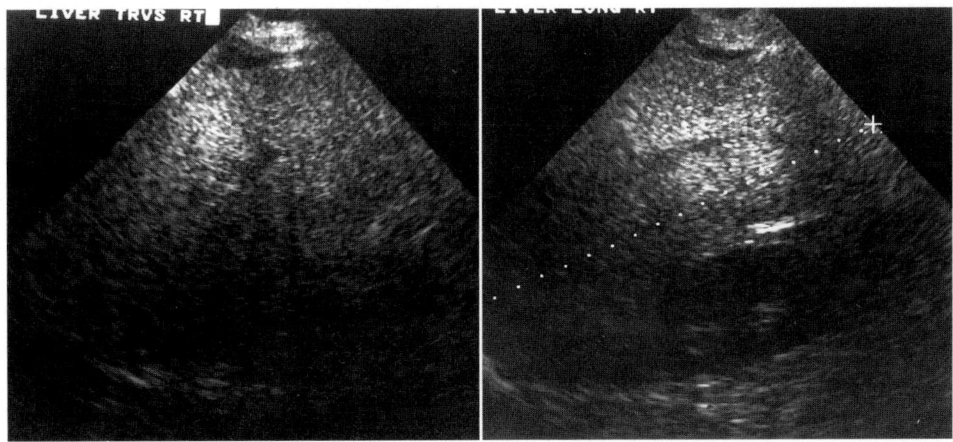

FIG. 5-37 Transverse and longitudinal scans of the liver show increased echogenicity and attenuation in this patient with fatty infiltration.

DIFFUSE DISEASE ULTRASOUND FINDINGS

Fatty Liver Ultrasound
Increased echogenicity
Increased attenuation of sound
Impaired visualization of borders of intrahepatic vessels
Hepatomegaly

Focal Fatty Infiltration Ultrasound
Patchy distribution
Nonspherical
Poorly marginated
Fan-shaped
No "mass effect" produced (normal portal vascular preserved)

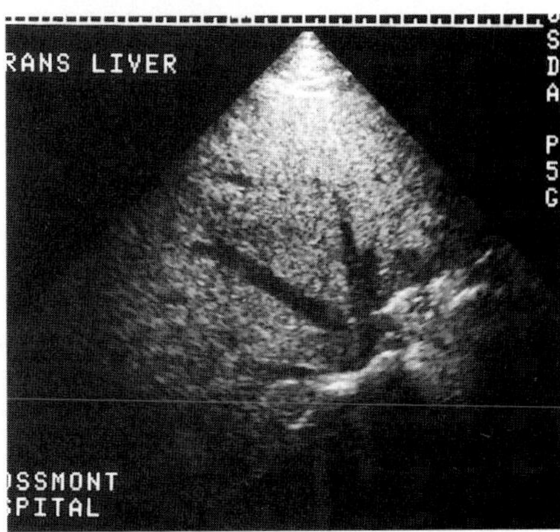

FIG. 5-38 Transverse scan of grade I fatty infiltration of the liver. There is a slight diffuse increase in fine echoes in the liver parenchyma with normal visualization of the vessels and diaphragm.

liver or a systemic disorder leading to impaired or excessive metabolism of fat. Fatty infiltration is a benign process and may be reversible. Common causes of fatty liver are alcoholic liver disease, diabetes mellitus, obesity, severe hepatitis, chronic illness, and steroids.

Moderate to severe fatty infiltration shows increased echogenicity on ultrasound (Fig. 5-37). Enlargement of the lobe affected by the fatty infiltration is evident. The portal vein structures may be difficult to visualize because of the increased attenuation of the ultrasound. Thus it becomes more difficult to see the outline of the portal vein and hepatic vein borders. Authors have stated that this increase in echo texture may result from increased collagen content of the liver or increases in lipid accumulation. The following three grades of liver texture have been defined in sonography for classification of fatty infiltration:

- Grade 1: a slight diffuse increase in fine echoes in the hepatic parenchyma with normal visualization of the diaphragm and intrahepatic vessel borders (Fig. 5-38).
- Grade 2: a moderate diffuse increase in fine echoes with slightly impaired visualization of the intrahepatic vessels and diaphragm (Fig. 5-39).
- Grade 3: a marked increase in fine echoes with poor or no visualization of the intrahepatic vessel borders, diaphragm, and posterior portion of the right lobe of the liver (Fig. 5-40).

Fatty infiltration is not always uniform throughout the liver parenchyma. It is not uncommon to see patchy distribution of fat, especially in the right lobe of the liver. The fat does not displace normal vascular architecture.

The other characteristics of fatty infiltration is focal sparing. This condition should be suspected in patients who have masslike hypoechoic areas in typical locations in a liver that is otherwise increased in echogenicity. The most common areas are anterior to the gallbladder or the portal vein and the posterior portion of the left lobe of the liver (Fig. 5-41).

Hepatitis

Hepatitis involves general inflammation of the liver. In the United States, about 60% of acute viral hepatitis is type B, about 20% is type A, and about 20% is type non-A, non-B. Type A hepatitis is transmitted primarily by the fecal-oral route. Type B is transmitted through a chronic carrier or via a parenteral inoculation.

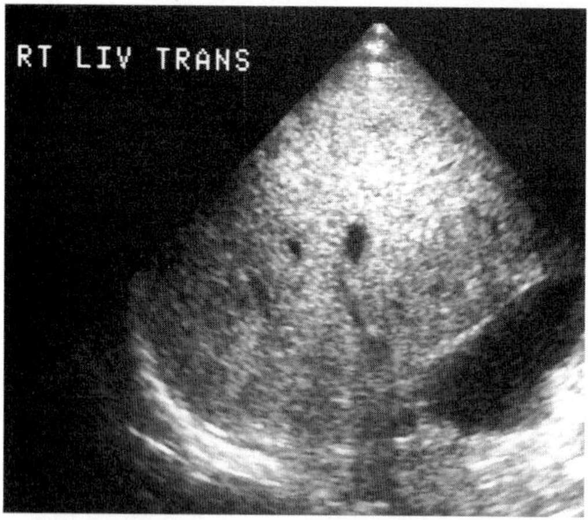

FIG. 5-39 Transverse scan of grade II fatty infiltration shows a moderate diffuse increase in the fine echoes with a slightly impaired visualization of the intrahepatic vessels and diaphragm.

Clinical symptoms. Patients with hepatitis may initially present with flu and gastrointestinal symptoms, including loss of appetite, nausea, vomiting, and fatigue. Jaundice may occur in severe cases. Lab values show abnormal liver function tests with increases in the SGOT, SGPT, and bilirubin. Leukopenia is present.

Acute hepatitis. In acute hepatitis, damage to the liver may range from mild disease to massive necrosis and liver failure. The pathologic changes seen include the following: (1) liver cell injury, swelling of the hepatocytes, and hepatocyte degeneration, which may lead to cell necrosis; (2) reticuloendothelial and lymphocytic response with Kupffer cells enlarging; and (3) regeneration. On ultrasound the portal vein borders are more prominent than usual and the liver parenchyma is slightly more echogenic than normal (Fig. 5-42). Hepatosplenomegaly is present and the gallbladder wall is thickened.

Chronic hepatitis. Chronic hepatitis exists when there is clinical or biochemical evidence of hepatic inflammation for at least 3 to 6 months. In chronic active hepatitis there are more extensive changes than in chronic persistent hepatitis, with inflammation extending across the limiting plate,

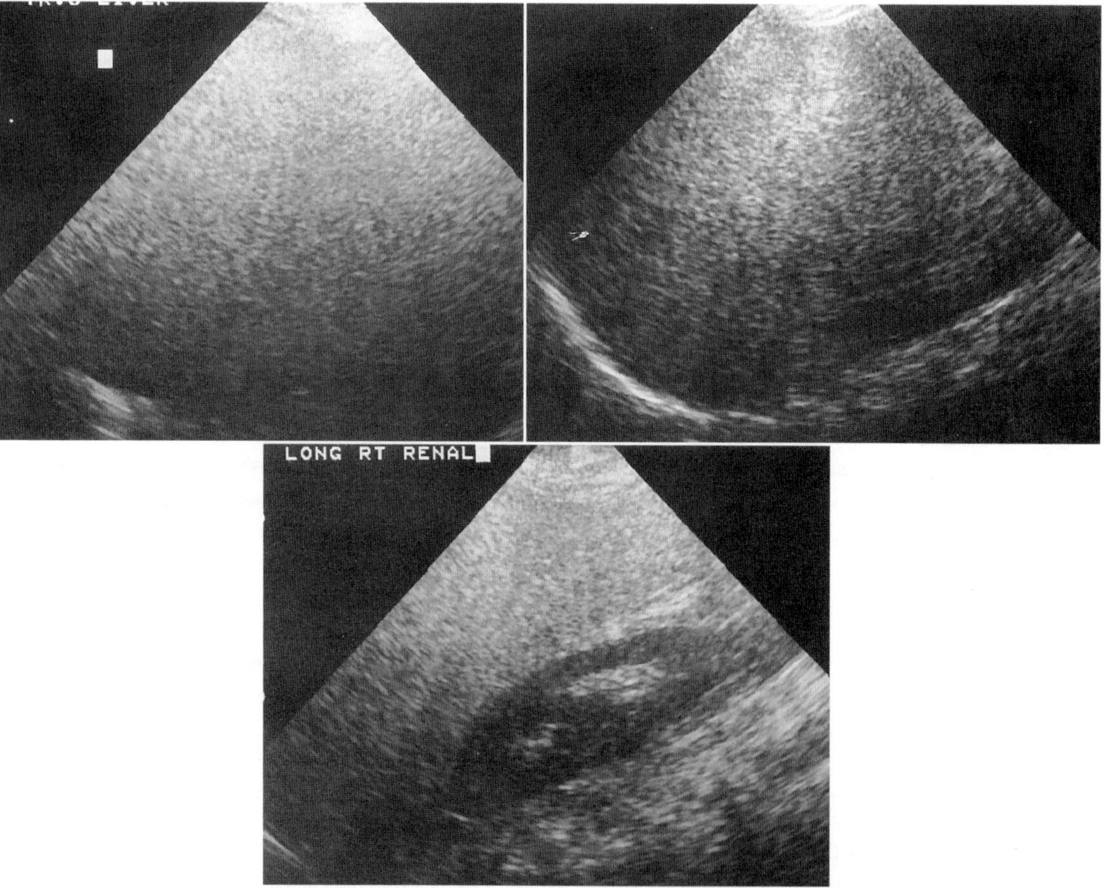

FIG. 5-40 Transverse and longitudinal scans of grade III fatty infiltration of the liver show a marked increase in the fine echoes with poor visualization of the intrahepatic vessel borders, diaphragm, and posterior lobe of the liver.

spreading out in a perilobular fashion, and causing piecemeal necrosis, which is frequently accompanied by fibrosis. Chronic persistent hepatitis is a benign, self-limiting process. Chronic active hepatitis usually progresses to cirrhosis and liver failure. On ultrasound the liver parenchyma is coarse with decreased brightness of the portal triads, but the degree of attenuation is not as great as is seen in fatty infiltration (Fig. 5-43). The liver does not increase in size with chronic hepatitis. Fibrosis may be evident, which may produce "soft shadowing" posteriorly.

Cirrhosis. Cirrhosis is a chronic degenerative disease of the liver in which the lobes are covered with fibrous tissue, the parenchyma degenerates, and the lobules are infiltrated with fat. The essential feature is simultaneous parenchymal necrosis, regeneration, and diffuse fibrosis resulting in disorganization of lobular architecture. The process is chronic and progressive with liver cell failure and portal hypertension as the end stage. Cirrhosis is most commonly the re-

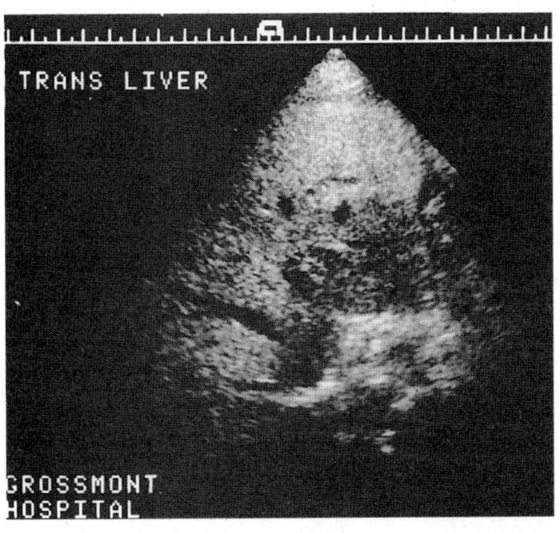

FIG. 5-41 Focal sparing of the caudate lobe.

HEPATITIS ULTRASOUND FINDINGS
Acute Hepatitis • Findings may be nonspecific and variable • Decreased echogenicity if severe • Increased brightness of portal vein borders • Hepatosplenomegaly
Chronic Hepatitis • Findings may be nonspecific • Coarse hepatic parenchyma echo pattern • Increased echogenicity • Decreased visualization of vessels

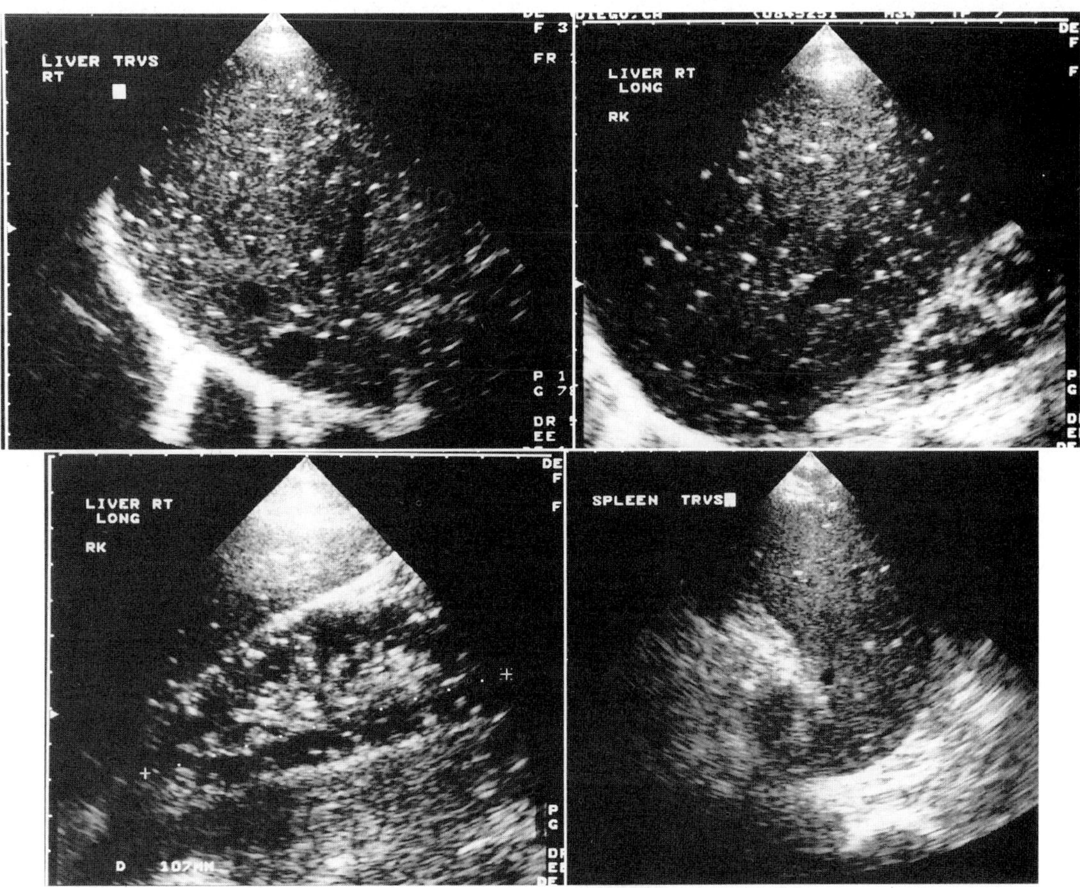

FIG. 5-42 A 32-year-old male with AIDS and acute hepatitis. The scans also show signs of pneumocystic disease with multiple areas of calcification throughout the liver, kidney, and spleen.

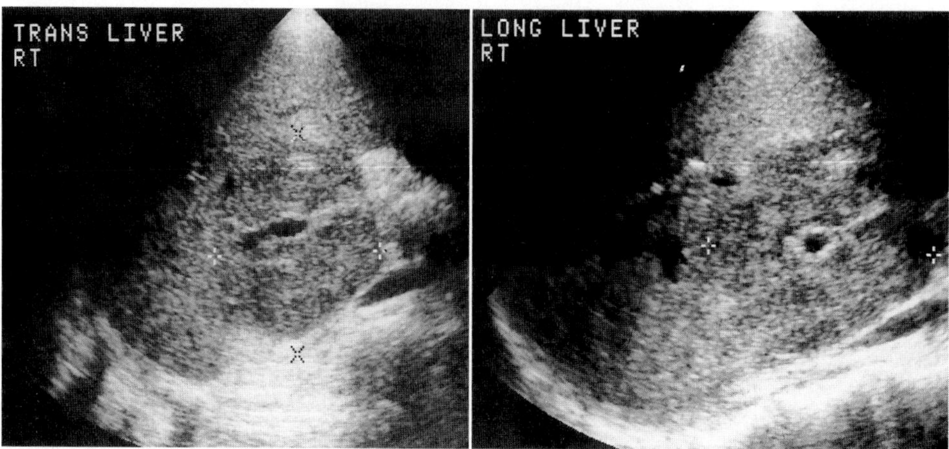

FIG. 5-43 A 45-year-old male with HIV, jaundice, and chronic hepatitis. A large hypoechoic mass was found within the hilum of the liver. The mass had irregular borders. The portal vein was patent. Intrahepatic biliary dilation was seen in other scans not shown. The liver texture was coarse with increased echogenicity.

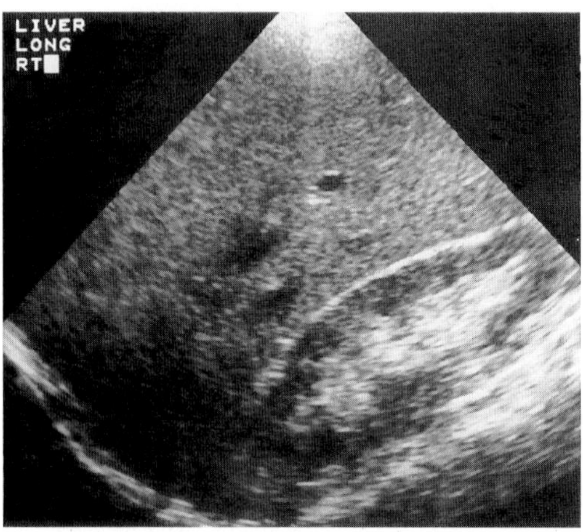

FIG. 5-44 A 54-year-old male with liver cirrhosis. The liver is enlarged with increased attenuation.

sult of chronic alcohol abuse but can be the result of nutritional deprivation or hepatitis or other infection.

Clinical symptoms include nausea, flatulence, anorexia, weight loss, ascites, light-colored stools, weakness, abdominal pain, varicosities, and spider angiomas.

There are several types of cirrhosis: biliary cirrhosis, fatty cirrhosis, and posthepatic cirrhosis.

The diagnosis of cirrhosis by ultrasound may be difficult. Specific findings may include coarsening of the liver parenchyma secondary to fibrosis and nodularity. Increased attenuation may be present with decreased vascular markings (Fig. 5-44). Hepatosplenomegaly may be present with ascites surrounding the liver (Fig. 5-45). Chronic cirrhosis may show nodularity of the liver edge, especially if ascites is present (Figs. 5-46 and 5-47). The hepatic fissures may be accentuated. The isoechoic regenerating nodules may be seen throughout the liver parenchyma. Portal hypertension may be present with or without abnormal Doppler flow patterns. Patients who have cirrhosis have an increased incidence of hepatoma tumors within the liver parenchyma (Figs. 5-48 and 5-49).

CIRRHOSIS ULTRASOUND FINDINGS

- Increased echogenicity
- Increased attenuation
- Decreased vascular markings
- Hepatosplenomegaly with acute; shrunken liver size with chronic
- Ascites
- Nodularity or regenerating nodules
- Accentuation of fissures
- Portal hypertension
- Increased incidence of hepatoma

Glycogen Storage Disease

There are six categories of glycogen storage disease, which are divided on the basis of clinical symptoms and specific enzymatic defects. The most common is type I, or von Gierke's disease. This is a form of glycogen storage disease in which abnormally large amounts of glycogen are deposited in the liver and kidneys.

On ultrasound, patients with this disease present with hepatomegaly, increased echogenicity, and slightly increased attenuation. The disease is associated with hepatic adenomas, focal nodular hyperplasia, and hepatomegaly (Figs. 5-50 and Fig. 5-51). The adenomas present as round, homogeneous, echogenic tumors. If the tumor is large, it may be slightly inhomogeneous.

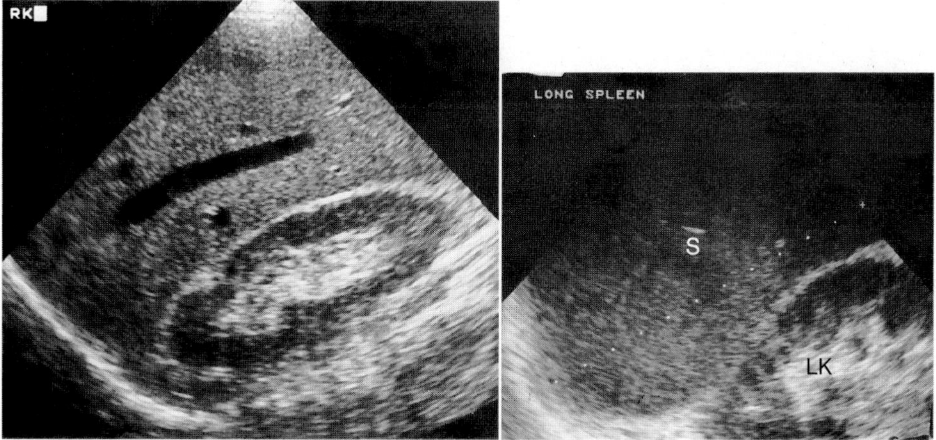

FIG. 5-45 A patient with cirrhosis shows hepatosplenomegaly and abnormal liver function tests.

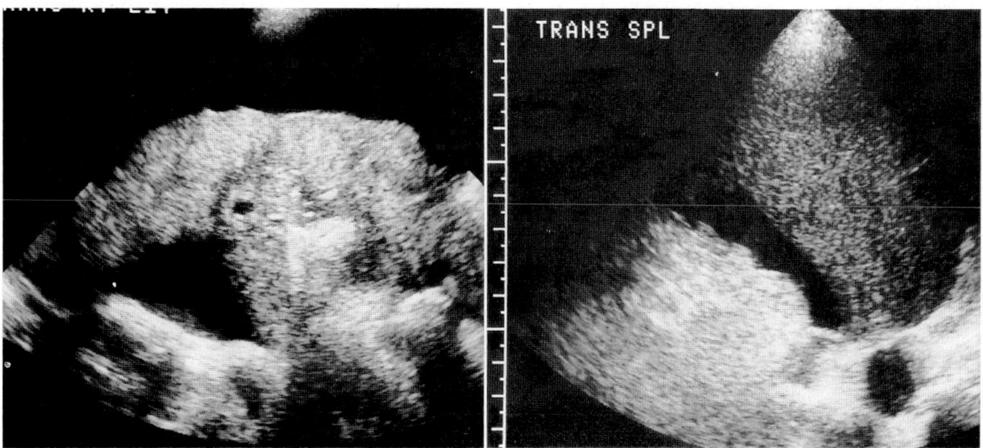

FIG. 5-46 Chronic cirrhosis shows ascites with nodularity of the liver edge.

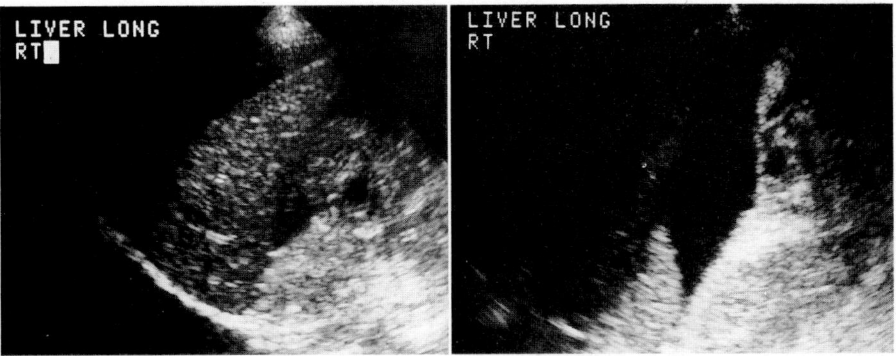

FIG. 5-47 Longitudinal scan of a patient with chronic cirrhosis shows ascites and a small shrunken liver parenchyma.

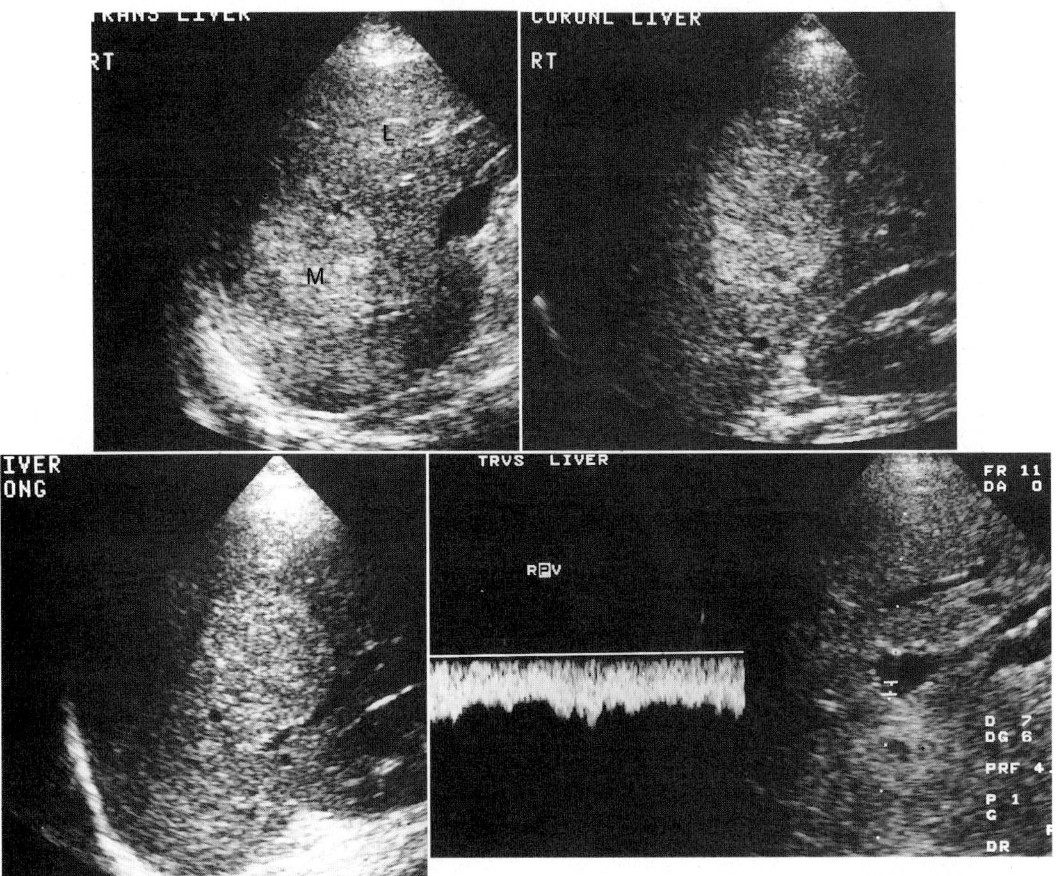

FIG. 5-48 A 48-year-old male with cirrhosis and a hepatoma within the right lobe of the liver. The right portal vein showed normal flow.

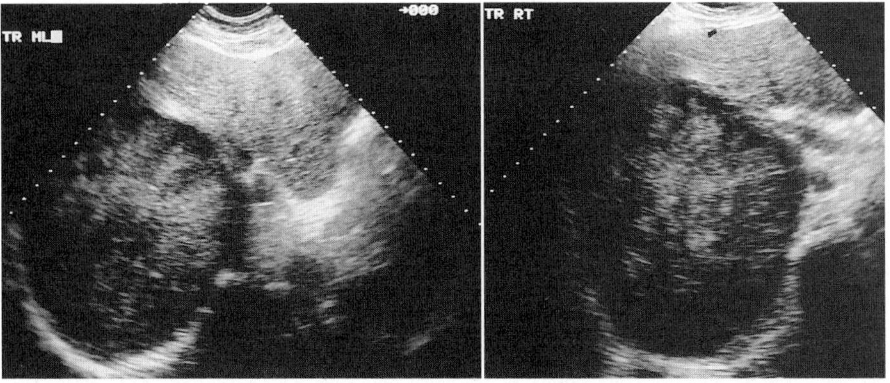

FIG. 5-49 A 56-year-old male with a palpable abdominal mass (hepatoma) and chronic cirrhosis.

Hemochromatosis

Hemochromatosis is a rare disease of iron metabolism characterized by excess iron deposits throughout the body. This disorder may lead to cirrhosis and portal hypertension. Ultrasound does not show specific findings other than hepatomegaly and cirrhotic changes. Some increased echogenicity may be seen uniformly throughout the hepatic parenchyma.

Diffuse Abnormalities of the Liver Parenchyma

Abnormalities such as biliary obstruction, common duct stones and stricture, extrahepatic mass, and passive hepatic congestion are discussed as each lesion is seen on the ultrasound.

Biliary obstruction. Biliary obstruction proximal to the cystic duct can be caused by carcinoma of the common bile duct or metastatic tumor invasion of the porta hepatis. Clin-

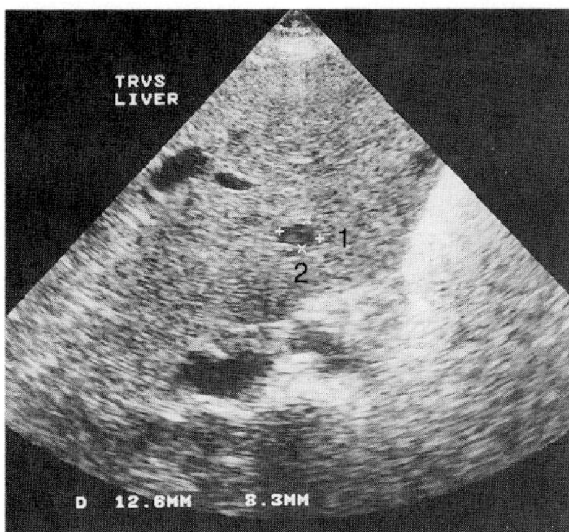

FIG. 5-50 Patient with von Gierke's disease with hepatic adenoma in the caudate lobe of the liver.

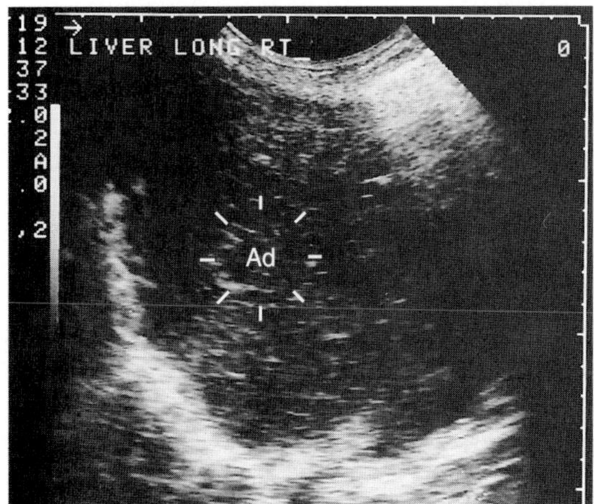

FIG. 5-51 A 31-year-old female with von Gierke's disease and hepatic adenoma in the right lobe of the liver.

ically the patient may be jaundiced with pruritus (itching). Liver function tests show an elevation in the direct bilirubin and alkaline phosphatase levels. Sonographically, carcinoma of the common duct shows as a tubular branching with dilated intrahepatic ducts best seen in the periphery of the liver (Fig. 5-52). It may be difficult to image a discrete mass lesion. The gallbladder is of normal size, even after a fatty meal is administered.

A biliary obstruction distal to the cystic duct may be caused by stones in the common duct (Fig. 5-53), an extrahepatic mass in the porta hepatis, or stricture of the common duct. Clinically, common duct stones cause right upper quadrant pain, jaundice, and pruritus, as well as an increase in direct bilirubin and alkaline phosphatase. On ultrasound the dilated intrahepatic ducts are seen in the periphery of the liver (Fig. 5-54). The gallbladder size is variable, usually small. Gallstones are often present and appear as hyperechoic lesions along the posterior floor of the

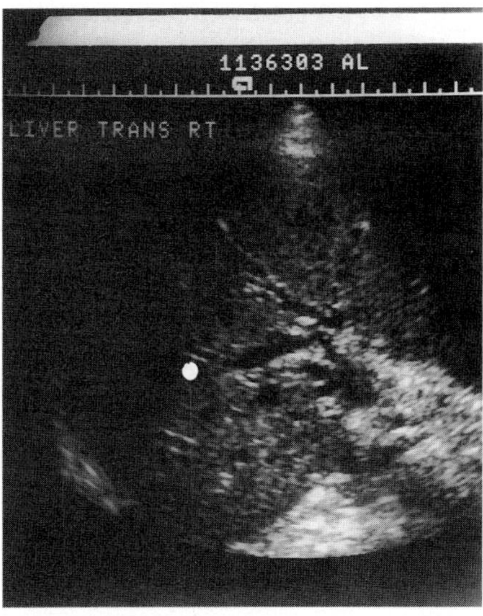

FIG. 5-52 Biliary obstruction proximal to the cystic duct can be caused by carcinoma of the common bile duct or metastatic tumor invasion of the porta hepatis. This patient had a metastatic invasion of the porta hepatis with intrahepatic biliary distension.

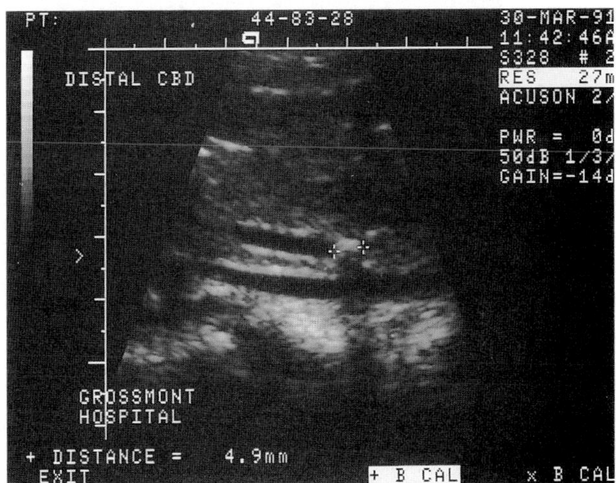

FIG. 5-53 A biliary obstruction distal to the cystic duct may be caused by stones in the common duct. The distal cystic duct is enlarged with a large stone within. The inferior vena cava is posterior.

gallbladder with a sharp posterior acoustic shadow. Careful evaluation of the common duct may show shadowing stones within the dilated duct.

Extrahepatic mass. An extrahepatic mass in the area of the porta hepatis causes the same clinical signs as seen in biliary obstruction. On ultrasound an irregular, ill-defined, hypoechoic and inhomogeneous mass lesion may be seen in the area of the porta hepatis. There is intrahepatic ductal dilation with a hydropic gallbladder. The lesion may arise from the lymph nodes, pancreatitis, pseudocyst, or carcinoma in the head of the pancreas.

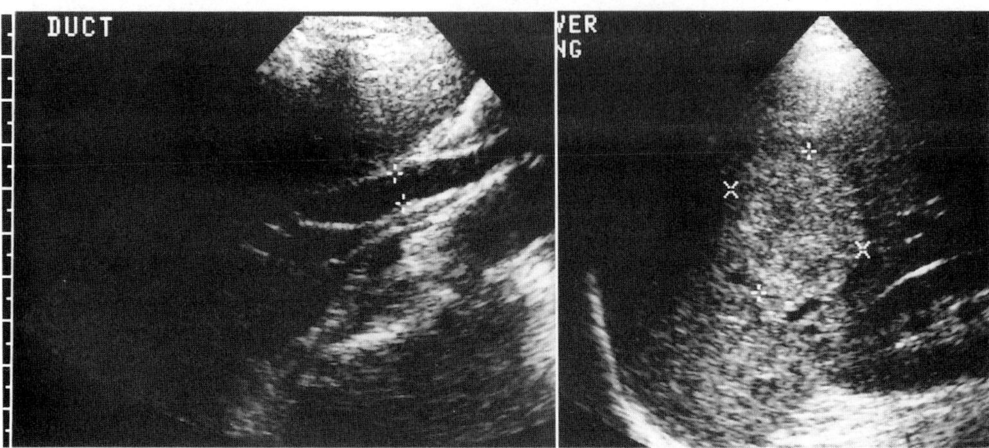

FIG. 5-54 A large mass in the area of the porta hepatis has caused obstruction of the common bile duct.

Common duct stricture. A common duct stricture would present as dilated intrahepatic ducts with absence of a mass in the porta hepatis on ultrasound. Clinically the patient would be jaundiced with a previous cholecystectomy. Laboratory values would show an increase in the direct bilirubin and alkaline phosphatase.

Passive hepatic congestion. Passive hepatic congestion develops secondary to congestive heart failure with signs of hepatomegaly. Laboratory data indicates normal to slightly elevated liver function tests. On ultrasound, dilation of the inferior vena cava, superior mesenteric, hepatic, portal, and splenic veins are noted. The venous structures may decrease in size with expiration and increase with inspiration.

Focal Liver Disease

Very few hepatic lesions have specific sonographic features. Therefore it is important to know the patient's clinical history and the sonographic patterns associated with various lesions. The knowledge of laboratory values in liver function tests also helps determine the hepatic lesions. The differential diagnosis for focal diseases of the liver includes cysts, abscess, hematoma, primary tumor, and metastases. The sonographer should be able to differentiate whether the mass is extrahepatic or intrahepatic. Intrahepatic masses may cause the following findings on ultrasound: displacement of the hepatic vascular radicles, external bulging of the liver capsule, or a posterior shift of the inferior vena cava. An extrahepatic mass may show internal invagination or discontinuity of the liver capsule, formation of a triangular fat wedge, anteromedial shift of the inferior vena cava, or anterior displacement of the right kidney.

Cystic Lesions

Hepatic cysts may be congenital or acquired, solitary or multiple. Patients are often asymptomatic, except patients who have large cysts, which can compress the hepatic vasculature or ductal system.

Cystic lesions within the liver include the following: simple or congenital hepatic cysts, traumatic cysts, parasitic cysts, inflammatory cysts, polycystic disease, and pseudocysts.

Simple Hepatic Cysts

The ultrasound finding of a simple hepatic cyst is usually incidental because most patients are asymptomatic. As the cyst grows, it may cause pain or a mass effect to suggest a more serious condition, such as infection, abscess, or necrotic lesion. Hepatic cysts occur more often in females than in males. On ultrasound the cyst walls are thin, with well-defined borders, and anechoic with distal posterior enhancement (Figs. 5-55 and 5-56). Infrequently cysts contain fine linear internal septae. Complications, such as hemorrhage, may occur and cause pain. Calcification may be seen within the cyst wall, which may cause shadowing.

Congenital Hepatic Cysts

A solitary congenital cyst of the liver is rare and usually is an incidental lesion. This abnormality arises from developmental defects in the formation of bile ducts. The mass is usually solitary and may vary in size from tiny to as large as 20 cm (Fig. 5-57). The cyst is usually found on the anterior undersurface of the liver. It usually does not cause liver enlargement and is found in the right lobe of the liver more often than the left lobe.

Polycystic Liver Disease

Polycystic liver disease is autosomal-dominant and affects one person in 500. At least 25% to 50% of patients with polycystic renal disease have one to several hepatic cysts. Of patients with polycystic liver disease, 60% have associated polycystic renal disease. The cysts are small, under 2 to 3 cm, and multiple throughout the hepatic parenchyma. Cysts within the porta hepatis may enlarge and cause biliary obstruction. Histologically they appear similar to simple hepatic cysts. It may be very difficult to as-

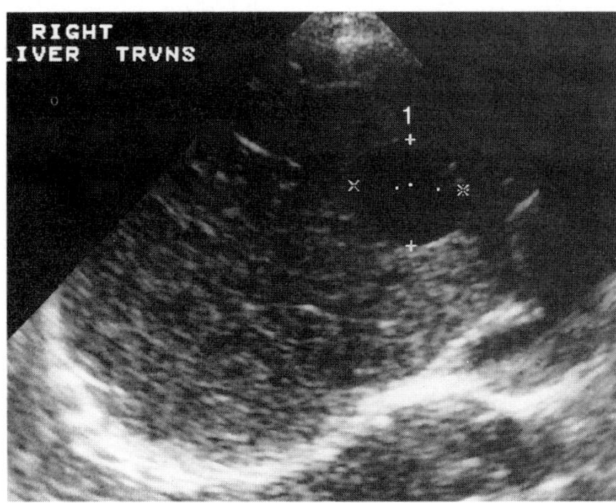

FIG. 5-55 A simple hepatic cyst has smooth, uniform borders with no internal echoes.

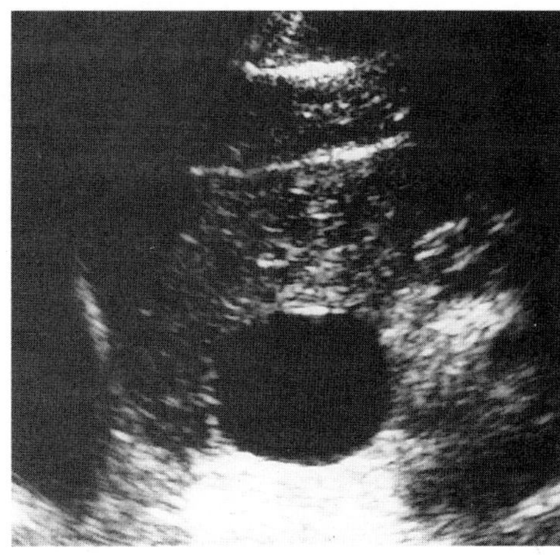

FIG. 5-57 A solitary hepatic cyst in the left lobe of the liver. Good through-transmission is noted beyond the mass.

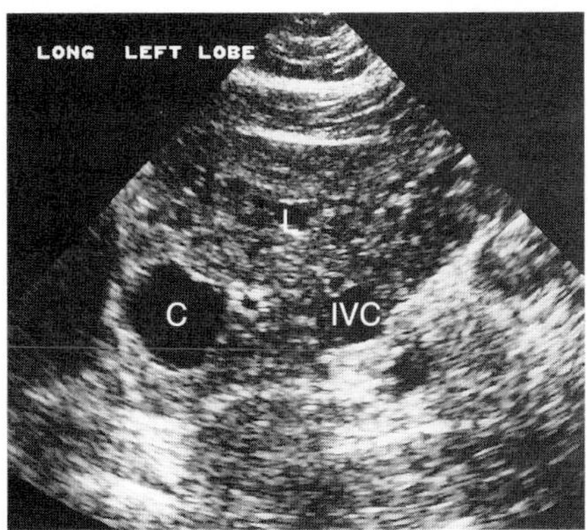

FIG. 5-56 An asymptomatic patient with a solitary hepatic cyst in the right lobe of the liver.

sess an abscess formation or neoplastic lesion in a patient with polycystic liver disease.

On ultrasound the cysts generally present as anechoic, well-defined borders with acoustic enhancement (Fig. 5-58). The differential diagnosis for a cystic lesion includes the following: necrotic metastasis, echinococcal cyst, hematoma, hepatic cystadenocarcinoma, and abscess. Ultrasound may be used to direct the needle if percutaneous aspiration is needed to obtain specific diagnostic information.

Inflammatory Hepatic Lesions

Hepatic abscesses have occurred most often as complications of biliary tract disease, surgery, or trauma. The following three basic types of abscess formation occur in the liver: intrahepatic, subhepatic, and subphrenic. Generally, the patient presents with fever, elevated white cell counts, and right upper quadrant pain. The search for an abscess must be made to locate solitary or multiple lesions within the liver or to search for abnormal fluid collections in Morison's pouch, in the subdiaphragmatic or subphrenic space.

The following infectious processes are discussed: pyogenic abscess, hepatic candidiasis, chronic granulomatous disease, amebic abscess, and echinococcal disease.

Pyogenic Abscess

A pyogenic abscess is a "pus-forming" abscess formation. There are many routes for bacteria to gain access to the liver—through the biliary tree, the portal vein, or the hepatic artery; through a direct extension from a contiguous infection; and, rarely, through hepatic trauma. Sources of infection include cholangitis, portal pyemia secondary to appendicitis, diverticulitis, inflammatory disease, or colitis; direct spread from another organ; trauma with direct contamination; or infarction after embolization or from sickle cell anemia.

Clinically the patient presents with fever, pain, pleuritis, nausea, vomiting, and diarrhea. Elevated liver function tests, leukocytosis, and anemia are present. The abscess formation is multiple in 50% to 67% of patients. The most frequent organisms are *E. coli* and anaerobes.

The ultrasound appearance of a pyogenic abscess may be variable depending on the internal consistency of the mass. The size varies from 1 cm to very large. The right central lobe of the liver is the most common site for abscess development. The abscess may be hypoechoic with round or ovoid margins and acoustic enhancement, or it may be complex with some debris along the posterior margin and irregular walls (Fig. 5-59). It may have a fluid level; if gas is present, it can be hyperechoic with dirty shadowing.

Hepatic Candidiasis

Hepatic candidiasis is caused by a species of *Candida*. It usually occurs in immunocompromised hosts, such as patients undergoing chemotherapy, organ transplantation, or HIV infection. The *Candida* fungus invades the bloodstream and may affect any organ, with the more perfused kidneys, brain, and heart affected the most.

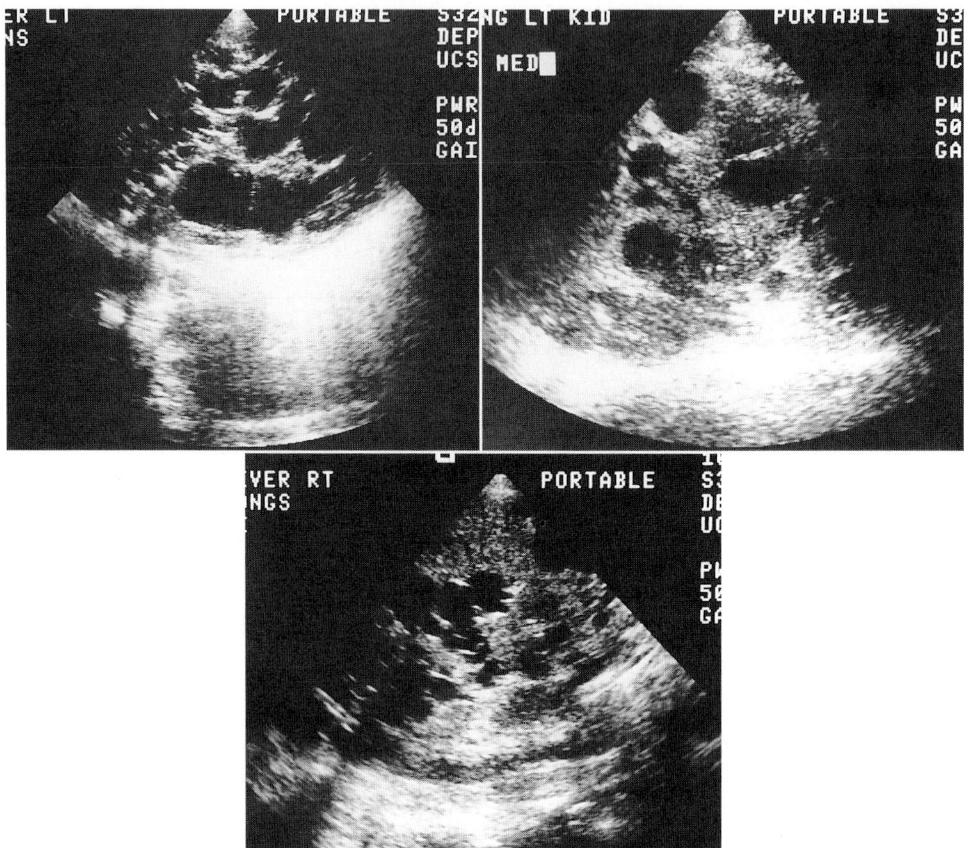

FIG. 5-58 Polycystic liver and renal disease shows multiple cysts throughout the liver and kidney.

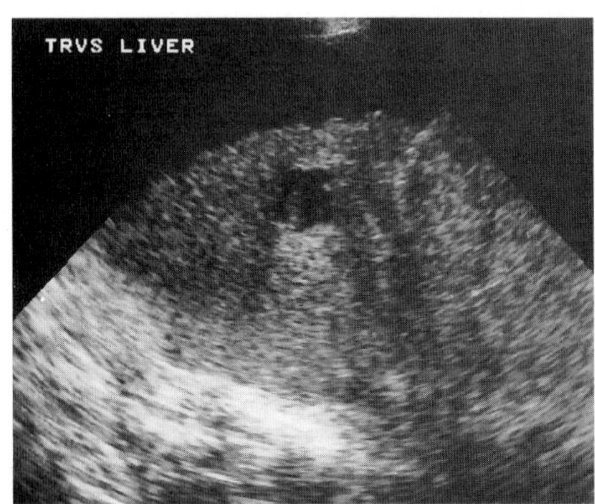

FIG. 5-59 A 49-year-old male with cirrhosis, abdominal pain, and fever presented in the emergency room. An irregular, ill-defined mass is seen in the right lobe of the liver. This abscess presented as a complex lesion.

Clinically the patient may present with nonspecific findings, such as fever and localized pain. On ultrasound, candidiasis within the liver may present as multiple small hypoechoic masses with echogenic central cores, referred to as *bull's-eye* or *target* lesions. Other sonographic patterns

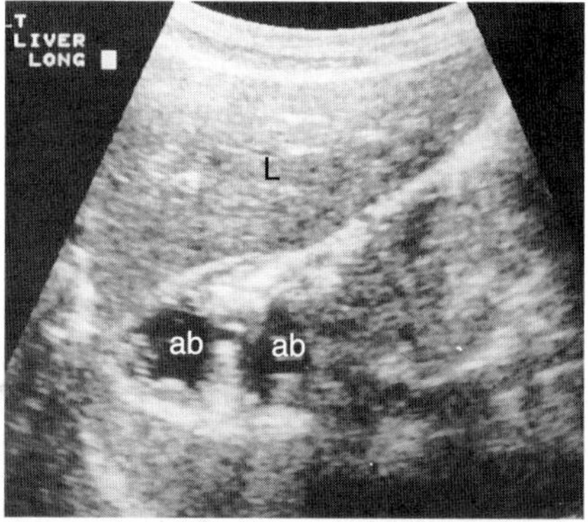

FIG. 5-60 A 6-year-old female presented in the emergency room with high fever and right upper quadrant pain for 3 days. A complex lesion was seen in the right lobe of the liver. This represented a hepatic abscess *(ab)*.

have been described as "wheel-within-wheel" patterns, or multiple small hypoechoic lesions (Fig. 5-60). Specific diagnosis can only be made with fine-needle aspiration.

Chronic Granulomatous Disease

Chronic granulomatous disease is a recessive trait related to a congenital defect in the leukocyte that renders it unable to inactivate catalase-positive, previously phagocytized bacteria. A pediatric patient may present with recurrent respiratory infections. On ultrasound a poorly marginated, hypoechoic mass is seen with posterior enhancement. Calcification may be present with posterior shadowing. Aspiration is necessary to specifically classify the mass as granulomatous disease.

Amebic Abscess

Amebic abscess is a collection of pus formed by disintegrated tissue in a cavity, usually in the liver, caused by the protozoan parasite *Entamoeba histolytica*. The infection is primarily a disease of the colon, but it can also spread to the liver, lungs, and brain. The parasites reach the liver parenchyma via the portal vein. Amebiasis is contracted by ingesting the cysts in contaminated water and food. The ameba usually affects the colon and cecum and the organism remains within the gastrointestinal tract. If the organism invades the colonic mucosa, it may travel to the liver via the portal venous system.

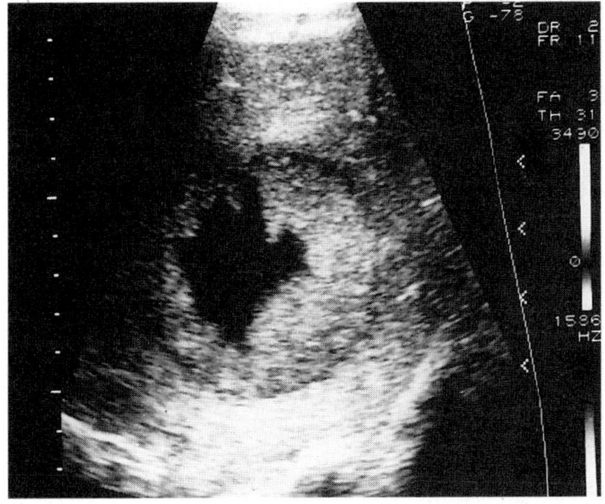

FIG. 5-61 A 16-year-old female returned from Mexico with right upper quadrant pain, fever, and nausea. A large, complex mass was seen in the right lobe of the liver consistent with an amebic abscess.

Patients may be asymptomatic or may present with gastrointestinal symptoms of abdominal pain, diarrhea, leukocytosis, and low fever. The ultrasound appearance of amebic abscess is variable and nonspecific. The abscess may be round or oval in shape and lack significant defined wall echoes. The lesion is hypoechoic compared with normal liver parenchyma, with low-level echoes at higher sensitivity. There may be some internal echoes along the posterior margin secondary to debris (Figs. 5-61 and 5-62). Distal enhancement may be seen beyond the mass lesion. Some organisms may rupture through the diaphragm into the hepatic capsule.

Echinococcal Cyst

Hepatic echinococcosis is an infectious cystic disease common in sheep-herding areas of the world but seldom encountered within the United States. The echinococcus is a tapeworm that infects man as the intermediate host. The worm resides in the small intestine of dogs. The ova from the adult worm are shed through canine feces into the environment where the intermediate hosts ingest the eggs. After entering the proximal portion of the small intestine in humans, the larvae burrow through the mucosa, enter the portal circulation, and travel to the liver. The echinococcal cyst has two layers, the inner layer and outer or inflammatory reaction layer. The smaller, daughter cysts may develop from the inner layer. The cysts may enlarge and rupture. The cysts may also impinge on the blood vessels and lead to vascular thrombosis and infarction.

On ultrasound, several patterns may occur, from a simple cyst to a complex mass with acoustic enhancement. The shape may be oval or spherical with regularity of the walls. Calcifications may occur. Septations are very frequent and include: honeycomb appearance with fluid collections, "water lily" sign, which shows a detachment and collapse of the germinal layer, or "cyst within a cyst." Sometimes the

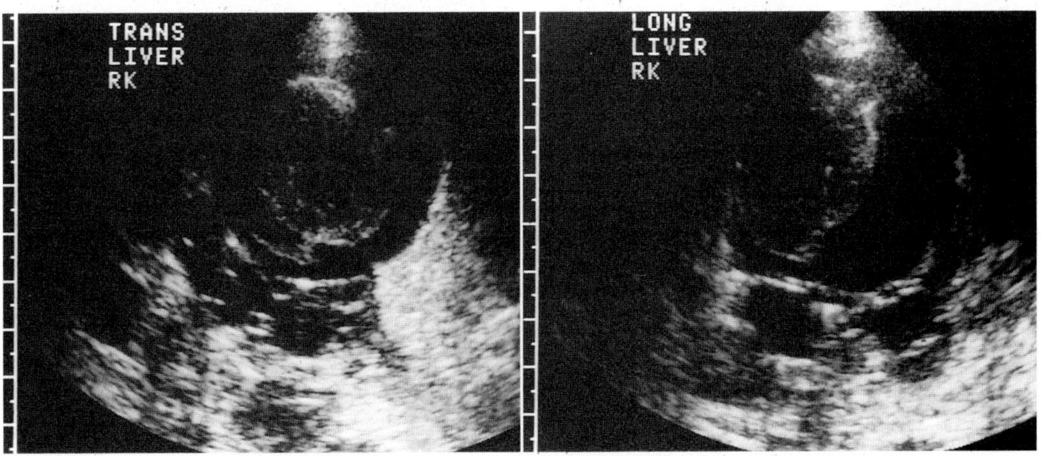

FIG. 5-62 The amebic abscess is complex, with internal echoes along the posterior margin secondary to debris.

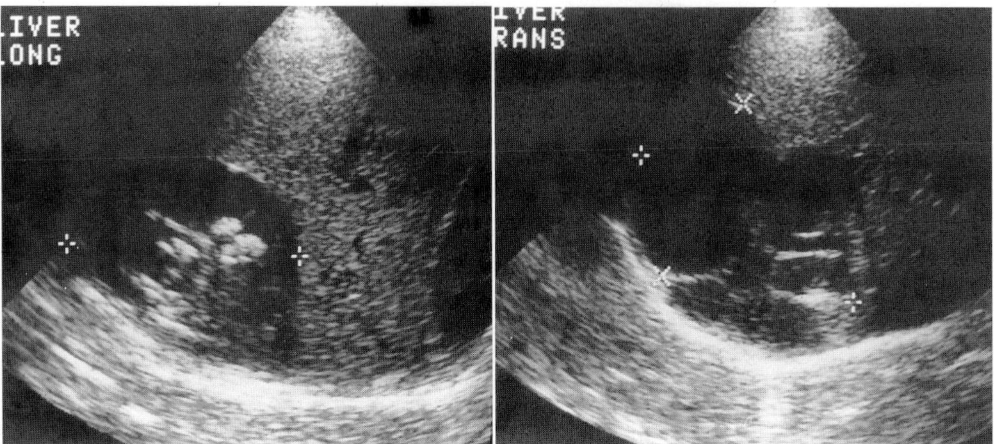

FIG. 5-63 A 58-year-old female with an echinococcal cyst in the right lobe of the liver. The ultrasound pattern is complex, with oval walls and multiple echogenic foci within.

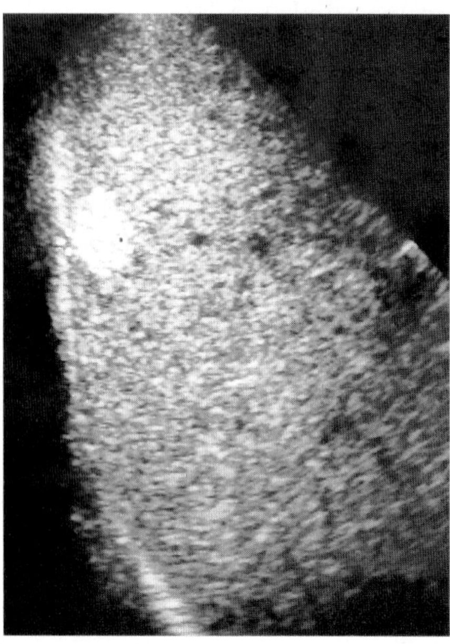

FIG. 5-64 A 71-year-old asymptomatic male with a solitary hyperechoic mass in the dome of the right lobe of the liver consistent with a cavernous hemangioma.

liver contains multiple parent cysts in both lobes of the liver; the cyst with the thick walls occupies a different part of the liver (Fig. 5-63). The tissue between the cysts indicates that each cyst is a separate parent cyst and not a daughter cyst. If a daughter cyst is found, it is specific for echinococcal disease.

Hepatic Tumors

A neoplasm is any new growth of new tissue, either benign or malignant. A benign growth occurs locally but does not spread or invade surrounding structures. It may push surrounding structures aside or adhere to them. A malignant mass is uncontrolled and is prone to metastasize to nearby or distant structures via the bloodstream and lymph nodes. Thus it is important not only to recognize the tumor mass itself but also to appreciate which structures the malignancy may invade.

Benign Hepatic Tumors of the Liver

Cavernous Hemangioma

A hemangioma is a benign, congenital tumor consisting of large, blood-filled cystic spaces. Cavernous hemangioma is the most common benign tumor of the liver. The tumor is found more frequently in females. Patients are usually asymptomatic, although a small percentage may bleed, causing right upper quadrant pain. Hemangiomas enlarge slowly and undergo degeneration, fibrosis, and calcification. They are found in the subcapsular hepatic parenchyma or in the posterior right lobe more than the left lobe of the liver.

The ultrasound appearance is typical; most are hyperechoic with acoustic enhancement (Figs. 5-64 and 5-65). Many authors have speculated that the echo-dense pattern results from the multiple interfaces between the walls of the cavernous sinuses and blood within them. They are round, oval, or lobulated with well-defined borders. The larger hemangiomas may have a mixed pattern resulting from necrosis (Fig. 5-66). Hemangiomas may become more heterogeneous as they undergo degeneration and fibrous replacement. They may also project with calcifications or a complex or anechoic echo pattern (Fig. 5-67). The differential diagnosis for hemangioma should include metastases, hepatoma, focal nodular hyperplasia, and adenoma.

Liver Cell Adenoma

An adenoma is a tumor of the glandular epithelium in which the cells of the tumor are arranged in a recognizable glandular structure. The liver cell adenoma is composed of normal or slightly atypical hepatocytes frequently containing areas of bile stasis and focal hemorrhage or necrosis. The lesion is found more commonly in women and has been related to oral contraceptive usage. Patients may present with right upper quadrant pain secondary to rupture with

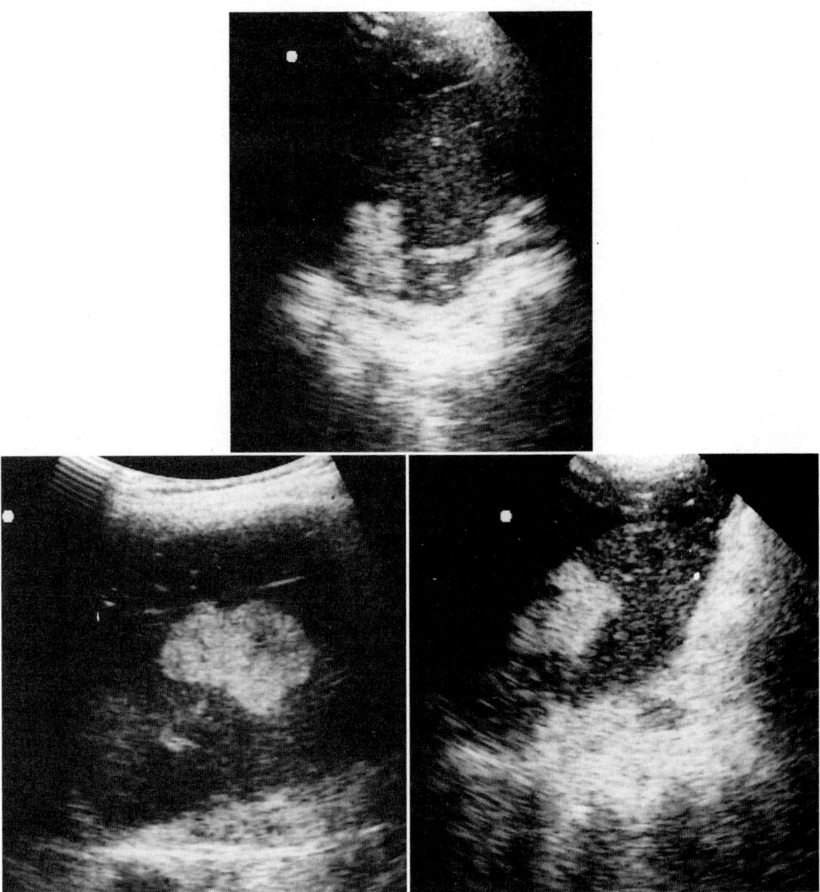

FIG. 5-65 A 43-year-old male with vague abdominal pain. A large, irregular, echogenic mass is seen in the right lobe of the liver. The hemangioma may be painful if it begins to hemorrhage.

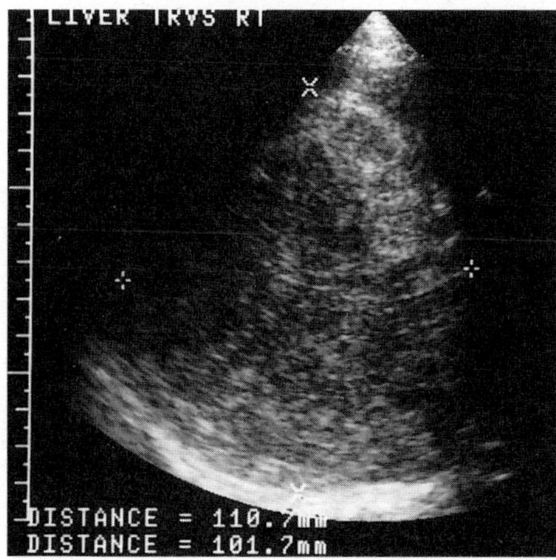

FIG. 5-66 A 62-year-old male with a palpable abdominal mass in the right upper quadrant. A large mass was seen to fill the right lobe of the liver. The larger hemangiomas have a mixed pattern resulting from necrosis and degeneration.

bleeding into the tumor. The incidence is increased in patients with type I glycogen storage disease or von Gierke's disease.

On ultrasound the mass can look similar to focal nodular hyperplasia. It is hyperechoic with a central hypoechoic area caused by hemorrhage (Figs. 5-68 to 5-70). The lesion may be solitary or multiple. If the lesion ruptures, fluid should be found in the peritoneal cavity.

Hepatic Cystadenoma

Hepatic cystadenoma contains cystic structures within the lesion. This adenoma is a rare neoplasm occurring in middle-aged women. Most present with a palpable abdominal mass. The lesions may be multilocular with mucinous fluid.

Focal Nodular Hyperplasia

Focal nodular hyperplasia is found in younger women under 40 years of age. An increased incidence is seen in women using oral contraceptive pills, and there is increased bleeding within the tumors in these patients. The patient is asymptomatic. The lesions occur more in the right lobe of the liver. There may be more than one mass; many are located along the subcapsular area of the liver, some are pendunculated, and many have a central scar. The lesion is composed of normal hepatocytes, Kupffer's cells, bile duct elements, and fibrous connective tissue. The multiple nodules are separated by bands of fibrous tissue.

On ultrasound the lesions appear well-defined with hy-

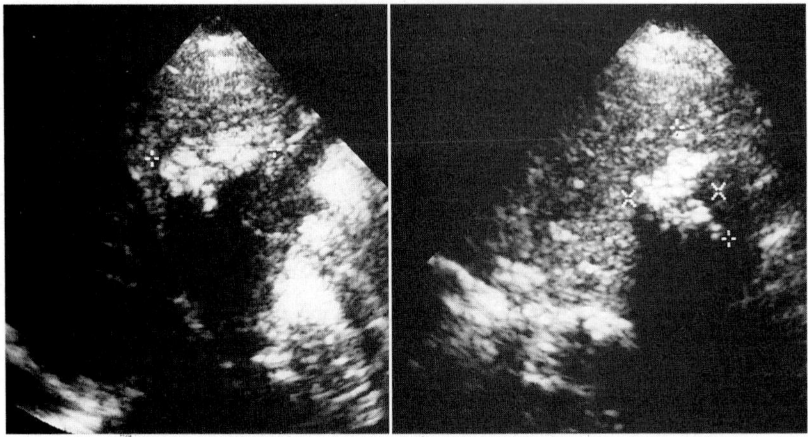

FIG. 5-67 Cavernous hemangioma with calcifications and shadowing beyond.

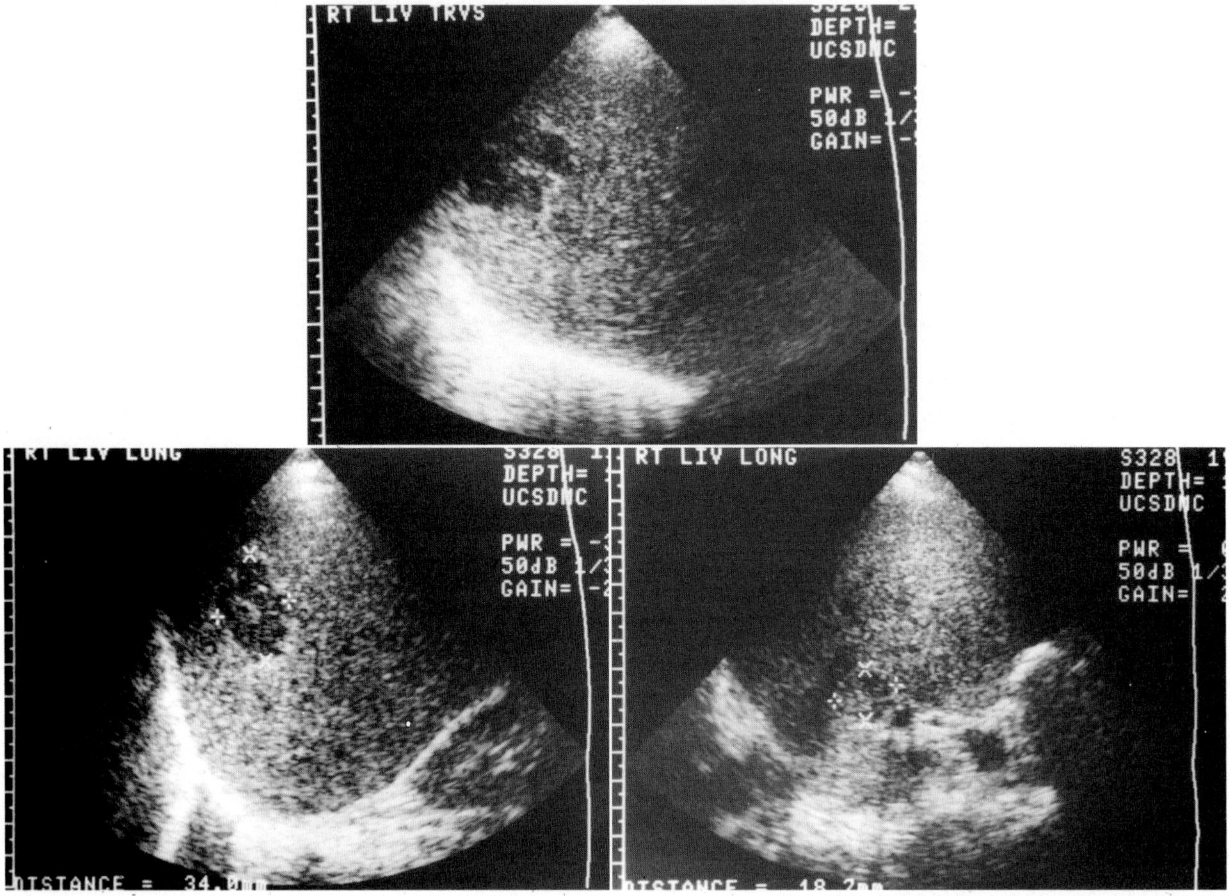

FIG. 5-68 Hepatic adenoma may appear similar to focal nodular hyperplasia.

perechoic to isoechoic patterns compared with the liver (Fig. 5-71). The internal linear echoes may be seen within the lesions if multiple nodules occur together (Fig. 5-72).

Malignant Disease

Hepatocellular Carcinoma

The pathogenesis of hepatocellular carcinoma is related to cirrhosis (80% of patients with preexisting cirrhosis develop hepatocellular carcinoma), chronic hepatitis B virus infection, and hepatocarcinogens in foods. This tumor comprises 90% of all primary liver malignancies. It occurs more frequently in men.

The carcinoma may present in one of three patterns: solitary massive tumor, multiple nodules throughout the liver, or as diffuse infiltrative masses in the liver. All of the patterns cause hepatomegaly. The carcinoma can be very in-

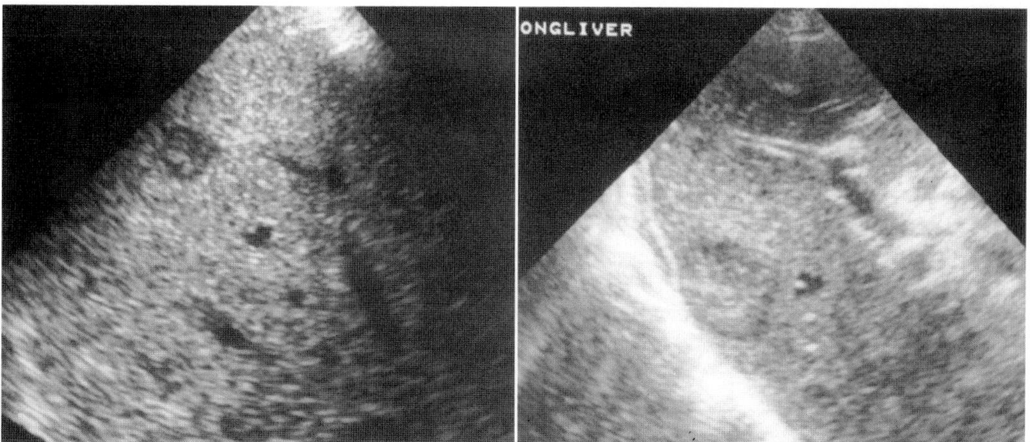

FIG. 5-69 Small adenoma with a central isoechoic area secondary to old hemorrhage.

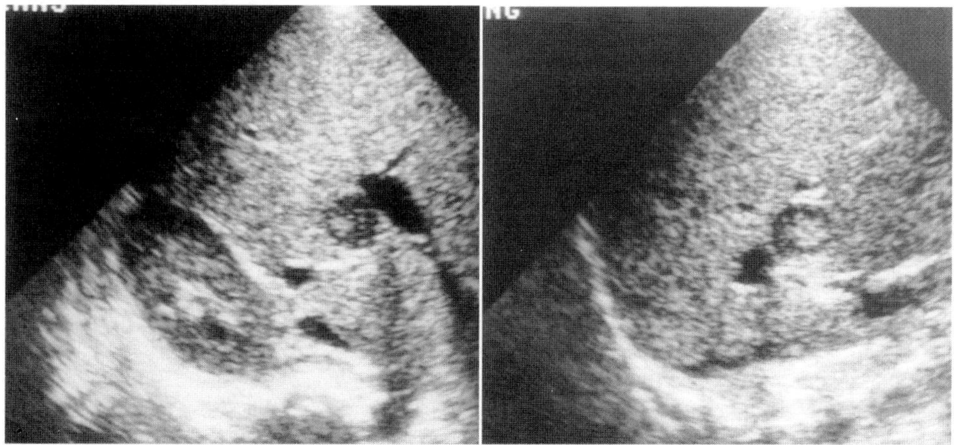

FIG. 5-70 A 32-year-old female on birth control pills presents with right upper quadrant pain. A small hepatic adenoma is seen in the right lobe of the liver.

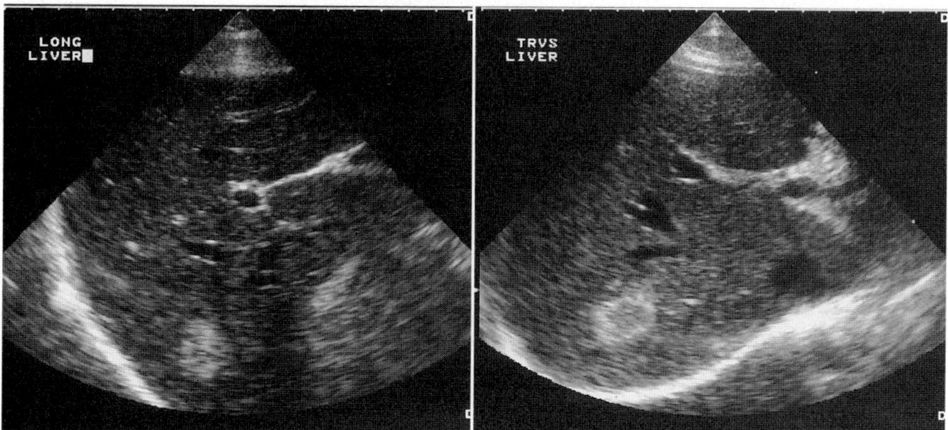

FIG. 5-71 A 41-year-old female on birth control pills presents with an echogenic focus in the right lobe of the liver consistent with focal nodular hyperplasia.

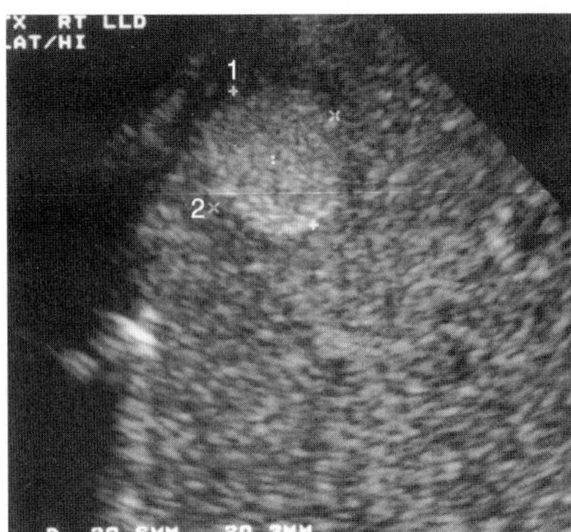

FIG. 5-72 Focal nodular hyperplasia appears well-defined with a hyperechoic internal structure.

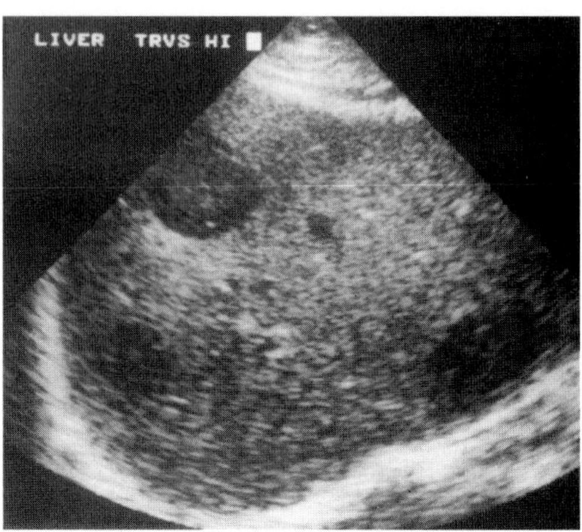

FIG. 5-73 Hepatocellular carcinoma: discrete multiple lesions shown to be isoechoic with a halo surrounding the lesion.

vasive and is seen to invade the hepatic veins to produce Budd-Chiari syndrome. The portal venous system may also be invaded with tumor or thrombosis. The hepatocellular carcinoma has a tendency to destroy the portal venous radicle walls with invasion into the lumen of the vessel.

Clinically the patient presents with a palpable mass in the liver, hepatomegaly, unexplained fever, and signs of cirrhosis. Hepatocellular carcinoma produces no abnormalities in liver function tests other than indications of cirrhosis, although 70% of the patients have an elevated alpha-fetaprotein level.

On ultrasound a variable appearance is noted with discrete lesions, either solitary or multiple, which are usually hypoechoic or hyperechoic. Sometimes they may area isoechoic and a halo surrounds the lesion (Fig. 5-73). Another pattern presents as diffuse parenchymal involvement with inhomogeneity throughout the liver without distinct masses (Fig. 5-74). The last pattern is a combination of discrete and diffuse echoes (Figs. 5-75 and 76). One cannot differentiate hepatocellular carcinoma from metastases on ultrasound.

Internal echoes within the portal veins, hepatic veins, or inferior vena cava indicate tumor invasion or thrombosis within the vessel. The evaluation of the vascular structures with color Doppler helps to rule out the presence of clot or tumor invasion. Hepatic flow is abnormal if an obstruction is present.

Metastatic Disease

Metastatic disease is the most common form of neoplastic involvement of the liver. The primary sites are the colon, breast, and lung. The majority of metastases arise from a primary colonic malignancy or a hepatoma. Metastatic spread to the liver occurs as the tumor erodes the wall and travels through the lymphatic system or through the bloodstream to the portal vein or hepatic artery to the liver.

Clinically the patient presents with hepatomegaly, abnormal liver function tests, weight loss, and decreased appe-

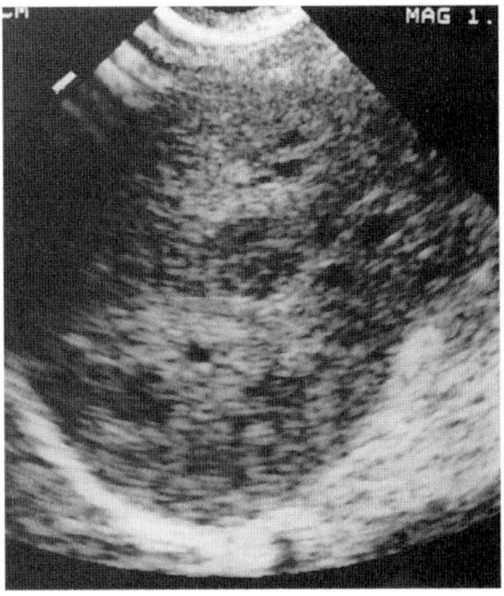

FIG. 5-74 Hepatocellular carcinoma: diffuse parenchymal involvement with inhomogeneity throughout the liver without distinct masses.

tite. It is typical to have multiple nodes throughout both lobes of the liver.

The ultrasound patterns of metastatic tumor involvement in the liver vary. The following three specific patterns have been described: (1) a well-defined hypoechoic mass (Figs. 5-77 and 5-78), (2) a well-defined echogenic mass (Figs. 5-79 and 5-80), and (3) diffuse distortion of the normal homogeneous parenchymal pattern without a focal mass (Figs. 5-81 to 85). The hypovascular lesions produce hypoechoic patterns in the liver because of necrosis and ischemic areas from neoplastic thrombosis. Most cases of hypervascular lesions correspond to hyperechoic patterns. The common primary masses include renal cell carcinoma, carcinoid, choriocarcinoma, transitional cell carcinoma, islet cell carcinoma, and hepatocellular carcinoma. The echogenic lesions are common with primary colonic tumors and may present with calcification. Target types of metastases or bull's-eye patterns are the result of edema around the tumor or necrosis or hemorrhage within the tumor (Fig. 5-86). As the nod-

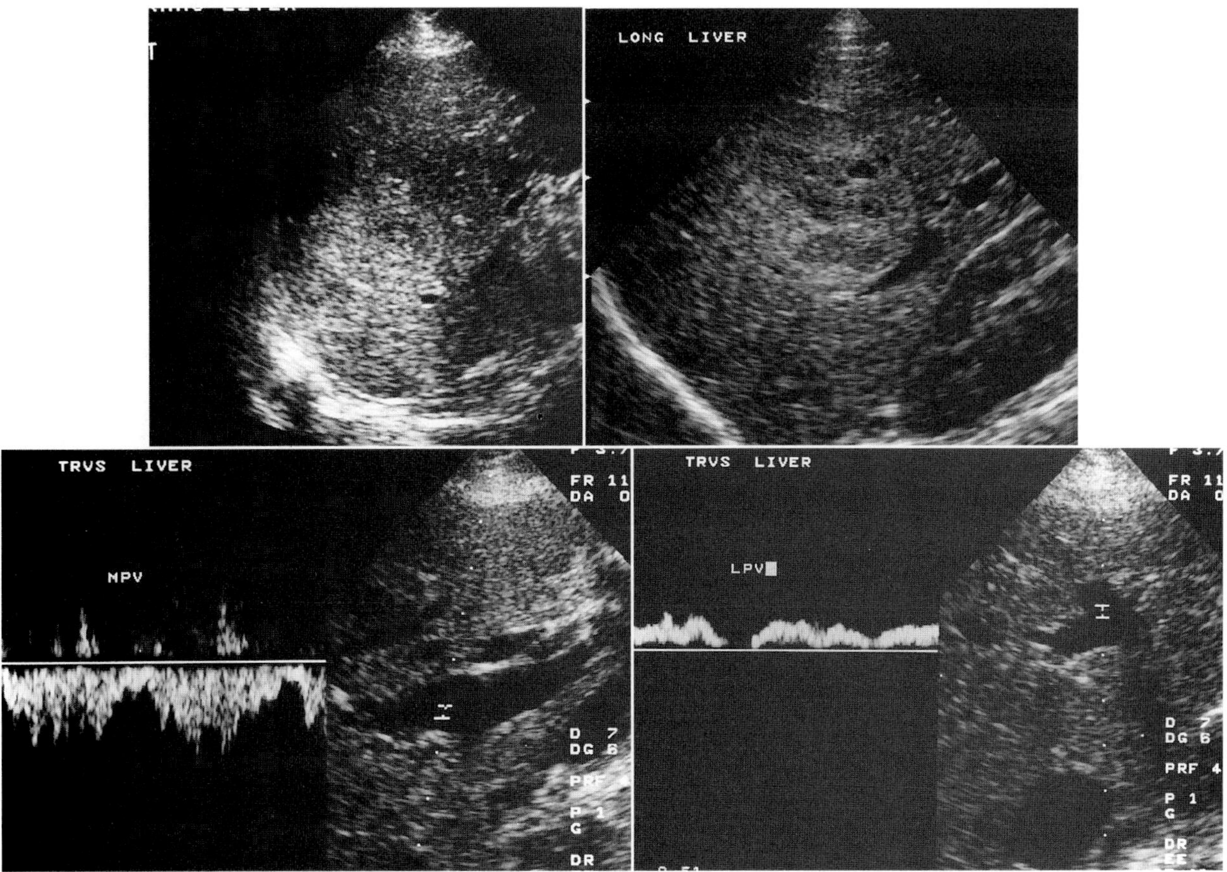

FIG. 5-75 Hepatocellular carcinoma is difficult to distinguish from metastases on ultrasound. This patient had a large lesion in the right lobe of the liver. The portal vein was evaluated to assure patency.

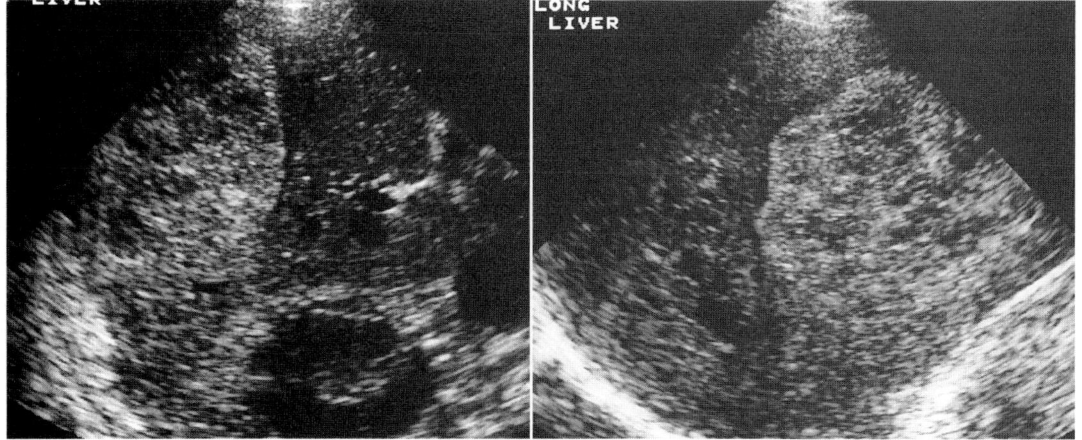

FIG. 5-76 A 58-year-old male with hepatocellular carcinoma shows hepatomegaly with diffuse abnormal lesions throughout the liver parenchyma.

ules increase rapidly in size and outgrow their blood supply, central necrosis and hemorrhage may result.

Various combinations of these patterns can be seen simultaneously in a patient with metastatic liver disease. The first abnormality is hepatomegaly or alterations in contour, especially on the lateral segment of the left lobe. The lesions may be solitary or multiple, variable in size and shape, and have sharp or ill-defined margins. Metastases may be extensive or localized to produce an inhomogeneous parenchymal pattern.

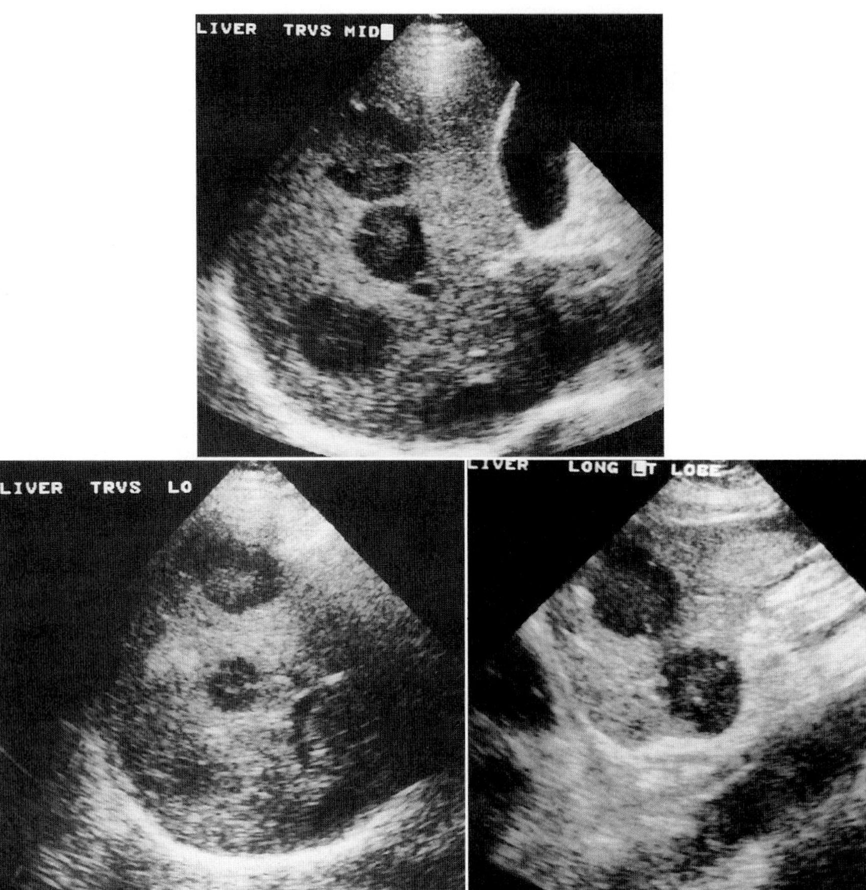

FIG. 5-77 Metastatic disease: well-defined complex lesions throughout the both lobes of the liver.

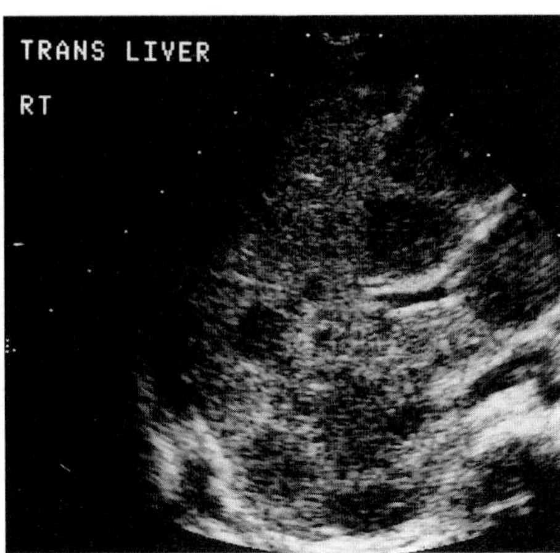

FIG. 5-78 Metastatic disease: well-defined hypoechoic lesions throughout the right lobe of the liver.

Ultrasound may be useful to follow patients after surgery. After a baseline hepatic ultrasound has been performed, the sonographer can assess regression or progression of tumor and change in parenchymal pattern, if any.

Lymphoma

Patients with lymphoma have hepatomegaly with a normal or diffuse alternation of parenchymal echoes. A focal hypoechoic mass is sometimes seen. The presence of splenomegaly or retroperitoneal nodes may help confirm the diagnosis of lymphadenopathy.

Hodgkin's lymphoma presents with hypoechoic and diffuse ultrasound patterns in the liver. Non-Hodgkin's lymphoma may appear with target and echogenic mass lesions. Burkitt's lymphoma may appear intrahepatic and lucent. Patients with leukemia present with multiple small discrete hepatic masses that are solid with no acoustic enhancement (Fig. 5-87). A bull's-eye appearance with a dense central core may be present as a result of tumor necrosis.

In the pediatric population the most common malignancies are neuroblastomas, Wilms' tumor, and leukemia. The neuroblastoma tumor presents as a densely reflective echo pattern with liver involvement similar to that of a hepatoma. In patients with a Wilms' tumor, metastases generally invade the lung; however the liver may be a secondary site. These lesions present as a densely reflective pattern with lucencies resulting from necrosis.

HEPATIC TRAUMA

The liver is the third most common organ injured in the abdomen after the spleen and kidney. Laceration of the liver occurs in 3% of trauma patients and is frequently associated with other injured organs. The need for surgery is de-

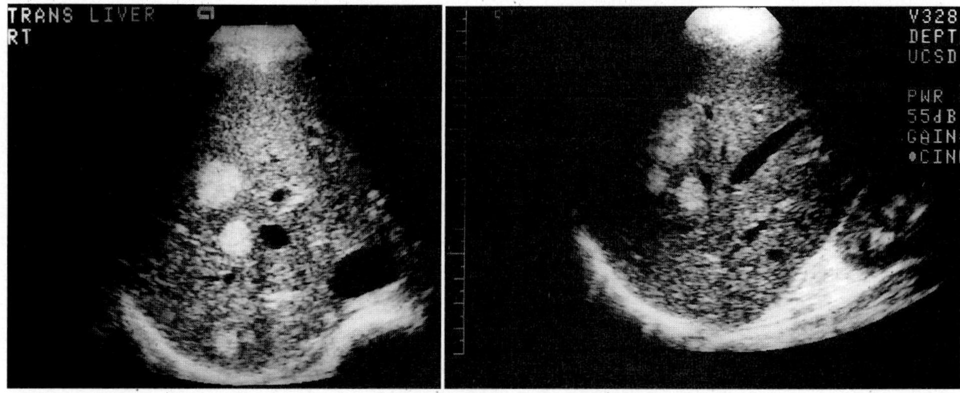

FIG. 5-79 Metastatic disease: well-defined echogenic lesions throughout the liver.

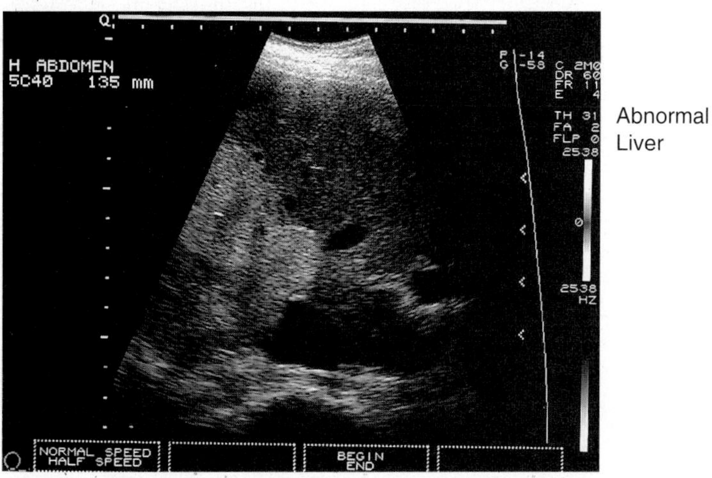

FIG. 5-80 Metastatic disease: well-defined echogenic lesion in the right lobe of the liver.

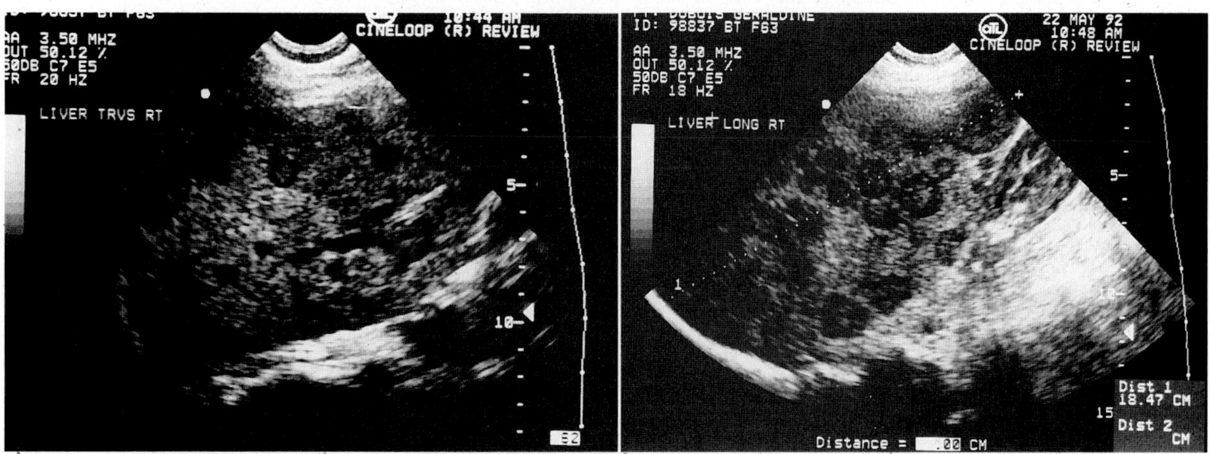

FIG. 5-81 Metastatic disease: multiple diffuse area of "target" bull's-eye lesions throughout the liver.

termined by the size of the laceration, the amount of hemoperitoneum, and the patient's clinical status. The right lobe is more affected than the left. The degree of trauma can vary, with a small laceration, large laceration with a hematoma, subcapsular hematoma, or capsular disruption.

Ultrasound is not used as commonly as other imaging modalities to localize the extent of the laceration. Ultrasound has difficulty detecting small lacerations in the dome of the right lobe of the liver. Intraperitoneal fluid should be assessed along the flanks and into the pelvis. Intrahe-

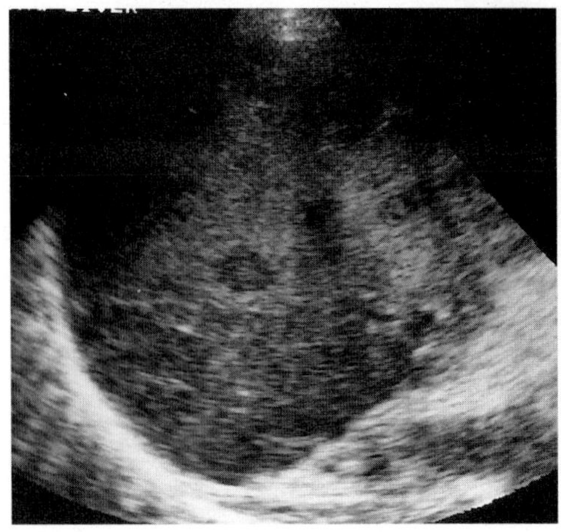

FIG. 5-82 Metastatic disease: hepatomegaly with multiple hypoechoic areas throughout the liver parenchyma.

patic hematomas are hyperechoic in the first 24 hours and hypoechoic and sonolucent thereafter because of the resolution of the blood within the area. Septations and internal echoes develop 1 to 4 weeks after the trauma (Figs. 5-88 and 5-89). A subcapsular hematoma may appear as anechoic, hypoechoic, septated lenticular, or curvilinear. It may be differentiated from ascitic fluid in that it occurs unilaterally, along the area of laceration. The degree of homogenicity depends on the age of the laceration.

LIVER TRANSPLANTATION

Ultrasound can play a significant role in the preoperative and postoperative evaluation of hepatic transplantation. The primary function of the ultrasound examination is to evaluate the portal venous system, the hepatic artery, the inferior vena cava, and the liver parenchymal pattern. The vascular structures should be assessed for size and patency in the preoperative evaluation. The liver parenchyma should be examined to rule out the presence of hepatic architec-

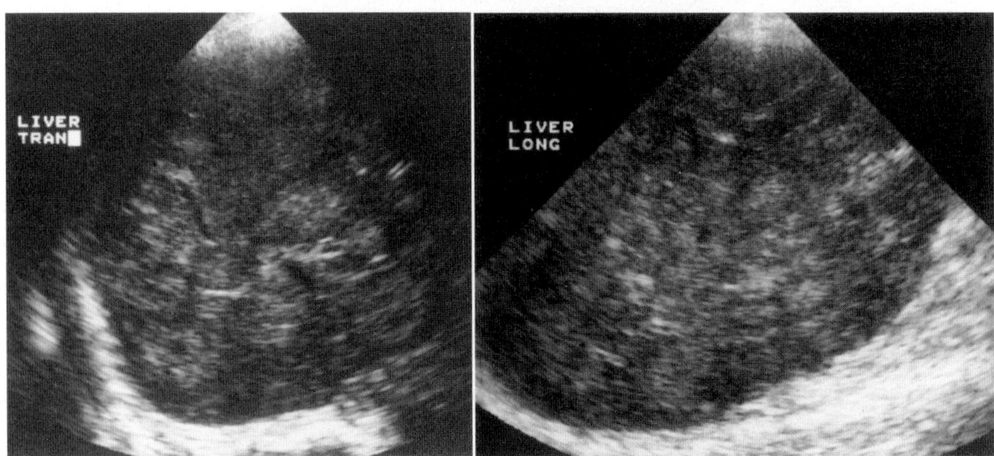

FIG. 5-83 Metastatic disease: hepatomegaly with diffuse lesions throughout the liver parenchyma.

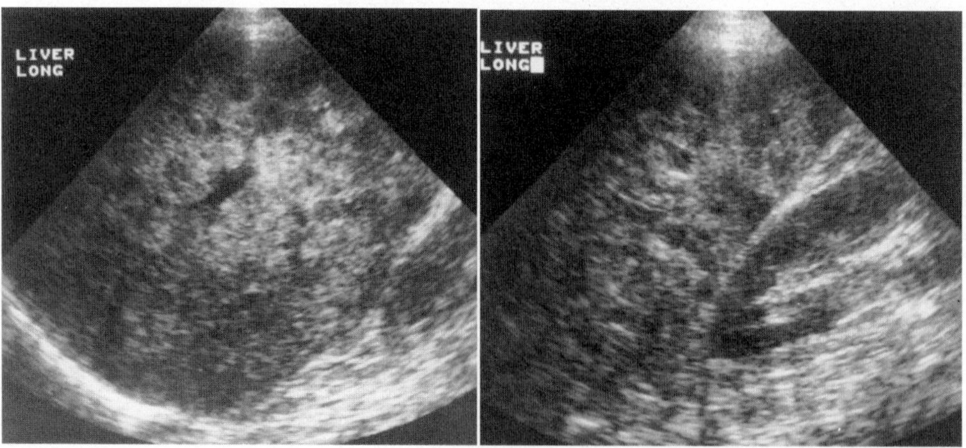

FIG. 5-84 Metastatic disease: hepatomegaly with multiple small hypoechoic lesions throughout the liver.

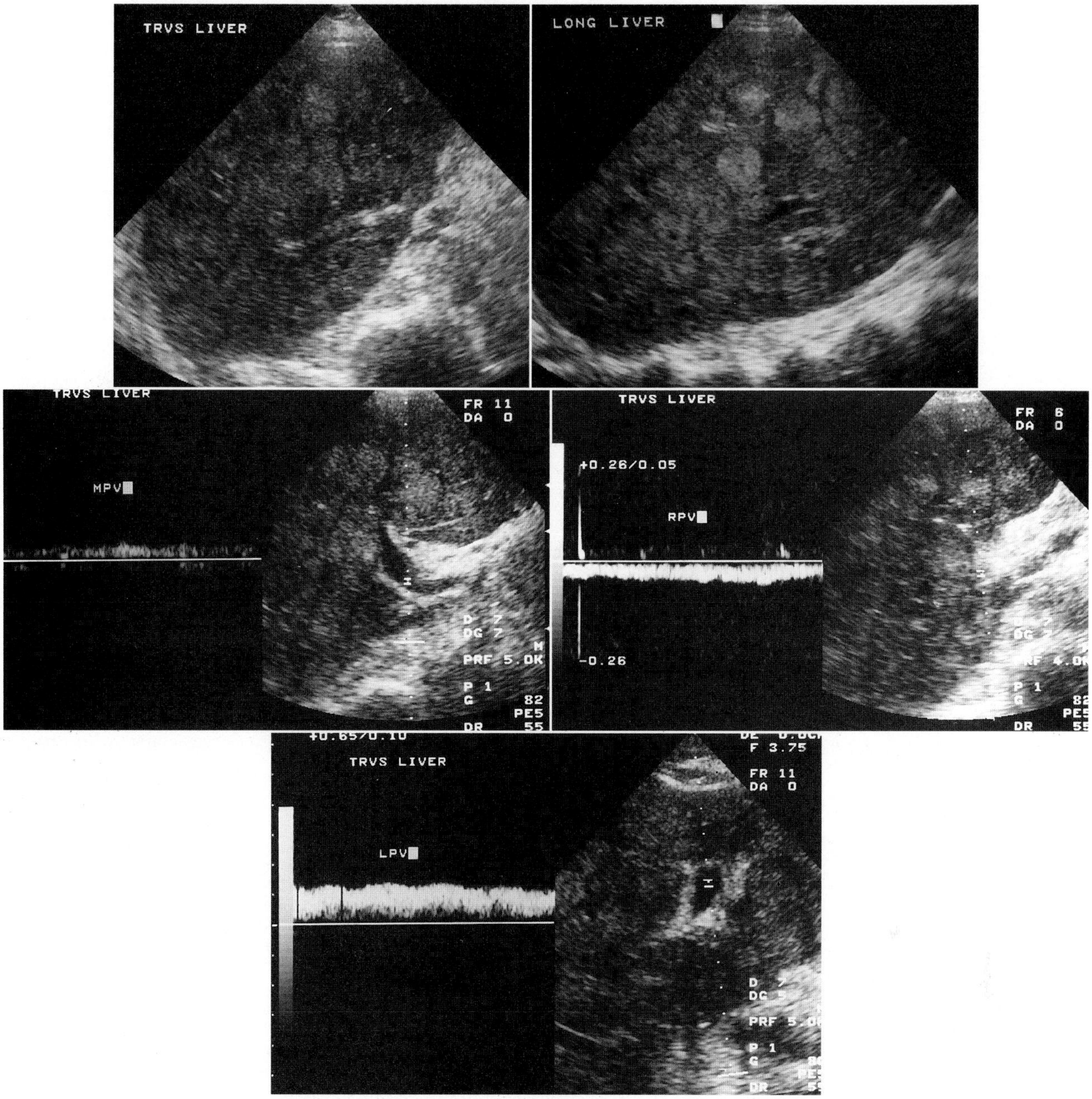

FIG. 5-85 Metastatic disease: hepatomegaly with diffuse isoechoic lesions throughout the liver parenchyma. Decreased flow is noted in the main portal vein secondary to compression of the portal system from the multiple lesions.

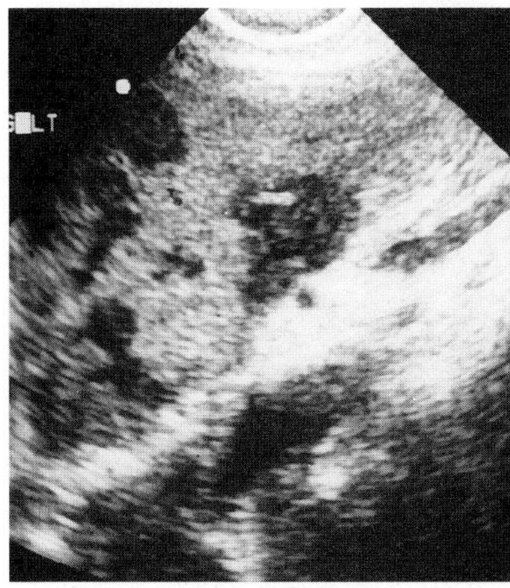

FIG. 5-86 Metastatic disease: the target-type of bull's-eye patterns are the result of edema around the tumor, or necrosis or hemorrhage within the tumor.

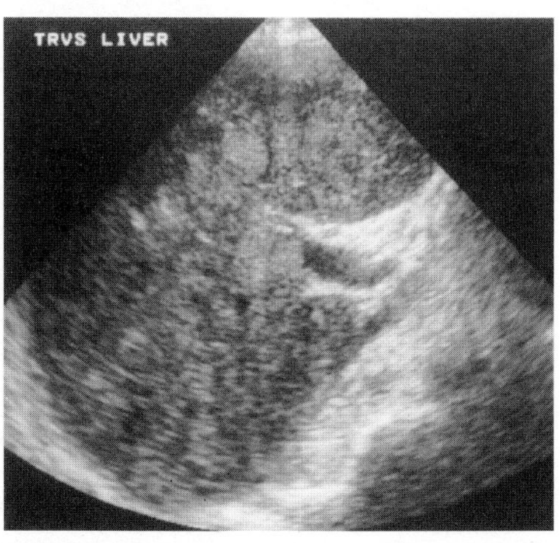

FIG. 5-87 Patient with leukemia presents with hepatosplenomegaly and multiple small discrete hepatic masses that are solid with no acoustic enhancement.

ture disruption. The sonographer should also evaluate the biliary system, to look for dilation, and the portosystemic collateral vessels.

In the pediatric patient the most common reason for liver transplantation is biliary atresia and associated anomalies of the spleen, hepatic vasculature, and kidneys. Therefore, in addition to the examination described above, both kidneys and the spleen must be evaluated.

In the postoperative period, hepatic artery thrombosis is the most serious complication of liver transplantation. The hepatic artery is evaluated with Doppler and color-flow ultrasound in the area of the porta hepatis. The normal hepatic artery flow is a low-resistance arterial signal. Thrombosis may be detected when this signal is absent. In the adult patient collateral vessels in the region of the hepatic artery have not developed. However, in children, collateral hepatic artery circulation may have developed. Thus the scans should be made within 24 hours after surgery, 48 hours after surgery, and weekly thereafter to assess for changes in the velocity-flow pattern.

The development of anastomotic stenoses is another problem in the transplant patient. This flow pattern is a turbulent, high-velocity signal indicative of hepatic artery stenosis. Portal vein thrombosis may also occur in the postoperative period. Air in the portal vein may be seen as brightly echogenic moving targets within the portal venous system. Compromise of the inferior vena cava is another complication of transplantation. A fatal complication is hepatic necrosis associated with thrombosis of the hepatic artery or portal vein. Massive necrosis

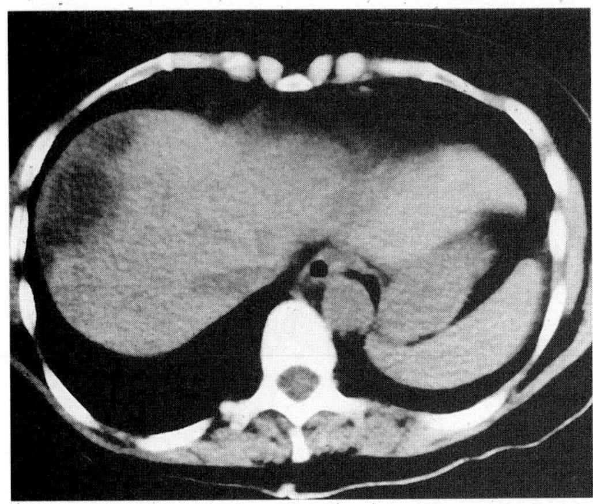

FIG. 5-88 CT of a 54-year-old female with pain in her right upper quadrant for 3 years. The liver function tests were normal. The patient had been involved in a car accident 7 years before the scan. The transverse scan shows old blood along the lateral border of the liver.

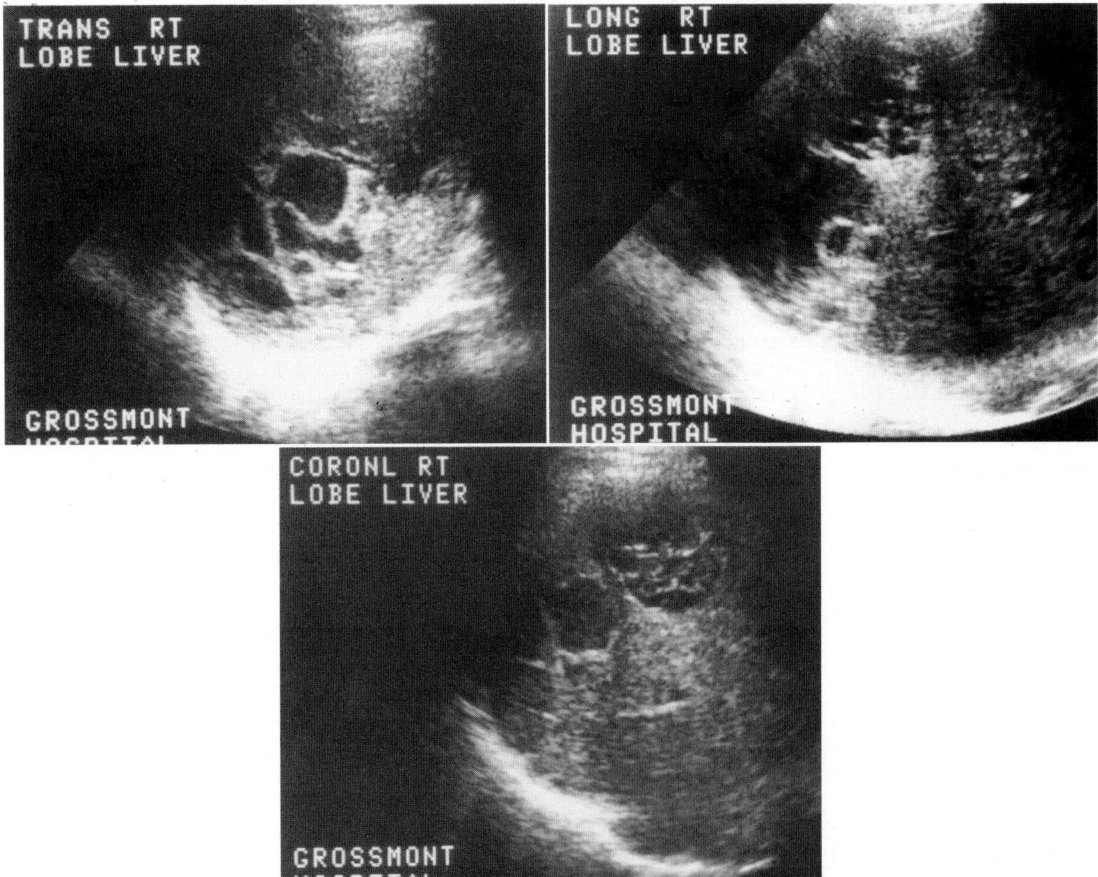

FIG. 5-89 Ultrasound of the patient in Fig. 5-88 shows a complex, septated mass in the right lobe of the liver.

produces gangrene of the liver and air in the hepatic parenchyma.

HEPATIC VASCULAR FLOW ABNORMALITIES

Portal Venous Hypertension

The development of increased pressure in the portal-splenic venous system is the cause of portal hypertension. The hypertension develops when hepatopedal flow (toward the liver) is impeded by thrombus or tumor invasion. The blood becomes obstructed as it passes through the liver to the hepatic veins and is diverted to collateral pathways in the upper abdomen.

Portal hypertension may develop along two pathways. One entails increased resistance to flow and the other entails increased portal blood flow. The most common mechanism for increased resistance to flow occurs in patients with cirrhosis. This disease process produces areas of micro and macro nodular regeneration, atrophy, and fatty infiltration, which makes it difficult for the blood to perfuse. This condition may be found in patients with liver disease or diseases of the cardiovascular system. Patients who present with increased portal blood flow may have an arteriovenous fistula or splenomegaly secondary to a hematologic disorder.

Collateral circulation develops when the normal venous channels become obstructed. This diverted blood flow causes embryologic channels to reopen; blood flows hepatofugally (away from the liver) and is diverted into collateral vessels. The collateral channels may be into the gastric veins (coronary veins), esophageal veins, recanalized umbilical vein, or splenorenal, gastrorenal, retroperitoneal, hemorrhoidal, or intestinal veins. The most common collateral pathways are through the coronary and esophageal veins, as occurs in 80% to 90% of patients with portal hypertension. Varices, tortuous dilations of veins, may develop because of increased pressure in the portal vein, usually secondary to cirrhosis. Bleeding from the varices occurs with increased pressure.

Clinically the patient would present with ascites, hepatosplenomegaly, gastrointestinal bleeding, elevated liver enzymes, jaundice, and hematemesis.

The most definitive way to diagnose portal hypertension is with arteriography. Ultrasound may be very useful in these patients to define the presence of ascites, hepatosplenomegaly, and collateral circulation; the cause of jaundice; and the patency of hepatic vascular channels.

LIVER DISEASES
Cirrhosis—all types
Congenital hepatic fibrosis
Schistosomiasis (parasitic worms)
Idiopathic portal hypertension
Sarcoidosis
Alcoholic hepatitis

DISEASES OF THE CARDIOVASCULAR SYSTEM
Portal vein occlusion
Splenic vein occlusion
Hepatic vein occlusion
Thrombosis of the inferior vena cava
Congestive right heart failure

Color Doppler Evaluation of Collateral Circulation

On ultrasound the dilated venous structures near the superior mesenteric-splenic vein confluence, the main portal vein, and the gastric veins should be evaluated. As one scans in the longitudinal plane, medial to the superior mesenteric and splenic vein confluence, the right and left gastric veins may be seen as collateral circulation. If the gastric veins are serving as collateral circulation, their diameter should be enlarged to 4 to 5 mm (Figs. 5-90 and 5-91; see color images of Fig. 5-90).

The umbilical vein may become recanalized secondary to portal hypertension (Fig. 5-92). This vessel is best seen on the longitudinal plane near the midline, as a tubular structure coursing posterior to the medial surface of the left lobe of the liver (Fig. 5-93). On transverse scans a bull's-eye is seen within the ligamentum teres as the enlarged umbilical vein. Color Doppler helps the sonographer identify this vascular structure.

Other vessels that may become collaterals include the esophageal vessels, which are best seen in the midline transverse plane as the transducer is angled in a cephalic direction through the left lobe of the liver. The dilated gastrorenal, splenorenal, and short gastric veins are seen in the transverse and longitudinal planes near the splenic hilum (Fig. 5-94).

As you recall, the normal portal venous blood flows toward the liver, with the main portal vein flowing in a hepatopedal direction into the liver. Color Doppler would show this flow as a red or positive color pattern. The portal branches running posteriorly, or away, would appear as blue or negative flow. Thus the right portal vein would appear blue, the left portal vein would appear red. The normal portal vein waveform is monophasic with low velocity. There should be little change with the patient's respiration and cardiac motion. The flow should be smooth and laminar. The normal diameter of the portal vein is 1.0 to 1.6 mm (Fig. 5-95). The superior mesenteric vein and splenic vein are more influenced by respiration and patient position; thus, if they appear larger it may not be as a result of portal hypertension. Flow reversal is seen both with spectral waveform patterns below the baseline in the main portal vein and with reversed color direction. Obstruction

FIG. 5-90 A 43-year-old female with a history of chronic hepatitis and cirrhosis. The liver was within normal size limits, but small compared with the spleen. Diffuse coarsening with focal parenchymal lesions were seen in the liver. Cavernous transformation of the portal vein is identified, with multiple small periportal collaterals seen on color-flow imaging. Multiple collateral channels and varices are also identified on the surface of the left lobe of the liver. See color images.

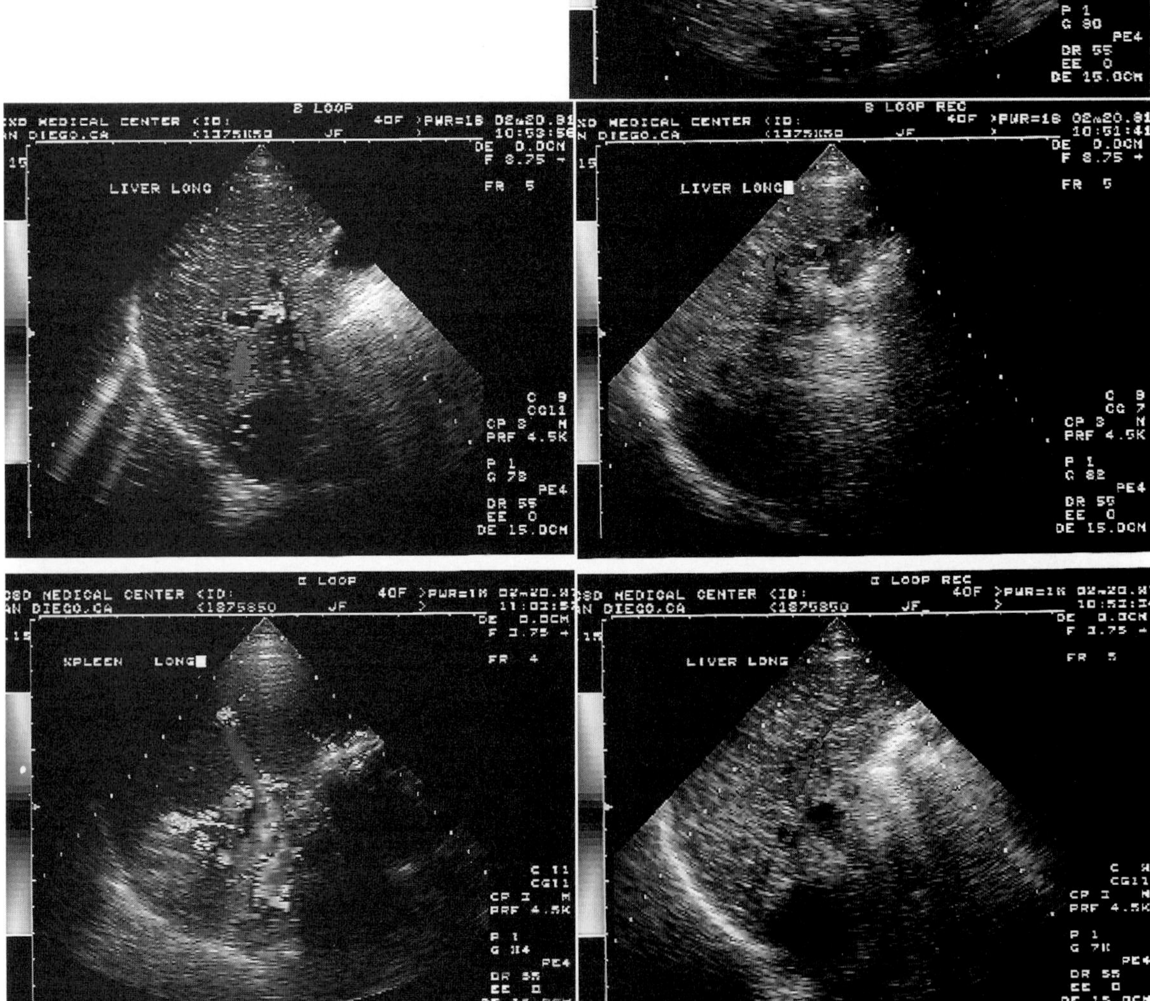

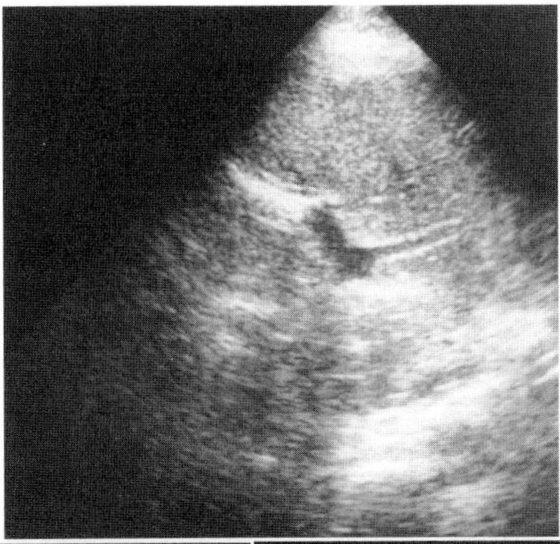

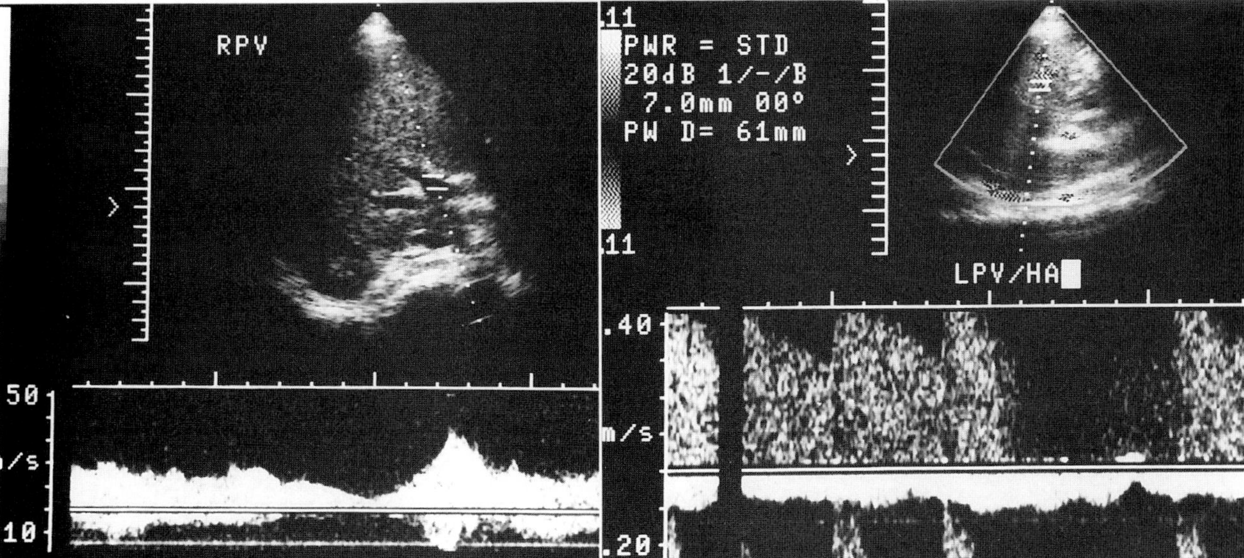

FIG. 5-91 A 37-year-old male suffered a stab wound of the right upper quadrant with laceration of the portal vein. Doppler flow patterns were normal in the right and main portal veins. Thrombus formation was seen in the left portal vein.

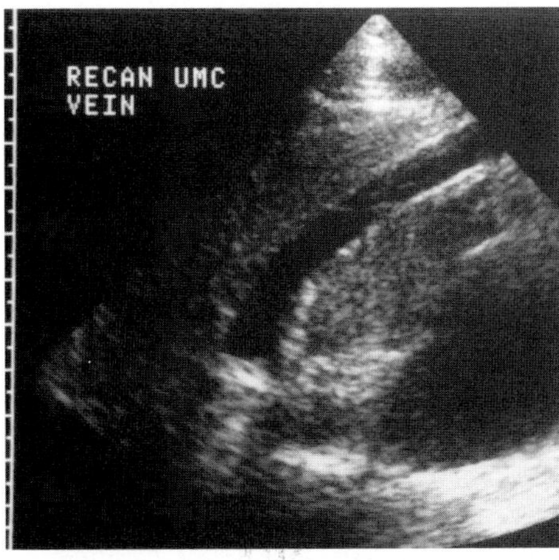

FIG. 5-92 The umbilical vein may become recanalized secondary to portal hypertension. The longitudinal scan shows the left lobe of the liver with the recanalized umbilical vein flowing under its posterior surface.

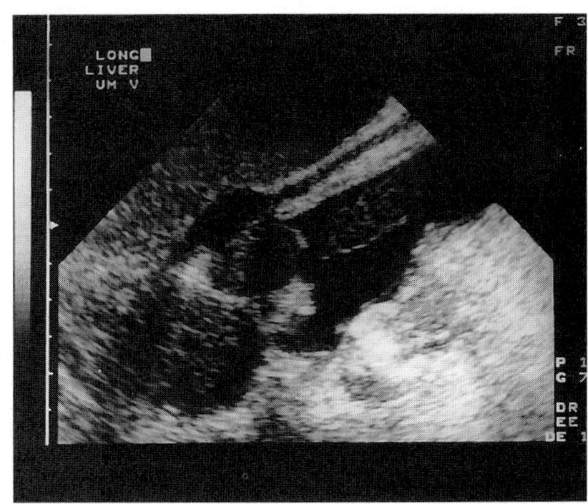

FIG. 5-93 A recanalized umbilical vein is seen in this patient with ascites and cirrhosis.

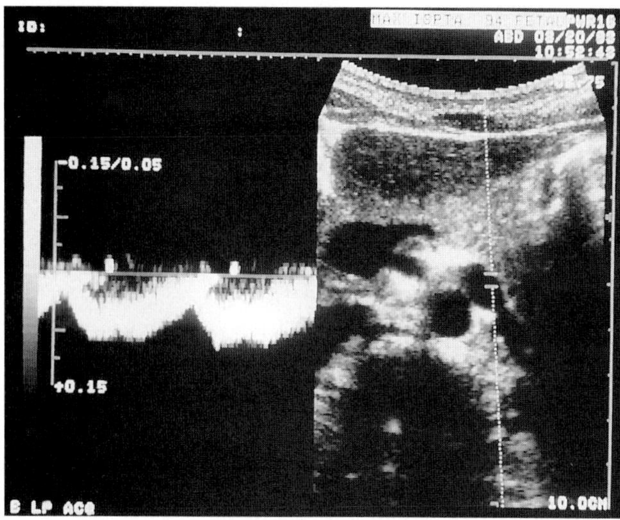

FIG. 5-94 The splenic vein shows flow reversal in this patient with portal hypertension and thrombosis of the main portal vein.

of the portal venous system is recognized by turbulence within the vessel.

Portal Hypertension Secondary to Portal Vein Thrombosis

The invasion of the portal system with tumor or thrombosis may cause portal hypertension if the vessel is significantly occluded so blood cannot flow into the liver. The clinical symptoms are very different from those of intrahepatic disease; ascites is the primary complaint. The patient does not have jaundice or a tender, enlarged liver. Splenomegaly may be present, as well as bleeding varices.

Portal vein thrombosis may develop secondary to trauma, sepsis, cirrhosis, or hepatocellular carcinoma (Fig. 5-96; see color images). The definitive diagnosis is made with a liver biopsy and positive findings of portal hypertension. On ultrasound, portal flow is absent and the vessel may be filled with hypoechoic thrombus.

Portal Vein Hypertension and Portal Caval Shunts

If the portal hypertension becomes extensive, the portal system can be decompressed by shunting blood to the sys-

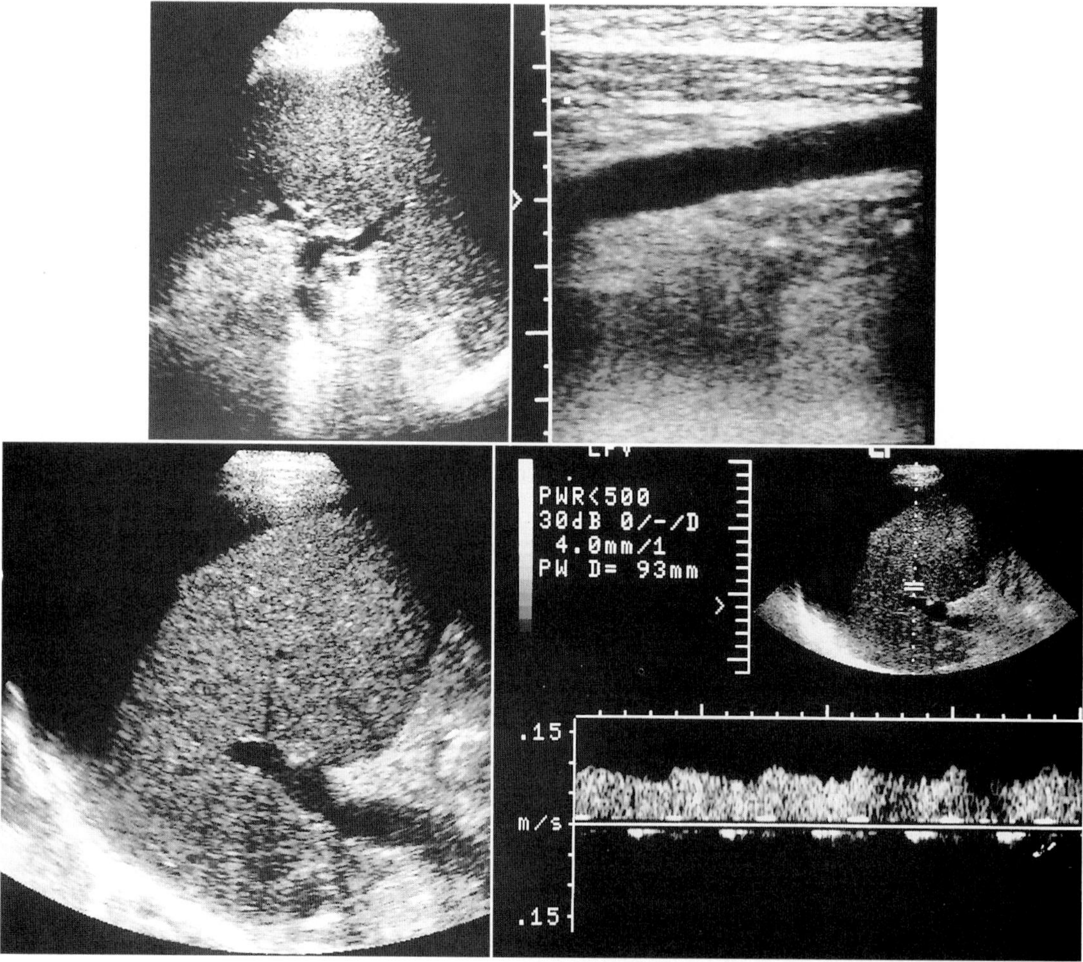

FIG. 5-95 A patient with cirrhosis and hepatosplenomegaly shows a recanalized umbilical vein with normal flow in the left portal vein.

temic venous system. There are basically the following three types of shunts: portacaval, mesocaval, and splenorenal. It is the responsibility of the sonographer to know specifically which type of shunt the patient has in place to image the flow patterns correctly. The portacaval shunt attaches the main portal vein at the superior mesenteric vein-splenic vein confluence to the anterior aspect of the inferior vena cava (Fig. 5-97). The mesocaval shunt attaches the middistal superior mesenteric vein to the inferior vena cava (Figs. 5-98 to 5-100; see color image of Fig. 5-99). This shunt may be difficult to image if overlying bowel gas is present. The splenorenal shunt attaches the splenic vein to the left renal vein. The shunt and connecting vessel should be documented with real time pulsed Doppler and color Doppler to determine flow patterns and patency.

Budd-Chiari Syndrome

Budd-Chiari syndrome is an uncommon, often dramatic illness caused by thrombosis of the hepatic veins or inferior vena cava. It was first described by Budd in 1846 and by Chiari in 1899. In 1959, Parker reviewed 164 patients with this disorder, including 18 from his own hospital.

Budd-Chiari syndrome is characterized by abdominal pain, massive ascites, and hepatomegaly. It has a poor prognosis. It may present acutely or as a chronic illness lasting from a few weeks to several years. Extensive hepatic vein occlusion is usually fatal within weeks or months of the onset of symptoms.

Ultrasonography has proven useful in diagnosing this syndrome. Doppler sonography may be used to evaluate blood-flow patterns in the hepatic venous system in patients with suspected hepatic vein thrombosis. Here we discuss the etiology, clinical manifestations, diagnosis, and sonographic features of this disease.

Etiology

Budd-Chiari syndrome may be classified as primary or secondary on the basis of its pathophysiology. The primary

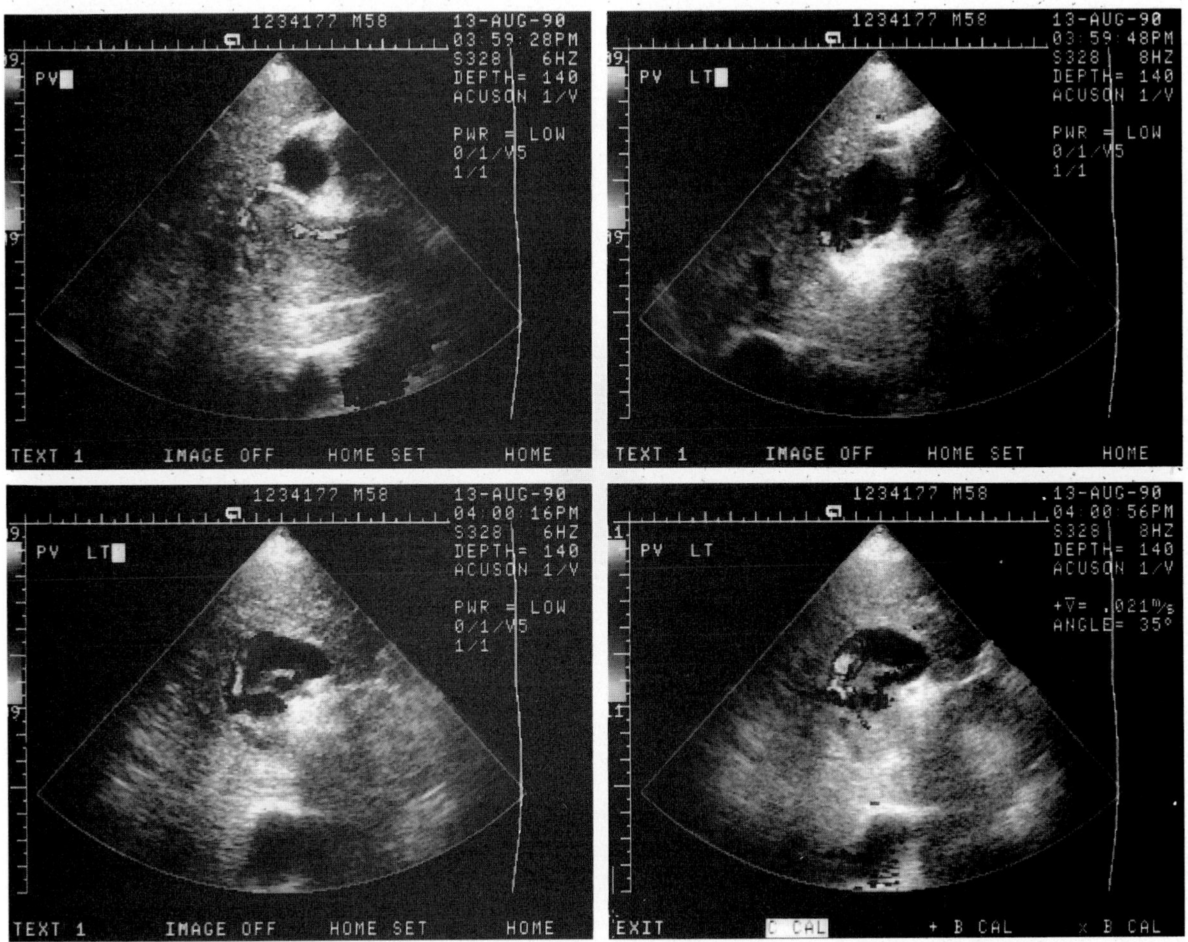

FIG. 5-96 A 60-year-old male 5 years after portacaval shunt. Ultrasound findings revealed hepatomegaly with diffusely abnormal liver architecture and thrombus within the portal venous system, porta caval shunt, and inferior vena cava. These findings were consistent with diffuse hepatoma invading the portal venous system. The portacaval shunt was patent with turbulent flow. The portal vein flow was hepatofugal. There was hepatopedal flow in the superior mesenteric vein and splenic vein. See color images.

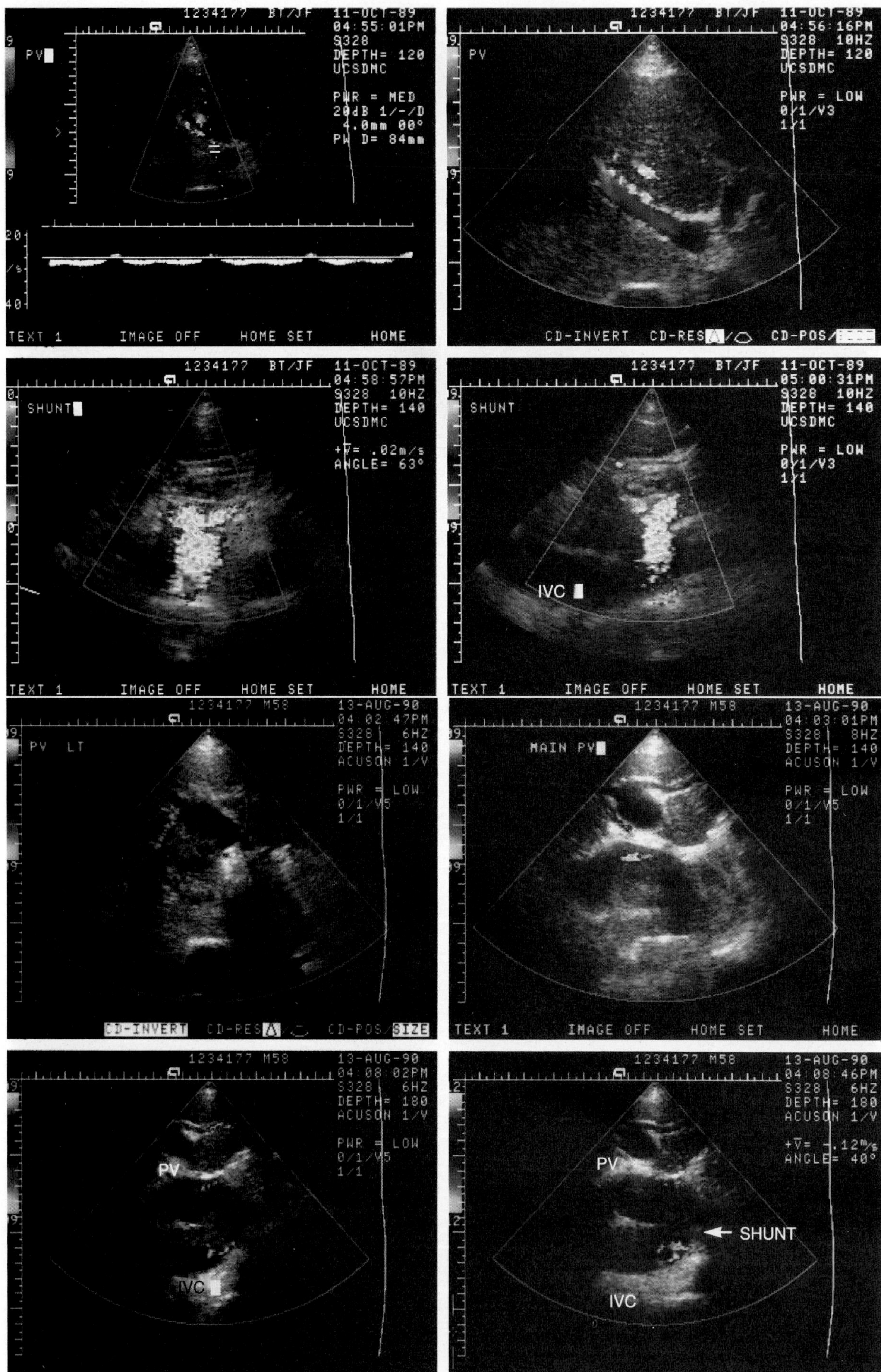

FIG. 5-96, cont'd.

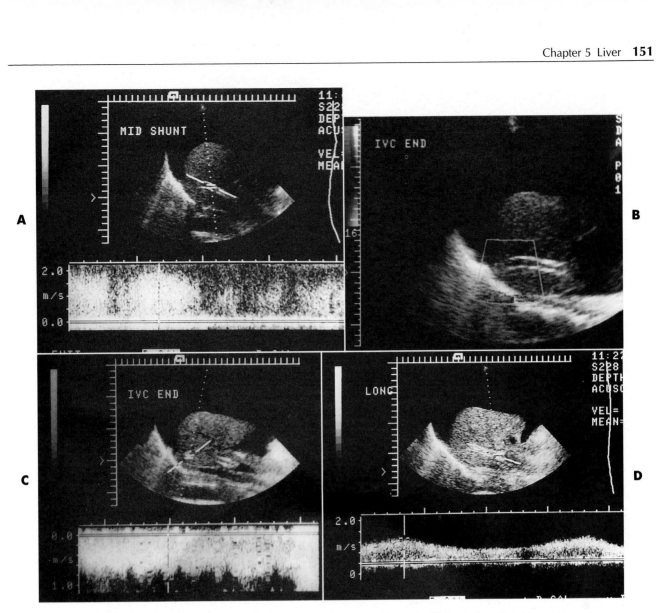

FIG. 5-97 A 54-year-old male after portacaval shunt. The shunt should be evaluated at its proximal, middle, and distal ends to make sure turbulent flow is present. The bright, echogenic tubular structure, **B,** represents the Gore-Tex shunt material.

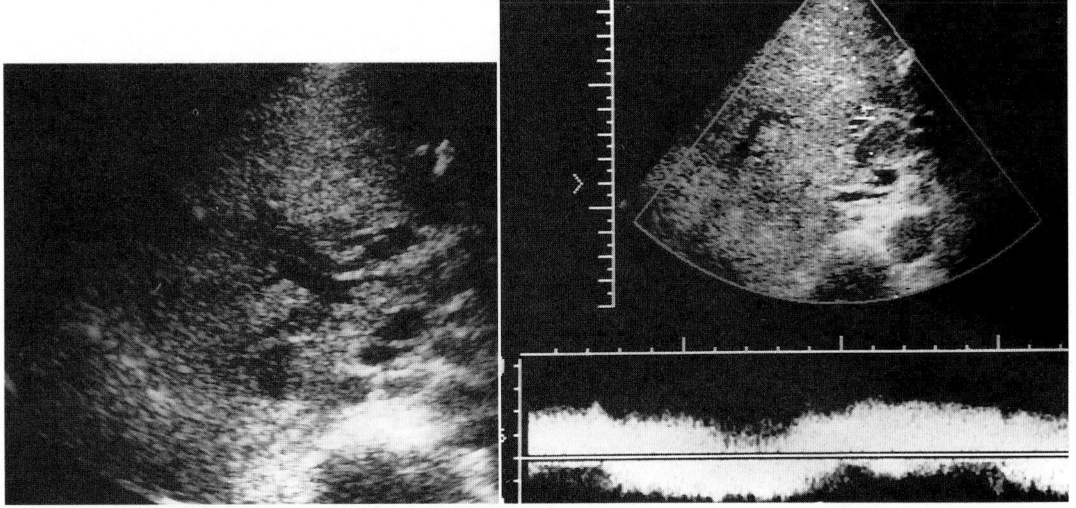

FIG. 5-98 The mesocaval shunt attaches the middistal superior mesenteric vein to the inferior vena cava. This patient showed thrombosis at its distal end with to-and-fro flow reversal.

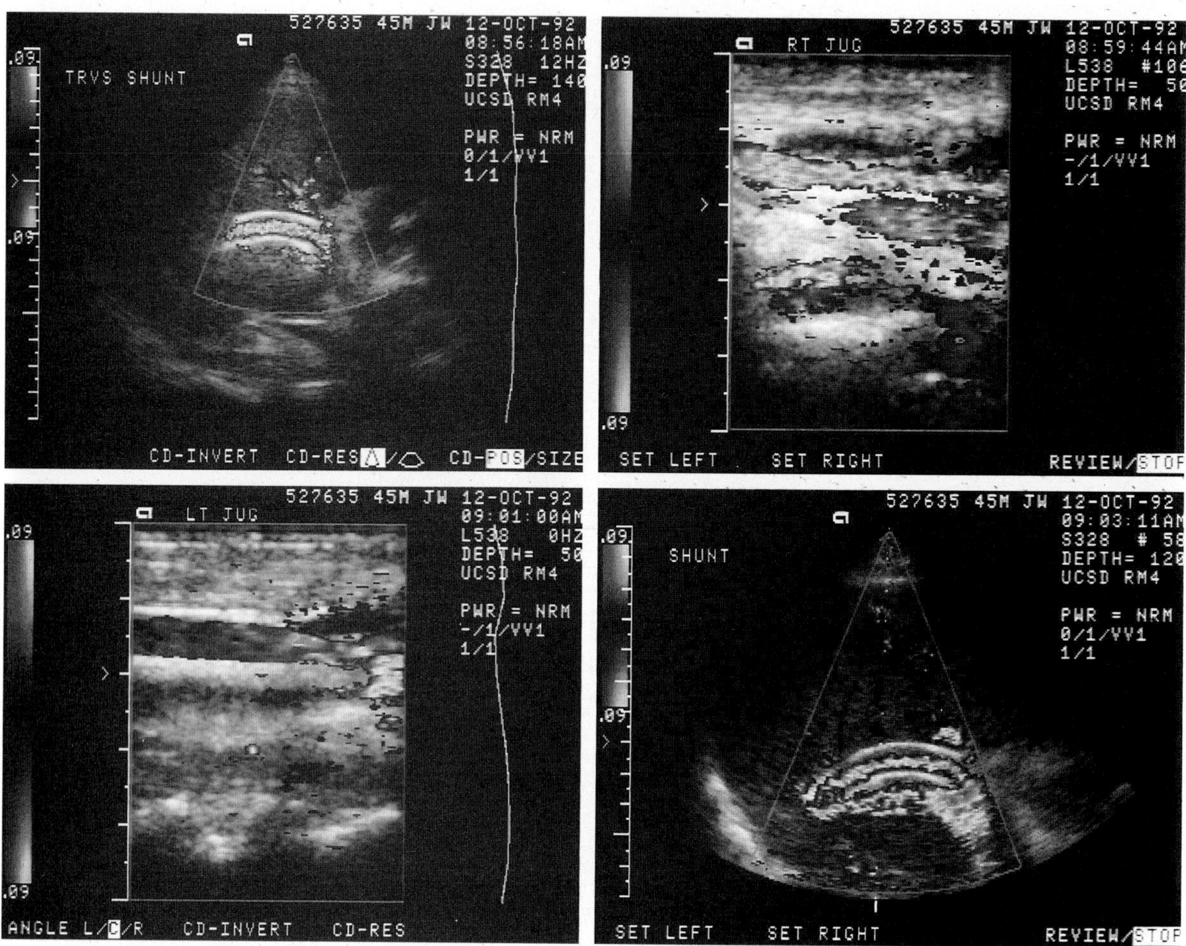

FIG. 5-99 Color flow is very helpful to determine the patency of the shunt and direction of flow. This patient showed turbulence within the patent shunt. The jugular vessels were evaluated as well. See color image.

type is caused by congenital obstruction of the hepatic veins or inferior vena cava by membranous webs across the upper vena cava at or just above the entrance of the left and middle hepatic veins. This lesion has been found to be most common in Asia.

The secondary type results from thrombosis in the hepatic veins or inferior vena cava. It often occurs in patients with predisposing posing conditions, such as polycythemia rubra vera, paroxysmal nocturnal hemoglobinuria, prolonged use of oral contraceptives, pregnancy tumors (hepatocellular carcinoma, renal cell carcinoma, adrenal carcinoma, leiomyosarcoma of the inferior vena cava), infections, and in rare cases, trauma. In approximately 25% to 30% of all cases the exact cause is never determined.

Clinical Manifestations

Ascites is the most characteristic clinical feature of this disease. Other symptoms are abdominal pain, hepatosplenomegaly, jaundice, vomiting, and diarrhea. Rarely, patients present with acute illness with abdominal pain, hepatomegaly, and shock. This condition often occurs in patients with an underlying disease, such as renal cell carcinoma, primary cancer of the liver, thrombophlebitis migrans, or polycythemia. More commonly, patients present with vague illness and abdominal distress weeks or months in duration, followed by the appearance of ascites and hepatomegaly. Jaundice is mild or absent. As portal hypertension increases, the spleen becomes palpable. When thrombus is found in the inferior vena cava, edema of the legs is gross and there is venous distension over the abdomen, flanks, and back. Albuminuria may be found.

Laboratory Values

Routine biochemical determinations of aminotransferases and alkaline phosphate indicate mild or moderate impairment of hepatic function, depending on the stage of disease. Clinically apparent jaundice is unusual.

Diagnosis

The following are three important diagnostic steps in managing hepatic vein thrombosis: imaging the liver, liver biopsy, and angiography and venography. Several imaging techniques have been used to evaluate patients with suspected hepatic vein thrombosis, including liver scintigra-

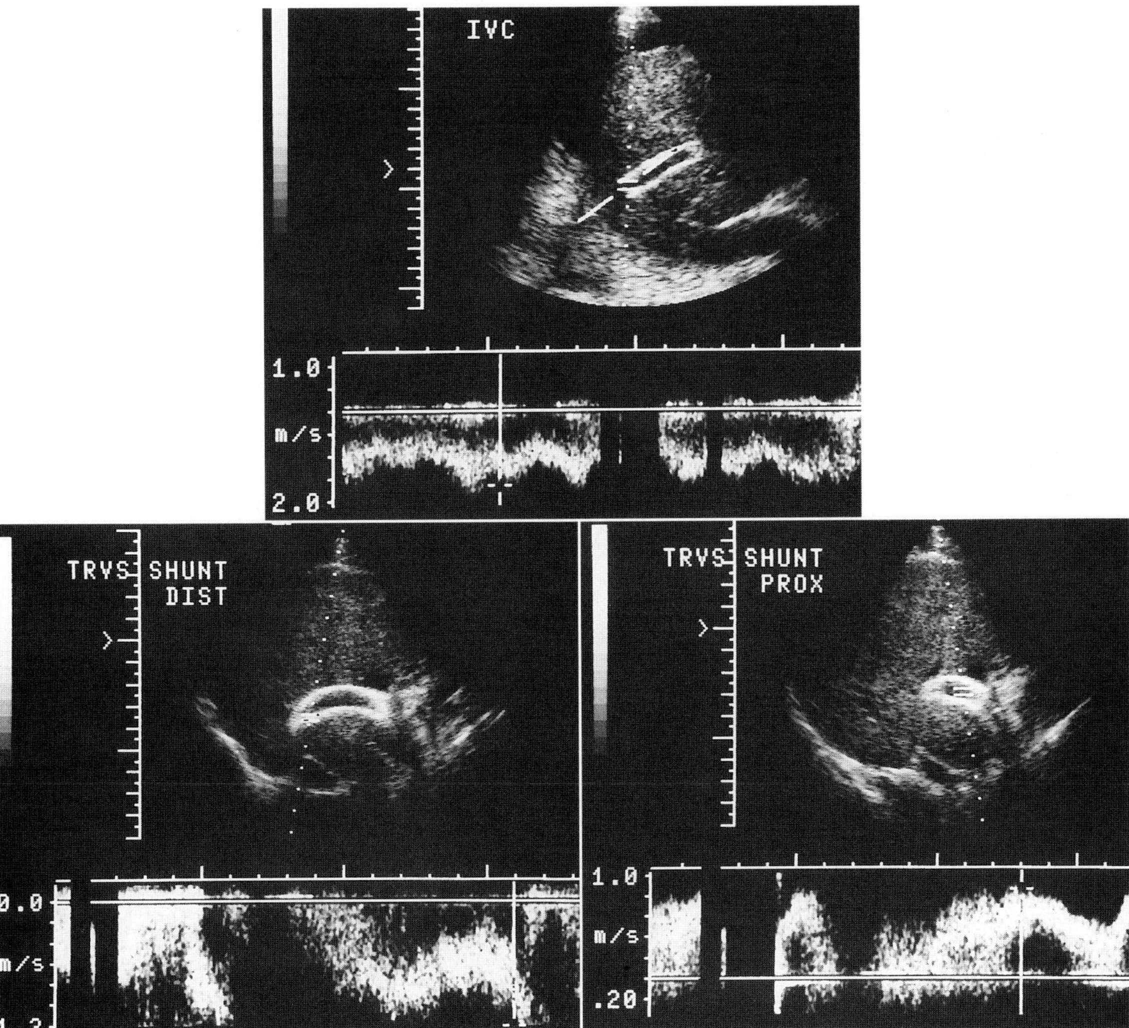

FIG. 5-100 A 50-year-old male after TIPS procedure. Ultrasound evaluation of the liver and TIPS stent revealed patency of the stent and normal flow direction from the portal vein to the inferior vena cava. No evidence of thrombosis was seen.

phy, computed tomography, magnetic resonance imaging, and ultrasound.

Liver Biopsy

A needle liver biopsy is essential to the actual diagnosis of Budd-Chiari syndrome. Characteristic pathologic features found in the liver biopsy are intense centrilobar congestion and extravasation of red cells into the Disse's spaces. Cell atrophy and necrosis secondary to local ischemia are often present. Hepatic metastases are distinguished clinically and by the liver biopsy.

Hepatic Angiography and Venography

Hepatic angiography is critical in establishing the diagnosis and the presence of additional vascular involvement. Arteriography demonstrates an enlarged liver with stretching and bowing of the hepatic arteries. Hepatic venography may fail or show narrow occluded veins. It is imperative to search the inferior vena cava for the presence of membranous webs, thrombosis, and extrinsic compression.

Sonographic Features

Ultrasonography is useful in imaging patients with hepatic vein thrombosis and has proven to be diagnostic in 87% of cases. The caudate lobe of the liver, seen in longitudinal and transverse scans, has an independent vascular supply. In Budd-Chiari syndrome the caudate lobe becomes enlarged and there is often atrophy of the right hepatic lobe, probably as a result of sparing of caudate lobe hepatic veins when there is thrombosis of the right, middle, and left hepatic veins.

The liver appears hypoechoic in the early stages of acute thrombosis; it appears hyperechoic and inhomogeneous with fibrosis in later stages. The thrombosed hepatic veins become enlarged. In chronic cases of Budd-Chiari syndrome the hepatic veins are usually not visualized. Demonstration of at least one major vein may show abnormalities in the vessel suggestive of this syndrome: stenosis, dilation, thick wall echoes, abnormal course, extrahepatic anastomoses, and thrombosis.

Doppler sonography may show altered blood-flow patterns in the hepatic veins and inferior vena cava. In normal subjects the Doppler signal in the hepatic veins is triphasic with wide variations in flow velocity and direction (Fig. 5-101). Abnormal Doppler patterns with slow, continuous flow probably indicate partial obstruction. The absence of flow signals suggests subtotal or total occlusion. Turbulent flow may be observed beyond the area of stenosis.

Color flow Doppler is an excellent technique for evaluating the hepatic venous system. Flow direction and velocities and areas of turbulent flow can be demonstrated with color. Patency of the hepatic veins and inferior vena cava can be determined with color flow Doppler, which compares very favorably with angiography.

Ascites

The presence of ascites can be confirmed by ultrasound; it is present in more than 90% of patients with this syndrome.

Splenomegaly

Splenomegaly is present in 30% of patients. It may be secondary to portal hypertension or to an underlying myeloproliferative disorder.

Treatment

The mortality rate for patients with hepatic vein thrombosis is high, but with the routine use of imaging, this syndrome has been diagnosed more often and in milder forms. Anticoagulants and streptokinase may be of value, although there is no definite evidence that this therapy promotes resolution of established thrombosis.

Surgical construction of portosystemic shunts is consid-

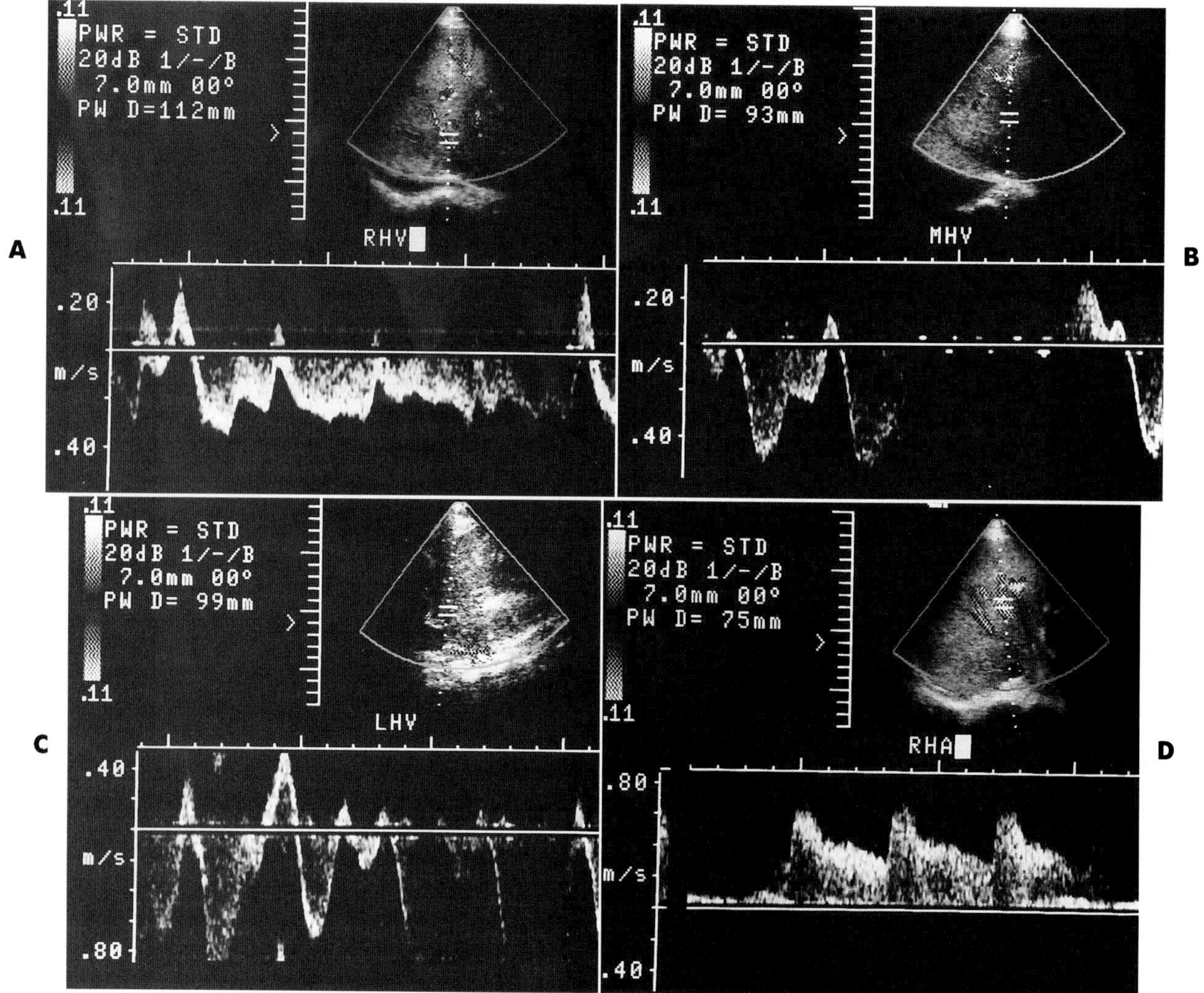

FIG. 5-101 Normal flow patterns in the hepatic veins show a triphasic flow with wide variations in flow velocity and direction. Abnormal Doppler patterns with slow, continuous flow indicate partial obstruction. **A,** Right hepatic vein. **B,** Middle hepatic vein. **C,** Left hepatic vein. **D,** Right hepatic artery.

ered in symptomatic patients who have a patent portal vein. These include portacaval, mesocaval and splenorenal shunts. The aim of these shunts is to decompress the congested liver and reverse portal venous flow.

Budd-Chiari syndrome may be managed with side-to-side portocaval shunting but is best treated by liver transplantation in patients with end-stage liver disease. Long-term anticoagulant therapy is mandatory for patients with this syndrome after liver transplantation, since there is an increased risk of thrombotic complications.

Membranous webs may be surgically corrected by resection. Transluminal angioplasty has also been used to dilate webs.

Recently nonsurgical treatments have been performed using interventional techniques. A percutaneous portocaval shunt is placed using a wall-stent prosthesis and right internal jugular approach to relieve portal hypertension. This may provide an attractive alternative to surgery since many patients with Budd-Chiari syndrome are poor surgical risks.

Budd-Chiari syndrome is a rare disorder characterized by right upper quadrant pain, hepatomegaly, and ascites. Although biopsy and venography are essential to diagnose this disease, ultrasonography is a noninvasive technique that provides valuable information. Thorough knowledge of liver anatomy and the characteristics of hepatic vein thrombosis enable the sonographer to better evaluate hepatic vasculature in the patient with Budd-Chiari syndrome.

REVIEW QUESTIONS

1. How would you describe the echogenicity of the liver compared to that of the spleen, pancreas, and kidney?
2. Describe the anatomic position of the liver as it relates to the nine abdominal sections.
3. Describe the three lobes of the liver.
4. What are the tributaries of the portal venous system and what is the relationship of these vessels to other structures in the upper abdomen?
5. What are the distinguishing characteristics of hepatic and portal veins?
6. Name the segments of the right and left lobes of the liver.
7. Describe the location and usefulness of the following intrahepatic structures:
   a. Right hepatic vein
   b. Middle hepatic vein
   c. Left hepatic vein
   d. Right anterior portal vein
   e. Right posterior portal vein
   f. Left portal vein (initial)
   g. Left ascending portal vein
   h. Inferior vena cava fossa
   i. Gallbladder fossa
   j. Ligamentum teres
   k. Fissure of ligamentum venosum
8. Describe the relational anatomy of the liver.
9. Name the functions of the liver.
10. What are the important hepatic enzymes found in the liver?
11. Describe the laboratory differences and similarities between hepatocellular disease and obstructive disease of the liver (bilirubin, serum albumin, SGOT, SGPT, alkaline phosphatase).
12. What is the difference between direct and indirect bilirubin?
13. Discuss bile as the excretory product of the liver.
14. What happens to blood flow in a patient with portal hypertension?
15. What is the difference between hepatopedal and hepatofugal flow in the liver?
16. Describe the relationship of the hepatic artery, common bile duct, and portal vein.
17. What technique is used to properly set your ultrasound system controls for a liver examination?
18. Define the criteria used for "adequate scanning technique."
19. Define the protocol for a normal liver examination.
20. In hepatocellular disease, what happens to the bilirubin and alkaline phosphatase levels?
21. What is the ultrasound appearance of fatty infiltration of the liver?
22. Are there specific differences between acute and chronic hepatitis on ultrasound? What are they?
23. Describe the ultrasound characteristics of cirrhosis.
24. What are the causes for biliary obstruction proximal to the cystic duct? Distal to the cystic duct?
25. Describe the types of cystic lesions found in the liver.
26. Define the characteristics of polycystic liver disease.
27. What are the primary causes and clinical symptoms of hepatic abscesses?
28. What are the ultrasound appearances of pyogenic abscess and hepatic candidiasis?
29. Discuss the course of amebic abscess in the liver and its ultrasound findings.
30. What are the ultrasound characteristics of echinococcal disease in the liver?
31. Describe the ultrasound appearance of a cavernous hemangioma.
32. Discuss the causes of hepatic adenoma.
33. What liver lesions are associated with the use of oral contraceptives?
34. What is the most common malignant liver tumor? Describe the tumor patterns, clinical course, and ultrasound appearance.
35. What are the primary sites of tumor that metastasize to the liver?
36. Name the ultrasound patterns of liver metastases.
37. Discuss trauma to the right upper quadrant and its effect on the liver. What are the ultrasound findings?
38. What structures should the sonographer scan in a liver transplant patient before and after surgery?

39. Name the collateral pathways developed in patients with portal hypertension.
40. What structures should be evaluated with color and Doppler flow in patients with portal hypertension?
41. Name the three basic surgical shunts in the portal venous system.
42. Describe the primary and secondary types of Budd-Chiari syndrome.
43. What are the sonographic features of Budd-Chiari syndrome?

BIBLIOGRAPHY

Liver

Auh YH, Rubenstein WA, Zirinsky K, et al: Accessory fissures of the liver: CT and sonographic appearance, Am J Roentgenol 143:565, 1984.

Berland LL: Focal areas of decreased echogenicity in the liver at the porta hepatis, J Ultrasound Med 5:157, 1986.

Brown BM, Filly RA, and Callen, PW: Ultrasonographic anatomy of the caudate lobe, JUM 1:189, 1982.

Budd G: On diseases of the liver, pg 147, London, 1845, Churchill.

Callen PW, Filly RA, and Demartini WJ: The left portal vein: a possible source of confusion on ultrasonograms, Radiology 130:205, 1979.

Chiari H: Ueber die Selbstandige Phlebitis Obliterans der Haupstamme der Vanae Hepaticae als Todesur sache, Beitr Z Pathol Anat 26:1, 1899.

Donoso L, Noguera Am, Zidan A, et al: Papillary process of the caudate lobe of the liver: sonographic appearance, Radiology 173:631, 1989.

Feigin RD, Glickson M, Varstending A, et al: Famial Budd-Chiari syndrome due to membranous obstruction of the hepatic vein treated with transluminal angioplasty. Am J Gastroenterology, 85(1):94-7, 1990.

Filly RA, Allen B, Menton M, et al: In vitro investigation of the origin of echoes within biliary sludge, J Clin Ultrasound 8:193, 1980.

Fried AM, Kreel L, and Cosgrove DD: The hepatic interlobar fissure, Am J Radiol 143:561, 1984.

Gips CH: Membranous obstruction of the suprahepatic segment of the inferior vena cava, Folia Med Neerl 15:228, 1972.

Grant EG: Budd-Chiari syndrome: the results of duplex and color Doppler imaging, Am J Roentgenol 142:377, 1989.

Kimura C, Shirotani H, Hirooka M, et al: Membranous obliteration of the inferior vena cava in the hepatic portion, J Cardiovasc Surg 4:87, 1963.

Leopold GR: Ultrasonography of jaundice, Radiol Clin North Am 17:127, 1979.

Marchal G, Kint E, Nijssens M, et al: Variability of the hepatic arterial anatomy, J Clin Ultrasound 9:377, 1981.

Marks WM, Filly RA, and Callen PW: Ultrasonic anatomy of the liver: a review with new applications, J Clin Ultrasound 7:137, 1979.

Martinoli C, Cittadini G, Conzi R, et al: Sonographic characterization of an accessory fissure of the left hepatic lobe determined by omental infolding, J Ultrasound Med 11:103, 1992.

Matsui O, Kadoya M, Kameyama T, et al: Benign and malignant nodules in cirrhotic livers: distinction based on blood supply, Radiology 178:493, 1991.

Mattrey RF, Strich G, Shelton RE, et al: Perfluorochemicals as US contrast agents for tumor imaging and hepatosplenography, Radiology 163:339, 1987.

Mitchell MC, Boitnott JK, Kaufman S, et al: Budd-Chiari syndrome: etiology, diagnosis and management, Medicine, 61: 199, 1982.

Murphy FB: The Budd-Chiari syndrome: a review. Am J Roentgenol 147:9, 1986.

Oldhafer KJ, Ringe B, Wittekind C, et al: Budd-Chiari syndrome: portacaval shunt and subsequent liver transplantation, Surgery 107:471, 1990.

Parker RGF: Occlusion of the hepatic veins in man, Medicine 38:369, 1959.

Pompili M: U.S.-Doppler diagnosis of Budd-Chiari syndrome, J Clin Gastroenterol 12:591, 1990.

Powell-Jackson, et al: Ultrasound scanning and 99mTC sulphur colloid scintigraphy in diagnosis of Budd-Chiari syndrome, Gut 27:1502, 1986.

Raby N, et al: Budd-Chiari syndrome: shunt selection and postoperative assessment, Clinical Radiol 40:586, 1989.

Radin DR, Colletti PM, Ralls PW, et al: Agenesis of the right lobe of the liver, Radiology 164:639, 1987.

Ring EJ: Percutaneous portacaval shunts. Presented at the Third Interventional Symposium on Peripheral Vascular Intervention, Miami, Fla, January 1991.

Rubenstein WA, Yong HA, Whalen JP, et al: The perihepatic spaces, Radiology 149:231, 1983.

Sherlock S: Diseases of the liver and biliary system, London, 1989, Blackwell Scientific Publications.

Tavill AS, Wood EJ, Kreel L, et al: The Budd-Chiari syndrome. Correlation between hepatic scintigraphy and the clinical, radiological and pathological findings in nineteen cases of hepatic venous outflow obstruction, Gastroenterology 68:508, 1975.

Weill F, Eisenscher A, Aucant D, et al: Ultrasonic study of venous patterns in the right hypochondrium: an anatomical approach to differential diagnosis of obstructive jaundice, J Clin Ultrasound 3:23, 1974.

Zimmerman H: Current perspectives in hepatology, New York and London, 1989 Plenum Medical Book.

Diffuse Disease

Abbitt PL and Teates CD: The sonographic appearance of extramedullary hematopoiesis in the liver: J Clin Ultrasound 17:280, 1989.

Bisset RA and Khan AN: Differential diagnosis in abdominal ultrasound, pp. 23-24, Philadelphia, 1990, Bailliere Tindall, W.B. Saunders.

Garra BS, Insana MF, Shawker TH, et al: Quantitative ultrasonic detection and classification of diffuse liver disease comparison with human observer performance, Invest Radiol 24(3):196-203, 1989.

Giorgio A, Amoroso P, Fico P, et al: Ultrasound evaluation of uncomplicated and complicated acute viral hepatitis, J Clin Ultrasound 14:675, 1986.

Giorgio A, Amoroso P, Lettieri G, et al: Cirrhosis: value of caudate to right lobe ratio in diagnosis with US, Radiology 161:443, 1986.

Giorgio A, Francica G, de Stefano G, et al: Sonographic recognition of intraparenchymal regenerating nodules using high-frequency transducers in patients with cirrhosis, J Ultrasound Med 10:355, 1991.

Gosink BB, Lemon SK, Scheible W, et al: Accuracy of ultrasonography in diagnosis of hepatocellular disease, Am J Roentgenol 133:19, 1979.

Gosink BB and Leymaster CE: Ultrasonic determination of hepatomegaly, J Clin Ultrasound 9:37, 1981.
Ishak KG, Zimmerman HJ, and Ray MB: Alcoholic liver disease: pathologic, pathogenetic and clinical aspects, Alcohol Clin Exp Res 15:45, 1991.
Kudo M, Tomita S, Minowa K, et al: Color Doppler flow imaging of hepatic focal nodular hyperplasia, J Ultrasound Med 11:553, 1992.
Ljubicic N and Bilic A: Effect of verapamil on portal blood flow in patients with liver cirrhosis, J Ultrasound Med 11:517, 1992.
Miller JH, Stanley P, and Gates GF: Radiography of glycogen storage diseases, Am J Roentgenol 132:379, 1979.
Mori H, Aikawa A, Hirao K, et al: Exophytic spread of hepatobiliary disease via perihepatic ligaments: demonstration with CT and US, Radiology 172:41, 1989.
Needleman L, Kurtz AB, Rifkin MD, et al: Sonography of diffuse benign liver disease, Am J Roentgenol 146:1011, 1986.
Nomura F, Ohnishi K, Ochiai T, et al: Obesity-related nonalcoholic fatty liver, Radiology 162:845, 1987.
Quinn SF and Gosink BB: Characteristic sonographic signs of hepatic fatty infiltration, Am J Roentgenol 145:753, 1985.
Sauerbrei EE and Lopez M: Pseudotumor of the quadrate lobe in hepatic sonography, Am J Roentgenol 147:923, 1986.
Scatariage JC, Scott WW, Donovan PJ, et al: Fatty infiltration of the liver, J Ultrasound Med 3:9, 1984.
Schapiro BL, Newburger PE, Klempner MS, et al: Chronic granulomatous disease presenting in a 69-year-old man, New Eng J Med 1991.
Yoshikawa J, Matsui O, Takashima T, et al: Focal fatty change of the liver adjacent to the falciform ligament, Am J Roentgenol 149:491, 1987.
Zoli M, Cordiani MR, Marchesini G, et al: Ultrasonographic follow-up of liver cirrhosis, J Clin Ultrasound 18:91, 1990.

Abscess

Hadidi A: Sonography of hepatic echinococcal cysts, Gastrointest Radiol 7:349, 1982.
Hussain S: Diagnostic criteria of hydatid disease on hepatic sonography, J Ultrasound Med 4:603, 1985.
Mircea PA, Cucu A, and Vlaicu R: Contained rupture of a liver hydatid cyst, J Ultrasound Med 6:339, 1987.
Nordestgaard AG, Stapleford L, Worthen N, et al: Contemporary management of amebic liver abscess, Am Surg 58:315, 1992.
Ralls PW, Barnes PF, Radin DR, et al: Sonographic features of amebic and pyogenic liver abscesses, Am J Roentgenol 149:499, 1987.
Steinhart AH, Simons M, Stone R, et al: Multiple hepatic abscesses: cholangiographic changes simulating sclerosing cholangitis and resolution after percutaneous drainage, Am J Gastroenterol 85:306, 1990.
Sukov RJ, Cohen LJ, and Sample WF: Sonography of hepatic amebic abscesses, Am J Roentgenol 134:911, 1980.
Teefey SA and Wechter DG: Sonographic evaluation of pericholecystic abscess with intrahepatic extension, J Ultrasound Med 6:659, 1987.

Benign Disease

Bowerman RA, Samuels BI, and Silver TM: Ultrasonographic features of hepatic adenomas in Type I glycogen storage disease, J Ultrasound Med 2:51, 1983.
Bree RL, Schwab RE, and Neiman HL: Solitary echogenic spot in the liver: is it diagnostic of a hemangioma? Am J Roentgenol 140:41, 1983.
Bulas DI, Johnson D, Allen JF, et al: Fetal hemangioma, J Ultrasound Med 11:499, 1992.
Freeny PC, Vimont TR, and Barnett DC: Cavernous hemangioma of the liver, Radiology 132:143, 1979.
Gabow PA, Johnson AM, Kaehny WD, et; al: Risk factors for the development of hepatic cysts in autosomal dominant polycystic kidney disease, Hepatology 11:1033, 1990.
Gandolfi L, Leo P, Solmi L, et al: Natural history of hepatic haemangiomas: clinical and ultrasound study, Gut 32:677, 1991.
Gibney RG, Hendin AP, and Cooperberg PL: Sonographically detected hepatic hemangiomas, Am J Roentgenol 149:953, 1987.
Levine E, Cook LT, Grantham JJ: Liver cysts in autosomal-dominant polycystic kidney disease, Am J Roentgenol 145:229, 1985.
Low V and Khangure MS: Hepatic adenoma and focal nodular hyperplasia: a diagnostic dilemma, Austral Rad 44:124, 1990.
Marks F, Thomas P, Lustig I, et al: In utero sonographic description of a fetal liver adenoma, J Ultrasound Med 9:119, 1990.
Menu Y, Lorphelin JM, Scherrer A, et al: Sonographic and CT evaluation of intrahepatic calculi, Am J Roentgenol 145:579, 1985.
Mirk P, Rubaltelli L, Bazzocchi M, et al: Ultrasonographic patterns in hepatic hemangiomas, J Clin Ultrasound 10:373, 1982.
Tait N, Richardson AJ, Muguti G, et al: Hepatic cavernous haemangioma: a 10 years review, Austr NZ J Surg 62:521, 1992.
Wernecke K, Vassallo P, Bick U, et al: The distinction between benign and malignant liver tumors on sonography: value of a hypoechoic halo, Am J Roentgenol 159:1005, 1992.
Wyngaarden JB, Smith LH, and Bennett JC: Textbook of Medicine, ed 19, Philadelphia, 1991, WB Saunders.

Malignant Disease

Belghiti J, Panis Y, Farges O, et al: Intrahepatic recurrence after resection of hepatocellular carcinoma complicating cirrhosis, Ann Surg 214:2, 1991.
Bolondi L, Gaiani S, Benzi G, et al: Ultrasonography and guided biopsy in the diagnosis of hepatocellular carcinoma, Ital J Gastroenterol 24:46, 1992.
Cecchetto BL, Noventa F, Tremolada F, et al: Space-occupying lesions of the liver detected by ultrasonography and their relation to hepatocellular carcinoma in cirrhosis, Liver 12:80, 1992.
Karak PK, Mukhopadhyay S, and Berry M: Hepatocellular carcinoma, Trop Gastroenterol 13:21, 1992.
Lin ZY, Chang WY, Wang LY, et al: Doppler sonography in the differential diagnosis of hepatocellular carcinoma and other common hepatic tumors, Br J Radiol 65:202, 1992.
Miller WJ, Federle MP, and Campbell WL: Diagnosis and staging of hepatocellular carcinoma, Am J Roentgenol 157:303, 1991.
Sautereau D, Berry P, Cessot F, et al: Hepatocellular carcinoma, J Hepatol 14:413, 1992.
Scheible W, Gosink BB, Leopold GR: Gray scale echographic patterns of hepatic metastatic disease, Am J Roentgenol 129: 983, 1977.
Shibata T, Kubo S, Itoh K, et al: Recurrent hepatocellular carcinoma, J Clin Ultrasound 19:8, 1991.
Yasuyuki Y, Takahashi M, Baba Y, et al: Hepatocellular carcinoma with or without cirrhosis: a comparison of CT and angiographic presentations in the US and Japan, Abdom Imaging 18:168, 1993.
Yoshida T, Matsue H, Okazaki N, et al: Ultrasonographic differentiation of hepatocellular carcinoma from metastatic liver cancer, J Clin Ultrasound 15:431, 1987.
Yoshikawa J, Matsui O, Takashima T, et al: Fatty metamorphosis in hepatocellular carcinoma, Am J Roentgenol 151:717, 1988.

AIDS

Grumbach K, Coleman BG, Gal AA, et al: Patients with AIDS, J Ultrasound Med 8:247, 1989.

Tower MJ, Withers CE, Rachlis AR, et al: Ultrasound diagnosis of hepatic kaposi sarcoma, J Ultrasound Med 10:701, 1991.
Townsend RR, Laing FC, Jeffrey RB, et al: Abdominal lymphoma in AIDS: evaluation with US, Radiol 171:719, 1989.
Wetton EWN, McCarty M, Tomilinson D, et al: Ultrasound findings in hepatic mycobacterial infections in patients with acquired immune deficiency syndrome (AIDS), Clin Radiol 47: 36, 1993.

Hepatic Vascular System and Doppler

Chalmers N, Redhead DN, Simpson KJ, et al: Transjugular intrahepatic portosystemic stent shunt (TIPSS), Clin Radiol 46:166, 1992.
Chezmar JL, Nelson RC, and Bernardino ME: Portal venous gas after hepatic transplantation, Am J Roentgenol 153:1203, 1989.
Eidt JF, Harward T, and Cook JM: Current status of doppler ultrasound in the examination of abdominal vasculature, Am J Surg 160:604, 1990.
Furuse J, Matsutani S, Yoshikawa M, et al: Diagnosis of portal vein tumor thrombus by pulsed doppler ultrasonography, J Clin Ultrasound 20:439, 1992.
Goyal AK, Pokharna DS, and Sharma SK: Ultrasonic measurements of portal vasculature in diagnosis of portal hypertension, J Ultrasound Med 9:45, 1990.
Grant EG: Budd-Chiari syndrome, Am J Roentgenol 142:377, 1989.
Harter LP, Gross BH, St Hilaire J, et al: CT and sonographic appearance of hepatic vein obstruction, Am J Roentgenol 139: 176, 1982.
Kreigshauser JS, Reading CC, King BF, et al: Combined systemic and portal venous gas, Am J Roentgenol 154:1219, 1990.
Lev-Toaff AS, Friedman AC, Cohen LM, et al: Hepatic infarcts, Am J Roentgenol 149:87, 1987.
Mittelstaedt CA: General ultrasound, pp. 191-197, New York, 1992, Churchill Livingstone.
Murphy FB: The Budd-Chiari syndrome, Am J Roentgenol 147:9, 1986.
Pompili M: Ultrasound doppler diagnosis of Budd-Chiari syndrome, J Clin Gastroenterol 12:591, 1990.
Subramanyam BR, Balthazar EJ, Madamba MR, et al: Sonography of portosystemic venous collaterals in portal hypertension, Radiology 146:161, 1983.
Sugiura N, Karasawa E, Saotome N, et al: Portosystemic collateral shunts originating from the left portal veins in portal hypertension: demonstration by color Doppler flow imaging, J Clin Ultrasound 20:427, 1992.
Trigaux JP, Van Beers B, Melange M, et al: Alcoholic liver disease: value of the left-to-right portal vein ratio in its sonographic diagnosis, Gastrointestinal Radiol 16:215, 1991.
Wyngaarden JB, Smith LH, and Bennet JC: Cecil textbook of medicine, pp. 791-793, Philadelphia, 1992, WB Saunders.

Transplantation and Intraoperative

Dominguez R, Young LW, Ledesma-Medina J, et al: Pediatric liver transplantation, Radiol 157:339, 1985.
Flint EW, Sumkin JH, Zajko AB, et al: Duplex sonography of hepatic artery thrombosis after liver transplantation, Am J Roentgenol 151:481, 1988.
Igawa S, Sakai K, Kinoshita H, et al: Intraoperative sonography, Radiol 156:473, 1985.
Letourneau JG, Day DL, Ascher NL, et al: Abdominal sonography after hepatic transplantation, Am J Roentgenol 149:299, 1987.
Longley DG, Skolnick ML, Zajko AB, et al: Doppler sonography in the evaluation of adult patients before and after liver transplantation, Am J Roentgenol 151:687, 1988.
Thomas BL, Krummel TM, Parker GA, et al: Use of intraoperative ultrasound during hepatic resection in pediatric patients, J Ped Surgery 24:690, 1989.

CHAPTER 6

Gallbladder and the Biliary System

Sandra L. Hagen-Ansert

Ultrasonic evaluation of the gallbladder and biliary system has been effective in diagnosing gallbladder disease such as cholelithiasis, cholecystitis, and dilation of the ductal system.

ANATOMY OF THE EXTRAHEPATIC BILIARY SYSTEM

The extrahepatic biliary apparatus consists of the right and left hepatic ducts, the common hepatic duct, the common bile duct, the gallbladder, and the cystic duct (Fig. 6-1).

Hepatic Ducts

The right and left hepatic ducts emerge from the right lobe of the liver in the porta hepatis and unite to form the common hepatic duct, which then passes caudally and medially. The hepatic duct runs parallel with the portal vein. Each duct is formed by the union of bile canaliculi from the liver lobules.

The common hepatic duct is approximately 4 mm in diameter and descends within the edge of the lesser omentum. It is joined by the cystic duct to form the common bile duct.

Common Bile Duct

The normal common bile duct has a diameter of up to 6 mm. The first part of the duct lies in the right free edge of the lesser omentum (Fig. 6-2). The second part of the duct is situated posterior to the first part of the duodenum. The third part lies in a groove on the posterior surface of the head of the pancreas. It ends by piercing the medial wall of the second part of the duodenum about halfway down the duodenal length. There the common bile duct is joined by the main pancreatic duct, and together they open through a small ampulla (the ampulla of Vater) into the duodenal wall. The end parts of both ducts (common bile duct and main pancreatic duct) and the ampulla are surrounded by circular muscle fibers known as the *sphincter of Oddi*.

The proximal portion of the common bile duct is lateral to the hepatic artery and anterior to the portal vein. The duct moves more posterior after it descends behind the duodenal bulb and enters the pancreas. The distal duct lies parallel to the anterior wall of the vena cava.

Within the liver parenchyma the bile ducts follow the same course as the portal venous and hepatic arterial branches. The hepatic and bile ducts are encased in a common collagenous sheath forming the portal triad.

Cystic Duct

The cystic duct is about 4 cm long and connects the neck of the gallbladder with the common hepatic duct to form the common bile duct. It is usually somewhat S shaped and descends for a variable distance in the right free edge of the lesser omentum.

Gallbladder

The gallbladder is a pear-shaped sac in the anterior aspect of the right upper quadrant closely related to the visceral surface of the liver. It is divided into the fundus, body, and neck (Fig. 6-3). The rounded fundus usually projects below the inferior margin of the liver, where it comes into contact with the anterior abdominal wall at the level of the ninth right costal cartilage. The body generally lies in contact with the visceral surface of the liver and is directed upward, backward, and to the left. The neck becomes continuous with the cystic duct, which turns into the lesser omentum to join the right side of the common hepatic duct to form the common bile duct.

The neck of the gallbladder is oriented posteromedially toward the porta hepatis; and the fundus is situated lateral, caudal, and anterior to the neck. Occasionally the gallbladder lies in an intrahepatic or other anomalous location, and it may be difficult to detect by sonography if the entire upper abdomen is not examined.

The size and shape of the gallbladder are variable. Generally the normal gallbladder measures about 3 cm in diameter and 7 to 10 cm long. The walls are less than 2 mm thick.

Several anatomic variations may occur within the gallbladder to give rise to its internal echo pattern on the sonogram. The gallbladder may fold back on itself at the neck, forming Hartmann's pouch. Other anomalies include partial septation, complete septation (double gallbladder), and folding of the fundus (phrygian cap) (Figs. 6-4 and 6-5).

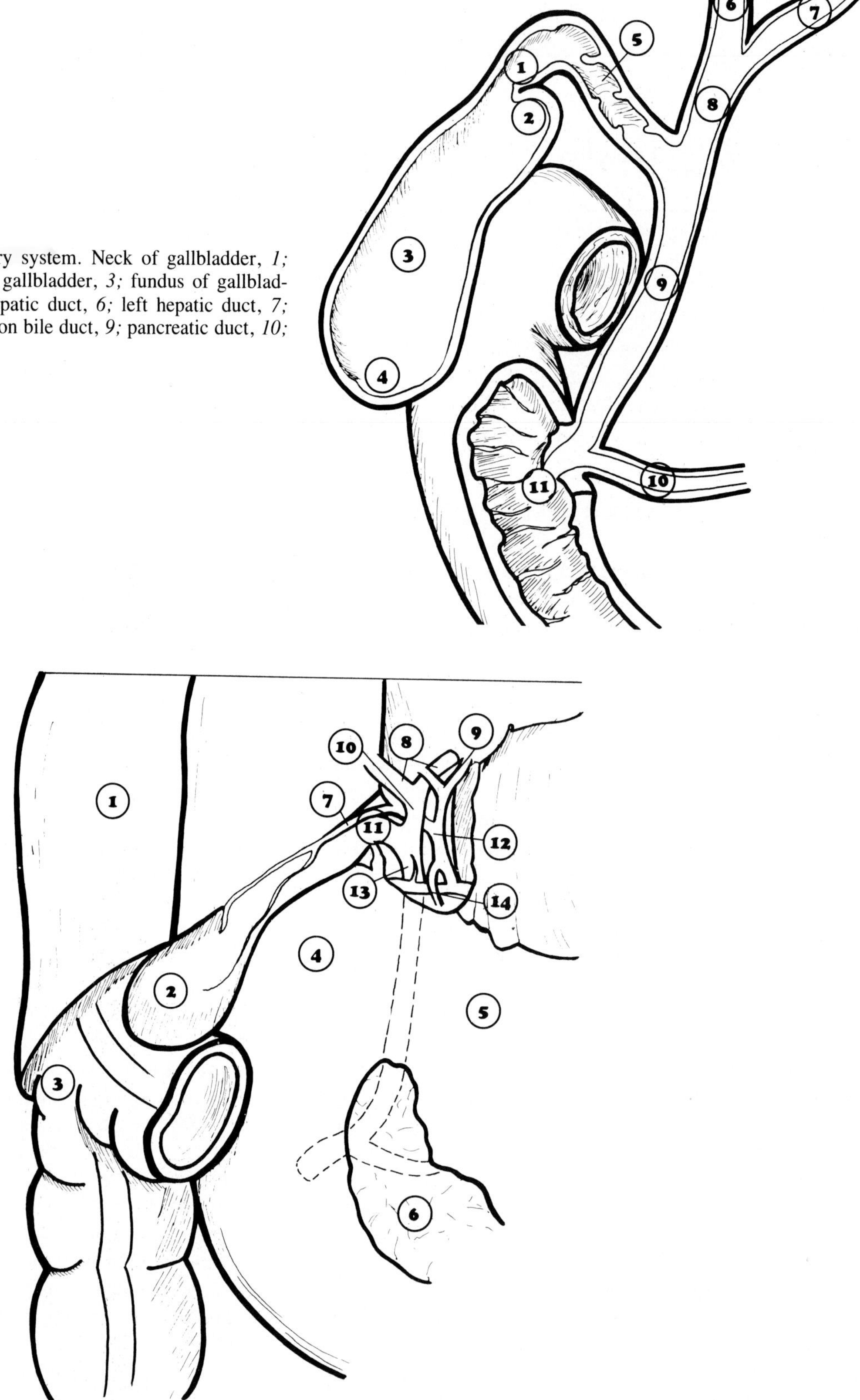

FIG. 6-1 Gallbladder and biliary system. Neck of gallbladder, *1;* Hartmann's pouch, *2;* body of gallbladder, *3;* fundus of gallbladder, *4;* cystic duct, *5;* right hepatic duct, *6;* left hepatic duct, *7;* common hepatic duct, *8;* common bile duct, *9;* pancreatic duct, *10;* papilla of Vater, *11*.

FIG. 6-2 Relationships within the porta hepatis. Liver, *1;* gallbladder, *2;* colon, *3;* duodenum, *4;* stomach, *5;* pancreas, *6;* cystic artery, *7;* right and left hepatic ducts, *8;* right and left hepatic arteries, *9;* common hepatic duct, *10;* cystic duct, *11;* proper hepatic artery, *12;* common bile duct, *13;* right gastric artery, *14*.

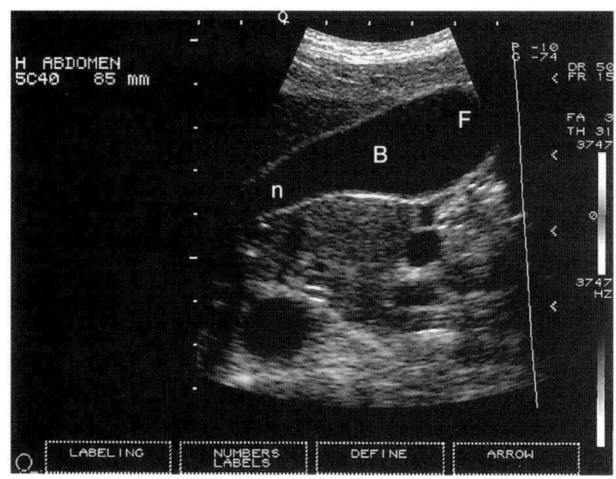

Gallbladder
Normal

FIG. 6-3 Longitudinal scan of the gallbladder in its fasting state. The walls are thin, measuring less than 2 mm. The gallbladder is divided into fundus, *F,* body, *B,* and neck, *n.*

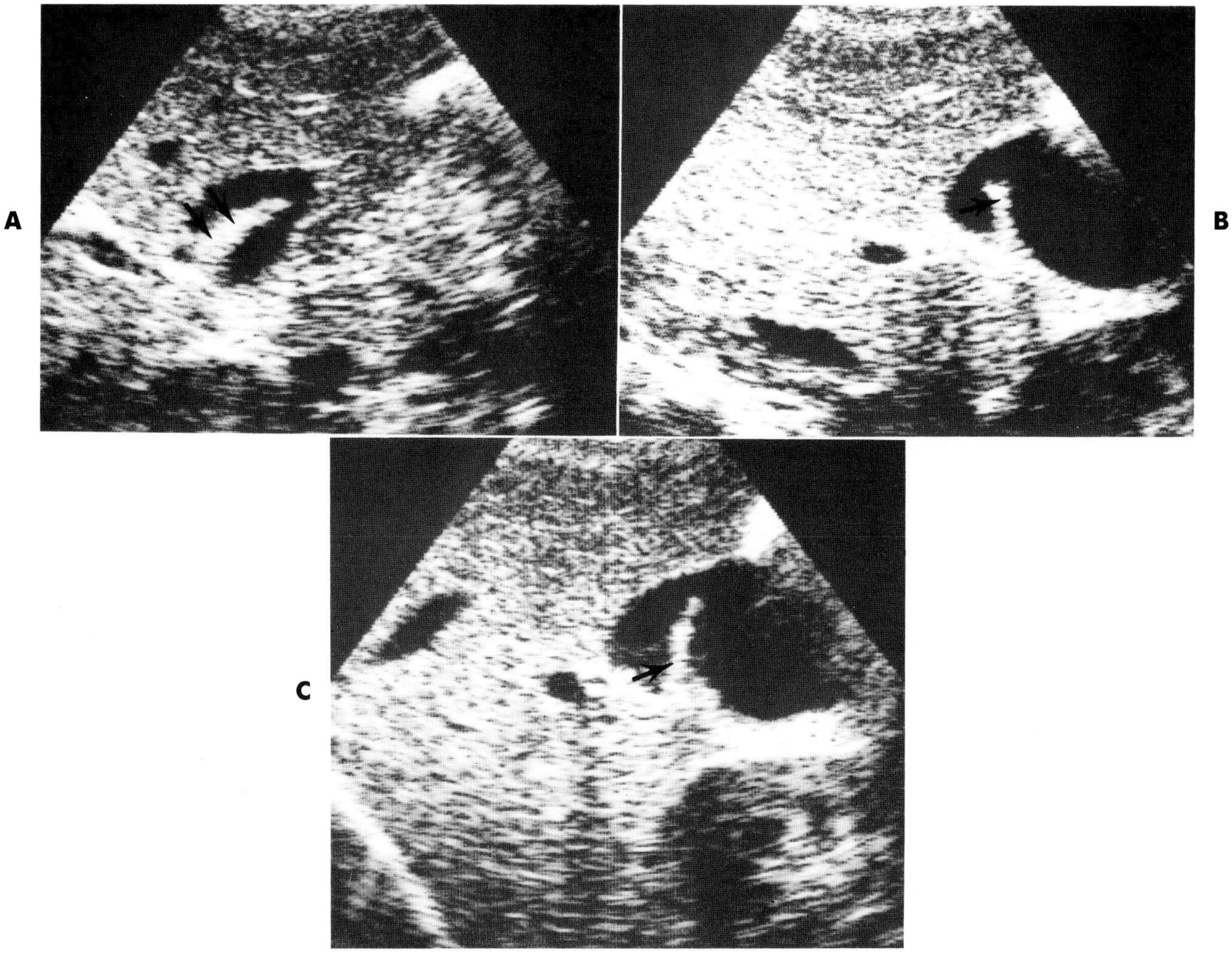

A

B

C

FIG. 6-4 A, Transverse, **B** and **C,** sagittal scans of a neonate with a partial septation within the gallbladder *(arrows).*

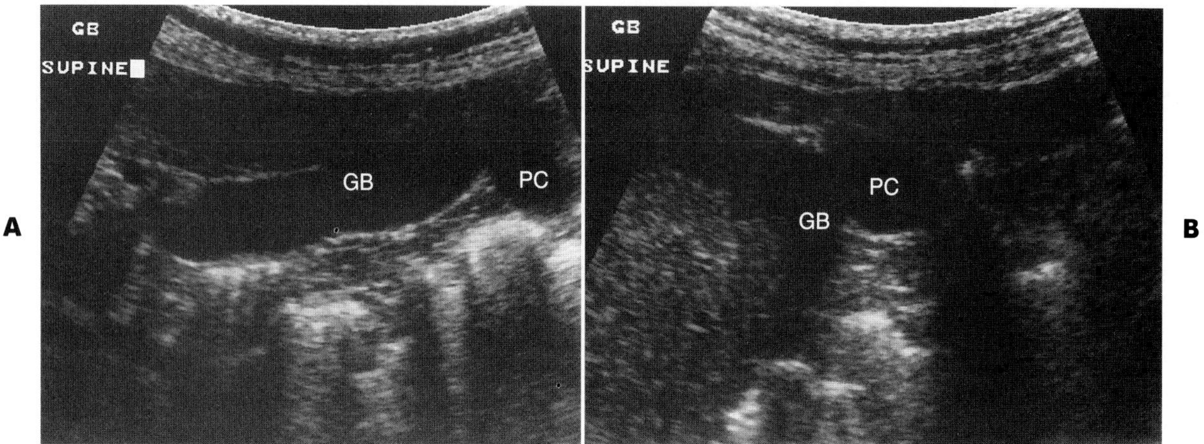

FIG. 6-5 An anatomic variation of the gallbladder is the phrygian cap, *Pc,* shown here with the folding of the fundus.

With a capacity of 50 ml, the gallbladder serves as a reservoir for bile. It also has the ability to concentrate the bile. To aid this process, its mucous membrane contains folds that unite with each other, giving the surface a honeycomb appearance. The Heister's valve in the neck of the gallbladder helps to prevent kinking of the duct (Fig. 6-6).

The arterial supply of the gallbladder is from the cystic artery, which is a branch of the right hepatic artery. The cystic vein drains directly into the portal vein. A number of smaller arteries and veins run between the liver and the gallbladder.

GALLBLADDER PHYSIOLOGY

The primary function of the extrahepatic biliary tract is the transportation of bile from the liver to the intestine and the regulation of its flow. Since the liver secretes approximately 1 to 2 L of bile per day, this is an important function.

When the gallbladder and bile ducts are functioning normally, they respond in a fairly uniform manner in various phases of digestion. Concentration of bile in the gallbladder occurs during a state of fasting. It is forced into the gallbladder by an increased pressure within the common bile duct that is produced by the action of the sphincter of Oddi at the distal end of the gallbladder.

During the fasting state, very little bile flows into the duodenum. Stimulation produced by the influence of food causes the gallbladder to contract resulting in an outpouring of bile into the duodenum. When the stomach is emptied, duodenal peristalsis diminishes, the gallbladder relaxes, the tonus of the sphincter of Oddi increases slightly, and thus very little bile passes into the duodenum. Small amounts of bile secreted by the liver are retained in the common duct and forced into the gallbladder.

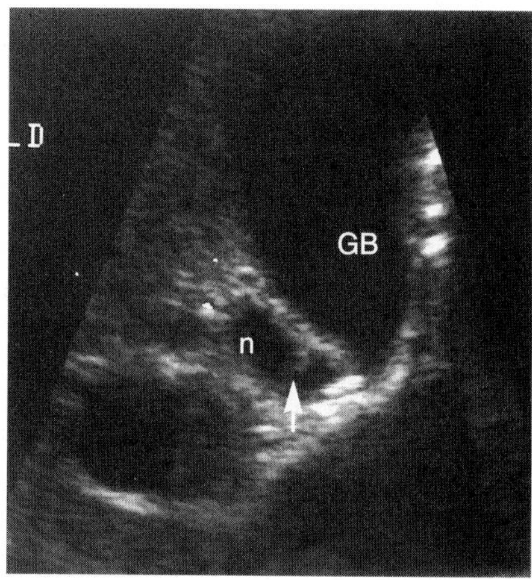

FIG. 6-6 The Heister's valve *(arrows)* in the neck of the gallbladder helps to prevent kinking of the duct.

Removal of the Gallbladder

When the gallbladder is removed, the sphincter of Oddi loses tonus, and pressure within the common bile duct drops to that of intraabdominal pressure. Bile is no longer retained in the bile ducts but is free to flow into the duodenum during fasting and digestive phases. Dilation of the extrahepatic bile ducts (usually less than 1 cm) occurs after cholecystectomy.

Secretion is largely caused by a bile salt–dependent mechanism and ductal flow is controlled by secretion. Bile salts form micelles, solubilize triglyceride fat and assist in its absorption and that of calcium, cholesterol, and fat-soluble vitamins from the intestine.

Bile is the principle route for excretion of bilirubin and cholesterol. The products of steroid hormones are also excreted in the bile, as are drugs and poisons (e.g., salts of heavy metals). The bile salts from the intestine stimulate

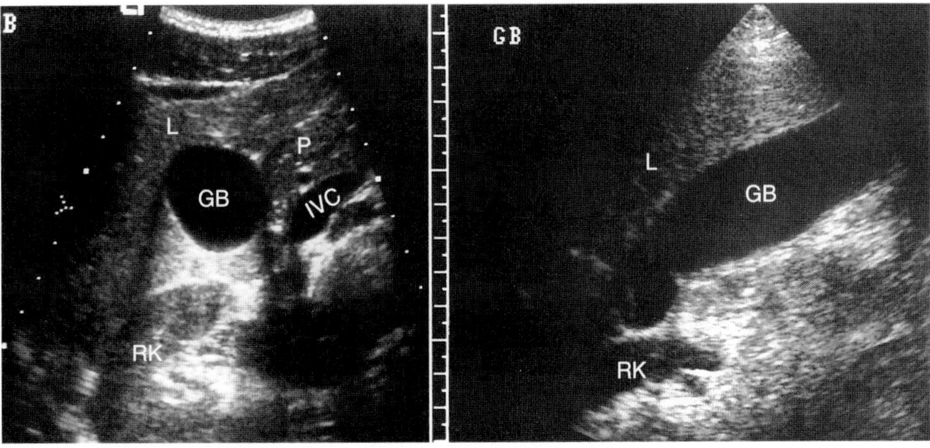

FIG. 6-7 The gallbladder, *GB*, is identified as a sonolucent oblong structure located anterior to the right kidney, *RK*, and inferior vena cava, *IVC*, lateral to the head of the pancreas, *P*, and duodenum, and indenting the inferior to medial aspect of the right lobe of the liver, *L*.

the liver to make more bile. Bile salts activate intestinal and pancreatic enzymes.

SONOGRAPHIC EVALUATION OF THE NORMAL GALLBLADDER AND BILIARY SYSTEM

Gallbladder

To ensure maximum dilation of the gallbladder, the patient should be given nothing to eat for at least 8 to 12 hours before the ultrasound examination. The patient is initially examined in the supine position with a real time sector scanner. Transverse, oblique, and sagittal scans are made over the upper abdomen to identify the gallbladder, biliary system, liver, right kidney, and head of the pancreas. The patient should also be rolled into a steep decubitus or upright position in an attempt to separate small stones from the gallbladder wall or cystic duct.

The gallbladder may be identified as a sonolucent oblong structure located anterior to the right kidney, lateral to the head of the pancreas and duodenum, indenting the inferior to medial aspect of the right lobe of the liver (Fig. 6-7). The sagittal scans show the right kidney posterior to the gallbladder. The fundus is generally oriented slightly more anterior, and on sagittal scans often reaches the anterior abdominal wall.

Carter et al. reported seeing on sagittal scans a bright linear echo within the liver connecting the gallbladder and the right or main portal vein in a high percentage of patients (Fig. 6-8).[2] They stated that the neck of the gallbladder usually comes into contact with the main segment of the portal vein near the origin of the left portal vein. The gallbladder commonly resides in a fossa on the medial aspect of the liver. Because of fat or fibrous tissue within the main lobar fissure of the liver (which lies between the gallbladder and the right portal vein), this bright linear reflector was a reliable indicator of the location of the gallbladder. The gallbladder lies in the posterior and caudal aspect of the fissure. The caudal aspect of the linear echo "pointed" directly to the gallbladder.

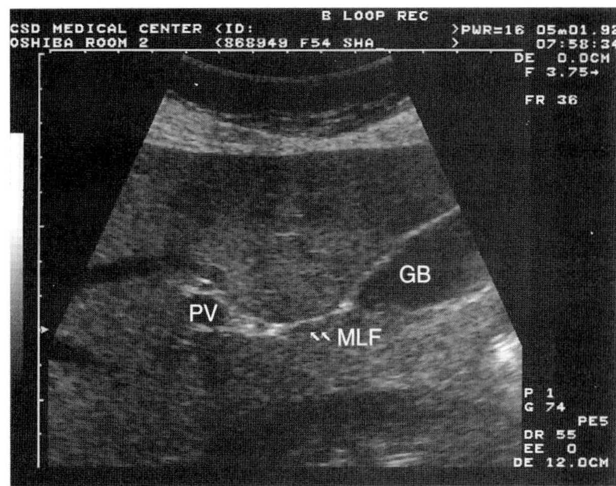

FIG. 6-8 On sagittal scans, the bright linear echo band within the liver connecting the gallbladder, *GB*, and the right or main portal vein, *PV*, is the main lobar fissure, *MLF*.

A small echogenic fold has been reported to occur along the posterior wall of the gallbladder at the junction of the body and infundibulum. It may be very small (3 to 5 mm) but may give rise to an acoustic shadow in the supine position. It is not duplicated in the oblique position. The causes for such a junctional fold are the incisurae between the body and infundibulum or the Heister's valve, which is a spiral fold beginning in the neck of the gallbladder and lining the cystic duct.

A prominent gallbladder may be normal in some indi-

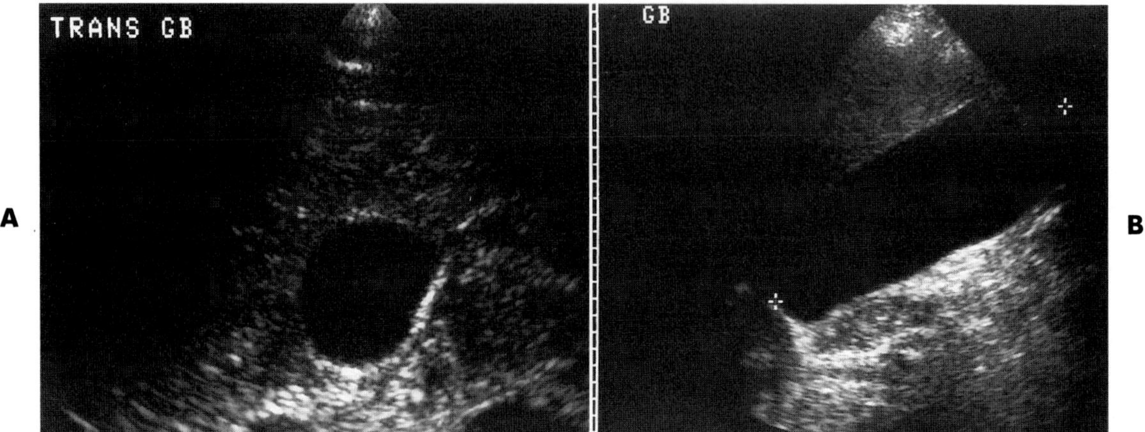

FIG. 6-9 **A,** Transverse and, **B,** longitudinal scans of the distended gallbladder. The gallbladder size may be quite variable from patient to patient. A good rule of thumb is to compare the size of the gallbladder with the transverse view of the right kidney. The width should always be smaller, under 5 cm.

viduals because of their fasting state (Fig. 6-9). A large gallbladder has been detected in patients with diabetes, patients who are bedridden with protracted illness or pancreatitis, and those who are taking anticholinergic drugs. A large gallbladder may even fail to contract after a fatty meal, or intravenous cholecystokinin; other studies may be needed to make the diagnosis of obstruction.

If a gallbladder appears too large, a fatty meal may be administered and further sonographic evaluation made to detect whether the enlargement is abnormal or normal. If the gallbladder fails to contract during the examination, the pancreatic area should be investigated further. Courvoisier's sign indicates an extrahepatic mass compressing the common bile duct, which can produce an enlarged gallbladder (Fig. 6-10). In addition, the liver should be carefully examined for the presence of dilated bile ducts.

In a well-contracted gallbladder the wall changes from a single to a double concentric structure with the following three components recognized as reported by Marchal et al.[15]: (1) a strongly reflective outer contour, (2) a poorly reflective inner contour, and (3) a sonolucent area between both reflecting structures.

Bile Ducts

Sonographically the common duct lies anterior and to the right of the portal vein in the region of the porta hepatis and gastrohepatic ligament (Fig. 6-11; see color image). The hepatic artery lies anterior and to the left of the portal vein. On a transverse scan the common duct, hepatic artery, and portal vein have been referred to as the *Mickey Mouse sign* by Bartrum and Crow (Fig. 6-12).[1] The portal vein serves as Mickey's face, with the right ear the common duct and the left ear the hepatic artery. To obtain such a cross section, the transducer must be directed in a slightly oblique path from the left shoulder to the right hip.

On sagittal scans the right branch of the hepatic artery usually passes posterior to the common duct. The common duct is seen just anterior to the portal vein before it dips posteriorly to enter the head of the pancreas (Fig. 6-13). The patient may be rotated into a slight (45-degree) or steep (90-degree) right anterior oblique position with the beam directed posteromedially to visualize the duct. This enables the examiner to avoid cumbersome bowel gas and to use the liver as an acoustic window.

When the right subcostal approach is used, the main portal vein may be seen as it bifurcates into the right and left branches. As the right branch continues into the right lobe of the liver, the right branch can be followed laterally in a longitudinal plane. The portal vein appears as an almond-shaped sonolucent structure anterior to the inferior vena cava. The common hepatic duct is seen as a tubular structure anterior to the portal vein. The right branch of the hepatic artery can be seen between the duct and the portal vein as a small circular structure.

The small cystic duct is generally not identified; since this landmark is needed to distinguish the common hepatic from the common bile duct, a more general term of common duct is used to refer to these structures (Figs. 6-14 and 6-15).

CLINICAL SYMPTOMS OF GALLBLADDER DISEASE

The most classic symptom of gallbladder disease is right upper quadrant abdominal pain, usually occurring after ingestion of greasy foods. Nausea and vomiting sometimes occur and may indicate the presence of a stone in the common bile duct. A gallbladder attack may cause pain in the right shoulder, with inflammation of the gallbladder often causing referred pain in the right shoulder blade.

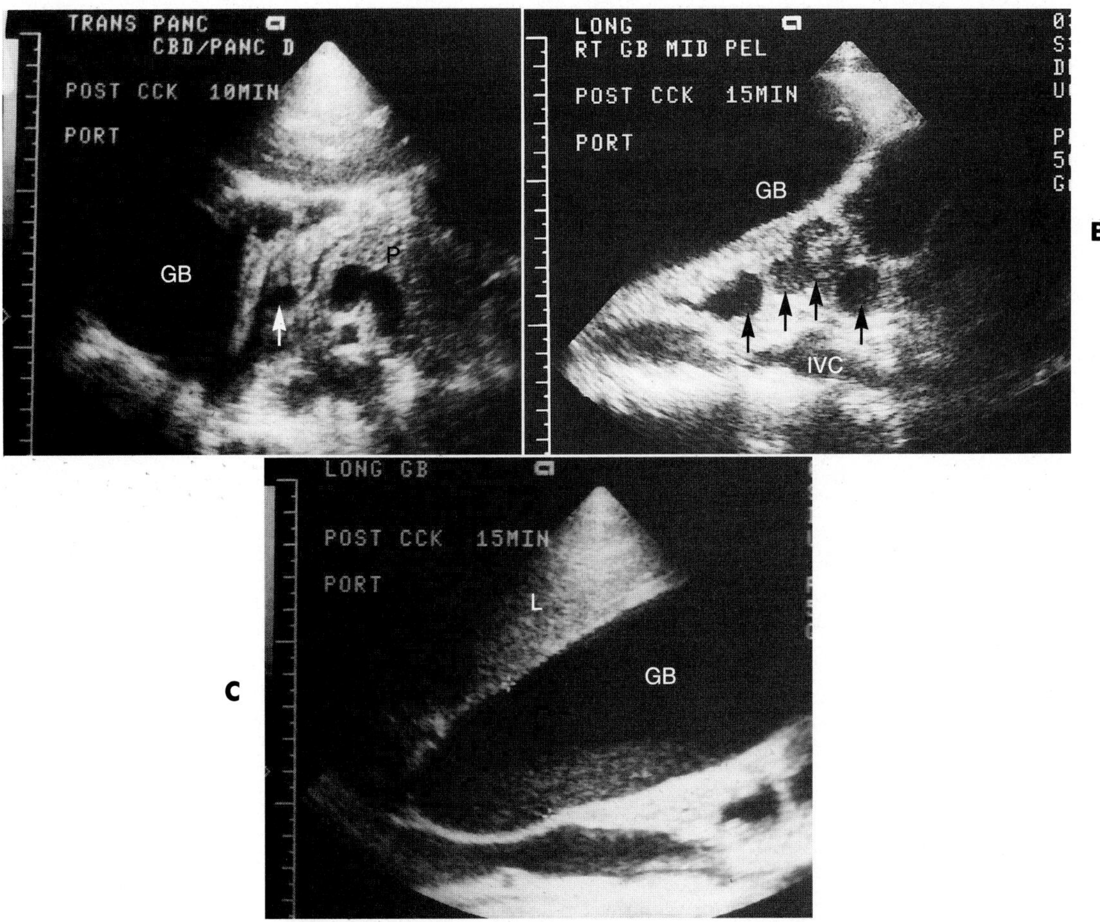

FIG. 6-10 A patient who presents with jaundice and a palpable abdominal mass in the right upper quadrant is sent to ultrasound to rule out an obstructive versus nonobstructive cause of jaundice. A pancreatic mass was found in the head of the gland, causing obstruction of the common bile duct, with distention of the gallbladder, *GB* (Courvoisier's sign). **A,** Transverse: Pancreas, *P;* common duct *(arrow)*. **B,** Longitudinal: Inferior vena cava, *IVC;* gallbladder, *GB;* **C,** Longitudinal: Distended gallbladder, *GB;* liver, *L.*

Gallstones

After a fatty meal the gallbladder contracts to release bile; and if the outflow tract is blocked by gallstones, pain results. As the bile is being stored in the gallbladder, small crystals of bile salts precipitate and may form gallstones varying from pinhead size to the size of the organ itself. There may be a single large gallstone or hundreds of tiny ones. The tiny stones are the most dangerous, since they can enter the bile ducts and obstruct the outflow of bile.

Jaundice

Jaundice is characterized by the presence of bile in the tissues with resulting yellow-green color of the skin. It may develop when a tiny gallstone blocks the bile ducts between the gallbladder and the intestines, producing pressure on the liver and forcing bile into the blood.

Cholecystitis

Inflammation of the gallbladder usually is a chronic illness punctuated by intermittent acute episodes, which occur when the cystic duct is obstructed by a calculus. Calculi (gallstones) are almost always associated with cholecystitis, although rare cases of acalculus cholecystitis are believed to occur. About 85% of gallstones are composed entirely of cholesterol; 10% are bile pigment stones, and 5% are a combination of bile pigments and cholesterol. Varying degrees of calcification may be superimposed, with the result that some stones are visible radiographically. Gallstones occur commonly in whites (more than 25% of persons over 40 years of age) and occur with even higher incidence in specific populations, such as Swedes and American Indians.

The relationship of gallstones to the pathogenesis of cholecystitis has long been a point of debate. Which comes first, the stone or the inflammation? The current tendency is to regard cholecystitis as a result of gallstone formation rather than a cause of it. This view is supported by the discovery of lithogenic bile, a form of bile supersaturated with cholesterol that is found in some individuals but not in others. Lecithin and bile salts keep

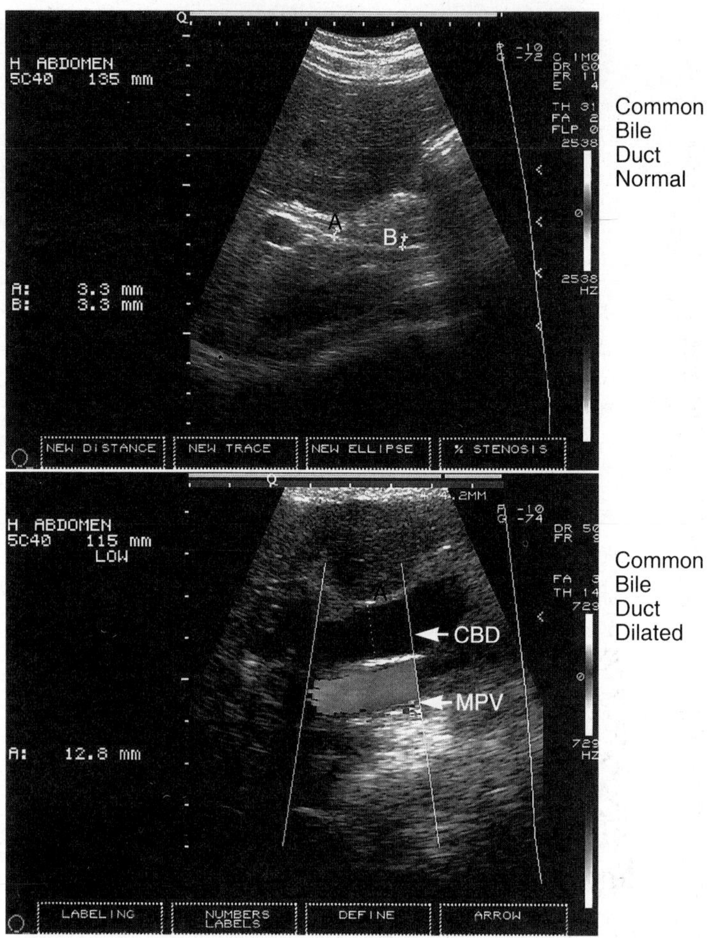

FIG. 6-11 Longitudinal oblique scans of the common bile duct as it lies anterior to the portal vein. The bottom image shows the distinction between the dilated common duct, *CBD,* and color-filled portal vein. The ductal structures will not fill with color, thus helping the sonographer to separate distended ducts from vascular structures. See color image.

cholesterol in solution in bile; hence the relative concentration of these elements may determine whether cholesterol precipitates and forms stones. In patients with lithogenic bile the liver secretes too much cholesterol relative to the amount of lecithin and bile salts present. It is believed that precipitated cholesterol crystals in such patients aggregate and grow, forming stones. Gallstones may result in inflammation of the gallbladder mucosa through direct contact or by intermittent obstruction of the cystic duct. In the latter case, overdistension is believed to stretch the gallbladder wall excessively and produce ischemia. Obstruction also causes stasis, which promotes bacterial growth in the bile. Both ischemia and stasis are believed to account for the inflammation and scarring that occur in cholecystitis.

The gallbladder is not an essential organ. When the gallbladder is removed surgically, the common duct is believed to distend in some cases and take over the reservoir function.

PATHOLOGIC PATTERNS OF GALLBLADDER DISEASE

Gallbladder Sludge

Occasionally a patient presents sonographically with a prominent gallbladder containing low-level internal echoes that may be attributed to thick or inspissated bile.[3] Filly et al. state that the source of echoes in biliary sludge is particulate matter (predominantly pigment granules with lesser amounts of cholesterol crystals).[6] They report that the viscosity does not appear to be important in the generation of internal echoes in fluids. The particles can be small and still produce perceptible echoes (Fig. 6-16).

Some gallbladders may be so packed with bile that the gallbladder is confused with the liver parenchyma. Occasionally the thick bile is also found in the common duct.[4] Sludge is gravity dependent. With alterations in patient position, one may be able to separate sludge from occasional artifactual echoes found in the gallbladder. Filly et al. state that sludge should be considered an abnormal finding, be-

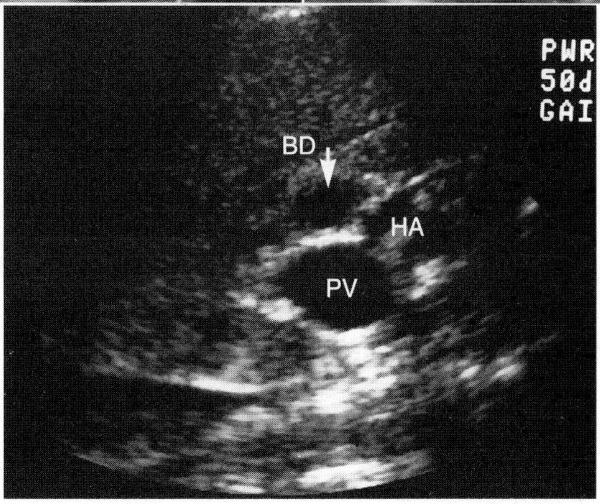

FIG. 6-12 A, The transverse view of the right upper quadrant shows the common duct, *1,* to be anterior and lateral to the portal vein, *PV.* The hepatic artery, *2,* is anterior and medial to the portal vein. The longitudinal scan shows the common duct between the gallbladder, *GB,* and portal vein, *PV.* **B,** The dilated common bile duct, *BD,* is well seen in this transverse view.

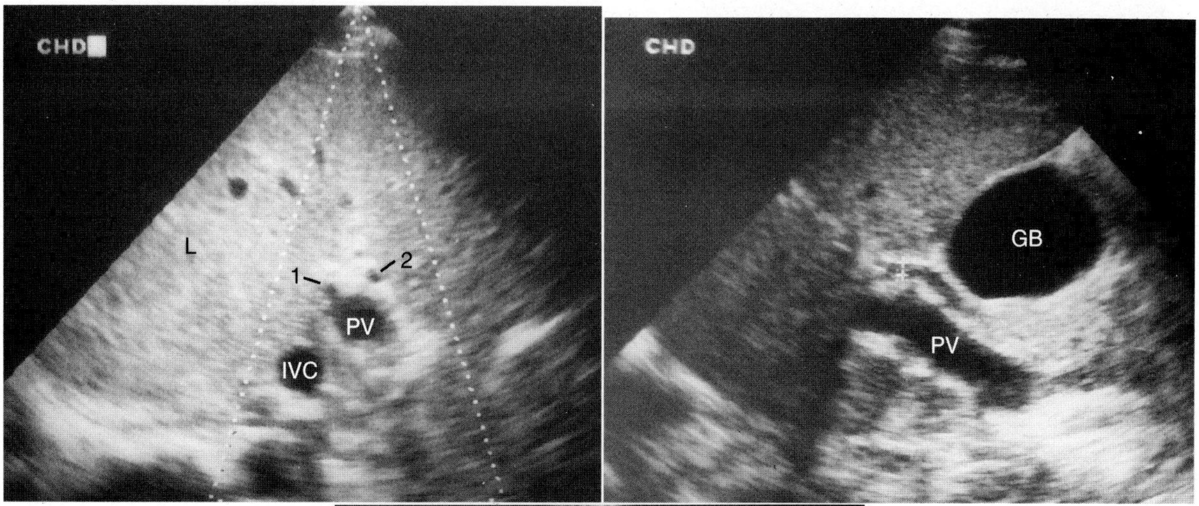

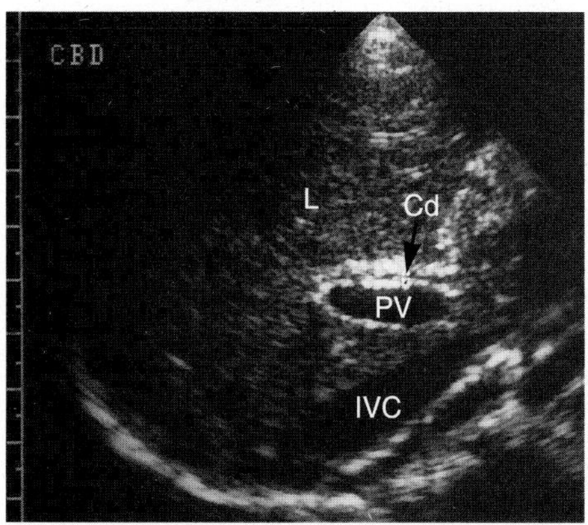

FIG. 6-13 Longitudinal scan of the common bile duct, *cd,* as it lies anterior to the portal vein, *PV.* When seen, the common hepatic artery is shown as a circle, crossing posterior to the common bile duct at the level of the portal vein.

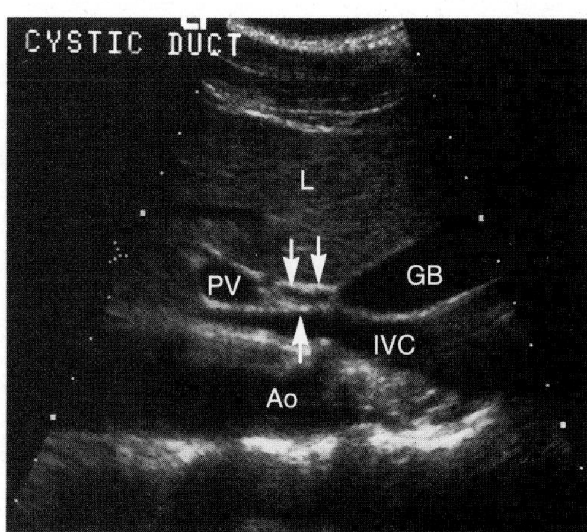

FIG. 6-14 The cystic duct is sometimes seen to arise from the neck of the gallbladder *(arrows).* This coronal decubitus view shows the aorta, *Ao,* inferior vena cava, *IVC,* gallbladder, *GB,* portal vein, *PV,* and liver, *L.*

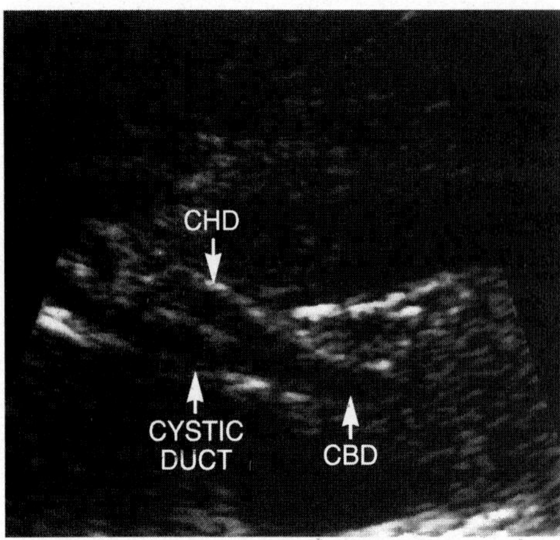

FIG. 6-15 Oblique longitudinal view of the common bile duct, *CBD*, cystic duct, and common hepatic duct, *CHD*.

cause either a functional or a pathologic abnormality exists when calcium bilirubin or cholesterol precipitates in bile (Figs. 6-17 and 6-18).[6]

Wall Thickness

The normal wall thickness of the gallbladder is 1 to 2 mm. Sonographically it may be underestimated when the wall has extensive fibrosis or is surrounded by fat (Fig. 6-19).[8]

The sonographic appearance of acute cholecystitis has been identified as a gallbladder with an irregular outline of a thickened wall (Fig. 6-20). In addition, Marchal et al. have found a sonolucent area within the thickened wall probably caused by edema.[14,15] A study by Engel et al. of wall thickness indicated that 98% of patients whose gallbladder walls were thick had disease, whereas 50% with gallbladder disease had a wall thickness of less than 3 mm (Fig. 6-21).[5]

Sanders states that the wall is not always thick in acute cholecystitis.[17] Some walls will be thicker because of pericholecystic abscesses (Fig. 6-22). Occasionally a thickened gallbladder wall is seen in normal individuals. It seems to be related to the degree of contraction of a normal gallbladder. Sanders found the gallbladder wall thickened symmetrically with smooth outlines in patients with acute cholecystitis without abscess or ascites (Figs. 6-23 and 6-24). If the thickened wall is localized and irregular, one should consider cholecystosis or carcinoma of the gallbladder.

Another condition wherein the gallbladder wall may be thickened is gangrenous cholecystitis. The wall is also edematous with focal areas of exudate, hemorrhage, and necrosis. In addition, there may be ulcerations and perforations resulting in pericholecystic abscesses or peritonitis. Gallstones or fine gravel occur in 80% to 95% of the patients. Kane states that the common echo features of gangrene are the presence of diffuse medium-to-coarse echogenic densities filling the gallbladder lumen in the absence of bile duct obstruction.[12] This echogenic material has the following three characteristics: (1) it does not cause shadowing, (2) it is not gravity dependent, and (3) it does not show a layering effect. The lack of layering is attributed to increased viscosity of the bile.

Fiski et al. have stated that a thickened wall is a nonspecific sign and is not necessarily related to gallbladder disease.[9] It may be found in the following conditions beside those previously discussed: hepatitis, adenomyomatosis, gallbladder tumor, or severe hypoalbuminemic states (Figs. 6-25 and 6-26).

GALLBLADDER PERILS

Gallbladder Wall Thickness

Common Causes of Thickening (More Than 2 mm) of the Gallbladder Wall

Hypoalbuminemia
Acquired Immune Deficiency Syndrome
Congestive Heart Failure
Cholecystitis
Nonfasting status
Hepatitis
Tumor
Ascites
Drugs
Hydration (rapid)

Gallstones, False Positive Findings

Polyp
Adenomyosis
Sludge ball
Duodenal gas
Clips
Biliary air
Porcelain gallbladder
Gallbladder agenesis

Gallstones, False Negative Findings

Contracted gallbladder
Very small stones
Geographic location/technique
Sludge
Gallstone in fundal cap

Choledochal Cysts

Choledochal cysts are possibly the result of pancreatic juices refluxing into the bile duct because of an anomalous junction of the pancreatic duct into the distal common bile duct, causing duct wall abnormality, weakness, and outpouching of the ductal walls.

They are rare; the incidence is more common in females

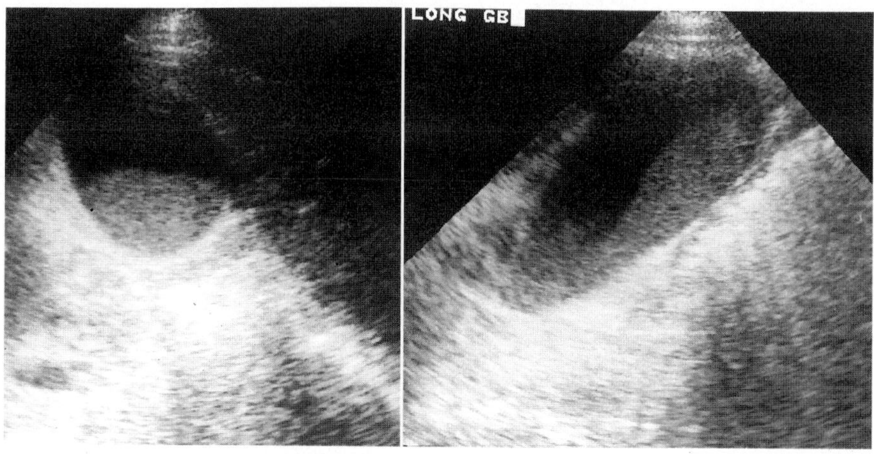

FIG. 6-16 Transverse and longitudinal scans of the distended gallbladder with low-level echoes representing inspissated bile or sludge along the posterior border.

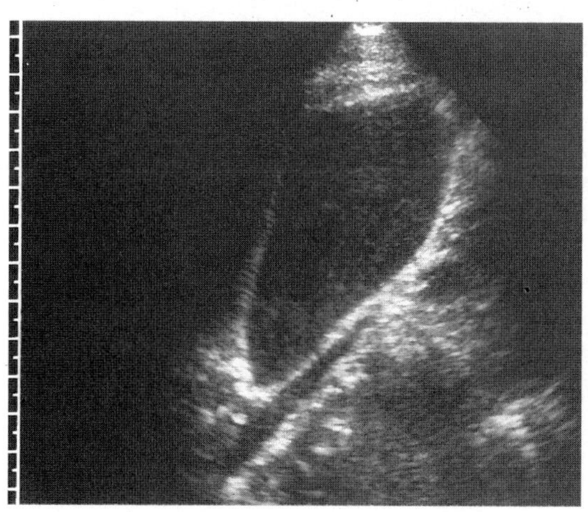

FIG. 6-17 Longitudinal view of a patient with low-level echoes nearly filling the entire gallbladder. Sometimes this pattern of thick sludge is so viscous that it takes several minutes for the sludge to change positions as the patient is rotated.

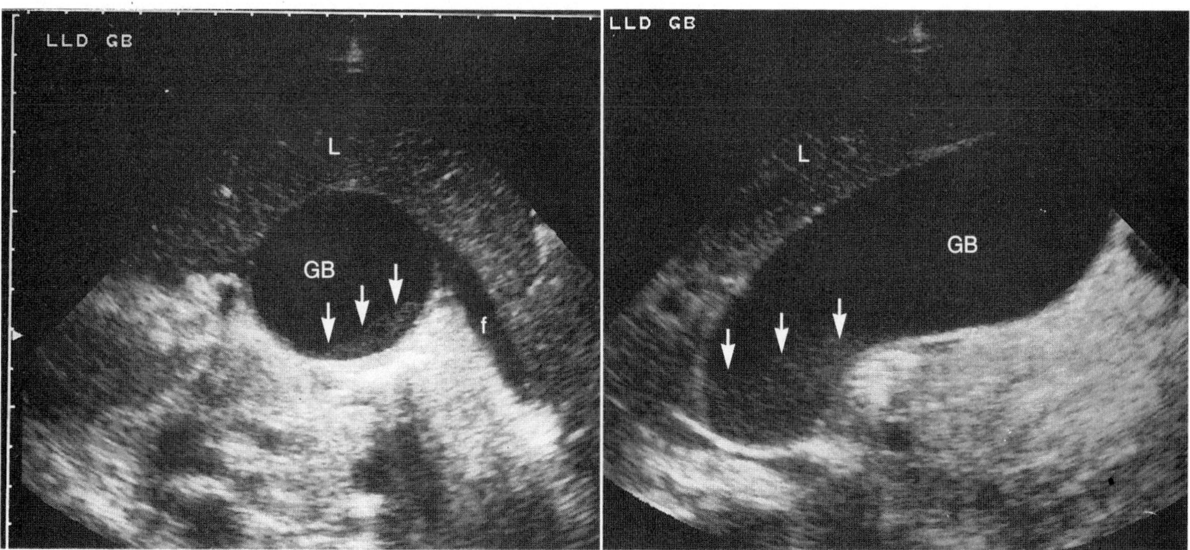

FIG. 6-18 Transverse view of the distended gallbladder, *GB*, with a small amount of sludge *(arrows)* along the posterior border. A small amount of ascitic fluid, *f*, is seen medial to the gallbladder.

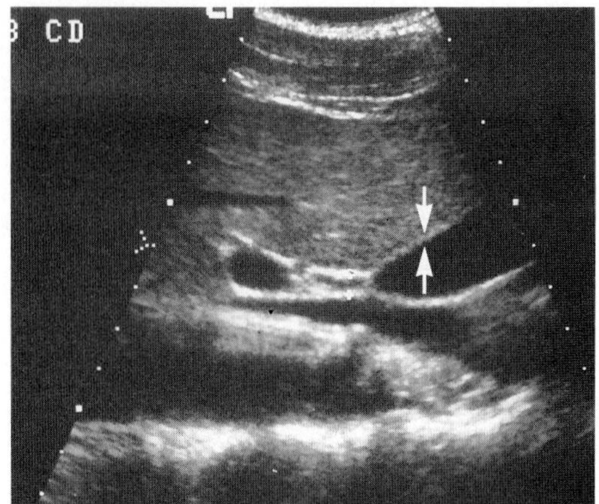

FIG. 6-19 The normal gallbladder wall thickness measures under 2 mm *(arrows)*.

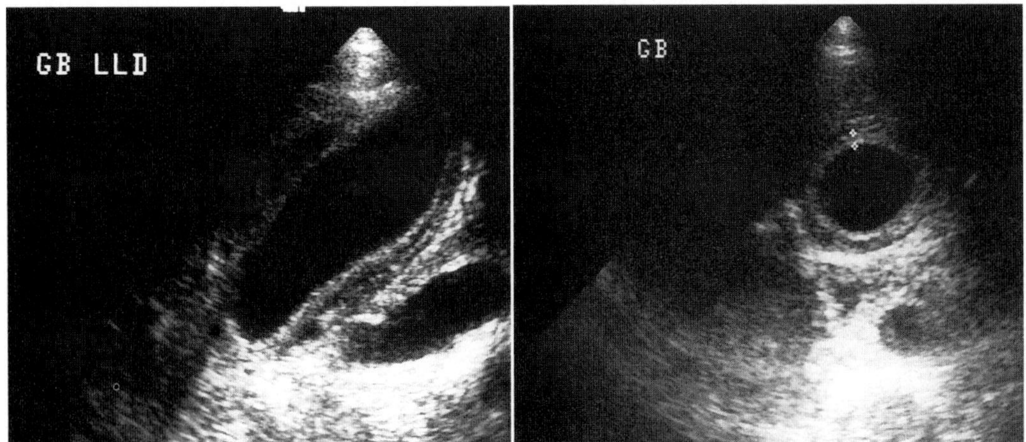

FIG. 6-20 The sonographic appearance of acute cholecystitis is shown in this patient with a distended gallbladder and thickened, irregular wall. The wall measures 3.5 mm.

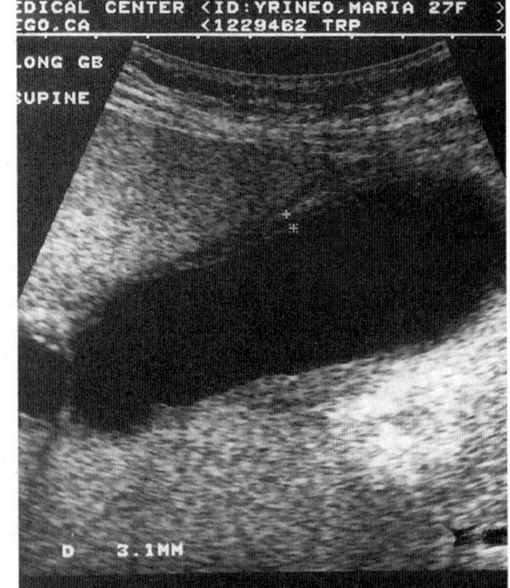

FIG. 6-21 Longitudinal view of the distended gallbladder in a patient with acute cholecystitis. Edema of the wall is shown, with the wall measuring 3.1 mm.

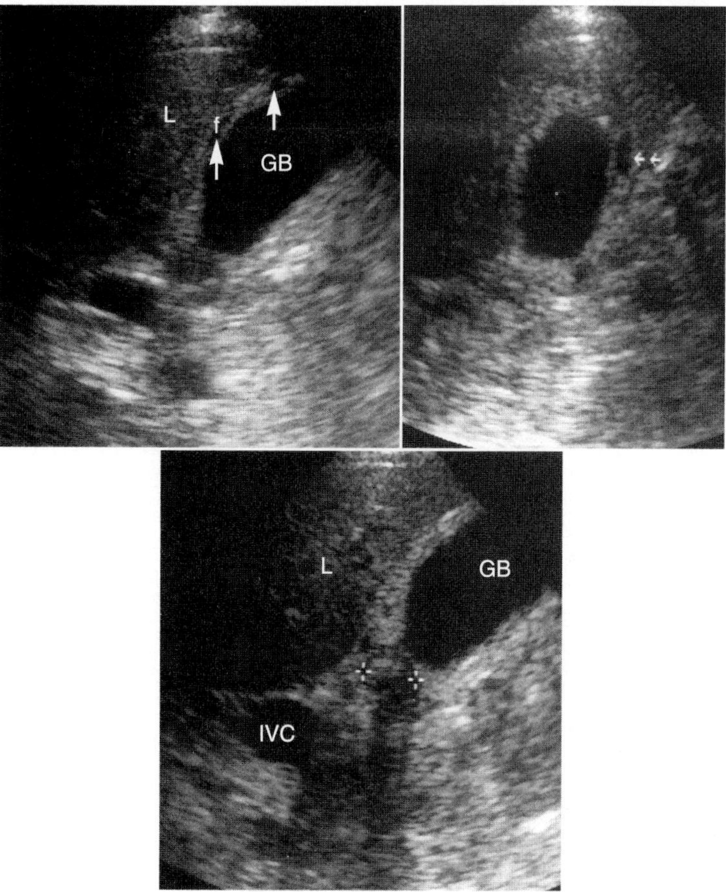

FIG. 6-22 A complication of acute cholecystitis is a pericholecystic abscess *(arrows)*. This patient had a large stone in the neck of the gallbladder *(crossbars)* with a sharp shadow posterior.

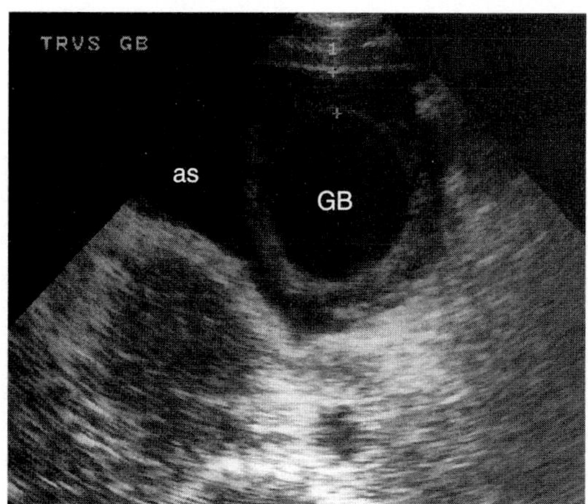

FIG. 6-23 Ascitic fluid causes the gallbladder wall to appear thickened.

than males (4:1), with an increased incidence in infants (although the condition may occur in adults). Choledochal cysts may be associated with gallstones, pancreatitis, or cirrhosis. The patient presents with an abdominal mass, pain, fever, or jaundice. The diagnosis may be confirmed with a nuclear medicine HIDA scan.

The majority of cases are thought to be congenital and result from bile reflux. The mass presents as a cystic dilation of the biliary system.

Sonographic Appearance. Choledochal cysts appear as true cysts in the right upper quadrant with or without apparent communication with the biliary system (Fig. 6-27). The cysts are classified by anatomy:

I. Localized cystic dilation of the common bile duct
II. Diverticulum from the common bile duct
III. Invagination of the common bile duct into the duodenum
IV. Dilation of the entire common bile duct and the common hepatic duct

Cholelithiasis

The evaluation of gallstones in real time has proven to be an extremely useful procedure in patients who present with symptoms of cholelithiasis (Fig. 6-28). The gallbladder is evaluated for increased size, wall thickness, presence of internal reflections within the lumen, and posterior acoustic shadowing (Fig. 6-29). Frequently patients with gallstones have a dilated gallbladder. Stones that are less than 1 to 2 mm may be difficult to separate from one another by ultrasound evaluation and thus are reported as gall-

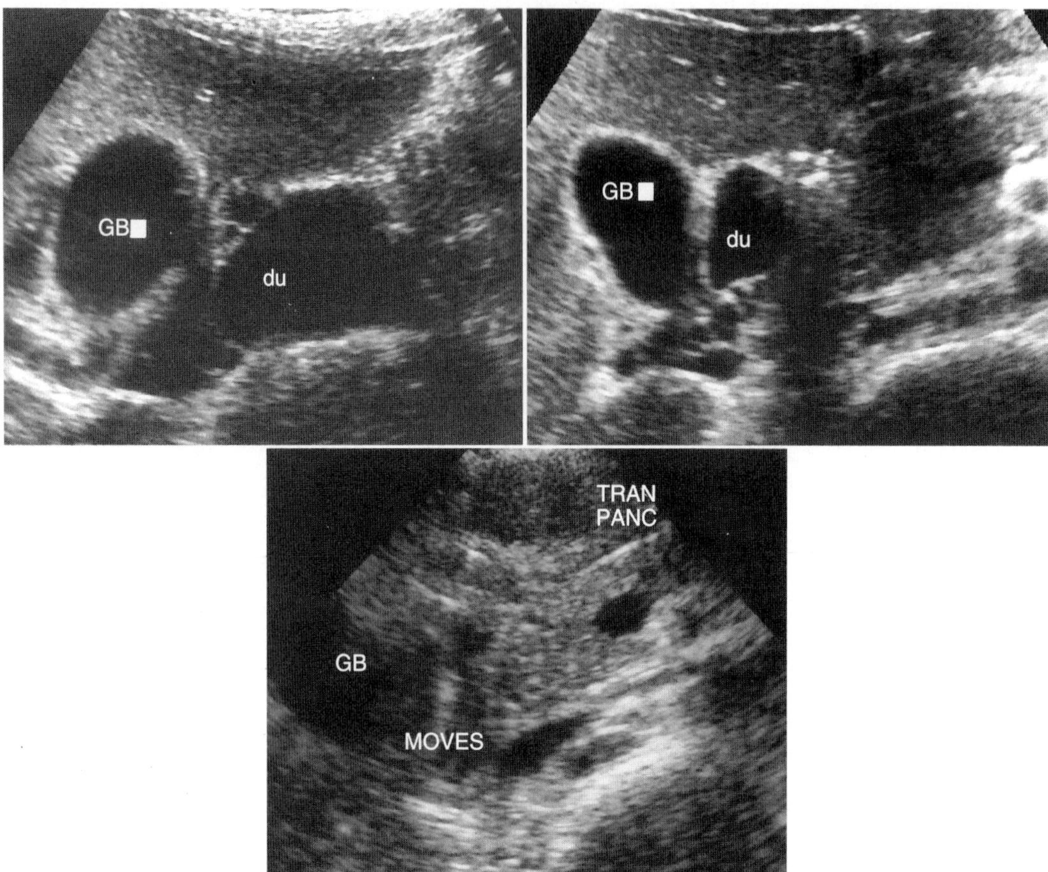

FIG. 6-24 Other fluid collections in the right upper quadrant should be observed by the sonographer for signs of change, or peristalsis, as illustrated in these images. The large collection of fluid was in the antrum and duodenum; with time, the fluid collection changed shape and distinct peristaltic movement could be seen with real time.

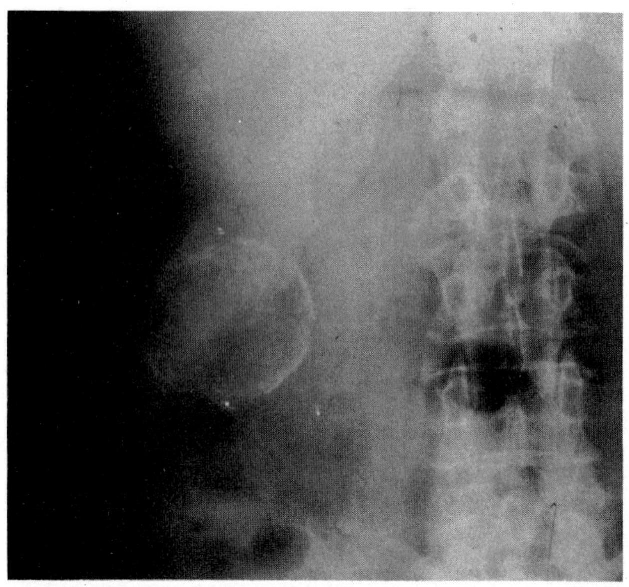

FIG. 6-25 Radiography of the calcified porcelain gallbladder.

stones without comment on the specific number that may have been seen on the scan (Fig. 6-30).

The patient's position should be shifted during the procedure to demonstrate the presence of the stones. Patients should be scanned in the left decubitus, right lateral, or upright position. The stones should shift to the most dependent area of the gallbladder. In some cases the bile has a thick consistency and the stones remain near the top of the gallbladder. Thus the density of the stones and the shadow posterior will be the sonographic evidence for stones (Figs. 6-31 to 6-36).

Gonzalez and MacIntyre have evaluated the theory for acoustic shadowing formed from gallstones and discovered that scattered reflections do not affect shadowing as much as specular reflections do.[10] The factors that produced a shadow were attributed to acoustic impedance of the gallstones; refraction through them or diffraction around them; their size, central or peripheral location, and position in relation to the focus of the beam; and the intensity of the beam.

Filly et al. found in their in vitro phantom studies that all stones cast acoustic shadows regardless of the specific

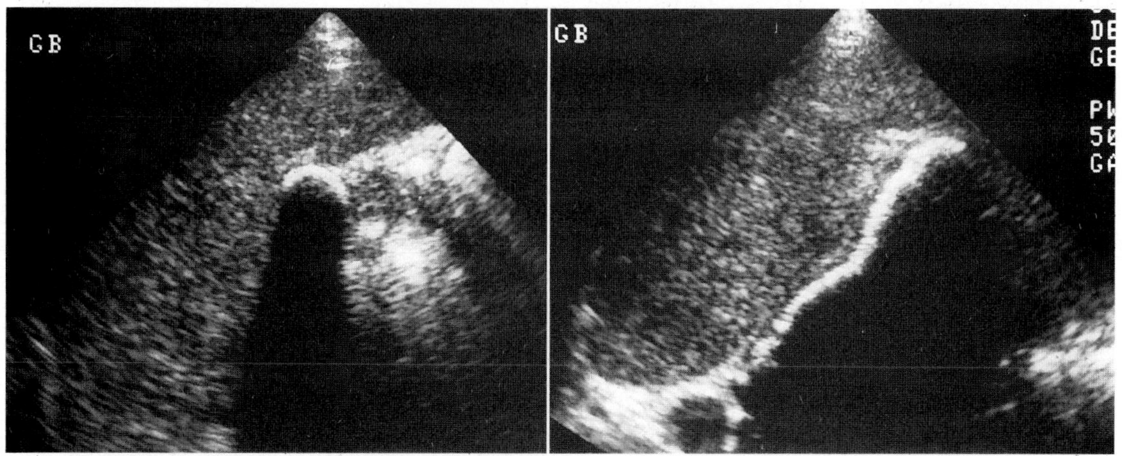

FIG. 6-26 The porcelain gallbladder is so calcified that only the anterior border of the gallbladder is seen. A sharp, well-demarcated shadow is seen beyond. This image is more difficult than a "packed bag" gallbladder full of stones.

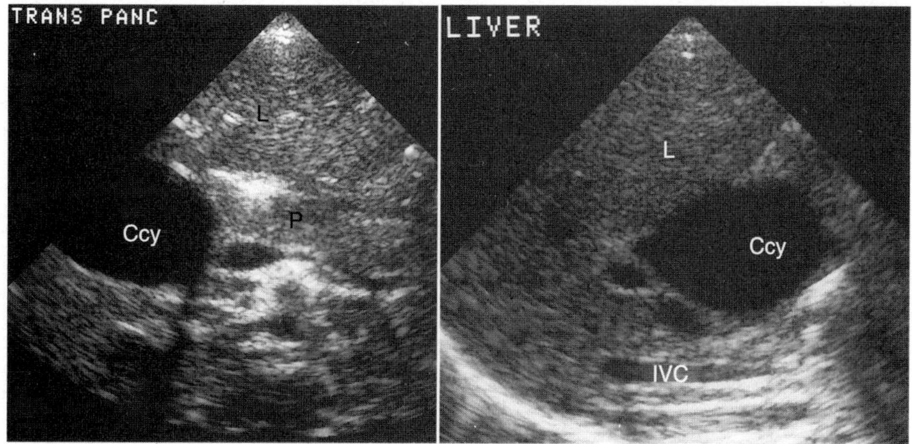

FIG. 6-27 Transverse and longitudinal scan of a young patient with a choledochal cyst in the right upper quadrant. Liver, *L;* pancreas, *P;* inferior vena cava, *IVC*.

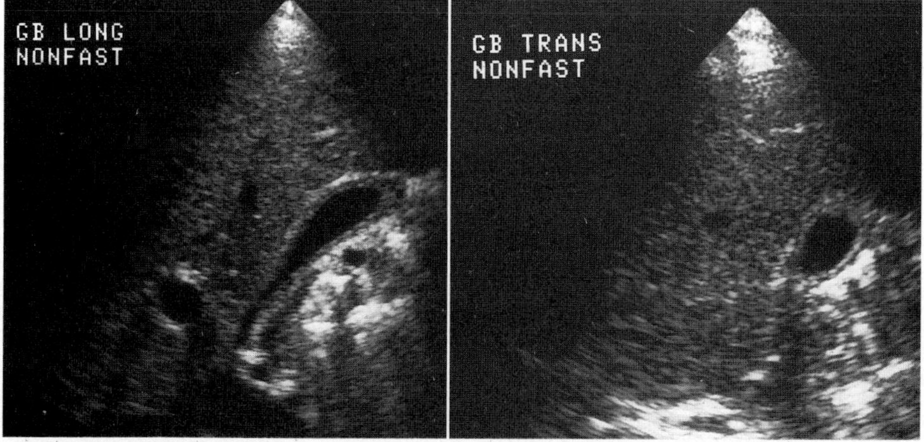

FIG. 6-28 The sonographer must be careful to obtain a complete history before the ultrasound examination. This patient forgot about his fasting instructions before the examination. Although the gallbladder is imaged, the walls appear thickened and the size diminished.

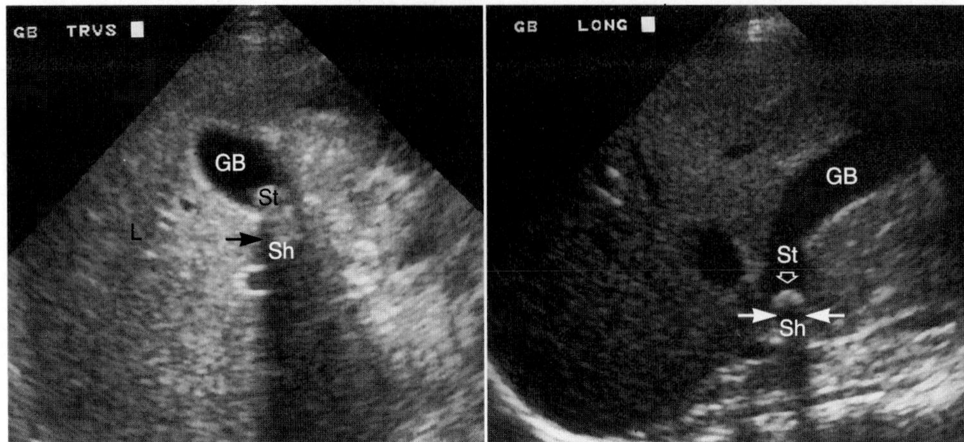

FIG. 6-29 A 45-year-old female with right upper quadrant pain and increased bilirubin. Large echogenic calculus, *st,* is seen in the dependent neck of the gallbladder. Acoustic shadowing is present beyond the stone, *sh.*

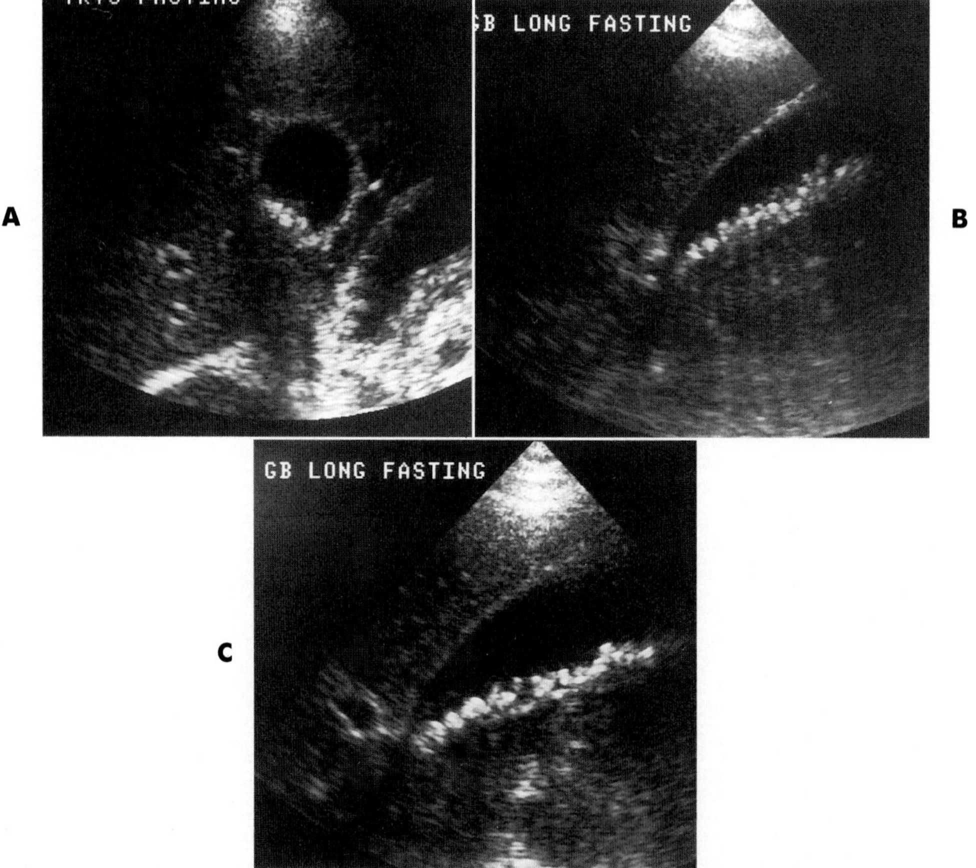

FIG. 6-30 A, Multiple small stones are layered along the posterior wall of the gallbladder. These bright echogenic foci give acoustic shadowing beyond. **B,** A higher frequency transducer would outline the stones and the shadowing even more clearly **C,** If the transducer is not exactly perpendicular to the stones, no shadow will be present.

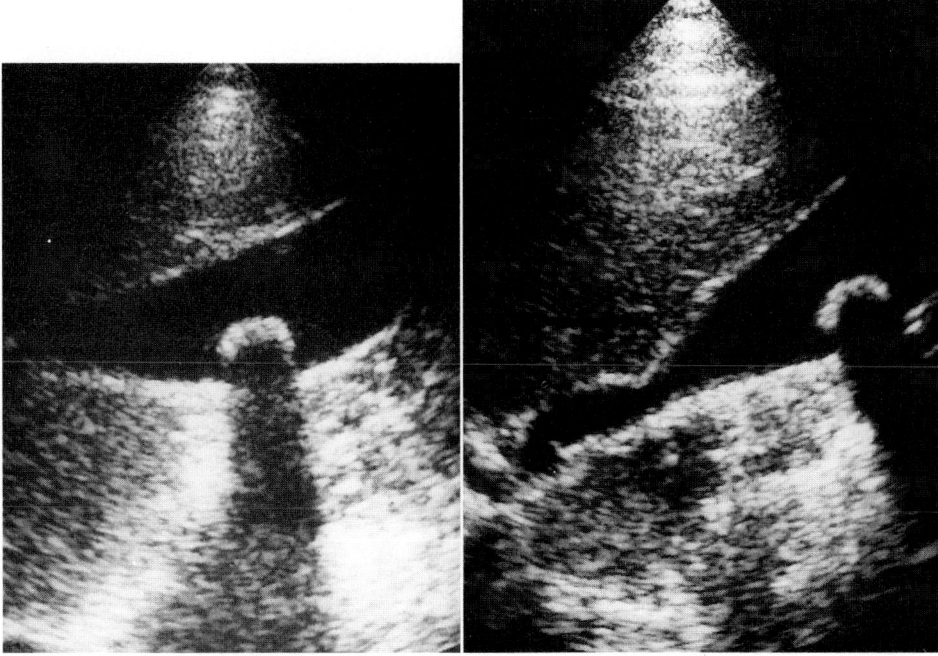

FIG. 6-31 Longitudinal scans of a patient with a single large echogenic focus in the body of the gallbladder. A change in the patient position will show a movement of the stone to a more dependent position. If the bile is very thick, the stone may take several minutes to change its position.

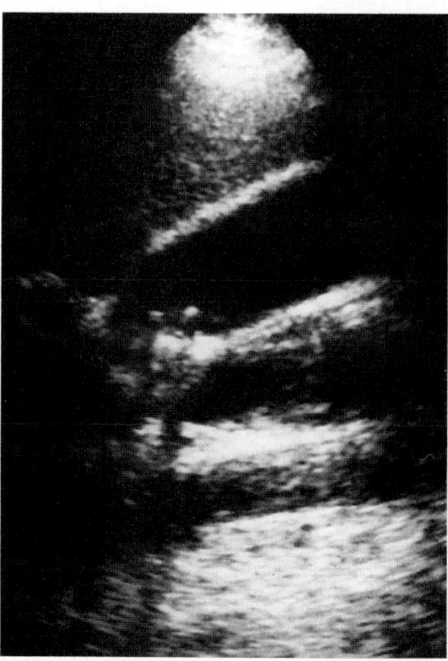

FIG. 6-32 Longitudinal scan of a distended gallbladder with two distinct gallstones lying in a bed of sludge. Two distinct shadows may be seen.

properties of the stones.[6,7] The size of the stone was important, with stones greater than 3 mm always casting a shadow and those smaller than 3 mm sometimes not casting one. They found that any stone scanned two or more times with the same transducer and machine settings might or might not generate a shadow even though the scans were within seconds of each other. The shadow was highly dependent on the relationship between the stone and the acoustic beam. If the central beam was at or near the stone, a shadow would be seen. Thus some critical ratio between the stone diameter and the beam width must be achieved before shadowing is seen.

Floating Gallstones

Some stones are seen to float when contrast material from an oral cholecystogram is present. This is because of the higher specific gravity of the contrast material than of the bile. The gallstones seek a level where their specific gravity equals that of the mixture of bile and contrast material (Fig. 6-37).[18]

Choledocholithiasis

The majority of stones in the common bile duct have migrated from the gallbladder. Common duct stones are usually associated with calculous cholecystitis. Stones tend to impact in the ampulla of Vater and may project into the duodenum. This is why it is important for the surgeons to check the common bile duct when removing the gallbladder (Fig. 6-38).

Gas in the Biliary Tree Shadow

Another cause of shadowing in the right upper quadrant is gas in the biliary tree. This is a spontaneous occurrence resulting from the formation of a biliary enteric fistula in chronic gallbladder disease (Fig. 6-39).[8]

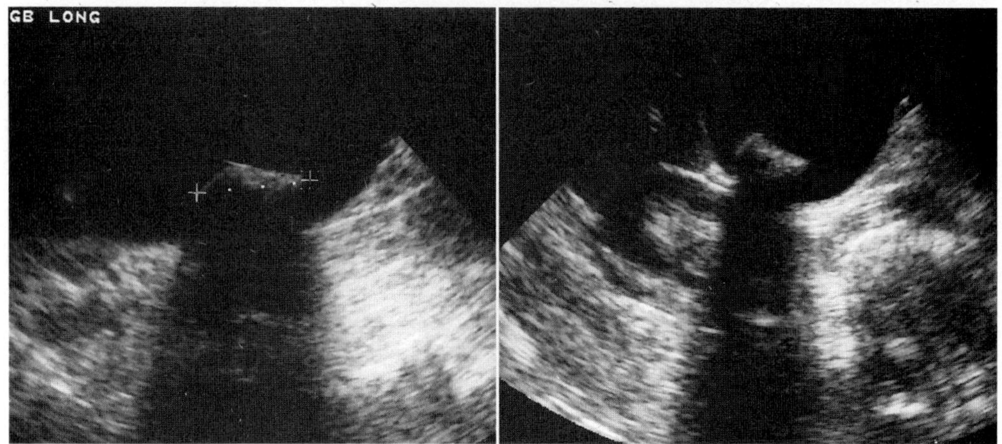

FIG. 6-33 Gallstones may take several different shapes and sizes. This patient presented with a huge gallstone measuring more than 3 cm.

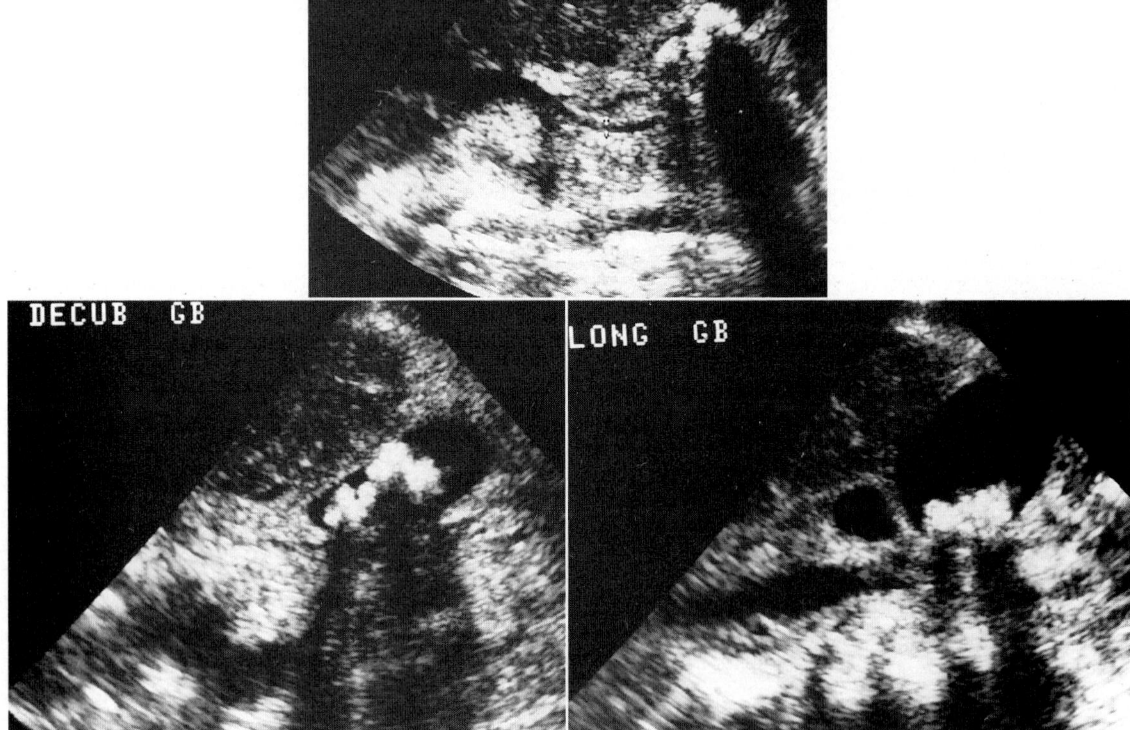

FIG. 6-34 A 55-year-old male with several episodes of right upper quadrant pain, radiating to his right shoulder. Multiple echogenic foci were seen within the gallbladder. The common bile duct *(crossbars)* was normal in size. The gallbladder wall was upper normal in size.

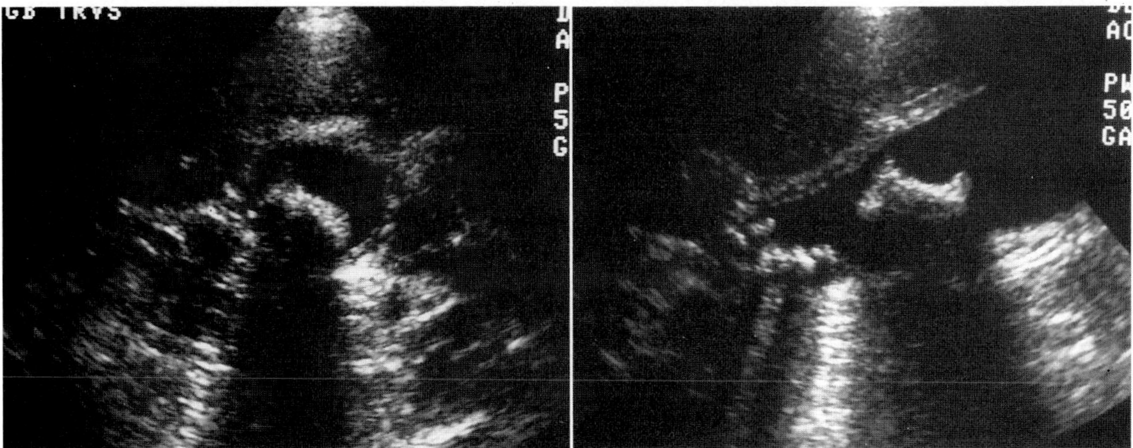

FIG. 6-35 A 95-year-old female with abdominal pain. Cholelithiasis is present with gallbladder wall thickening and a positive Murphy's sign. In addition, stones were seen in the mid common hepatic duct; there was common bile duct dilation measuring 1 cm in size.

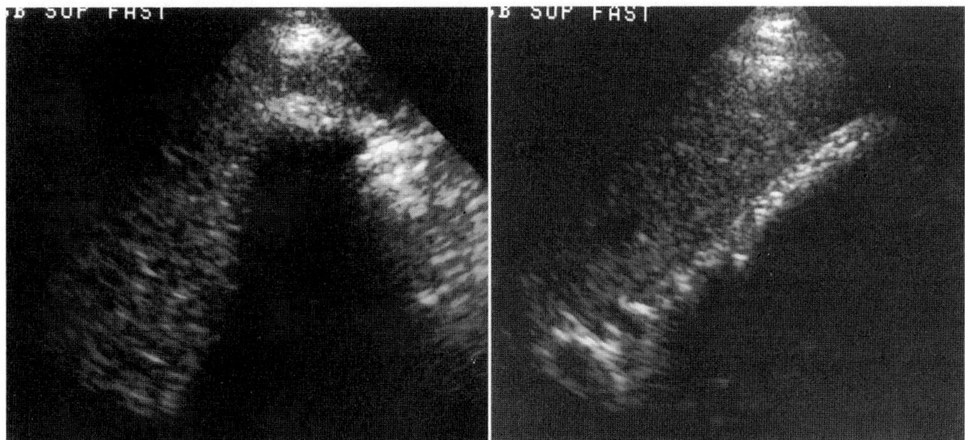

FIG. 6-36 A 45-year-old female with right upper quadrant pain and distention. The "wall-echo-shadow" ("WES") sign was visualized and indicated that the gallbladder was a packed bag. Note the sharp posterior shadow. This appearance is different than that of the porcelain gallbladder because the anterior wall is not as bright or echogenic.

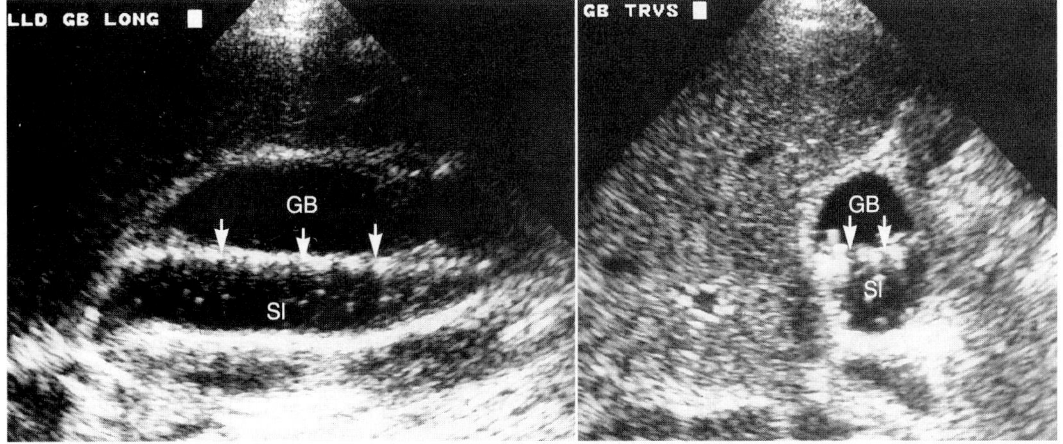

FIG. 6-37 Longitudinal and transverse scans of the gallbladder, *GB*, with a layer of stones "floating" *(arrow)* along the thick bile layer of sludge, *sl*.

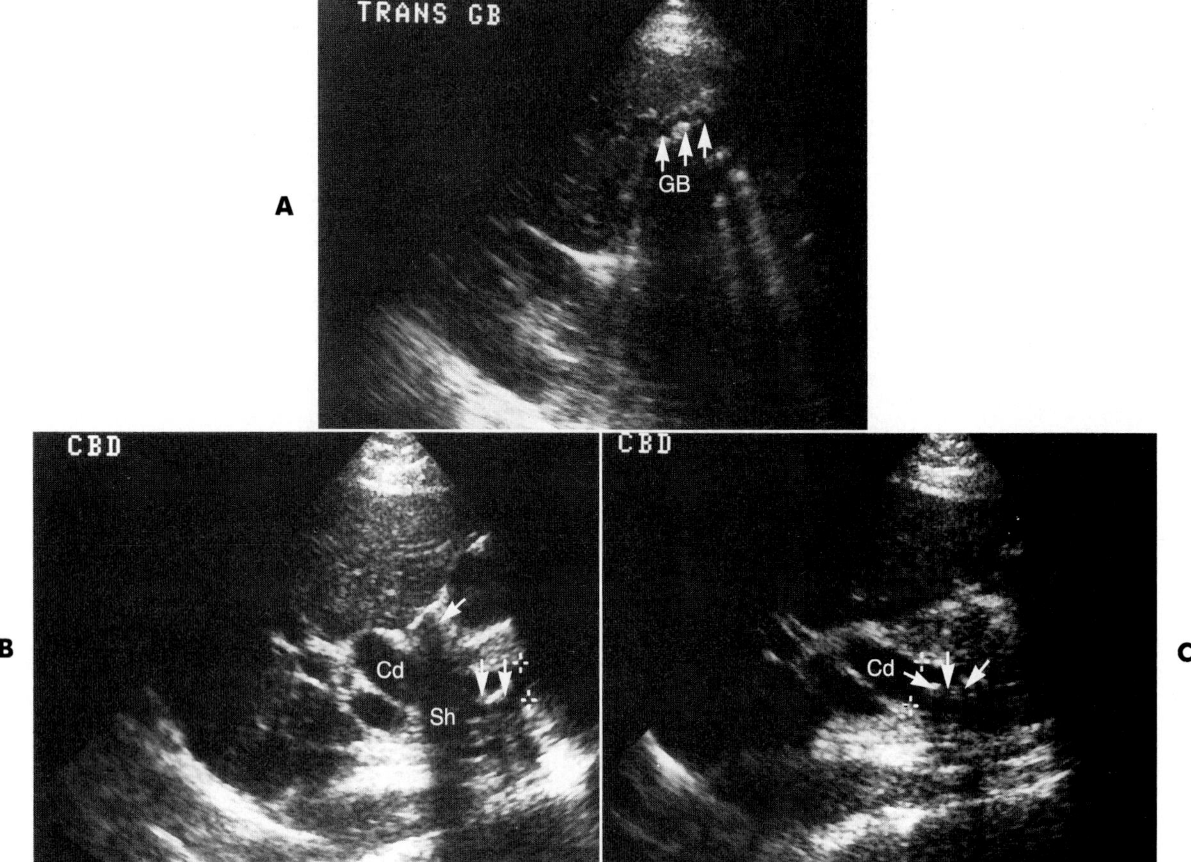

FIG. 6-38 In patients with choledocholithiasis the majority of stones have migrated from the gallbladder. **A,** Transverse: gallstones *(arrow)*. **B,** Longitudinal: common duct, *cd;* stone *(arrows);* gallstone *(single arrow);* shadow, *sh*. **C,** Longitudinal: dilated common duct with stone *(arrows)*.

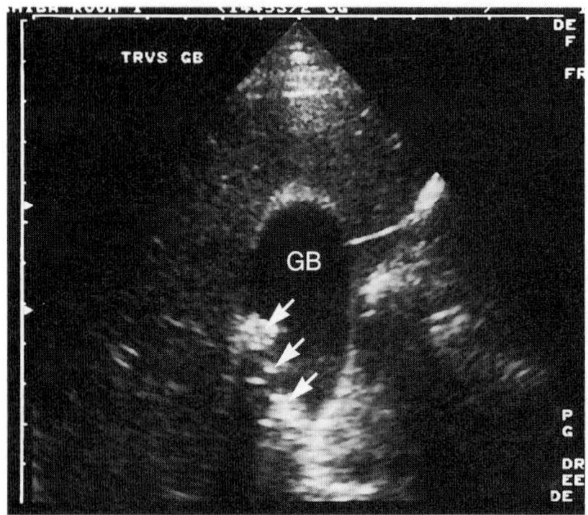

FIG. 6-39 Gas in the right upper quadrant may cause shadowing in the area of the gallbladder *(arrows)*.

Biliary Dyspepsia

Biliary dyspepsia consists of a feeling of fullness, indigestion, and belching that occurs soon after the ingestion of food. Dyspepsia may occur whether or not the gallbladder is infected. It may be that the amount of bile present in the duodenum at the beginning of a meal is insufficient to produce proper fat digestion. Removal of the diseased gallbladder is accompanied by a loss of tonus of the sphincter of Oddi, and the unimpaired flow of bile into the duodenum both in the fasting state and during feeding provides an adequate amount of bile in the duodenum to permit proper digestion. This seems to be a logical explanation for relief of dyspepsia. Mild forms of dyspepsia can be relieved by the oral feeding of bile salts.

Biliary Dyskinesia

Biliary dyskinesia is a functional disorder of the biliary tract, especially spasm of the sphincter of Oddi. Biliary colic without jaundice or fever results from the contraction of the gallbladder. Treatment is with antispasmodics.

Cholangitis

Bile may become infected because of the intestines turning dark brown and opaque. The common bile duct is thickened and dilated, especially in the ampulla of Vater (Fig. 6-40). Cholangitis abscesses are seen in severe or prolonged infection. Malaise and fever followed by sweating and shivering develop during cholangitis. In severe cases the patient is lethargic, prostrate, and in shock.

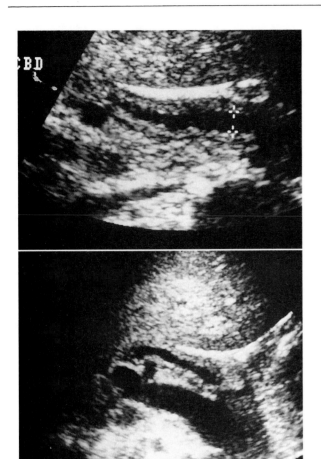

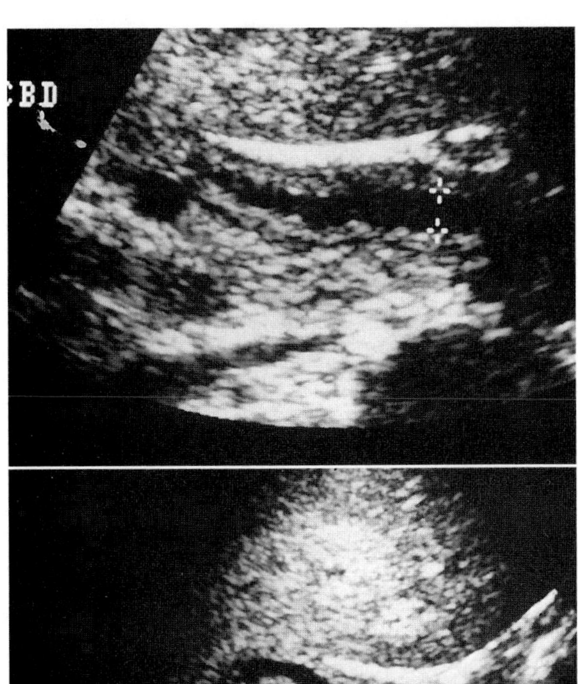

FIG. 6-40 Sclerosing cholangitis appears as dilated ducts with thickened walls. This may be seen in patients with severe or prolonged infections, such as AIDS.

Because of increasing pressure in the biliary tree, pus accumulates. Decompression of the common bile duct is necessary.

Biliary Fistula

After a cholecystostomy or T-tube choledochotomy, a biliary fistula may occur. Only under certain circumstances does a fistula occur after gallstones, carcinoma of the gallbladder, or trauma. If possible, the bile lost should be returned to the patient. Hemorrhage into the biliary tree may follow trauma, aneurysms of the hepatic artery or one of its branches, liver biopsy, tumors of the tract, gallstones, or inflammation of the liver.

Strictures

A stricture may develop if biliary pressure is raised, perhaps by a residual common duct stone. Usually after biliary tract surgery, benign strictures of the common bile duct appear. Prolonged T-tube drainage of the common bile duct, cholecystotomy, rough probing of the bile duct for calculi, and attempts at operative cholangiography, especially with a normal-sized duct, have resulted in infected bile.

NEOPLASMS OF THE GALLBLADDER

Benign Tumors

Adenomas. True benign tumors of the gallbladder are very rare. Adenomas are the most common type. These tumors occur as flat elevations located in the body of the gallbladder. They almost always occur in or near the fundus and must be distinguished pathologically from adenomyomatosis.

Adenomyomatosis is a hyperplastic change in the gallbladder wall. Papillomas may occur singly or in groups and may be scattered over a large part of the mucosal surface of the gallbladder. These papillomas are not precursors to cancer. On the oral cholecystogram, the tumor is better seen after partial contraction of the gallbladder. Various patient positions and compression show the lesion to be immobile within the gallbladder (Figs. 6-41 to 6-44).

Pseudotumors of the Gallbladder

Cholesterol polyp is the most common pseudotumor of the gallbladder. Other masses that occur are mucosal hyperplasia, inflammatory polyps, mucous cysts, and granulomata (resulting from parasitic infections).

Ultrasound Findings. Benign tumors appear as small elevations in the gallbladder lumen. These elevations maintain their initial location during positional changes, and there is no acoustic shadow behind a papillomatous elevation. An intraparietal diverticulum would suggest an adenomyomatosis (Figs. 6-45 to 6-47).

Malignant Tumors

Primary carcinoma of the gallbladder is nearly always a rapidly progressive disease, with a mortality rate approaching 100%. It is associated with cholelithiasis in about 80% to 90% of cases (although there is no direct proof that gallstones are the carcinogenic agent).

Porcelain gallbladder patients have an increased incidence of cancer. It is twice as common as cancer of the bile ducts and occurs most frequently in women 60 years of age and older.

Carcinoma

Carcinoma of the gallbladder is very rare. The tumor arises in the body of the gallbladder or, rarely, in the cystic duct (Fig. 6-48). The tumor infiltrates the gallbladder locally or diffusely and causes thickening and rigidity of the wall. The adjacent liver is often invaded by direct continuity extending through tissue spaces, the ducts of Luschka, the lymph channels, or some combination of these. Obstruction of the cystic duct results from direct extension of the tumor or extrinsic compression by involved lymph nodes (this obstruction occurs early) (Fig. 6-49).

A small tumor in the neck may not be evident on sonography if secondary signs of obstruction and ductal dilation are absent. The most frequent sonographic sign is a large, irregular, fungating mass that contains low-intensity echoes within the gallbladder. The mass may completely fill the gallbladder, obscuring the gallbladder walls (Figs.

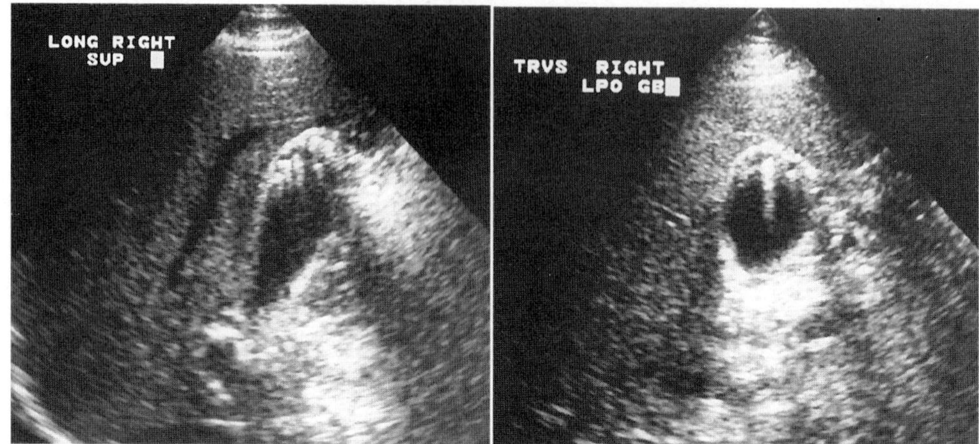

FIG. 6-41 Adenomyomatosis is a hyperplastic change in the gallbladder wall. Multiple papillomas are seen along the anterior wall of the gallbladder, causing a "ring down" of echoes to occur.

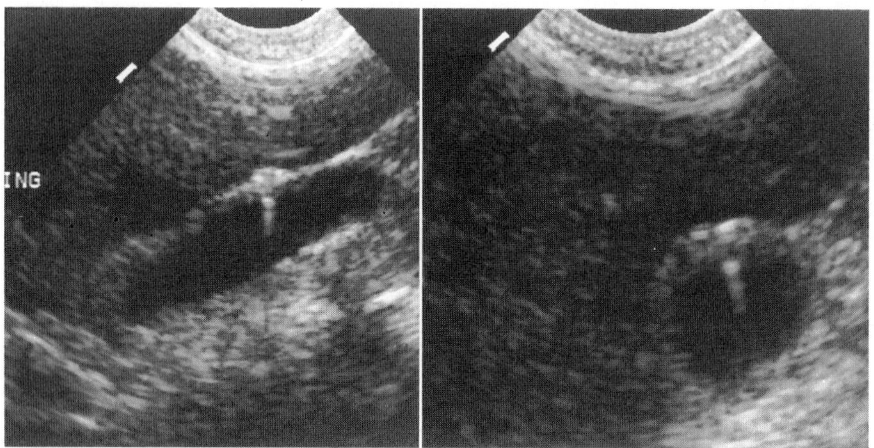

FIG. 6-42 Adenomyomatosis is very typical in its appearance. Changes in the patient position does not alter the position of the papilloma.

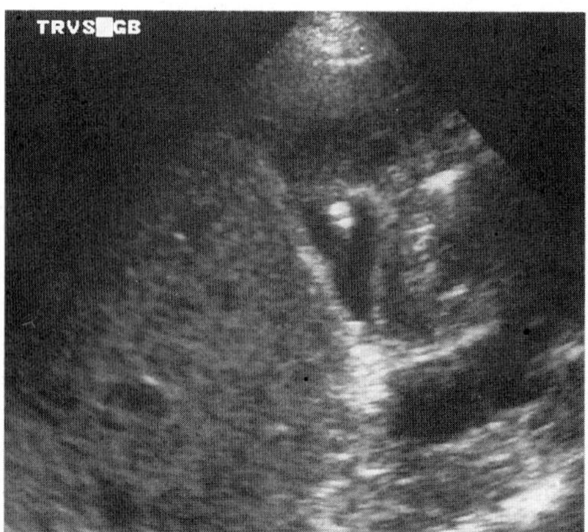

FIG. 6-43 A 37-year-old male with incidental findings of adenomyomatosis along the anterior wall of the gallbladder.

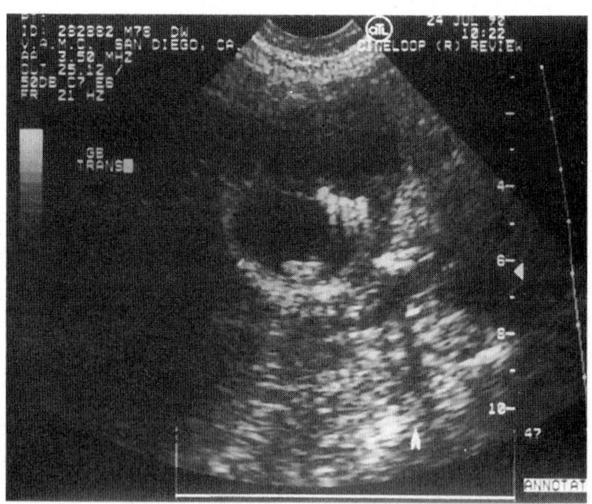

FIG. 6-44 A 37-year-old female with cholelithiasis and adenomyomatosis in the gallbladder. The stones are along the posterior wall, the papillomas along the anterior wall.

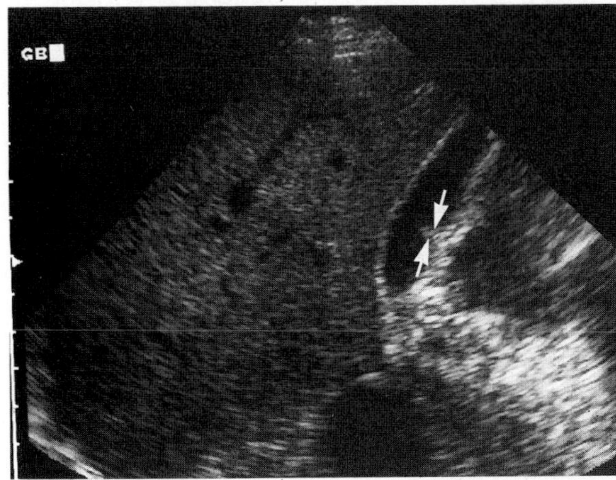

FIG. 6-45 A cholesterol polyp is the most common benign tumor of the gallbladder. This mass is immobile with change in position and usually does not shadow.

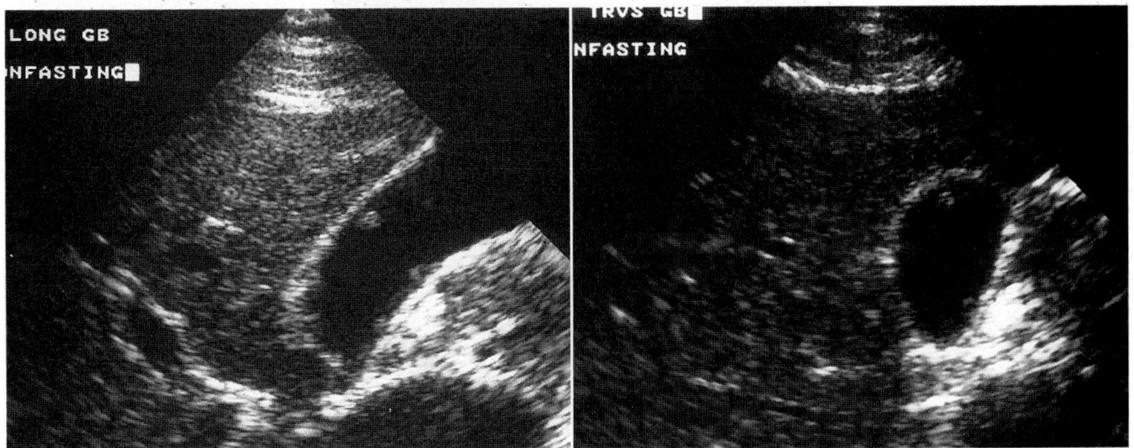

FIG. 6-46 A patient with a distended gallbladder showing multiple low-level echo reflections from polyps attached to the gallbladder wall.

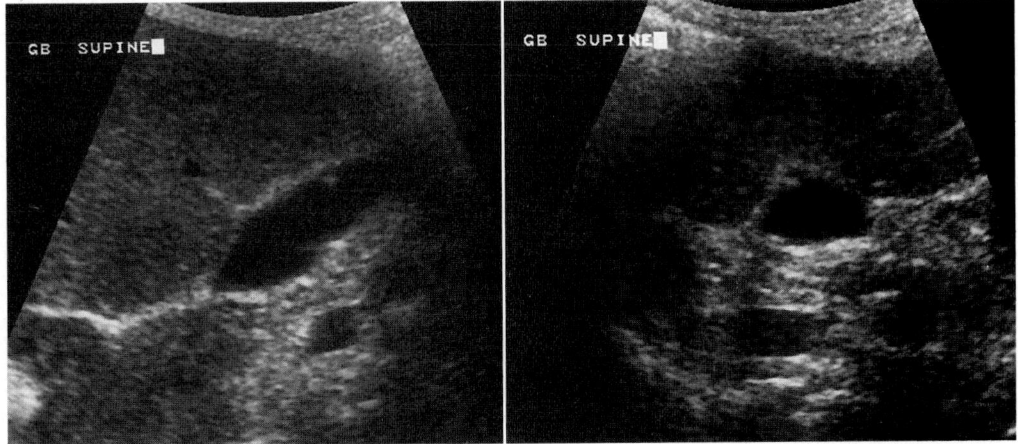

FIG. 6-47 The polyp presents differently than the adneomyomatosis papilloma. The lesion is more well defined, softer in its echo appearance, and has no "ring-down" comet-tail appearance.

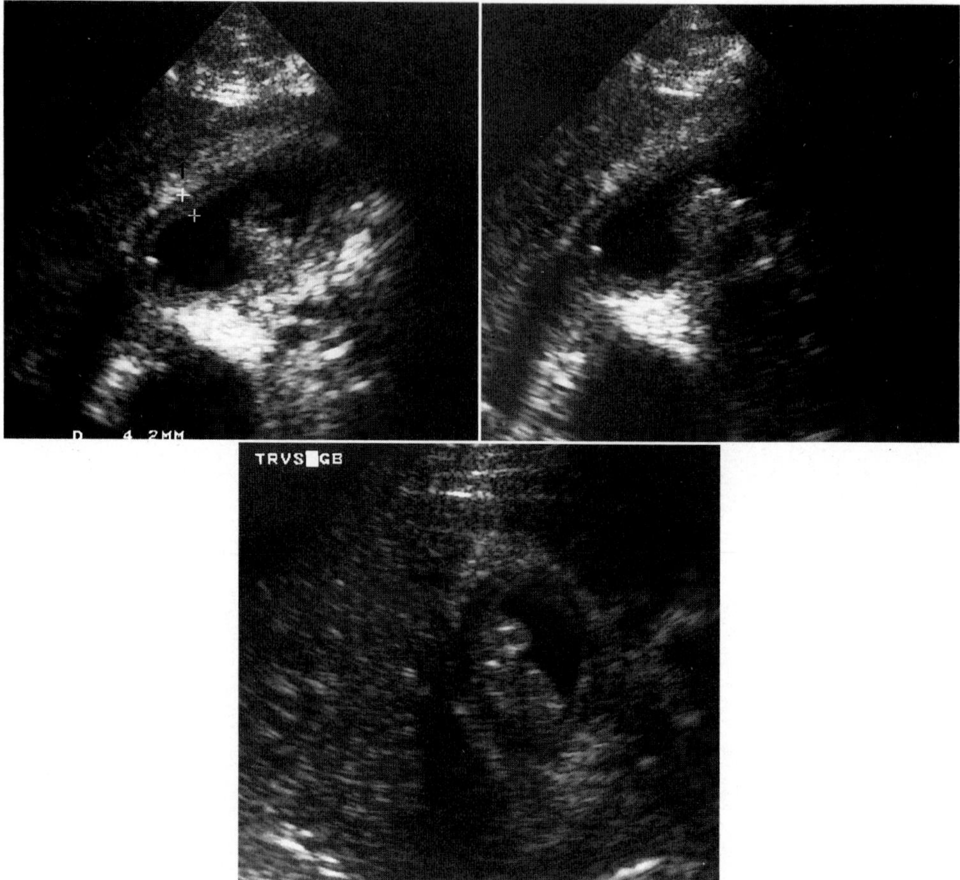

FIG. 6-48 Carcinoma of the gallbladder arises usually in the body of the gallbladder and rarely in the cystic duct. The tumor infiltrates the gallbladder and causes thickening and rigidity of the wall.

6-50). There may be stones along with the tumor, causing posterior shadowing.

The differential diagnosis of carcinoma, empyema, and xanthogranulomatous cholecystitis is virtually impossible by ultrasound, and surgical intervention may be the only recourse (Fig. 6-51).

Carcinoma of the gallbladder is almost never detected at a resectable stage. Obstruction of the cystic duct by the tumor or lymph nodes occurs early in the course of the disease and causes nonvisualization of the gallbladder on oral cholecystogram.

The gallbladder tumor is usually columnar cell adenocarcinoma, sometimes mucinous in type. Squamous cell carcinoma occurs but is unusual. Metastatic carcinoma to the gallbladder may occur secondary to melanoma. It usually is accompanied by liver metastases. Most patients have no symptoms that relate to the gallbladder unless there is complicating acute cholecystitis.

Characteristics of Malignant Gallbladder Masses

The global shape of malignant gallbladder masses is similar to that of the gallbladder. The mass has a heterogeneous, solid, or semisolid echotexture. The gallbladder wall is markedly abnormal and thickened. The adjacent liver tissue, in the hilar area, is often heterogeneous because of direct tumoral spread. There may be dilated biliary ducts within the liver parenchyma, causing the "shotgun" sign (a "double barrel" of portal veins and dilated ducts).

Tumors Arising from Extrahepatic Bile Ducts

Tumors arising from the common bile duct and ampullar carcinoma have the same ultrasonic features as pancreatic tumors. A specific pattern exists when the ampulloma bulges inside a dilated common bile duct. Cancer of the biliary convergence or of the hepatic duct usually infiltrates the ductal wall without bulging outside. It may be difficult to image these tumors—the diagnosis is indirect, based on biliary dilation above the tumor.

Tumors Arising from Intrahepatic Bile Ducts

These tumors have the same features as primary tumors of the liver (infiltrative or nodular). They may be associated with dilation of the intrahepatic ducts and a pattern of rare cystic cholangiocarcinoma.

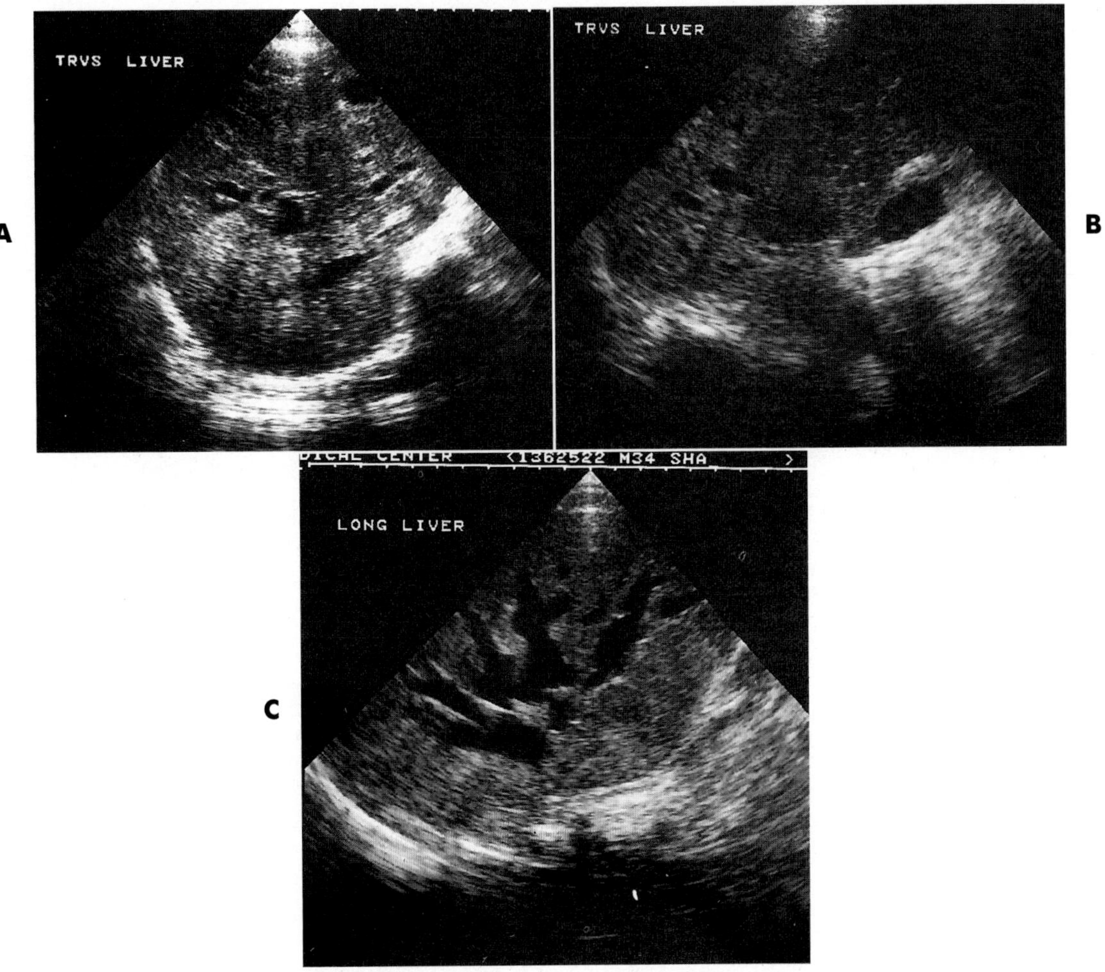

FIG. 6-49 Carcinoma of the gallbladder may extend into the cystic duct either by direct extension of the tumor or extrinsic compression by the involved lymph nodes. **A,** A transverse scan of the liver shows dilated ducts with an inhomogeneous liver parenchyma. **B,** A transverse scan of the inhomogeneous liver parenchyma. **C,** A transverse scan of the dilated ducts within the liver.

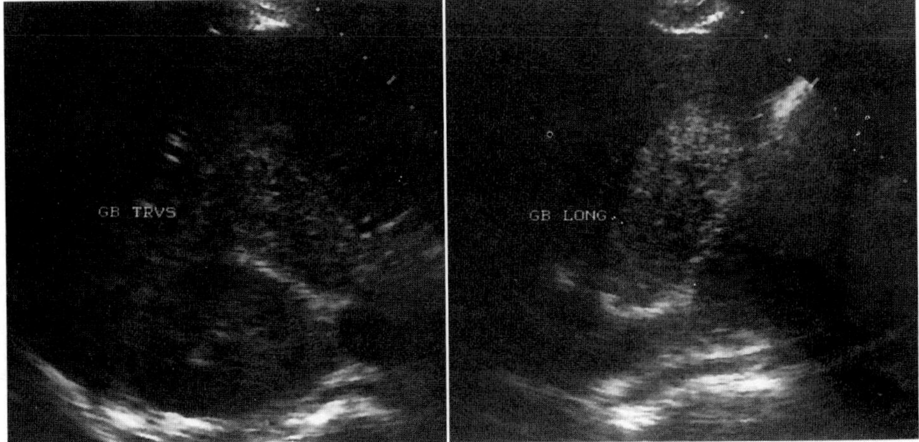

FIG. 6-50 The most frequent sonographic finding in gallbladder carcinoma is a large, irregular, fungating mass that contains low-intensity echoes within the gallbladder, causing obscurity of the gallbladder wall.

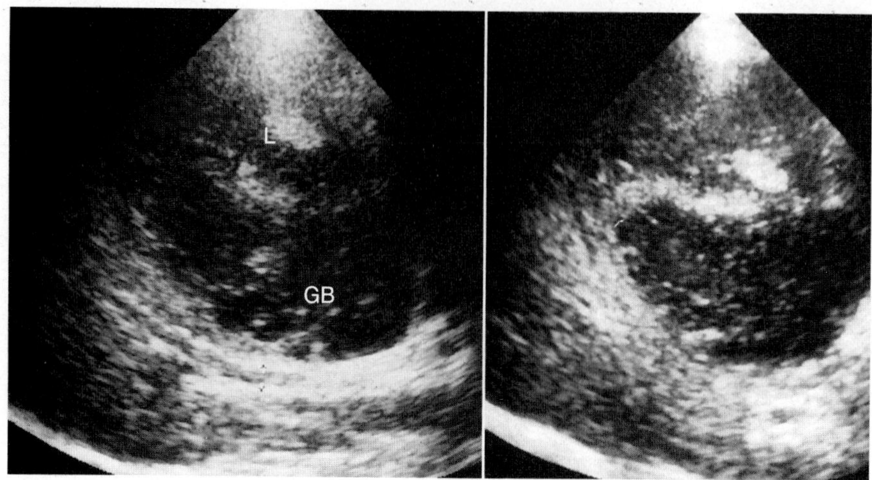

FIG. 6-51 The area of the gallbladder shows a complex pattern that could represent diffuse tumor infiltration, perforation, or abscess. This patient was febrile and very tender over the right upper quadrant. At surgery the gallbladder was perforated with gangrenous pus.

Dilated Ducts

The common hepatic duct has an internal diameter of less than 4 mm.[10,11] A duct diameter of 5 mm is borderline, and 6 mm requires further investigation. A patient may have a normal-sized hepatic duct and still have distal obstruction. The distal duct is often obscured by gas in the duodenal loop.

The common bile duct has an internal diameter slightly greater than that of the hepatic duct. Generally a duct over 6 mm is considered borderline, and over 10 mm is dilated (Fig. 6-52). Minimal dilation may be seen in nonjaundiced patients with gallstones or pancreatitis or in jaundiced patients with a common duct stone or tumor (Figs. 6-53 to 6-56). However, a diameter of more than 11 mm suggests obstruction by stone or tumor of the duct or pancreas or some other source (Fig. 6-57). Parulekar measured the common duct at 7.7 mm in nonjaundiced patients who had undergone cholecystectomy.[16]

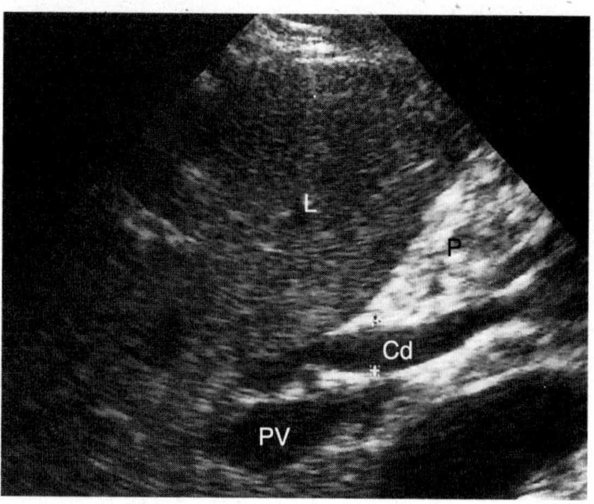

FIG. 6-52 Sagittal scan of a prominent common bile duct as it runs anterior to the portal vein, *PV,* and posterior to the head of the pancreas, *P*.

Dilated ducts may also be found in the absence of jaundice. The patient may have biliary obstruction involving one hepatic duct, an early obstruction secondary to carcinoma, or gallstones causing intermittent obstruction resulting from a ball-valve effect (Figs. 6-58 and 6-59).

In an excellent study, Laing, London, and Filly give the following five characteristics that distinguish bile ducts from other intrahepatic structures (parasagittal scans provided the best visualization of the ducts)[13]:

1. Alteration in the anatomic pattern adjacent to the main (right) portal vein segment and the bifurcation. This was more pronounced in individuals who displayed greater degrees of dilation of the intrahepatic bile ducts.
2. Irregular walls of dilated bile ducts. As the intrahepatic biliary system dilates, the course and caliber of ducts become increasingly tortuous and irregular.
3. Stellate confluence of dilated ducts. This was noted at the points where the ducts converge. Dilated ducts look like spokes of a wheel.
4. Acoustic enhancement by dilated bile ducts. Both portal veins and ducts have high-amplitude reflections surrounding them.
5. Peripheral duct dilation. It is normally unusual to visualize hepatic ducts in the liver periphery, whereas dilated bile ducts may be observed.

REVIEW QUESTIONS

1. Describe the composition of the biliary system.
2. What are the normal dimensions of the common hepatic duct and common bile duct?
3. Describe the course of the common bile duct as it relates to the head of the pancreas and portal vein.

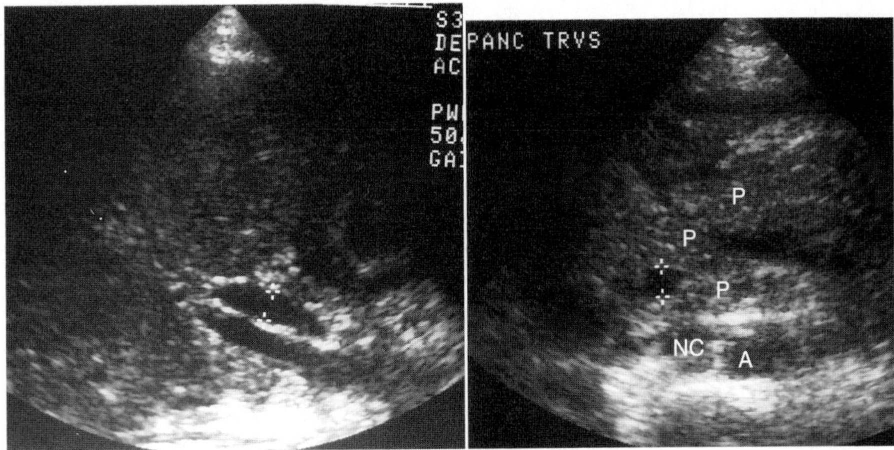

FIG. 6-53 Inflammation of the pancreas may cause the common duct to dilate. This patient had acute pancreatitis, *P*, and dilation of the common duct *(crossbars)*.

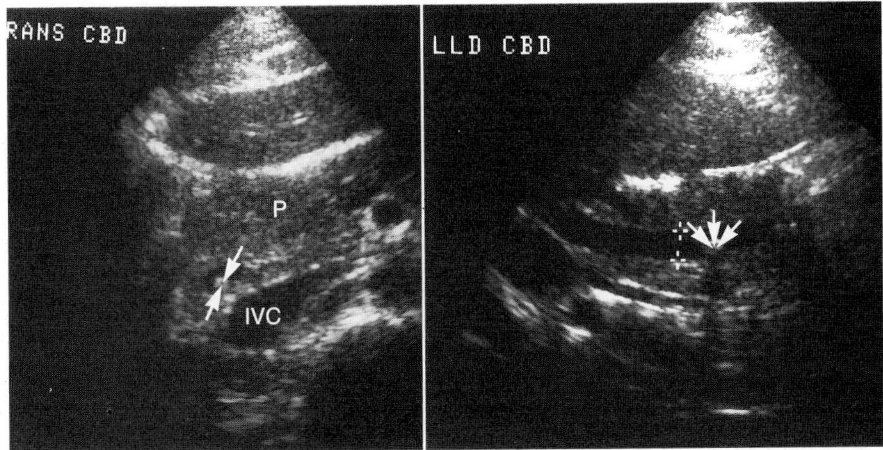

FIG. 6-54 Stones within the common duct are seen if the duct is dilated. The small echogenic focus *(arrows)* is well seen within the duct in this transverse view.

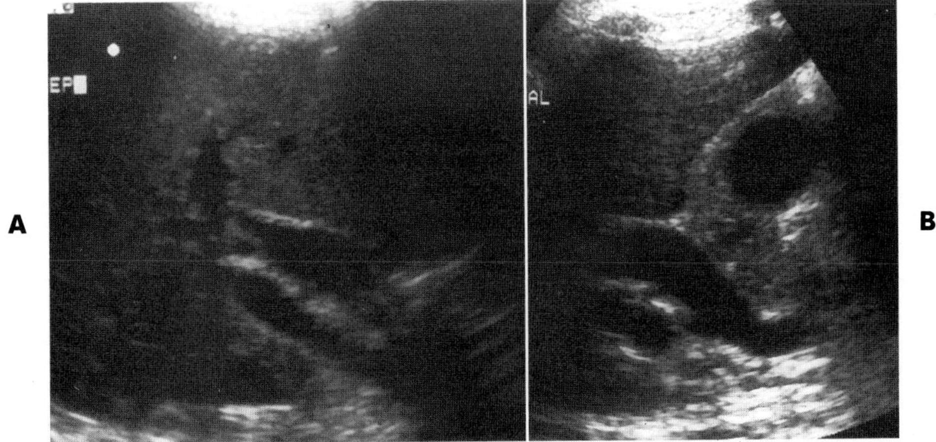

FIG. 6-55 A mass in the head of the pancreas may cause obstruction of the common bile duct, with subsequent intrahepatic ductal dilation. **A,** Liver with intrahepatic ductal dilation. **B,** Longitudinal scan of the dilated common duct.

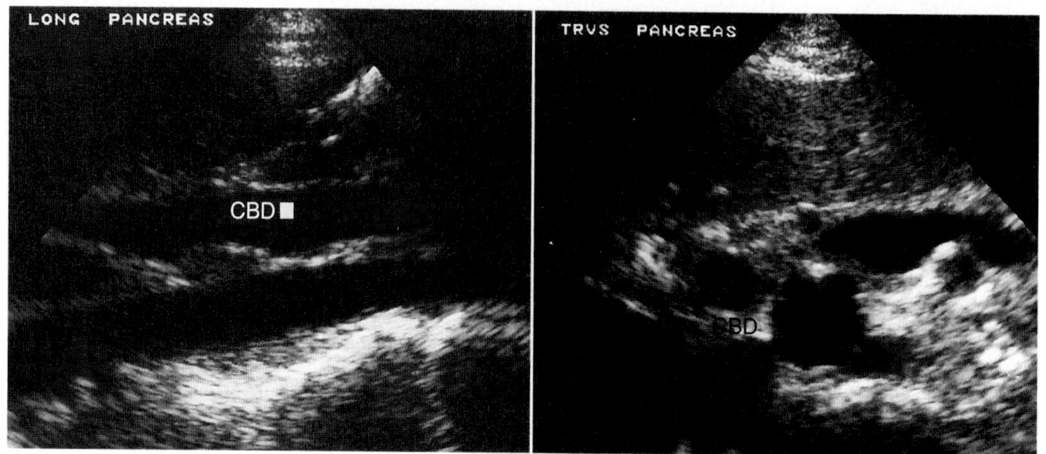

FIG. 6-56 Carcinoma of the head of the pancreas with obstruction of the common bile duct.

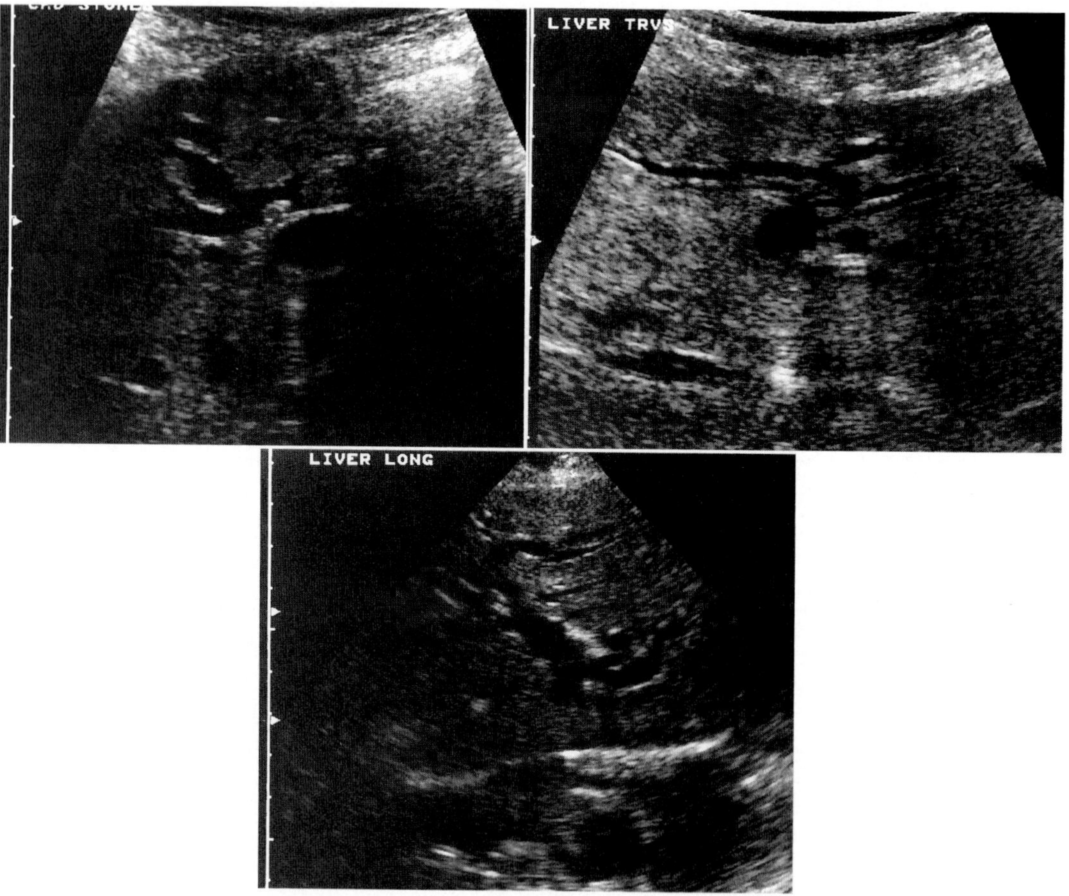

FIG. 6-57 A 60-year-old female with a history of cholecystectomy several years ago. The patient was known to have had previous hepatic calculi and now presents with right upper quadrant pain. Moderate diffuse dilation of the right and left intrahepatic ducts is present. Echogenic ovoid structures seen in the distal right hepatic and left hepatic ducts represent calculi or sludge balls. The intrahepatic duct was minimally dilated.

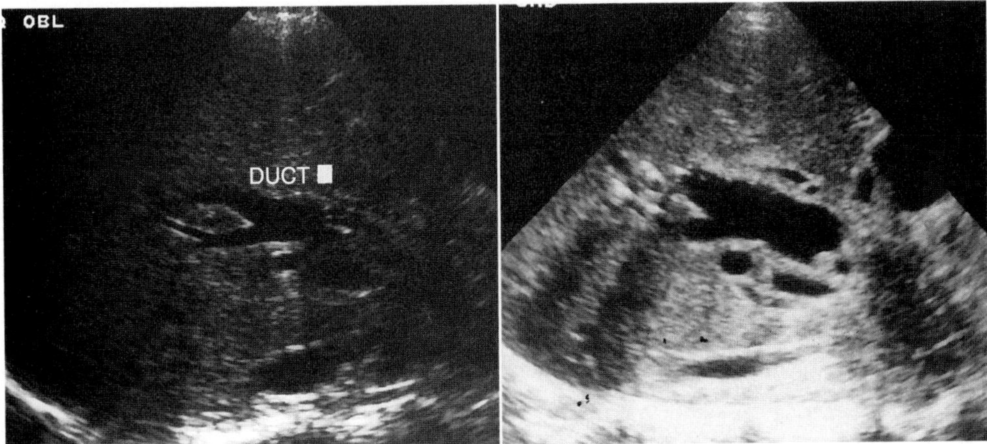

FIG. 6-58 Dilated intrahepatic ducts secondary to a mass in the area of the porta hepatis.

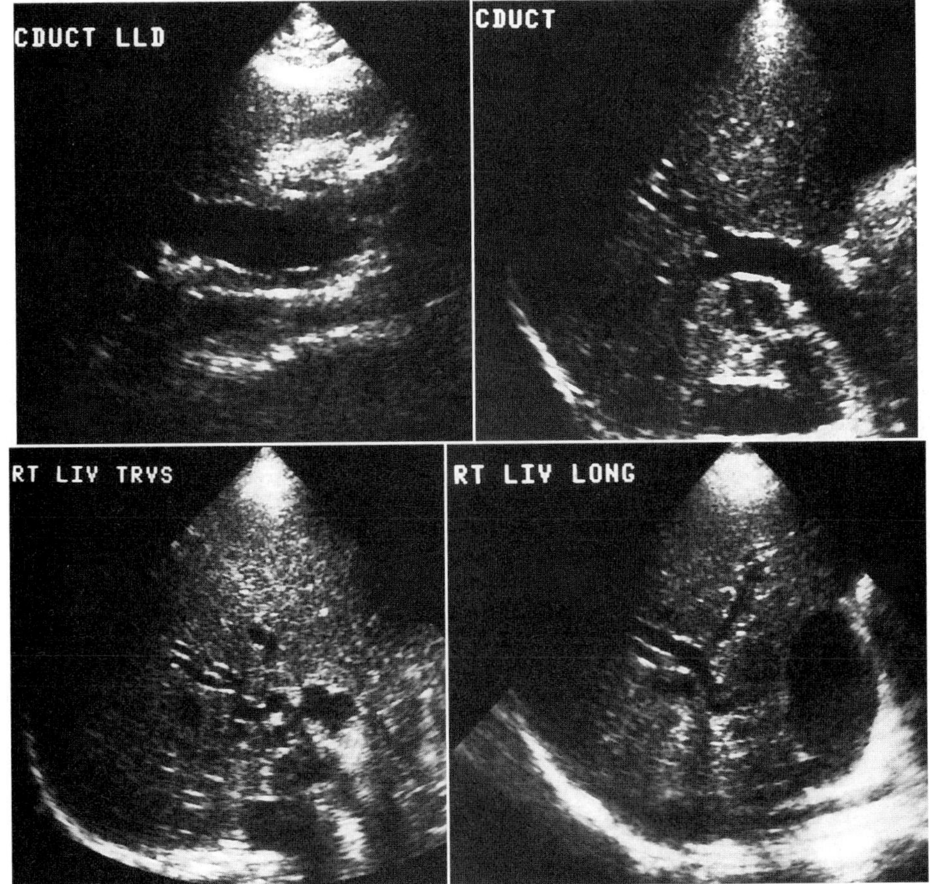

FIG. 6-59 A 58-year-old male with carcinoma of the head of the pancreas; shows dilation of the common duct with mild dilation of the intrahepatic ducts.

4. What are the three sections of the gallbladder?
5. Describe the Heister's valve and where it is found.
6. What is a Phrygian cap?
7. Why does the patient need to fast before a gallbladder ultrasound?
8. What landmark should the sonographer look for on a sagittal scan to find the gallbladder?
9. What are the clinical symptoms of gallstones?
10. Describe the process and formation of gallstones.
11. What is jaundice?

12. What is cholecystitis?
13. Describe the appearance of gallbladder sludge on ultrasound.
14. What conditions cause gallbladder wall thickening?
15. Distinguish between cholelithiasis and choledocholithiasis.
16. Define adenomyomatosis and describe its appearance on the ultrasound image.
17. How can the sonographer differentiate a polyp from a gallstone?
18. What is a porcelain gallbladder?
19. What is the appearance of gallbladder carcinoma on ultrasound?
20. Describe the appearance of carcinoma of the bile ducts and its influence on other structures in the upper abdomen.

REFERENCES

1. Bartrum RJ and Crow HC: Inflammatory diseases of the biliary system, Semin Ultrasound 1, 1980.
2. Carter SJ, Rutledge J, Hirch JH, et al: Papillary adenoma of the gallbladder; ultrasonic demonstration, J Clin Ultrasound 6:433, 1978.
3. Conrad MR, James JO, and Dietchy J: Significance of low level echoes within the gallbladder, Am J Roentgenol 132:967, 1979.
4. Conrad MR, Landay MJ, and James JO: Sonographic parallel channel sign of biliary tree enlargement in mild to moderate obstructive jaundice, Am J Roentgenol 130:279, 1978.
5. Engel JM, Deitch EA, and Sikkema W: Gallbladder wall thickness: sonographic accuracy and relation to disease, Am J Roentgenol 134:907, 1980.
6. Filly RA, Allen B, Minton MJ, et al: In vitro investigation of the origin of echoes within biliary sludge, J Clin Ultrasound 8:193, 1980.
7. Filly RA, Moss AA, and Way LW: In vitro investigation of gallstone shadowing with ultrasound tomography, J Clin Ultrasound 7:255, 1979.
8. Finberg JJ and Birnholz JC: Ultrasound evaluation of the gallbladder wall, Radiology 133:693, 1979.
9. Fiski CE, Laing FC, and Brown TW: Ultrasonographic evidence of gallbladder wall thickening in association with hypoalbuminemia, Radiology 135:713, 1980.
10. Gonzalez L and MacIntyre WJ: Acoustic shadow formation by gallstones, Radiology 135:217, 1980.
11. Graham MF, Cooperberg PL, Cohen MM, et al: The size of the normal common hepatic duct following cholecystectomy; an ultrasonic study, Radiology 135:137, 1980.
12. Kane RA: Ultrasonographic diagnosis of gangrenous cholecystitis and empyema of the gallbladder, Radiology 134:191, 1980.
13. Laing FC, London LA, and Filly RA: Ultrasonographic identification of dilated intrahepatic bile ducts and their differentiation from portal venous structures, J Clin Ultrasound 6:73, 1978.
14. Marchal GJF, Casaer M, Baert AL, et al: Gallbladder wall sonolucency in acute cholecystitis, Radiology 133:429, 1979.
15. Marchal G, Van de Voorde P, Van Dooren W, et al: Ultrasonic appearance of the filled and contracted normal gallbladder, J Clin Ultrasound 8:439, 1980.
16. Parulekar SG: Ultrasound evaluation of common bile duct size, Radiology 133:703, 1979.
17. Sanders RC: The significance of sonographic gallbladder wall thickening, J Clin Ultrasound 8:143, 1980.
18. Scheske GA, Cooperberg PL, Cohen MM, et al: Floating gallstones; the role of contrast material, J Clin Ultrasound 8:227, 1980.

BIBLIOGRAPHY

Amberg JR and Leopold GR: Is oral cholecystography still useful? Am J Roentgenol 151:73, 1988.

Behan M and Kazam E: Sonography of the common bile duct: value of the right anterior oblique view, Am J Roentgenol 130:701, 1978.

Bloom RA, Libson E, and Lebensart PD: The ultrasound spectrum of emphysematous cholecystitis, J Clin Ultrasound, 17:251, 1989.

Bressler EL, Rubin JM, McCracken S, et al: Sonographic parallel channel sign: a reappraisal, Radiology 164:343, 1987.

Bret PM, de Stempel JV, Atri M, et al: Intrahepatic bile duct and portal vein anatomy revisited, Radiology 169:405, 1988.

Byung IC, Lim JH, Han MC, et al: Biliary cystadenoma and cystadenocarcinoma: computed tomography and sonographic findings, Radiology 171:57, 1989.

Callen PW and Filly RA: Ultrasonographic localization of the gallbladder, Radiology 133:687, 1979.

Carroll BA and Oppenheimer DA: Sclerosing cholangitis: sonographic demonstration of bile duct wall thickening, Am J Roentgenol 139:1016, 1982.

Cerri GG, Leite GJ, Simoes JB, et al: Ultrasonographic evaluation of ascaris in the biliary tract, Radiology 146:753, 1983.

Chen HH, Zhang WH, and Wang SS: Twenty-two year experience with the diagnosis and treatment of intrahepatic calculi, Surg Gynecol Obstet 159:519, 1984.

Childress MH: Sonographic features of milk calcium cholecystitis, J Clin Ultrasound 14:312, 1986.

Chun GH, Deutsch AL, and Scheible W: Sonographic findings in milk of calcium bile, Gastrointest Radiol 7:371, 1982.

Cooperberg PL and Burhenne HJ: Real-time ultrasonography: an approach to the nonvisualized gallbladder, Radiology 103:645, 1972.

Crade M, Taylor KJW, Rosenfield AT, et al: Surgical and pathological correlation of cholecystosonography and cholecystography, Am J Roentgenol 131:227, 1978.

Desai RK, Paushter DM, and Armistead J: Intrahepatic arterial calcification mimicking pneumobilia, J Ultrasound Med 8:333, 1989.

Dong B and Chen M: Improved sonographic visualization of choledocholithiasis, J Clin Ultrasound 15:185, 1987.

Ferin P and Lemer RM: Contracted gallbladder: a finding in hepatic dysfunction, Radiology 154:769, 1985.

Fiske CE, Filly RA: Pseudo-sludge: a spurious ultrasound appearance within the gallbladder, Radiology 144:631, 1982.

Fitzgerald EJ and Toi A: Pitfalls in the ultrasonographic diagnosis of gallbladder diseases, Postgrad Med J 63:525, 1987.

Gabaldon A, Mofidi C, Moskovskij S, et al: Control of ascariasis, World Health Organization. Technical Report Series 379:6, 1967.

Gibson RN, Yeung E, Thompson J, et al: Bile duct obstruction: radiologic evaluation of level, cause, and tumor resectability, Radiology 160:43, 1986.

Han BK, Babcock DS, and Gelfand MH: Choledochal cyst with bile duct dilatation: sonography and 99mTc-IDA cholescintigraphy, Am J Roentgenol 136:1075, 1981.

Jeanty P, Ammann W, Cooperberg P, et al: Mobile intraluminal masses of the gallbladder, J Ultrasound Med 2:65, 1983.

Jeffrey RB, Laing FC, Wong W, et al: Gangrenous cholecystitis; diagnosis by ultrasound, Radiology 148:219, 1983.

Kane RA, Jacobs R, Katz J, et al: Porcelain gallbladder: ultrasound and computed tomography appearance, Radiology 152:137, 1984.

Klatskin G: Adenocarcinoma of the hepatic duct at its bifurcation within the porta hepatis: an unusual tumor with distinctive clinical and pathologic features, Am J Med 38:241, 1965.

Laing FC: Ultrasound diagnosis of choledocholithiasis, Sem Ultrasound, CT and MR 8:103, 1987.

Laing FC, Jeffrey RB Jr, and Wing VW: Biliary dilatation: defining the level and cause by real-time ultrasound, Radiology 160:39, 1986.

Lewandowski BJ, Withers C, and Winsberg F: The air-filled left hepatic duct: the saber sign as an aid to the radiographic diagnosis of pneumobilia, Radiology 153:329, 1984.

Lim JH, Ko YT, Lee DH: Clonorchiasis: sonographic findings in 59 proved cases, Am J Roentgenol 152:761, 1989.

Lim JH, Ryu KN, Ko YT, et al: Anatomic relationship of intrahepatic bile ducts to portal veins, J Ultrasound Med 9:137, 1990.

Lin HH, Changchien CS, and Lin DY: Hepatic parenchymal calcifications: differentiation from intrahepatic stones, J Clin Ultrasound 17:411, 1989.

MacDonald FR, Cooperberg PL, and Cohen MM: The WES triad: a specific sonographic sign of gallstones in the contracted gallbladder, Gastrointest Radiol 6:39, 1981.

McGahan JP and Lindfors KK: Acute cholecystitis: diagnostic accuracy of percutaneous aspiration of the gallbladder, Radiology 167:669, 1988.

McGahan JP and Walter JP: Diagnostic percutaneous aspiration of the gallbladder, Radiology 155:619, 1985.

Machan L, Muller NL, Cooperberg PL: Sonographic diagnosis of Klatskin tumors, Am J Roentgenol 147:509, 1986.

Madrazo BL, Francis I, Hricak H, et al: Sonographic findings in perforation of the gallbladder, Am J Roentgenol 139:491, 1982.

Meyer DG, Weinstein BJ: Klatskin tumors of the bile ducts: sonographic appearance, Radiology 148:803, 1983.

Mitchell DG, Needleman L, Frauenhoffer S, et al: Gas containing gallstones: the sonographic "double echo sign," J Ultrasound Med 7:39, 1988.

Nemcek AA Jr, Gore RM, Vogelzang RL, et al: The effervescent gallbladder: a sonographic sign of emphysematous cholecystitis, Am J Roentgenol 150:575, 1988.

Niederau C, Muller J, Sonnenberg A, et al: Extrahepatic bile ducts in healthy subjects, in patients with cholelithiasis, and in postcholecystectomy patients: a prospective ultrasonic study, J Clin Ultrasound 11:23, 1983.

Parulekar SG: Ultrasound evaluation of common bile duct size, Radiology 133:703, 1979.

Parulekar SG: Sonographic findings in acute emphysematous cholecystitis, Radiology 145:117, 1982.

Parulekar SG: Sonography of the distal cystic duct, J Ultrasound Med 8:367, 1989.

Phillips G, Pochaczevsky R, Goodman J, et al: Ultrasound patterns of metastatic tumors in the gallbladder, J Clin Ultrasound 10:379, 1982.

Raghavendra BN, Subramanyam BR, Balthazer EJ, et al: Sonography of adenomyomatosis of the gallbladder, Radiology 146:747, 1983.

Ralls PW, Mayekawa, Lee KP, et al: The use of color Doppler sonography to distinguish dilated intrahepatic ducts from vascular structures, Am J Roentgenol 152:291, 1988.

Ralls PW, Quinn MF, and Juttner HU: Gallbladder wall thickening: patients without intrinsic gallbladder disease, Am J Roentgenol 137:65, 1981.

Romano AJ, VanSonnenberg E, Casola G, et al: Gallbladder and bile duct abnormalities in AIDS: sonographic findings in eight patients, Am J Roentgenol 150:123, 1988.

Rubaltelli L, Talenti E, Rizzatto G, et al: Gas-containing gallstones: their influence on ultrasound images, J Clin Ultrasound 12:279, 1984.

Schulman A: Non-Western patterns of biliary stones and the role of ascariasis, Radiology 162:425, 1987.

Schulman A, Loxton AJ, Heydenrych JJ, et al: Sonographic diagnosis of biliary ascariasis, Am J Roentgenol 139:485, 1982.

Shlaer WJ, Leopold GR, and Scheible FW: Sonography of the thickened gallbladder wall: a nonspecific finding, Am J Roentgenol 136:337, 1981.

Simeone JF, Brink JA, Mueller PR, et al: The sonographic diagnosis of acute gangrenous cholecystitis: importance of the Murphy sign, Am J Roentgenol 152:289, 1989.

Sukov RJ, Sample WF, Sarti DA, et al: Cholecystosonography: the junctional fold, Radiology 133:435, 1979.

Takada T, Yasuda H, Uchiyama K, et al: Pericholecystic abscess: classification of ultrasound findings to determine the proper therapy, Radiology 172:693, 1989.

Willson SA, Gosink BB, and vanSonnenberg E: Unchanged size of a dilated common bile duct after fatty meal: results and significance, Radiology 160:29, 1986.

Wing VW, Laing FC, and Jeffrey RB: Sonographic differentiation of enlarged hepatic arteries from dilated intrahepatic bile ducts. Am J Roentgenol 145:57, 1985.

Wu CC, Ho YH, and Chen CY: Effect of aging on common bile duct diameter: a real-time ultrasonographic study, J Clin Ultrasound 12:473, 1984.

Yeh HC, Goodman J, and Rabinowitz JG: Floating gallstones in bile without added contrast material, Am J Roentgenol 146:49, 1986.

CHAPTER 7

Pancreas

Sandra L. Hagen-Ansert

With the advent of each new medical procedure, efforts to visualize the pancreas have met with varying degrees of success. Before the relatively recent use of diagnostic ultrasound, computerized tomography, and magnetic resonance, other noninvasive procedures were unsuccessful in visualization of the pancreas. The plain film of the abdomen is diagnostic of pancreatitis if calcification is visible in the pancreatic area; however, calcification does not occur in all cases. Localized ileus ("paralyzed gut," gas, and fluid accumulation near the area of inflammation) may be shown on the plain radiograph in patients with pancreatitis. The upper gastrointestinal test series provides indirect information about the pancreas when the widened duodenal loops are visualized. Other diagnostic methods, such as hypotonic duodenography, isotope examination, arteriography, fiberoptic gastroscopy, and intravenous cholangiography, all provide indirect information about the pancreas or prove limited in their diagnostic ability. Thus investigators have been striving to develop an examination that will be accurate, readily repeatable, and safe. Diagnostic ultrasound appears to be such an examination in many patients who are very slender in stature. The more obese patient images much better with computerized tomography.

The normal pancreas can be visualized in the majority of patients by using the neighboring organs and vascular landmarks as an aid in localization. The gland appears echographically as dense as or slightly denser than the hepatic parenchyma. Variations in patient positioning or use of contrast media through the stomach may aid in visualizing the entire gland.

NORMAL ANATOMY

The pancreas is a multilobular gland located in the retroperitoneal cavity. It lies anterior to the first and second lumbar bodies located deep in the epigastrium and left hypochodrium behind the lesser omental sac (Fig. 7-1). The pancreas extends from the second portion of the duodenum to the splenic hilum. Other variations in the lie of the pancreas are transverse, horseshoe, sigmoid, L-shaped, or inverted V. The normal length of the pancreas is about 15 cm. The gland appears larger or thicker in children than in adults. It becomes smaller with advancing age.

The pancreas is divided into the following four areas: head, neck, body, and tail (Fig. 7-2). We discuss each area as it relates to its surrounding anatomy.

Head

The head of the pancreas is anterior to the inferior vena cava and left renal vein, inferior to the caudate lobe of the liver and portal vein, and lateral to the second portion of the duodenum as it "lies in the lap" of the duodenum. The stomach is the anterior border. The superior mesenteric vessels cross anterior to the uncinate part of the gland and posterior to the neck of the pancreas. The common bile duct passes through a groove posterior to the pancreatic head, and the gastroduodenal artery is the anterolateral border. The head measures 2.0 to 2.5 cm in its anterior-to-posterior dimension.

Neck

The neck of the pancreas is directly anterior to the superior mesenteric vein. The portal vein is formed behind the neck by the junction of the superior mesenteric vein and the splenic vein. It measures about 1.0 cm in its anteroposterior dimension.

Body

The body is the largest section of the pancreas. It rests anterior to the aorta, superior mesenteric artery, and the left renal vein, adrenal gland, and kidney. The tortuous splenic artery is the superior border of the gland. The anterior border is the posterior wall of the antrum of the stomach. The neck of the pancreas forms the right lateral border. The splenic vein courses across the posterior surface. The body measures 2 cm in anteroposterior dimension.

Tail

The tail is more difficult to image because it lies anterior to the left kidney and posterior to the left colic flexure and transverse colon. The tail begins to the left of the lateral border of the spine and extends toward the splenic hilum. The splenic vein is the posterior border of the body and tail. The splenic artery and stomach are the anterior borders. The tail measures approximately 1.0 to 2.0 cm.

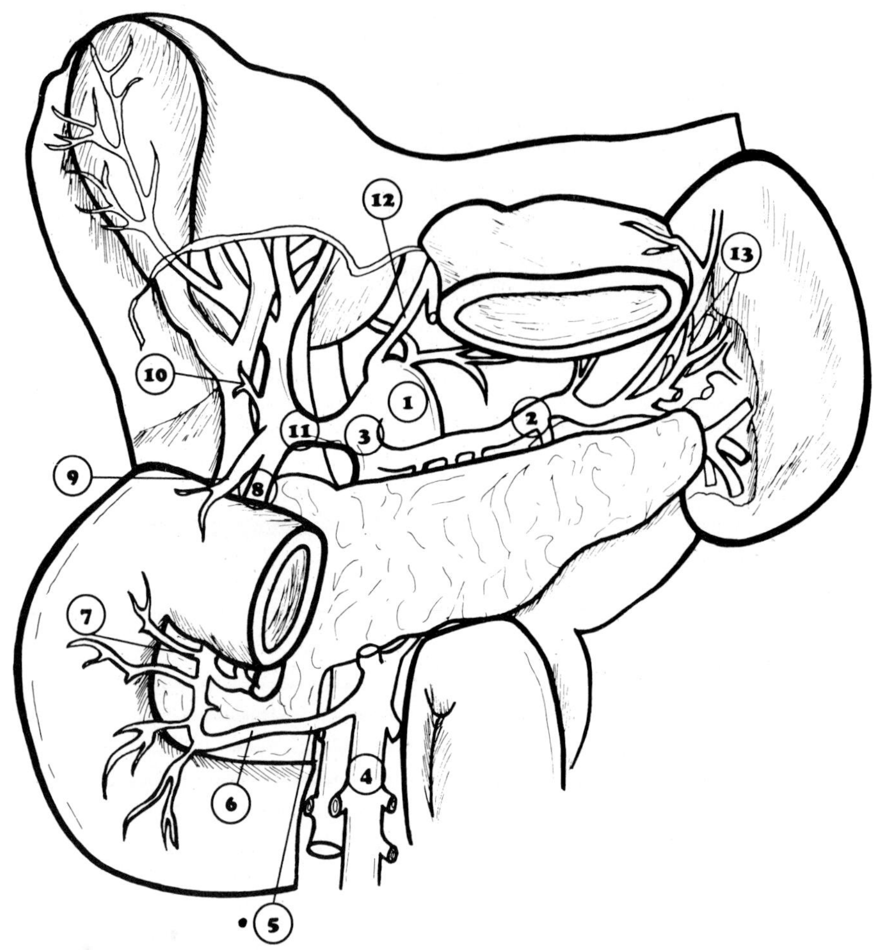

FIG. 7-1 Anterior view of the pancreas and its vascular structures. Aorta, *1;* splenic artery, *2;* celiac trunk, *3;* superior mesenteric artery, *4;* inferior pancreaticoduodenal artery, *5;* anterior inferior pancreaticoduodenal artery, *6;* anterior superior pancreaticoduodenal artery, *7;* gastroduodenal artery, *8;* supraduodenal artery, *9;* right gastric artery, *10;* common hepatic artery, *11;* left gastric artery, *12;* short gastric arteries, *13*. (From Hagen-Ansert SL: The anatomy workbook, Philadelphia, 1986, JB Lippincott).

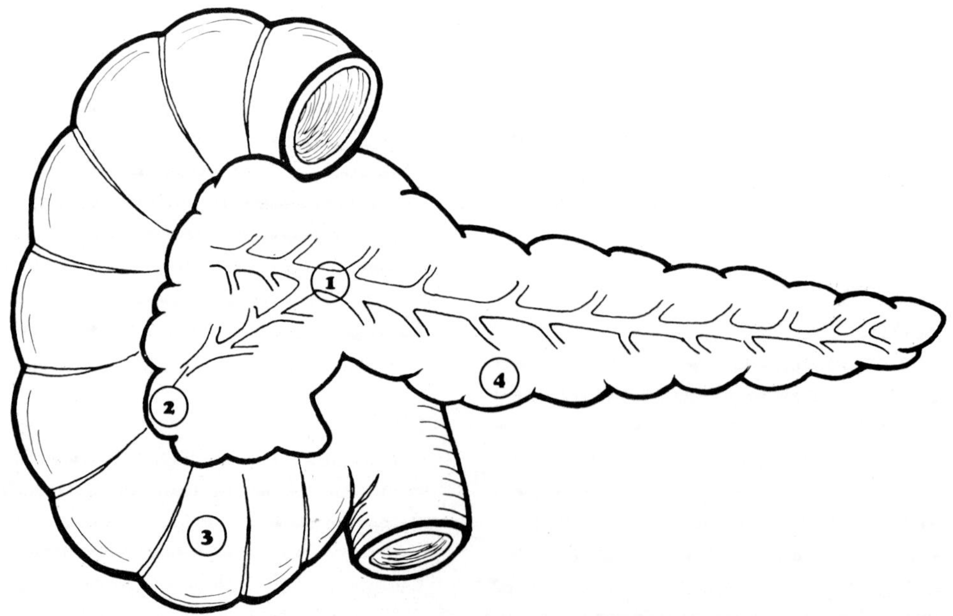

FIG. 7-2 The pancreatic gland is divided into four areas: head, uncinate process (neck), body, and tail. Accessory pancreatic duct, *1;* main pancreatic duct, *2;* duodenum, *3;* pancreas, *4*.

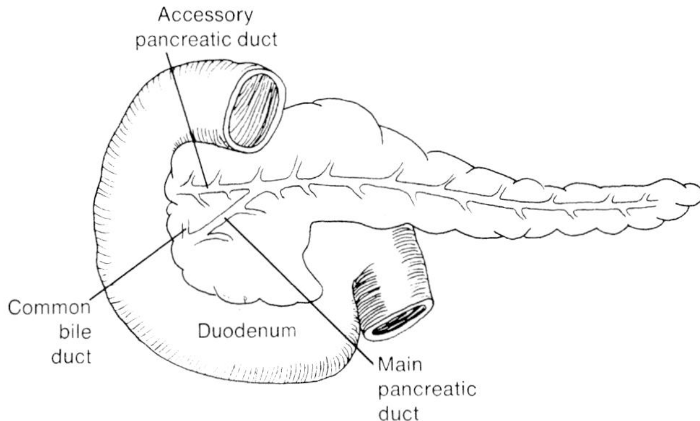

FIG. 7-3 The duct of Wirsung is the main pancreatic duct that extends the entire length of the gland. It receives tributaries from lobules at right angles and enters the medial second part of the duodenum with the common bile duct at the ampulla of Vater. The duct of Santorini is an accessory pancreatic duct that drains the upper anterior head of the gland.

Pancreatic Duct

Two ducts are seen in the pancreas, the duct of Wirsung and the duct of Santorini. To aid in the transport of pancreatic fluid, the ducts have smooth muscle surrounding them. The duct of Wirsung is a primary duct extending the entire length of the gland (Fig. 7-3). It receives tributaries from lobules at right angles and enters the medial second part of the duodenum with the common bile duct at the ampulla of Vater (guarded by the sphincter of Oddi). The duct of Santorini is a secondary duct that drains the upper anterior head. It enters the duodenum at the minor papilla about 2 cm proximal to the ampulla of Vater.

The sonographer has an easier time seeing the pancreatic duct as it courses through the midline of the body of the gland. It appears as an echogenic line or lucency bordered by two echogenic lines. The ducts should measure under 2 mm, with tapering as they reach the tail. Color Doppler may help distinguish the dilated pancreatic duct from the vascular structures in the area.

Blood Supply

The blood supply is from the splenic artery, gastroduodenal artery, and superior mesenteric artery. Venous drainage is through tributaries of the splenic and superior mesenteric veins (Fig. 7-4).

VASCULAR AND DUCTAL LANDMARKS TO THE PANCREAS

Portal Vein and Tributaries

The main portal vein is formed behind the neck of the pancreas by the junction of the superior mesenteric vein and splenic vein. The splenic vein runs from the splenic hilum along the posterosuperior aspect of the pancreas. The superior mesenteric vein runs posterior to the lower neck of the pancreas and anterior to the uncinate process.

Splenic Artery

The splenic artery arises from the celiac artery and runs along the superior margin of the gland, slightly anterior and superior, to follow the splenic vein.

Common Hepatic Artery

The common hepatic artery arises from the celiac artery and courses along the superior margin of the first portion of the duodenum to divide into the proper hepatic artery and gastroduodenal artery, usually when it crosses onto the front of the portal vein. In some patients the right hepatic artery arises from the superior mesenteric artery and courses posterior to the medial portion of the splenic vein.

Gastroduodenal Artery

The gastroduodenal artery is seen in a small percentage of patients as it travels a short distance along the anterior aspect of the head just to the right of the neck before it divides into the superior pancreaticoduodenal branches; they join with the inferior pancreaticoduodenal branches, which arise from the superior mesenteric artery.

Superior Mesenteric Artery

The superior mesenteric artery arises from the aorta behind the lower portion of the body and courses anterior to the third portion of the duodenum to enter the small bowel mesentery.

Common Bile Duct

The common bile duct crosses the anterior aspect of the portal vein to the right of the proper hepatic artery. The portal vein is found anterior to the inferior vena cava. The duct passes along the anterior border of the portal vein and travels posterior to the first portion of the duodenum to course inferior and somewhat posterior in the parenchyma of the head of the pancreas. It joins the pancreatic duct close to the ampulla of Vater.

PHYSIOLOGY

The pancreas is both an exocrine and an endocrine gland. Its exocrine function is to produce pancreatic juice, which enters the duodenum together with bile. The exocrine secretions of the pancreas and those of the liver, which are delivered into the duodenum through duct systems, are essential for normal intestinal digestion and absorption of food. Pancreatic secretion is under the control of the vagus nerve and two hormonal agents, secretin and pancreozymin, that are released when food enters the duodenum. The endocrine function is to produce the hormone insulin. Failure of the pancreas to furnish sufficient insulin leads to diabetes mellitus.

The enzymes of the pancreatic juice are lipase, amylase, carboxypeptidase, trypsin, and chymotrypsin. The last three are secreted as inactive enzyme precursors to be activated

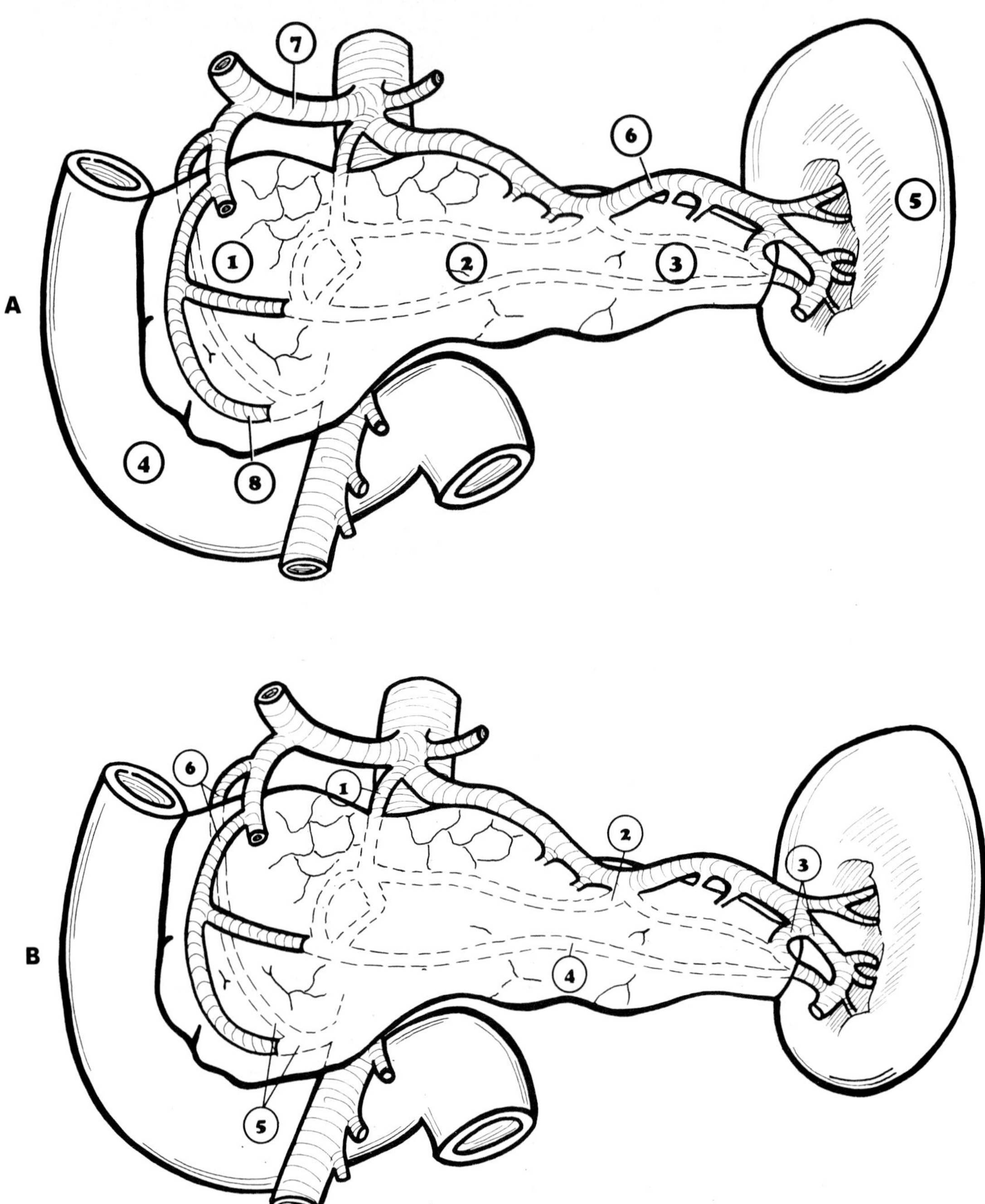

FIG. 7-4 A, Arterial supply surrounding the pancreas. Head of the pancreas, *1;* body, *2;* tail, *3;* duodenum, *4;* spleen, *5;* splenic artery, *6;* hepatic artery, *7;* gastroduodenal artery, *8.* **B,** Pancreas and its main arterial supply. Dorsal pancreatic artery, *1;* great pancreatic artery, *2;* caudal pancreatic artery, *3;* inferior pancreatic artery, *4;* posterior and anterior inferior pancreaticoduodenal arteries, *5;* posterior and anterior superior pancreaticoduodenal arteries, *6.* (From Hagen-Ansert SL: The anatomy workbook, Philadelphia, 1986, JB Lippincott.)

when they have entered the duodenum. The pancreas contains acinar cells, exocrine secretory cells that are arranged in saclike clusters (acini) connected by small intercalated ducts to larger excretory ducts. The excretory ducts converge into one or two main ducts, which deliver the exocrine secretion of the pancreas into the duodenum.

Pancreatic juice is the most versatile and active of the digestive secretions. Its enzymes are capable of nearly completing the digestion of food in the absence of all other digestive secretions. Because the digestive enzymes that are secreted into the lumen of the small intestine require an almost neutral pH for best activity, the acidity of the contents entering the duodenum must be reduced. Thus the pancreatic juice contains a relatively high concentration of sodium bicarbonate, and this alkaline salt is largely responsible for the neutralization of gastric acid.

The nervous secretion of pancreatic juice is thick and rich in enzymes and proteins. The chemical secretion, resulting from pancreozymin activity, also is thick, watery, and rich in enzymes. Pancreatic juice is alkaline and becomes more so with increasing rates of secretion. This is because of a simultaneous increase in bicarbonates and decrease in chloride concentration.

The proteolytic enzyme trypsin may hydrolyze protein molecules to polypeptides. Chymotrypsinogen is activated by trypsin. Amylase causes hydrolysis of starch with the production of maltose, which is further hydrolyzed to glucose. Lipase is capable of hydrolyzing some fats to monoglycerides and some to glycerol and fatty acids. Although lipases are also secreted by the small intestine, what is secreted by the pancreas accounts for 80% of all fat digestion. Thus impaired fat digestion is an important indicator of pancreatic dysfunction.

LABORATORY TESTS

Amylase is a digestive enzyme for carbohydrates. It is secreted by the pancreas, parotid glands, gynecologic system, and bowel. Lipase is excreted specifically by the pancreas and parallels the elevation in amylase levels.

Amylase

In certain types of pancreatic disease the digestive enzymes of the pancreas escape into the surrounding tissue, producing necrosis with severe pain and inflammation. Under these circumstances there is an increase in serum amylase. A serum amylase level of twice normal usually indicates acute pancreatitis. In chronic pancreatitis the serum amylase is not elevated. Other conditions that may cause an increase in amylase are mumps, ischemic bowel disease, and pelvic inflammatory disease.

Lipase

The lipase test is performed to assess damage to the pancreas. Lipase is secreted by the pancreas, and small amounts pass into the blood. The lipase level rises in acute pancreatitis and in carcinoma of the pancreas. Both amylase and lipase rise at the same rate, but the elevation in lipase concentration persists for a longer period.

Glucose

The glucose tolerance test is performed to discover whether there is a disorder of glucose metabolism. An increased blood glucose level is found in severe diabetes, chronic liver disease, and overactivity of several of the endocrine glands. There may be a decreased blood sugar level in tumors of the islets of Langerhans in the pancreas.

NORMAL PANCREATIC TEXTURE

The echogenicity of the pancreas is discussed in terms of how it relates to the liver's homogeneous soft echo pattern. The normal pancreas has an echo pattern that is homogeneous and finer in texture than that of the surrounding retroperitoneum. The echo intensity of the pancreas is usually slightly less than that of surrounding soft tissues and slightly greater than that of the liver.

The parenchymal texture of the pancreas depends on the amount of fat between the lobules, and to a lesser extent on the interlobular fibrous tissue. The internal echoes of pancreas consist of closely spaced elements of the same intensity with uniform distribution throughout the gland.

Filly and London note that retroperitoneal fat is strongly echogenic and that extensive fatty infiltrations of the pancreas are difficult to visualize by ultrasound because the pancreas blends in with the surrounding retroperitoneal fat. A lesser degree of fatty infiltration may not render the pancreas invisible but may raise the amplitude of returning pancreatic echoes, resulting in the clinical observation that the pancreas returns stronger echoes than the liver.[1]

Marks et al. investigated the echogenicity of the gland, observing that a higher-amplitude echogenicity from the pancreas is the result of more than fat infiltration alone. Fibrous tissue may account for the portion of increased echogenicity.[4]

SONOGRAPHIC TECHNIQUES FOR THE PANCREAS

The pancreas is one of the most difficult of all abdominal organs to image with ultrasound. To help visualize the pancreas the patient should fast 6 to 8 hours, since this promotes dilation of the gallbladder and ducts and ensures an empty stomach. Real time visualization of peristalsis and movement within the duodenum and the stomach can be useful to help outline the head, body, and tail of the pancreas.

Ultrasound techniques may vary. For adult patients, use a 3- to 5-MHz transducer with a midfocal zone; for pediatric patients, use a 5- to 7.5-MHz transducer.

Ultrasound Scan Technique

The patient is usually examined in the supine, RAO or LAO, or upright positions (Fig. 7-5). The sonographer should identify the head, neck, body, and tail in the supine, longitudinal, and transverse planes. They should evaluate the shape, contour, lie, and texture (compare with liver parenchyma). The coronal scans may improve visualization of the pancreas and peripancreatic region. The following surrounding structures should be identified: superior mesenteric artery and vein, portal and splenic vein, aorta and

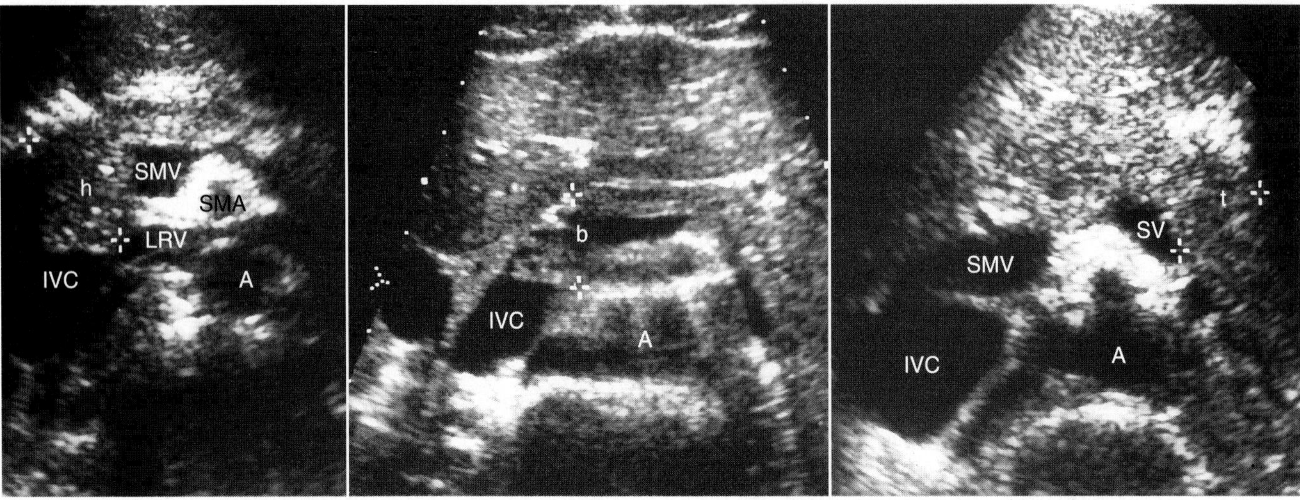

FIG. 7-5 The normal transverse scan of the pancreas showing the head, *h;* body, *b;* and tail, *t,* of the gland. The vascular structures are used as landmarks to identify the gland. Aorta, *A;* inferior vena cava, *IVC;* superior mesenteric artery *SMA;* superior mesenteric vein, *SMV;* left renal vein, *LRV;* splenic vein, *SV.*

inferior vena cava, common bile duct, gastroduodenal artery, left renal vein, duodenal bulb, posterior wall of the stomach, and the pancreatic duct.

Windows for Visualization. Difficulties in visualization of the pancreas may result from bowel gas, a transverse stomach obscuring the anatomy, or a small left lobe of the liver (Fig. 7-6). A left lobe measuring 2 to 2.5 cm makes an excellent sonic window for imaging the pancreatic area. This view can be used with a slight caudal angle of the transducer (15 to 20 degrees).

If the sonographer is unable to image the pancreas, the water ingestion technique may be effective as a window to image the gland (Fig. 7-7). The initial scans of the biliary system should be made before asking the patient to drink 32 to 300 ml of fluids through a straw in the erect or left lateral decubitus position. In the upright position, use the stomach as a window; if the patient is unable to sit up, the exam can be done in the decubitus position. This method fills the body and antrum of the stomach initially to help outline the body and tail of the pancreas. The fluid then fills the duodenal cap to outline the lateral margin of the head of the pancreas. The upright position allows the air to move from the gastric antrum to the fundus of the stomach and causes the upper viscera to move downward for a better sonic window. The upright position also results in distention of the venous structures, which further aids in the localization of the pancreas.

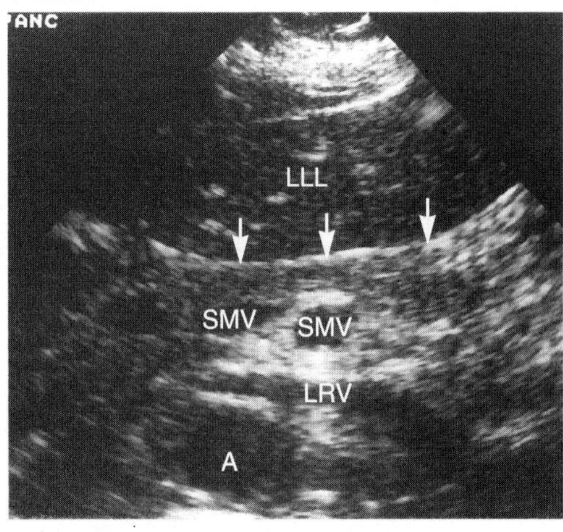

FIG. 7-6 Transverse scan of the left lobe of liver, *LLL.* If the left lobe measures at least 2 to 3 cm, it may serve as an ideal window to visualize the pancreas posterior *(arrows).* Aorta, *A;* left renal vein, *LRV;* superior mesenteric vein, *SMV;* superior mesenteric artery, *SMA.*

Transverse Scans. Generally the pancreas is imaged first in the transverse plane. The patient should be in full inspiration to distend the venous structures that serve as landmarks to visualize the pancreas. The sonographer should use the left lobe of the liver and angle the transducer slightly toward the feet to image the aorta and celiac axis. This is the superior border of the pancreas. Often the splenic artery may be seen arising from the celiac axis and demarcating the superior border of the pancreas (Figs. 7-8 and 7-9). The body and tail of the gland should be imaged as the transducer is slowly angled inferiorly from the celiac axis. Visualization of the superior mesenteric vessels, left renal vein, and inferior vena cava also helps delineate the borders of the pancreas (Figs. 7-10 to 7-12). The stomach may be seen as the walls are collapsed because it lies anterior to the pancreas (Fig. 7-13). The duodenum, gastroduodenal artery, and common bile duct are useful landmarks in identifying the head of the gland (Fig. 7-14). The sonographer may watch for peristalsis or fluid to pass through

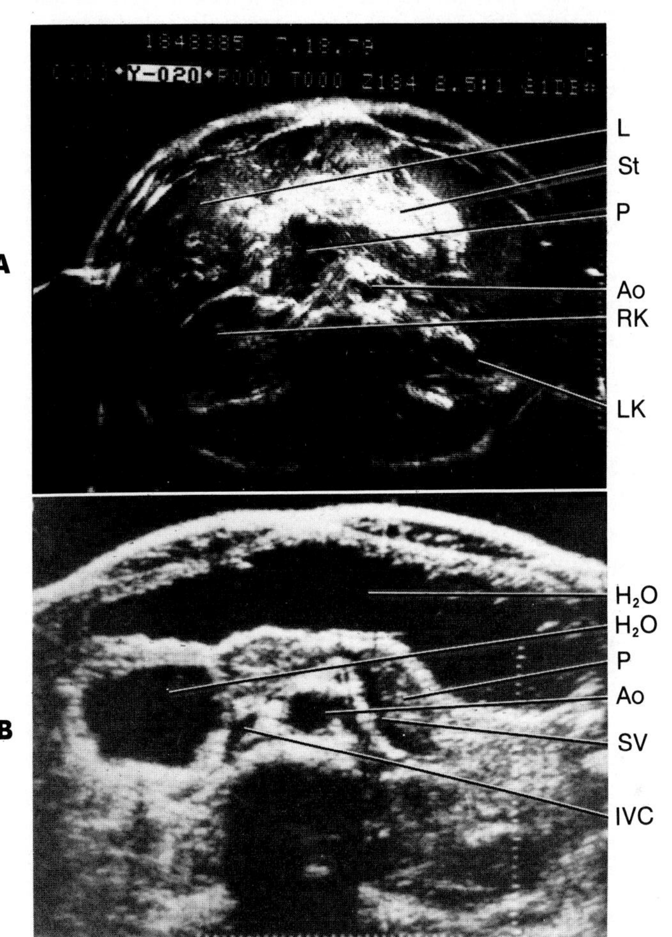

FIG. 7-7 A, The stomach, *St,* can serve as an acoustic impediment or an acoustic enhancement if the patient is properly hydrated. This transverse scan shows the collapsed walls of a stomach that has just enough fluid within to permit adequate visualization of the posterior pancreas. **B,** This scan shows an extremely distended stomach, which helps to visualize the pancreas and prevertebral vessels posterior to its border. Water, H_2O; pancreas, *P;* aorta, *Ao;* inferior vena cava, *IVC;* splenic vein, *SV,* liver, *L;* left kidney, *LK;* right kidney, *RK.* (Courtesy John Deitz, Philadelphia, Penn.)

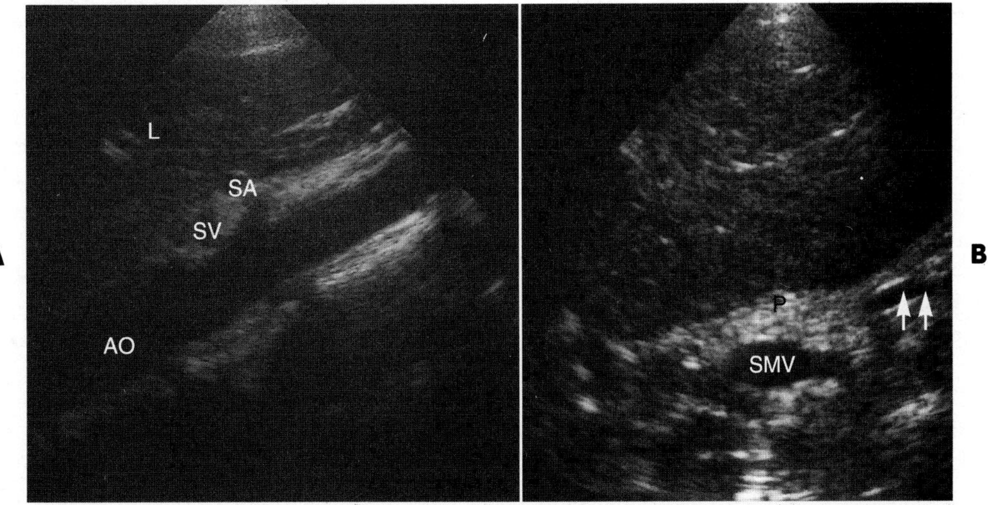

FIG. 7-8 A, Longitudinal. **B,** Transverse. The splenic artery demarcates the superior border of the body and tail of the pancreas. This vessel is usually quite tortuous and may be seen to course throughout the upper part of the pancreatic gland. Pancreas, *P;* superior mesenteric vein, *SMV;* splenic artery *(arrows).*

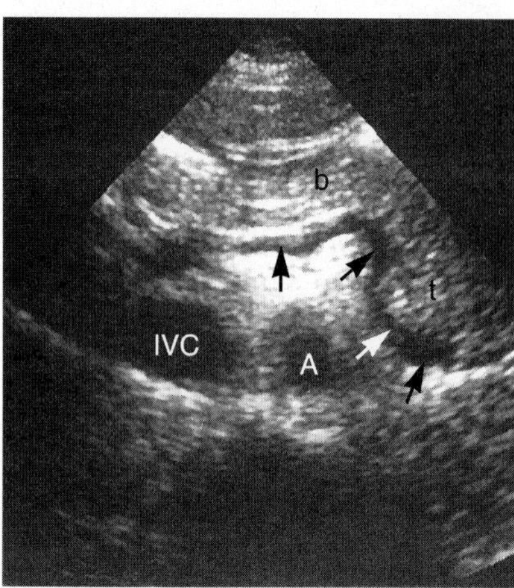

FIG. 7-9 Transverse scan of the tortuous splenic artery in this patient demarcates the posterior border of the tail and body of the pancreas. Aorta, *A;* inferior vena cava, *IVC;* splenic artery *(arrows),* body, *b,* tail, *t.*

the second part of the duodenum as it forms the lateral border of the head of the gland.

Sagittal. The initial scan should be made slightly to the right of midline with the patient in full inspiration. The dilated inferior vena cava is seen as the posterior border (Fig. 7-15). The main portal vein, or right branch of the portal vein, is the next landmark seen anterior to the cava. The pancreas lies just inferior to the portal vein, and anterior to the inferior vena cava. As the pancreas enlarges, a slight indentation is apparent on the anterior border of the cava. This view is also good to image the common bile duct, since it lies anterior to the portal vein before dropping posterior to enter the head of the pancreas (Fig. 7-16). The hepatic artery is sometimes visible as a circular tube when the common duct is seen (Fig. 7-17). The use of color Doppler may help the sonographer separate the hepatic artery from the common duct. Subsequent scans are made slightly to the left of midline to image the aorta and superior mesenteric artery and vein, since they form the posterior border of the body of the pancreas. The superior mesenteric vein flows cephalad to join the portal vein and may be seen as a long, tubular structure posterior to the neck of the pancreas and anterior to the uncinate process (Fig. 7-18). The tail of the pancreas is more difficult to see, but as the sonographer angles slightly to the left of the aorta, the tail may be imaged.

The antrum of the stomach appears as a collapsed bull's-eye and may be identified anterior and slightly caudal to the body of the pancreas. The splenic vein is a circular sonolucent structure posterior to the cephalic portion of the gland. The left renal vein is a slitlike sonolucency between the aorta and the superior mesenteric artery.

Pancreatic Duct. The pancreatic duct may be imaged on transverse scans because it courses through the body of the gland (Fig. 7-19). The sonographer should identify pancreatic tissue on both sides of the duct so as not to confuse it with vascular structures that may lie near it. The splenic vein is usually too posterior and the hepatic artery too anterior to be confused with the duct. Color Doppler may be used to help distinguish a dilated duct from vascular structures. The duct appears as an echo-free area sharply marginated by two parallel echogenic lines. A thin strip of retroperitoneal fat may underlie the anterior aspect of the pancreas. This sonolucent linear pattern should not be mistaken for duct. On transverse scans the posterior wall of the antrum can be seen overlying the pancreas. Care should be taken to distinguish the antrum of the collapsed stomach from the small pancreatic duct.

CLINICAL SIGNS AND PATHOLOGIC CONDITIONS OF THE PANCREAS

Congenital Abnormalities

Congenital abnormalities of the pancreas are uncommon. The following abnormalities are presented: ectopic pancreatic tissue, annular pancreas, fibrocystic disease, and congenital cysts.

Ectopic Pancreatic Tissue. Ectopic pancreatic tissue is the most common pancreatic anomaly, usually in the form of intramural nodules. The ectopic tissue may be found in various places in the gastrointestinal tract. Frequent sites are the stomach, duodenum, small bowel, and large bowel. On palpation these lesions may seem polypoid, and they characteristically have a central dimple. They are composed of elements of the pancreas, usually the acinar and ductal structures and less frequently the islets of Langerhans. They are generally small (0.5 to 2 cm), and acute pancreatitis or tumor may occur in them.

Annular Pancreas. Annular pancreas is a rare anomaly in which the head of the pancreas surrounds the second portion of the duodenum. It is more common in males than in females, and all grades (from an overlapping of the posterior duodenal wall to a complete ring) may be found. It may be associated with complete or partial atresia of the duodenum and is susceptible to any of the diseases of the pancreas.

Fibrocystic Disease of the Pancreas. Fibrocystic disease of the pancreas is a hereditary disorder of the exocrine glands seen frequently in children and young adults. The pancreas is usually firm and of normal size. Cysts are very small but may be present in the advanced stages. The acini and ducts are dilated. The acini are usually atrophic and may be totally replaced by fibrous tissue in many of the lobules. Nausea and vomiting may also occur, leading to malnourishment. The pancreatic secretion is gradually lost. With advancing pancreatic fibrosis, jaundice may develop from the common duct obstruction. A late manifestation is diabetes. Grossly the pancreas is found to be somewhat nodular and firm. There may be edema and fat necrosis, but gradually fibrous replacement occurs in much of the parenchyma. The duct may enlarge and contain calculi.

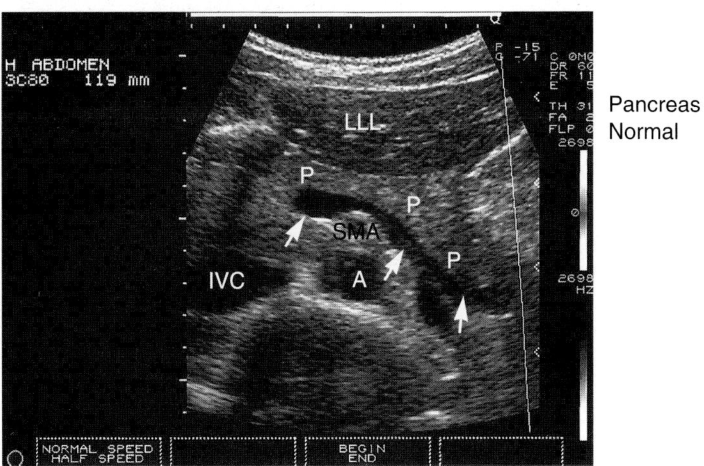

FIG. 7-10 Transverse scan of the normal pancreas and its vascular landmarks. Aorta, *A;* inferior vena cava, *IVC;* superior mesenteric artery, *SMA;* splenic vein *(arrows);* pancreas, *P;* left lobe liver, *LLL.*

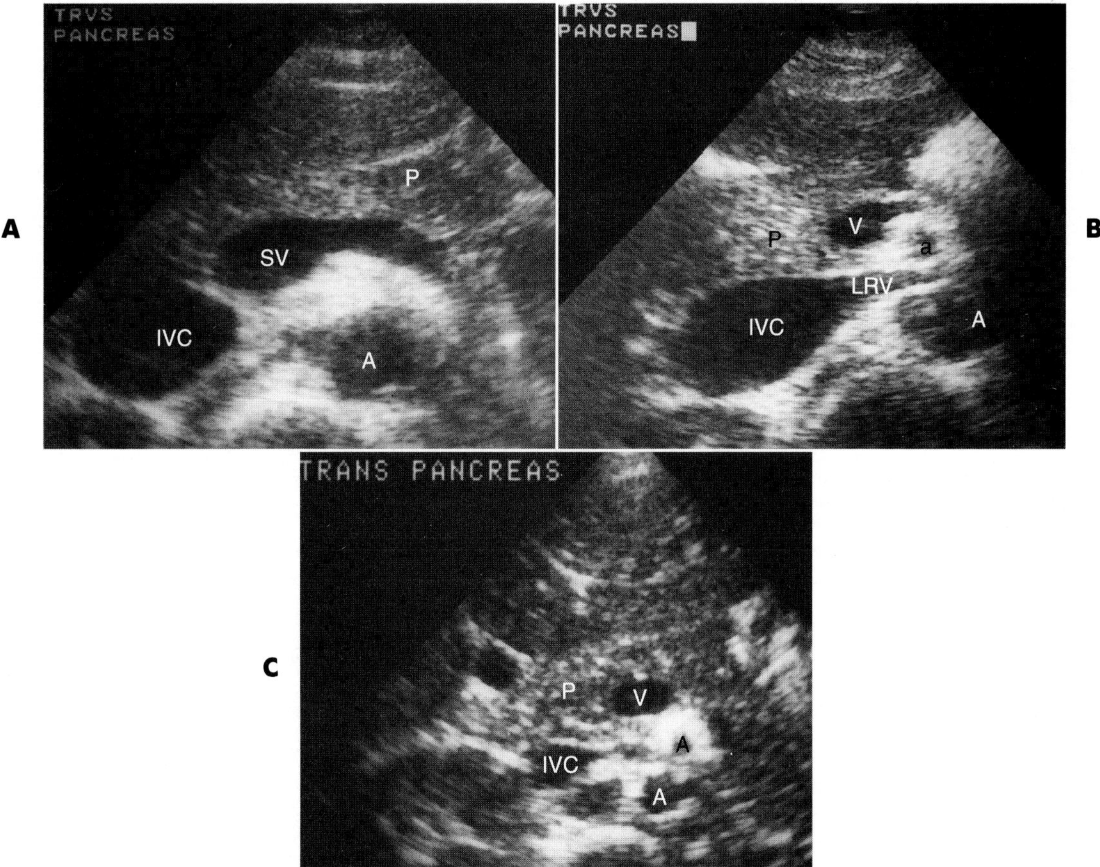

FIG. 7-11 Transverse scans of variations in vascular anatomy and the pancreas. **A,** The splenic vein, *sv,* is considered the posterior medial border of the pancreas, *P,* the aorta, *A,* and inferior vena cava, *IVC,* are posterior. **B,** The left renal vein is shown as it crosses anterior to the aorta, *A,* and posterior to the superior mesenteric artery, *a,* to enter the lateral wall of the inferior vena cava, *IVC.* The superior mesenteric vein, *v,* lies posterior to the body of the pancreas, *P,* and anterior to the uncinate process of the gland. **C,** Transverse scan of the aorta, *A,* inferior vena cava, *IVC,* superior mesenteric artery, *a,* superior mesenteric vein, *v,* and pancreas, *P.*

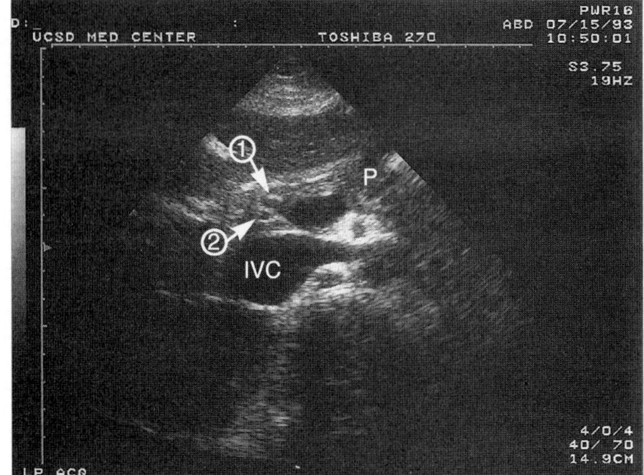

FIG. 7-12 Transverse scan of the head of the pancreas, *P*. The gastroduodenal artery, *1*, is the anterolateral border, the common bile duct, *2*, the posterior border. The air-filled duodenum is the far lateral border of the gland. Inferior vena cava, *IVC*.

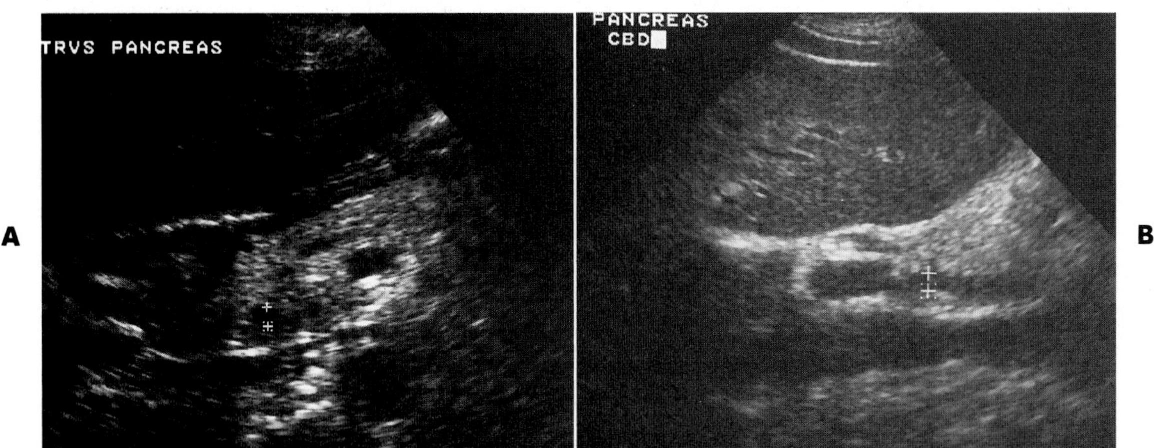

FIG. 7-13 A, Transverse. **B,** Longitudinal. The common bile duct courses along the posterior margin of the pancreatic head before it joins with the main pancreatic duct to empty into the duodenum. The normal common duct should measure under 6 mm if the patient is under 60 years old.

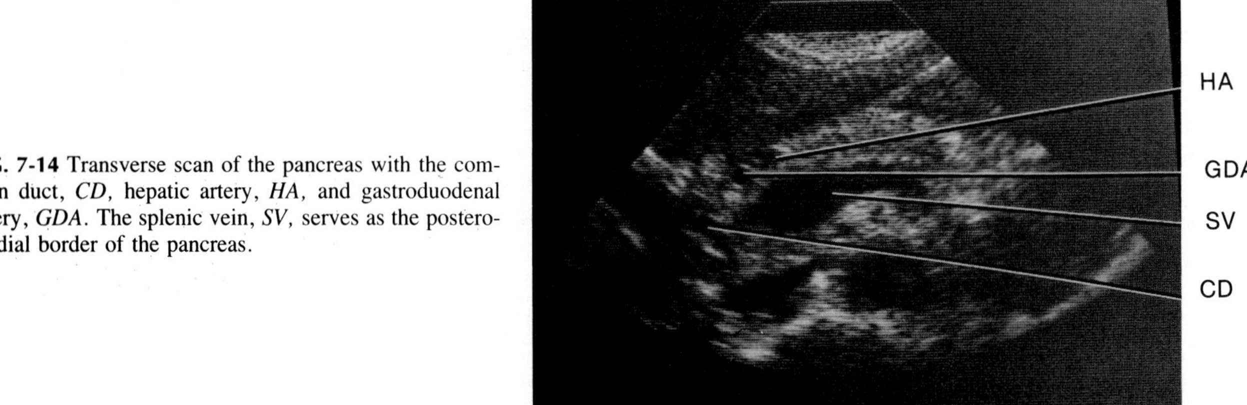

FIG. 7-14 Transverse scan of the pancreas with the common duct, *CD*, hepatic artery, *HA*, and gastroduodenal artery, *GDA*. The splenic vein, *SV*, serves as the posteromedial border of the pancreas.

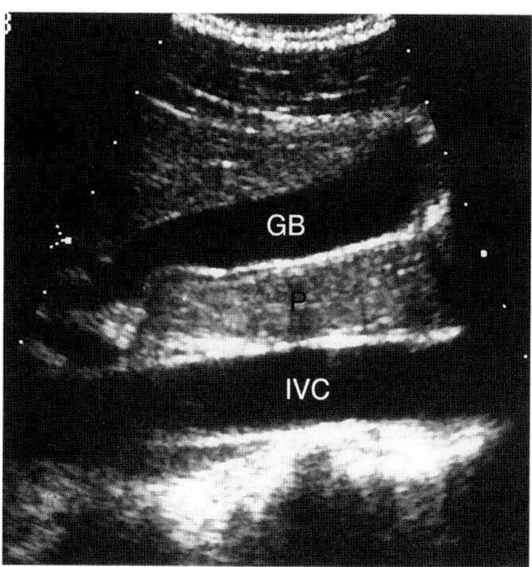

FIG. 7-15 Sagittal oblique scan of the dilated inferior vena cava, *IVC,* as it demarcates the posterior border of the pancreas, *P*. The gallbladder, *GB,* is seen anterior.

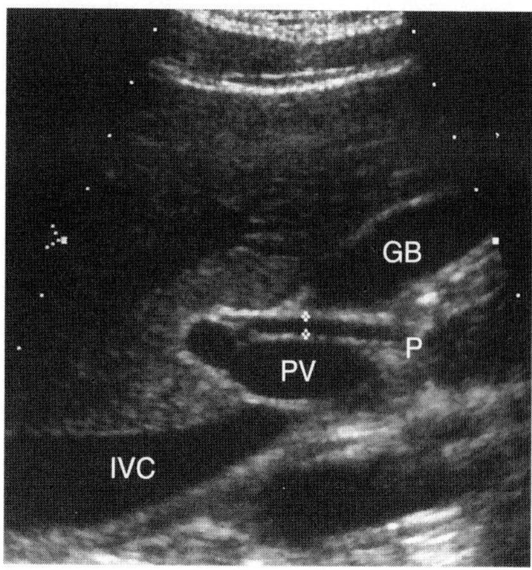

FIG. 7-16 On the sagittal scan, the patient should be in full inspiration to dilate the venous structures. The pancreas, *P,* is seen anterior to the inferior vena cava, *IVC,* and inferior to the portal vein, *PV*. The common bile duct *(cross-marks)* lies anterior to the portal vein before dipping posterior to enter the pancreas. Gallbladder, *GB*.

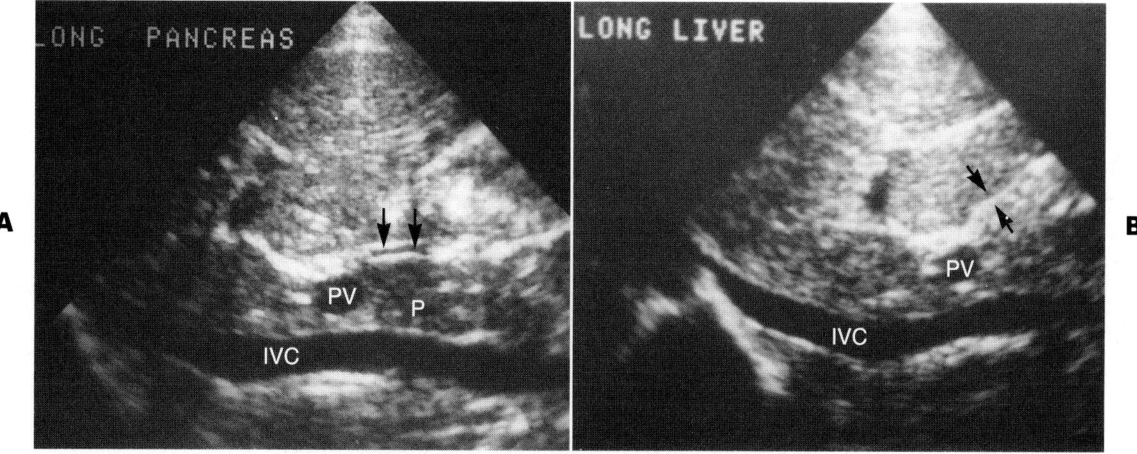

FIG. 7-17 A, On sagittal scans, the hepatic artery *(arrows)* can be seen as a small pulsatile structure that runs along the anterior border of the pancreas, *P*. Color flow may help to distinguish this vessel from other structures in the abdomen. **B,** The stomach may be seen in various phases of filling and peristalsis. The arrows demarcate the collapsed walls of the stomach.

Congenital Cysts. Congenital cysts of the pancreas result from anomalous development of the pancreatic ducts. They are usually multiple and range from small to 3 to 5 cm in size.

Acute Pancreatitis

An acute attack of pancreatitis is related to biliary tract disease and alcoholism. The most common cause of pancreatitis in the United States is biliary tract disease. Gallstones are present in 40% to 60% of patients, and 5% of patients with gallstones present with acute pancreatitis. Gallstone pancreatitis causes a relatively sudden onset of constant biliary pain. As the pancreatic parenchyma is further damaged, the pain becomes more severe and the abdomen becomes rigid and tender.

Alcohol abuse is the second most common cause of pancreatitis. Other causes include trauma, inflammation from adjacent peptic ulcer or abdominal infection, vascular thrombosis and embolism, and drugs.

The laboratory analysis of pancreatic enzymes (protease, lipase, and elastase) are keys to pancreatic destruction. The following are morphologic changes in acute pancreatitis:

1. Proteolytic destruction of pancreatic substance
2. Necrosis of blood vessels with subsequent hemorrhage
3. Necrosis of fat by lipolytic enzymes
4. Accompanying inflammatory reaction

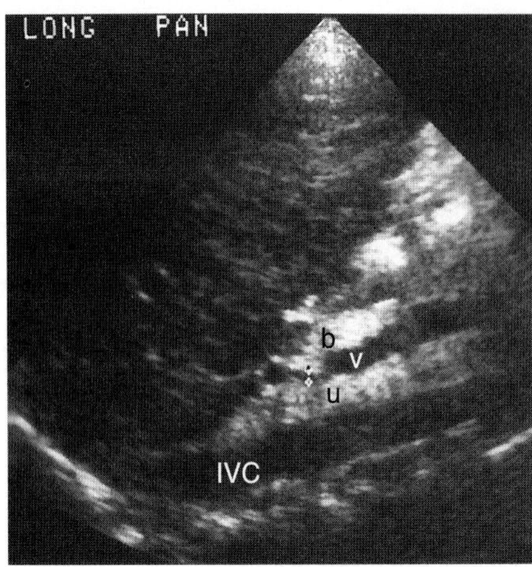

FIG. 7-18 Sagittal scan of the right upper quadrant shows the superior mesenteric vein, *v,* as it flows anterior to the uncinate process, *u,* and posterior to the body, *b,* of the pancreas.

The process may be severe. Damage to the acinar tissue and duct system results in exudation of pancreatic juice into the interstitium of the gland, leakage of secretions into the peripancreatic tissues, or both. After the acini or duct disrupts, the secretions migrate to the surface of the gland. The common course is for fluid to break through the pancreatic connective tissue layer and thin posterior layer of the peritoneum and enter the lesser sac.

The pancreatic juice enters the anterior pararenal space by breaking through the thin layer of the fibrous connective tissue, or the fluid might migrate to the surface of the gland and remain within the confines of the fibrous connective tissue layer.

Collections of fluid in the peripancreatic area generally retain communication with the pancreas. A dynamic equilibrium is established so that fluid is continuously absorbed from the collection and replaced by additional pancreatic secretions. The drainage of juices may cease as the pancreatic inflammatory response subsides and the rate of pancreatic secretions returns to normal. The collections of extrapancreatic fluid should be reabsorbed or, if drained, should not recur with recovery of proper drainage through the duct.

Clinical Signs of Acute Pancreatitis. The patient may present with moderate-to-severe tenderness in the epigastrium radiating to the back. The pain may be persistent. Fever is present, along with leukocytosis. The abdomen may be distended secondary to an ileus. Generally jaundice is not present. The pancreatitis may be localized, associated with biliary disease or trauma, or generalized, associated with alcoholism. The patient may be at risk for abscess and hemorrhage secondary to the pancreatitis.

Clinical Course. The symptoms begin with severe pain that usually occurs after a large meal or alcohol binge. The serum amylase increases within 24 hours and serum lipase increases within 72 to 94 hours.

Other Complications. Patients with acute pancreatitis may go on to develop other complications, such as pseudocyst formation (10%), phlegmon (18%), abscess (1% to 9%), hemorrhage (5%), or duodenal obstruction.

Ultrasound Findings. In the early stages of acute pancreatitis the gland may not show swelling (Figs. 7-20 to 7-22). When swelling does occur the gland is hypoechoic to anechoic and is less echogenic than the liver because of the increased prominence of lobulations and congested vessels. The borders may be somewhat indistinct but smooth. On the longitudinal scan the anterior compression of the inferior vena cava by the swollen head of the pancreas may be apparent.

If localized enlargement is present, it may be difficult to separate from neoplastic involvement of the gland (Fig. 7-23). Analysis of the patient history and laboratory values should enable the clinician to make the distinction.

The pancreatic duct may be obstructed in acute pancreatitis as a result of inflammation, spasm, edema, swelling of the papilla, or pseudocyst formation.[5]

Hemorrhagic Pancreatitis

Hemorrhagic pancreatitis is a rapid progression of acute pancreatitis. In hemorrhagic pancreatitis, there is a diffuse enzymatic destruction of the pancreatic substance caused by a sudden escape of active pancreatic enzymes into the glandular parenchyma. These enzymes cause focal areas of fat necrosis in and about the pancreas, which leads to rupture of the pancreatic vessels and hemorrhage. Nearly half of the patients have sudden necrotizing destruction of pancreas after an alcoholic binge or an excessively large meal.

Clinical Signs. Symptoms may include intense and severe pain radiating to the back, with subsequent shock and ileus. Lab values may show a decreased hemocrit and serum calcium level. Patients may be hypotensive despite volume replacement with metabolic acidosis and adult respiratory distress syndrome.

Ultrasound Findings. Specific ultrasound findings depend on the age of the hemorrhage. A well-defined homogeneous mass in the area of the pancreas may be seen with areas of fresh necrosis (Fig. 7-24). Foci of extravasated blood and fat necrosis are also seen. Further necrosis of the blood vessels results in the development of hemorrhagic areas referred to as Grey Turner's sign (discoloration of the flanks).

At one week the mass may appear cystic with solid elements or septation. After several weeks the hemorrhage may appear cystic.

Phlegmonous Pancreatitis

A phlegmon is a spreading area of diffuse inflammatory edema of soft tissues that may proceed to necrosis and suppuration. Extension outside the gland occurs in 18% to 20% of patients with acute pancreatitis. It appears hypoechoic with good through-transmission. The phlegmon usually involves the lesser sac, left anterior pararenal space, and

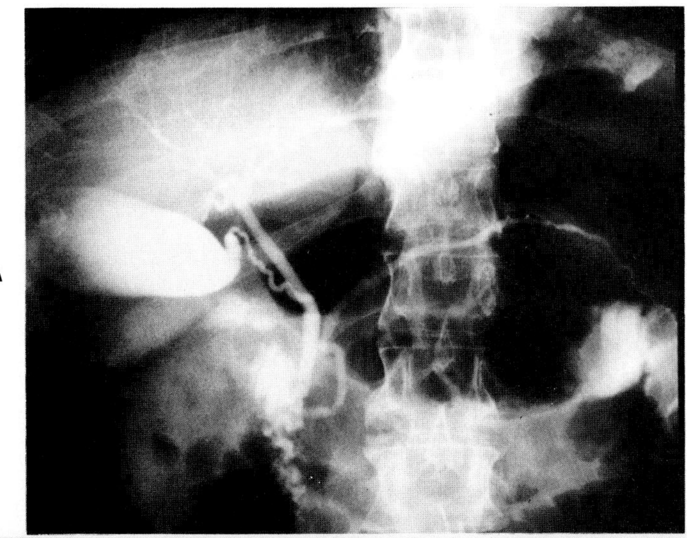

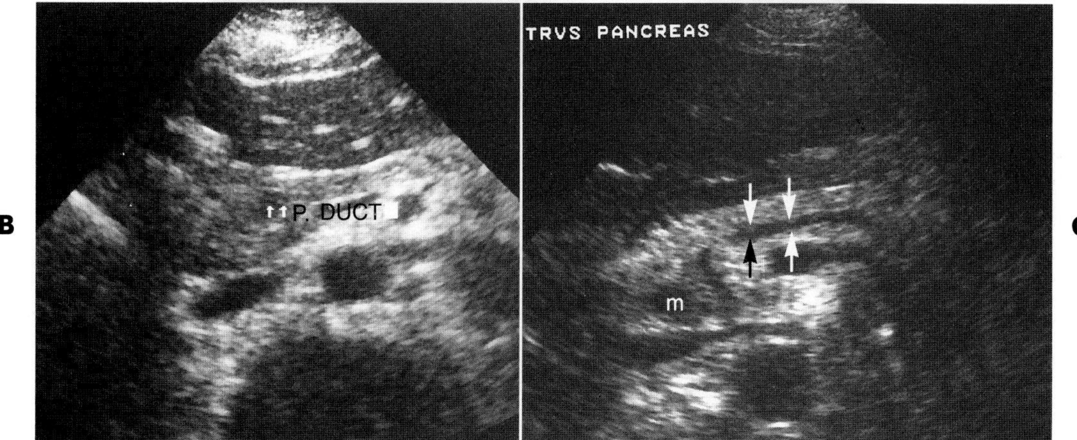

FIG. 7-19 A, Endoscopic retrograde pancreatogram demonstrating the pancreatic duct, common bile duct, and hepatic ducts. **B,** The pancreatic duct may be imaged on transverse scans as it courses through the body of the gland. The normal duct should measure under 2 mm. **C,** The enlarged pancreatic duct is very easy to identify on the transverse scan. This duct measured 3.5 mm and was dilated *(arrows)* secondary to a mass, *m,* in the head of the pancreas.

transverse mesocolon. Less commonly, it involves the small bowel mesentery, lower retroperitoneum, and pelvis.

Acute Pancreatitis in Children

The pediatric pancreas is more easily seen because there is less body fat to interfere with visualization (Fig. 7-25). Often the left lobe of the liver is more prominent and the gland is more isosonic than hyperechoic. In acute pancreatitis the gland is increased in size with a hypoechoic pattern and an indistinct outline. Acute pancreatitis may result from trauma, drugs, infection, or congenital anomalies, or it may be familiar or idiopathic.

Complications of Pancreatitis

Abscess. Pancreatic abscess has a low incidence; the condition is related to the degree of tissue necrosis. The majority of patients develop abscess secondary to pancreatitis that develops from postoperative procedures. A very high mortality rate is associated with this condition if left untreated.

An abscess may arise from a neighboring infection, such as a perforated peptic ulcer, acute appendicitis, or acute cholecystitis.

A pancreatic abscess may be unilocular or multilocular and can spread superiorly into the mediastinum, inferiorly into the transverse mesocolon, or down the retroperitoneum into the pelvis.

Clinical patterns. Patients present with persistent fever and leukocytosis. The patient may have chills, hypotension, and a tender abdomen with a growing mass. It may develop 7 to 14 days after the onset of symptoms to acute necrotizing pancreatitis.

Ultrasound findings. A pancreatic abscess is imaged on ultrasound as a hypoechoic mass with smooth or irregular thick walls, causing few internal echoes; it may be echo-free to echodense. The sonographic appearance depends on

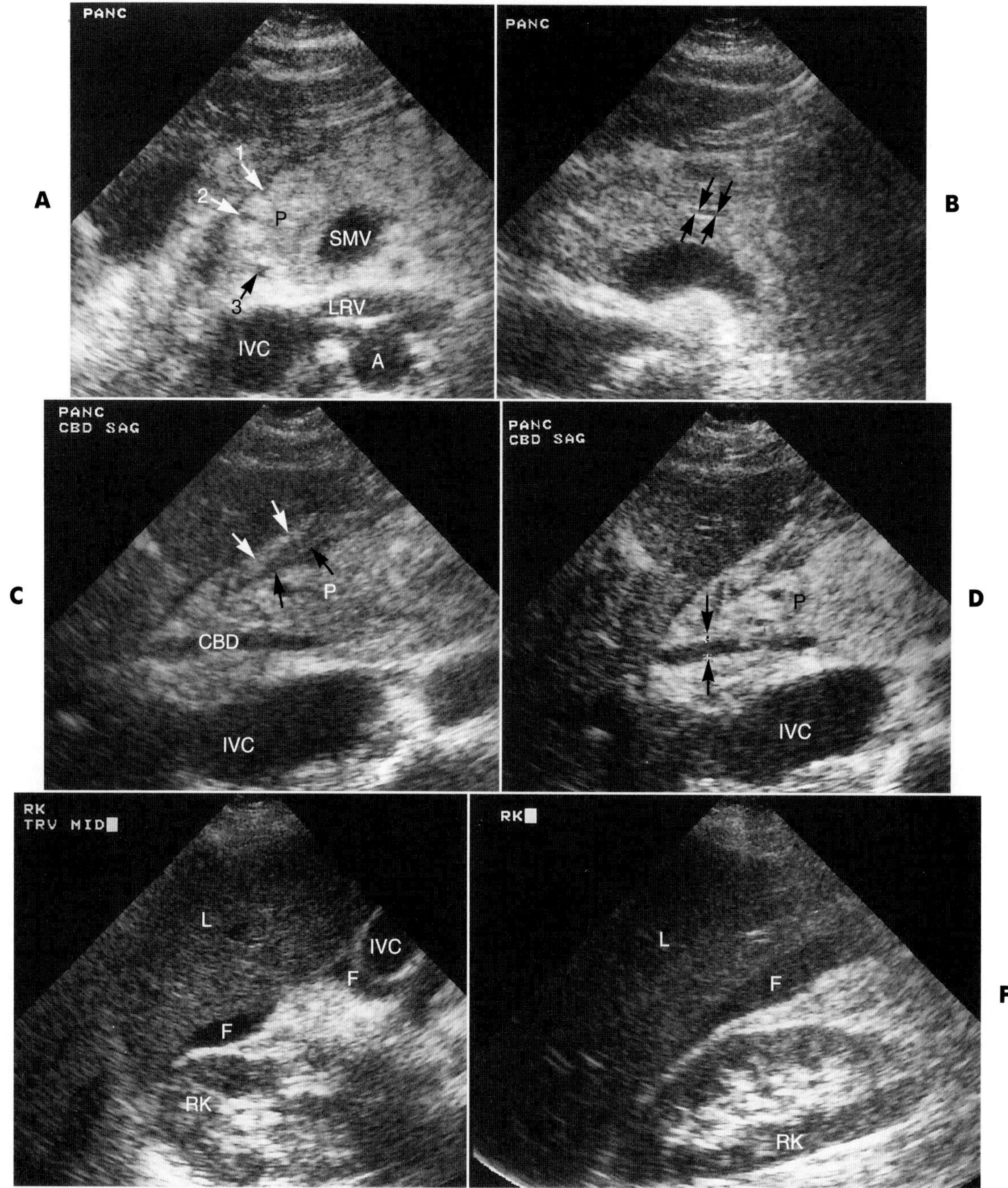

FIG. 7-20 A fifty-year-old female with acute abdominal pain and elevated amylase shows a prominent pancreatic head with increased echogenicity within the head compatible with pancreatitis. The pancreatic duct is mildly dilated, 2.6 mm. **A,** Transverse: aorta, *A;* inferior vena cava, *IVC;* superior mesenteric vein, *SMV;* left renal vein, *LRV;* pancreas, *P;* hepatic artery, *1;* gastroduodenal artery, *2;* common bile duct, *3*. **B,** Transverse scan of the enlarged pancreatic duct *(arrows)*. **C,** Sagittal scan of the collapsed stomach *(arrows);* common bile duct, *CBD;* pancreas, *P;* inferior vena cava, *IVC*. **D,** Sagittal scan of the common bile duct *(arrows)* as it enters the body of the pancreas, *P*. **E** and **F,** A small amount of intraperitoneal fluid is seen within Morison's pouch and around the right kidney. Liver, *L;* right kidney, RK; inferior vena cava, *IVC;* fluid, *f*.

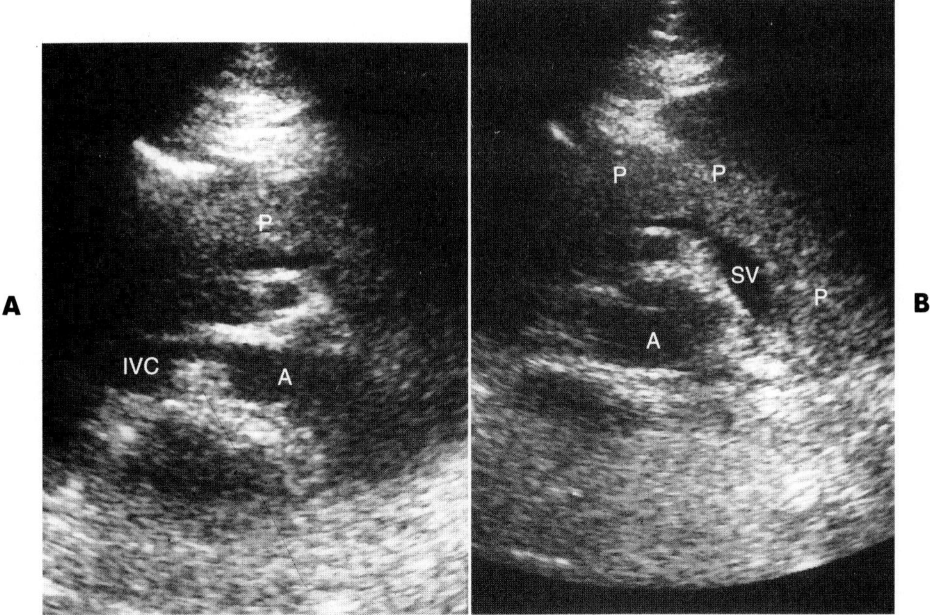

FIG. 7-21 A 45-year-old male presented with midepigastric pain, elevated amylase and lipase, and tenderness. The pancreas is diffusely enlarged representing acute pancreatitis. **A** and **B,** Transverse scans over the upper abdomen show the inflamed pancreatic tissue. Aorta, *A;* inferior vena cava, *IVC;* pancreas, *P;* splenic vein, *SV*.

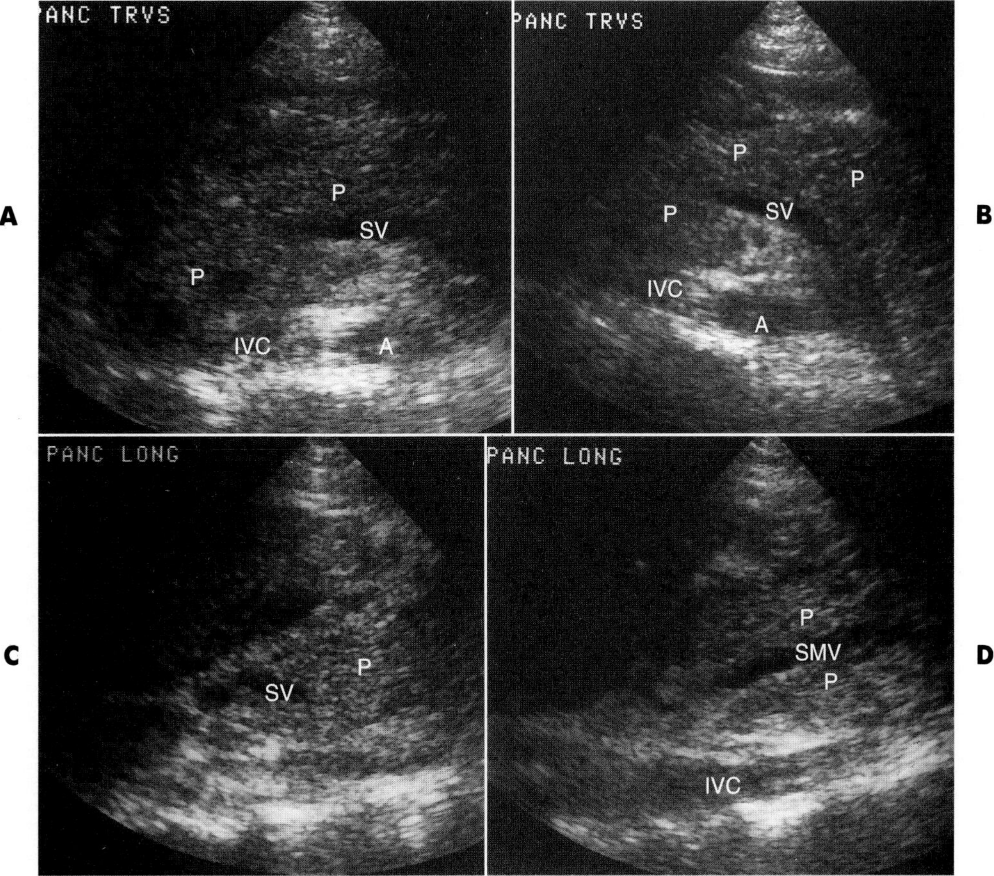

FIG. 7-22 A 29-year-old female presented with back pain, nausea, and vomiting for 1 week, and elevated lipase. The pancreas was found to be diffusely enlarged with decreased echogenicity representing pancreatitis. **A** and **B,** Transverse; aorta, *A;* inferior vena cava, *IVC;* splenic vein, *SV;* pancreas, *P*. **C** and **D,** Sagittal; splenic vein, *SV;* pancreas, *P;* inferior vena cava, *IVC*.

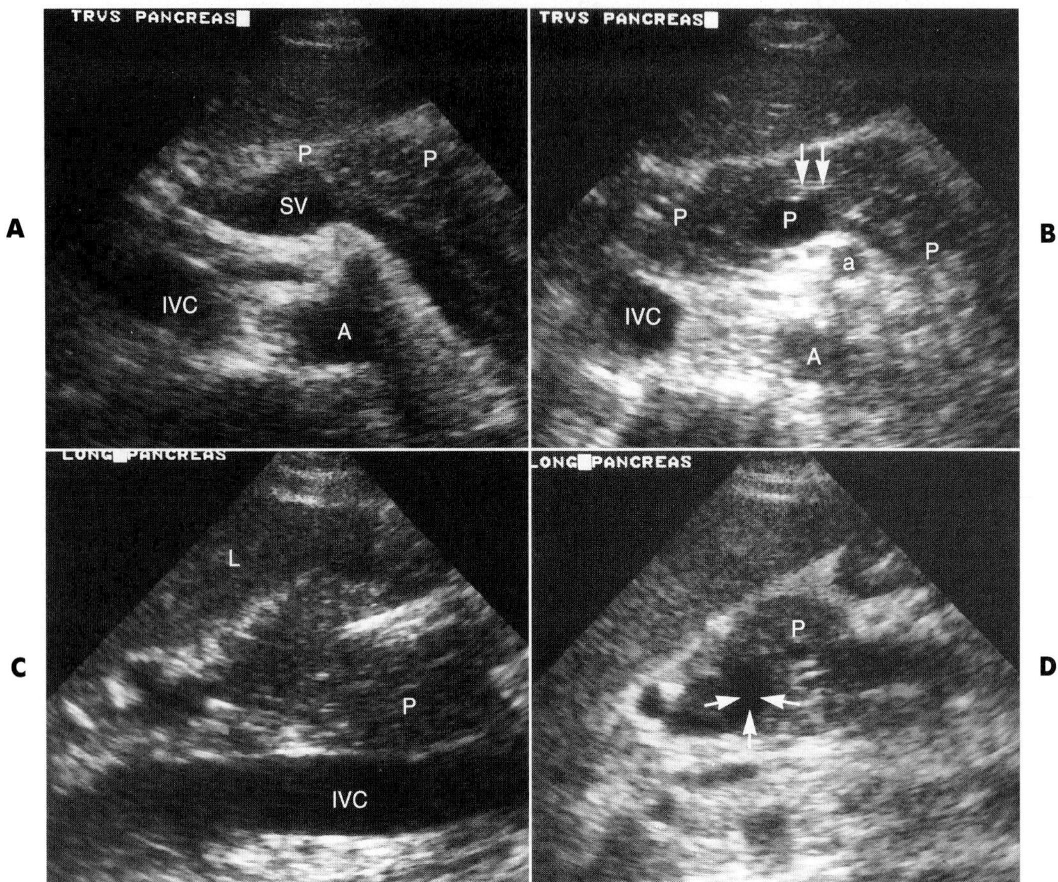

FIG. 7-23 A 37-year-old male patient with AIDS presents with pancreatitis, hepatosplenomegaly, peripancreatic adenopathy, and small polyps in the gallbladder. **A** and **B,** Transverse scans; aorta, *A;* inferior vena cava, *IVC;* splenic vein, *SV;* pancreas, *P;* pancreatic duct, *(arrow);* superior mesenteric artery, *a.* **C** and **D,** Sagittal scans of the enlarged pancreas with the peripancreatic adenopathy *(arrows).* Inferior vena cava, *IVC;* pancreas, *P;* liver, *L.*

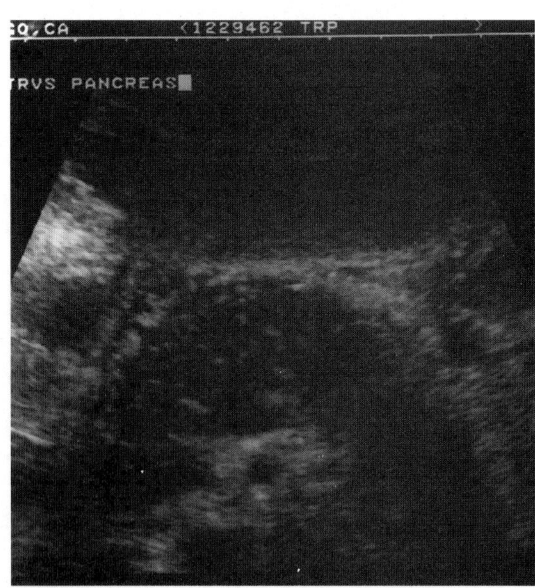

FIG. 7-24 Transverse scan of the right upper quadrant shows an edematous swollen gland. Hemorrhagic pancreatitis would show irregular borders with hemorrhagic areas usually developing in the flank areas known as Grey Turner's sign.

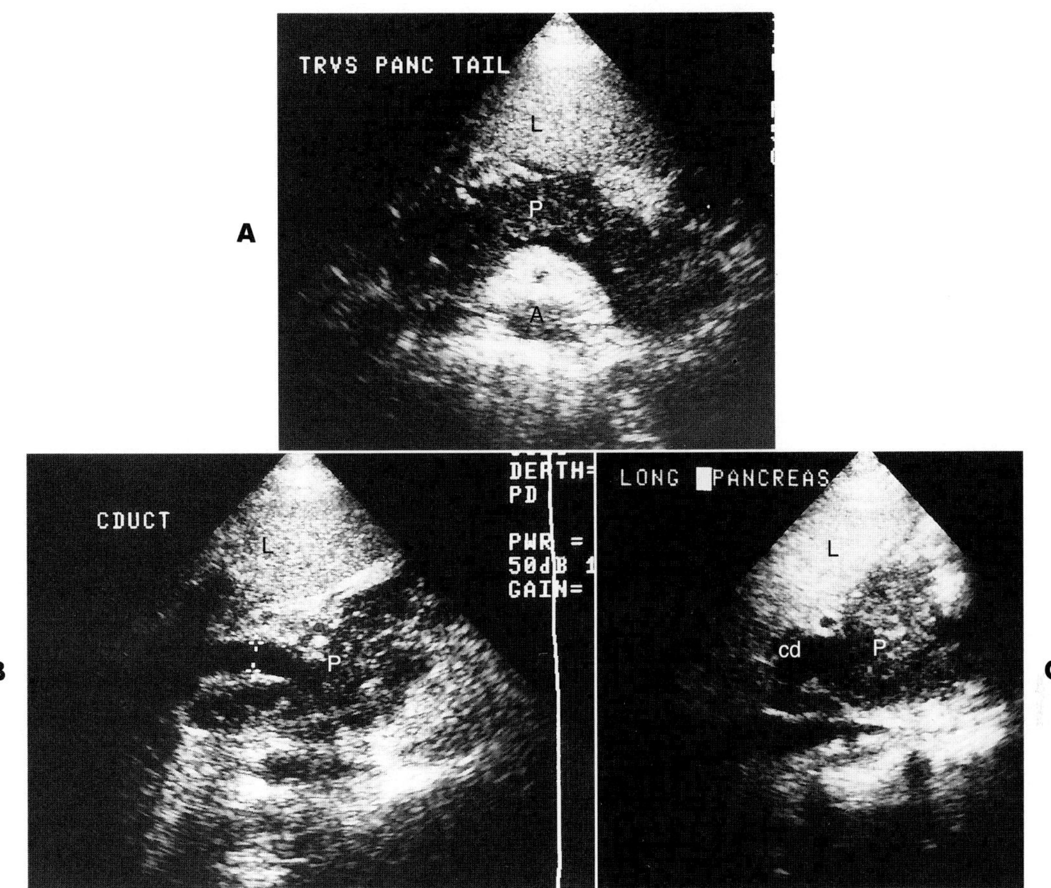

FIG. 7-25 A 9-year-old female with pancreatitis and prominent common bile duct. **A,** Transverse; aorta, *A;* pancreas, *P;* liver, *L.* **B** and **C,** Sagittal; liver, *L;* common bile duct *(cross bars);* pancreas, *P.*

the amount of debris present. If air bubbles are present, an echogenic region with a shadow posterior is imaged.

Chronic Pancreatitis

Chronic pancreatitis results from recurrent attacks of acute pancreatitis and causes continuing destruction of the pancreatic parenchyma. It generally is associated with chronic alcoholism or biliary disease, although patients with hypercalcemia and hyperlipidemia are more predisposed to chronic pancreatitis.

On pathology the pancreas shows an increase in the interlobular fibrous tissue and chronic inflammatory infiltration changes. Stones of calcium carbonate may be found inside the ductal system, and pseudocysts are common.

Clinical Signs. Patient symptoms may include epigastric pain progressing with the disease, gastrointestinal problems, and jaundice secondary to common-duct obstruction. The pancreatic duct may dilate and contain calculi. There is calcification of the gland in 20% to 40% of the patients.[5]

Ultrasound Findings. Chronic pancreatitis may appear as a diffuse or localized involvement of the gland (Fig. 7-26). Echogenicity of the pancreas is increased beyond

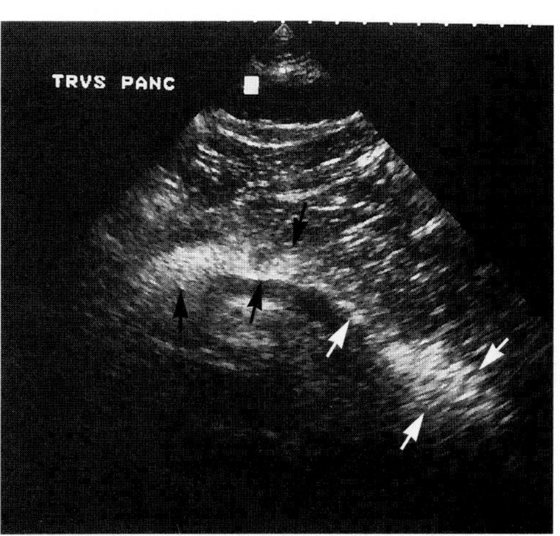

FIG. 7-26 A 56-year-old male with right upper quadrant pain. The pancreas is atrophic and increased in echogenicity suggestive of chronic pancreatitis *(arrows).*

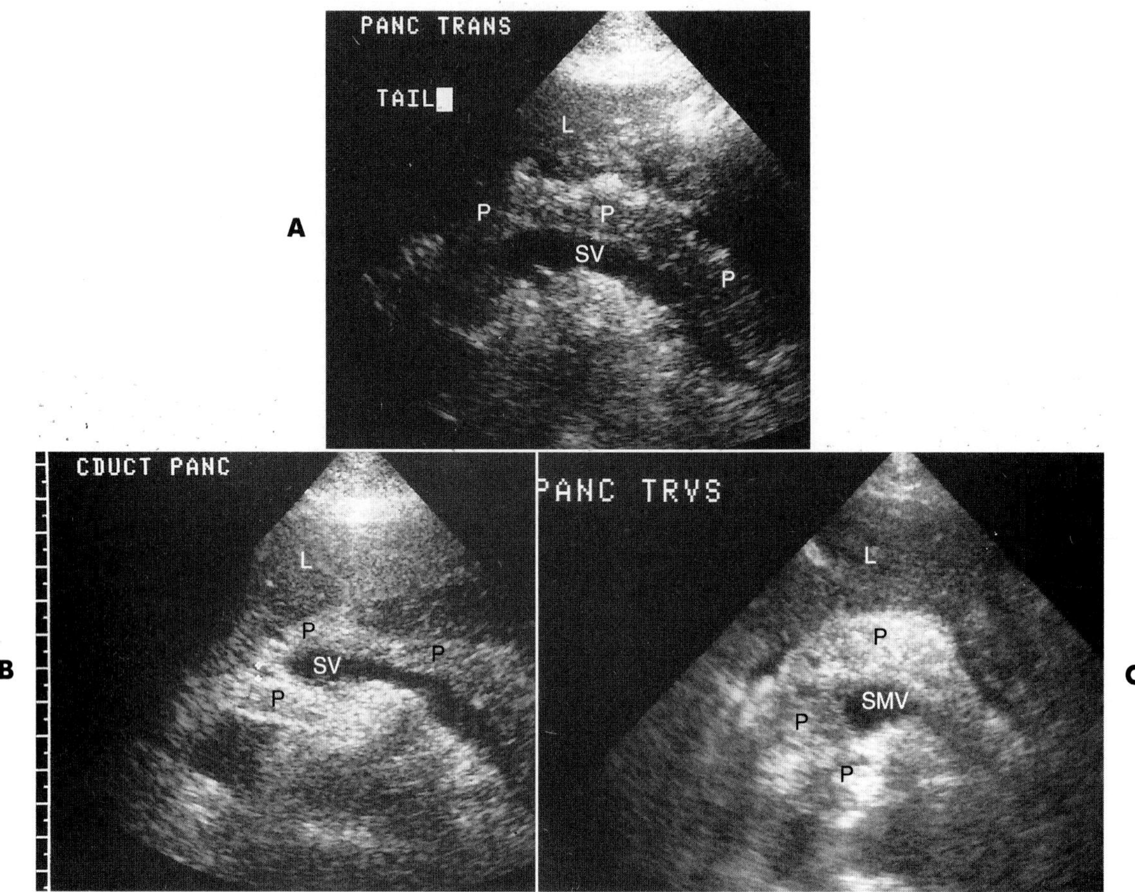

FIG. 7-27 A 43-year-old male with a history of alcohol abuse presents with an echogenic pancreas representing chronic pancreatitis. **A, B,** and **C,** Transverse scan of the echogenic pancreas. Liver, *L;* pancreas, *P;* splenic vein, *SV;* superior mesenteric vein, *v*.

normal because of fibrotic and fatty changes (Fig. 7-27). The borders are irregular and the duct may be dilated secondary to stricture or as the result of an extrinsic stone moving from a smaller pancreatic duct into a major duct (Fig. 7-28). With ductal lithiasis shadowing may be present. The most common site of obstruction is at the papilla. The incidence of carcinoma with pancreatic calcification is 25%.

Complications. Patients with chronic pancreatitis may go on to develop pseudocysts (20%) or thrombosis of the splenic vein, portal vein, or both (Fig. 7-29).

Pancreatic Cyst

There are two types of pancreatic cysts: true cysts and pseudocysts. The cysts may be unilocular or multilocular.

True Cysts. True cysts are microscopic sacs, which may be congenital or acquired. The congenital cysts are the result of anomalous development of the pancreatic duct and may be single but are usually multiple and without septation. Acquired cysts are retention cysts, parasitic cysts, or neoplastic cysts.

The cysts arise from within the gland, usually in the head first, then in the body and tail. They have a lining epithelium, which may be lost with inflammation. The cysts contain pancreatic enzymes or may be found to be continuous with the pancreatic duct.

Both pseudocysts and true cysts may protrude anteriorly in any direction, although the true cyst is generally associated directly with the pancreatic area. Pseudocysts usually develop through the lesser omentum, displacing the stomach or widening the duodenal loop.

Pseudocysts. Pancreatic pseudocysts are always acquired; they result from trauma to the gland or from acute or chronic pancreatitis. Approximately 11% to 18% of patients with acute pancreatitis develop a pseudocyst. A pseudocyst may be defined as a collection of fluid that arises from the loculation of inflammatory processes, necrosis, or hemorrhage. The pancreatic enzymes that escape the ductal system cause enzymatic digestion of the surrounding tissue and pseudocyst development. The walls of the pseudocyst form in the various potential spaces in which the escaped pancreatic enzymes are found. The pseudocyst usually presents few symptoms until it becomes large enough to cause pressure on the surrounding organs.

Locations of a pseudocyst. The most common location

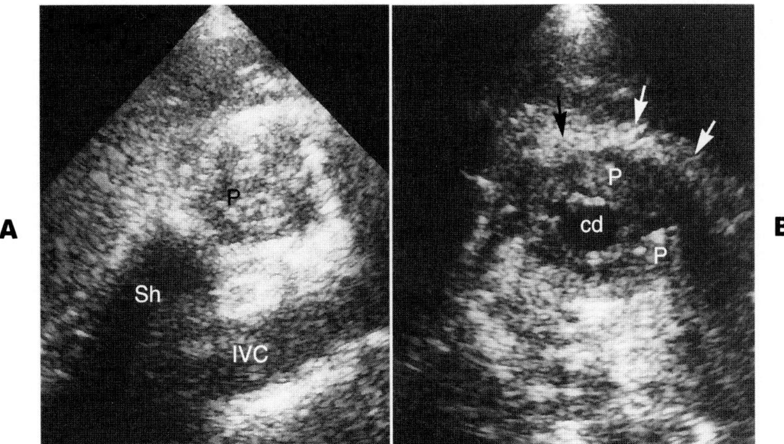

FIG. 7-28 A 31-year-old female with repeated episodes of pancreatitis. **A,** Sagittal scan of the pancreatic area shows an enlarged gland with very bright internal echoes, *P*. The shadow, *sh,* from gallstones, was present. **B,** Transverse scan of the enlarged common bile duct, *cd;* the calcifications are seen within the pancreas *(arrows).*

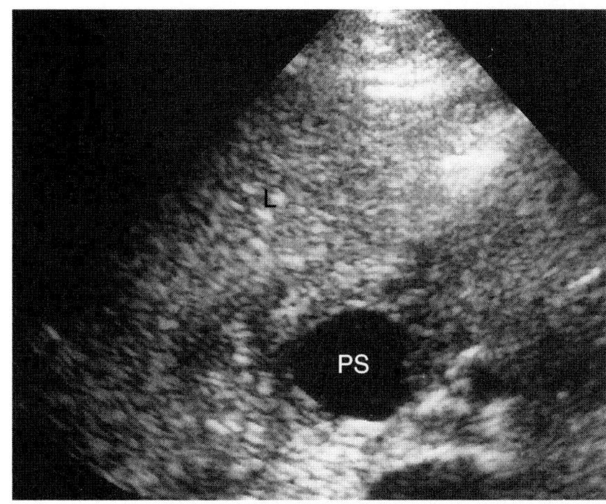

FIG. 7-29 About 20% of patients with chronic pancreatitis go on to develop pseudocysts. Liver, *L;* pseudocyst, *pc.*

of a pseudocyst is in the lesser sac anterior to the pancreas and posterior to the stomach. The second most common location is in the anterior pararenal space (posterior to the lesser sac, bounded by Gerota's fascia). The spleen is the lateral border of the anterior pararenal space on the left. Fluid occurs more commonly in left pararenal space than the right. Sometimes the posterior pararenal space is fluid-filled; fluid spreads from the anterior pararenal space to the posterior pararenal space on the same side. Fluid may enter the peritoneal cavity via the foramen of Winslow or by disrupting the peritoneum in the anterior surface of the lesser sac. It may extend into the mediastinum by extending through the esophageal or aortic hiatus or it may extend into small bowel mesentery or down into the retroperitoneum into the pelvis and groin.

A pseudocyst develops when pancreatic enzymes escape from the gland and break down tissue to form a sterile abscess somewhere in the abdomen. Its walls are not true cyst walls; hence the name *pseudo-* or false cyst. They generally take on the contour of the available space around them and therefore are not always spherical, as are normal cysts (Fig. 7-30). There may be more than one pseudocyst, so the sonographer should search for daughter collections when performing an echogram.

Sonographic findings. Sonographically pseudocysts usually appear as well-defined masses with essentially sonolucent echo-free interiors. Because of debris, scattered echoes may be seen at the bottom of the cysts, and increased through-transmission is present (Fig. 7-31). The borders are very echogenic, and the cysts usually are thicker than other simple cysts (Fig. 7-32). When a suspected pseudocyst is located near the stomach, the stomach should be drained so the cyst is not mistaken for a fluid-filled stomach. If the patient has been on continual drainage before the ultrasonic examination, this problem is eliminated.

Unusual sonographic patterns. Laing et al. have reported a series of pseudocysts found to contain unusual internal echoes.[2] There were three classifications: (1) septated, which presented with multiple internal septations; (2) excessive internal echoes, caused by an associated inflammatory mass, hemorrhage, or clot formation; and (3) pseudocyst, with absence of posterior enhancement resulting from the rim of calcification.

Spontaneous rupture. Spontaneous rupture is the most common complication of a pancreatic pseudocyst, occurring in 5% of patients.[3] In half of this 5% the drainage is directly into the peritoneal cavity. Clinical symptoms are sudden shock and peritonitis. The mortality rate is 50%. Ascites developing as a consequence of spontaneous rupture may be differentiated from that associated with cirrhosis in patients who have known rupture of a pseudocyst by

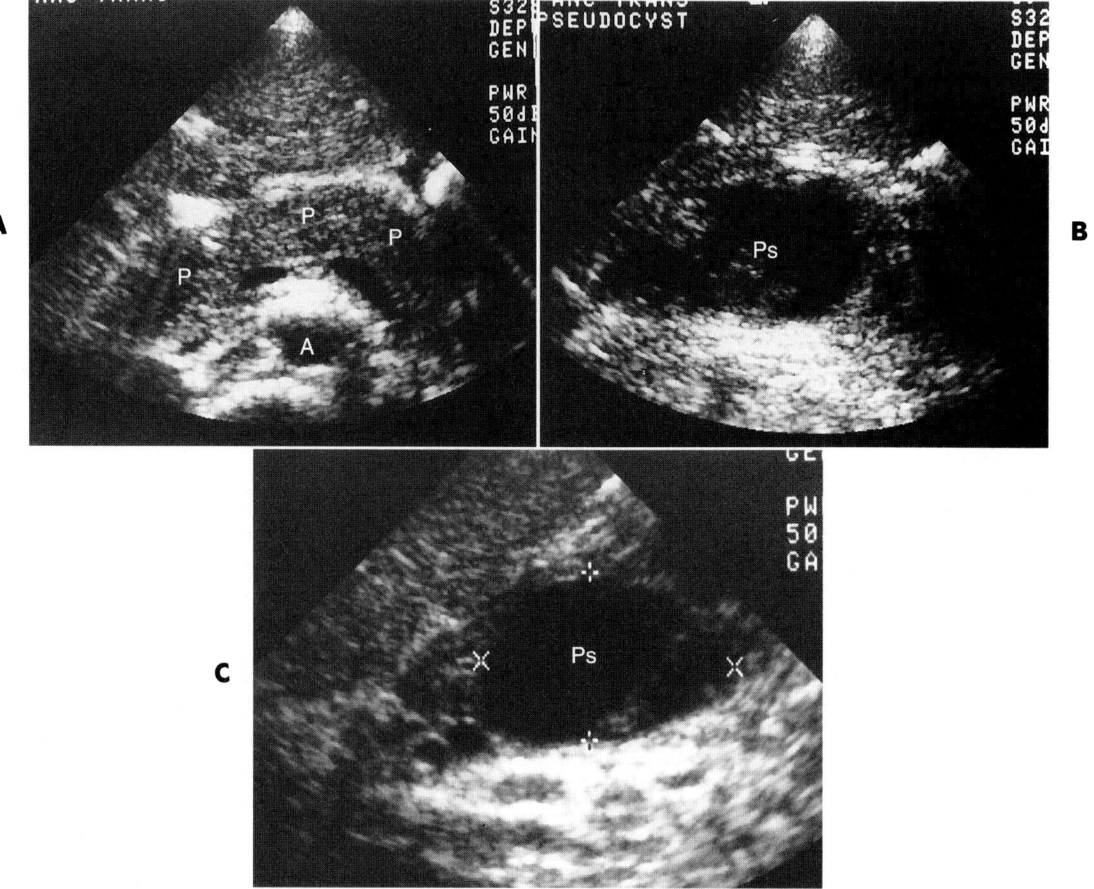

FIG. 7-30 Pancreatic pseudocyst usually develops near the lesser sac anterior to the pancreas and posterior to the stomach. **A,** Transverse; Aorta, *A;* pancreas, *P*. **B,** Transverse of the pseudocyst, *ps,* shows the somewhat irregular borders with internal debris. **C,** Sagittal view of the pseudocyst.

analysis of the fluid for elevated amylase and protein content.[7]

In the other half of the 5% of patients the rupture is into the gastrointestinal tract. Such patients may present a confusing picture sonographically. The initial scan shows a typical pattern for a pseudocyst formation, but the patient may develop intense pain secondary to the rupture, and consequent examination shows the disappearance of the mass.

Pancreatic Tumors

Cystadenoma and Cystadenocarcinoma

Cystadenocarcinoma. Cystadenocarcinoma (macrocystic adenoma) is an uncommon, slow-growing tumor that arises from the ducts as a cystic neoplasm. It is composed of a large cyst with or without septations and has a significant malignant potential. Patients present with epigastric pain or a palpable mass. Many patients have concurrent diseases: diabetes, calculous disease of biliary tract, or arterial hypertension. It occurs more in middle-aged females, with 60% in the tail, 35% in the body, and 5% in the head. Frequently foci of calcification may be seen within the pancreas.

Cystadenocarcinoma may be difficult to separate from carcinoma arising in a true cyst or cystic degeneration of a solid carcinoma. It is an irregular, lobulated cystic tumor with thick cellular walls. Metastases arise most commonly in the lymph nodes and liver. The course of this tumor may be slowly progressive with a tendency for the recurrent disease to remain localized.

Cystadenoma. Cystadenoma (microcystic adenoma) is a rare benign disease found more often in females. Tiny cysts are found primarily in the body and tail (60%). The coarsely lobulated cystic tumors sometimes present sonographically with cyst walls thicker than the membranes between multilocular cysts.

These cystic neoplasms look similar to pseudocysts and may have one of the following four ultrasound patterns:

1. Anechoic mass with posterior enhancement and irregular margins
2. Anechoic mass with internal homogeneous echoes
3. Anechoic mass with irregular internal vegetations protruding into the lumen and showing no movement
4. Completely echogenic mass with nonhomogeneous pattern (Fig. 7-33)

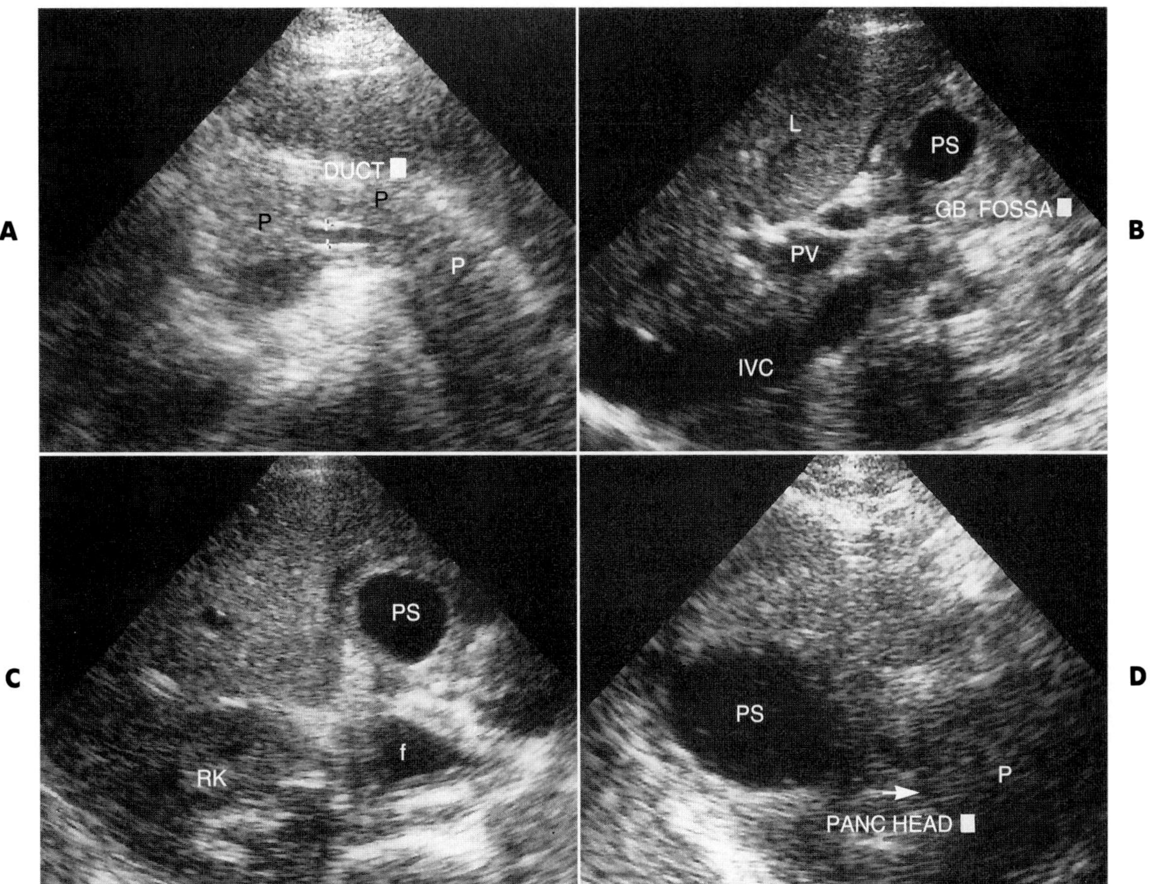

FIG. 7-31 A 32-year-old female with a history of pancreatic pseudocyst and persistent abdominal pain. A fluid collection is seen to the right of the pancreatic head, near the gallbaldder fossa. The gallbladder has been surgically removed. The pancreatic duct and common bile duct are dilated. **A,** Transverse of the dilated pancreatic duct *(crossbars),* and *pancreas, p.* **B,** Sagittal scan of the pseudocyst, *ps;* liver, *L;* inferior vena cava, *IVC;* portal vein, *PV.* **C,** Transverse scan of the pseudocyst, *ps;* fluid in Morison's pouch, *f;* right kidney, *RK.* **D,** Transverse scan of pseudocyst, *ps,* located just lateral to the head of the pancreas, *P.*

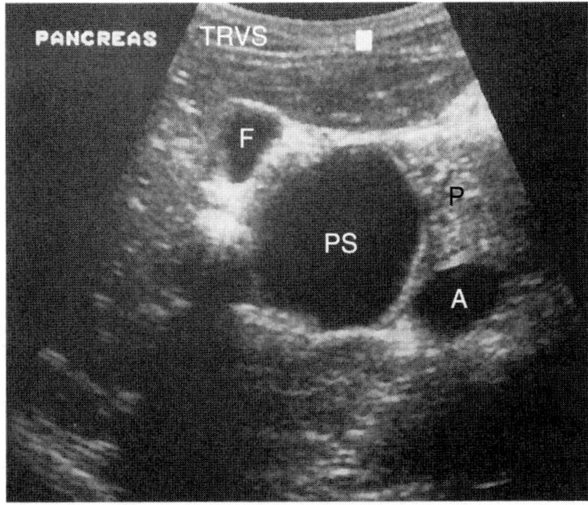

FIG. 7-32 Transverse scan of a large pseudocyst, *ps,* located just lateral to the head of the pancreas, *P.* Fluid is seen in Morison's pouch, *f;* aorta, *A.*

Adenocarcinoma. The most common primary neoplasm of the pancreas is adenocarcinoma. This fatal tumor involves the exocrine portion of the gland and accounts for 95% of all malignant pancreatic tumors. It usually occurs in 60- to 80-year-old males and occurs less often in females. The most frequent site of occurrence is in the head of the gland, (60% to 70%) with 20% to 30% in the body and 5% to 10% in the tail. One fifth of the tumors are diffuse. The tumors in the head present early, causing obstruction of the common bile duct and hydrops of the pancreas.

Clinical signs. Symptoms usually occur late. The time from symptoms until diagnosis is 4 months; the time to death is 8 months to 1.6 years. The most common symptom is pain radiating to the back or a dull, steady aching midepigastric pain. Weight loss, painless jaundice, nausea, vomiting, and changes in stools are also clinical symptoms. The painless jaundice usually appears first, followed by nausea and vomiting. The presence of a dilated gallbladder

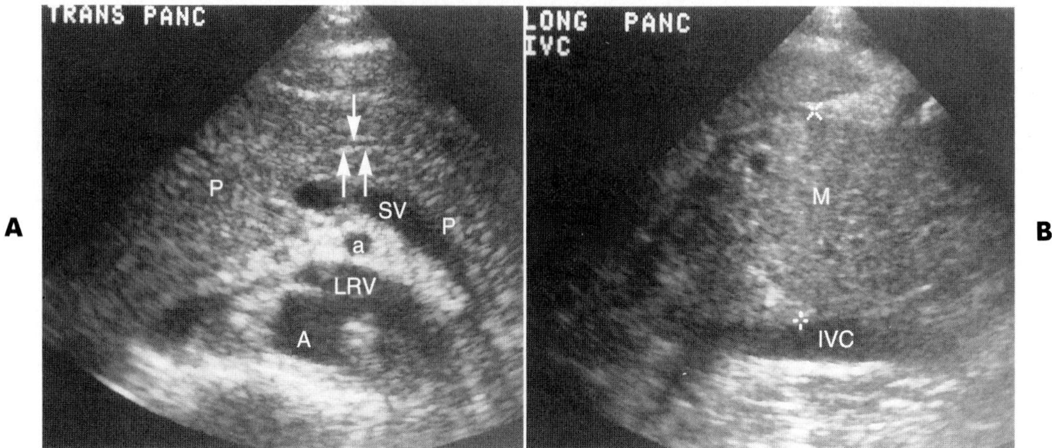

FIG. 7-33 A 65-year-old patient with cystadenoma in the head of the pancreas without causing obstruction of the pancreatic duct. **A,** Transverse of the pancreas, pancreatic duct *(arrow),* splenic vein, *sv,* superior mesenteric artery, *a;* left renal vein, *LRV;* aorta, *A.* **B,** Large mass in the head of the pancreas seen compressing the inferior vena cava, *IVC.*

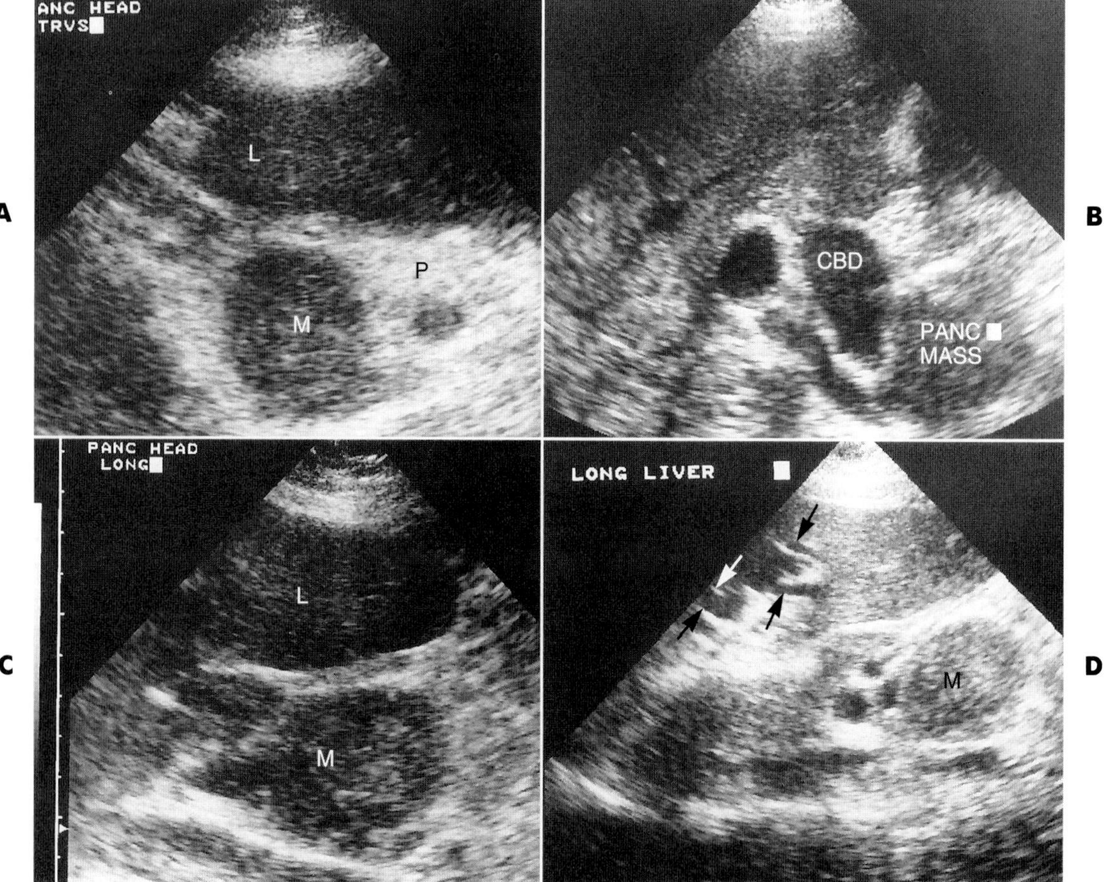

FIG. 7-34 A 63-year-old male presents with back pain, weight loss, and painless jaundice. A large hypoechoic mass is seen in the head of the pancreas with a dilated common bile duct. **A,** Transverse; adenocarcinoma of the head of the pancreas, *m;* pancreas, *P;* liver, *L.* **B,** Transverse of the pancreatic mass compressing the dilated common bile duct. **C,** Sagittal of the pancreatic mass, *m.* **D,** Sagittal of the pancreatic mass, *m;* intrahepatic ductal dilation, *(arrows).*

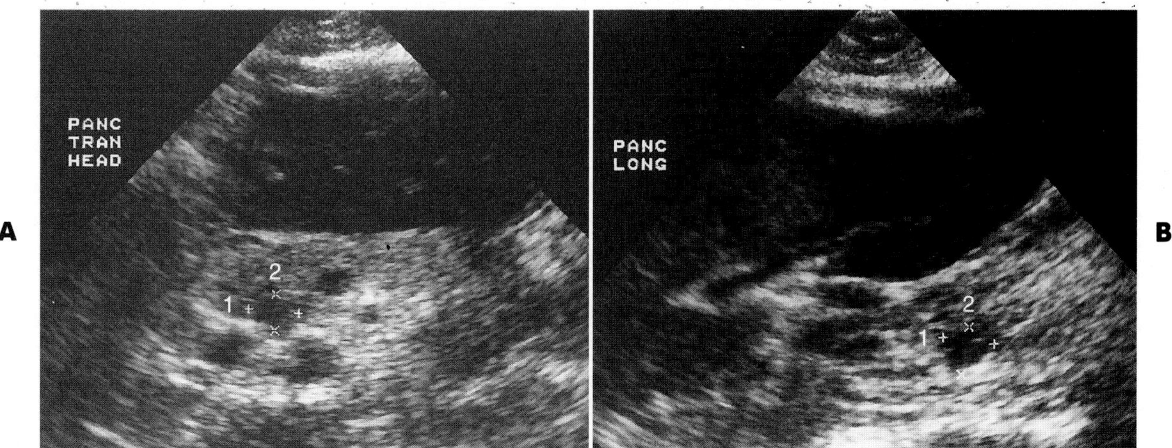

FIG. 7-35 The ultrasound appearance of adenocarcinoma is a loss of the normal pancreatic parenchymal pattern. If the mass is under 3 cm, it becomes more difficult to image with ultrasound techniques. **A,** Transverse scan of a patient with a small adenocarcinoma in the head of the pancreas. **B,** Sagittal scan of the hypoechoic mass lesion.

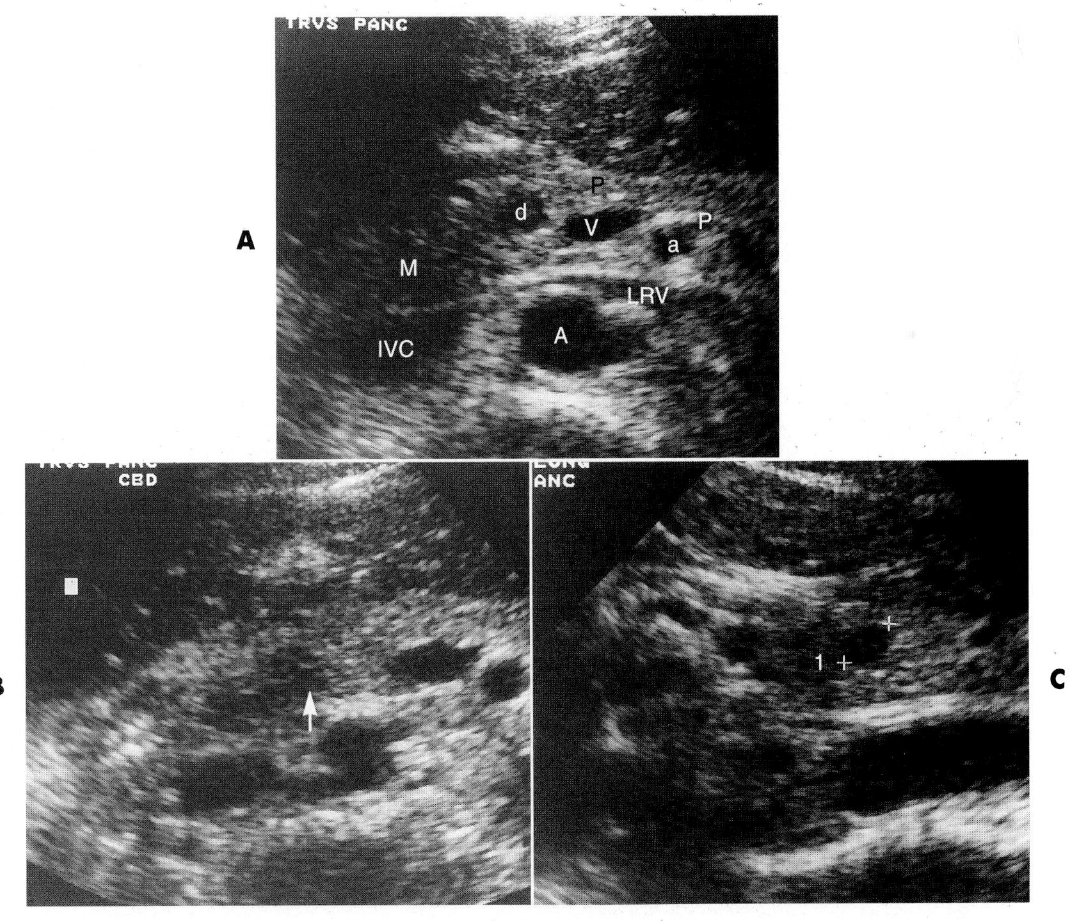

FIG. 7-36 A 65-year-old male presents with weight loss and pain radiating to the back. The pancreatic duct is dilated and the head of the pancreas is very hypoechoic representing adenocarcinoma of the pancreas. **A,** Transverse; aorta, *A;* inferior vena cava, *IVC;* pancreatic duct, *d;* superior mesenteric vein, *v;* superior mesenteric artery, *a;* left renal vein, *LRV.* **B,** Transverse; *arrow* points to the hypoechoic abnormal tissue in the head of the pancreas. **C,** Sagittal scan of the dilated pancreatic duct *(crossbars).*

and a palpable mass is strongly suggestive of carcinoma (Courvoisier's law). A cyst or pancreatitis may occur behind the neoplastic obstruction of the duct. With obstruction the enzymes will be absent or present in only small amounts.

Ultrasound findings. The sonographic appearance of adenocarcinoma is a loss of the normal pancreatic parenchymal pattern (Figs. 7-34 to 7-36). The lesions represent localized change in the echodensity of the pancreas. The echopattern is hypoechoic or less dense than the pancreas or liver. The borders become irregular and there may be pancreatic enlargement. There may be secondary enlargement of the common duct resulting from edema or tumor invasion of the pancreatic head. Usually there is dilation of the pancreatic duct. The sonographer should look for metastatic spread into the liver, the paraortic nodes (abnormal displacement of the superior mesenteric artery), or the portal venous system. The superior mesenteric vessels may be displaced posteriorly by the pancreatic mass; anterior displacement is present when the carcinoma is in the uncinate process, and posterior displacement when the tumor is in the head or body. A soft tissue thickening caused by neoplastic infiltration of perivascular lymphatics may be seen surrounding the celiac axis or superior mesenteric artery; this occurs more with carcinoma of the body and tail.

Most patients have obstructive jaundice and anterior wall compression of the inferior vena cava when the tumor involves the head of the pancreas. A tumor in the tail can compress the splenic vein, producing secondary splenic enlargement. A tumor may displace or invade the splenic or portal vein or produce thrombosis.

Islet Cell Tumors. There are several types of islet cell tumors; they may be functional or nonfunctional. The tumors may be benign adenomas or malignant tumors. The nonfunctioning islet cell tumors comprise one third of all islet cell tumors, 92% being malignant.

The most common functioning islet cell tumor is insulinoma (60%) followed by the gastrinoma (18%). The tu-

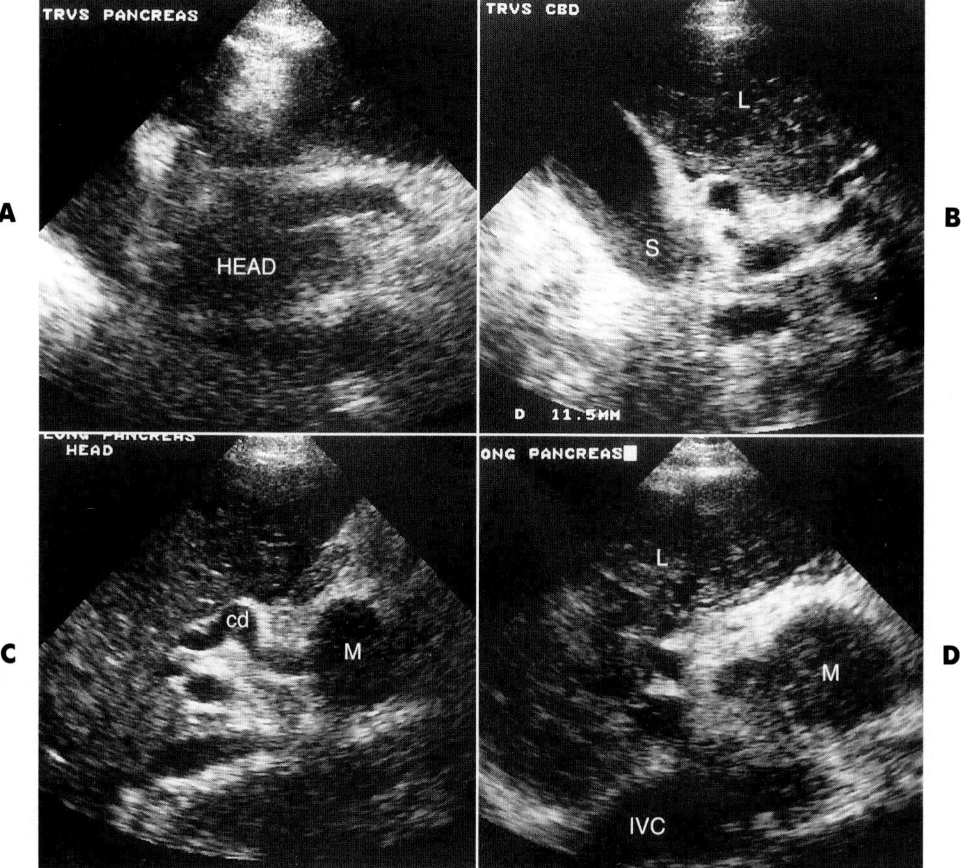

FIG. 7-37 A 46-year-old female presents with sweating and insulin shock. An ill-defined mass is seen in the head of the pancreas, compressing the common bile duct. This was an islet cell tumor of the pancreas. **A,** Transverse scan of the head of the pancreas shows the irregularly margined mass. **B,** The dilated common bile duct *(crossbars)* measures 11.5 mm. The distended gallbladder is half filled with sludge, *s.* **C,** Sagittal scan of the distended common duct, *cd,* and mass in the head of the pancreas, *m.* **D,** Sagittal scan of the liver, *L,* mass in the pancreas, *m,* and inferior vena cava, *IVC.*

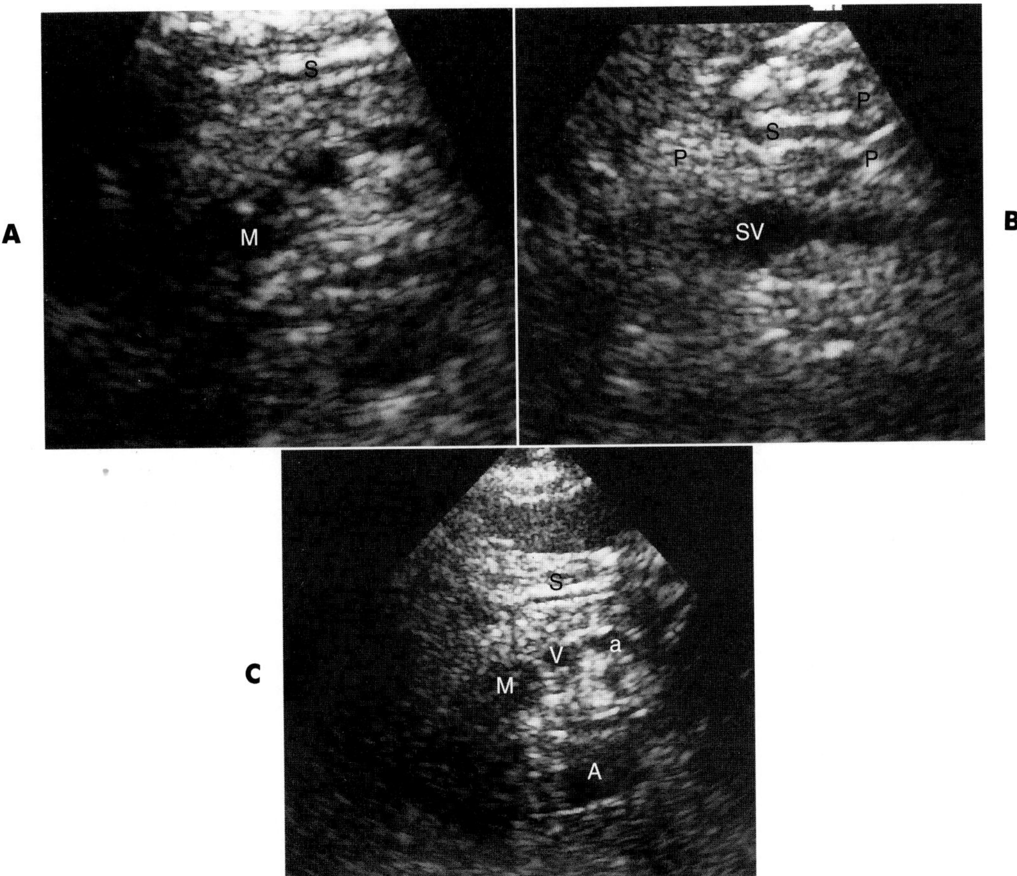

FIG. 7-38 A 61-year-old female with obstructive jaundice and stasis after biliary stent insertion. The patient was evaluated for bile duct carcinoma and to rule out hepatic metastases. Within the pancreatic head, a 1.5 × 1.2 cm hypoechoic lesion was seen close to the biliary stent. Sludge was seen in the gallbladder. **A,** Transverse; splenic vein, *SV;* stent, *s;* pancreas, *P*. **B,** Transverse; stent, *s;* mass, *m*. **C,** Transverse; stent, *s;* mass, *m;* superior mesenteric vein, *v;* superior mesenteric artery, *a;* aorta, *A*.

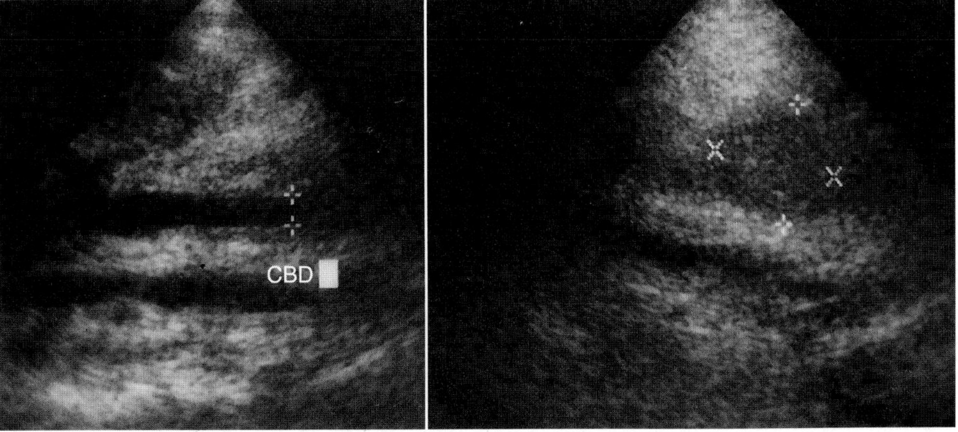

FIG. 7-39 A mass in the head of the pancreas is sometimes difficult to separate from enlarged retroperitoneal nodes. Careful evaluation of the superior mesenteric vessels (compression or abnormal angulation) may help to distinguish whether the mass is intrapancreatic or extrapancreatic.

mor size is small (1 to 2 cm), and they are well encapsulated with a good vascular supply. The tumors may be multiple and occur mostly in the body and tail, where there is the greatest concentration of Langerhans islets (Fig. 7-37). A large percentage occurs in patients with hyperinsulinism and hypoglycemia. Sonographically the islet cell tumors are difficult to image because of their small size. The greatest success is when they are located in the head of the pancreas.

Metastatic Disease to the Pancreas. An intraabdominal lymphoma may cause a hypoechoic mass in the pancreas (Figs. 7-38 and 7-39). The superior mesenteric vessels may be displaced anterior instead of posterior as seen with a primary pancreatic mass. Multiple nodes are seen along the pancreas, duodenum, porta, and superior mesenteric vessels; they may be difficult to distinguish from a pancreatic mass. The enlarged nodes appear hypoechoic and well defined.

REVIEW QUESTIONS

1. The pancreas is divided into four sections. Name them, describe their relationship with vascular structures, and define their dimensions.
2. Name the two pancreatic ducts. What is their relationship to the ampulla of Vater, sphincter of Oddi, and the common bile duct?
3. What is the vascular supply to the pancreas?
4. What are the enzymes of the pancreatic juice? How can they help determine if the patient has pancreatic disease?
5. Name the laboratory tests used in defining pancreatic disease.
6. Describe the normal texture of the pancreatic gland.
7. What are the best patient positions and windows to image the pancreas?
8. In what part of the pancreas does the pancreatic duct appear on ultrasound?
9. Describe an annular pancreas and explain its problems with duodenal atresia.
10. What effect does cystic fibrosis have on the pancreas?
11. How does acute pancreatitis develop? What are the patient signs and symptoms? How would it appear on ultrasound? What are the complications?
12. Define phlegmon.
13. What is the difference between a pseudocyst and a true cyst in the pancreas? What are the characteristics of a pseudocyst and how is it formed?
14. Define chronic pancreatitis. What are the ultrasound findings?
15. What are the most common benign tumors of the pancreas?
16. What is the most common primary tumor of the pancreas? Why is it so often fatal? What is the sonographic criterion for pancreatic carcinoma?
17. What is an islet cell tumor and where is it found?
18. What is Courvoisier's law?

REFERENCES

1. Filly RA and London SS: The normal pancreas: acoustic characteristics and frequency of imaging, J Clin Ultrasound 7:121, 1979.
2. Laing FC, Gooding GAW, Brown T, and Leopold GR: Atypical pseudocysts of the pancreas: an ultrasonographic evaluation, J Clin Ultrasound 7:27, 1979.
3. Leopold GR, Berg RN, and Reinke RT: Echographic-radiological documentation of spontaneous rupture of a pancreatic pseudocyst into the duodenum, Radiology 120:699, 1972.
4. Marks WM, Filly RA, and Callen PW: Ultrasonic evaluation of normal pancreatic echogenicity and its relationship to fat deposition, Radiology 137:475, 1980.
5. Weinstein BJ, Weinstein DP, and Brodmerkel GJ: Ultrasonography of pancreatic lithiasis, Radiology 134:185, 1980.

BIBLIOGRAPHY

Aquino NM, Mortan R, and Singh H: Carcinoma of the pancreas metastasizing to the tunica vaginalis testis, J Clin Ultrasound 17:287, 1989.

Arger PH, Mulhern CB, Bonavita JA, et al: Analysis of pancreatic sonography in suspected pancreatic disease, J Clin Ultrasound 7:91, 1979.

Bolondi L, Bassi, SL, and Gaiani S: Sonography of chronic pancreatitis, Radiol Clin North Am 27:815, 1989.

Cavallini G, Bovo P, Zamboni M, et al: Exocrine and endocrine functional reserve in the course of chronic pancreatitis as studied by maximal stimulation tests, Dig Dis Sci, 37:215, 1992.

de Graaff CS, Taylor KJW, Simonds BD, et al: Gray-scale echography of the pancreas: re-evaluation of normal size, Radiology 129:157, 1978.

Eisenscher A and Weill F: Ultrasonic visualization of Wirsung's duct: dream or reality? J Clin Ultrasound 7:41, 1979.

Filly RA and Freimanis AK: Echographic diagnosis of pancreatic lesions, Radiology 96:575, 1970.

Gosink BB and Leopold GR: The dilated pancreatic duct: ultrasonic evaluation, Radiology 126:475, 1978.

Gumaste VV, Dave PB, Weissman D, and Messer J: Lipase/amylase ratio, Gastroenterology, 101:1361, 1991.

Gupta AK, Arenson A, and McKee JD: Effect of steroid ingestion on pancreatic echogenicity, J Clin Ultrasound 15:171, 1987.

Hadidi A: Pancreatic duct diameter: sonographic measurement in normal subjects, J Clin Ultrasound 11:17, 1983.

Hassani SN, Smulewicz JJ, and Bard R: Pattern of pancreatic carcinoma by real time and gray scale ultrasonography, Appl Radiol, September-October 1977.

Jeffrey RB, Laing FC, and Wing VW: Ultrasound in acute pancreatic trauma, Gastrointest Radiol 11:4448, 1986.

Macmahon H, Bowie JD, and Beezhold C: Erect scanning of pancreas using a gastric window, Am J Roentgenol 132:587, 1979.

Niederau C, Muller J, Sonnenberg A, et al: Extrahepatic bile ducts in healthy subjects, in patients with cholelithiasis, and in postcholecystectomy patients: a prospective ultrasonic study, J Clin Ultrasound 11:23, 1983.

Odo Op den Orth J: Tubeless hypotonic duodenograpy with water: a simple aid in sonography of the pancreatic head, Radiology 154:826, 1985.

Patti MG and Pellegrini CA, Gallstone pancreatitis, Surg Clin North Am, 70:1277, 1990.

Sample WF, Po JB, Gray RK, and Cahill PJ: Gray scale in ultrasonography techniques in pancreatic scanning, Appl Radiol, September-October, 1975.

Sarti DA: Rapid development and spontaneous regression of pancreatic pseudocysts documented by ultrasound, Radiology 125:789, 1977.

So CB, Cooperberg PL, Gibney RG, et al: Sonographic findings in pancreatic lipomatosis, Am J Roentgenol 149:67, 1987.

Sokoloff J, et al: Pitfalls in the echographic evaluation of pancreatic disease, J Clin Ultrasound 2:321, 1974.

Stott MA, Farrands PA, Guyer PB, et al: Ultrasound of the common bile duct in patients undergoing cholecystectomy, J Clin Ultrasound 19:73, 1991.

Swobodnik W, Wolf A, Wechsler JG, et al: Ultrasound characteristics of the pancreas in children with cystic fibrosis, J Clin Ultrasound 13:469, 1985.

Warner RL, Othersen HB, and Smith CD: Traumatic pancreatitis and pseudocyst in children: current management, J Trauma, 29:597, 1988.

Weighall SL, Wolfman NT, and Watson N: The fluid-filled stomach: a new sonic window, J Clin Ultrasound 7:353, 1979.

Weizman Z and Durie PR: Acute pancreatitis in childhood, J Pediatr 113:24, 1988.

Wright CH, Maklad F, and Posenthal S: Grey scale in ultrasonic characteristics of carcinoma of the pancreas, Br J Radiol 52:281, 1979.

CHAPTER 8

Gastrointestinal Tract

Sandra L. Hagen-Ansert

The gastrointestinal tract may be difficult to image with ultrasound in most patients unless they ingest fluids or some other acoustic transmittable contrast agent. Many laboratories have begun to investigate various contrast agents in pursuit of the ideal medium for imaging the stomach, duodenum, small bowel, and colon.

ANATOMY

Intraluminal air is echogenic. The scattering effect of gas in the gastrointestinal tract often produces an incomplete or mottled distal acoustic shadow. The rim of lucency represents the wall (i.e., intima, media, and serosa), and its periserosal fat produces the outer echogenic border of the tract wall (Fig. 8-1). The wall should measure less than 5 mm, when distended 3 mm. The sonographer should measure from the edge of the echogenic core (intraluminal gas) to the outer border of the anechoic halo (bowel wall).

If the colon is dilated, measure from the fluid to the outside of the wall. Distention is considered adequate if the stomach diameter is greater than 8 cm, the small bowel is greater than 3 cm, and the lower bowel is greater than 5 cm; the entire halo should measure less than 2 cm (target sign).

TECHNIQUE

The technique used to observe the upper gastrointestinal tract is for the patient to drink 10 to 40 ounces of water through a straw after a baseline ultrasound study of the upper abdomen. The straw helps avoid excess air being ingested when the water is consumed. It is helpful to examine the patient in an upright position; this causes the air to rise to the fundus of the stomach and not interfere with the ultrasound beam. The lower gastrointestinal tract requires no preparation. To image the lower colon, it may be useful to give the patient a water enema to help delineate the colon better.

Stomach

The esophagogastric junction is seen on the sagittal scan to the left of the midline as a bull's-eye or target structure anterior to the aorta, posterior to the left lobe of the liver, and next to the hemidiaphragm. The left lobe of the patient's liver must be large enough to be able to image the esophagogastric junction.

The gastric antrum can be seen as a target in the midline (Fig. 8-2). The remainder of the stomach usually is not visualized unless dilated with fluid.

When pathology is present, the serosal layer of the normal gastric wall is seen running toward the serous side of a tumor, which allows differentiation of intramural from extraserosal tumors. If a serosal bridging layer (three layers are seen on the mucosal side of the tumor and at least two of them are continuous with layers 1 and 2 of normal gastric wall) is present, the tumor lies within the gastric wall. If mucosal bridging is continuous with the mucosal layers of the normal gastric wall, intramucosal or deeply infiltrated carcinoma can be excluded. The sonographer needs to orient the transducer vertical to the area of transition between the lesion and stomach wall in order to show their relationship.

Cystic mass in the left upper quadrant. If a patient presents with a cystic mass in the left upper quadrant, several measures can be taken to determine if the mass is the fluid-filled stomach or another mass arising from the adjacent organs (Fig. 8-3). The sonographer may give the patient a carbonated drink to see bubbles in the stomach; ask the clinician to place a nasogastric tube for drainage; watch for a change in the shape or size of the "stomach" mass with the ingestion of fluids; alter the patient's position by scanning in an upright or left or right lateral decubitus position; watch for peristalsis; or ask the patient to drink water to see the swirling effect.

Duodenum

Usually only the gas-filled duodenal cap is seen to the right of the pancreas. The duodenum is divided into the following four portions (Fig. 8-4):

1. A superior portion that courses anteroposteriorly from the pylorus to the level of the neck of the gallbladder
2. A sharp bend in the duodenum into the descending portion that runs along the inferior vena cava at the level of L4
3. A transverse portion that passes right to left with a slight inclination upward in front of the great vessels and crura
4. An ascending portion that rises to the right of the aorta

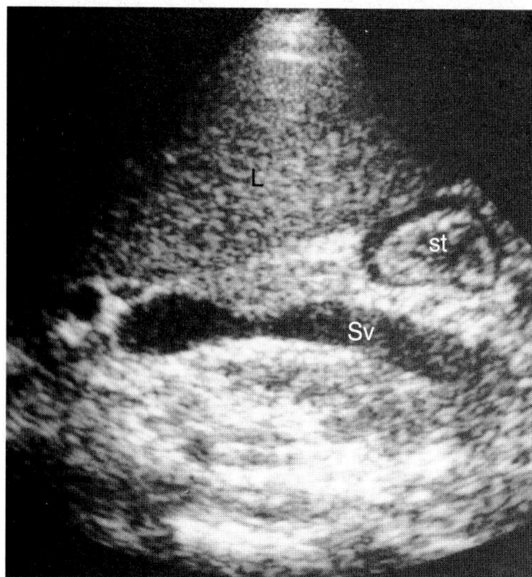

FIG. 8-1 Transverse view of the left lobe of the liver, *L*. The antrum of the stomach, *st*, is seen posterior to the liver and anterior to the splenic vein, *sv*.

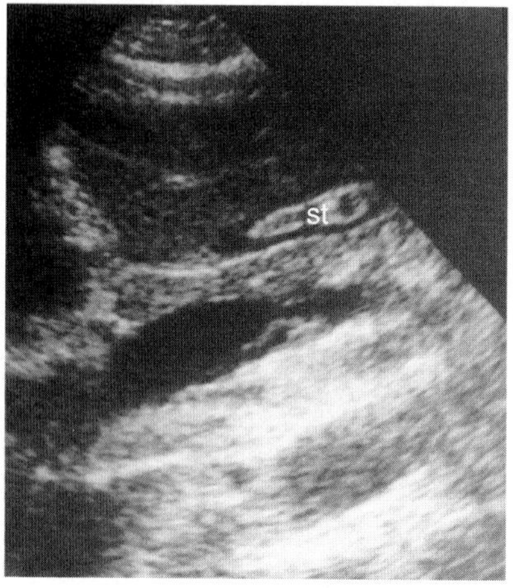

FIG. 8-2 Transverse view of the collapsed gastric antrum, *st*.

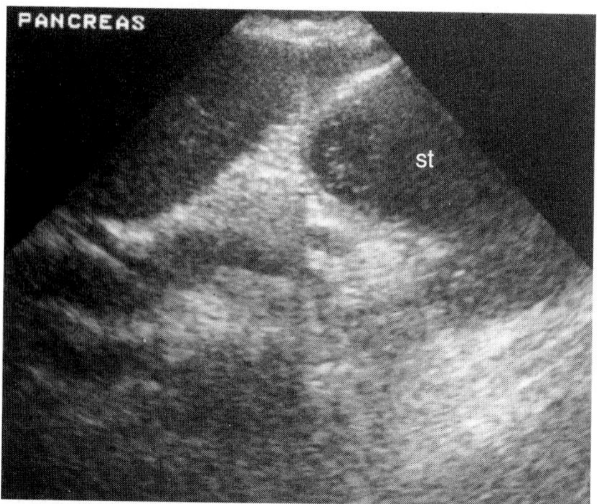

FIG. 8-3 Transverse view of the fluid-filled stomach. Real time shows movement throughout the stomach, *ST*.

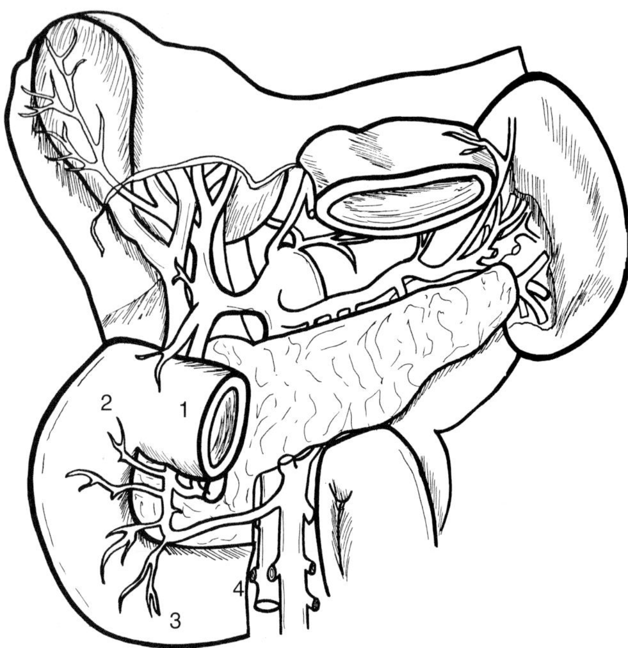

FIG. 8-4 The duodenal cap is an excellent landmark for the head of the pancreas. The duodenum is divided into four sections; see text for explanation. (From Hagen-Ansert SL: The anatomy workbook. Philadelphia, JB Lippincott, 1986.)

and reaches the upper border at L2, where, at the duodenojejunal flexure, it turns forward to become the jejunum (usually not seen with ultrasound)

The duodenum can be outlined easily with water ingestion or a change in position (Fig. 8-5). Generally the right lateral decubitus position allows the fluid to drain from the antrum of the stomach into the duodenum. Observation of peristalsis is useful to delineate the duodenum.

Small Bowel

The small bowel is more difficult to image with ultrasound. If there is fluid in the bowel loops, the sonographer may be able to look for peristalsis, air movement, or movement of intraluminal fluid contents (Fig. 8-6).

The sonographer usually cannot see the small bowel with ultrasound; the valvulae conniventes may be seen as linear echo densities spaced 3 to 5 mm apart. This is called the *keyboard sign* and can be seen in the duodenum and jejunum. The ileum is smooth walled and the small bowel wall is under 3 mm thick.

Appendix

The vermiform appendix is a remnant of what was originally the apex of the cecum. It is a long, tubular structure extending from the cecum in one of several directions; it may lie superiorly behind the cecum, medially behind the ileum and mesentery, or downward and medial into the true pelvis (Fig. 8-7).[3,9] It is located on the abdominal wall under McBurney's point. McBurney's point is located by drawing a line from the right anterior superior iliac spine

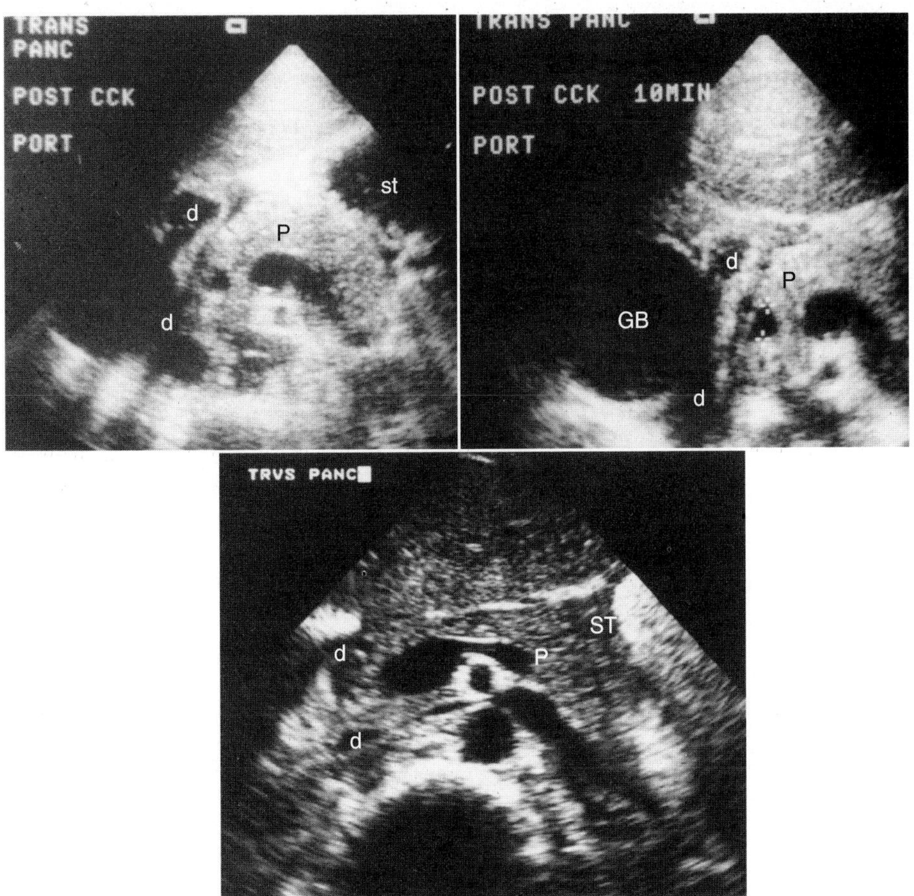

FIG. 8-5 Transverse views of the fluid-filled stomach, *st,* and duodenum, *d,* as they outline the body and head of the pancreas, *P.*

to the umbilicus.[9] At approximately the midpoint of this line lies the root of the appendix. The appendix varies from 1 to 9 inches in length, averaging 3 inches. It is retained in position by a fold of the peritoneum that forms a mesentery for it, which is derived from the left leaf of the mesentery. This triangular-shaped structure covers two thirds of the appendix, leaving the distal one third completely uncovered by peritoneum. A branch of the ileocolic artery lies between the layers of this mesentery, the artery of the appendix. This artery runs the entire length of the appendix.

Its small canal communicates with the cecum by an orifice, which is below and behind the ileocecal opening. The cellular layers that constitute the appendix are the serous, muscular, submucous, and mucous, the same layers as in the intestine. An abundant amount of retiform tissue is found in the mucosa layer, especially in younger ages.[3]

The appendix has no known physiologic significance. It is stated that the appendix tends to undergo obliteration as a result of involution.[3]

Colon

A fluid-filled colon may present as a mass (Figs. 8-8 and 8-9). The water-enema technique should be used to help delineate if the mass is within the colon, separate from the colon, or just the colon itself. The patient should be scanned with a full bladder to help push the small bowel out of the pelvis. The water in the enema should be lukewarm with the patient rolled into the left lateral decubitus position. Only a small amount of water needs to be given as the sonographer follows the rectum and rectosigmoid colon. The normal wall thickness measures 4 mm. There are five layers in the colon: from the inside out, the first two layers are mucosa, the third is submucosa, the fourth is muscularis propria, and the fifth is subserosal fatty tissue (Fig. 8-10).

PATHOLOGY OF THE UPPER GASTROINTESTINAL TRACT

Duplication Cysts

Duplication cysts are embryologic mistakes. They may cause symptoms, depending on their size, location, and histology. The criteria for a duplication cyst are as follows: (1) the cyst is lined with alimentary tract epithelium; (2) the cyst has a well-developed muscular wall, and (3) the cyst is contiguous with the stomach. It may arise from the

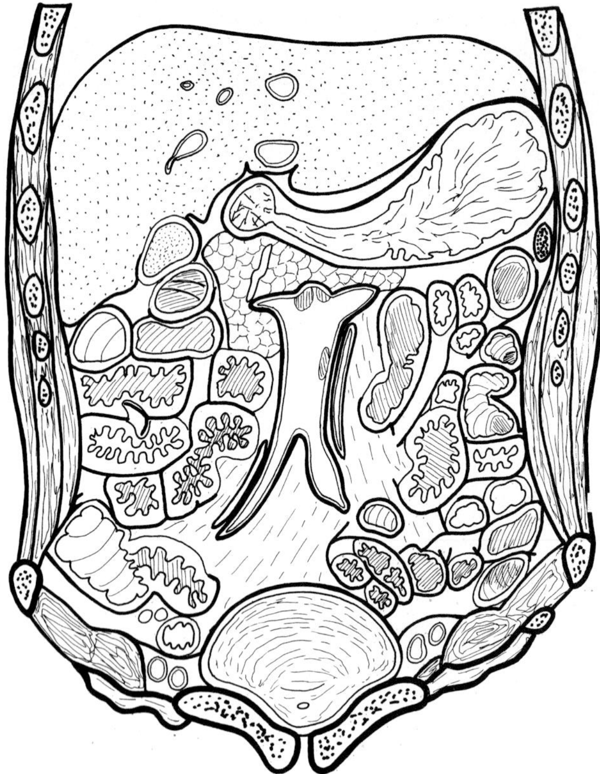

FIG. 8-6 Coronal view of the stomach, ascending and descending colon, and multiple loops of small bowel. (From Hagen-Ansert SL: The anatomy workbook. Philadelphia, JB Lippincott, 1986.)

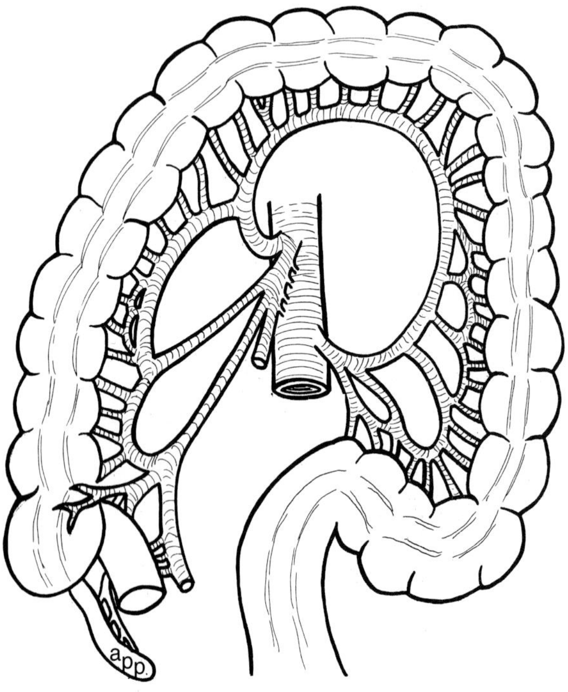

FIG. 8-7 The appendix is a long, tubular structure extending from the cecum in one of three directions. It may lie superiorly behind the cecum, medial behind the ileum and mesentery, or downward and medial into the true pelvis. (From Hagen-Ansert SL: The anatomy workbook. Philadelphia, JB Lippincott, 1986.)

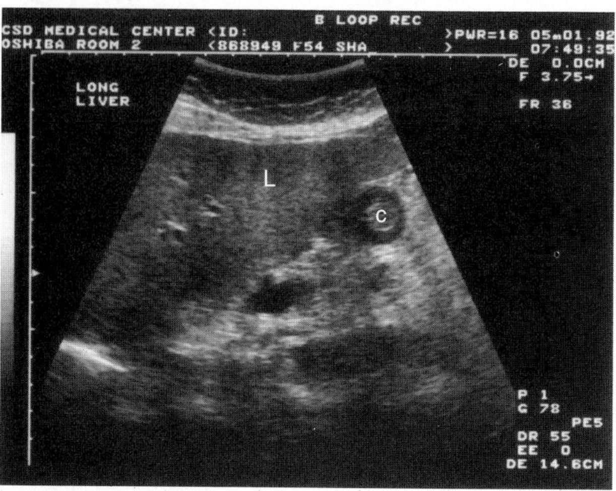

FIG. 8-8 Longitudinal scan of the typical bull's-eye appearance of the transverse colon, *c*.

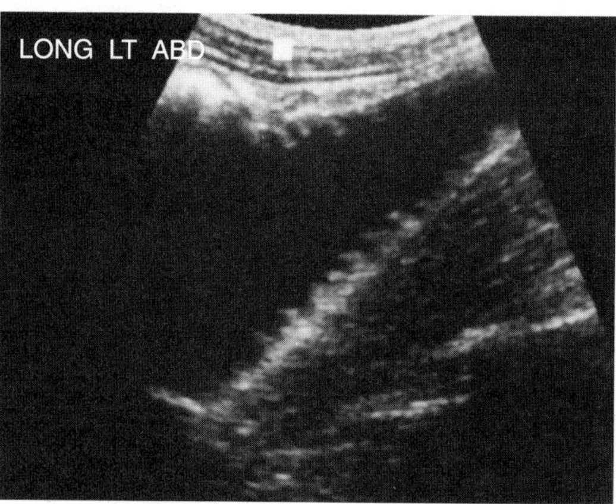

FIG. 8-9 Longitudinal scan of a fluid-filled loop of colon. The tiny cilla may be seen to move on the real-time examination.

pancreas or duodenum and occurs more often in females than in males. It usually is found on the greater curvature of the stomach.

Clinical symptoms are of high intestinal obstruction—distention, vomiting, and abdominal pain; hemorrhage and fistula formation may also occur.

Ultrasound appears as anechoic with a thin inner echogenic rim (mucosa) and wider outer hypoechoic rim (muscle layer). The differential diagnosis includes mesenteric or omental cyst, pancreatic cyst or pseudocyst, enteric cyst, renal cyst, splenic cyst, congenital cyst of the left lobe of the liver, or gastric distention.

Gastric Bezoar

Bezoars are divided into the following three categories: (1) trichobezoars—hair balls in young women, (2) phytobezoars—vegetable matter (unripe persimmons), and (3) concretions—inorganic materials (i.e., sand, asphalt, and shellac).

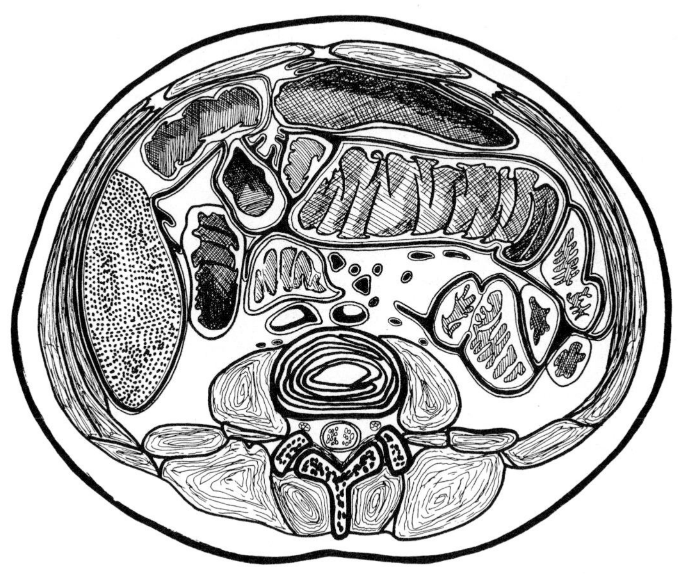

FIG. 8-10 The normal colon wall thickness measures 4 mm. The five layers in the colon are the mucosa, submucosa, muscularis propria, serosa, and subserosal fatty tissue. (From Hagen-Ansert SL: The anatomy workbook. Philadelphia, JB Lippincott, 1986.)

Gastric Bezoars

Gastric bezoars are movable intraluminal masses of congealed ingested materials that are seen on upper gastrointestinal radiographs. Clinically, patients present with nausea, vomiting, and pain. Their symptoms may simulate those of a tumor. On ultrasound a complex mass is seen with internal mobile echogenic components. In the fasting patient the sonographer would see a broad band of high-amplitude echoes or a hyperechoic curvilinear dense strip at the anterior margin.

Benign Tumors

Polyps. Polyps are seen with fluid distention of the stomach and appear as solid masses that adhere to the gastric wall. The polyp has variable echogenicity. A large polyp may be inhomogeneous; its contours may or may not be sharply defined, depending on the nature of the surface; the detection of a pedicle may be possible.

Leiomyomas. Leiomyoma is the most common tumor of the stomach. Leiomyoma is seen as a mass similar to carcinoma; it is usually small and asymptomatic for the patient. It is often associated with other gastrointestinal abnormalities, such as cholelithiasis, peptic ulcer disease, adenocarcinoma, and leiomyosarcoma. On ultrasound the mass is seen as hypoechoic and continuous with the muscular layer of the stomach. It may also be seen as a circular or oval space-occupying lesion with a homogeneous echo pattern and hemispheric bulging into the lumen, frequently separated from the lumen by two or three layers continuous with those of normal wall. The mass may appear as a solid with cystic areas that represent necrosis.

Malignant Tumors

Gastric carcinoma. At least 90% to 95% of malignant tumors of the stomach are carcinomas. Gastric carcinoma is the sixth leading cause of death; it occurs more in older males. One half of the tumors occur in the pylorus, with one fourth occurring in the body and fundus of the stomach. The lesions may be fungating, ulcerated, diffuse, polypoid, superficial, or some combination of these. On ultrasound the sonographer should look for the target or pseudokidney sign; the patient may have gastric wall thickening (Figs. 8-11 and 8-12).

Lymphoma. Lymphoma can occur as a primary tumor of the gastrointestinal tract (3% of stomach tumors). In patients with disseminated lymphoma a primary tumor occurs as a multifocal lesion in the gastrointestinal tract. The stomach has enlarged and thickened mucosal folds, multiple submucosal nodules, ulceration, and a large extraluminal mass. Clinical symptoms include nausea and vomiting with weight loss. On ultrasound, one sees a large and poorly echogenic (hypoechoic) mass, thickening of gastric walls, and a spoke-wheel pattern within the mass.

Leiomyosarcoma. Leiomyosarcoma is the second most common gastric sarcoma (1% to 5% of tumors). It occurs in the fifth to sixth decades of life. The mass is generally globular or irregular; it may become huge, outstripping blood supply, with central necrosis leading to cystic degeneration and cavitation. On ultrasound, there is a target lesion, although the pattern is variable; hemorrhage and necrosis may occur causing irregular echoes or a cystic cavity.

Metastatic disease. Metastatic disease to the stomach is rare; it may arise from melanoma or lung or breast cancer. The tumor is found in the submucosal layer, forming circumscribed nodules or plaques. On ultrasound, there is a target pattern, circumscribed thickening, or uniform widening of wall without layering.

PATHOLOGY OF THE LOWER GASTROINTESTINAL TRACT

Obstruction and/or dilation. A small bowel obstruction is associated with dilation of the bowel loops proximal to

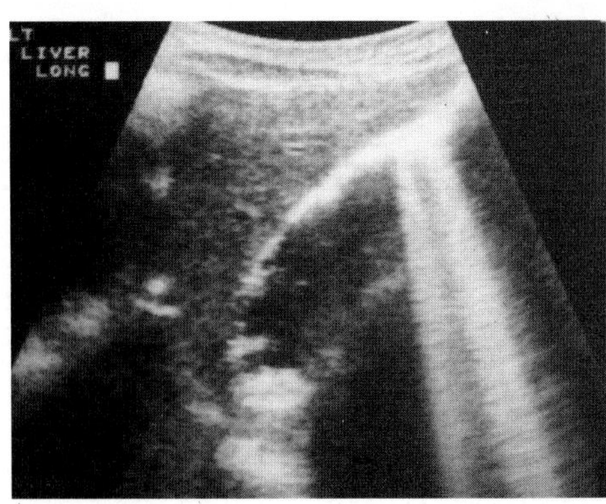

FIG. 8-11 Longitudinal scan of a patient with a fluid-filled stomach. The bright echo reflections are the result of air bubbles within the stomach cavity. Analysis of the wall thickness, through-transmission characteristics, and internal echo architecture determines the nature of the mass in the stomach. This patient would be given fluid to help outline the internal structure of the stomach better. Upright scans would help eliminate the air interference. Gastric carcinoma was found.

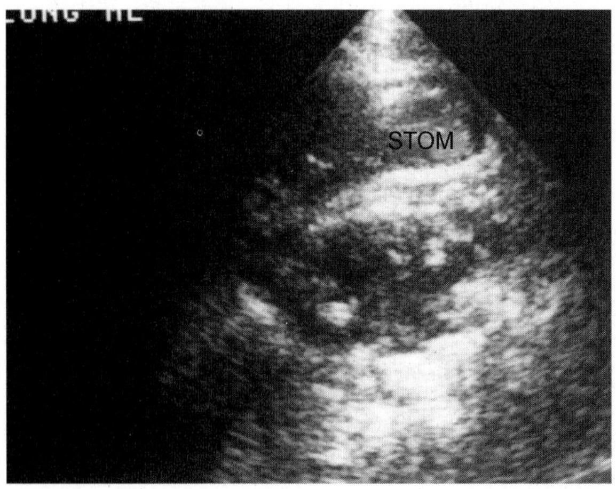

FIG. 8-12 A 32-year-old male with coffee-ground emesis, epigastric pain, and elevated liver function tests. In the region of the gastric antrum and duodenum an irregular inhomogeneous round 3.5-cm structure is identified. This may represent a very edematous, ulcerated antral or duodenal wall or an extraluminal collection, possibly related to the pancreas.

the site of the obstruction. In 6% of cases the dilated loops are filled with fluid and can be mistaken for a soft tissue mass on x ray. The dilated loops have a tubular or round echo-free appearance. In adynamic ileus the dilated bowel has normal to somewhat increased peristaltic activity and less distention than with dynamic ileus. In dynamic ileus the loops are round with minimal deformity at the interfaces with adjacent loops of distended bowel; valvulae conniventes and peristalsis are seen. The fluid loops are not always associated with obstruction; they can occur with gastroenteritis and paralytic ileus (Fig. 8-13). The sonographer should demonstrate pliability and compressibility of bowel wall (Fig. 8-14).

Closed-loop obstruction or volvulus. With volvulus the involved loop is doubled back on itself abruptly, so that a U appearance is seen on sagittal scan and a C-shaped anechoic area with a dense center is seen on a transverse scan; the dense center represents medial bowel wall and mesentery.

Abnormalities of the Appendix

Acute appendicitis. Acute appendicitis is the result of luminal obstruction and inflammation, leading to ischemia of the vermiform appendix. This may produce necrosis, perforation, and subsequent abscess formation and peritonitis.[4] The appendix lumen may be obstructed by fecal material, a foreign body, carcinoma of the cecum, stenosis, inflammation, kinking of the organ, or even lymphatic hypertrophy resulting from systemic infection.[3,14] Obstruction results in edema, which can compromise the vascular supply to the appendix. Subsequently, the permeability of the mucosa increases and bacterial invasion of the wall of the appendix results in infection and inflammation.[4] The increased intraluminal pressure may cause occlusion of the appendicular end artery.[9] If the condition persists, the appendix may necrose, leading to gangrene, rupture, and subsequent local or generalized peritonitis. Periappendiceal abscess or peritonitis does not necessarily mean perforation; the organism may permeate the wall in the absence of perforation to cause these extraappendiceal complications.

The symptoms of acute appendicitis are pain and rebound tenderness, which is usually localized over McBurney's point. Typically, the pain is followed by nausea and vomiting, anorexia, diarrhea, and systemic signs of inflammation, such as leukocytosis and fever.[4] Acute appendicitis can occur at any age, but it is more prevalent at younger ages. Diagnosis of even the classic case of appendicitis is complicated by the fact that many disorders present with a similar clinical picture of an acute abdomen.[1] Differential diagnosis may include the following: (1) acute gastroenteritis; (2) mesenteric lymphadenitis in children; (3) ruptured ectopic pregnancy; (4) Mittelschmerz; (5) inflammation of Meckel's diverticulum; (6) regional enteritis; and (7) right ovarian torsion. Progression of acute appendicitis to frank perforation is more rapid in the younger child, sometimes occurring within 6 to 12 hours. The rate of perforation in the preschool child can be as high as 70%, compared with the overall figure of 30% for children and 21% to 22% for adults.[5] Women in the age range of 20 to 40 years are at high risk of being misdiagnosed on initial physical examination.[11]

Acute appendicitis is one of the most frequent causes of abdominal surgery in nearly all age groups. Abdominal ultrasound has proven to be useful in diagnosing acute appendicitis and its complications. Before high-resolution sonography, no noninvasive imaging technique was available to enable direct visualization of the inflamed vermiform appendix.[11] Barium enema examination traditionally has been

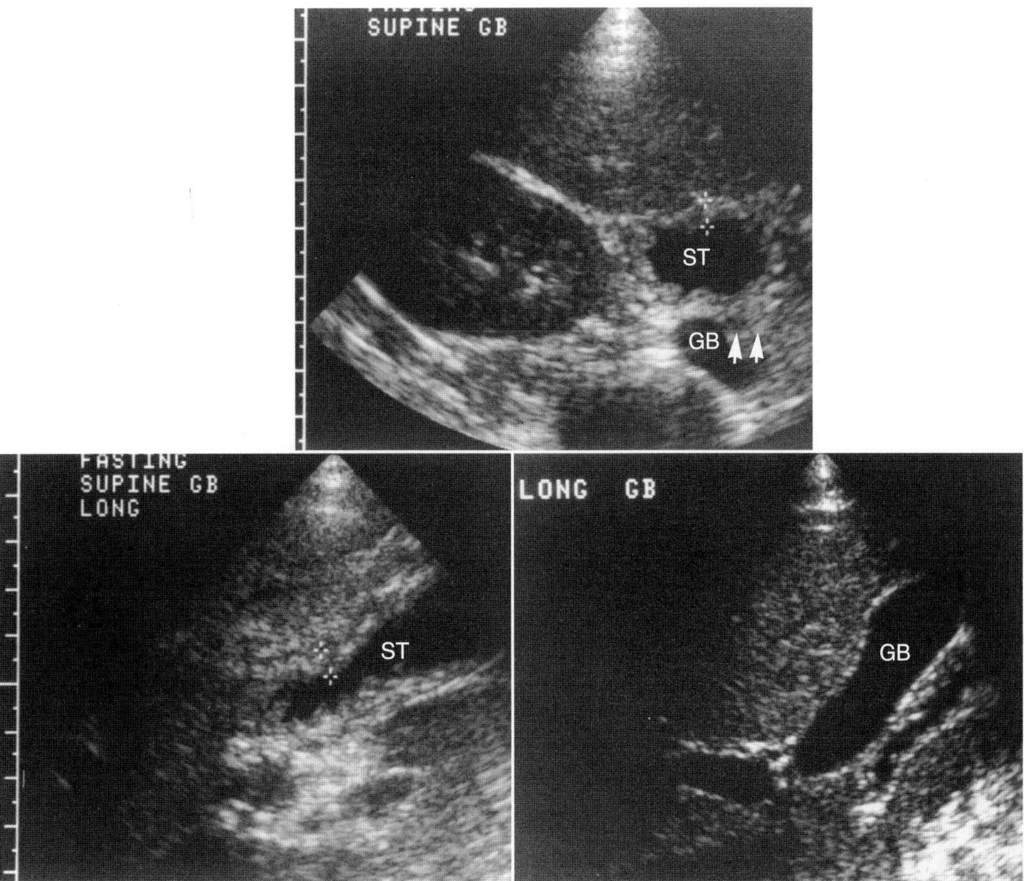

FIG. 8-13 This young patient presented with right upper quadrant pain and nausea. The collection anterior to the gallbladder, *GB*, was originally thought to be a thick-walled gallbladder. However, with real-time observation and fluid ingestion, the stomach was found to be filled and clearly separate from the gallbladder.

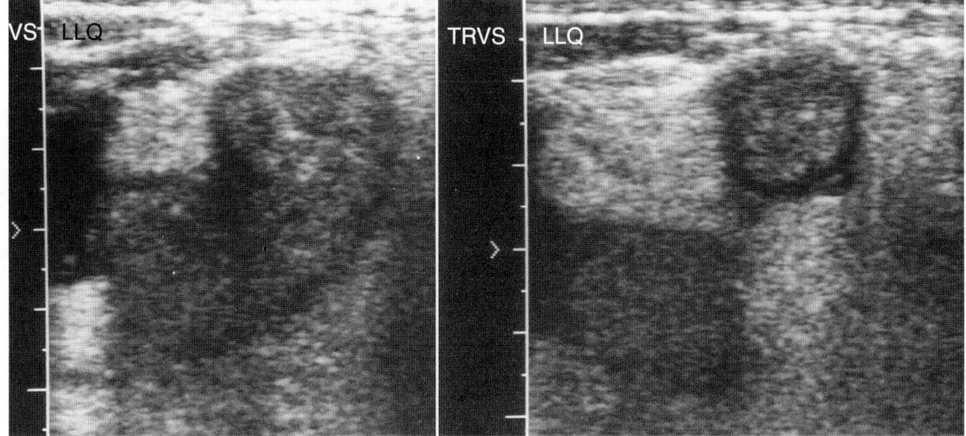

FIG. 8-14 A 17-year-old male with cystic fibrosis with meconium ileus equivalent. He was sent to ultrasound to rule out abscess. A large hyperechoic structure was seen just to the left of the umbilicus in the region of the palpable abnormality. This probably represents a bowel loop with inspissated stool.

used to aid diagnosis, but the appendix does not fill with barium in 15% of patients.[12]

The normal appendix can occasionally be visualized by graded compression sonography. The maximal outer diameters of the normal appendix can measure up to 6 mm.[7] Abu-Yosef et al. noted that the wall of the inflamed appendix is greater than 2 mm thick and also proposed diagnosis of perforation when asymmetric wall thickening was seen.[15] In inflamed specimens, both the integrity and the stratification of wall layers were altered. The distinction of layers is impaired and each layer sonographically inhomogeneous. Only the sum of the two opposite wall measurements shows a statistical increase in thickness. The sum of the wall thickness in vitro may be similar to measurements of the overall appendix thickness when gentle external compression is applied.

Wall appearance should not be the only criteria for confirmation of appendicitis.[13] The ultrasound pattern of acute appendicitis is characterized by a so-called targetlike appearance of the appendix in transverse view.[7,11] Views of the appendix in the transverse plane should demonstrate a thickened muscular wall and increased appendiceal diameter (Fig. 8-15).[15] The typical target lesion consists of a hypoechoic, fluid-distended lumen, a hyperechoic inner ring representing mainly the mucosa and submucosa, and an outer hypoechoic ring representing the muscularis externa. The inflamed appendix is further characterized by a lack of peristalsis and compressibility and demonstration of its blind end tip.[10] It is important to carefully survey the entire length of the appendix to avoid a false-negative examination.

Retrocecal appendicitis represents approximately 28% of pediatric appendicitis patients. Retrocecal appendicitis is easy to diagnose by ultrasound. There are no bowel loops interposed between the appendix and the lateral wall of the abdomen. The inflamed appendix is identified on cross sections as a target image underneath the abdominis muscle. The incidence of complex masses is greater in retrocecal appendicitis, reflecting a higher incidence of perforation. The sonographic appearance of an appendiceal abscess is a complex mass. Sometimes you can recognize the appendix inside the mass. The omentum wrapping the appendix is in the form of an echogenic band and some bowel loops.[1]

The initial inflammatory changes in appendicitis are more pronounced in the distal half of the appendix and may be focally confined to the appendiceal tip. Ulcerations and necrosis may cause loss of the echogenic submucosal layer in the tip of the appendix. The appendix should be compressed to the tip and visualized longitudinally and transversely to its blind termination. Appendicoliths or calculi are seen as intraluminal foci of high-amplitude echoes with acoustic shadowing.[5]

In infancy and childhood the appendix frequently becomes decompressed after perforation and the inflammatory process may not wall off or form a well-defined abscess, as is typically seen in adults. With perforation and decompression and an abnormally thickened wall, a collapsed appendix may still be identified. In some patients, however, no appendix may be found and only questionable remnants remain. Supplemental findings, such as free abdominal fluid with debris or thickening of the adjacent abdominal wall, may suggest the diagnosis. However, the possibility of appendicitis cannot be ruled out even in a patient who lacks an abnormal appendix or a well-defined abscess. Radiographic contrast studies may help diagnosis.[9]

Gas collections within the appendix may be a pitfall in ultrasound diagnosis. Gas within the appendix is diagnosed on the basis of sonographic findings of high-amplitude echogenic foci, causing either distal reverberation artifacts (i.e., comet-tails or dirty acoustic shadowing). Although this is a relatively rare finding, its importance lies in the fact that it may be misconstrued as either a normal bowel

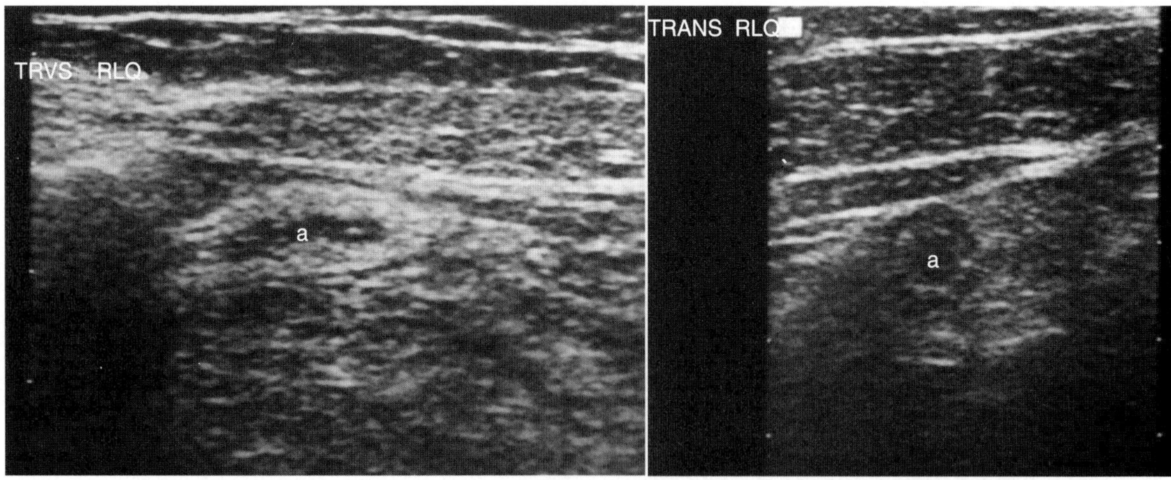

FIG. 8-15 Longitudinal and transverse scans of a thick-walled appendix that does not collapse with compression.

loop or a gas-forming appendiceal abscess. Gas collections from within the bowel loops should be distinguished from an inflamed appendix. The inflamed appendix is noncompressible and demonstrates other specific anatomic features.[14]

Graded compression ultrasound is an alternate technique for diagnosing appendicitis; it has a sensitivity of 88% and a specificity of 96%. Color Doppler ultrasound can be used to detect increased flow, demonstrating hyperperfusion associated with inflammation. Vessels can be seen coursing through the periphery of the dilated appendix. Addition of color Doppler alone did not increase the sensitivity for detecting appendicitis compared with ultrasound alone. Color Doppler is a simple means of confirming the gray-scale ultrasound findings.

Mucocele. Mucocele of the appendix is a rare pathologic entity.[6] This term designates gross enlargement of the appendix from accumulation of mucoid substance within the lumen. It was recognized in 0.2% to 0.3% of 45,000 appendectomies.[8] Scarring or fecalith after an appendectomy is the most common cause of mucocele,[5] although proximal obstruction of the lumen by inflammatory fibrosis, cecal carcinoma, carcinoid polyp, and even endometriosis have been reported.[5,7] More recently, mucoceles have been classified into three distinct entities: mucosal hyperplasia, an innocuous hyperplastic process; mucinous cystadenoma, a benign neoplasm; and mucinous cystoadenocarcinoma, a malignant tumor.[6]

There are several classifications of mucoceles. If the tumor remains encapsulated and there are no malignant cells, this lesion could be called a *mucocele*. If the mucus spreads through the abdominal cavity without evidence of malignant cells, this condition is called *pseudomyxoma peritonei*. The pseudomyxoma assumes a malignant potential only when epithelial cells occur within the gelatinous peritoneal fluid in association with carcinoma.[5]

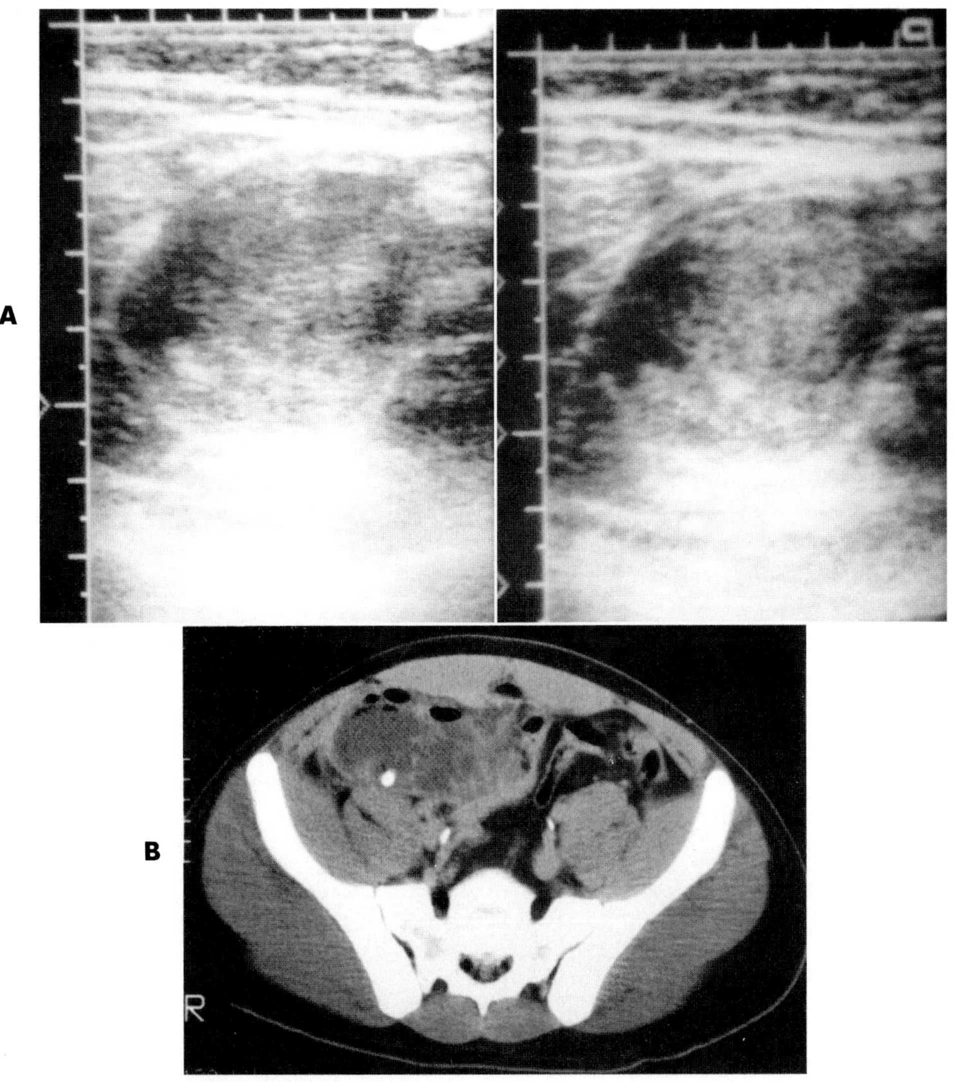

FIG. 8-16 A, Ultrasound of a mucocele. This patient shows a complex mass with high-level echoes. **B,** CT of the mucocele.

Appendiceal mucoceles reportedly show a female-to-male predominance of four to one with an average age at presentation of 55 years.[6,8] The most common clinical complaint is right lower quadrant pain.[6] About 25% are asymptomatic.[6,7] Other known symptoms are right iliac fossa mass, sepsis, and urinary symptoms.[8] Bloating of the abdomen is specific to patients with pseudomyxoma peritonei. Laboratory values show an increased erythrocyte sedimentation rate and an elevated leukocyte count. Also, elevated levels of carcinoembryonic antigen have been reported.[8] Pseudomyxoma peritonei significantly decreases survival of patients with appendiceal cystadenocarcinomas.[6,8]

Preoperative diagnosis of mucocele is helpful. If a mucocele is suspected, needle aspiration is not advised. Careful mobilization surgically may reduce the possibility of rupture, peritoneal contamination, and development of pseudomyxoma peritonei.[6-8] Radiographically, a mucocele is seen as a soft-tissue mass, with typically a rimlike, curvilinear calcification of the mucocele wall.[6,8] A barium enema examination classically describes nonfilling of the appendix and an extrinsic or submucosal mass at the cecal tip with intact overlying mucosa.[6] CT appearance varies. The contents of the cystic mass, with or without calcifications or septations, range from near-water attenuation to soft-tissue attenuation, depending on the presence of mucin or debris within the mucocele.[6] On CT, anteriorly situated septated ascites and scalloping of the liver are two criteria specific for pseudomyxoma peritonei.[8] On ultrasound the examiner should locate the appendix in the right lower quadrant, using the psoas muscle and iliac vessels.

Ultrasound varies according to the content of the mucocele, which may be anechoic when mucoid material is more fluid.[2] The following patterns have been defined: (1) a purely cystic lesion with anechoic fluid; (2) a hypoechoic mass containing fine internal echo; and (3) a complex mass with high-level echoes (Fig. 8-16).[6] As it enlarges, inspissation of the mucoid material creates this internal echo pattern.[7] This mass has an irregular inner wall caused by mucinous debris with varying degrees of epithelial hyperplasia.[5] Calcification of the rim can produce acoustic shadowing.[7] Internal, thin septations have been seen, as well as variable degrees of mucosal atrophy and ulceration.[6]

Pseudomyxoma peritonei is seen as septated ascites with numerous suspended echoes that do not mobilize as the patient changes position.[8] Combined with ultrasound, paracentesis may accurately establish the diagnosis of gelatinous ascites.

Meckel's diverticulitis

Meckel's diverticulitis is located on the antimesenteric border of the ileum approximately 2 ft from the ileocecal valve. It is present in 2% of the population. Adults may present with intestinal obstruction, rectal bleeding, or diverticular inflammation. Acute appendicitus and acute Meckel's diverticulum may not be distinguished clinically. The wall of Meckel's diverticulum is composed of

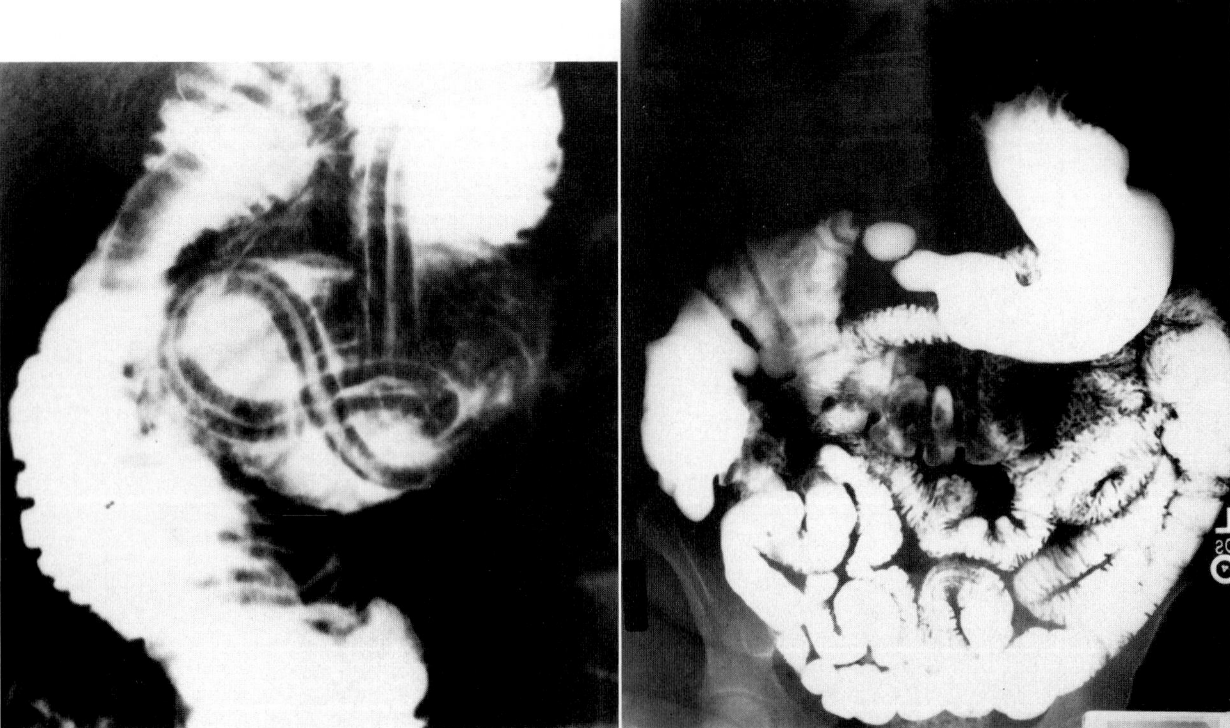

FIG. 8-17 Barium studies of the stomach, small bowel, and colon show filling defects secondary to ascaris.

mucosal, muscular, and serosal layers. Noncompressibility of the obstructed inflamed diverticulum indicates that the intraluminal fluid is trapped. The area of maximum tenderness is evaluated with its distance from the cecum.

Crohn's disease

Crohn's disease is regional enteritis, a recurrent granulomatous inflammatory disease that affects the terminal ileum, colon, or both at any level. The reaction involves the entire thickness of the bowel wall. Clinical symptoms include diarrhea, fever, and right lower quadrant pain. On ultrasound a symmetrically swollen bowel target pattern with preserved parietal layers around the stenotic and hyperdense lumen is seen. The findings are most prominent in ileocolonic disease, with uniformly increased wall thickness involving all layers, but especially the mucosa and submucosa. A matted-loop pattern is found in the late states. Patients with Crohn's disease show rigidity to pressure exerted with the transducer. Peristalsis is absent or sluggish (Fig. 8-17).

Tumors

Lymphoma. Lymphoma is a tumor that usually occurs late in life, near the sixth decade; it is also the most common tumor of the gastrointestinal tract in children under 10 years of age. The intraperitoneal masses frequently involve the mesenteric vessels that encase them. Clinical signs include intestinal blood loss, weight loss, anorexia, and abdominal pain. The patient may have an intestinal obstruction or palpable mass. On ultrasound the sonographer may see a large discrete mass with a target pattern, an exoenteric pattern with a large mass on the mesenteric surface of bowel, and small anechoic mass representing subserosal nodes or mesenteric nodal involvement.

Lymphomatous involvement of the intestinal wall may lead to pseudokidney or hydronephrotic pseudokidney. The lumen may be dilated with fluid with a lack of peristalsis. The bowel wall is uniformly thickened, with homogeneous low echogenicity between the well-defined mucosal and serosal surfaces that contain a persistent, echo-free, wide, and long lumen.

Leiomyosarcoma. Leiomyosarcoma represents 10% of primary small bowel tumors. Approximately 10% to 30% of these occur in the duodenum, 30% to 45% in the jejunum, and 35% to 55% in the ileum. The patients are in their fifth to sixth decades of life. On ultrasound a large solid mass containing necrotic areas anterior to solid viscus may be found.

REVIEW QUESTIONS

1. What effect do the stomach, small bowel, and colon have on the ultrasound beam?
2. Describe the technique frequently used to image the gastrointestinal tract.
3. What is the esophagogastric junction and how does it present on the ultrasound image?
4. How does the gastric antrum appear on sonography?
5. Describe the technique used to rule out a cystic mass in the left upper quadrant. What would your differential diagnosis be?
6. Describe the four divisions of the duodenum.
7. How can the sonographer determine if the fluid-filled structure is small bowel or a mass lesion?
8. What is the keyboard sign?
9. Where is the appendix located and how does it appear on ultrasound?
10. How can a water enema help define colon lesions?
11. Define the five layers of the colon.
12. What is the ultrasound appearance of a duplication cyst?
13. What is a gastric bezoar? How would it present on ultrasound?
14. Describe the most common tumor of the stomach and its appearance on ultrasound.
15. What are some of the gastric malignant tumors found by ultrasound and their characteristic appearance?
16. How would the sonographer determine if a lower gastrointestinal tract is obstructed?
17. What are the clinical symptoms of appendicitis?
18. Describe the ultrasound technique for evaluating a patient with suspected appendicitis.
19. Describe the pseudokidney sign.
20. What are some of the lower gastrointestinal tumors found by ultrasound?

REFERENCES

1. Ceres L, Alonso I, Lopez P, et al: Ultrasound study of acute appendicitis in children with emphasis upon the diagnosis of retrocecal appendicitis, Pediatr Radiol 20:258, 1990.
2. Dubbins PA: Ultrasound demonstration of bowel wall thickness in inflammatory bowel disease, Clin Radiol 35:227, 1984.
3. Gray HFRS: Anatomy: descriptive and surgical, pp. 722-923, London, 1989, Crown.
4. Groer M and Shekelton M: Basic pathophysiology: a conceptual approach, pp. 360-361, St Louis, 1979, Mosby.
5. Hayden K, Kuchelmeister J, and Lipscomb T: Sonography of acute appendicitis in childhood: perforation versus nonperforation, J Ultrasound Med 11:209, 1992.
6. Landen S, Bertrand C, Maddern GJ, et al: Appendiceal mucoceles and pseudomyxoma peritonei, Surg Gynecol Obstet 175:401, 1992.
7. Macek D, Jafri SZ, and Madrazo BL: Ultrasound case of the day: mucocele of the appendix, Radiographics 12:1247, 1992.
8. Mittelstaedt C: Abdominal ultrasound. New York, 1987, Churchill Livingstone.
9. Poljak A, Jeffrey RB Jr, and Kernberg ME: The gas-

containing appendix: potential sonographic pitfall in the diagnosis of acute appendicitis, J Ultrasound Med 10:625, 1991.
10. Price S and Wilson L: Pathophysiology and clinical concepts of disease processes, pp. 240-241. New York, 1982, McGraw-Hill.
11. Quillin SP and Siegel MJ: Appendicitis in children: color Doppler sonography, Radiology 184:745, 1992.
12. Schwerk WB, Wichtrup B, Rothmund M, and Ruschoff J: Ultrasonography in the diagnosis of acute appendicitis: a prospective study, Gastroenterol 97:630, 1989.
13. Sivit CJ, Newman KD, Boenning DA, et al: Appendicitis: usefulness of ultrasound in the diagnosis in a pediatric population, Radiology 185:549, 1992.
14. Spear R, Kimmey MB, Wang KY, et al: Appendiceal ultrasound scans: histologic correlation, Radiology 183:831, 1992.
15. Tortora G and Anagnostakes N: Principles of anatomy and physiology, pp. 632-633. New York, 1981, Harper & Row.

BIBLIOGRAPHY

Abu Ziden FM, al-Hilaly MA, and a-Atrabi N: Torsion of a mucocele of the appendix in a pregnant woman, Acta Obstet Gynecol Scand 71:140, 1992.

Abu-Yousef MM: Sonography of the right iliac fossa, Ultrasound Q 8:73, 1990.

Bidula MM, Rifkin MD, and McCoy RI: Ultrasonography of gastric phytobezoar, J Clin Ultrasound 14:49, 1986.

Borushok KF, Jeffrey RB Jr, Laing FC, et al: Sonographic diagnosis of perforation in patients with acute appendicitis, Am J Roentgenol 154:275, 1990.

Derchi LE, Bandereali A, Bossi MC, et al: Sonographic appearance of gastric lymphoma, J Ultrasound Med 3:251, 1984.

DiCandio G, Mosca F, Campatelli A, et al: Sonographic detection of postsurgical recurrence of Crohn's disease, Am J Roentgenol 146:523, 1986.

Fakhry JR and Berk RN: The "target" pattern: characteristic sonographic features of stomach and bowel abnormalities, Am J Roentgenol 137:969, 1981.

Frager DH, Frager JD, Brandt LJ, et al: Gastrointestinal complications of AIDS: radiologic features, Radiology 158:597, 1986.

Gaensler EHL, Jeffrey RB Jr, Laing FC, et al: Sonography in patients with suspected acute appendicitis: value in establishing alternative diagnoses, Am J Roentgenol 152:49, 1989.

Jeffrey RB Jr, Laing FC, and Lewis FR: Acute appendicitis: high-resolution real-time ultrasound findings, Radiology 163:11, 1987.

Jeffrey RB Jr, Laing FC, and Townsend RR: Acute appendicitis: sonographic criteria based on 250 cases, Radiology 67:327, 1988.

Kaftori JK, Aharon M, and Kleinhaus U: Sonographic features of gastrointestinal leiomyosarcoma, J Clin Ultrasound 9:11, 1981.

Kimmey MB, Martin RW, Haggitt RC, et al: Histologic correlates of gastrointestinal ultrasound images, Gastroenterology 96:433, 1989.

Lee DH, Lim JH, Ko YT, et al: Sonographic detection of pneumoperitoneum in patients with acute abdomen, Am J Roentgenol 154:107, 1990.

Limberg B: Diagnosis of inflammatory and neoplastic large bowel diseases by conventional abdominal and colonic sonography, Ultrasound Q 6:151, 1988.

Limberg B: Sonographic features of colonic Crohn's disease: comparison of in vivo and in vitro studies, J Clin Ultrasound 18:161, 1990.

Maglinte DDT, Lappas JC, and NG AC: Sonography of Boveret's syndrome, J Ultrasound Med 6:675, 1987.

Malpani A, Ramani SK, and Wolverson MK: Role of sonography in trichobezoars, J Ultrasound Med 7:661, 1988.

Mittelstaedt CA: Gastrointestinal tract. In Mittelstaedt CA: General ultrasound, pp. 449-588. New York, Churchill Livingstone, 1992.

Miyamoto Y, Tsujimoto F, and Tada S: Ultrasonographic diagnosis of submucosal tumors of the stomach: the "bridging layers" sign, J Clin Ultrasound 16:251, 1988.

Nghiem HV and Jeffrey RB Jr: Acute appendicitis confined to the appendiceal tip: evaluation with graded compression sonography, J Ultrasound Med 11:205, 1992.

Peterson LR and Cooperberg PL: Ultrasound demonstration of lesions of the gastrointestinal tract, Gastrointest Radiol 3:303, 1978.

Puylaert JBCM: Acute appendicitis: ultrasound evaluation using graded compression, Radiology 158:355, 1986.

Rubesin SE and Levine MS: Omental cakes: colonic involvement by omental metastases, Radiology 54:593, 1985.

Seibert JJ, Williamson SL, Golladay ES, et al: The distended gasless abdomen: a fertile field for ultrasound, J Ultrasound Med 5:301, 1986.

Seitz K and Rettenmaier G: Inflammatory bowel disease. In Pharma F: Sonographic diagnostics. West Germany: GmbH, 1988.

Shirahama M, Morita SI, Koga T, et al: Gastrointestinal amyloidosis associated with multiple myeloma: sonographic features, J Clin Ultrasound 19:493, 1991.

Siegel MJ: Acute appendicitis in childhood: the role of ultrasound, Radiology 185:341, 1992.

Telerman A, Gerend B, Van der Heul B, et al: Gastrointestinal metastases from extra-abdominal tumors, Endoscopy 17:99, 1985.

Tennenhouse JE and Wilson SR: Sonographic detection of a small bowel bezoar, J Ultrasound Med 9:603, 1990.

Wilson SR and Toi A: The value of sonography in the diagnosis of acute diverticulitis of the colon, Am J Roentgenol 154:1199, 1990.

Worlicek H, Dunz H, and Engelhard K: Ultrasonic examination of the wall of the fluid-filled stomach, J Clin Ultrasound 17:5, 1989.

Worlicek H, Lutz H, Heyder N, et al: Ultrasound findings in Crohn's disease and ulcerative colitis: a prospective study, J Clin Ultrasound 15:153, 1987.

Worrell JA, Drolshagen LF, Kelly TC, et al: Graded compression ultrasound in the diagnosis of appendicitis: a comparison of diagnostic criteria, J Ultrasound Med 9:145, 1990.

Wright LL, Baker KR, and Meny RG: Ultrasound demonstration of gastroesophageal reflux, J Ultrasound Med 7:471, 1988.

CHAPTER 9

Urinary System

Sandra L. Hagen-Ansert

The urinary system has two principal functions: excreting wastes and regulating the composition of blood. Blood composition must not be allowed to vary beyond tolerable limits or the conditions in tissues necessary for cellular life will be lost. Regulating blood composition involves not only removing harmful wastes but conserving water and metabolites in the body.

The urinary system is composed of two large kidneys, which remove wastes from the blood and produce urine, and two ureters, which act as tubal ducts leading from the hilus of the kidneys that drain into the urinary bladder. The bladder collects and stores urine, which is eventually discharged through the urethra. The urinary system is located behind the peritoneum lining the abdominal cavity in an area called the *retroperitoneum.*

Evaluating the kidneys with ultrasound is a noninvasive approach to diagnosing renal problems. Generally sonography is used after an intravenous pyelogram has disclosed the need to investigate the acoustic properties of a mass or to further delineate an abnormal lie of the kidney resulting from an extrarenal mass or other renal anomaly. In patients who cannot tolerate an intravenous pyelogram because of an allergic reaction or some other reason, sonography may be selected as the examination of choice to rule out renal disease.

In addition to delineating a renal mass, ultrasound can define perirenal fluid collections such as a hematoma or abscess, determine renal size and parenchymal detail, detect enlarged ureters and hydronephrosis, as well as image renal congenital anomalies.

The function of the kidney is to excrete urine. More than any other organ, the kidneys adjust the amounts of water and electrolytes leaving the body so that these equal the amounts of substances entering the body.

EXCRETION

Cells in the body continually carry on metabolic activities that produce waste products. If permitted to accumulate, metabolic wastes eventually reach toxic concentrations and threaten homeostasis. To prevent this, metabolic wastes must be quickly excreted. The process of excretion entails separating and removing substances harmful to the body. Excretion is carried out by the skin, lungs, liver, large intestine, and kidneys.

The principal metabolic waste products are water, carbon dioxide, and nitrogenous wastes (including urea, uric acid, and creatinine). Nitrogen is derived from amino acids and nucleic acids. Amino acids break down in the liver, and the nitrogen-containing amino group is removed. The amino group is then converted to ammonia, which is chemically converted to urea. Uric acid is formed from the breakdown of nucleic acids. Both urea and uric acid are carried away from the liver into the kidneys by the vascular system. Creatinine is a nitrogenous waste produced from phosphocreatine in the muscles.

Anatomy of the Kidneys

The kidneys lie in the retroperitoneal cavity near the posterior body wall just below the diaphragm (Fig. 9-1). Both kidneys are protected by the lower ribs. The right kidney lies slightly lower than left kidney because the large right lobe of the liver pushes it inferiorly. With deep inspiration, both kidneys move downward approximately 1 inch.

Both kidneys are dark red, bean-shaped organs that measure 9 to 12 cm long, 5 cm wide, and 2.5 cm thick. The outer cortex of the kidney is darker than the inner medulla because of the increased perfusion of blood. The inner surface of the medulla is folded into projections, called *pyramids,* which empty into the renal pelvis. Numerous collecting tubules bring the urine from its sites of formation in the cortex to the pyramids. The renal tubules, or nephrons, are the functional units of the kidney.

On the medial surface of each kidney is a vertical slit called the *hilus.* Within the hilus of the kidney are found a number of vascular structures, a ureter, and the lymphatics. The renal vein is the most posterior and superior structure. The two branches of the renal artery are anterior to the renal vein (Fig. 9-2). The ureter is located slightly inferior to the renal artery. When present, the third branch of the renal artery may be seen to arise from the hilus. The lymph vessels and sympathetic fibers also are found within the renal hilus.

The kidney is surrounded by a fibrous capsule, called the *true capsule,* that is closely applied to renal cortex. Outside of this fibrous capsule is a covering of perinephric fat.

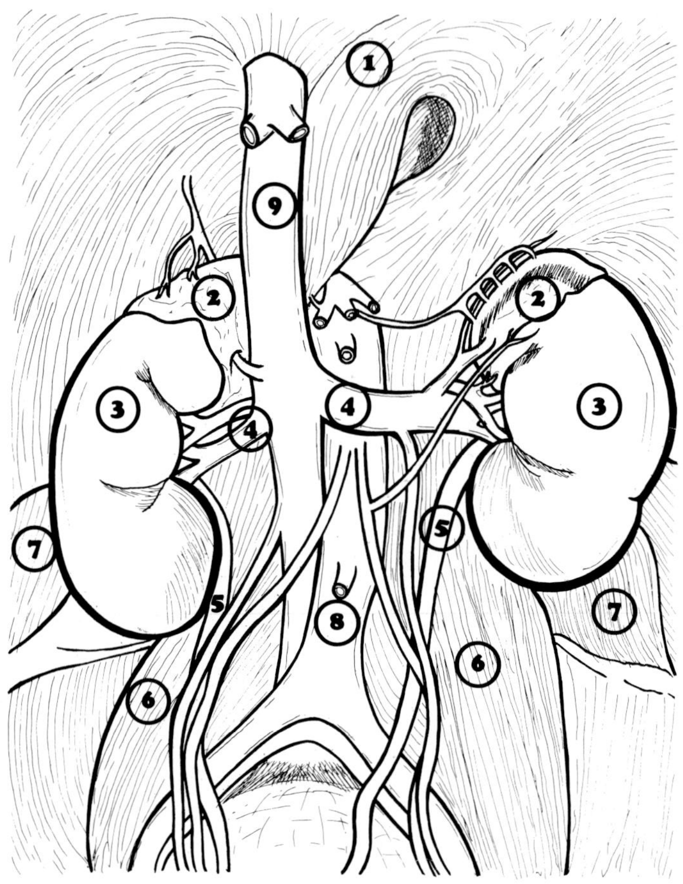

FIG. 9-1 Relationship of the kidneys, suprarenal glands (adrenal), and vascular structures to one another. Diaphragm, *1;* suprarenal gland, *2;* kidney, *3;* renal vein, *4;* ureter, *5;* psoas major muscle, *6;* quadratus lumborum muscle, *7;* aorta, *8;* inferior vena cava, *9.*

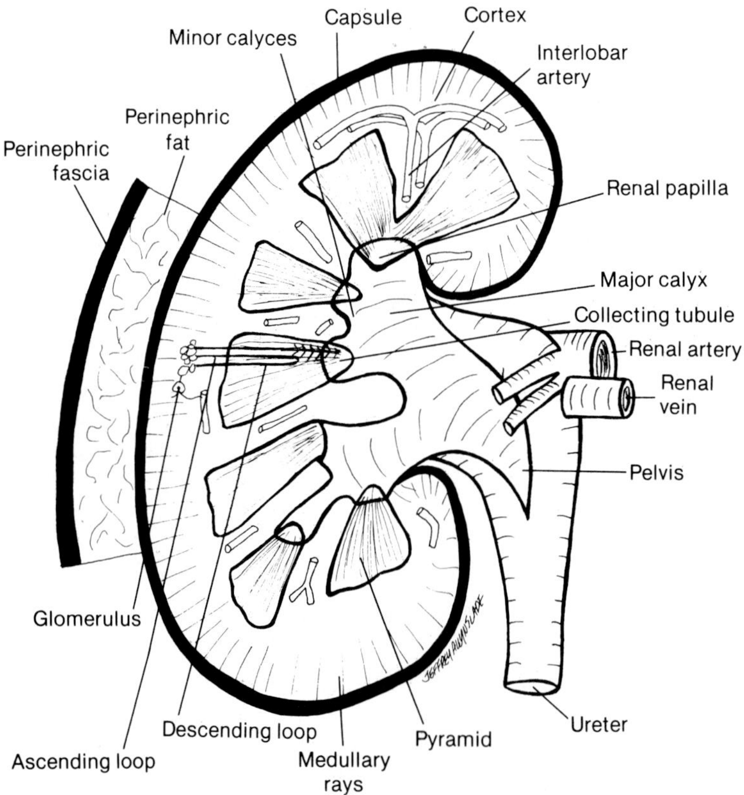

FIG. 9-2 The kidney cut longitudinally to show the internal structure.

The perinephric fascia surrounds the perinephric fat and encloses the kidneys and adrenal glands. The perinephric fascia is a condensation of areolar tissue, which is continuous laterally with the fascia transversalis. The renal fascia, known as *Gerota's fascia,* surrounds the true capsule and perinephric fat.

Relationships

Anterior to the right kidney are the adrenal gland, liver, second part of the duodenum, and the right colic flexure (Fig. 9-3). Anterior to the left kidney are the adrenal gland, spleen, stomach, pancreas, left colic flexure, and coils of jejunum.

Posterior to the right kidney are the diaphragm, costodiaphragmatic recess of the pleura, twelfth rib, psoas muscle, quadratus lumborum, and transversus abdominis muscles. The subcostal (T12), iliohypogastric, and ilioinguinal nerves (L1) run downward and laterally. Posterior to the left kidney are the diaphragm, costodiaphragmatic recess of the pleura, eleventh and twelve ribs, psoas muscle, quadratus lumborum, and transversus abdominis muscles. The same nerves are seen near the left kidney as in the right.

Within the kidney, the upper expanded end of the ureter, known as the *pelvis* of the ureter, divides into two or three major calyces, each of which divides further into two or three minor calyces (see Fig. 9-2). Each minor calyx is indented by the apex of a medullary pyramid called the *renal papilla*. The kidney is composed of an internal medullary portion and an external cortical substance. The medullary substance consists of a series of striated conical masses, called the *renal pyramids,* which vary from 8 to 18 in number, and their bases are directed toward the outer circumference of the kidney. Their apices converge toward the renal sinus, where their prominent papillae project into the lumina of the minor calyces. Spirally arranged muscles surround the calyces and may exert a milking action on these tubes, aiding in the flow of urine into the renal pelvis. As the pelvis leaves the renal sinus, it rapidly becomes smaller and ultimately merges with the ureter.

Vascular Supply

The arterial supply to the kidney is through the main renal artery. This vessel is a lateral branch of the aorta and arises just inferior to the superior mesenteric artery (Fig. 9-4). Each artery divides into three branches to enter the hilus of the kidney, two in front and one behind the pelvis of the ureter. The branches of the renal artery may vary in size and number. In most cases the renal artery divides into two primary branches, a larger anterior and a smaller posterior. These arteries break down into smaller segmental arteries, then into interlobar arteries, and finally into tiny arcuate arteries.

Five or six veins join to form the main renal vein. This vein emerges from the renal hilus anterior to the renal artery. The renal vein drains into the lateral walls of the inferior vena cava.

The lymphatic vessels follow the renal artery to the lateral aortic lymph nodes near the origin of the renal artery. Nerves originate in the renal sympathetic plexus and are distributed along the branches of the renal vessels.

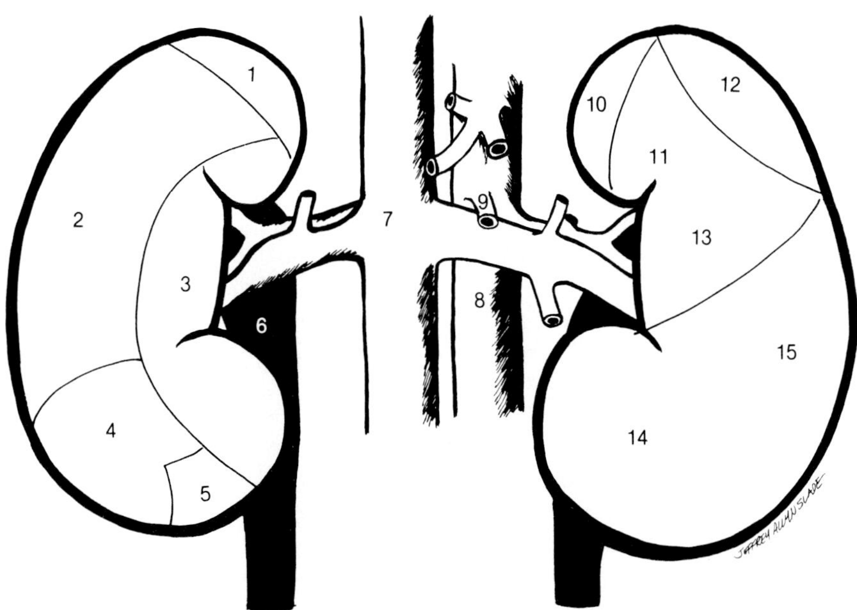

FIG. 9-3 Anatomic structures related to the anterior surfaces of the kidneys. Right adrenal gland, *1;* liver, *2;* duodenum, *3;* right colic flexure, *4;* small intestine, *5;* ureter, *6;* inferior vena cava, *7;* aorta, *8;* superior mesenteric artery, *9;* left adrenal gland, *10;* stomach, *11;* spleen, *12;* pancreas, *13;* jejunum, *14;* descending colon, *15*.

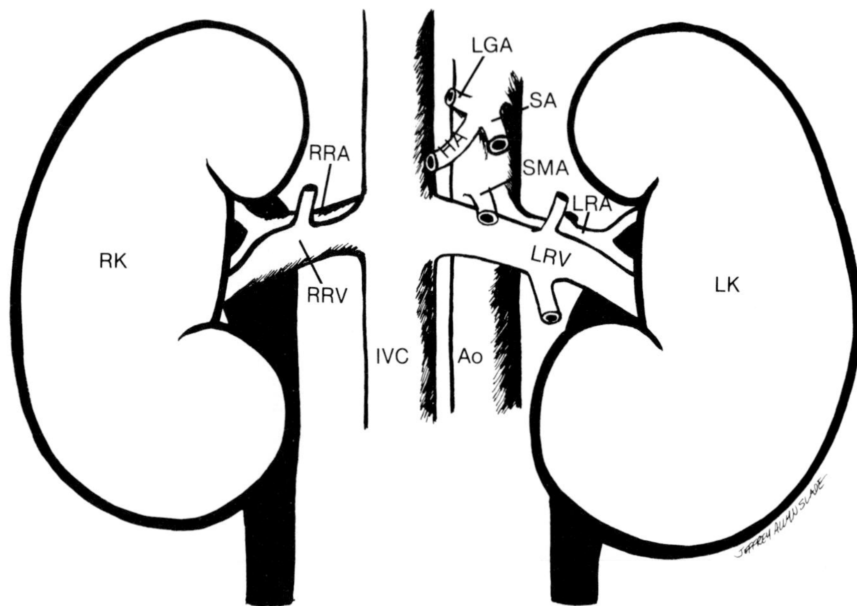

FIG. 9-4 Vascular relationship of the great vessels and their tributaries to the kidneys. Aorta, *Ao;* inferior vena cava, *IVC;* right renal vein, *RRV:* right renal artery, *RRA;* left renal vein, *LRV,* left renal artery, *LRA;* superior mesenteric artery, *SMA;* splenic artery, *SA;* hepatic artery, *HA;* left gastric artery, *LGA*.

Nephron

A nephron consists of two main structures—a renal corpuscle and a renal tubule. Nephrons filter the blood and produce urine. Blood is filtered in the renal corpuscle. The filtered fluid passes through the renal tubule. As the filtrate moves through the tubule, substances needed by the body are returned to the blood. Waste products, excess water, and other substances not needed by the body pass into the collecting ducts as urine.

The renal corpuscle consists of a network of capillaries, called the *glomerulus,* which is surrounded by a cuplike structure known as *Bowman's capsule*. Blood flows into the glomerulus through a small afferent arteriole and leaves the glomerulus through an efferent arteriole. This arteriole conducts blood to a second set of capillaries, the peritubular capillaries, which surround the renal tubule.

Bowman's capsule has an opening in its bottom through which filtrate passes into the renal tubule. The first part of the renal tubule is the coiled proximal convoluted tubule. After passing through the proximal convoluted tubule, filtrate flows into the loop of Henle and then into the distal convoluted tubule. Urine from the distal convoluted tubules of several nephrons drains into a collecting duct. A portion of the distal convoluted tubule curves upward and contacts the afferent and efferent arterioles. Some cells of the distal convoluted tubule and some cells of the afferent arteriole are modified to form the juxtaglomerular apparatus, a structure that helps regulate blood pressure in the kidney.

The renal corpuscle, the proximal convoluted tubule, and the distal convoluted tubule of each nephron are located within the renal cortex. Loops of Henle dip down into the medulla.

Blood supply to nephrons begins at the renal artery. The artery subdivides within the kidneys, and a small vessel (afferent arteriole) enters Bowman's capsule, where it forms a tuft of capillaries, the glomerulus, which entirely fills the concavity of the capsule. Blood leaves the glomerulus via the efferent arteriole, which subdivides into a network of capillaries that surrounds the proximal and distal tubules and eventually unites as veins, which become the renal vein.

The renal vein returns the cleansed blood to the general circulation. By movements of substances between the nephron and the capillaries of the tubules, the composition of the blood filtrate moving along in the tubules is changed. From the nephrons the fluid moves to collecting tubules and into the ureter, leading to the bladder where urine is stored.

Urine Formation. The formation of urine involves the following three processes: glomerular filtration, tubular reabsorption, and tubular secretion.

Ureter

The ureter is 25 cm long and resembles the esophagus in having the following three constrictions along its course: (1) where the ureter leaves the renal pelvis, (2) where it is kinked as it crosses the pelvic brim, and (3) where it pierces the bladder wall. The pelvis of the ureter is funnel-shaped in its expanded upper end of the ureter. It lies within the hilus of the kidney and receives major calyces.

The ureter emerges from the hilus of the kidney and runs

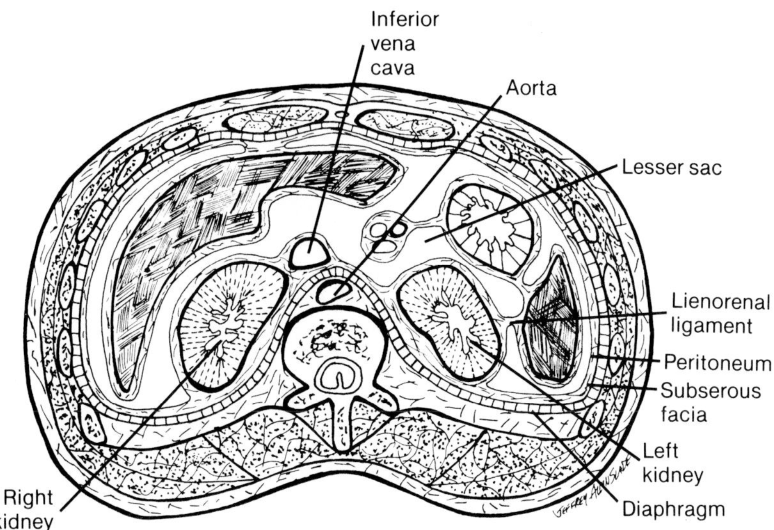

FIG. 9-5 Transverse section of the abdominal cavity through the epiploic foramen.

vertically downward behind the parietal peritoneum along the psoas muscle, which separates it from the tips of the transverse processes of the lumbar vertebrae. It enters the pelvis by crossing the bifurcation of the common iliac artery in front of the sacroiliac joint. The ureter runs along the lateral wall of the pelvis to the region of the ischial spine and turns forward to enter the lateral angle of the bladder. The arterial supply to the ureter is from the following three sources: the renal artery, the testicular or ovarian artery, and the superior vesical artery.

Urinary Bladder

The urinary bladder is a large muscular bag. It has a posterior and lateral opening for the ureters and one anterior opening for the urethra. The interior of bladder is lined with highly elastic transitional epithelium. When the bladder is full, the lining is smooth and stretched; when it is empty, the lining is a series of folds. In the middle layer a series of smooth muscle coats distend as urine collects and contracts to expel urine through the urethra. Urine is produced almost continuously and accumulates in the bladder until the increased pressure stimulates the organ's nervous receptors.

Urethra

The urethra is a membranous tube that passes from the anterior part of the urinary bladder to the outside of the body. There are two sphincters—the internal sphincter and the external sphincter.

SONOGRAPHIC EVALUATION OF THE KIDNEYS

Normal Texture and Patterns

The kidneys are imaged by ultrasound as organs with smooth outer contours surrounded by reflected echoes of perirenal fat. The renal parenchyma surrounds the fatty central renal sinus, which contains the calyces, infundibula, pelvis, vessels, and lymphatics (Fig. 9-5). Because of the fat interface, the renal sinus is imaged as an area of intense echoes with variable contours. If two separate collections of renal sinus fat are identified, a double collecting system should be suspected.

Generally patients are given nothing by mouth before their ultrasound or intravenous program (IVP) examination. This state of dehydration causes the infundibula and renal pelvis to be collapsed and thus indistinguishable from the echo-dense renal sinus fat. If, on the other hand, the bladder is distended from rehydration, the intrarenal collecting system will also become distended.[11] An extrarenal pelvis may be seen as a fluid-filled structure medial to the kidney on transverse scans. Differentiation of the normal variant from obstruction is made by noting the absence of a distended intrasinus portion of the renal pelvis and infundibula.[9] Dilation of the collecting system has also been noted in pregnant patients. (The right kidney is generally involved with a mild degree of hydronephrosis. This distension returns to normal shortly after delivery.)

Patient Position and Technique

The most efficient way to evaluate the kidneys is through the liver for the right kidney (Figs. 9-6 and 9-7) or through the spleen for the left kidney (Fig. 9-8). The patient should be in a supine or decubitus position. The parenchymal echoes of the liver and spleen must be compared with the echo pattern of the renal parenchyma.

A proper adjustment of time gain compensation (TGC) with adequate sensitivity settings allows a uniform acoustic pattern throughout the image. The renal cortical echo amplitude should be compared with the liver parenchymal echo amplitude at the same depth to effectively set the TGC and sensitivity.

If the patient has a significant amount of perirenal fat, a

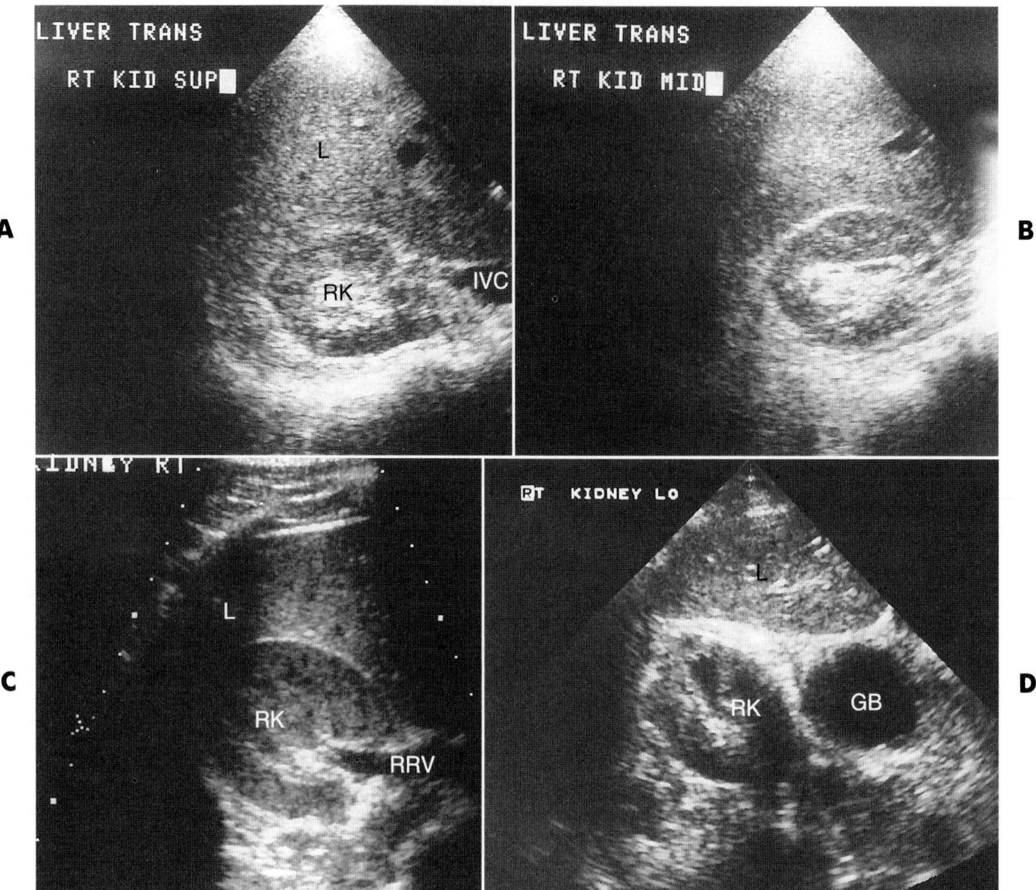

FIG. 9-6 **A** to **C**, Transverse scans of the normal right kidney, *RK*, as imaged through the homogeneous liver parenchyma, *L*. The inferior vena cava, *IVC*, is the medial border of the kidney. Scans are made from the upper pole, midpole to include right renal vein, *RRV*, to the lower pole. **D**, A slight decubitus allows the liver to roll anterior to the right kidney and gallbladder, *GB*, for better visualization.

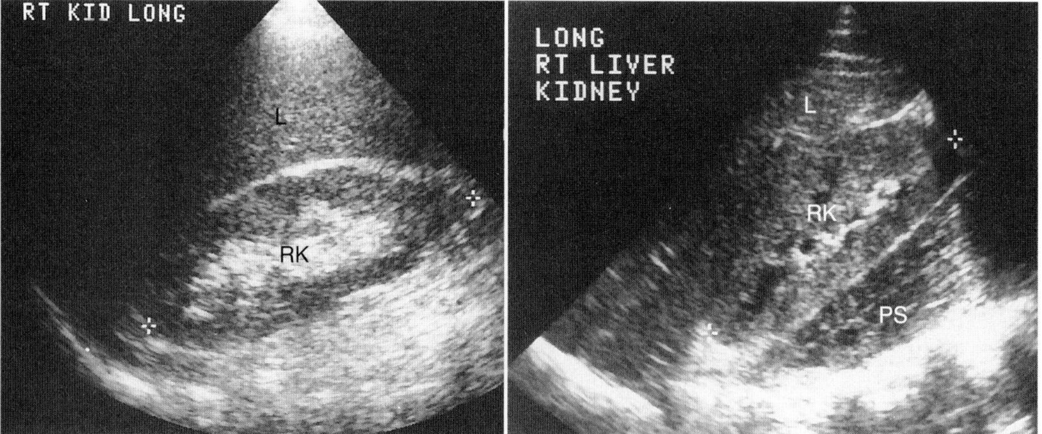

FIG. 9-7 Longitudinal scans through the long axis of the right kidney, *RK*, liver, *L*, and psoas muscle, *Ps*. Measurements are made along the maximum length of the kidney from upper pole to lower pole.

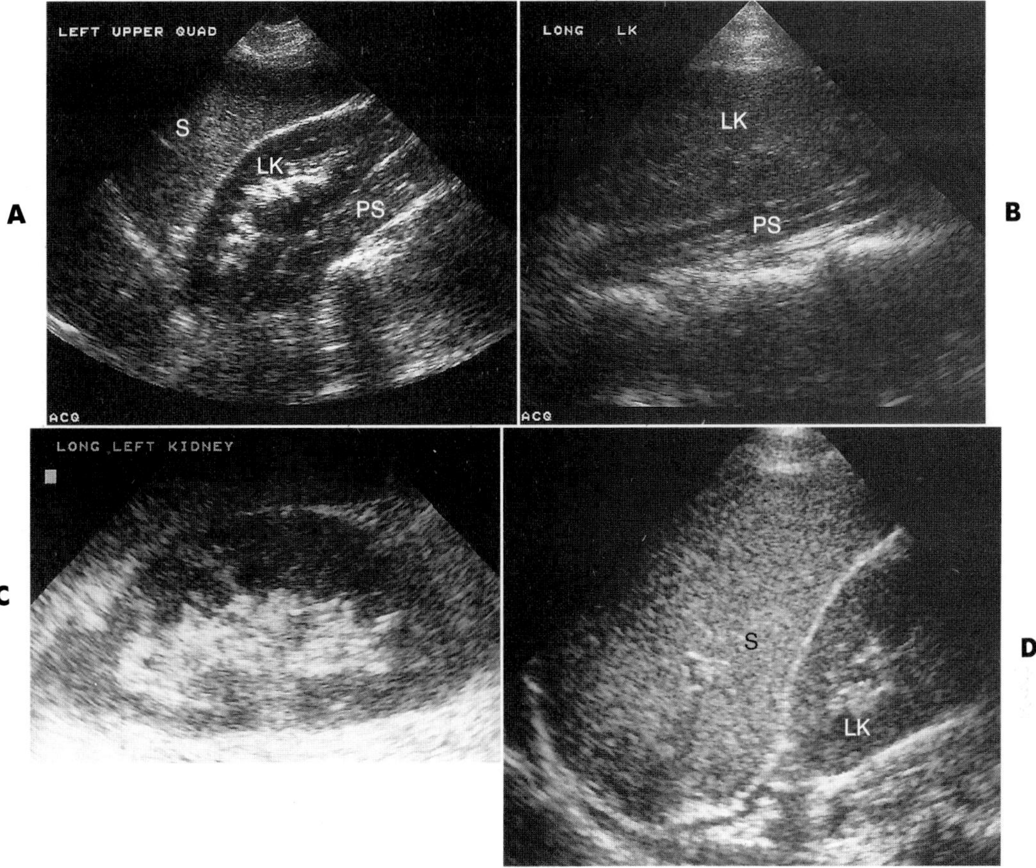

FIG. 9-8 A and **B,** Longitudinal scans of the normal left kidney, *LK*, as imaged through the homogeneous spleen, *S*. The psoas muscle, *Ps*, is the posterior medial border of the kidney. **C,** The patient may be rolled into a right lateral decubitus for better visualization of the renal parenchyma. **D,** Splenomegaly aids in the visualization of the upper pole of the left kidney.

high-frequency transducer may not penetrate the area properly and give the appearance as hypoechoic in the deeper areas of the kidney. Renal detail may also be obscured if the patient has hepatocellular disease, gallstones, rib interference (Fig. 9-9), or other abnormal mass collections between the liver and kidney.

There are several alternate scanning windows to image the kidney. These include the right posterior oblique, the right lateral decubitus, and the left lateral decubitus views.

Renal Parenchyma

The parenchyma is the area from the renal sinus to the outer renal surface (Fig. 9-10). The arcuate and interlobar vessels are found within and are best demonstrated as intense specular echoes in cross section or oblique section at the corticomedullary junction.[13]

The cortex generally is echo producing (Fig. 9-11) (although its echoes are less intense than those from normal liver), whereas the medullary pyramids are echo free (Fig. 9-12). The two are separated from each other by bands of cortical tissue, called *columns of Bertin,* that extend inward to the renal sinus.

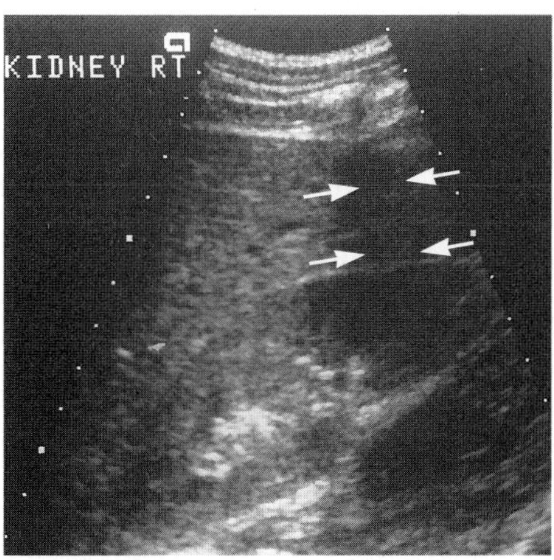

FIG. 9-9 Interference from the ribs may interfere with uniform visualization of the kidney. Variations in respiration help the sonographer find the best window to image the renal parenchyma without rib interference.

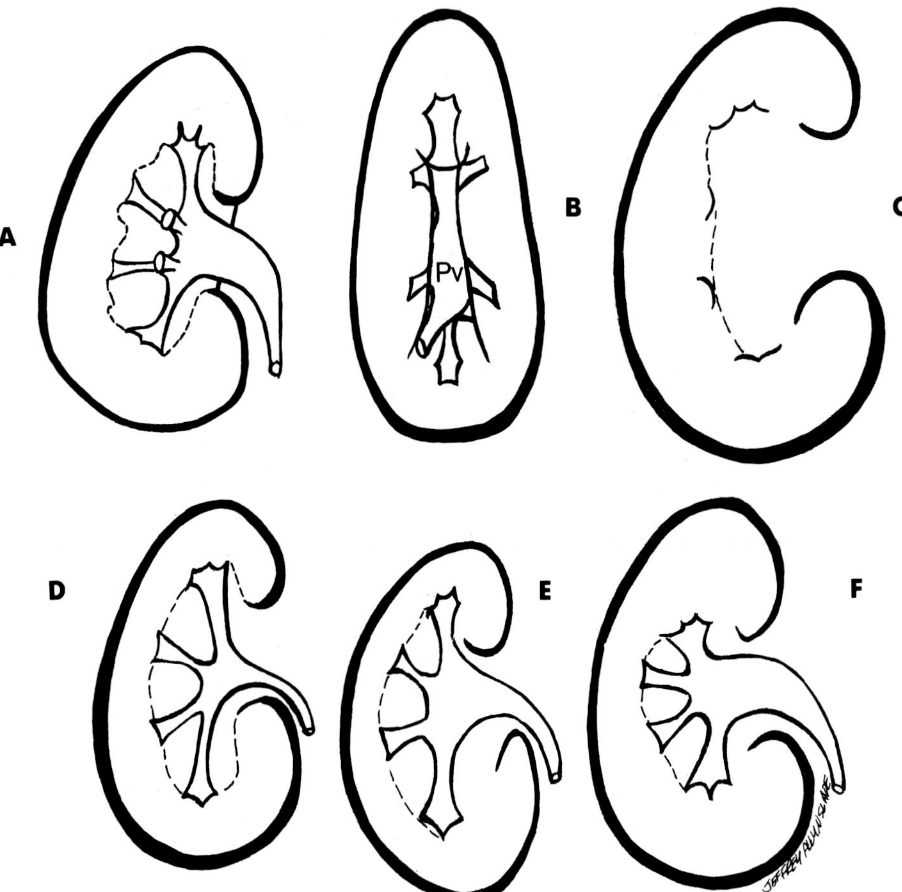

FIG. 9-10. Thickness of the renal substance. **A,** Maximal in the polar regions, medium in the middle zone. **B,** Medial plane showing the pelvis, *PV,* emerging through the hilum and minimal thickness anteriorly and posteriorly. **C,** Hypertrophy. **D,** Normal adult proportions of the renal substance. **E,** Senile atrophy. **F,** Normal appearance in a 2-year-old child.

Rosenfield et al. divided diseases of the renal parenchyma into those that accentuate cortical echoes but preserve or exaggerate the corticomedullary junction (Type I) and those that distort the normal anatomy, obliterating the corticomedullary differentiation in either a focal or diffuse manner (Type II).[8b]

The criteria for Type I changes were that (1) the echo intensity in the cortex be equal to or greater than that in the adjacent liver or spleen and (2) the echo intensity in the cortex equal that in the adjacent renal sinus. Minor signs would include the loss of identifiable arcuate vessels or the accentuation of corticomedullary definition.

Type II changes can be seen in a focal disruption of normal anatomy with any mass lesion, including cysts, tumors, abscesses, and hematomas.

Renal Vessels

The renal arteries are located on the posterolateral aortic wall (Fig. 9-13). The arteries are best seen with the supine and left lateral decubitus views. The right renal artery extends from the posterior lateral wall of the aorta to enter the central renal sinus (Fig. 9-14). On the longitudinal scan the right renal artery can be seen as a circular structure posterior to the inferior vena cava (Fig. 9-15). The right renal vein extends from the central renal sinus directly into the inferior vena cava (Fig. 9-16). Both vessels appear as tubular structures in the transverse plane.

The renal arteries have an echo-free central lumen with highly echogenic borders that consist of vessel wall and surrounding retroperitoneal fat and connective tissue. They lie posterior to the veins and can be demonstrated with certainty if their junction with the aorta is seen.

The left renal artery flows from the posterior lateral wall of the aorta to the central renal sinus (Fig. 9-17). The left renal vein flows from the central renal sinus, anterior to the aorta, and posterior to the superior mesenteric artery to join the inferior vena cava (Fig. 9-18). It is seen as a tubular structure on the transverse scan.

The diaphragmatic crura run transversely in the paraaortic region. The crura lie posterior to the renal arteries and should be identified by their lack of pulsations and absence of Doppler flow (Fig. 9-19). They vary in echogenicity, depending on the amount of surrounding retroperitoneal fat. They may appear hypoechoic, like lymph nodes.

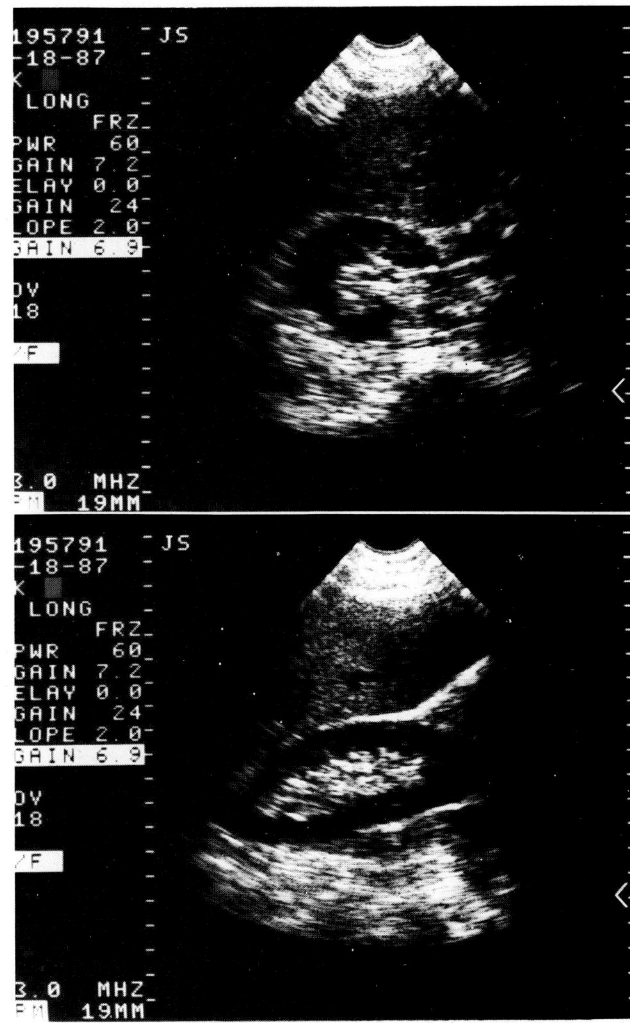

FIG. 9-11 A and **B,** Sagittal scans of the normal kidney. The cortex is the brightest of the echoes within the renal parenchyma. The medullary pyramids are echo free. The pyramids are separated from the cortex by bands of cortical tissue, the columns of Bertin, that extend inward to the renal sinus.

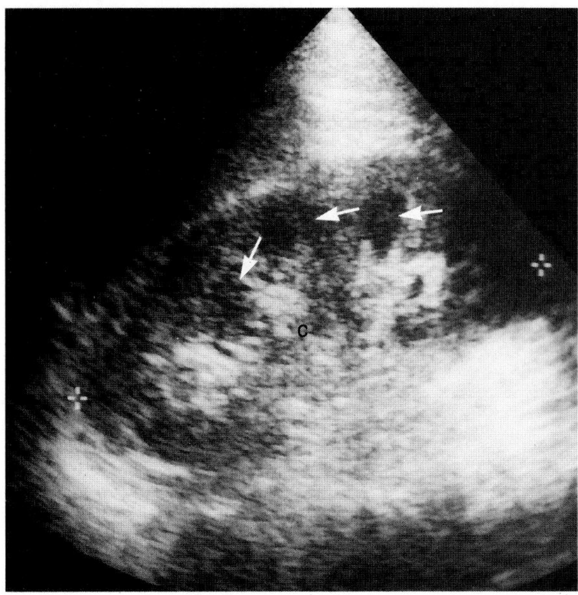

FIG. 9-12 Longitudinal scan of the hypoechoic renal pyramids *(arrows).*

Renal Medulla

The renal medulla consists of hypoechoic pyramids disbursed in a uniform distribution, separated by bands of intervening parenchyma that extend toward the renal sinus. The pyramids are uniform in size, shape (triangular), and distribution. The apex of the pyramid points toward the sinus and the base lies adjacent to the renal cortex. The arcuate vessels lie at the base of the pyramids. The pyramids are located at the junction between the more-peripheral renal cortex and the central sinus (see Fig. 9-2).

Renal Variants

Column of Bertin

The columns of Bertin are prominent invaginations of the cortex located at varying depths within the medullary substance of the kidneys. These areas are normal cortex. The columns may be the fusion of two septa into a single col-

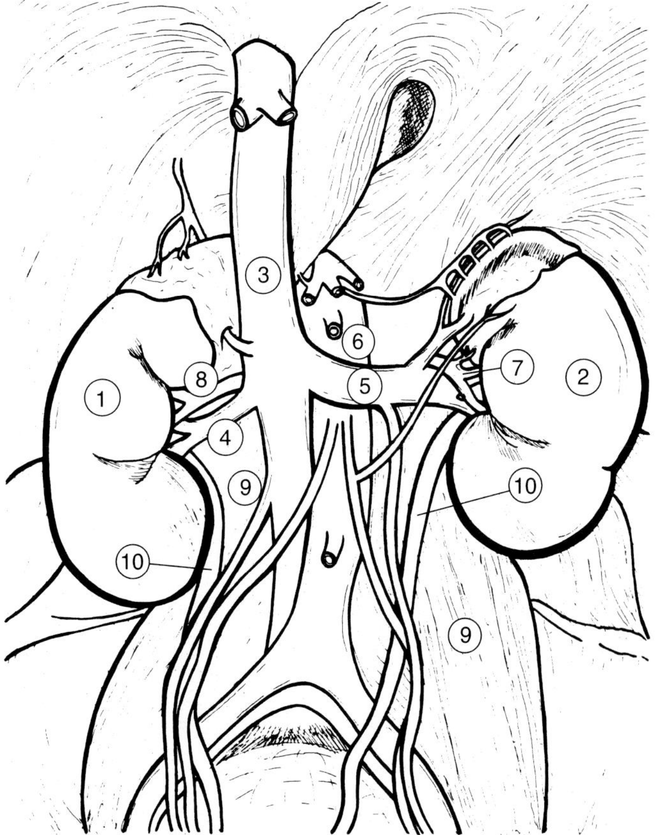

FIG. 9-13 The kidneys and their vascular relationships. Right kidney, *1;* left kidney, *2;* inferior vena cava, *3;* right renal vein, *4;* left renal vein, *5;* aorta, *6;* left renal artery, *7;* right renal artery, *9;* psoas muscle, *9;* ureter, *10.* (From Hagen-Ansert SL: The anatomy workbook. Philadelphia, 1986, JB Lippincott.)

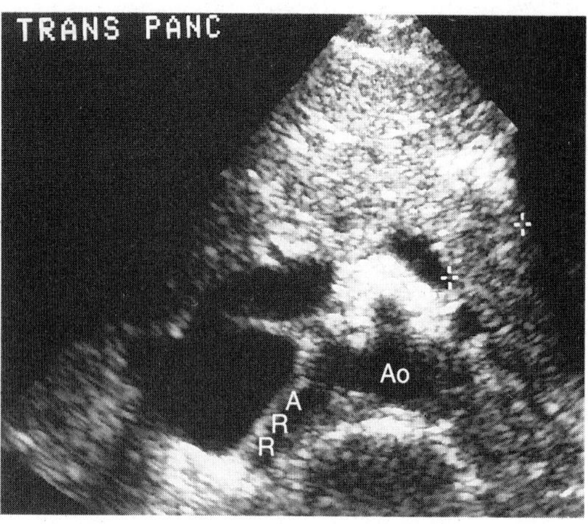

FIG. 9-14 Transverse scan of the right renal artery, *RRA*, as it extends from the posterior lateral wall of the aorta to enter the central renal sinus.

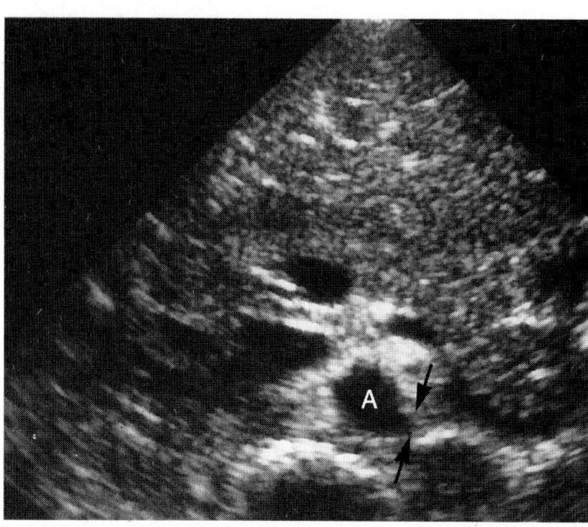

FIG. 9-17 The left renal artery *(arrows)* flows from the posterior lateral wall of the aorta, *A*, to the central renal sinus.

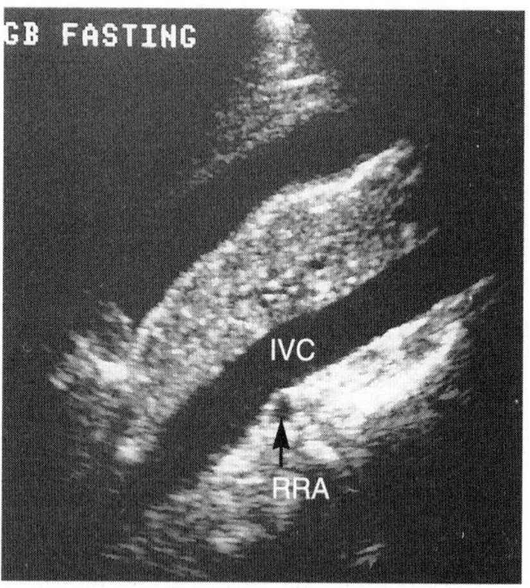

FIG. 9-15 On the longitudinal scan, the right renal artery, *RRA*, can be seen as a circular structure posterior to the inferior vena cava, *IVC*.

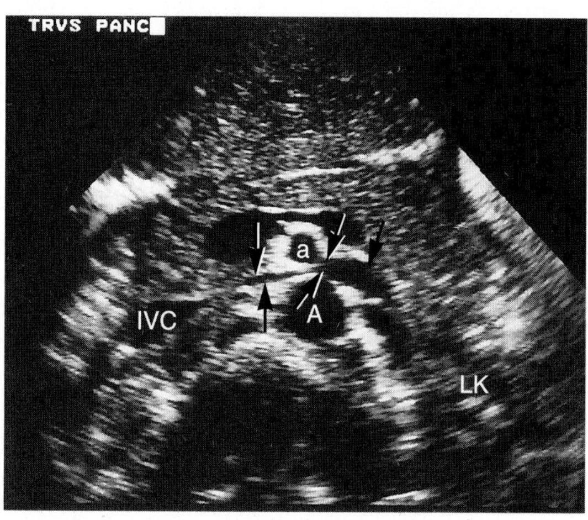

FIG. 9-18 The left renal vein *(arrows)* flows from the central renal sinus, anterior to the aorta, *A*, and posterior to the superior mesenteric artery, *a*, to join the inferior vena cava, *IVC*.

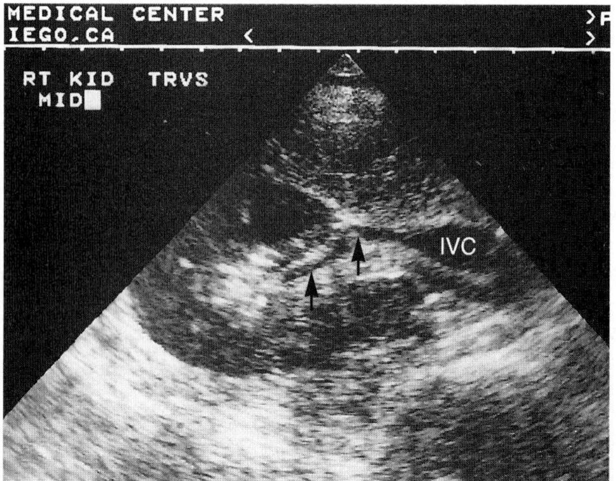

FIG. 9-16 The right renal vein *(arrows)* extends from the central renal sinus directly into the inferior vena cava, *IVC*.

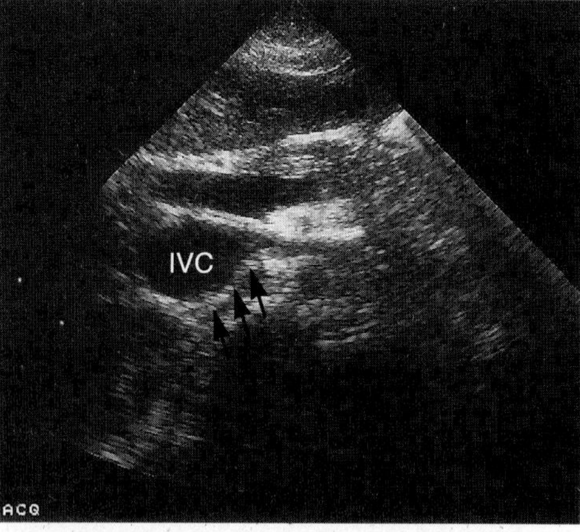

FIG. 9-19 The crura of the diaphragm lie posterior to the renal arteries and should be identified by their lack of pulsations and no Doppler flow *(arrows)*.

umn of twice normal thickness. The columns are most exaggerated in patients with complete or partial duplication (Fig. 9-20).

Sonographic features of a renal mass effect produced by a hypertrophied column of Bertin include the following: a lateral indentation of the renal sinus, a clear definition from the renal sinus, or a maximum dimension that does not exceed 3 cm. There is contiguity with the renal cortex and the overall echogenicity is similar to that of the renal parenchyma.

Dromedary Hump

The dromedary hump is a cortical bulge that occurs on the lateral border of the kidney, typically more on the left (Fig. 9-21). In some patients, it may be so prominent that it looks like a neoplasm. It probably results from pressure on the developing fetal kidney by the spleen. The echogenicity is identical to that of the rest of the renal cortex.

Junctional Parenchymal Defect

A junctional parenchymal defect is a triangular echogenic area in the upper pole of the renal parenchyma that can be seen during normal scanning (Fig. 9-22). The defect results from the normal extensions of the renal sinus in cases where there is distinct division between the upper and lower poles of the kidney.

The kidneys develop from fusion of two embryonic parenchymatous masses referred to as *renunculi*. In cases of partial fusion, parenchymal defects occur at the junction of the renunculi and are best demonstrated on sagittal scans.

Duplex Collecting System

The duplex collecting system is a common normal variant. Usually the sonographer cannot tell if it is complete or incomplete because it is difficult to see the ureters well. The duplex kidney is usually enlarged with smooth margins. The central renal sinus appears as two echogenic regions

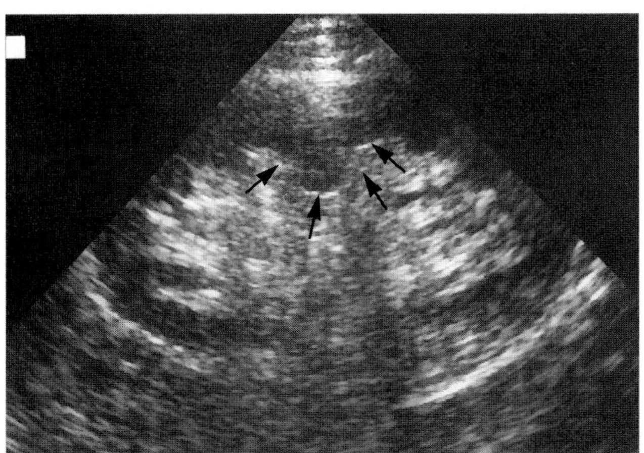

FIG. 9-20 Longitudinal scan of a kidney with a prominent column of Bertin *(arrows)*.

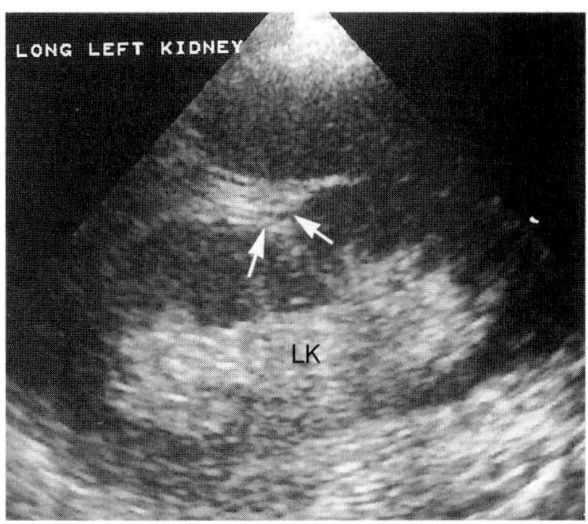

FIG. 9-22 A junctional parenchymal defect *(arrows)* is a triangular echogenic area in the upper pole of the renal parenchyma.

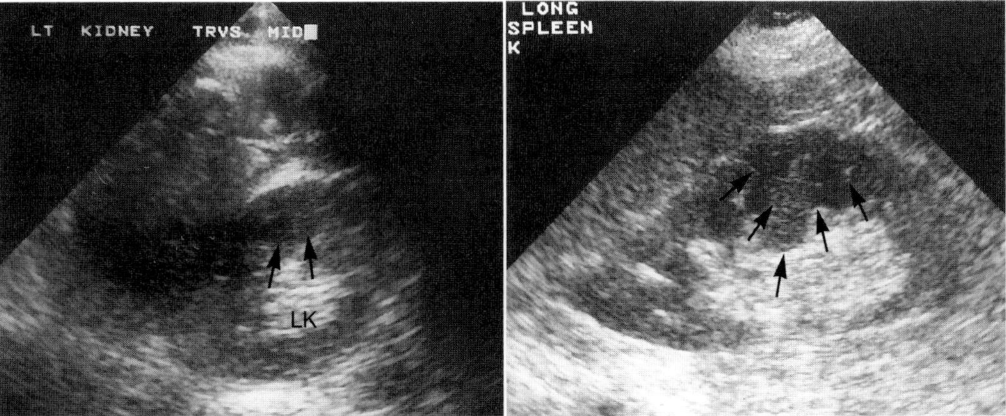

FIG. 9-21 The dromedary hump *(arrow)* is a cortical bulge that occurs on the lateral border of the kidney, typically more on the left than the right.

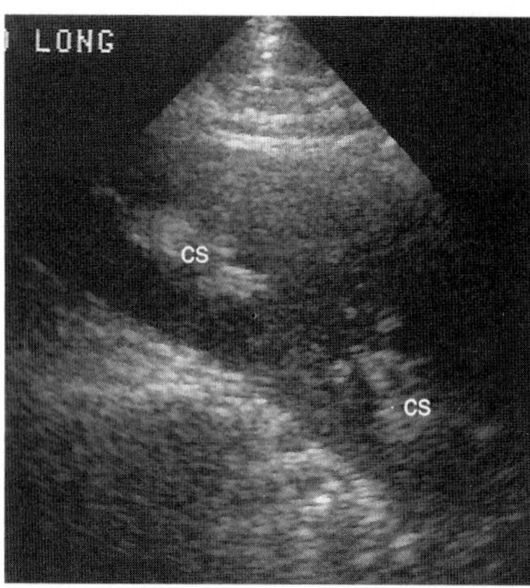

FIG. 9-23 Duplex collecting system. The central renal sinus, *cs*, appears as two echogenic regions separated by a cleft of moderately echogenic tissue similar in appearance to the normal renal parenchyma.

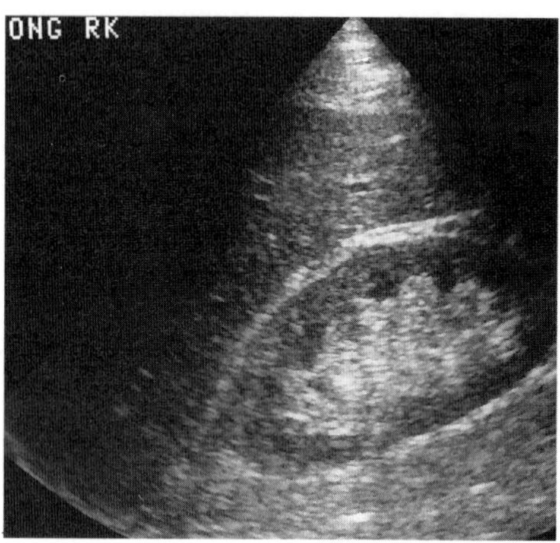

FIG. 9-24 Longitudinal scan of the right kidney showing increased renal sinus fat consistent with the renal sinus lipomatosis.

separated by a cleft of moderately echogenic tissue similar in appearance to the normal renal parenchyma (Fig. 9-23). The pelvis of the lower pole is usually larger than the upper pole.

Sinus Lipomatosis

Sinus lipomatosis is a condition characterized by deposition of a moderate amount of fat in the renal sinus (Figs. 9-24 and 9-25). The degree of proliferation of fibrofatty tissue varies. The renal sinus is composed of fibrous tissue, fat, lymphatic vessels, and renal vascular structures. On normal kidneys, this central zone appears as a bright area. In sinus lipomatosis the abundant fibrous tissue may cause enlargement of the sinus region, as well as increased echogenicity.

Extrarenal Pelvis

The normal renal pelvis is a triangular structure. Its axis points inferiorly and medially. An intrarenal pelvis lies almost completely within the confines of the central renal sinus. This is usually small and foreshortened. The extrarenal pelvis tends to be larger with long major calyces (Fig. 9-26). On sonography the pelvis appears as a central cystic area that is either partially or entirely beyond the confines of the bulk of the renal substance. Transverse views are best to see continuity with the renal sinus.

Renal Anomalies

Renal anomalies are abnormalities in number, size, position, structure, or form (Fig. 9-27). Anomalies in number include agenesis or dysgenesis and supernumerary kidneys. Agenesis of the kidney is the absence or failure of formation of the organ. Dysgenesis is the defective embryonic development of the kidney. A supernumerary kidney is a complete duplication of the renal system.

Solitary Kidney

A solitary kidney results from unilateral renal agenesis. It is very rare. The sonographer must look for a small, nonfunctioning kidney before making the diagnosis. Renal enlargement generally occurs with a solitary kidney.

Pelvic Kidney

If the kidney is not seen in the normal position in the renal fossa, the retroperitoneum and pelvis should be scanned. Most true ectopic kidneys are located in the bony pelvis and may be malrotated. The pelvic kidney may simulate a solid adnexal mass. It may be associated with other abnormalities, such as vesicoureteral reflux and anomalous extrarenal pelvis.

Horseshoe Kidney

Fusion anomalies of the kidneys include crossed renal ectopia and horseshoe kidney (most common). In a patient with a horseshoe kidney, there is fusion of the polar regions of the kidneys during fetal development that almost invariably involves the lower poles. Usually it is associated with improper ascent and malrotation of the kidneys, usually in a lower retroperitoneal position. The renal pelves and ureters are more ventrally located. These kidneys usually lie closer to the spine. The inferior poles lie more medially. The isthmus of the kidney lies anterior to the spine and may simulate a solid pelvic mass (Fig. 9-28). Associated pathologic conditions are pyelocaliectasis, anomalous extrarenal pelvis, and urinary calculi.

LABORATORY TESTS FOR RENAL DISEASE

Clinical Signs and Symptoms

A patient with a renal infection or disease process may present with any of the following symptoms: flank pain,

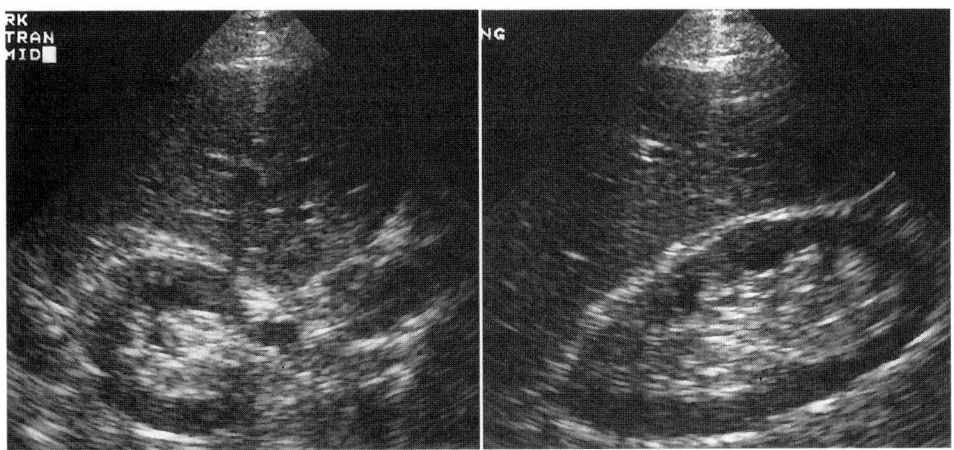

FIG. 9-25 Transverse and longitudinal scan of a patient with renal sinus lipomatosis.

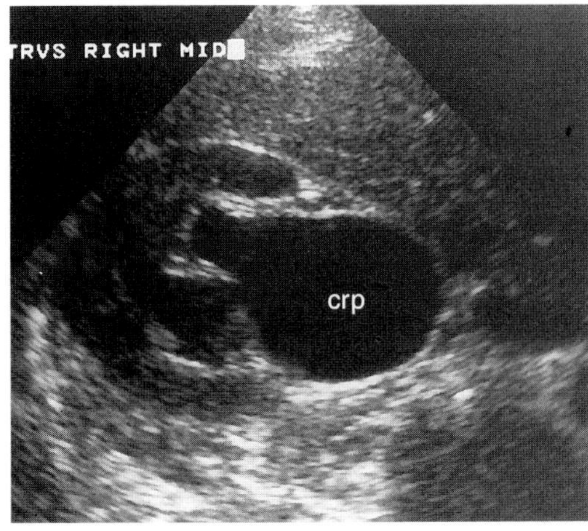

FIG. 9-26 Extrarenal pelvis. Transverse scan of the right kidney showing the renal pelvis appearing as a cystic area, *erp*, that extends beyond the confines of the bulk of the renal substance.

hematuria, polyuria, oliguria, fever, urgency, or generalized edema.

Diagnostic Laboratory Tests

A patient who presents with symptoms of renal infection or disease may undergo a number of laboratory tests to help the clinician determine the cause of the problem.

Urinalysis

Urinalysis is essential to detect urinary tract disorders in patients whose renal function is impaired or absent. Most renal inflammatory processes introduce a characteristic exudate for a specific type of inflammation into the urine. The presence of an acute infection causes hematuria, red blood cells in the urine; pyuria causes pus in the urine.

Urine pH

Urine pH is very important in managing diseases such as bacteriuria and renal calculi. The pH refers to the strength of the urine as a partly acidic or alkaline solution. The abundance of hydrogen ions in a solution is called *pH*. If urine contains an increased concentration of hydrogen ions, the urine is acidic. The formation of renal calculi partly depends on the pH of urine. Other conditions, such as renal tubular acidosis and chronic renal failure, are also associated with alkaline urine.

Specific Gravity

The specific gravity is the measurement of the kidney's ability to concentrate urine. The concentration factor depends on the amount of dissolved waste products. An excessive intake of fluids or a decrease in perspiration may cause a large output of urine and a decrease in the specific gravity. A low fluid intake, excessive perspiration, or diarrhea causes the output of urine to be low and the specific gravity to increase. The specific gravity is especially low in cases of renal failure, glomerular nephritis, and pyelonephritis. These diseases cause renal tubular damage, which affects the ability of the kidneys to concentrate urine.

Blood

Hematuria is the appearance of blood cells in the urine; it can be associated with early renal disease. An abundance of red blood cells in the urine may suggest renal trauma, calculi, pyelonephritis, or glomerular or vascular inflammatory processes, such as acute glomerulonephritis and renal infarction.

Leukocytes may be present whenever there is inflammation, infection, or tissue necrosis originating from anywhere in the urinary tract.

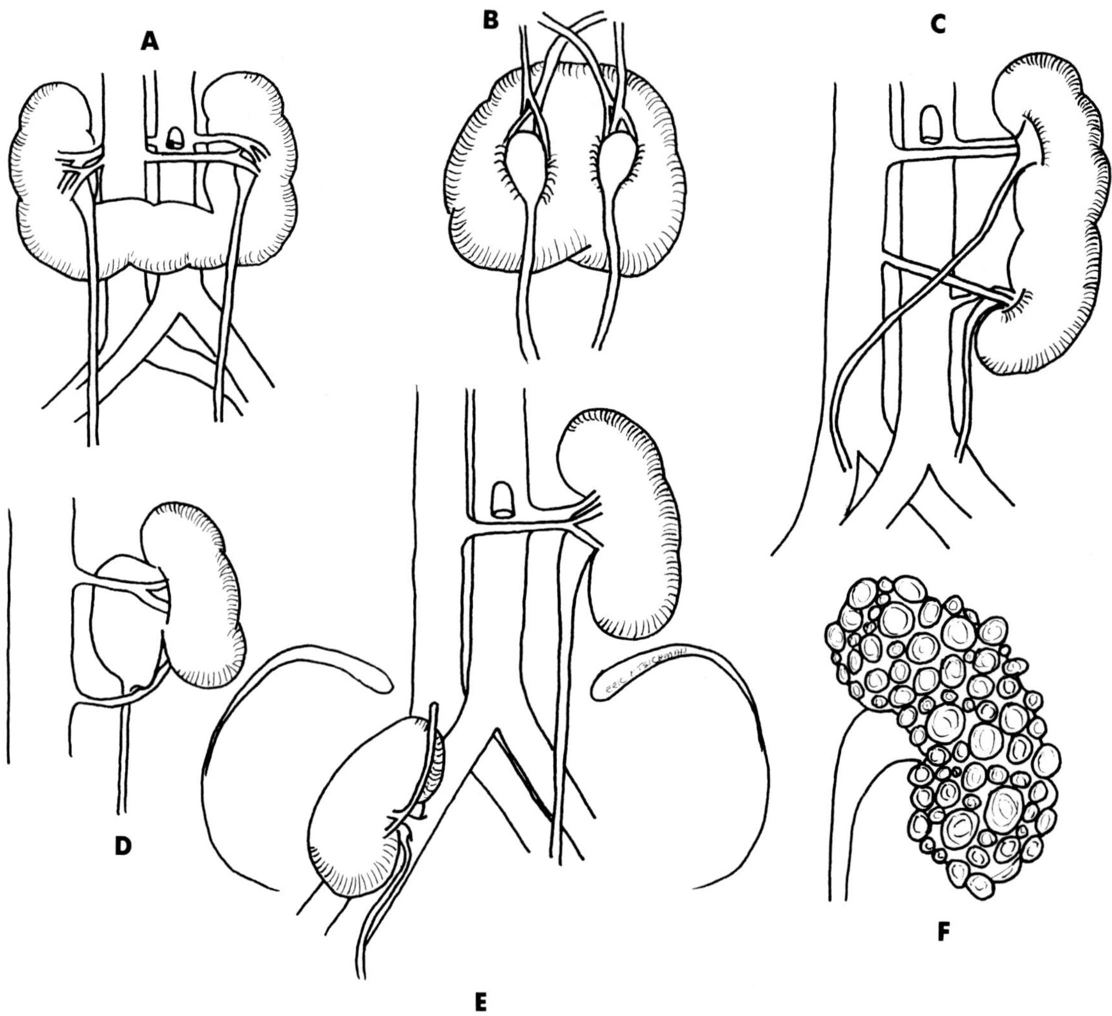

FIG. 9-27 Variations of renal anatomy, position within the retroperitoneal cavity, and pathology. **A,** Horseshoe kidney shown as two kidneys connected by an isthmus anterior to the great vessels and inferior to the inferior mesenteric artery. **B,** Cake kidney with a double collecting system. **C,** Double collecting system in a single kidney. **D,** Obstruction of the renal pelvis resulting in hydronephrosis. **E,** Pelvic kidneys with one kidney in the normal retroperitoneal position. **F,** Polycystic kidney.

Hematocrit

The hematocrit is the relative ratio of plasma to packed-cell volume in the blood. A decreased hematocrit occurs with acute hemorrhagic processes secondary to disease or blunt trauma.

Hemoglobin

The presence of hemoglobin in urine occurs whenever there is extensive damage or destruction of the functioning erythrocytes. This condition injures the kidney and can cause acute renal failure.

Protein

When glomerular damage is evident, albumin and other plasma proteins may be filtered in excess, allowing the overflow to enter the urine, which lowers the blood serum albumin concentration. Albuminuria is commonly found with benign and malignant neoplasms, calculi, chronic infection, and pyelonephritis.

Creatinine Clearance

Specific measurements of creatinine concentrations in urine, as well as blood serum, are considered an accurate index for determining the glomerular filtration rate. Creatinine is a by-product of muscle energy metabolism, which is normally produced at a constant rate as long as the body muscle mass remains relatively constant. Creatinine goes through complete glomerular filtration without normally being reabsorbed by the renal tubules. A decreased urinary creatinine clearance indicates renal dysfunction because it prevents the normal excretion of creatinine.

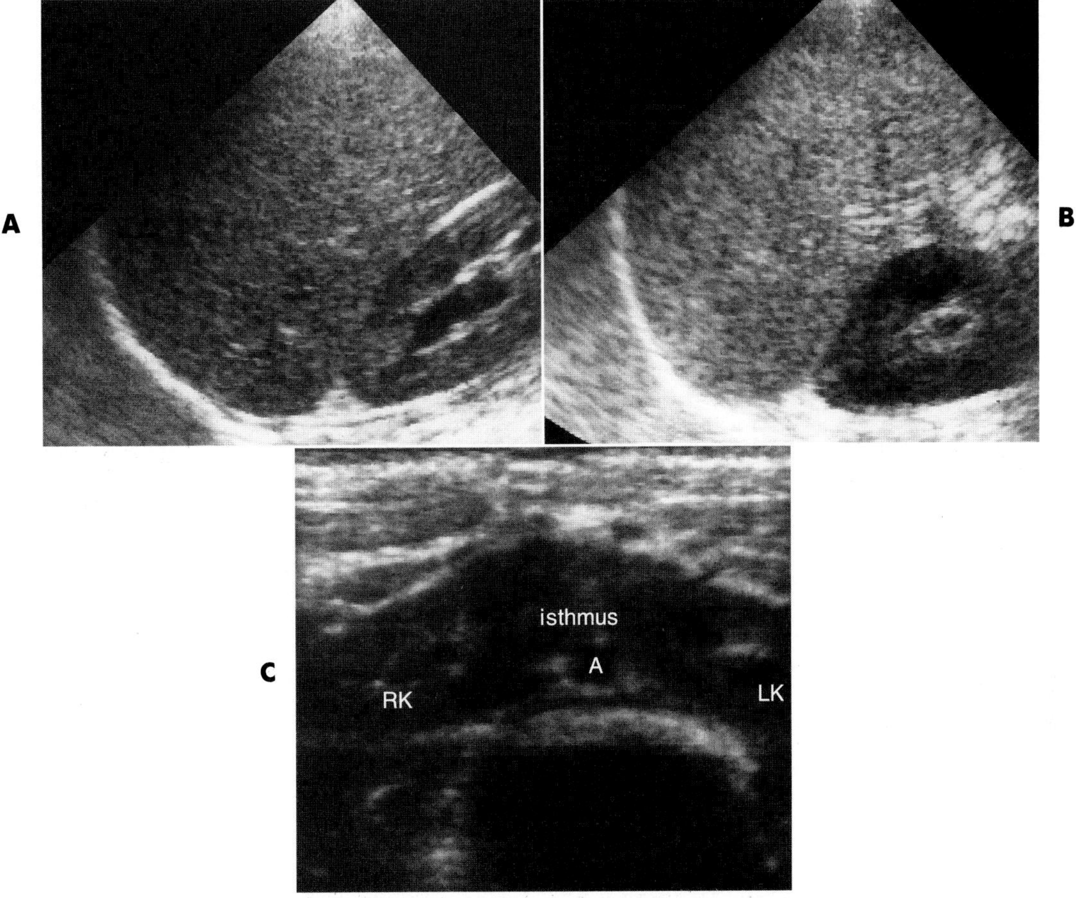

FIG. 9-28 **A** and **B**, Longitudinal scans of the right and left kidney in a pediatric patient. It was very difficult to record the lower poles of both kidneys. **C**, Transverse scan of the renal area shows a hypoechoic tissue mass connected to both kidneys. This represents the isthmus of the horseshoe kidney.

Blood Urea Nitrogen

The blood urea nitrogen (BUN) is the concentration of urea nitrogen in blood and is the end product of cellular metabolism. Urea is formed in the liver and carried to the kidneys through the blood to be excreted in urine. Impairment of renal function and increased protein catabolism result in BUN elevation that is relative to the degree of renal impairment and rate of urea nitrogen excreted by the kidneys.

Serum Creatinine

Renal dysfunction also results in serum creatinine elevation. Blood serum creatinine levels are said to be more specific and more sensitive in determining renal impairment than BUN.

EVALUATION OF A RENAL MASS

Before the ultrasound examination for the evaluation of a renal mass, the sonographer should make a complete review of the patient's chart and previous diagnostic examinations. Many patients have already had a previous imaging study, such as an intravenous pyelogram, CT, or MRI study. These films should be obtained before beginning the ultrasound study to tailor the examination to address the clinical problem. The sonographer should evaluate the films for the shape and size of the kidney, determine the location of the mass lesion, look for distortion of the renal or ureter structure, and look for calcium stones or gas within the kidney.

Renal masses are categorized as cystic, solid, or complex by ultrasound evaluation (box on p. 246). A cystic mass presents sonographically with several characteristic features (i.e., a smooth, well-defined circular border, a sharp interface between the cyst and renal parenchyma, and no internal echoes [anechoic]; it should also show excellent through-transmission beyond the posterior border).

A solid lesion projects as a nongeometric shape with irregular borders, a poorly defined interface between the mass and the kidney, low-level internal echoes, a weak posterior

SYMPTOMS IN DISEASES OF THE KIDNEY

Renal Cystic Disease

Inflammatory or Necrotic Cysts

Clinical symptoms include the following:
- Flank pain
- Hematuria
- Proteinuria
- White blood cells in urine
- Elevated protein

Renal Subcapsular Hematoma

Hematuria
Decreased hematocrit

Renal Inflammatory Processes

Abscess

Acute onset of symptoms
- Fever
- May have palpable mass

Elevated white blood cell count
Elevated pyuria

Acute Focal Bacterial Nephritis

Symptoms
- Fever
- Flank pain
- Pyuria

Increased BUN
Increased albumin
Increased total plasma proteins

Acute Tubular Necrosis

Symptoms (if caused by renal calculi)
- Moderate to severe intermittent flank pain
- Vomiting

Hematuria
Infection
Leukocytosis with infection

Chronic Renal Failure

Increased concentration of urea in blood
High urine protein excretion
Increased creatinine
Presence of granulocytes

Renal Cell Carcinoma

Erythrocytosis may occur
Leukocytosis
Red blood cells in urine
Pyuria
Elevated lactic acid dehydrogenase

border because of the increased attenuation of the mass, and poor through-transmission.

Areas of necrosis, hemorrhage, abscess, or calcification within the mass may alter the classification and cause the lesion to fall into the complex category. This means the mass shows characteristics associated with both the cystic and solid lesions.

Real time ultrasound allows the sonographer to carefully evaluate the renal parenchyma in many stages of respiration. If the mass is very small, respiratory motion may cause it to move in and out of the field of view. Careful evaluation of the best respiratory phase combined with use of the cine-loop feature, will adequately image most renal masses to determine their characteristic composition.

Renal Cystic Disease

Simple renal cystic disease encompasses a wide range of disease processes, which may be typical, complicated, or atypical. The disease may be acquired or inherited (e.g., von Hippel-Lindau disease or tuberous sclerosis). More complex cystic disease includes adult polycystic, infantile polycystic, or multicystic disease. There may be cystic disease in the renal medulla or sinus.

Simple Renal Cyst

The exact pathogenesis of a simple renal cyst is not known. Generally the cyst is believed to represent retention cysts that occur secondary to tubular obstruction, vascular occlusion, or focal inflammation. Simple renal cysts are common, occurring in half of adults over 50 years of age. Renal cysts may be located anywhere in the kidney and are not clinically significant unless they distort the adjacent calyces or produce hydronephrosis or pain.

Sonographic features of a simple renal cyst include a well-defined mass lesion, a smooth wall, and a circular anechoic mass with good through-transmission (Figs. 9-29 to 9-32). The tadpole sign may be seen as narrow bands of acoustic shadowing posterior to the margins of the cyst along the lateral borders of enhancement. A septum is occasionally seen within the cyst as a well-defined linear line. This would mean the cyst was not a simple cyst but a cyst with septations. Sometimes small sacculations or infoldings of the cystic wall produce wall irregularity; a cyst puncture or aspiration may be recommended to ascertain the pathology of the fluid within the mass.

Low-level echoes within a renal cyst may be artifacts (sensitivity too high or transducer frequency too low) or result from infection, hemorrhage, or a necrotic cystic tumor.

Parapelvic Cyst

The parapelvic cyst (renal sinus cyst) is found in the renal hilum but does not communicate with the renal collecting system (Fig. 9-33). Ultrasound shows a well-defined mass with no internal septations. It can have irregular borders because it may compress the adjacent renal sinus struc-

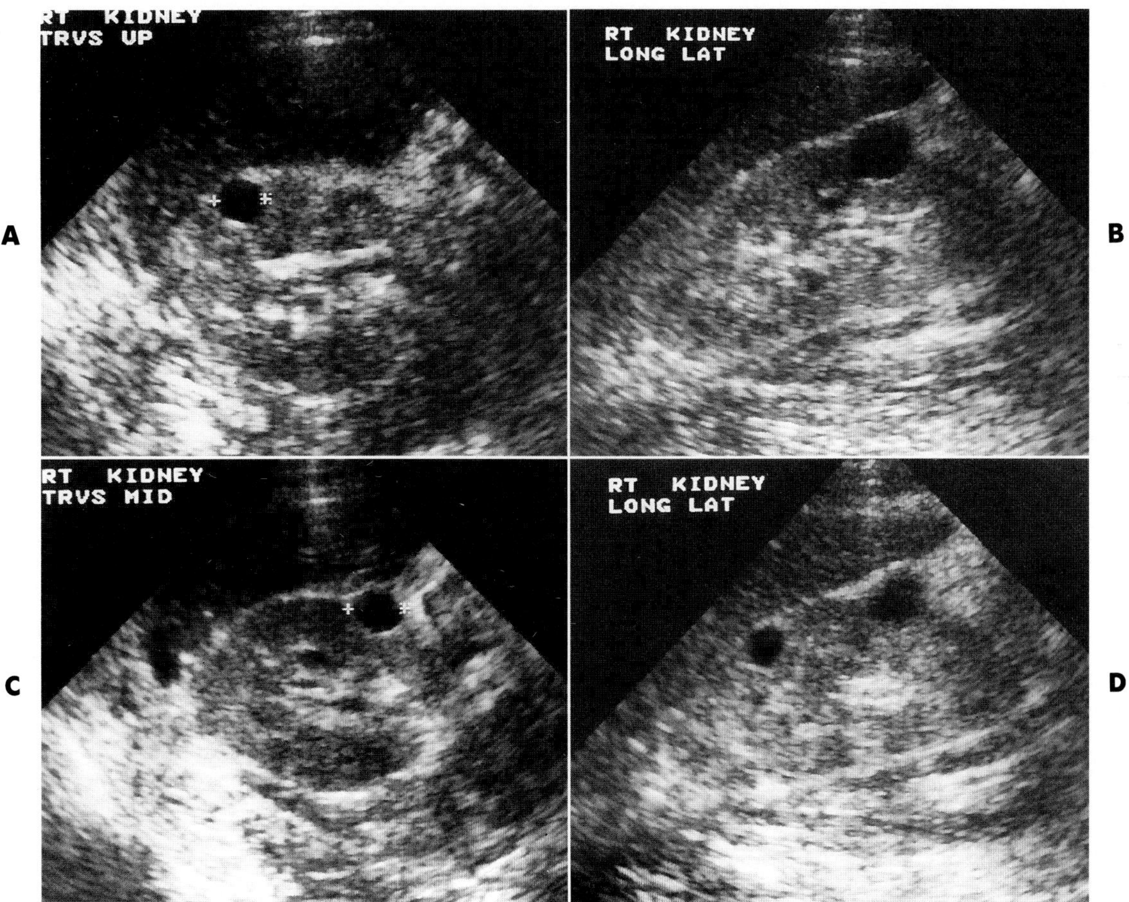

FIG. 9-29 A to **D,** Transverse and longitudinal scans of two small renal cysts along the lateral wall of the kidney. The borders are smooth and well defined. No internal echoes are seen.

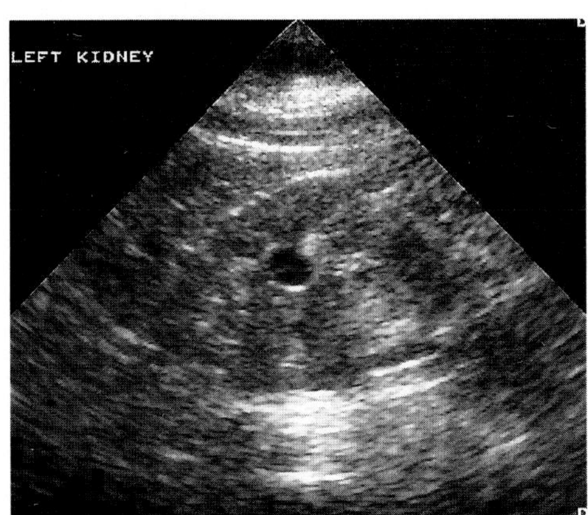

FIG. 9-30 Longitudinal scan of a small central renal cyst.

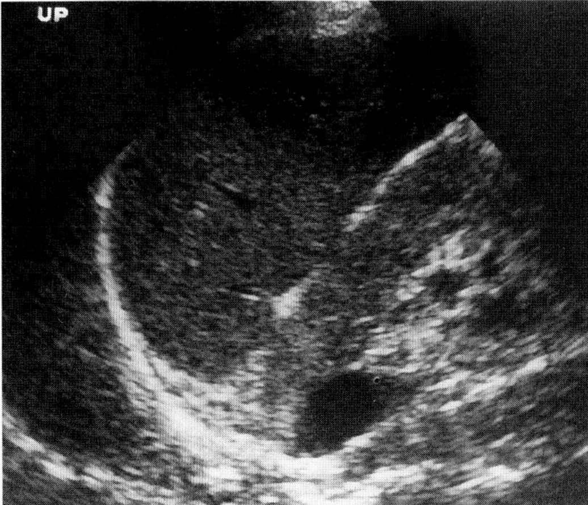

FIG. 9-31 Upper pole renal cyst.

tures. The parapelvic cyst may obstruct the kidney; the peripelvic cyst does not. Clinical symptoms are infrequent; the cyst can cause pain, hypertension, or obstruction. The sonographer should be able to differentiate the parapelvic cyst from hydronephrosis by trying to connect the dilated renal pelvis centrally. The dilated renal pelvis may present as a cauliflower appearance, whereas the parapelvic cyst is more spherical in appearance.

Ultrasonic aspiration techniques. Once a renal mass has met the criteria for a cystic mass, needle aspiration may be recommended to obtain fluid from the lesion to evaluate its internal composition.

The patient should be positioned with sandbags under the abdomen to help push the kidneys toward the posterior abdominal wall and provide a flat scanning surface. The cyst should be located in the transverse and longitudinal planes with scans performed at midinspiration. The depth of the mass should be noted from its anterior to posterior borders so that the exact depth can be given to aid in placement of the needle.

A beveled needle causes multiple echoes within the walls of the cyst. If the needle is slightly bent, many echoes appear until the bent needle is completely out of the transducer's path. The larger the needle gauge, the stronger the reflection.

Sterile technique is used for aspiration and biopsy procedures. The transducer must be gas sterilized. Sterile lubricant is used to couple the transducer to the patient's skin.

When the area of aspiration is outlined on the patient's back, the distance is measured from the anterior surface to the middle of the cyst.

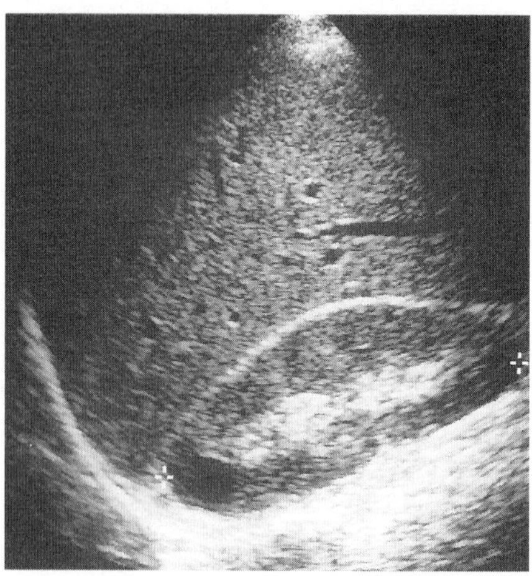

FIG. 9-32 Longitudinal scan of a upper pole renal cyst.

The volume of the cyst may be determined by measuring the radius of the mass and using the following formula:

$$V = \frac{4}{3}\pi r^3$$

The diameter of the mass can be applied to this formula:

$$V = d^3 \div 2$$

The patient's skin is painted with tincture of benzalkonium (Zephiran), and sterile drapes are applied. A local anesthetic is administered over the area of interest, and the sterile transducer is used to relocate the cyst. The needle is inserted into the central core of the cyst. The needle stop helps ensure that the needle does not go through the cyst. The fluid is then withdrawn according to the volume calculations.

Cysts Associated with Multiple Renal Neoplasms

Von Hippel-Lindau

Von Hippel-Lindau is an autosomal-dominant genetic disorder. Several areas of the body may be affected. Pathologic investigation has found retinal angiomas, cerebellar hemangioblastomas, and a variety of abdominal cysts and tumors, including renal and pancreatic cysts, renal adenomas, and frequent multiple and bilateral renal adenocarcinoma tumors.

Tuberous Sclerosis

Tuberous sclerosis is also an autosomal-dominant genetic disorder that may cause multiple renal cysts or angiomyolipomas, or cutaneous, retinal, and cerebral hamartomas.

Acquired Cystic Disease of Dialysis

Patients on renal dialysis have been shown to have an increased incidence of renal cysts, adenomas, and renal carcinoma. The incidence increases with time, particularly after the first 3 years of dialysis. Renal cysts can show spon-

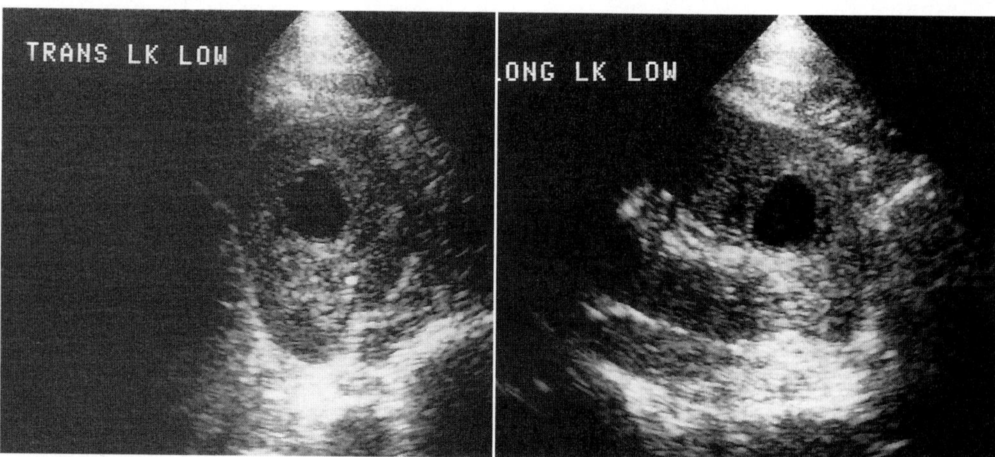

FIG. 9-33 Transverse scan of a renal sinus cyst. Good through-transmission is noted beyond the renal parenchyma.

taneous bleeding and hemorrhage, causing pain and flank discomfort.

Congenital Cystic Disease

Polycystic Renal Disease

Polycystic renal disease may present in one of two forms, the infantile autosomal-recessive form and the adult autosomal-dominant form. In the infantile form, the fetus may present with large echogenic kidneys and progress to renal failure and intrauterine demise.

The juvenile form presents with bile duct proliferation, periportal fibrosis, portal hepatic varices, and nephromegaly.

The adult form presents later in life with hypertension and renal failure that is less severe in onset. The kidneys are enlarged as they are replaced bilaterally with multiple cysts (Figs. 9-34 to 9-39). The cysts may grow large enough to obliterate the renal sinus. The cysts may have spontaneous bleeding, causing flank pain for the patient. Associated abnormalities include a circle of Willis aneurysm (20%), liver cysts (50%), splenic cysts (10%), and pancreatic cysts (10%).

Multicystic Dysplastic Kidney

Multicystic dysplastic kidney disease is nonhereditary renal dysplasia that usually occurs unilaterally. Bilateral disease is incompatible with life. In neonates and children the kidneys are enlarged; in adulthood, they may be small and calcified. The typical pattern is multiple cysts of varying size with no normal renal parenchyma. Other findings may also be present, including ureteral atresia (failure of the ureter to develop from the calyceal system), contralateral ureteropelvic obstruction in 30% of patients (development of the ureter from the bladder with retrograde filling), nonfunctioning kidney, or an atretic renal artery. This disease is the most common palpable abdominal mass in neonates.

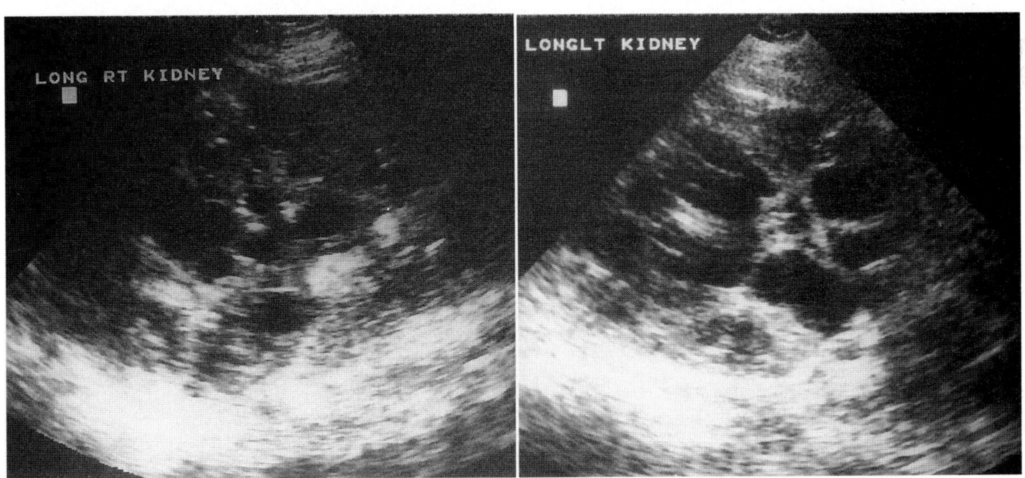

FIG. 9-34 A 54-year-old male with polycystic renal disease. Longitudinal scans of both kidneys are completely replaced with multiple small cystic structures.

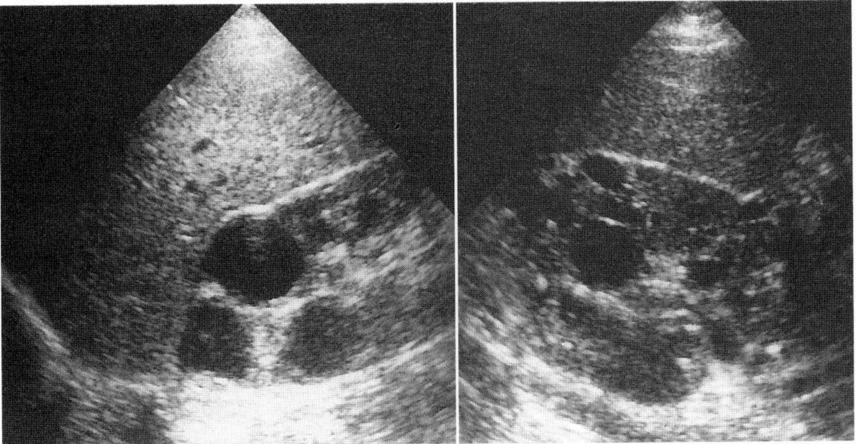

FIG. 9-35 Longitudinal and transverse scans of a patient with polycystic renal disease. The cysts are bilateral.

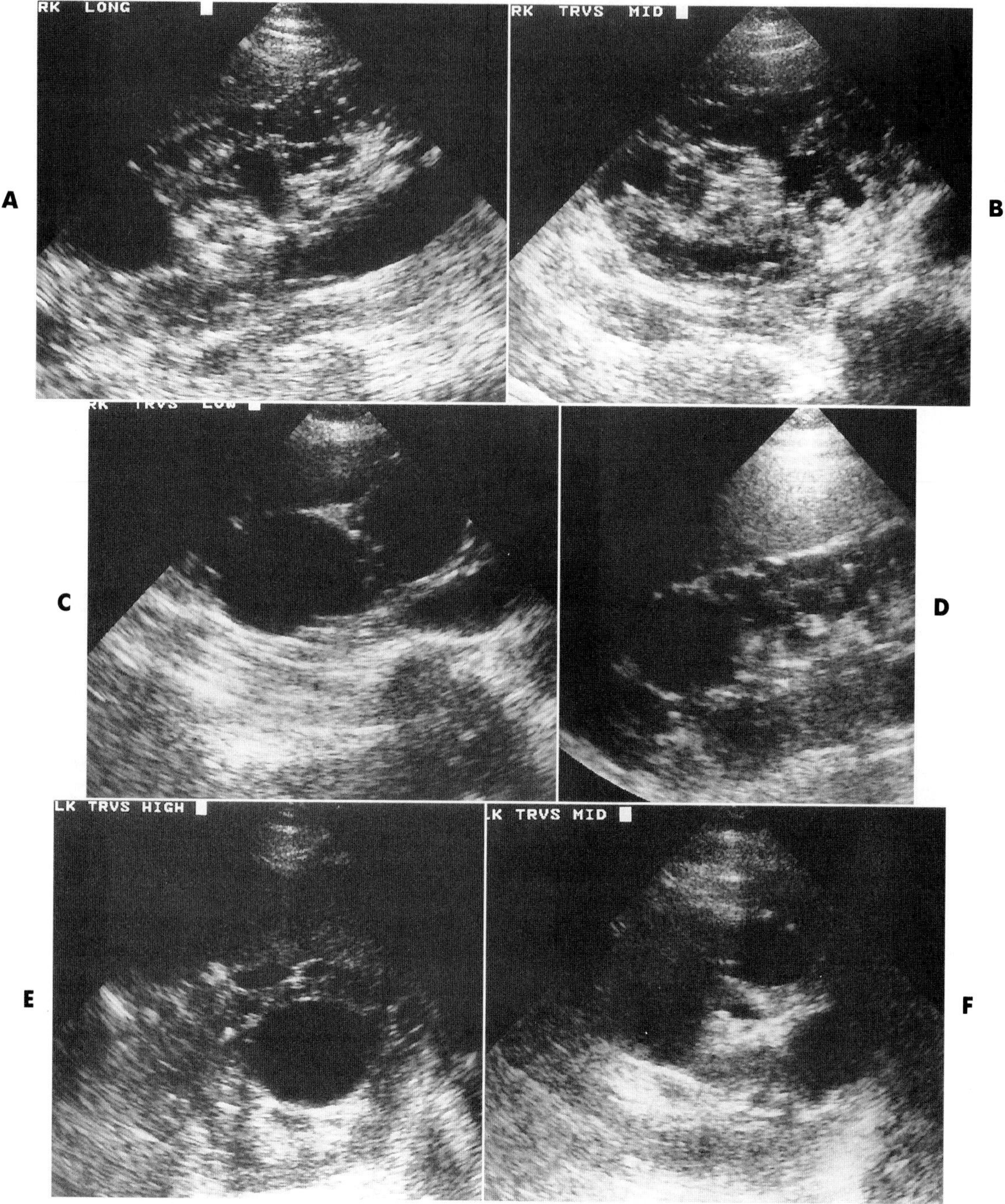

FIG. 9-36 Patients with polycystic disease show enlargement of both kidneys with multiple small cystic areas throughout. **A** to **C**, Right kidney. **D** to **F**, Left kidney.

Medullary Cystic Disease

Medullary Sponge Kidney

Medullary sponge kidney is a rare, nonhereditary, benign renal disease found in children. Common findings include tubular ectasia and calcium stones in 40% to 80% (nephrocalcinosis) (Figs. 9-40 and 41). It is also associated with Caroli's disease of the liver.

Medullary Cystic Disease (Nephronopthisis)

Medullary cystic disease is autosomal-recessive. It is characterized by salt-wasting nephropathy, presenting in young adults. The patient presents with small echo-dense kidneys, tubular atrophy, and glomerular sclerosis. There are multiple small cysts under 2 cm.

Renal Neoplasm

The sonographic appearance of most renal masses is nonspecific. Very often benign and malignant tumors cannot be differentiated from one another. In most clinical settings, ultrasound is usually the next step after the discovery of a renal mass on an intravenous pyelogram. If a solid mass is detected, abdominal scanning may be per-

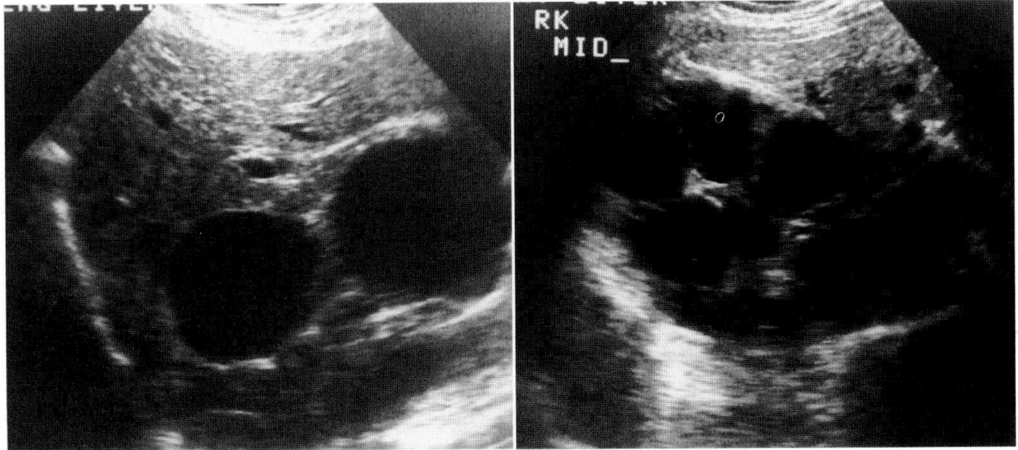

FIG. 9-37 A 45-year-old female with polycystic disease presented with huge cystic masses throughout the renal parenchyma. All of the cysts are distinct lesions and did not connect with the central renal sinus to indicate hydronephrosis.

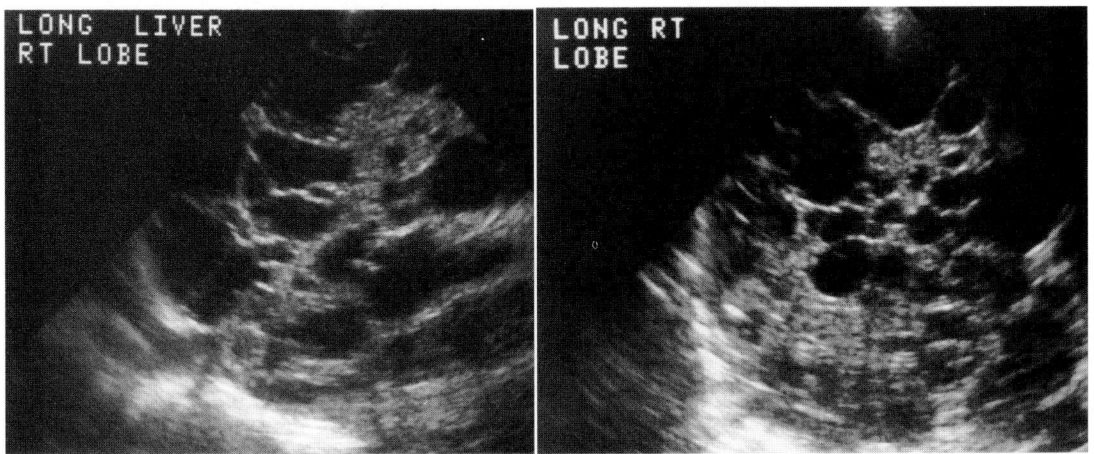

FIG. 9-38 About one third of the patients with polycystic renal disease also have polycystic liver disease. This severe case shows multiple cysts throughout the liver parenchyma. Often the cysts are so complex that it becomes difficult to distinguish the renal parenchyma from the liver.

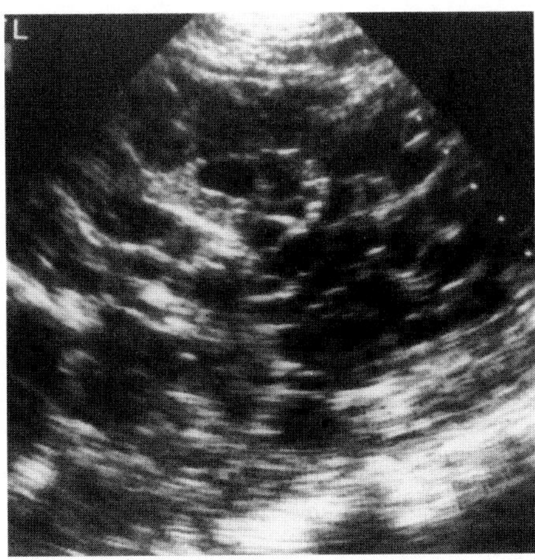

FIG. 9-39 A 30-year-old male with a solitary left polycystic kidney and hematuria was sent to rule out obstruction. It is very difficult to rule out obstruction with so many small cysts.

formed for staging purposes, although CT is superior in tumor staging.

Renal Cell Carcinoma

Renal cell carcinoma is the most common of all renal tumors, comprising 85% of all kidney tumors. It is twice as common in males as in females. The incidence usually does not peak until age 60 or 70. When found, it usually presents as a solid parenchymal mass, frequently with areas of hemorrhage and necrosis. Renal cell carcinoma is not usually echogenic unless calcification is present. Characteristically the mass is cystic or complex on ultrasound (Fig. 9-42). Occasionally renal cell carcinoma appears predominately as a cystic mass. Irregular tumor calcification can be seen in a small number of patients. Any calcified mass within the kidney indicates the possibility of tumor; a sonographer should define the extent of involvement by

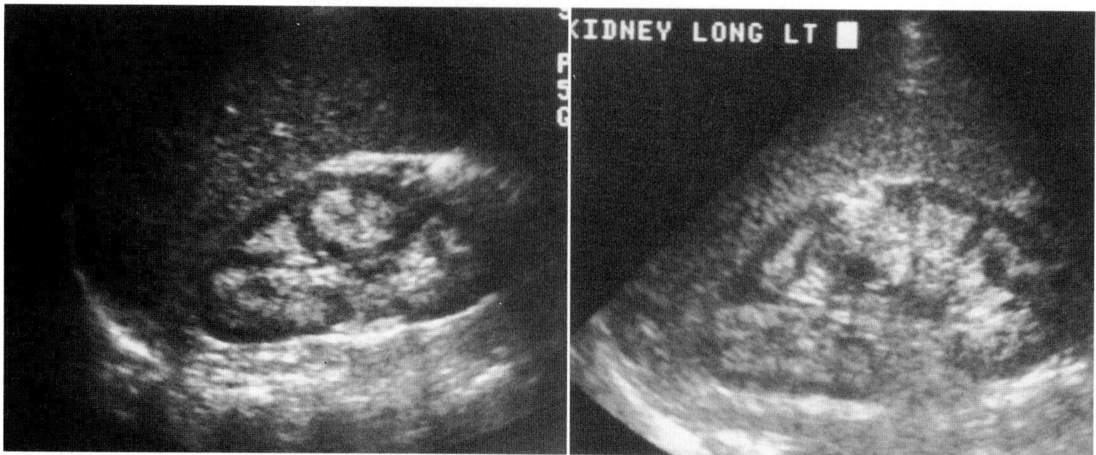

FIG. 9-40 Longitudinal scans of a young patient with medullary sponge kidney show nephrocalcinosis and an echogenic medullary renal parenchyma.

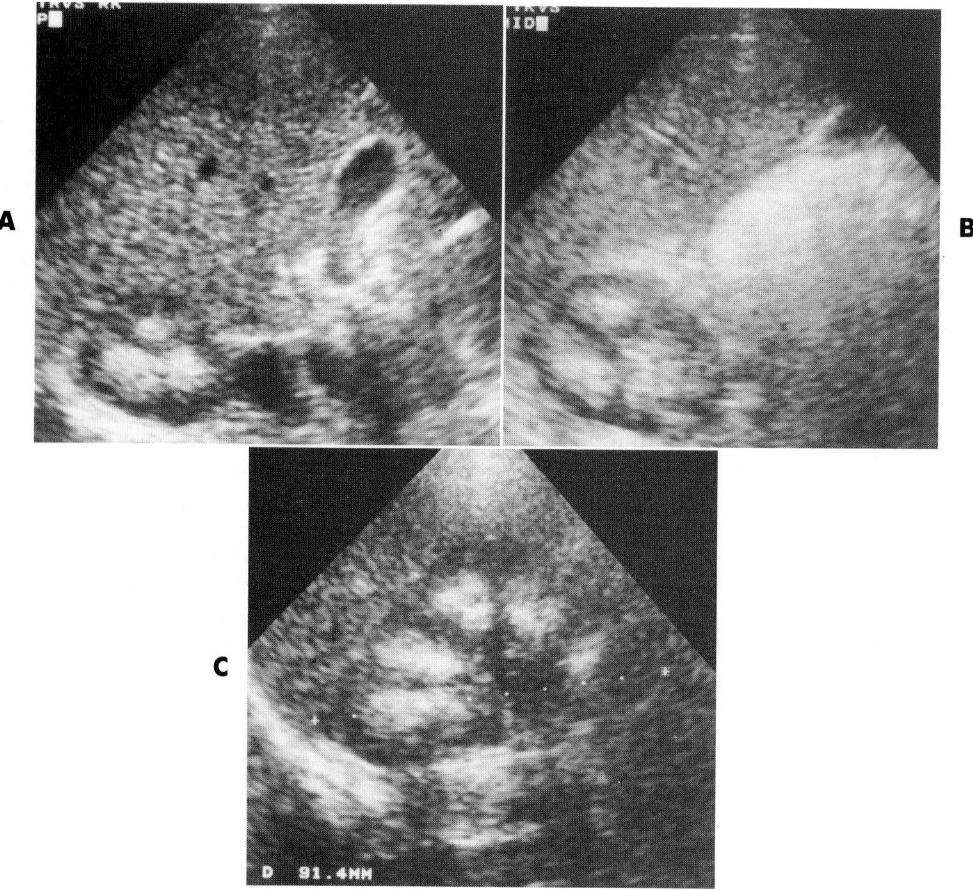

FIG. 9-41 A 6-year-old male with medullary sponge kidneys. **A** and **B,** Transverse scans. **C,** Longitudinal scan of the right kidney.

scanning the renal veins, inferior vena cava, and right atrium of the heart. Color-flow Doppler is useful to image the renal vein to observe flow rate—a low velocity may be seen if tumor obstruction is severe.

The incidence is increased in patients with Von Hippel-Lindau disease and patients on long-term dialysis. Tumors tend to be multiple and bilateral. The incidence of adenomas is increased. The tumor appears bilaterally in 0.1% to 1.5% of patients.

Staging of renal cell carcinoma is as follows:

I. Confined to kidney
II. Spread to perinephric fat but within Gerota's fascia

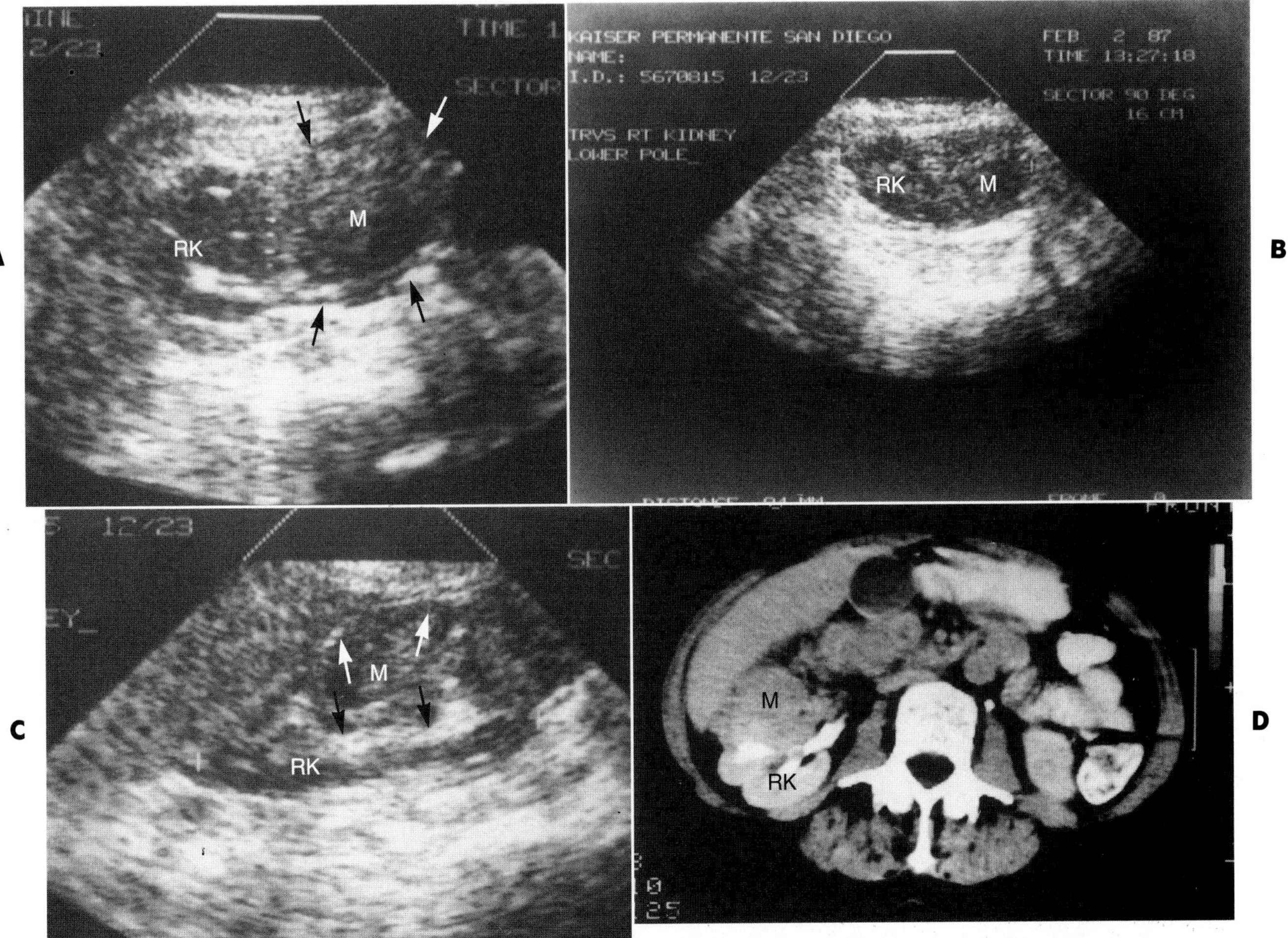

FIG. 9-42 Renal cell carcinoma is seen in this 62-year-old male who presented with hematuria. The mass is complex *(arrows),* distorting the renal parenchyma. **A,** Transverse scan with the large mass projecting from the medial border of the right kidney. **B,** Transverse scan of the renal cell carcinoma. **C,** Longitudinal scan of the mass as it distorts the central renal parenchyma. **D,** CT scan of the mass, *m,* arising from the right kidney, *RK.*

III. Spread to renal vein, inferior vena cava, or regional lymph nodes
IV. Invasion of neighboring structures; distant metastases

Transitional Cell Carcinoma

Transitional cell carcinoma is the most common tumor of the renal collecting system. The tumor is often multiple. The incidence is three to four times higher in males and increases with age.

On ultrasound the mass in the renal pelvis shows low-level echoes, widening of the central sinus echoes, and a hypoechoic central area (Fig. 9-43). Clinically the patient may present with a history of blood in the urine. The differential diagnosis includes other tumors of the renal pelvis, such as squamous cell tumor or adenoma, a blood clot, or a fungus ball.

Renal Lymphoma

The sonographic findings are not specific in patients with lymphoma involving the kidneys, although there is nonspecific enlargement of the kidney. The tumor is usually hypoechoic. The lymphomatous involvement of the kidneys is usually a secondary process, via either hematogenous spread or contiguous spread from the retroperitoneum. Non-Hodgkin's lymphoma is more common than Hodgkin's. Lymphoma is more common as a bilateral invasion with multiple nodules.

Metastases

Metastases to the kidneys are a relatively common finding at autopsy, but metastases may also present when the patient is alive. The most common primaries are from malignant melanoma, lymphoma, or carcinoma of the lungs, breast, stomach, cervix, colon, or pancreas.

Wilm's Tumor

Nephroblastoma or Wilm's tumor is the most common solid renal mass of childhood. It is rare in the newborn; the incidence peaks in the second year of life. Half of the tumors occur before the child's third birthday. The tumor

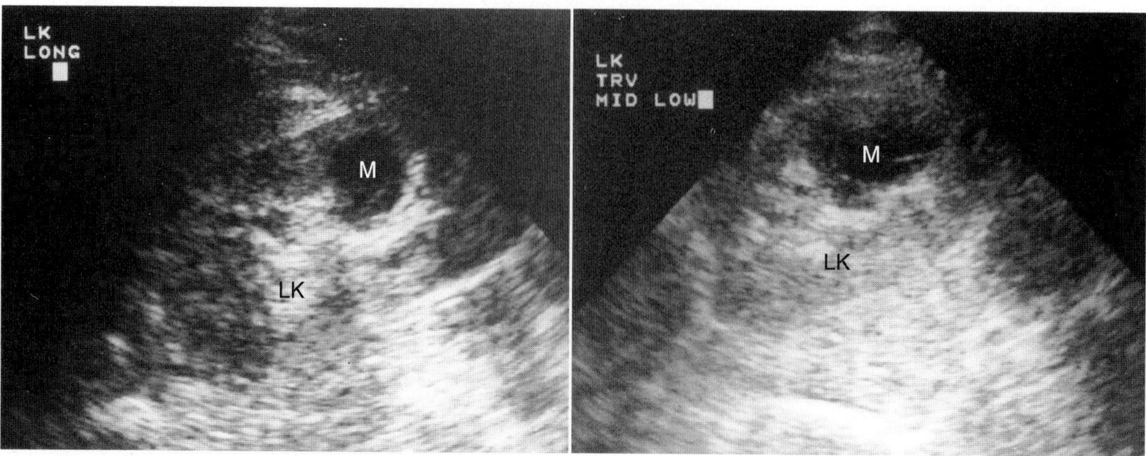

FIG. 9-43 Longitudinal and transverse scans of a transitional cell carcinoma. The mass is hypoechoic and is located near the renal sinus.

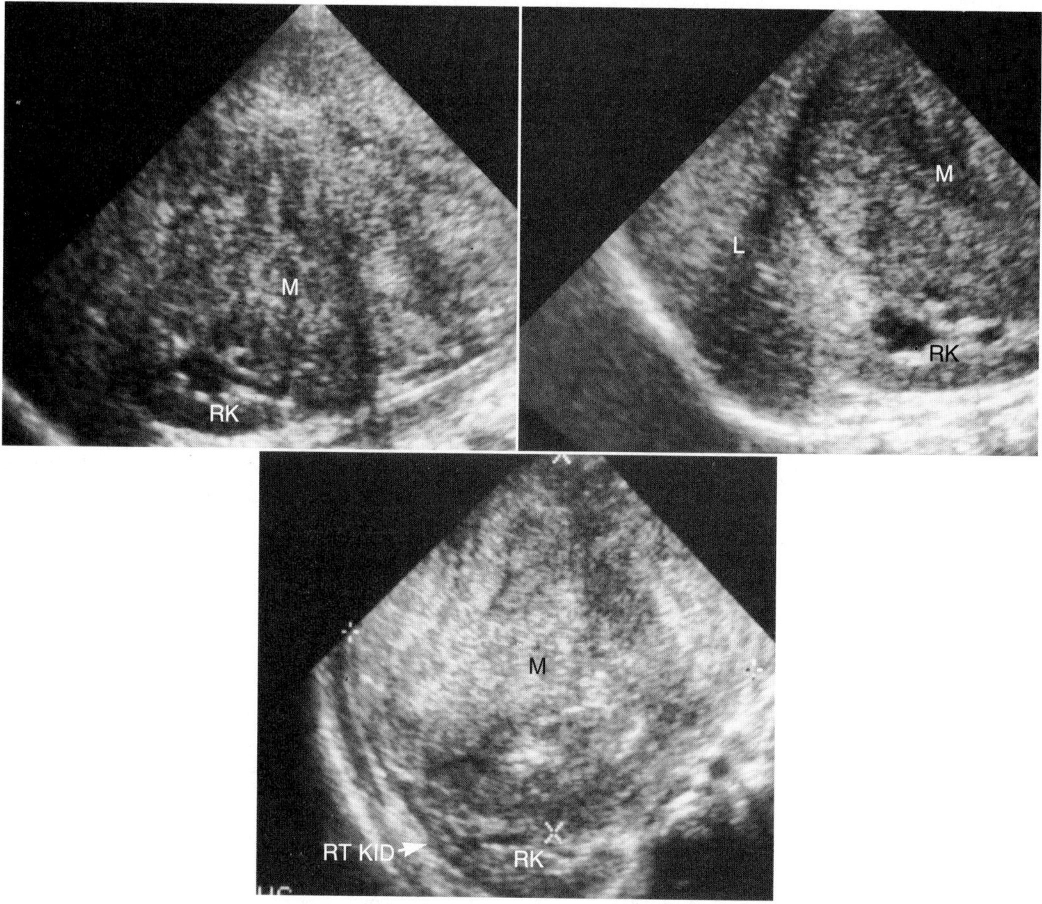

FIG. 9-44 This 2-year-old presented with a large palpable abdominal mass and nausea and vomiting. The tumor arises from the right kidney, *RK,* and compresses the renal sinus. It is clearly separate from the liver, *L.* This was a Wilm's tumor of the kidney.

may recur, so careful follow-up of the patient is important.

Wilm's tumor is associated with Beckwith-Wiedemann syndrome, sporatic aniridia (no color in the eye), omphalocele, and hemihypertrophy (one side of body is larger than other).

Most patients present with a palpable abdominal mass. Other clinical findings include abdominal pain, anorexia, nausea and vomiting, fever, and gross hematuria. Venous obstruction may result with findings of leg edema, varicocele, or Budd-Chiari syndrome. The tumor may spread beyond the renal capsule and invade the venous channel with tumor cells extending into the inferior vena cava and right atrium and eventual metastases into the lungs (Figs. 9-44 to 9-46). The tumor may be multifocal in a small percentage of patients.

Angiomyolipoma

Angiomyolipoma is an uncommon benign renal tumor composed mainly of fat cells. It is intermixed with smooth muscle cells and aggregates of thick-walled blood vessels. There may be hemorrhage in the tumor itself or in the subcapsular or perinephric space.

On ultrasound, a focal, solid hyperechoic mass is typical of an angiomyolipoma. There are two primary patterns of occurrence; the most common is the tumor that is solitary, nonhereditary, and found in young to middle-aged women (Figs. 9-47 and 9-48). The other, multiple tumors with bilateral renal involvement, are found in teenagers who have tuberous sclerosis.

Benign Renal Tumors

There are two common benign renal tumors—adenomas and oncocytomas. The adenoma can have calcifications. Oncocytomas resemble spoke-wheel patterns of enhancement with a central scar. To separate malignant from benign tumors the sonographer should look at the vascular flow patterns, the presence of nodes, or metastasis surrounding the structure or adjacent to the kidney. Ultrasound may distinguish the composition of a tumor, but it cannot indicate the histologic nature of the mass.

Malfunctioning Kidney

The excretory and regulatory functions of the kidneys are decreased in both acute and chronic renal failure. Acute renal failure is typically an abrupt, transient decrease in renal function often heralded by oliguria. The renal causes of acute azotemia include parenchymal disease (e.g., acute glomerulonephritis, acute interstitial nephritis, and acute tubular necrosis), renal vein thrombosis, and, rarely, renal artery occlusion. The etiologic basis of chronic renal failure includes obstructive nephropathies, parenchymal diseases, renovascular disorders, and any process that progressively destroys nephrons.

The pathophysiologic states that cause varying degrees of renal malfunction have been categorized as prerenal, postrenal, and renal. Decreased perfusion of the kidneys causes

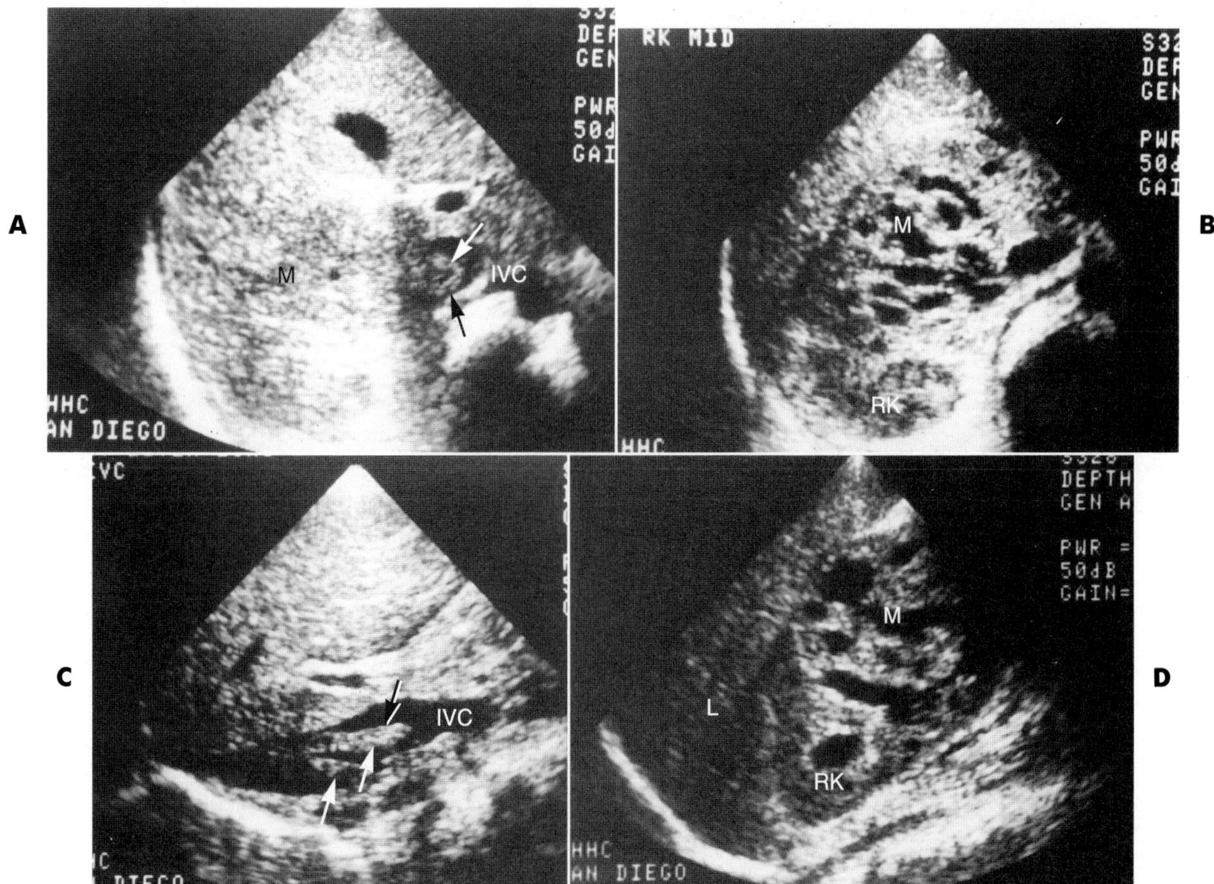

FIG. 9-45 One of the complications of a Wilm's tumor is the spread beyond the renal capsule into the renal vein and inferior vena cava. This eighteen-month-old child had a huge complex tumor with extension into the inferior vena cava *(arrows)*. **C** and **D,** longitudinal scan, showing the dilated IVC with tumor echoes along the posterior border. The tumor may extend into the right atrium of the heart.

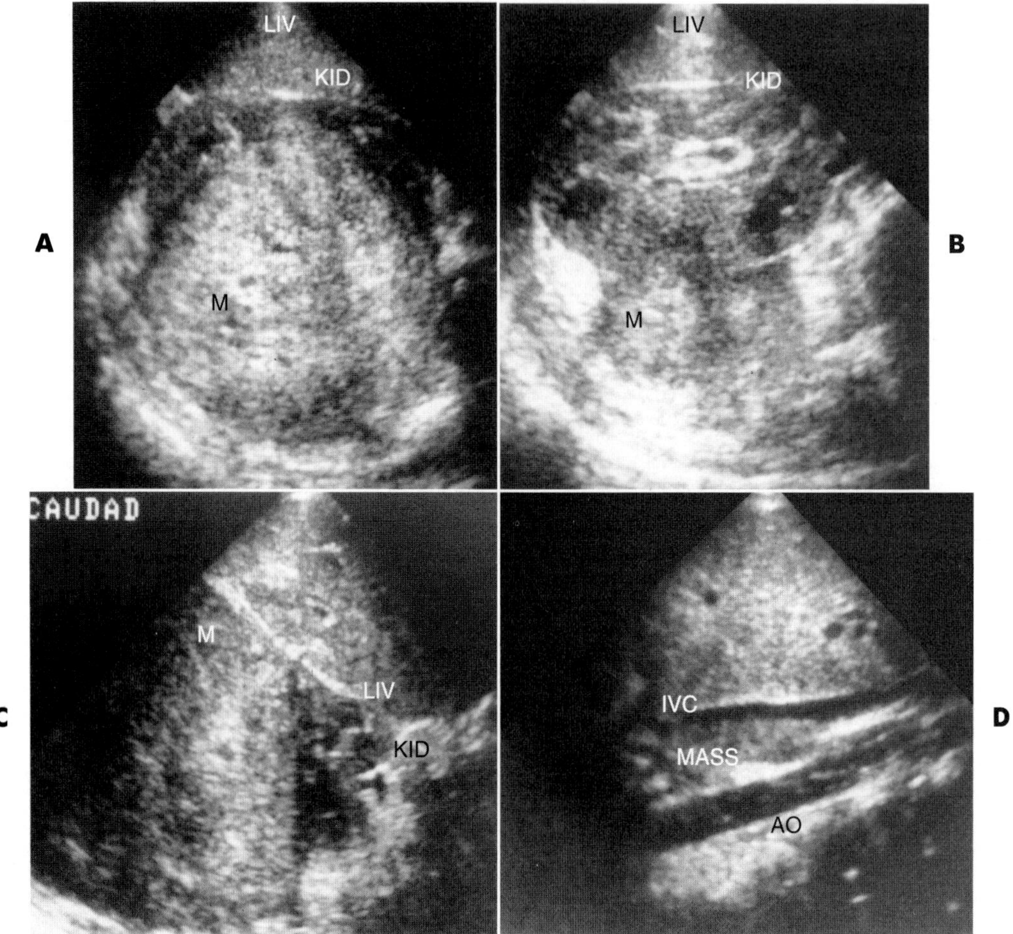

FIG. 9-46 A to **D,** A 14-month-old child with a huge Wilm's tumor, *M*, extending from the right kidney into the inferior vena cava. On the coronal scan, *D*, the tumor mass is seen within the IVC. The patient is rolled into a slight decubitus view to better image the IVC and aorta.

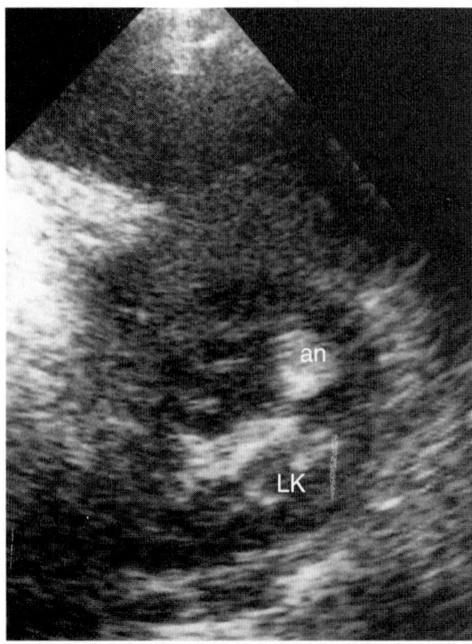

FIG. 9-47 An angiomyolipoma appears as a focal, bright, echogenic mass within the renal parenchyma.

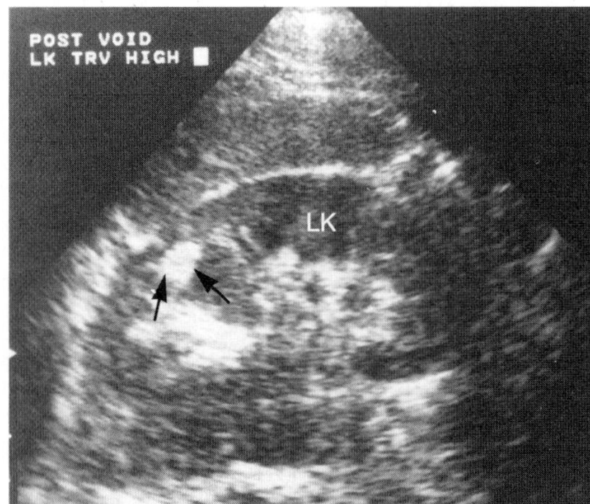

FIG. 9-48 A 29-year-old complained of right lower quadrant fullness. No adnexal masses were found. An incidental finding of an angiomyolipoma is seen in the upper pole of the left kidney *(arrows)*.

prerenal failure that can be diagnosed by clinical and laboratory data alone. Prompt diagnosis and treatment are crucial for postrenal failure, which is potentially reversible.

Numerous studies have previously documented that ultrasound is extremely sensitive in diagnosing hydronephrosis. Patients in whom laboratory test results indicate compromised renal function should receive rule-out-obstruction studies. Most agree that sonography is the initial procedure of choice in evaluating all patients with known or suspected renal failure.

Hydronephrosis is specific by various sonographic findings. The dilated pyelocalyceal system appears as separation of the renal sinus echoes by fluid-filled areas that conform anatomically to the infundibula, calyces, and pelvis. The renal sinus and parenchyma become compressed with progressive obstruction, and in end-stage hydronephrosis, only multiple cystic spaces may be seen (Fig. 9-49).

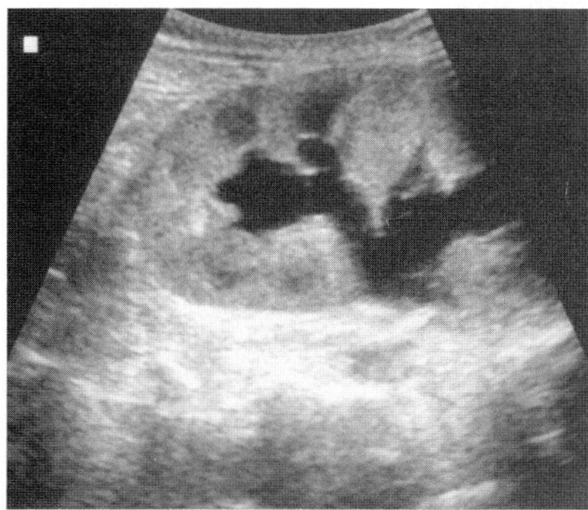

FIG. 9-49 Hydronephrosis of the kidney. The dilated pyelocaliceal system appears as separation of the renal sinus echoes by fluid-filled areas that conform anatomically to the infundibula, calyces, and pelvis.

It is possible to see the site of obstruction on ultrasound scans. A congenital obstruction of the ureteropelvic junction can be seen in utero. Whenever hydronephrosis is seen, the ureters and bladder are scanned because dilation of these structures indicates obstruction of the ureterovesical junction or of the urethra. A localized hydronephrosis occurs as a result of strictures, calculi, focal masses, or a duplex collecting system (Fig. 9-50).

When a mildly distended collecting system is seen, error can be caused by overhydration, underhydration, a normal variant of extrarenal pelvis, or a previous urinary diversion procedure (Fig. 9-51). Postvoid scanning techniques are helpful to avoid these errors.

Intrinsic renal disease can be demonstrated by examining the renal parenchyma with ultrasound. Two classifications of disease processes have been described. One group produces a generalized increase in cortical echoes, believed to result from deposition of collagen and fibrous tissue. This group includes interstitial nephritis, acute tubular necrosis, amyloidosis, diabetic nephropathy, systemic lupus erythematosus, and myeloma.

The second group of diseases causes loss of normal anatomic detail, resulting in the inability to distinguish the cortex and medullary regions of the kidneys. This group of diseases includes chronic pyelonephritis, renal tubular ectasia, and acute bacterial nephritis.

Lack of specificity and the overlapping appearances of different pathologic entities prevented this schematic from gaining wide acceptance. The end stage of many of these disease processes is renal atrophy, which can be seen on ultrasound by measuring renal length and cortical thickness. Some acute renal disorders can produce exactly the opposite findings—decreased parenchymal echogenicity and renal enlargement. Examples include renal-vein thrombosis, pyelonephritis, and renal-transplant rejection. Interstitial edema is thought to be the most likely cause of these findings.

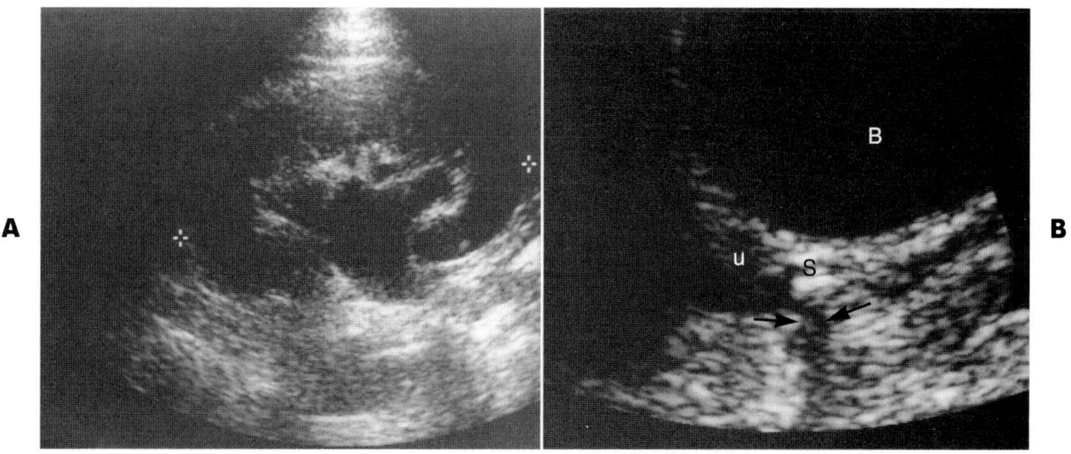

FIG. 9-50 A to **B,** A 40-year-old female presented with flank pain. **A,** Mild hydronephrosis is seen. The longitudinal scan of the full bladder shows a distended ureter with a large stone, *s*, obstructing the distal end of the ureter. The *arrows* demarcate the shadow posterior to the stone.

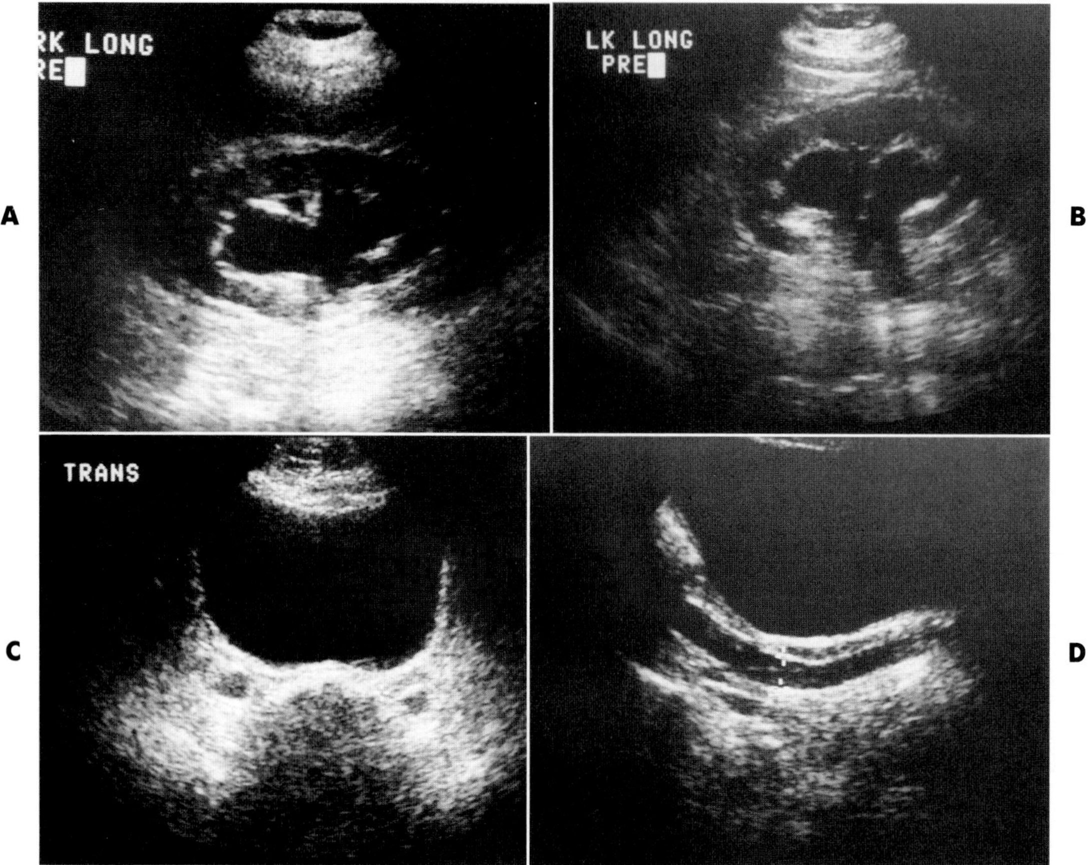

FIG. 9-51 **A** and **B,** A distended urinary bladder may cause pseudohydronephrosis of both kidneys and ureters. The patient should be scanned after the bladder has been emptied. **C** and **D** show the distended ureters in transverse and longitudinal sections.

Acute Glomerulonephritis

In acute glomerulonephritis, necrosis or proliferation of cellular elements (or both) occurs in the glomeruli. The vascular elements, tubules, and interstitium become secondarily affected; the end result is enlarged, poorly functioning kidneys.

Different forms of glomerulonephritis, including membranous, idiopathic, membranoproliferative, rapidly progressive, and poststreptococcal, can be associated with abnormal echo patterns from the renal parenchyma on ultrasound (Fig. 9-52). The increased cortical echoes probably result from changes within the glomerular, interstitial, tubular, and vascular structures. Patients have many symptoms, including nephrotic syndrome, hypertension, anemia, and peripheral edema.

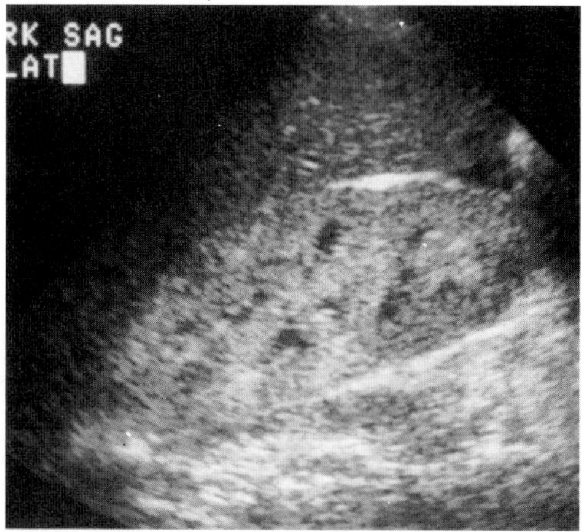

FIG. 9-52 Acute glomerulonephritis may be suspected when the echogenicity of the renal parenchyma exceeds that of the liver.

Acute Interstitial Nephritis

Acute interstitial nephritis has been associated with infectious processes—scarlet fever and diphtheria. It may be a manifestation of an allergic reaction to certain drugs. Patient signs and symptoms include uremia, proteinuria, hematuria, rash, fever, and eosinophilia.

The kidneys are enlarged and mottled. On ultrasound the renal cortical echogenicity is increased. The increase in echogenicity is greatest in cases of diffuse active disease. There is less increase in diffuse scarring.

Lupus Nephritis

Systemic lupus erythematosus is a connective-tissue disorder believed to result from an abnormal immune system.

Females are affected more, and the incidence peaks between 20 and 40 years of age. The kidneys are involved in more than 50% of patients.

The renal manifestations are hematuria, proteinuria, hypertension, renal vein thrombosis, and renal insufficiency. Sonography shows increased cortical echogenicity and renal atrophy (Fig. 9-53).

Acquired Immune Deficiency Syndrome

Acquired immune deficiency syndrome (AIDS) is a highly contagious disease, mainly spread by unprotected sexual activity or sharing infected needles. The virus destroys T cells and then replicates rapidly within the body. It affects many organs. Patients present with many various symptoms. Unexplained uremia or azotemia may indicate renal dysfunction resulting from AIDS. Focal segmental glomerulosclerosis may occur; it is not known if this is primary or secondary. An echogenic parenchymal pattern is present on ultrasound. Cortical echogenicity is increased. Kidneys are normal in size or enlarged (Figs. 9-54 to 9-56).

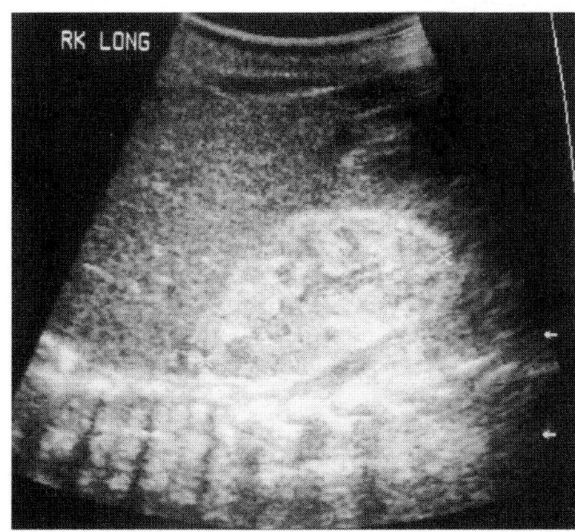

FIG. 9-53 Patients with lupus nephritis show a very echogenic renal parenchymal pattern as compared to the liver. Renal atrophy is usually present.

Sickle Cell Nephropathy

Renal involvement is common in patients with sickle cell disease. Abnormalities include glomerulonephritis, renal vein thrombosis, and papillary necrosis; hematuria is common.

The sonographic appearance depends on the type of pathologic disorder. In acute renal vein thrombosis the kidneys are enlarged with decreased echogenicity secondary to edema. In patients with subacute cases, renal enlargement is present with increased cortical echoes.

Hypertensive Nephropathy

Uncontrolled hypertension can lead to progressive renal damage and azotemia. Sonographically the kidneys are small with smooth borders. Superimposed scars of pyelonephritis or lobar infarction may distort the intrarenal anatomy. Bilateral small kidneys occur secondary to end-stage disease as a result of hypertension, inflammation, or ischemia (Fig. 9-57).

Papillary Necrosis

Many conditions may lead to papillary necrosis (e.g., sickle cell and diabetes). Necrosis may develop within weeks or months after transplantation. Patients previously treated for rejection and those with cadaveric kidney are at greatest risk. Ischemia is thought to have an important role in necrosis.

Symptoms suggest calculus or an inflammatory process. Complaints include hematuria, flank pain, dysuria, hypertension, and acute renal failure. Sonographic findings include one or more fluid spaces at the corticomedullary junction that correspond to the distribution of the renal pyramids. The cystic spaces may be round or triangular. Sometimes the arcuate vessels are seen.

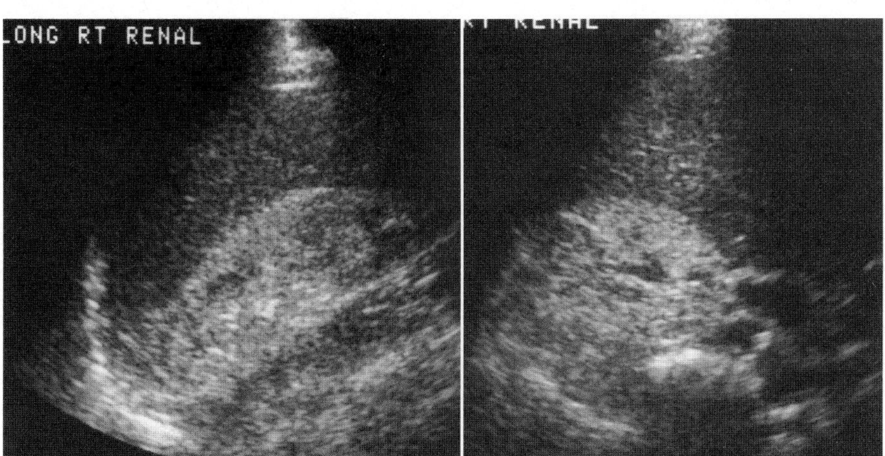

FIG. 9-54 Longitudinal and transverse scans in an AIDS patient show cortical echogenicity with normal to slightly increased renal size.

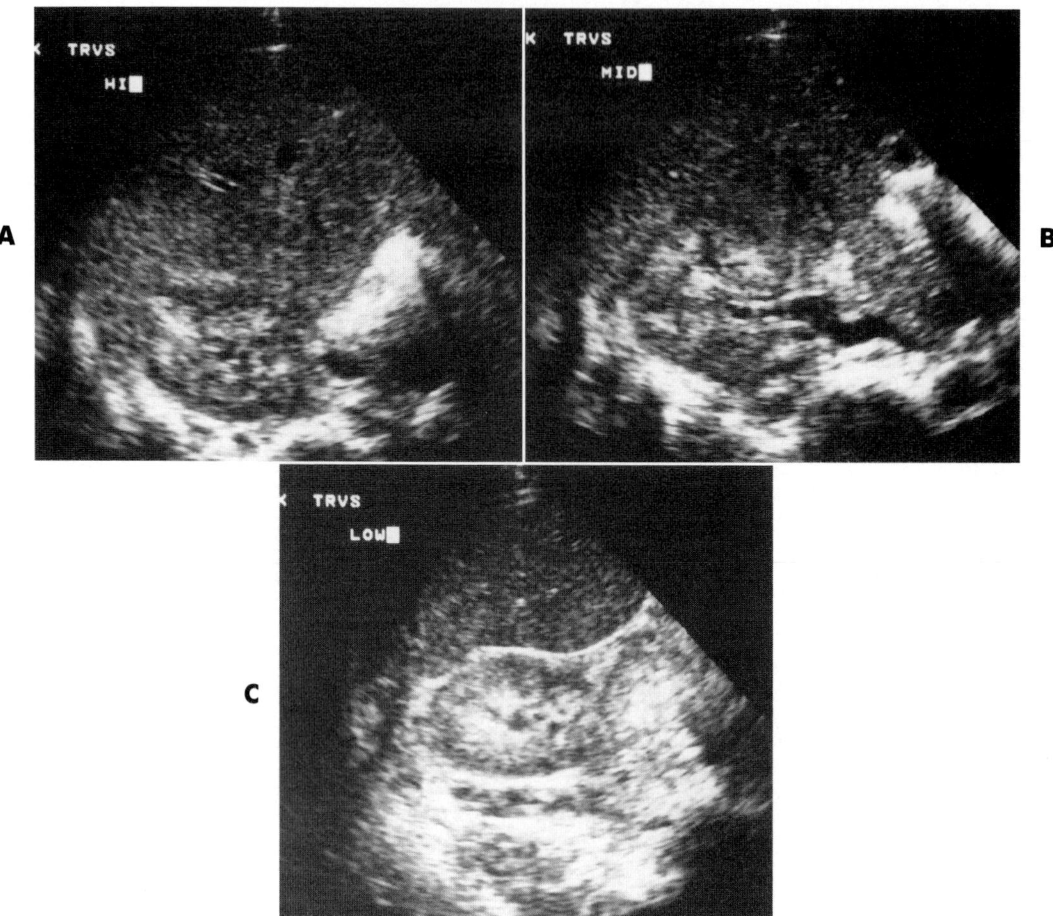

FIG. 9-55 A to **C,** Transverse scans of a young male with AIDS show a mildly echogenic renal parenchyma.

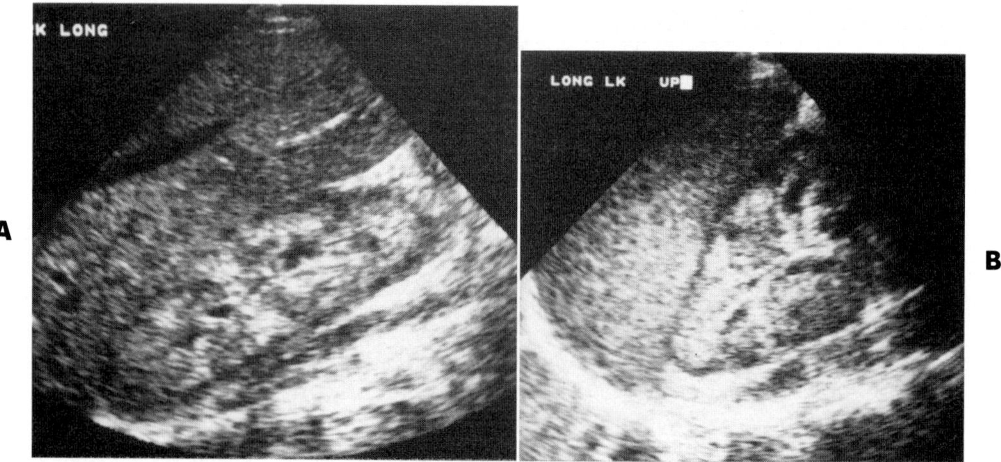

FIG. 9-56 A to **B,** Longitudinal scans of a 26-year-old male with AIDS.

The differential diagnosis includes congenital megacalyces, hydronephrosis, and postobstructive atrophy.

Renal Atrophy

Renal atrophy results from numerous disease processes. Intrarenal anatomy is preserved with uniform loss of renal tissue. Renal sinus lipomatosis occurs secondary to renal atrophy. More severe lipomatosis results from a tremendous increase in renal sinus fat content in cases of marked renal atrophy because of hydronephrosis and chronic calculus disease.

The kidneys appear enlarged with highly echogenic, en-

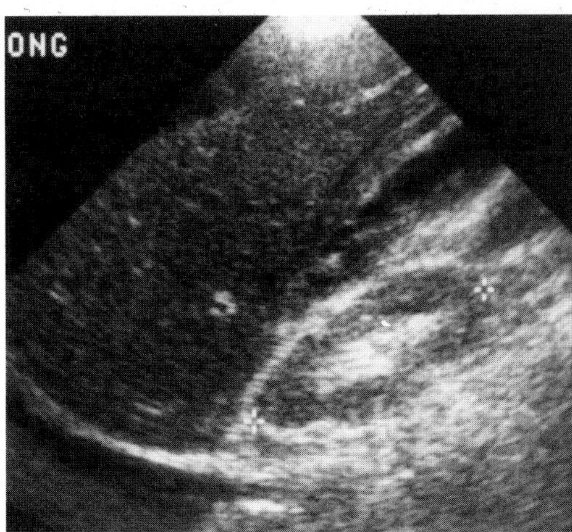

FIG. 9-57 Atrophy of the right kidney in a patient with renal ischemia.

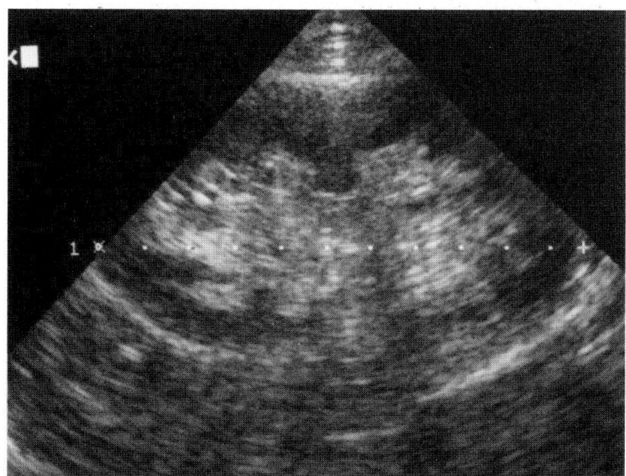

FIG. 9-58 Renal atrophy appears as enlarged kidneys with echogenic, enlarged renal sinus and a thin cortical rim. Renal sinus fat is easily seen on ultrasound as very echogenic reflections.

larged renal sinus and thin cortical rim. Renal sinus fat is easily seen on ultrasound as very echogenic reflections (Fig. 9-58).

Renal Failure, Infarction, and Infection

Acute Renal Failure

Acute renal failure may occur in prerenal, renal, or postrenal failure stages. The prerenal stage is secondary to the hypoperfusion of the kidney. The renal stages may be caused by parenchymal diseases (i.e., acute glomerulonephritis, acute interstitial nephritis, or acute tubular necrosis). It may also be caused by renal vein thrombosis or renal artery occlusion. In postrenal failure, radiologic imaging plays a major role. This condition is usually the result of outflow obstruction and is potentially reversible. Postrenal failure is usually increased in patients with a malignancy of the bladder, prostate, uterus, ovaries, or rectum.

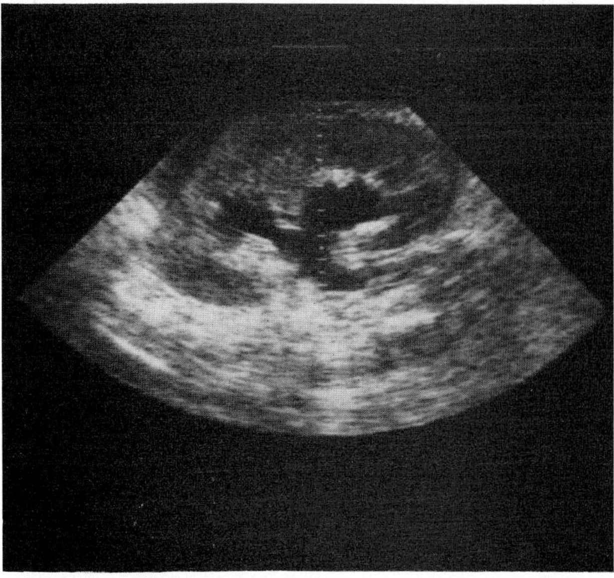

FIG. 9-59 Sagittal scan of the kidney with mild hydronephrosis of the pelvicalyceal system.

Less frequent causes include retroperitoneal fibrosis and renal calculi.

On ultrasound, urinary outflow obstruction can be differentiated from parenchymal disease. Obstruction is responsible for approximately 5% of acute renal failure. The most important issue is the presence or absence of urinary tract dilation. The degree of dilation does not necessarily reflect either the presence or severity of an obstruction. A sonographer should try to determine the level of obstruction. A normal ultrasound does not totally exclude urinary obstruction. In the clinical setting of acute obstruction secondary to calculi a nondistended collecting system can be present.

Hydronephrosis

Hydronephrosis is the separation of renal sinus echoes by interconnected fluid-filled areas. In patients with progressive obstruction the renal parenchyma is compressed. If hydronephrosis is suspected, the sonographer should evaluate the bladder. If it is full, a postvoid longitudinal scan of each kidney should be done to show that hydronephrosis has disappeared or remained the same. At the level of the obstruction, the sonographer should sweep the transducer back and forth in two planes to see if a mass can be distinguished.

There are three grades of hydronephrosis. Grade I entails a small separation of the calyceal pattern, also known as *splaying* (Fig. 9-59). The sonographer must be able to rule out a peripelvic cyst (the septations may be numerous) or renal vessels in the peripelvic area (color-flow Doppler is extremely useful). An extrarenal pelvis would protrude outside of the renal area, and the sonographer probably would not confuse this pattern with hydronephrosis (Fig. 9-60).

Grade II shows the bear-claw effect, with the fluid extending into the major and minor calyceal systems (Fig. 9-61). Grade III represents massive dilation of the renal pelvis with loss of renal parenchyma (Fig. 9-62).

In evaluating the patient for hydronephrosis, a sonographer must be sure to look for a dilated ureter (Fig. 9-63), an enlarged prostate (which may cause the ureter to become obstructed), or an enlarged bladder (this may be secondary to an enlarged prostate). Bladder carcinoma may obstruct the pathway of the urethra, causing urine to back into the ureter and renal pelvis. A ureterocele may also block urine output. This condition occurs where the ureter inserts into the bladder wall. The ureter can turn inside out and obstruct the orifice.

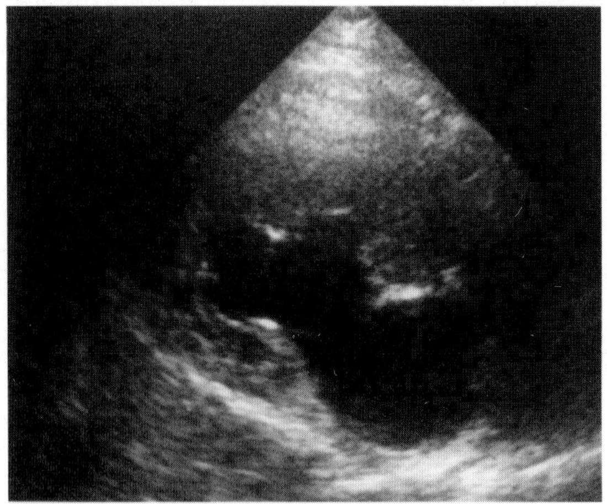

FIG. 9-60 An extrarenal pelvis should not be confused with hydronephrosis.

Nonobstructive hydronephrosis. Dilation of the renal pelvis does not always mean that obstruction is present. Several other factors may cause the renal pelvis to be dilated, such as reflux, infection, high flow states (polyuria), atrophy after obstruction (once obstruction is relieved the obstruction can remain), or pregnancy dilation (the enlarged uterus can compress the ureter; usually occurs more on the right).

Hydronephrosis—false-positive. Many conditions may mimic hydronephrosis, such as extrarenal pelvis, parapelvic cysts, reflux, transient diuresis, congenital megacalyces, papillary necrosis, renal artery aneurysm (color can help distinguish that this enlargement is vascular, not the renal pelvis), or an arteriovenous malformation (color can distinguish this abnormality).

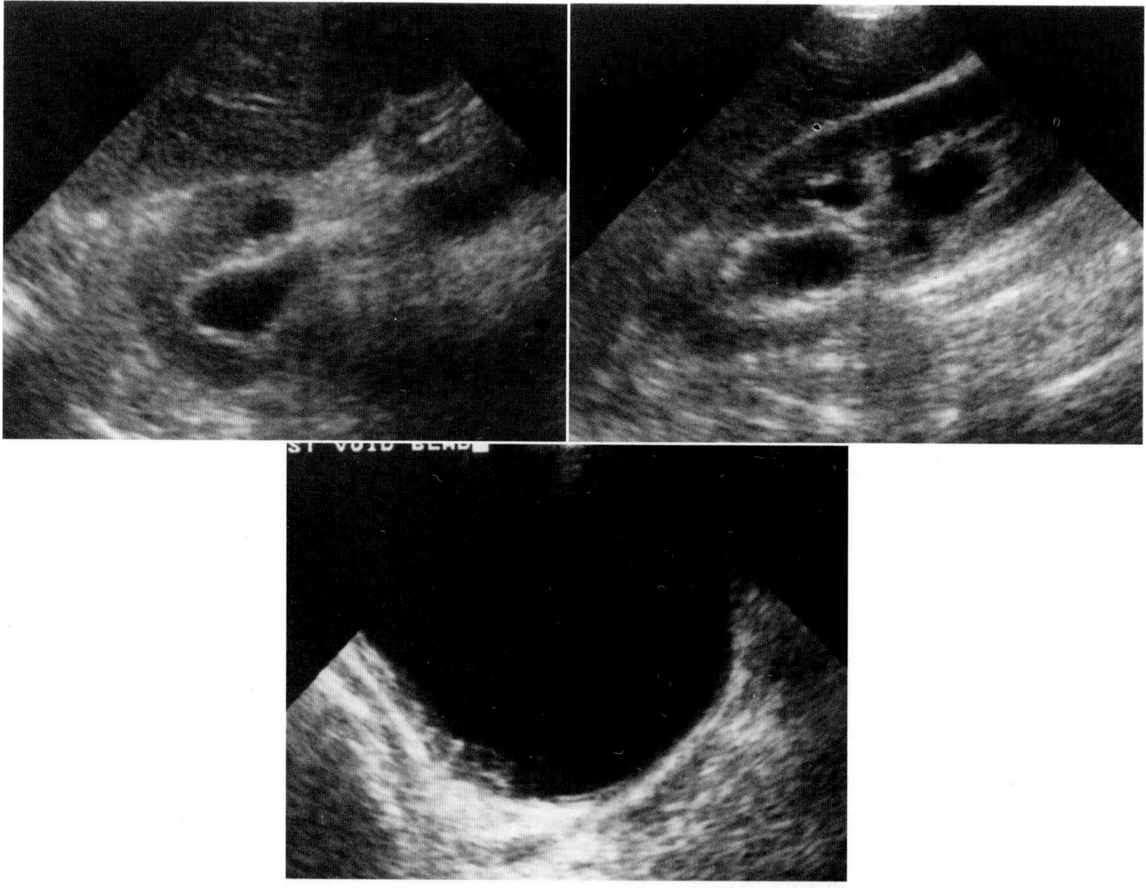

FIG. 9-61 Grade II hydronephrosis shows moderate splaying of the renal pelvis. The bladder was distended, so the patient voided and was rescanned, but the renal sinus remained prominent.

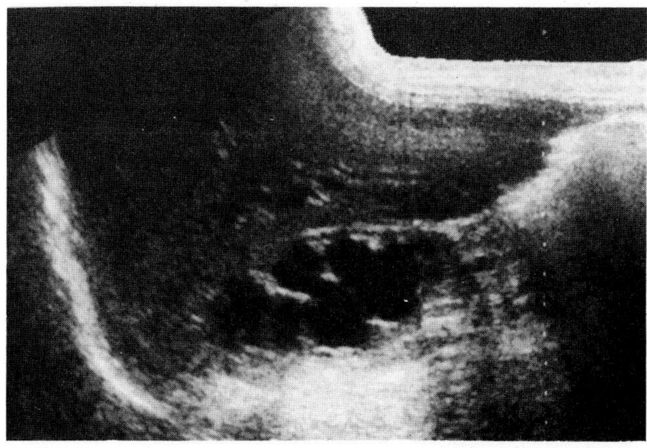

FIG. 9-62 Sagittal scan of a patient with right hydronephrosis. There is loss of the pelvicalyceal system with cysts of similar size representing the distended pelvis.

Localized hydronephrosis may be secondary to strictures, calculi, or focal masses (transitional). It can also occur in a duplex system when one of the systems can be obstructed because of an ectopic insertion of the ureter. In females it can insert below the external urinary sphincter and cause dribbling.

In patients with false-negative hydronephrosis, several techniques may be used to help distinguish the dilated renal pelvis from other conditions. In patients with retroperitoneal fibrosis or necrosis, give liquids to see if the renal pelvis dilates. In patients with a distal calculi, no obstruction can be seen unless the calculi has been there for several days. A staghorn calculus can mask an associated dilation.

Adult polycystic disease and multicystic renal disease with severe hydronephrosis may be confused. In patients with severe hydronephrosis the image shows dilated calyces as they radiate from a larger central fluid collection in the renal pelvis. The kidney usually retains a normal shape. The sonographer sees fluid-filled sacs in a radiating pattern or cauliflower configuration.

In patients with adult polycystic renal disease and multicystic renal disease the renal cysts are randomly distributed, the contour is disturbed, and the cysts are variable in size.

Once you have shown that renal failure is not the result of obstruction, consider renal medical disease, which is the leading cause of acute renal failure.

Renal Infarction

Infarcts within the renal parenchyma appear as irregular masses somewhat triangular in shape along the periphery of the renal border. The renal contour may be somewhat "lumpy-bumpy." Remember that lobulations in the pediatric patient may be normal, except for the dromedary hump variant. In the adult patient the renal contour should be smooth. In a patient with a renal infarct, the irregular area may be slightly more echogenic than the renal parenchyma.

Acute Tubular Necrosis

Acute tubular necrosis is the most common medical renal disease to produce acute renal failure, although it can be reversible. Ultrasound shows bilaterally enlarged kidneys with hyperechoic pyramids; this can revert to a normal appearance. The differential diagnosis includes nephrocalcinosis. In pediatric patients the renal pyramids are very echogenic without shadowing. The calculi may be too small to cause dilation and shadowing of the pyramids (Fig. 9-64). As renal function improves, the echogenicity decreases. This can occur in the medulla or cortex. If it reverses, it is probably acute tubular necrosis.

Chronic Renal Disease

Chronic renal disease is a diffusely echogenic kidney with loss of normal anatomy. It is a nonspecific ultrasound finding—chronic renal disease can be caused by multiple etiologies (AIDS can produce echogenic kidneys).

If chronic renal disease is bilateral, small kidneys are identified. This may result from hypertension, chronic inflammation, or chronic ischemia.

Renal Infections

There is a spectrum of severity in renal infections. The disease can progress from pyelonephritis to focal bacterial nephritis to an abscess. An abscess can be transmitted through the parenchyma into the blood. Most renal infections stay in kidney and are resolved with antibiotics (Fig. 9-65). A perirenal abscess occurs from a direct extension.

Pyonephrosis

Pyonephrosis occurs when pus is found within the obstructed renal system. It is often associated with severe urosepsis and represents a true urologic emergency that requires urgent percutaneous drainage. It usually occurs secondary to long-standing ureteral obstruction from calculus disease, stricture, or a congenital anomaly (Fig. 9-66).

The ultrasound findings include the presence of low-level echoes with a fluid debris level (Fig. 9-67). The sonographer should be aware that an anechoic dilated system can occur (ultrasound-guided aspiration or CT may be necessary).

Emphysematous Pyelonephritis

Emphysematous pyelonephritis occurs when there is air in the parenchyma (diffuse gas-forming parenchymal infection). It may be caused by *E. coli* bacteria. When this occurs in diabetic patients, they become very sick. It generally is found unilaterally and may be cause for an emergency nephrectomy. On ultrasound the enlarged kidneys appear hypoechoic and inflamed.

Xanthogranulomatous Pyelonephritis

Xanthogranulomatous pyelonephritis is an uncommon renal disease associated with chronic obstruction and infection. It involves destruction of renal parenchyma and infil-

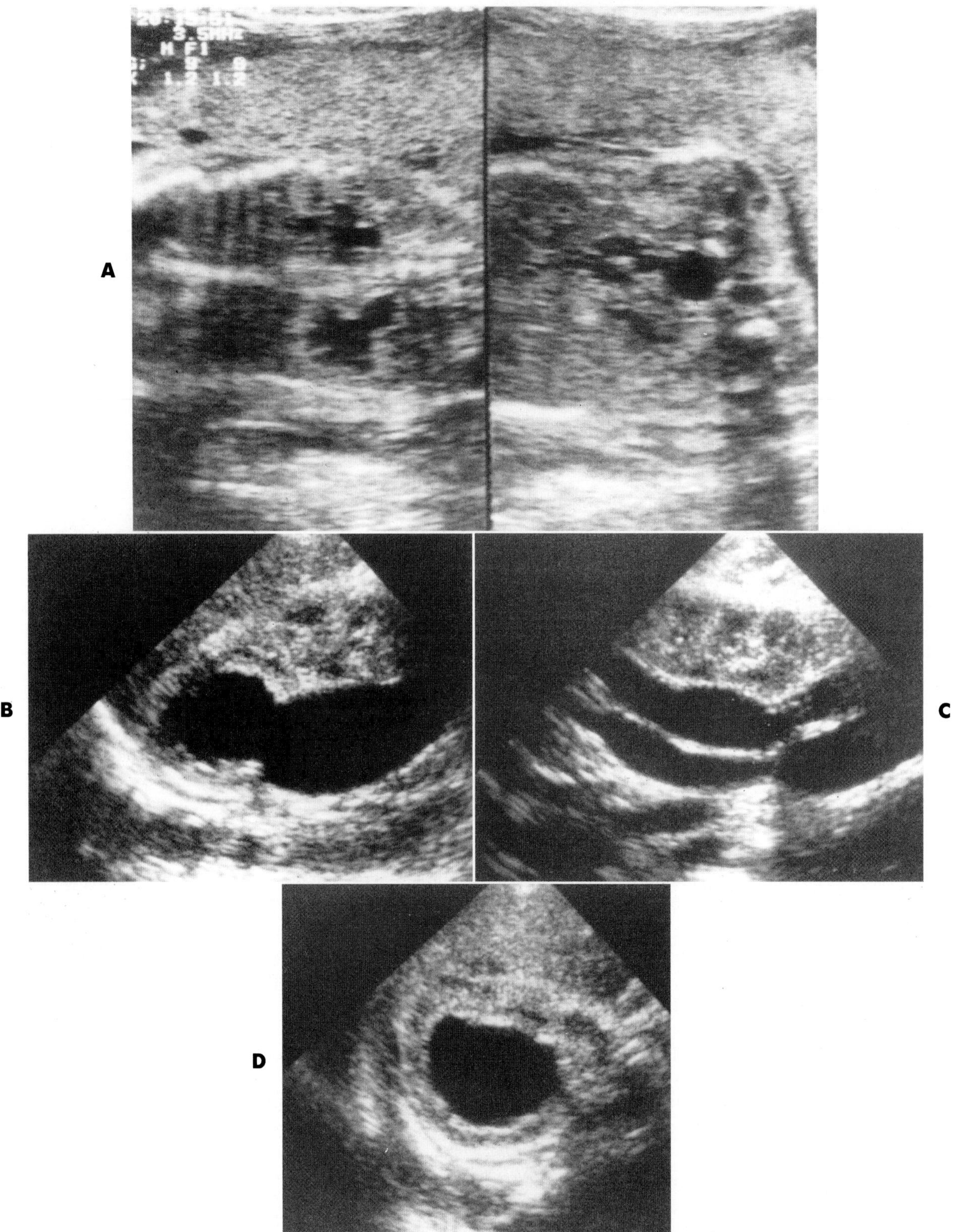

FIG. 9-63 A, Fetal renal study demonstrated bilateral dilation of the renal collecting system. **B,** Distended renal pelvis and ureter in the neonate. **C,** The left kidney and ureter were also distended. **D,** Transverse scan of the right kidney upper pole shows hydronephrosis of the renal pelvis.

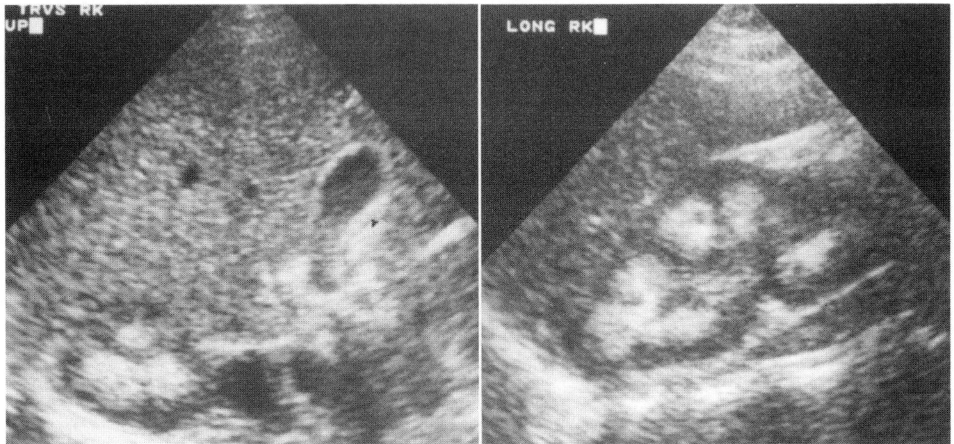

FIG. 9-64 Transverse and longitudinal scans of the pediatric patient with acute tubular necrosis and nephrocalcinosis. The echogenic renal pyramids are well seen.

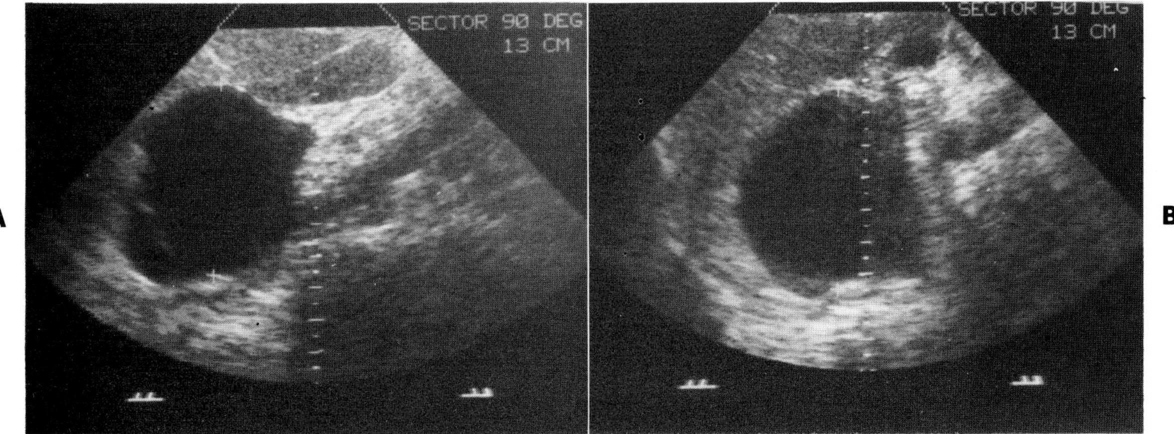

FIG. 9-65 This patient presented with an elevated white blood count and spiking fever. **A,** The supine sagittal scan reveals a homogeneous, slightly irregular mass arising from the upper pole of the right kidney. **B,** Transverse scan of the renal abscess. Note the decreased through-transmission posterior to the abscess wall.

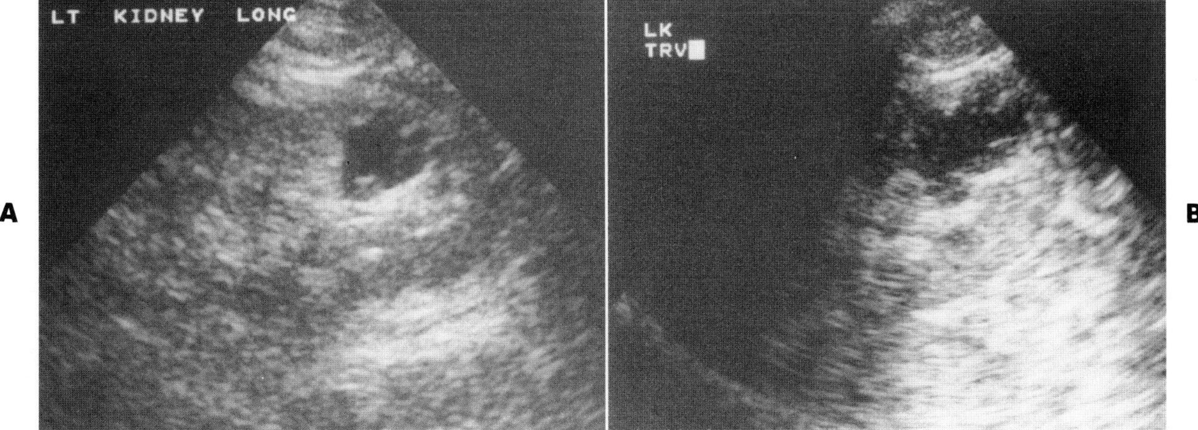

9-66 A, Longitudinal and transverse scans of the left kidney showing an irregular mass lesion in the lower pole. **B,** This patient was found to have pyonephrosis of the kidney secondary to ureteral obstruction.

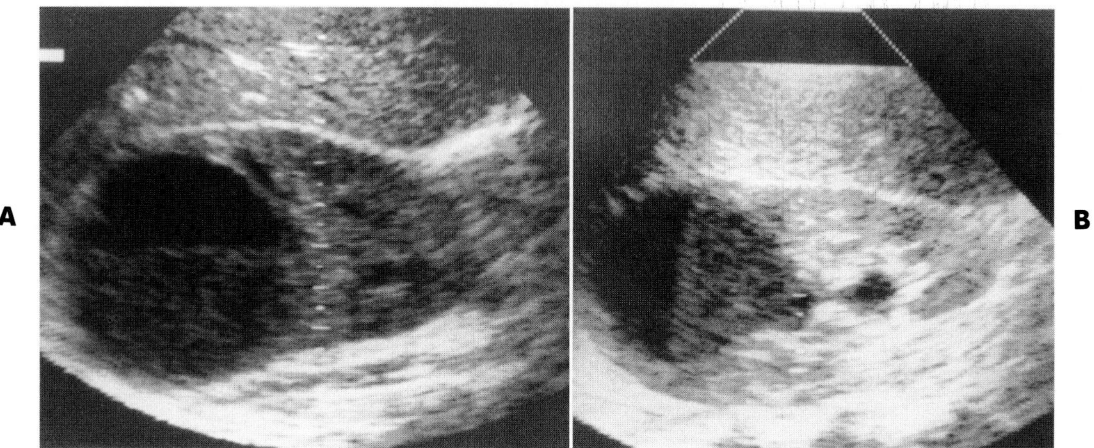

FIG. 9-67 A and **B,** Other findings in a patient with pyonephrosis include a fluid/debris level within a well-defined mass lesion.

tration of lipid-laden histiocytes. Clinically the patient presents with a large, nonfunctioning kidney, staghorn calculus, and multiple infections (Fig. 9-68). The disease is more common in females and is poorly understood. It is thought to be an impaired host responses to an infection in a chronically obstructed and infected kidney.

The ultrasound appearance may show the bright echogenicity from the staghorn calculus (peripelvic fibrosis can prevent the staghorn from shadowing). The renal parenchyma is replaced by cystic spaces. The overall renal size is increased. The disease process may be diffuse or segmental.

Nephrocalcinosis

The nephrocalcinosis disease process shows very echogenic pyramids with or without associated shadowing. Renal stones are very echogenic with shadowing posterior (Figs. 9-69 and 9-70). The patient may present with fever—this may indicate infection with hydronephrosis. When searching for renal stones, one should scan along the lines of the renal fat; usually the stones are small and may not shadow (Figs. 9-71 and 9-72).

Renal Transplant

Renal transplantation and dialysis are currently used to treat chronic renal failure or end-stage renal disease. Ultrasound has emerged as an excellent tool in monitoring such transplant patients and may complement nuclear medicine and laboratory values in distinguishing the course of rejection. Since the sonogram does not rely on the function of the kidney, serial studies can be readily incorporated in determining the diagnosis and the treatment to be administered.

A number of complications may arise after transplantation, including rejection, acute tubular necrosis (ATN), obstructive nephropathy, extraperitoneal fluid collections, hemorrhage or infarction, recurrent glomerulonephritis, graft rupture, and renal emphysema. Decreased renal function is commonly the main indication for ultrasonic evaluation.

The Procedure

Most renal transplant patients have had long-standing renal failure without obstructive nephropathy. Before the procedure, patient risk factors to be considered are age, primary diagnosis, secondary medical complications, and transplant source. It is found that recipients between 16 and 45 years of age with primary renal disease have the lowest risk for morbidity and mortality.

The major problem encountered with transplantation is graft rejection. The success of the transplant is directly related to the source of the donated kidney. Living relatives and cadavers are the two donor types.

The surgical procedure begins with removal of the donor's left kidney, which is then rotated and placed in the recipient's right iliac fossa or groin region. The renal artery is attached by an end-to-end anastomosis with either the common or the external iliac artery (Fig. 9-73).

The ureter is inserted into the bladder above the normal ureteral orifice through a submucosal tunnel in the bladder wall. The tunnel creates a valve in the terminal ureter to prevent reflux of urine into the transplanted kidney.

Although the kidney is more vulnerable to trauma when it is placed in the iliopelvic region, this has rarely been a problem. The advantage of such a location is its observation accessibility. Complications may arise after transplantation, however, so a variety of examinations may be incorporated to detect and follow the transplant. Useful information may be accumulated through laboratory tests, nuclear medicine, sonography, intravenous pyelography, and renal arteriography.

Sonographic Evaluation

As early as 48 hours after surgery a baseline sonographic examination is performed to determine renal size, calyceal pattern, and extrarenal fluid collections. Hydronephrosis

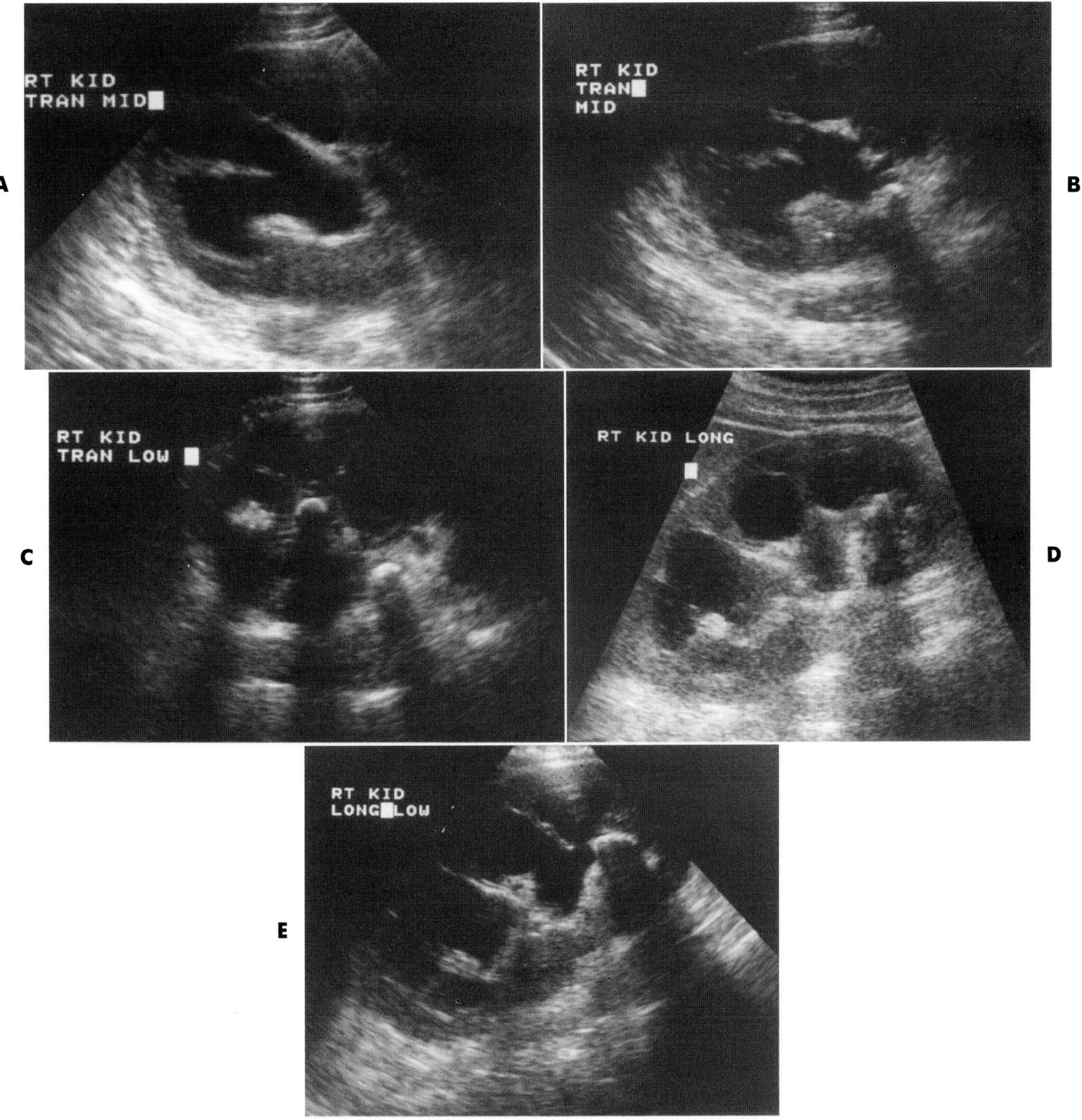

FIG. 9-68 A to **E,** Patient with xanthogranulomatous pyelonephritis shows a large, nonfunctioning right kidney secondary to a stone. Multiple areas of shadowing are seen within the renal parenchyma from the renal stones.

can be easily recognized sonographically with calyceal dilation. Perirenal fluid collections (hematoma, abscess, lymphocele, or urinoma) can be diagnosed reliably and differentiated from acute rejection. Serial scans at 3- to 6-month intervals may be made to detect fluid collections at an early asymptomatic stage. The patient should be examined at the first sign of tenderness in the graft area or mass development.

Technique for sonographic examination. To locate the kidney precisely by ultrasound, transverse supine scans are made from the pubic symphysis to above the level of the graft. Longitudinal and transverse scans are made parallel with and perpendicular to the long axis of the kidney. From these scans accurate measurements of the renal length, width, and anteroposterior dimensions can be determined (Figs. 9-74 and 9-75).

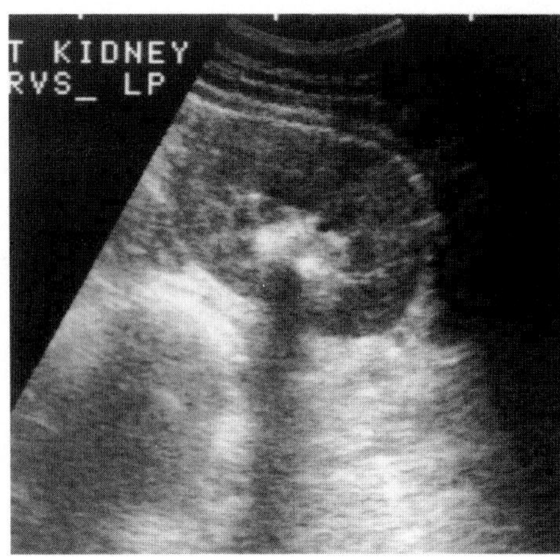

FIG. 9-69 A 29-year-old male presented with left flank pain and hematuria. The central renal parenchyma was echogenic with a shadow, representative of a renal stone.

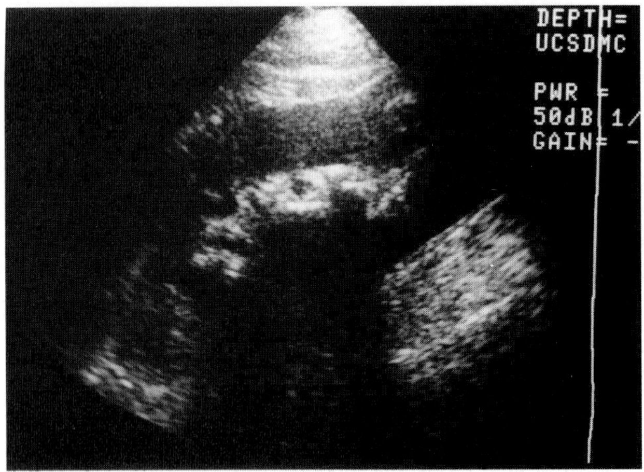

FIG. 9-70 This patient presented with multiple renal stones in the renal sinus.

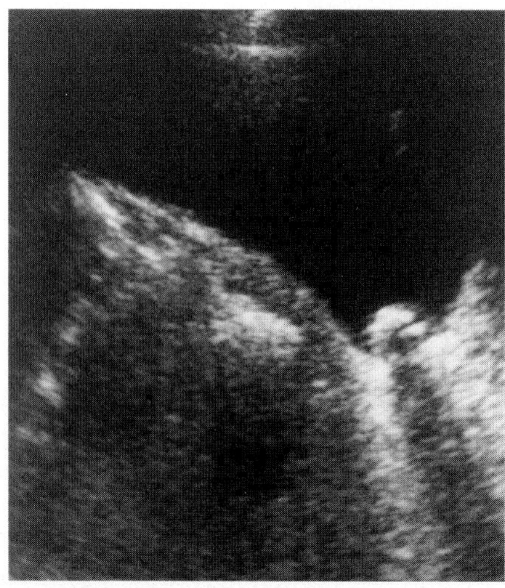

FIG. 9-71 An elderly male presented with a large stone at the dependent area of the bladder with posterior shadowing.

The normal transplant should appear as a smooth structure surrounding the homogeneous parenchymal pattern. A dense band of echoes in the midportion of the transplant represents the renal pelvis, calyces, blood vessels, and fatty fibrous tissues. The medullary pyramids are discrete sonolucent structures surrounded by the homogeneous grainy texture of the cortex (Fig. 9-76). The psoas appears as parallel linear echoes posterior to the kidney transplant (Fig. 9-77).

A sonolucent appearance of the anterior portion of the kidney and, at times, an increased echogenic band across the anterior kidney occur on some scans because of inaccurate settings in the near field. Decreased amplification of the near gain in the first few centimeters of the slope obliterates the decreased echoes of the near field and allows for better fill-in of the anterior portion of the kidney. This difference in anterior structure delineation is probably because of the attenuation of sound by subcutaneous fat, muscle thickness, skin texture, and scarring or the fact that some patients transmit the sound frequency more readily than others.

The opposite is true for the problem of increased echoes in the near field. By decrease in the near gain, suppression of the echoes in the near field yields an image with uniform texture. Thus it is important to maintain proper penetration and delineation of internal structures with a good outline of adjacent musculature.

To record echoes from the parenchyma and distinguish the cortex from the medulla, the sonographer should scan the patient with low-gain and high-gain settings. The scans include both kidneys and the pararenal area (i.e., iliac wing and iliopsoas).

Medical Complications

Renal transplant rejection. Rejection has always been the most difficult of the medical complications to accurately diagnose without percutaneous needle biopsy. No single imaging method permits accurate diagnosis with sufficient specificity and sensitivity to totally obviate renal biopsy.*

There are three types of rejection. Hyperacute rejection occurs within hours of transplantation and is caused by vasculitis leading to thrombosis and usually loss of the graft. Acute rejection occurs within days to months after transplant with rapid onset. The immunologic causes include preformed antibodies, immune complexes, and cell-mediated responses. Pathologically, acute rejection is separated into vascular and interstitial forms. Without aggressive therapy the graft can be lost. Lastly, chronic rejection can occur months after transplantation with gradual onset. It tends to be secondary to mononuclear infiltration and fibrosis. Steroid therapy and antilymphocyte serum are of little benefit in improving renal function and can lead to opportunistic infections.[1,5,6] Sonography can be useful in the

*References 2, 3, 4, 5, 6, 7.

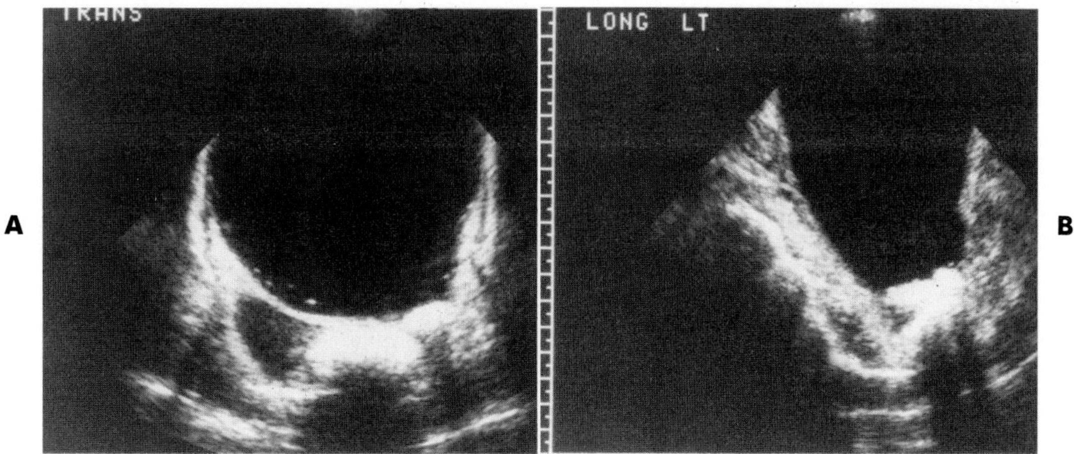

FIG. 9-72 A and **B**, Transverse and longitudinal scans of a patient with a ureterovesical stone (echogenic area with shadowing) at the distal segment of the ureter.

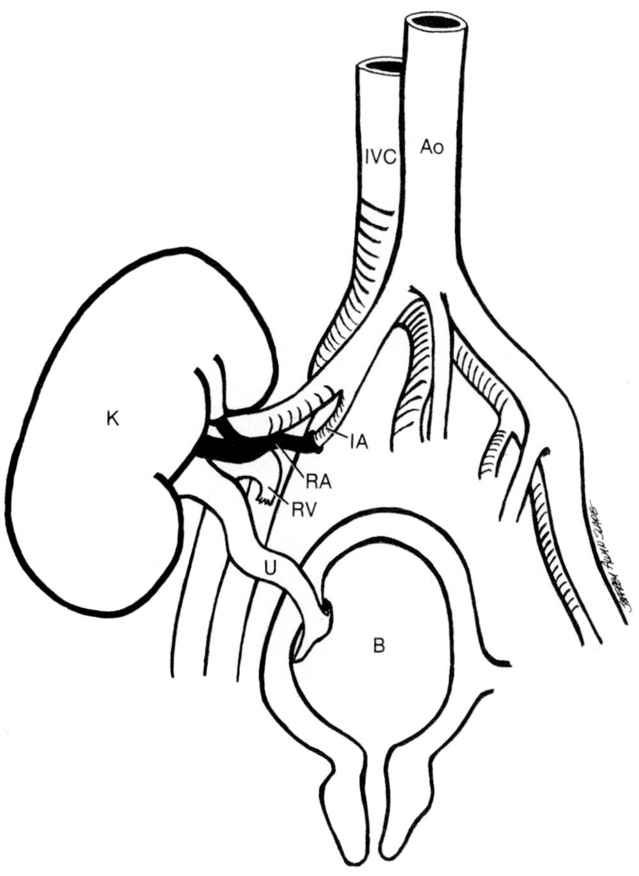

FIG. 9-73 Surgical placement of the renal transplant into the iliac fossa. Aorta, *Ao;* inferior vena cava, *IVC;* kidney, *K;* ureter, *U;* bladder, *B;* internal iliac artery, *IA;* renal artery, *RA;* renal vein, *RV*.

diagnosis of rejection. Care must be taken to observe the size and shape; the appearance of the pyramids, cortex, and parenchyma; and the presence of any surrounding fluid collections. Maklad et al.[8a] summarize the appearance of renal rejection by stating that the following five changes in the renal parenchymal echo pattern have been observed during the process of rejection:

1. Enlargement and decreased echogenicity of the pyramids. This appearance is not at all uniform, and only a few pyramids may appear as such (Fig. 9-78).
2. Hyperechogenic cortex. The swollen sonolucent pyramids stand out against the background of increased echogenicity of the outer and interpyramidal cortex (Fig. 9-79).
3. A localized area of renal parenchyma, including both the cortex and the medulla presenting an anechoic appearance, is very difficult to fill in even when high sensitivity and TGC settings are used. This is usually seen in polar regions (Fig. 9-80).
4. Distortion of the renal outline because of localized areas of swelling involving both the cortex and the pyramids. The renal sinus echoes may appear compressed and displaced (Fig. 9-81).
5. Patchy sonolucent areas involving both cortex and medulla with coalescence on follow-up studies. These areas can become quite extensive, affecting a large portion of the renal parenchyma.

In long-standing rejection, Maklad et al. state that two patterns have been observed: (1) a normal-sized renal transplant with very little differentiation between the parenchymal and renal sinus echoes, and (2) a small kidney with irregular margins and an irregular parenchymal echo pattern.[9]

These sonographic appearances correlate with the pathologic occurrences. When swelling with increased internal echoes within the cortex is present, rejection can be diagnosed. Edema, congestion, and hemorrhage of the interstitium produce swelling of the pyramids, which appears as decreased echogenicity (Fig. 9-82). Ischemia and cellular infiltration produce the increased echogenicity of the cortex. Increased areas of sonolucency may also occur in the cortex as a result of necrosis and infarction. These areas

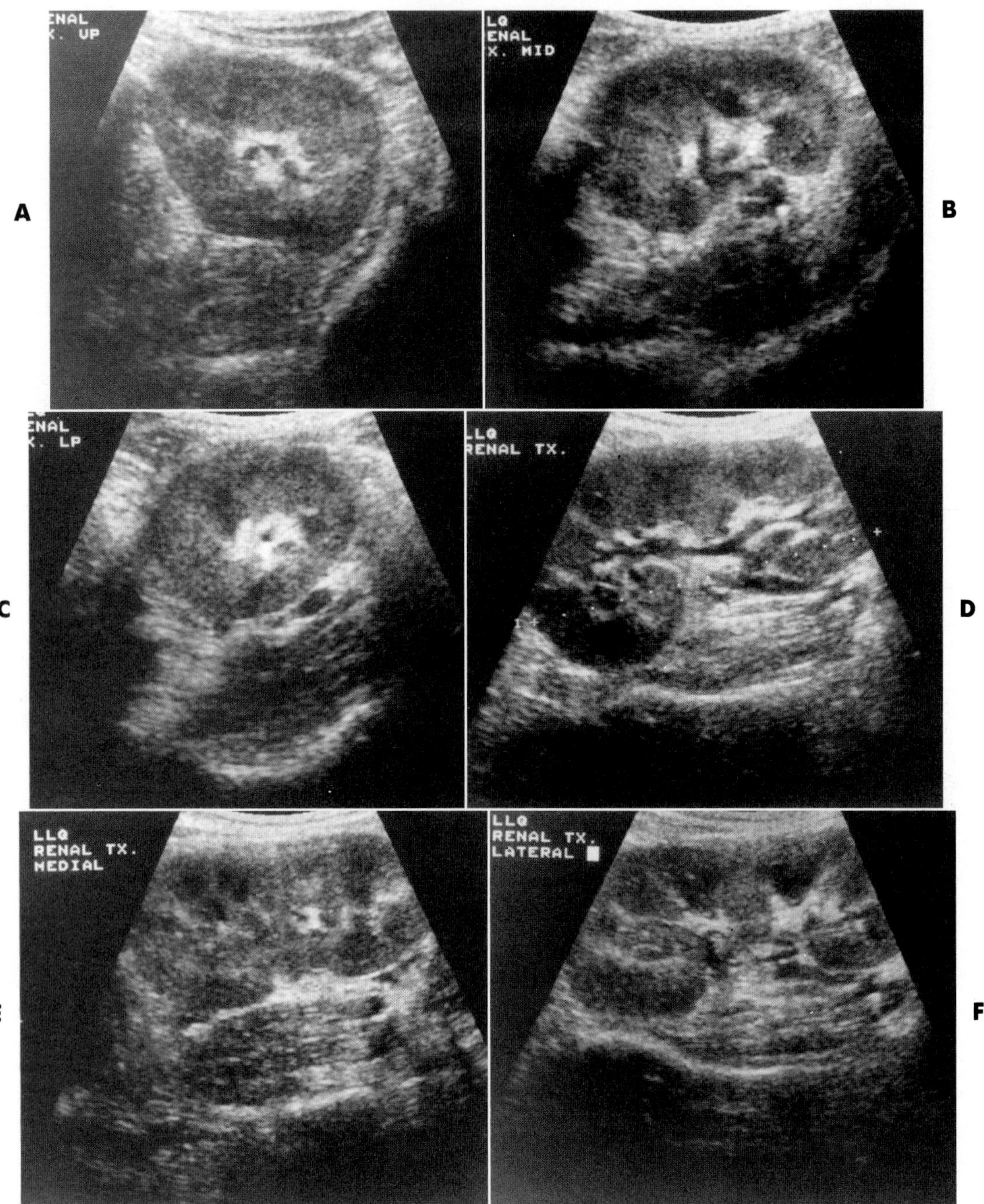

FIG. 9-74 **A** to **C**, Multiple transverse scans of the renal transplant taken in the transverse planes at the upper, middle, and lower segments. **D** to **F**, Longitudinal scans should be made along the longest axis of the kidney in the midline, medial, and lateral planes.

are usually seen in the polar regions of the transplant. If actual necrosis begins, the affected part appears as an area of decreased echogenicity, which suggests partial liquefaction. Irregular parenchymal echo patterns may result from parenchymal atrophy with fibrosis and shrinkage resulting from long-standing renal rejection.

Acute tubular necrosis. Acute tubular necrosis is a common cause of acute posttransplant failure. Some degree occurs in almost every transplant patient, and it has been stated that as many as 50% of the recipients of cadaver kidneys experience ATN after transplantation. The incidence of ATN is usually higher in cadaveric transplants than in donor-relative transplants or in kidneys that undergo warm ischemia or prolonged preservation, kidneys with multiple renal arteries, or kidneys obtained from elderly donors. ATN usually occurs as a medical complication after a loss

A B C D

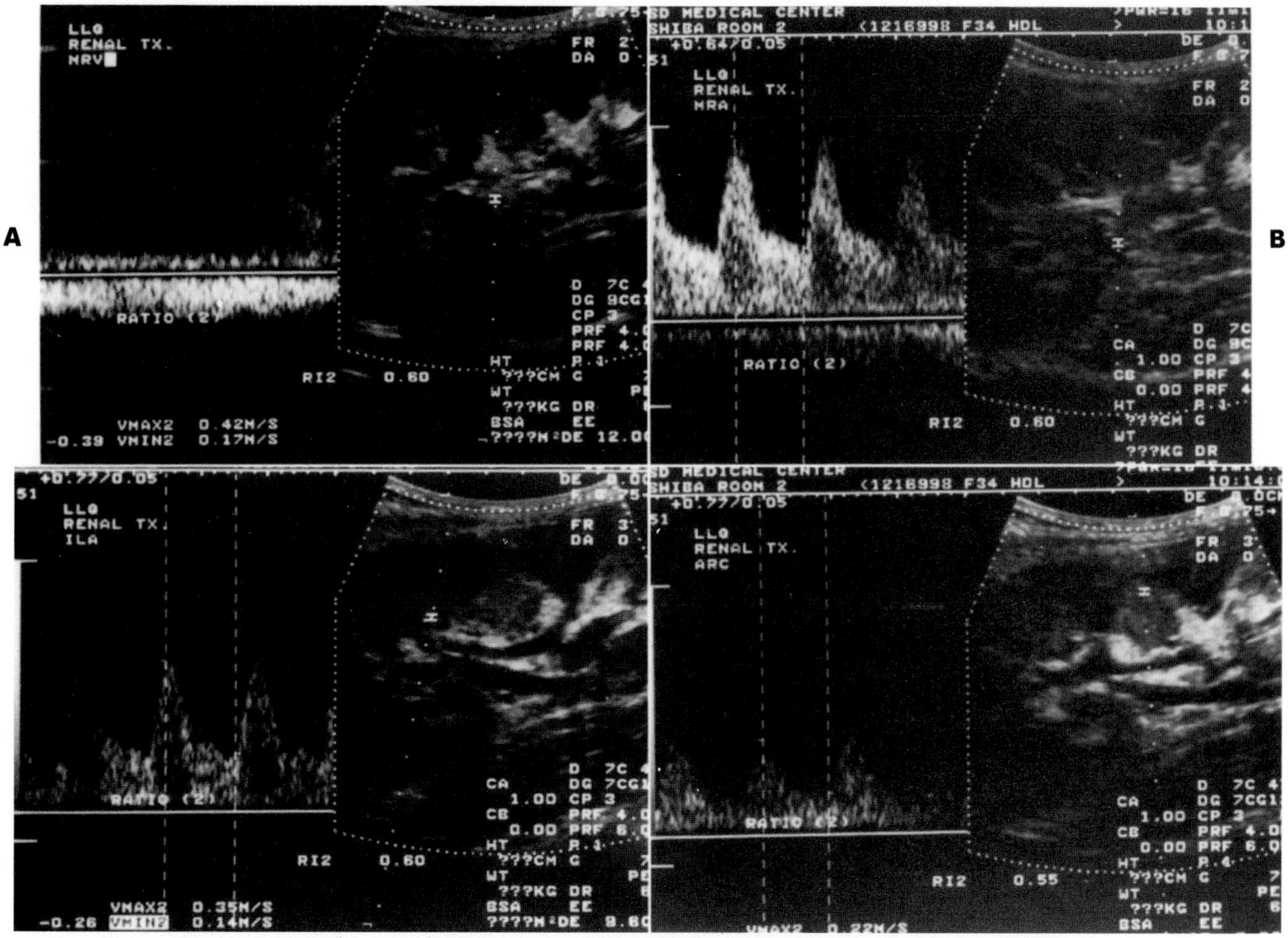

FIG. 9-75 Normal evaluation of the renal transplant includes evaluation of the size, renal parenchyma, the presence of abnormal fluid collections, and Doppler assessment of the renal vessels. **A,** Doppler evaluation of the main renal vein shows a smooth, continuous flow throughout the cardiac cycle with changes in respiratory motions. **B,** Evaluation of the main renal artery shows good perfusion in the systolic and diastolic segments. The resistive index measures 0.6, well within the normal range (resistive index measuring 0.7 or under is normal). **C,** Doppler of the interlobar renal artery with good perfusion in systole and diastole. The resistive index measured 0.6, within normal limits. **D,** Doppler of the arcuate artery shows normal flow and a normal resistive index.

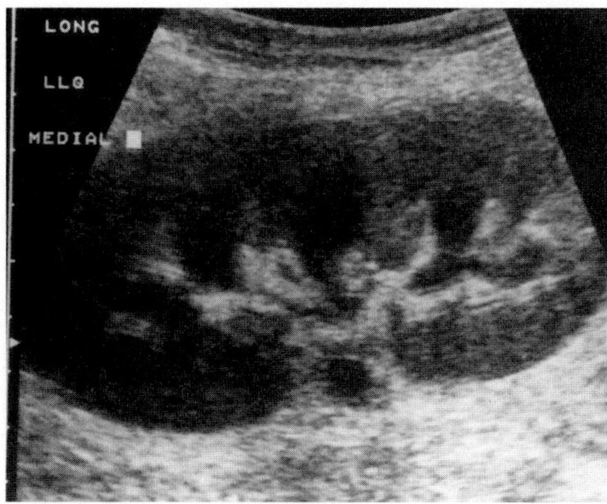

FIG. 9-76 The medullary pyramids are discrete sonolucent structures surrounded by the homogeneous grainy texture of the cortex.

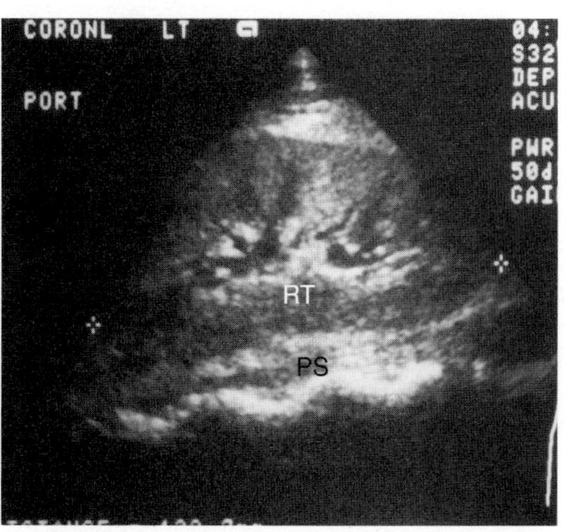

FIG. 9-77 The psoas muscle, *Ps,* is posterior to the renal transplant, *RT,* and appears as parallel linear echoes along the posterior border.

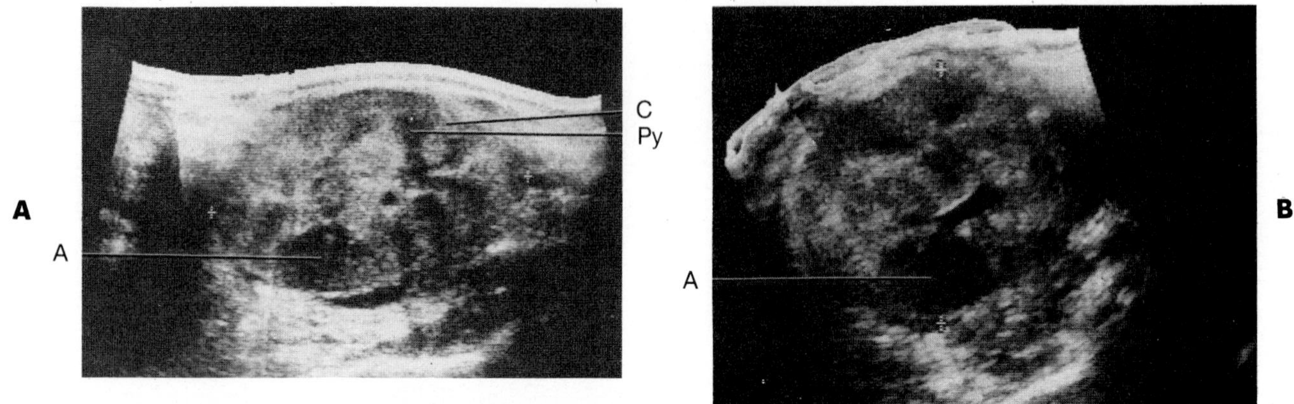

FIG. 9-78 A, Enlargement and decreased echogenicity of the pyramids, *Py,* due to edema and congestion with hemorrhage of the interstitial tissue. Ischemia and cellular infiltration (fibrosis) result in hyperechogenicity of the cortex, *C.* Anechoic, *A,* areas usually occur in the polar regions. **B,** Transverse scan of the same patient demonstrating the extent of the anechoic area.

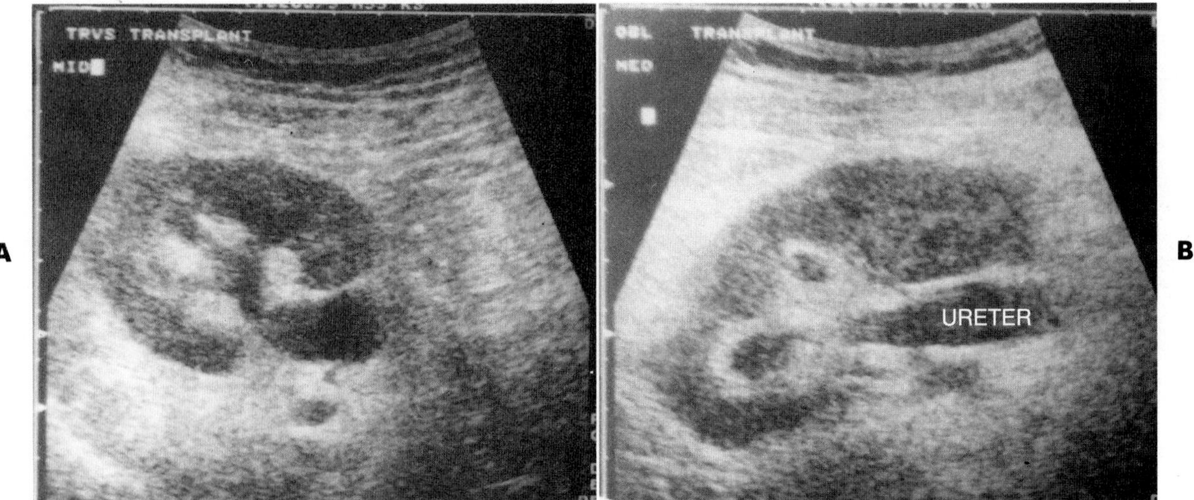

FIG. 9-79 A and **B,** The hyperechogenic cortex appears as swollen sonolucent pyramids against the background of increased echogenicity of the outer and interpyramidal cortex. In addition, this patient had obstruction near the distal ureter, causing mild dilation of the renal pelvis and ureter.

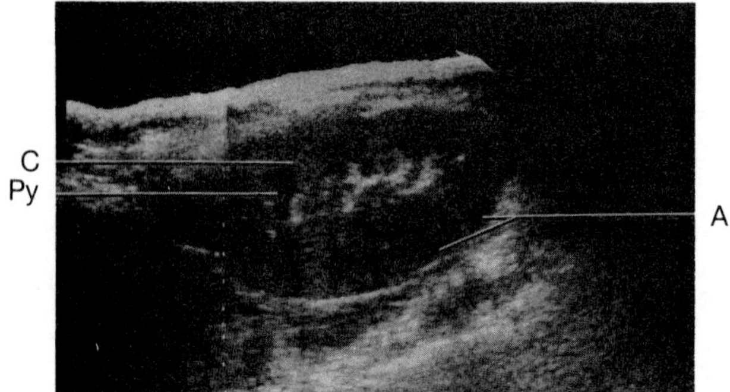

FIG. 9-80 This patient presented with enlargement and decreased echogenic pyramids, *Py,* hyperechogenic cortex, *C,* and a localized anechoic area of renal parenchyma, *A.* This correlated with pathology data on an edematous hemorrhagic cortex and medulla, with fibrin deposited throughout the kidney.

of blood supply to the transplant tissues. This can occur in the donor before harvesting the kidney; during the process of harvesting, preserving, and transportation; or during surgery or as a result of poor circulation after the transplant. Since ATN is associated with prolonged severe ischemia, the likelihood of it occurring after any incidence of cardiac arrest cannot be ruled out. This pertains to the donor and the recipient.[12]

ATN usually resolves early in the postoperative period. Uncomplicated ATN is often reversible and can be treated by immediate use of diuretics and satisfactory hydration. It is important to recognize uncomplicated ATN and distinguish it from acute rejection, because the therapy for the two conditions is very different.

Clinically ATN may present a variety of different patterns. Urine volumes may be good initially, followed by

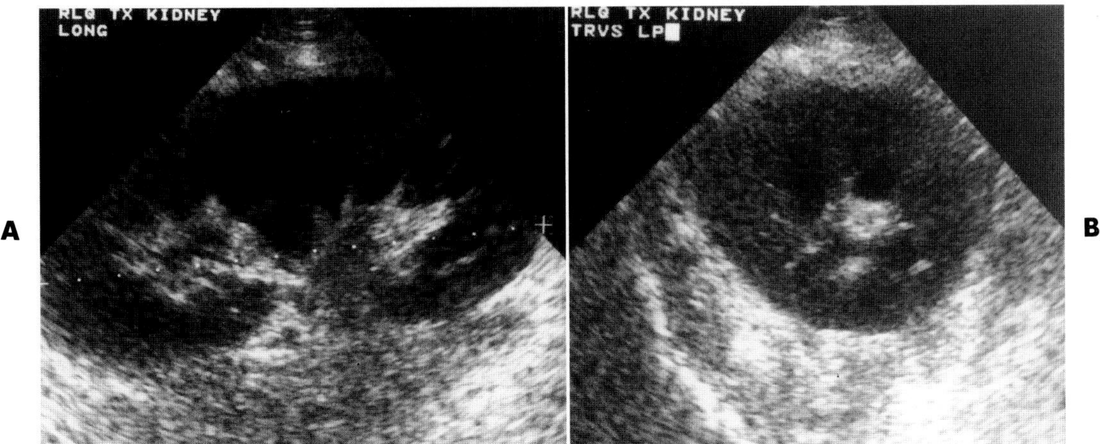

FIG. 9-81 **A** and **B,** Distortion of the renal outline because of localized areas of swelling involving both the cortex and the pyramids. The renal sinus echoes may appear compressed and displaced.

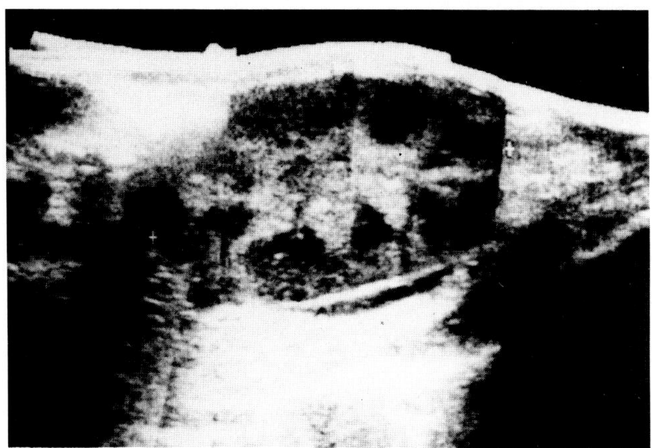

FIG. 9-82 Renal transplant rejection with prominent pyramids and echogenic renal cortex. A small amount of ascites is seen posterior to the transplant.

oliguria or anuria, or there may be low urine output from the time of transplantation. The serum creatinine level is always elevated. If urine output remains low and BUN and creatinine remain elevated, ATN may be difficult to distinguish from rejection. Other indications of rejection (e.g., hematuria, elevated eosinophil counts, or pain over the transplant) are helpful but may be late signs.

Sonographically there are usually no changes seen within the renal parenchyma. In the initial postoperative period the kidney may enlarge slightly as a result of secondary hypertrophy. This is believed to be a normal physiologic response of the newly transplanted kidney or is caused by swelling that often regresses within a week. However, if the swelling persists, then either ATN or rejection should be considered. With ATN the renal parenchymal pattern remains unchanged, in contrast to the earlier description of the parenchymal changes during rejection. If these changes are lacking and the transplant fails to function, the cause is most likely ATN, provided the radionuclide evaluation has confirmed the patency of the vascular supply to the transplant.

Cyclosporine toxicity. Cyclosporine A toxicity (drug toxicity) is a reaction to the antirejection drug cyclosporine A with azathioprine and steroids.[1,6] Over time, this drug can prove to be toxic to the transplant. At present biopsy best documents this diagnosis.[4,6]

Malignancy. Malignancy is a newly discovered delayed complication now becoming prevalent as the life of transplants has improved. A total of 55% of renal transplant recipients in a long-term (17-year) study developed at least one malignancy.[9] The two major types of neoplasms found in transplant patients are non-Hodgkin's lymphoma and skin cancer. Research on the incidence of occurrence of these malignancies has shown a strong correlation to the immunosuppressive drug used to maintain the transplant. A cyclosporine regimen has shown an increased incidence of non-Hodgkin's lymphoma (38% over azathioprine). Azathioprine produces an increased incidence of skin and lip tumors (40% over cyclosporine A). Cases have been documented of a neoplasm from a transplant primary, but this is uncommon. Even so, prescreening donor kidneys may reduce this occurrence.[9]

Extraperitoneal fluid collections. Numerous extraperitoneal fluid collections may occur after transplantation, including lymphoceles and lymph fistulas, urinary fistula and urinoma, perinephric abscess, and hematoma. These collections consist of lymph, blood, urine, pus, or a combination of the substances. A sign common to several of the complications is a decrease in renal function manifested by increased creatinine values. Sonographically the fluid collections may appear as round or oval structures with irregular and slightly thickened walls. Usually clinical or laboratory correlation suggests the etiology of the fluid. Because the transplant is superficial, scans can easily be made and, if necessary, sonographic guidance can be rendered for aspiration of the contents for further analysis.

Lymphocele. Lymphoceles are a common complication

of transplantation, occurring in approximately 12% of all transplant patients. The source of the lymph collection is probably vessels severed during the preparation of recipient vessels, or it may be the kidney itself in the form of leakage from injured capsular and hilar lymphatics. The lymph drains into the peritoneal cavity, provoking a fibrous reaction and eventually walling itself off. Primary clinical signs are deterioration of renal function (usually within 2 weeks to 6 months of transplantation), development of painless fluctuant swelling over the transplant, ipsilateral leg edema, or wound drainage of lymph cells. If an intravenous pyelogram was performed, a mass indenting the bladder, ureteral deviation, ureteral obstruction, or kidney deviation will be seen.

Sonographically the lymphocele is a well-defined anechoic area, occasionally with numerous septations (Fig. 9-83). Urinomas may appear similar to lymphoceles, although usually they appear early, whereas lymphoceles are more common chronically. If the mass is complex with solid components, hematoma or abscess must be considered. Percutaneous aspiration and drainage with ultrasound or CT guidance has a success rate of 80% with little risk of urinoma or abscess.[6] Lymphoceles often recur after catheter drainage and further surgery may be required.

Urinary fistula and urinoma. Abnormal collections of fluid surrounding the transplant may be readily detected by sonography.

Bladder leaks are derived from the anterior cystostomy or from the ureteroneocystostomy because of faulty surgical technique or bladder overdistension (Fig. 9-84). Clinical signs include local tenderness, fever, sudden decrease in urine output, or urine leakage from the wound. Most fistulas become manifest in the first 2 weeks after surgery, but presentation may be delayed for over a month.

A collection of urine may be present within the pelvis as either a walled-off urinoma or free fluid. These collections are usually echo free. Free urine can easily be differentiated from a loculated urinoma by shifting the patient's position and repeating the examination in the same plane to show redistribution of the fluid.

Perinephric abscess. Perinephric infections can be very hazardous to the transplant patient undergoing immunosuppressive therapy. It is an uncommon complication reported as early as 12 days or many months after transplantation. If the patient presents with a fever of unknown origin, care must be taken to rule out abscess formation. Sonographically an abscess may appear with septa in it. Edema and inflammation may be present around the mass, making the borders appear less distinct compared to those found with lymphoceles and hematomas.

Hematoma. A hematoma may develop shortly after surgery. One of the major indications for an ultrasound scan may be a drop in the hematocrit value. Other clinical findings pertinent to hematomas include signs of bleeding, perinephric hemorrhage, a palpable mass, hypertension, and impaired renal function, or the hematoma may be an incidental finding during scanning. Hematomas appear as walled-off, well-defined areas whose sonolucent echo production depends on the age or stage of the hematoma. It may appear sonolucent while the blood is fresh and be difficult to distinguish from a lymphocele or urinoma. As the clot becomes organized, the hematoma may tend to fragment and develop low-level internal echoes. The mass then appears complex and eventually solid. After a time it may revert to a sonolucent mass and form a seroma.

Obstructive Nephropathy

Early signs of obstruction are anuria or severe oliguria in a patient with satisfactory renal volumes. Numerous conditions may cause obstruction, such as ureteral necrosis, abscess, lymphocele, fungus ball, retroperitoneal fibrosis, stricture at the ureterovesical junction, ureteral calculus,

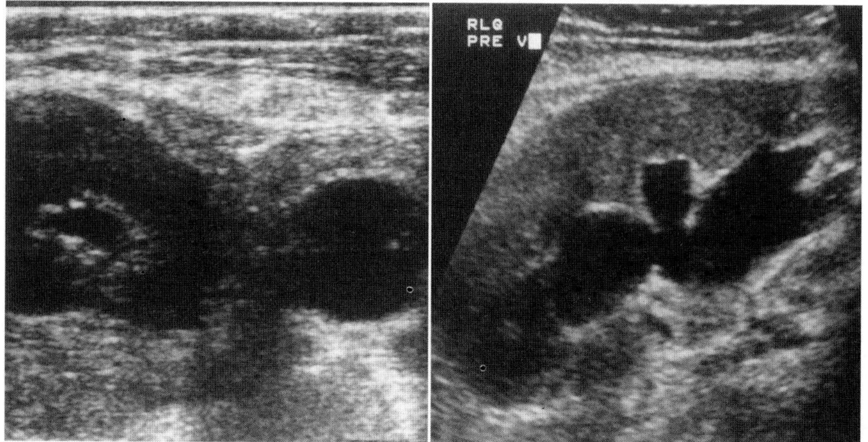

FIG. 9-83 A 30-year-old female with a renal transplant 14 years previously presents with right upper quadrant and midabdominal pain. She had rigors and chills but was afebrile. A tender cystic collection of fluid located above and to the right of the umbilicus and anterior to the IVC represented an infected lymphocele. She also had mild to moderate hydronephrosis.

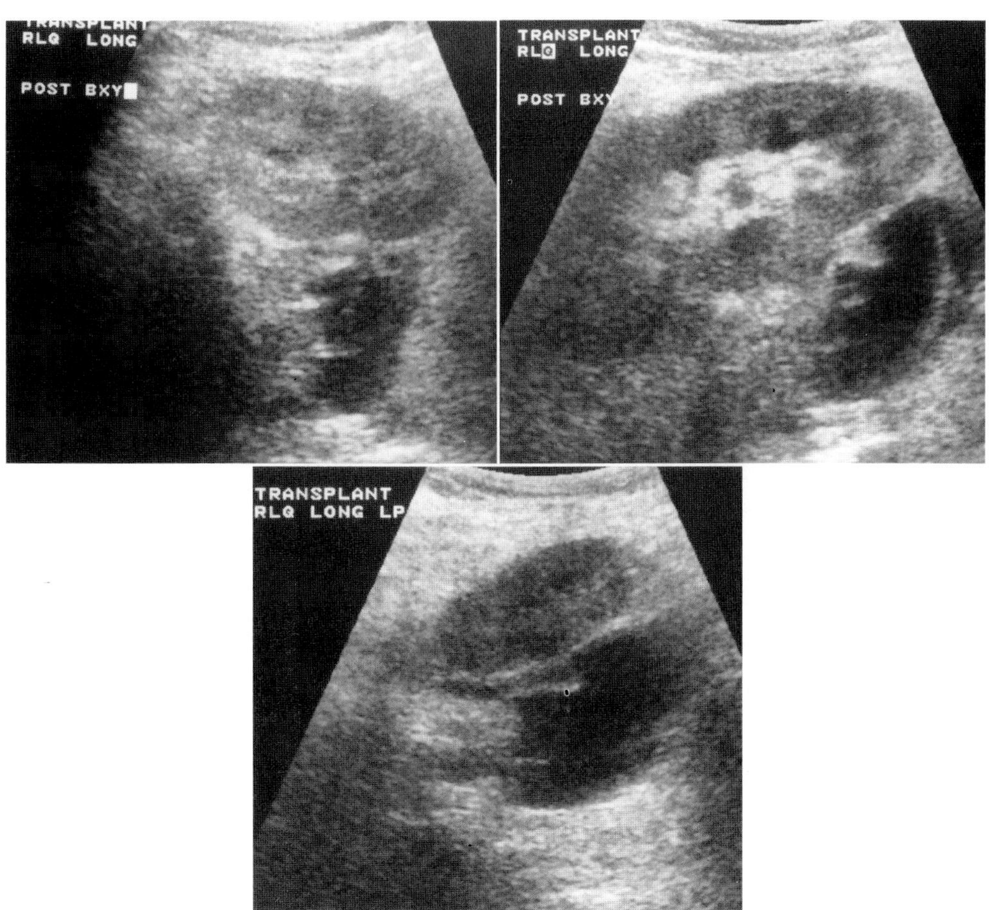

FIG. 9-84 A 29-year-old male with a right lower quadrant renal transplant. Two fluid collections were noted, one adjacent to the lower pole of the renal transplant and another within the anterior abdominal wall at the incision site.

and hemorrhage into the collecting system with obstruction from clots.

Obstruction can be identified sonographically as hydronephrosis.[14] There are many causes of obstruction after renal transplantation. In the early postoperative period, edema at the ureteric implantation site can cause temporary mild obstruction (Fig. 9-85; see color images), or extrinsic mass effect from perinephric fluid collections can impinge on and impair ureteral drainage (Fig. 9-86). In the later postoperative period, rejection or vascular insufficiency may predispose to distal ureteric stricture.[12,16,17] Ureteric blood clots or calculi can also cause the obstruction. A very common benign form of pelvic dilation of the collecting system, pyelocaliectasis, can mimic obstruction. Analysis of laboratory values and an increased resistive index help rule this out.[12,14,16] Finally, make sure to be wary of functional obstruction caused simply by an overdistended urinary bladder. Have the patient void and rescan to confirm.

Vascular insufficiency in the form of arterial stenosis or venous thrombus can be best diagnosed with color and duplex Doppler imaging.[12] When trying to rule out renal artery stenosis, look for a high-velocity jet with distal turbulence.[18]

Graft Rupture

Graft ruptures can occur in the first 2 weeks after surgery, presenting with an abrupt onset of pain and swelling over the graft, oliguria, and shock. Sonographically, graft ruptures appear as a gross distortion of the graft contour and a perinephric or paranephric hematoma.

Improvement of resistive index specificity. Perhaps the most confusing and frustrating problem presently is determining the use of the resistive index (Pourcelot index) to accurately determine and specify transplant disease.[10] Since so many transplant complications exhibit increased resistive indices, is there a way to help limit the differentials with time since transplant? Knowing that many transplant complications tend to surface at particular times after surgery,[1,5,6] a more holistic approach to interpretation of increased resistive indices may be the answer at present.

If there is high renovascular impedance immediately after surgery, patency of the renal vein must be tested. With the use of color and pulsed Doppler, renal thrombosis dis-

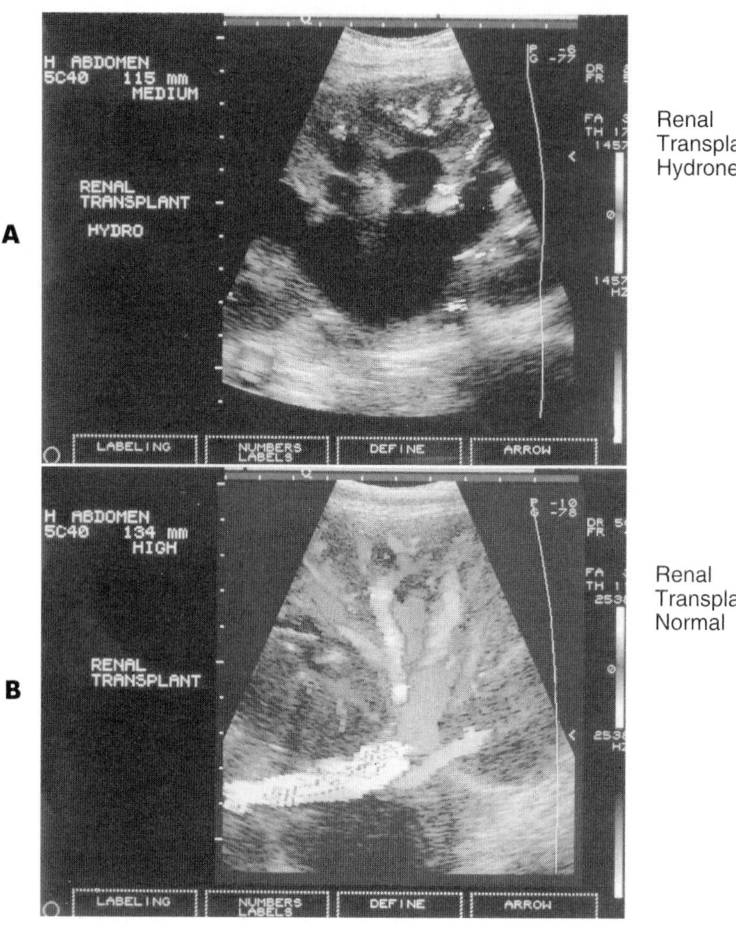

FIG 9-85 A and **B**, Images of the distended renal transplant with hydronephrosis versus a normal renal transplant.

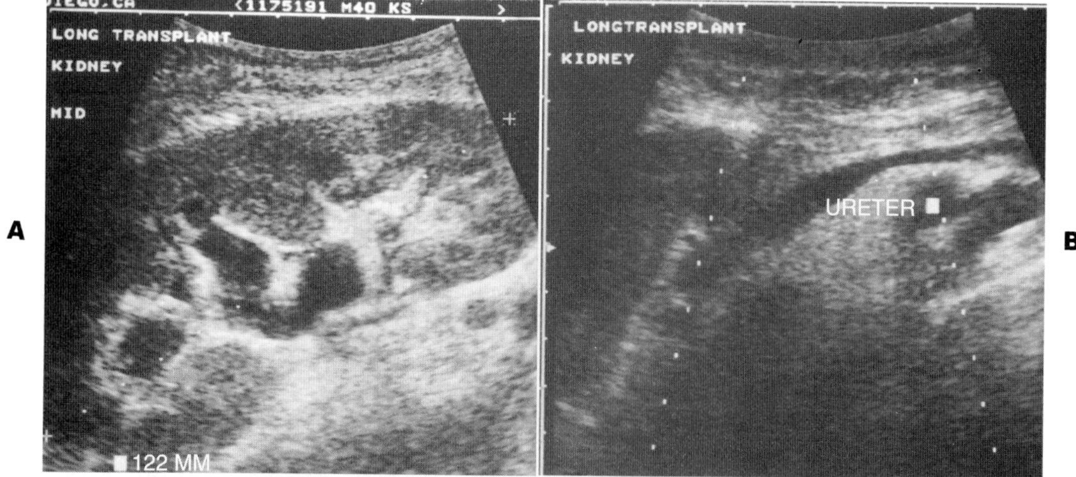

FIG. 9-86 A and **B**, In the early postoperative stages the ureter may be compressed by extrarenal fluid collections, mass effect, or kinks within the ureter. The result is mild obstruction, extending into the renal ureter.

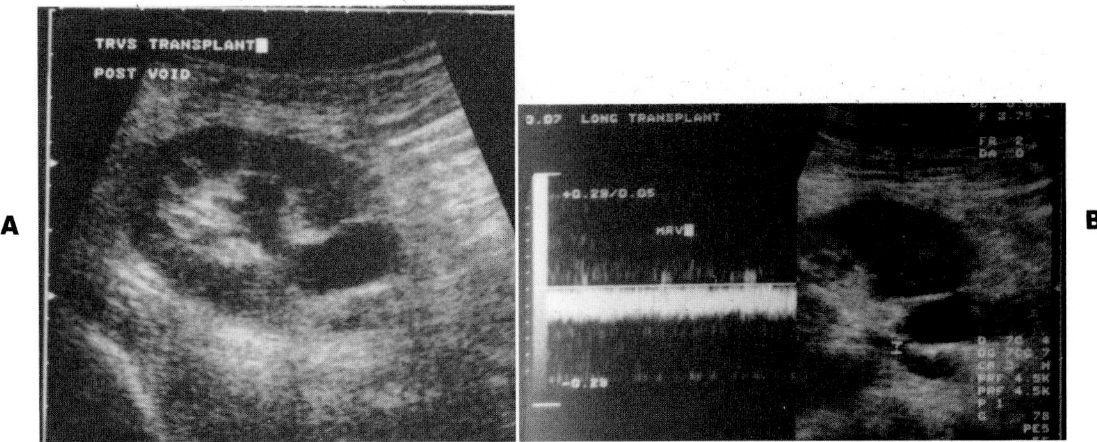

FIG. 9-87 A and **B,** Observation of renal vein patency is very important after renal transplantation. This patient showed a normal renal vein flow pattern.

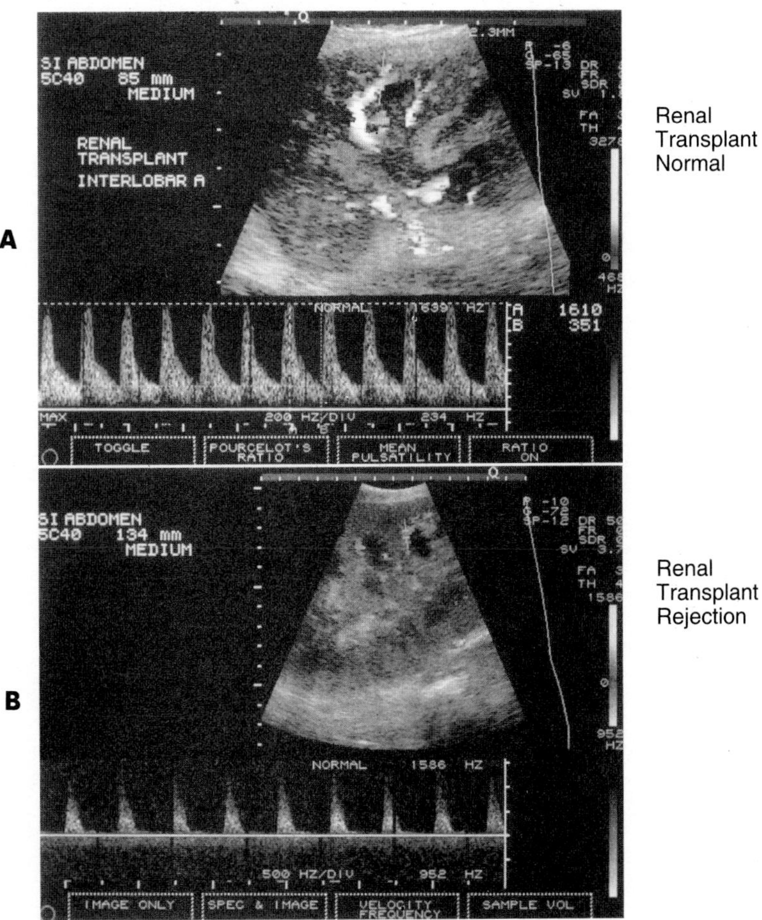

FIG. 9-88 A and **B,** Color flow and Doppler images of a normal flow pattern with good perfusion versus an abnormal flow pattern with no diastolic flow, as seen in a patient with rejection.

plays a distinctive spectral pattern with a plateaulike reversal of diastolic flow (accentuated at end diastole)[4,7,11] (Fig. 9-87). Renal artery stenosis exhibits a high-velocity jet with distal turbulence.[13] After venous patency has been established, one must question if the resistive index increase is caused by extrarenal compression (i.e., an adult allograft in a child is a common initial cause of extra renal compression; to evaluate this, change the child's position to alleviate vascular compromise).[14]

Although ATN does not commonly become abnormal until 24 hours after reperfusion of the graft,[14] this is still a possible cause of increased resistive index immediately after surgery (Figs. 9-88 to 9-90; see color images of Fig. 9-88) Percutaneous biopsy will confirm ATN or rejection (hyperacute or acute).[4,6] If there is an abnormally high renovascular impedance within the first few days after surgery (after a previous normal sonogram), obstructive uropathy should be suspected. The renal transplant should be evaluated with color (lack of color confirms hydronephrosis.[4,14] Pyelocaliectasis is common, and its appearance of hydronephrosis can lead to a false-positive diagnosis of ureteral obstruction.

Clinically the patient should next be evaluated for pyelonephritis, pyuria, and extrarenal compression. At this later period, fluid collections can be the cause of extrarenal compression. The patient should be evaluated for perial-lograft fluid collections.

When there is increased renovascular impedance in the second week after surgery, rejection is by far the most common cause, especially if rejection has a vascular component.* Biopsy is necessary to confirm rejection and to determine whether it is from a vascular or interstitial pathologic cause.[6,10]

Finally, if the creatinine levels increase in the first weeks after transplant, if resistive indices reveal increased renovascular impedance, and if no evidence of obstruction, compression, or infection can be found, the most common cause by far is acute rejection, which biopsy can confirm.[4,14]

New Discoveries

Arteriovenous malformations after biopsy, such as pseudoaneurysms and arteriovenous fistulas, can be readily seen using color Doppler. The color shows turbulent flow in the affected area. Duplex Doppler has not proven to be

*References 6, 7, 10, 11, 13, 14.

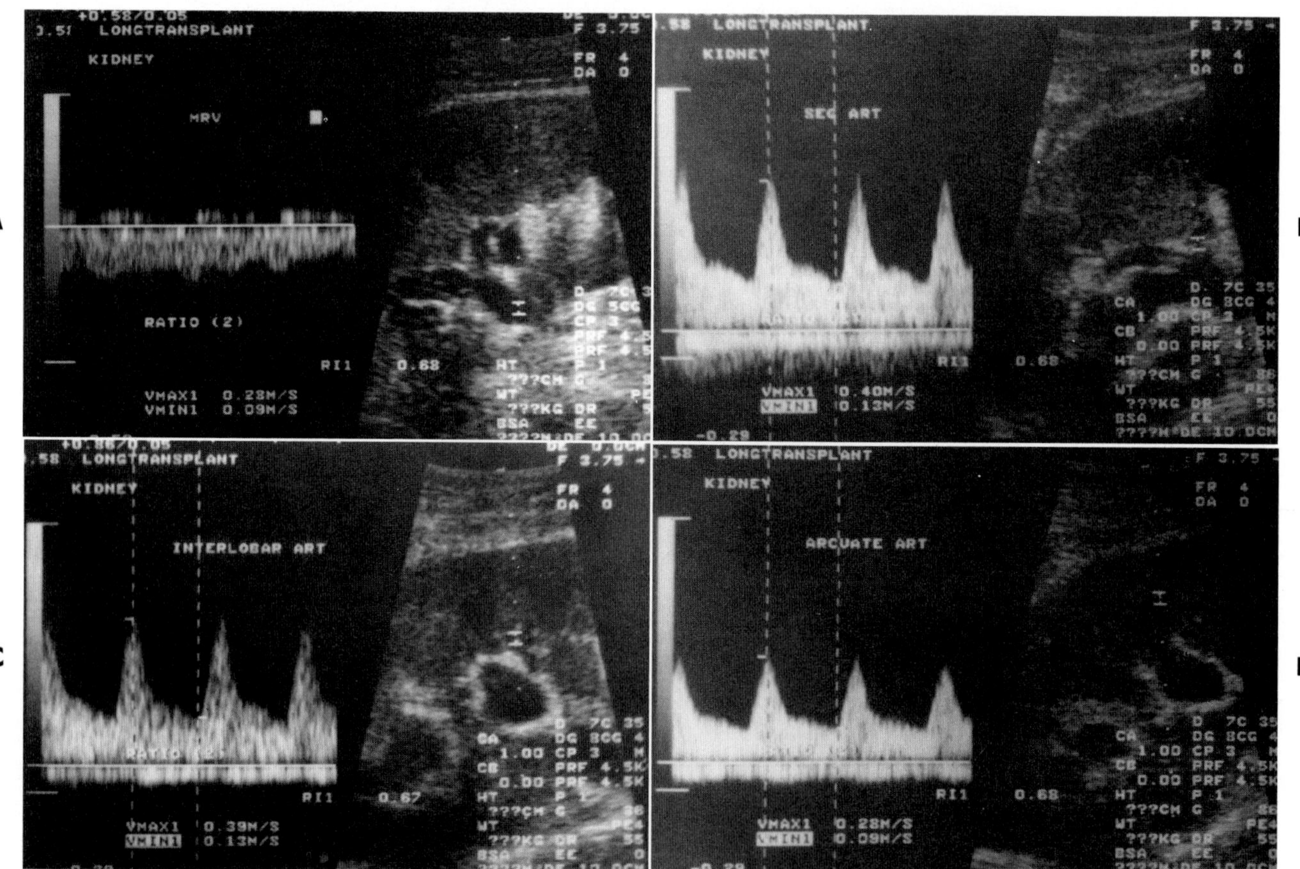

FIG. 9-89 Normal flow patterns in a recent renal transplant patient. **A,** Main renal vein. **B,** Main segmental renal artery. **C,** Interlobar artery. **D,** Arcuate aretery.

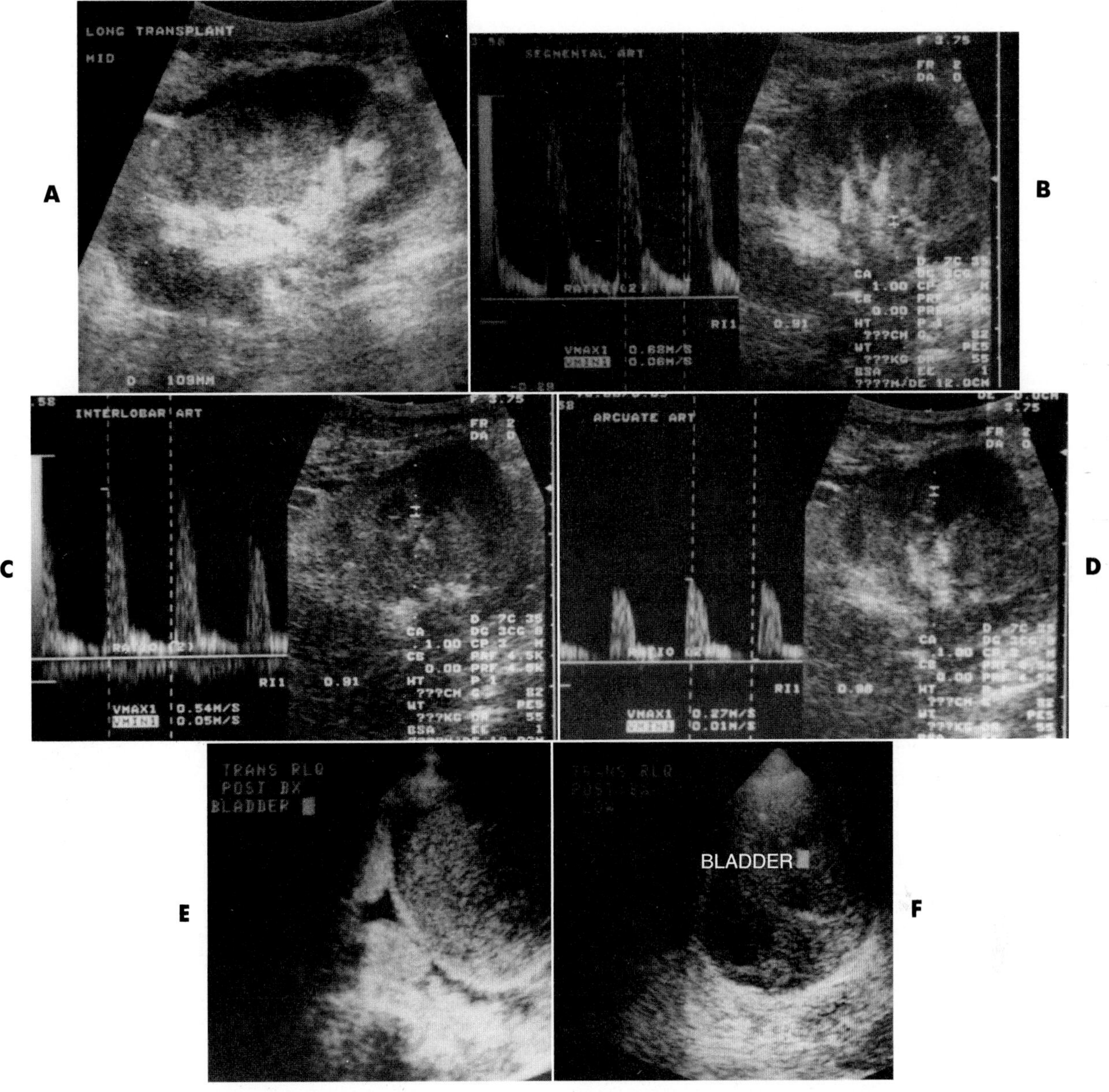

FIG. 9-90 Abnormal flow patterns in a patient with rejection. **A,** Large hypoechoic area along the anterior border of the kidney with compression of the calyceal system. **B,** Abnormal flow pattern in the segmental artery with decreased diastolic flow and increased resistive index to 0.9. **C,** Abnormal flow in the interlobar artery. **D,** Abnormal flow in the arcuate artery. **E** and **F,** The patient had a renal biopsy; status after biopsy shows fine stippled echoes throughout the bladder indicating hematoma within the bladder. Before and after biopsy, scans should routinely be made to search for hematoma collections around the kidney or within the bladder.

as sensitive for these arteriovenous malformations. Although color Doppler can identify them, it cannot distinguish one from the other.

Mostbeck et al. discovered that heart rate has a statistical significant effect on the resistive index in renal arteries.[8b] Increasing the heart rate of patients and taking measurements at paced rate intervals (70, 80, 90, 100, 120 bpm), the researchers found that the resistive index decreased with increasing heart rate in six of eight patients. They suggested that in interpreting resistive index in renal arteries, the actual heart rate must always be considered. They proposed a correction formula to overcome this effect on resistive index.

In conclusion, many factors must be considered when interpreting the meaning of increased resistive indices in the transplanted kidney. Knowledge of the different complications and their relation to postoperative time, patient history, donor history, and clinical findings plays an integral part in helping to understand and find the cause of an increased resistive index.

REVIEW QUESTIONS

1. Name the two principal functions of the urinary system.
2. Name the organs that help to carry out excretion.
3. What are the principal metabolic waste products from the kidney?
4. Draw the kidney, its capsule, and its internal anatomy.
5. Describe the sonographic texture of the kidneys.
6. Describe the following renal variants and their sonographic appearance: column of Bertin, dromedary hump, junctional parenchymal defect, duplex collecting system, sinus lipomatosis, and extrarenal pelvis.
7. If the kidney is not seen in its normal position, what other areas should be evaluated?
8. What is the sonographic appearance of a horseshoe kidney?
9. Describe the ultrasound evaluation of a renal mass in terms of its cystic, solid, or complex features.
10. What are the criteria for a simple renal cyst?
11. A renal sinus cyst may present several problems to the patient and the sonographer. Describe these problems.
12. How can a sonographer differentiate polycystic disease of the kidney from multicystic disease? What other organs may be affected?
13. What is the most common malignant tumor found in the kidney? Describe its ultrasound appearance.
14. Describe hydronephrosis of the kidney, its stages, and its ultrasound appearance.
15. How does acute glomerulonephritis affect the kidney?
16. AIDS affects many organs. Describe its effects and the ultrasound appearance it produces on the kidneys, liver, and gallbladder.
17. What is renal atrophy? What is its ultrasound appearance?
18. What are some causes of acute renal failure?
19. Name at least four conditions that mimic hydronephrosis.
20. Describe the ultrasound appearance of renal infarction.
21. What is the most common medical renal disease to produce acute renal failure?
22. Name the conditions that cause diffuse echogenicity of the renal parenchyma.
23. What is nephrocalcinosis and how would it appear on ultrasound?
24. Define the sonographic technique for evaluating a renal transplant.
25. What are some of the medical complications patients with a renal transplant may acquire?
26. How does the sonographer evaluate the renal transplant for rejection?
27. Define acute tubular necrosis.
28. What is the value of Doppler and color-flow Doppler in the renal transplant patient?

REFERENCES

1. Coyne SC, Walsh JW, Tisnado J, et al: Surgically correctable renal transplant complications: an integrated clinical and radiologic approach, Am J Roentgenol 136:1113, 1981.
2. Don S, Kopecky KK, Tuli MM, and Siddiqui AR: Detection of rejection in renal allografts, J Ultrasound Med 9:503, 1990.
3. Genkins SM, Sanfilippo FP, and Carroll BA: Duplex Doppler sonography of renal transplants: lack of sensitivity and specificity in establishing pathological diagnosis, Am J Roentgenol 152:535, 1989.
4. Grant EG and Perrella RR: Wishing won't make it so: duplex Doppler sonography in the evaluation of renal transplant dysfunction, Am J Roentgenol 155:538, 1990.
5. Kumar R, Wilson DD, and Santa-cruz FR: Postoperative urological complications of renal transplantation, Radiographics 4:531, 1984.
6. Letourneau JG, Day DD, and Ascher NL: Imaging of renal transplants, Am J Roentgenol 150:833, 1988.
7. Kaveggia LP, Perrella RR, Grant EG, et al: Duplex Doppler sonography in renal allografts: the significance of reversed flow in diastole, Am J Roentgenol 155:295, 1990.
8. Maklad NF, Wright CH, and Rosenthal SJ: Gray scale ultrasonic appearances of renal transplant rejection, Radiology 131:711, 1979.
9. Mostbeck GH, Gossinger HD, and Mallek R: Effect of heart rate on Doppler measurements of resistive index in renal arteries, Radiology 175:511, 1990.
10. Olcott ER, Goldstein RB, and Salvatierra O: Lymphoma presenting as allograft hematoma in a renal transplant recipient, J Ultrasound Med 9:239, 1990.
11. Platt JF, Ellis JH, and Rubin JM: Renal transplant pyelocaliecta sis: role of duplex Doppler US in evaluation, Radiology 179:425, 1991.
12. Reuther GR, Wanjukra D, and Bauer H: Acute renal vein thrombosis in renal allografts: detection with duplex Doppler US, Radiology 170:557, 1989.
13. Silver TM, Campbell D, Wicks JD, et al: Peritransplant fluid collections, Radiology 138:145, 1981.
14. Snider JF, Hunter DW, Moradian GP, et al: Transplant renal artery stenosis: evaluation with duplex sonography, Radiology 172:1027, 1989.
15. Taylor JW and Marks WH: Use of Doppler imaging for evaluation of dysfunction in renal allografts, Am J Roentgenol 155:536, 1990.
16. Taylor KJW, Morse SS, Rigsby CM, et al: Vascular complications in renal allografts: detection with duplex Doppler US, Radiology 162:31, 1987.

BIBLIOGRAPHY

Anatomy

Clements CD: Anatomy: a regional atlas of the human body, ed 3, p. 321. Baltimore, 1987, Urban & Schwarzenberg.

Bladder

Boag GS and Nolan RL: Sonographic features of urinary bladder involvement in regional enteritis, J Ultrasound Med 7:125, 1988.

Carroll BA: Lower urinary tract ultrasound, Journal Diagnostic Medical Sonography 2:74, 1986.

Cronan JJ, Simeone JF, Pfister RC, et al: Cystonography in the detection of bladder tumors, J Ultrasound Med 1:237, 1982.

Tsyb AF, Slesarev VI, and Komarevtsev VN: Transvaginal longitudinal ultrasonography in diagnosis of carcinoma of the urinary bladder, J Ultrasound Med 7:79, 1988.

Wan Y-L, Hsieh Ho, Lee T-Y: Wall defect as a sign of urinary bladder rupture in sonography, J Ultrasound Med 7:511, 1988.

Cystic Disease

Cronan JJ, Amis ES, Yodaer IC, et al: Peripelvic cysts, J Ultrasound Med 1:229, 1982.

Grossman H, Rosenberg ER, Bowie JD, et al: sonographic diagnosis of renal cystic diseases, AM J Roentgenol 140:81, 1983.

Kleiner B, Filly R, Mack L, et al: Multicystic dysplastic kidney, Radiology 161:27, 1986.

Lawson TL, McClennan BL, and Shirkhoda A: Adult polycystic kidney disease, J Clin Ultrasound 6:295, 1978.

Pretorius DH, Lee ME, Manco-Johnson ML, et al: Diagnosis of autosomal dominant polycystic kidney disease in utero and in the young infant, J Ultrasound Med 6:249, 1987.

Ralls PW, Esensten MK, Boger D, et al: Severe hydronephrosis and severe renal cystic disease, Am J Roentgenol 134:473, 1980.

Rego JD, Laing FC, Jeffrey RB: Ultrasonographic diagnosis of medullary cystic disease, J Ultrasound Med 2:433, 1983.

Rosenfield AT, Lipson MH, Wolf B, et al: Ultrasonography and nephrotomography in the presymptomatic diagnosis of dominantly inherited polycystic kidney disease, Radiology 135:423, 1980.

Taylor AJ, Cohen EP, Erickson SJ, et al: Renal imaging in long-term dialysis patients, AM J Rotentgenol 153:765, 1989.

Doppler

Berland LL, Lawson TL, Adams MB, et al: Evaluation of renal transplants with pulsed doppler duplex sonography. J Ultrasound Med 1:215, 1982.

Drake DG, Day DL, Letourneau JG, et al: Doppler evaluation of renal transplants in children: a prospective analysis with histopathologic correlation, Am J Roentgenol 154:785, 1990.

Kessler LS, Honeyman JC, Kaude JV, and Longmate JA: Intra- and interobserved variations in determining blood-flow indexes with Doppler sonography, Am J Roentgenol 156:1326, 1991.

Kier R, Taylor KJW, Feyock AL, et al: Renal masses: characterization with Doppler US, Radiology 176:703, 1990.

Mostbeck GH, Kain R, Mallek R, et al: Duplex Doppler sonography in renal parenchymal disease, J Ultrasound Med 10:189, 1991.

General

Afschrit M, deSy W, Voet D, et al: Fractured kidney and retroperitoneal hematoma diagnosed by ultrasound, J Clin Ultrasound 10:335, 1982.

Bisset RA and Kahn AN: Differential diagnosis in abdominal ultrasound. London, 1990, Bailliere Tindall.

Hubsch PJ, Mostbeck G, Barton PP, et al: Evaluation of arteriovenous fistulas and pseudoaneurysms in renal allografts following percutaneous needle biopsy. J Ultrasound Med 9:95, 1990.

Jones BE, Hoffer FA, Teele RL, et al: The compound renal pyramide, J Ultrasound Med 6:515, 1987.

Kay CJ, Rosenfield AT, and Armm M: Gray-scale ultrasonography in the evaluation of renal trauma, Radiology 134:461, 1980.

Marchal GJ, Desmer VJ, Proesmans WC, et al: Caroli's disease: high-frequency ultrasound and pathologic findings, Radiology 158:507, 1986.

Mittlestaedt C: Abdominal ultrasound. New York, 1992, Churchill Livingstone.

Lubat E, Schulman M, Genieser NB, et al: Sonography of the simple and complicated ipsilateral fused kidney, J Ultrasound Med 8:109, 1989.

Page JE and Dow J: Dilatation in the duplex kidney, Brit J Urol 66:459, 1990.

Patriquin H, Lefaivre JF, Lafortune M, et al: Fetal lobation, J Ultrasound Med 9:191, 1990.

Sanders R: Clinical sonography. Boston, 1991, Little, Brown & Co.

Hydronephrosis

Morin ME, Baker DA: The influence of hydration and bladder distension on the sonographic diagnosis of hydronephrosis, J Clin Ultrasound 7:192, 1979.

Infections

Allen HA, Walsh JW, Brewer WH, et al: Sonography of emphysematous pyelonephritis, J Ultrasound Med 3:533, 1984.

Goldman SM, Minkin SD, Naraval DC, et al: Renal carbuncle, J Urology 118:525, 1977.

Jeffrey RB, Laing FC, Wing VW, et al: Sensitivity of sonography in pyonephrosis: a re-evaluation, Am J Roentgenol 144:71, 1985.

Lee JK, McClennan BL, Melson GL, et al: Acute focal bacterial nephritis, Am J Roentgenol 135:87, 1980.

Van Kirk OC, Go RT, Wedel VJ: Sonographic features of xanthogranulomatous pyelonephritis, Am J Roentgenol 134:1035, 1980.

Laboratory Tests

Fischbach F: A manual of laboratory diagnostic tests. Philadelphia, 1980, JB Lippincott.

Starrett S: Laboratory values associated with renal function and disease processes. Journal Diagnostic Medical Sonography 2:206, 1986.

Neoplastic Disease

Birnbaum BA, Bosniak M, Megibow AJ, et al: Observations on the growth of renal neoplasms, Radiology 176:695, 1990.

Charboneau JW, Hattery RR, and Ernst EC: Spectrum of sonographic findings in 125 renal masses other than benign simple cyst, Am J Roentgenol 140:87, 1983.

Cunningham JJ: Ultrasonic demonstration of renal collecting system invasion by transitional cell cancer, J Clin Ultrasound 10:339, 1982.

Forer LE and Schaffer RM: Transitional cell carcinoma of a simple ureterocele, J Ultrasound Med 9:301, 1990.

Goldstein HM, Green B, and Weaver RM: Ultrasonic detection of renal tumor extension into the inferior vena cava, Am J Roentgenol 130:1083, 1978.

Grant DC, Dee GJ, Yoder IC, et al: Sonography in transitional cell carcinoma of the renal pelvis, Urol Radiol 89, 1986.

Janetschek G, Putz A, and Feichtinger H: J Ultrasound Med 7:83, 1988.

Lubat E, Schulman MH, and Genieser NB: Sonography of the simple and complicated ipsilateral fused kidney, J Ultrasound Med 8:109, 1989.

Schutz K, Siffring PA, Forrest TS, et al: Serial renal sonographic changes in preeclampsia, J Ultrasound Med 9:415, 1990.

Sisler CL and Siegel MJ: Malignant rhabdoid tumor of the kidney, Radiology 172:211, 1989.

Treiger BF, Humphrey LS, Peterson CV, et al: Transesophageal echocardiography in renal cell carcinoma, J of Urology 145:1138, 1991.

Renal Failure

Graif M, Shohet I, Strauss S, et al: Hemolytic uremic syndrome, J Ultrasound Med 3:563, 1984.

Ultrasound Technique

Brant TD, Neiman HL, and Dragowski MJ, et al: Ultrasound assessment of normal renal dimensions, J Ultrasound Med 1:49, 1982.

Brooke J Jr: CT and sonography of the acute abdomen pp. 181-194. New York, 1988, Raven Press.

Cook JH, Rosenfield At, and Taylor KJW: Ultrasonic demonstration of intrarenal anatomy, Am J Roentgenol 129:831, 1977.

Cronan JJ, Yoder IC, Amis ES, et al: The myth of anechoic renal sinus fat, Radiology 144:149, 1982.

Lewis E and Ritchie WGM: A simple ultrasonic method for assessing renal size, J Clin Ultrasound 8:417, 1980.

Rosenberg ER, Clair MR, and Bowie JD: The fluid-filled stomach as an acoustic window to left kidney, Am J Roentgenol 138:175, 1982.

Rosenfield AT, Taylor KJW, Crade M, et al: Anatomy and pathology of the kidney by gray ultrasound, Radiology 128:737, 1978.

Rosenfield AT, Taylor KJW, Dembner AG: Ultrasound of renal sinus, Am J Roentgenol 133:441, 1979.

Thompson IM, Kovac A, and Geshner J: Coronal renal ultrasound: II Urology 17:210, 1981.

Weill FS, Perriguey G, Rohmer P: Sonographic study of the juxtarenal retroperitoneal compartments, J Ultrasound Med 1:307, 1982.

CHAPTER 10
The Spleen

Sandra L. Hagen-Ansert

The spleen is the largest single mass of lymphoid tissue in the body. It is active in blood formation during the initial part of fetal life. This function decreases gradually by the fifth or sixth month when the spleen assumes its adult characteristics and discontinues its hematopoietic activities. The spleen plays an important role in the defense of the body. The spleen is rarely the primary site of disease, although it is often affected by systemic disease processes.

ANATOMY

The spleen lies in the left hypochrondrium, with its axis along the shaft of the tenth rib (Fig. 10-1). Its lower pole extends forward as far as the midaxillary line. The spleen is of variable size and shape, (i.e., "orange-segment," a tetrahedral, or triangular) but generally is considered to be ovoid with even borders and a convex superior and concave inferior surface. The spleen is an intraperitoneal organ covered with peritoneum over its entire extent except for a small area at its hilum (Fig. 10-2). Accessory spleens occasionally are found near the hilum of the spleen. An accessory spleen results from the failure of fusion of separate splenic masses forming on the dorsal mesogastrium; it is most commonly located in the splenic hilum or along the splenic vessels or associated ligaments. They have been reported from the diaphragm to the scrotum and are usually solitary. They usually remain small and do not present as a clinical problem. The accessory spleen may simulate a pancreatic, suprarenal, or retroperitoneal tumor.

Vascular Supply

Blood is supplied to the spleen by the splenic artery, which travels along the superior border of the pancreas (Fig. 10-3). On entering the splenic hilum, this artery immediately divides into about six branches to supply the organ with oxygenated blood.

The splenic vein leaves the hilum and joins the superior mesenteric vein to form the portal vein. The splenic vein travels along the posteromedial border of the pancreas.

The lymph vessels emerge from the splenic hilum, pass through other lymph nodes along the course of the splenic artery, and drain into the celiac nodes. The nerves to the spleen accompany the splenic artery and are derived from the celiac plexus.

Relational Anatomy

The spleen lies between the left hemidiaphragm and the stomach. The diaphragm may be seen as a bright curvilinear echogenic structure close to the proximal superolateral surface of the spleen. Posteriorly the diaphragm, left pleura, left lung, and ribs (8 to 11) are in contact with the spleen. The medial surface is related to the stomach, tail of the pancreas, left kidney, and splenic flexure of the colon.

Displacement of the Spleen

The spleen is held in place by the lienorenal, gastrosplenic, and phrenicolic ligaments. These ligaments are derived from the layers of peritoneum that form the greater and lesser sacs. A mass in the left upper quadrant may displace the spleen inferior. Caudal displacement may be secondary to a subclavian abscess, splenic cyst, or left pleural effusion. Cephalic displacement may result from volume loss in the left lung, left pneumonia, paralysis of the left hemidiaphragm, or a large intraabdominal mass. A normal spleen with medial lobulation between the pancreatic tail and left kidney may be confused with a cystic mass in the tail of the pancreas.

Wandering Spleen

A wandering spleen is a spleen that has migrated from its normal location in the left upper quadrant. It is the result of an embryologic anomaly of the supporting ligaments of the spleen. The patient presents with an abdominal or pelvic mass, intermittent pain, and volvulus (splenic torsion). The sonographer should use color Doppler to map the vascularity within the spleen. When torsion is complete, the vascular pattern shows decreased velocity.

Congenital Anomalies

Splenic Agenesis. Complete absence of the spleen (asplenia) or agenesis of the spleen is rare and by itself causes no difficulties. However it may occur as part of asplenic or polysplenia syndromes in association with complex cardiac malformations, bronchopulmonary abnormalities, or vis-

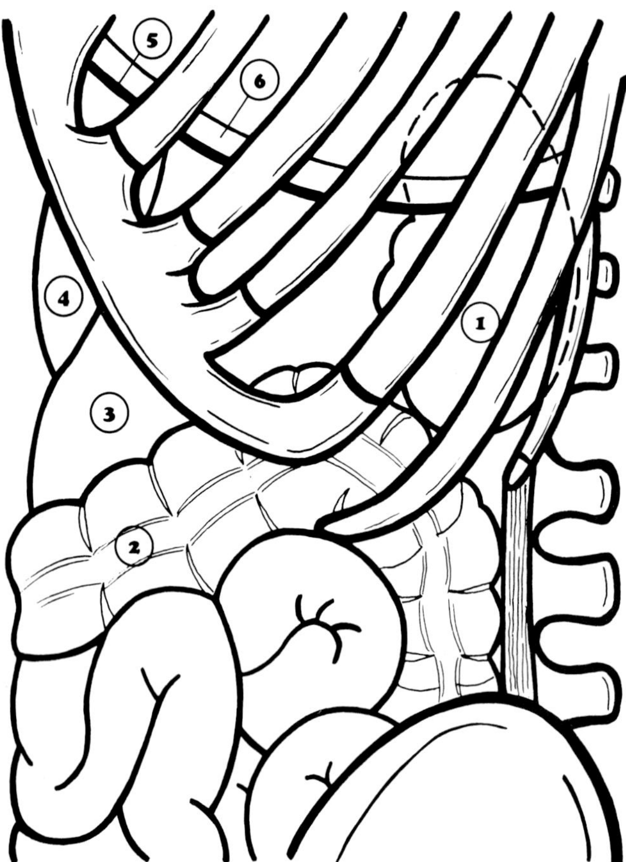

FIG. 10-1 The spleen and surrounding structures. *1,* Spleen; *2,* stomach; *3,* tail of pancreas; *4,* descending colon; *5,* splenic artery. (From Hagen-Ansert SL: The anatomy workbook, Philadelphia, 1986, JB Lippincott.)

ceral heterotaxis (anomalous placement of organs or major blood vessels, including a horizontal liver, malrotation of the gut, and interruption of the inferior vena cava with azygous continuation).

Splenic agenesis may be ruled out by demonstrating a spleen on ultrasound. The sonographer should be careful not to confuse the spleen with the bowel, which may lie in the area normally occupied by the spleen. Color Doppler helps determine the splenic vascular pattern and thus separate it from the colon.

Accessory Spleen. An accessory spleen is a more common congenital anomaly (Figs. 10-4 to 10-6). The accessory spleen may be difficult to demonstrate by sonography if it is very small. However, when it is seen, it appears as a homogeneous pattern like that of the spleen. It is usually found near the hilum or inferior border of the spleen but has been reported elsewhere in the abdominal cavity. Lesions affecting the normal spleen would also affect the accessory spleen.

Physiology

The red pulp of the spleen is composed of two principal elements—the splenic sinuses alternating with splenic cords. The sinuses are long irregular channels lined by endothelial cells or flattened reticular cells. There are pores or gaps between the lining cells, implying that the circulation is open and that blood cells can freely leave the sinuses to enter the intervening cords. The membrane shared by a cord and its adjacent sinuses is also perforated. Reticular cells with delicate processes sometimes bridge the cords. These highly phagocytic cells create an open meshwork with the cords. The blood that leaves the splenic sinuses to enter the reticular cords passes through a complex filter. The venous drainage of the sinuses and cords is not well defined, but it is assumed that tributaries of the splenic vein connect with the sinuses of the red pulp.

The white pulp of the spleen consists of the malpighian corpuscles, small nodular masses of lymphoid tissue attached to the smaller arterial branches. Extending from the splenic capsule inward are the trabeculae, containing blood vessels and lymphatics. The lymphoid tissue, or malpighian corpuscles, has the same structure as the follicles in the lymph nodes; but it differs in that the splenic follicles surround arteries, so that on cross section each contains a central artery. These follicles are scattered throughout the organ and are not confined to the peripheral layer or cortex, as are lymph nodes.

As part of the reticuloendothelial system, the spleen plays an important role in the defense mechanism of the body and is also implicated in pigment and lipid metabolism. It is not essential to life, and it can be removed with no ill effects. The functions of the spleen may be classified under two general headings—those that reflect the functions of the reticuloendothelial system and those that are characteristic of the organ itself.

The functions of the spleen as an organ of the reticuloendothelial system are (1) the production of lymphocytes and plasma cells, (2) the production of antibodies, (3) the storage of iron, and (4) the storage of other metabolites. The functions characteristic of the organ include (1) maturation of the surface of erythrocytes, (2) reservoir function, (3) culling function, (4) pitting function, and (5) disposal of senescent or abnormal erythrocytes; also included are functions related to platelet life span and leukocyte life span.

The role of the spleen as an immunologic organ concerns the production of cells capable of making antibodies (lymphocytes and plasma cells); however, it should be understood that antibodies are also produced at other sites.

Phagocytosis of erythrocytes and the breakdown of the hemoglobin occur throughout the entire reticuloendothelial system, but roughly half the catabolic activity is localized in the normal spleen. In splenomegaly the major portion of hemoglobin breakdown occurs in the spleen. The iron that is liberated is stored in the splenic phagocytes. In anomalies such as the hemolytic anemias, the splenic phagocytes become engorged with hemosiderin when erythrocyte destruction is accelerated.

In addition to storing iron, the spleen is subject to the storage diseases such as Gaucher's disease and Niemann-

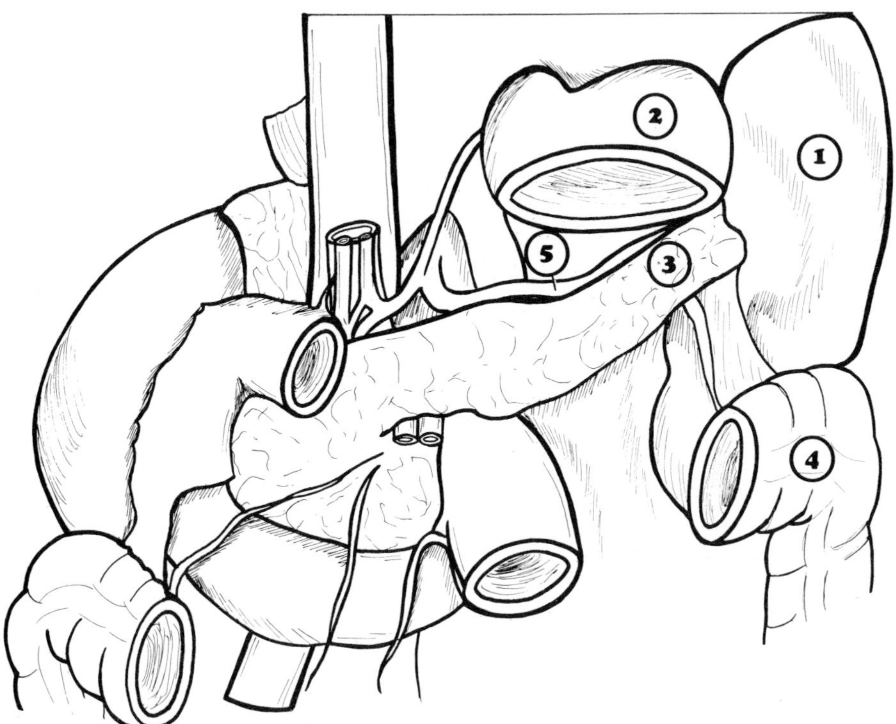

FIG. 10-2 Relationship of the spleen to adjacent structures as viewed from the left lateral position. *1,* Spleen; *2,* transverse colon; *3,* stomach; *4,* liver; *5,* diaphragm; *6,* costodiaphragmatic recess. (From Hagen-Ansert SL: The anatomy workbook, Philadelphia, 1986, JB Lippincott.)

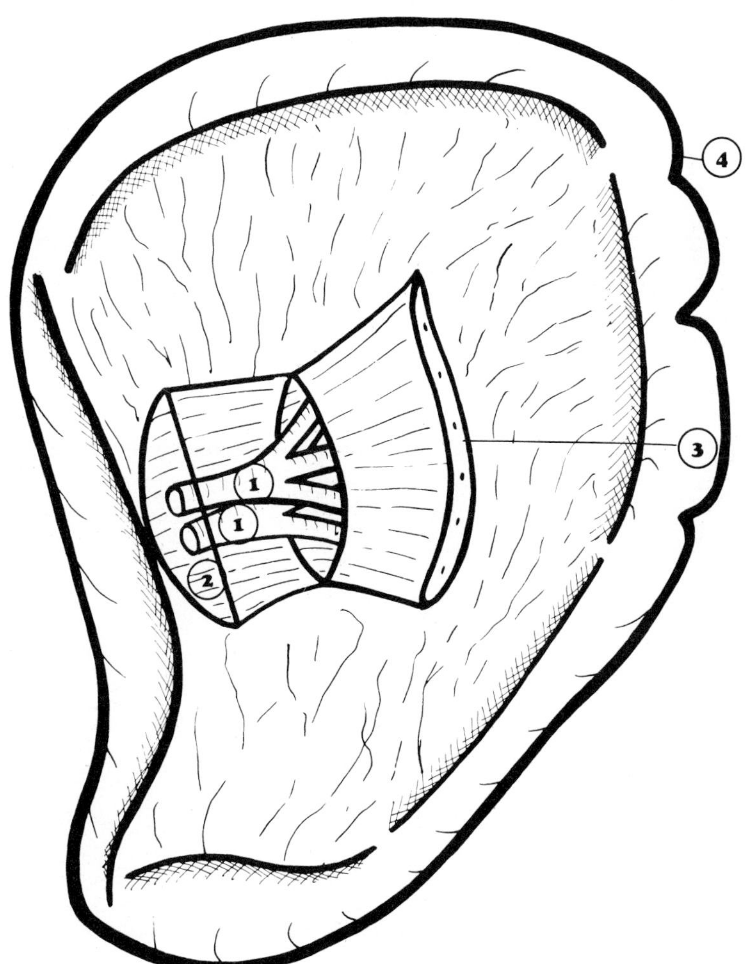

FIG. 10-3 Hilum of the spleen. *1,* Splenic vessels; *2,* lienorenal ligaments; *3,* gastrosplenic omentum; *4,* notched anterior border of spleen. (From Hagen-Ansert SL: The anatomy workbook, Philadelphia, 1986, JB Lippincott.)

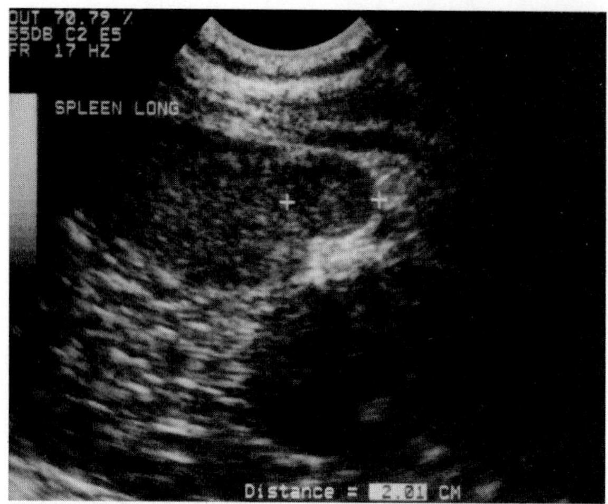

FIG. 10-4 An accessory spleen is a common congenital anomaly. The small spleen is seen lying at the tip of the splenic border, anterior to the kidney. (It measures 2 cm between the cross bars.)

Pick disease. Abnormal lipid metabolites accumulate in all phagocytic reticuloendothelial cells but may also involve the phagocytes in the spleen, producing gross splenomegaly.

The functions of the spleen that are characteristic of the organ relate primarily to the circulation of erythrocytes through it. In a normal individual the spleen contains only about 20 to 30 ml of erythrocytes. In splenomegaly the reservoir function is greatly increased, and the abnormally enlarged spleen contains many times this volume of red blood cells. The transit time is lengthened, and the erythrocytes are subject to destructive effects for a long time. In part, ptosis causes consumption of glucose, on which the erythrocyte depends to maintain normal metabolism, and the erythrocyte is destroyed. Selective destruction of abnormal erythrocytes is also accelerated by the splenic pooling.

As erythrocytes pass through the spleen, the organ inspects them for imperfections and destroys those it recognizes as abnormal or senescent. This is called the *culling*

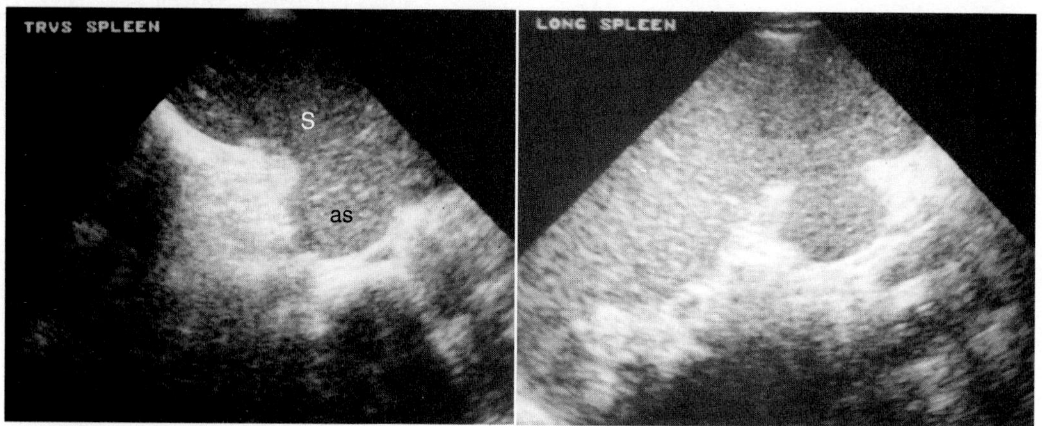

FIG. 10-5 Transverse and longitudinal scans of the accessory spleen. It takes on the same homogeneous pattern as the spleen.

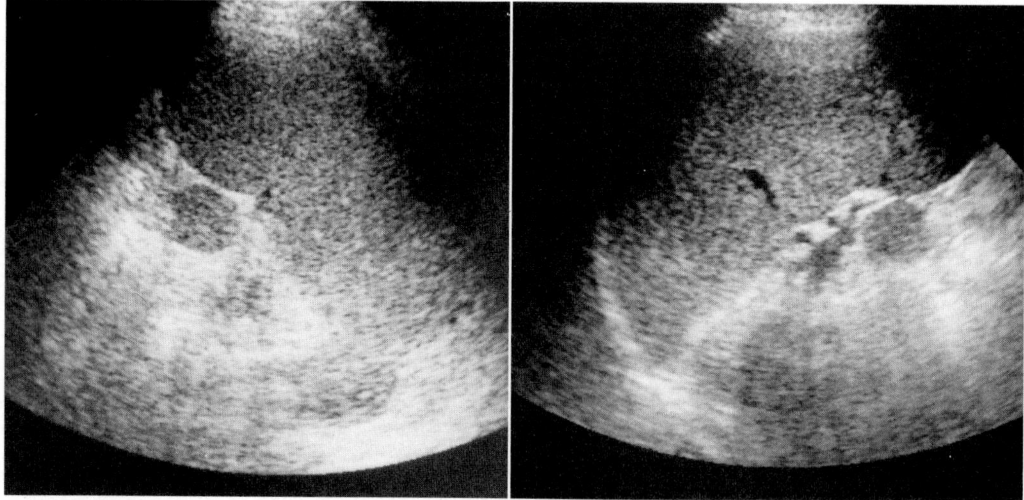

FIG. 10-6 Accessory spleen. These extra splenic tissue masses are usually found near the hilum or inferior border of the spleen. It may be confused with the tail of the pancreas or nodes in the splenic hilum.

function. The pitting function is a process by which the spleen removes granular inclusions without destroying the erythrocytes. The normal function of the spleen keeps the number of circulating erythrocytes with inclusions at a minimum.

The spleen also pools platelets in large numbers. The entry of platelets into the splenic pool and their return to the circulation are extensive. In splenomegaly the splenic pool may be so large that it produces thrombocytopenia. Sequestration of leukocytes in the enlarged spleen may produce leukopenia.

SONOGRAPHIC EVALUATION OF THE SPLEEN

Normal Texture and Patterns

Sonographically the splenic parenchyma should have a fine homogeneous low-level echo pattern as is seen within the liver parenchyma (Fig. 10-7). Cooperberg[1] states that the spleen has two components joined at the hilum. On transverse scans it has a crescentic appearance usually with a large medial component. As one moves inferiorly, only the lateral component is imaged. On longitudinal scans the superior component extends more medially than the inferior component. The irregularity of these components makes it difficult to assess mild splenomegaly accurately.

PATHOLOGY OF THE SPLEEN

Splenic Size

The spleen is normally measured along its long axis. The normal spleen is 8 to 12 cm long. Splenomegaly is diagnosed when the spleen measures over 12 cm.

REGRESSIVE CHANGES

Patient Position and Technique

Real time is fair to good for imaging the left upper quadrant. The sonographer can successfully manipulate the

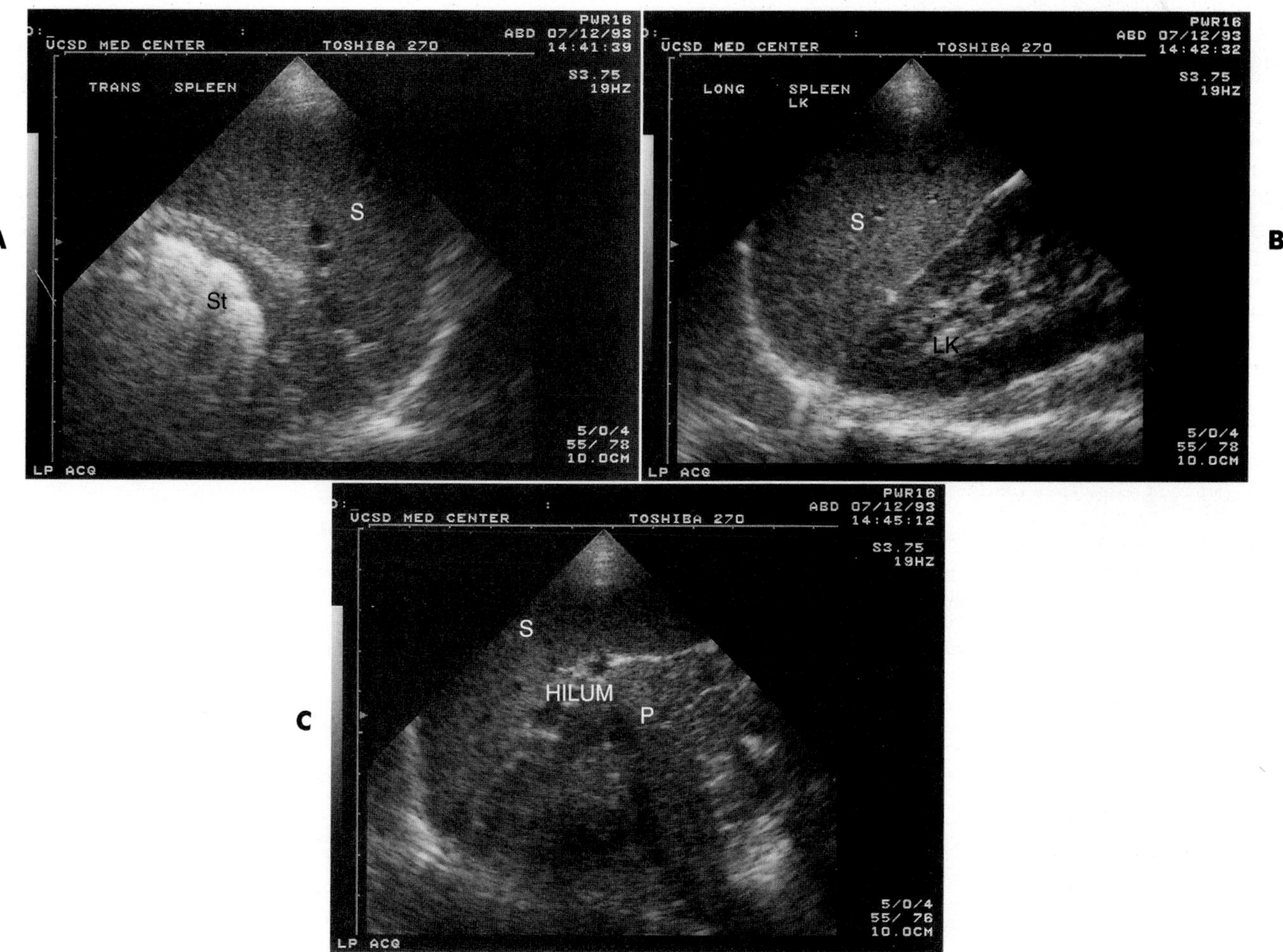

FIG. 10-7 A, Transverse scan of the normal spleen. The body of the stomach, *St,* is seen medial to the splenic hilum. **B,** Longitudinal scans of the splenic parenchyma. Sonographically, the splenic parenchyma should have a homogeneous, low-level echo pattern similar to the liver parenchyma. The upper pole of the left kidney is well seen, *LK*. **C,** Longitudinal decubitus view of the normal spleen, *S,* and its relationship to the tail of the pancreas, *P*.

transducer between costal margins to image the left kidney, spleen, and diaphragm adequately (Table 10-1) if bowel or stomach does not interfere.

The patient may be scanned in the supine, prone, or right lateral decubitus position. The supine scan may have the problem of overlying air-filled stomach or bowel anterior to the spleen; thus the patient may be rotated into a slight right decubitus position to permit better transducer contact without as much bowel interference. The right lateral decubitus, or axillary, position enables the sonographer to scan in an oblique fashion between the ribs.

PATHOLOGIC CONDITIONS

As the largest unit of the reticuloendothelial system the spleen is involved in all systemic inflammations and generalized hematopoietic disorders, and many metabolic disturbances (Figs. 10-8 and 10-9). It is rarely the primary site of disease. Whenever the spleen is involved in systemic disease, splenic enlargement usually develops; therefore splenomegaly is a major manifestation of disorders of this organ (Table 10-2).

Regressive Changes

Amyloidosis. In systemic diseases leading to amyloidosis the spleen is the organ most frequently involved. It may be of normal size or decidedly enlarged, depending on the amount and distribution of amyloid. Two types of involvement are seen—modular and diffuse. In the modular type, amyloid is found in the walls of the sheathed arteries and within the follicles but not in the red pulp (Fig. 10-10). In the diffuse type the follicles are not involved, the red pulp is prominently involved, and the spleen is usually greatly enlarged and firm.

Atrophy. Atrophy of the spleen is not uncommon in normal individuals. It may also occur in wasting diseases. In chronic hemolytic anemias, particularly sickle cell anemia, there is excessive loss of pulp, increasing fibrosis, scarring from multiple infarcts, and incrustation with iron and calcium deposits. In the final stages of atrophy the spleen may

TABLE 10-1 Ultrasonic-Pathologic Classification of Splenic Disorders

Uniform splenic sonodensity		Focal defects		
Normal sonodensity	**Low sonodensity**	**Sonodense**	**Sonolucent**	**Perisplenic defects**
Erythropoiesis (including myeloproliferative disorders) Reticuloendothelial hyperactivity Congestion	Granulocytopoiesis (excluding myelodisorders) Lymphopoiesis Other (multiple myeloma) Congestion	Nonspecific (metastasis)	Nonspecific (benign primary neoplasm, cyst, abscess, malignant neoplasm [lymphopoietic])	Nonspecific (hematoma)

From Mittelstraedt CA and Partain CL: Radiology 134:697, 1980.

TABLE 10-2 Pathologic Classification of Splenic Disorders

Hematopoietic	Reticuloendothelial hyperactivity (normal)

Granulocytopoiesis
  Reactive hyperplasia to acute and chronic infection (low sonodensity)
Noncaseous granulomatous inflammation
Myeloproliferative syndromes (normal)
Chronic myelogenous leukemia
Acute myelogenous leukemia
Lymphopoiesis (low sonodensity or focal sonolucent)
Chronic lymphocytic leukemia
  Lymphoma
  Hodgkin's disease
Erythropoiesis (normal)
Sickle cell disease
  Hereditary spherocytosis
  Hemolytic anemia
  Chronic anemia
  Myeloproliferative syndrome
Other
  Multiple myeloma (low sonodensity)
	Still's disease
	Wilson's disease
	Felty's syndrome
	Reticulum cell sarcoma
	
	Congestion (normal or low sonodensity)
	Hepatocellular disease
	
	Nonspecific
	Neoplasm-metastasis (focal sonodense)
	Cyst (focal sonolucent)
	Abscess (focal sonolucent)
	Malignant neoplasm (focal sonolucent)
	  Hodgkin's disease
	  Lymphoma
	Benign neoplasm (focal sonolucent)
	  Lymphangiomatosis
	Hematoma (perisplenic)

From Mittelstraedt CA and Partain CL: Radiology 134:697, 1980.

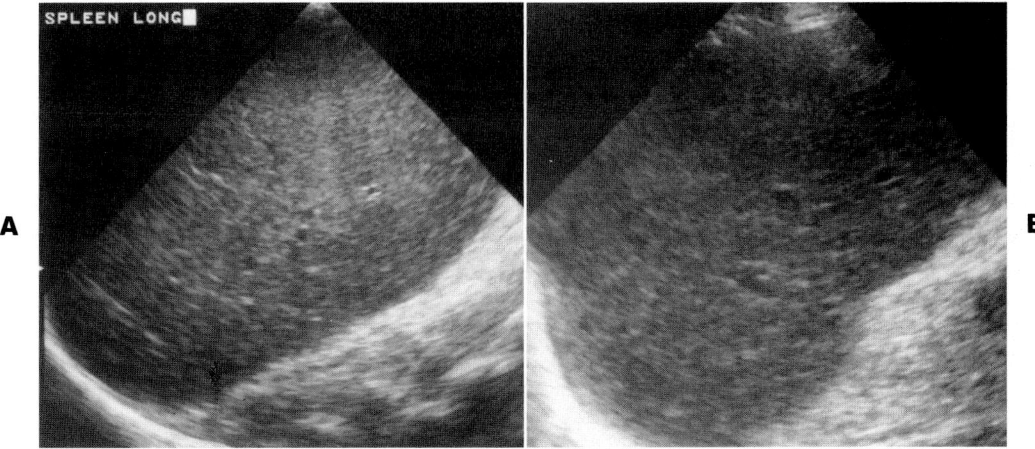

FIG. 10-8 A and **B,** Whenever the spleen is involved in systemic disease, splenic enlargement develops; therefore splenomegaly is a major manifestation of disorders of this organ. The normal spleen measures 9 to 12 cm along its long axis.

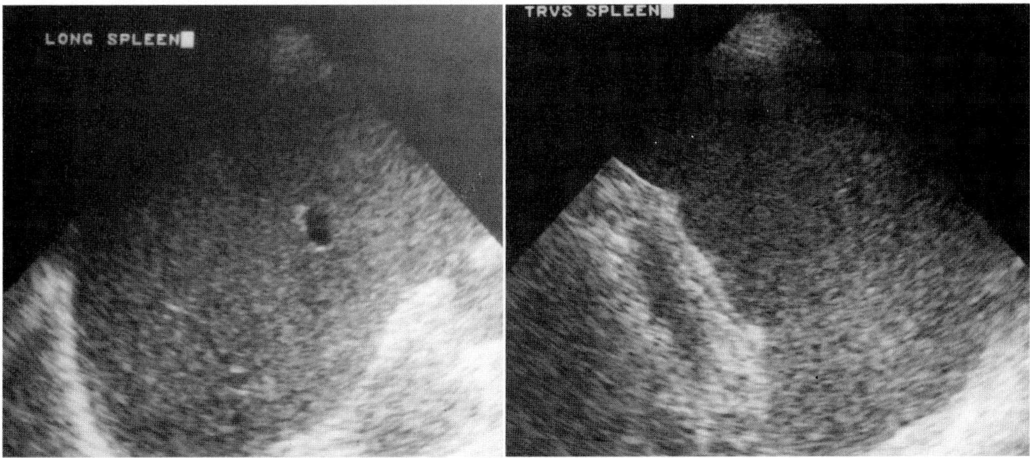

FIG. 10-9 Patient with sickle cell disease presents with splenomegaly.

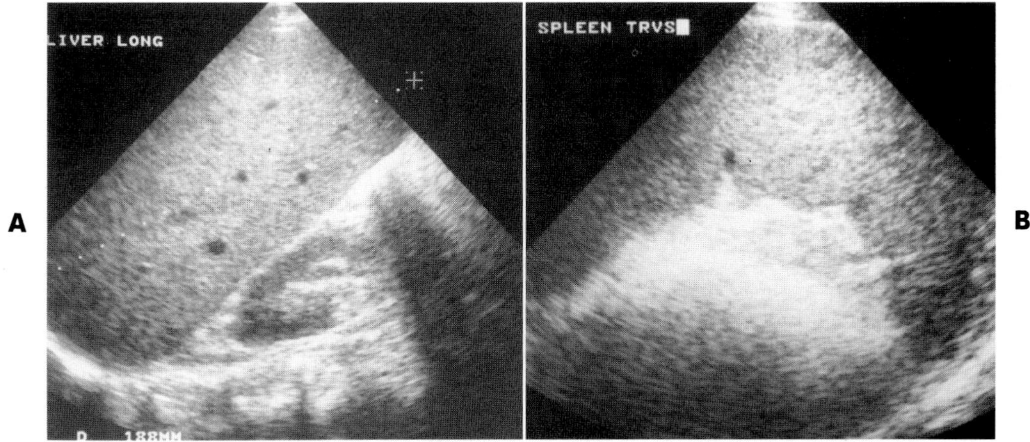

FIG. 10-10 A and **B,** Amyloidosis of the spleen. In system diseases leading to amyloidosis the spleen is the organ most frequently involved. This patient showed hepatosplenomegaly with increased congestion in the liver and splenic parenchyma.

be so small that it is hardly recognizable. Advanced atrophy is sometimes referred to as *autosplenectomy*.

CONGESTION OF THE SPLEEN

There are two types of splenic congestion, acute and chronic. In acute congestion, active hyperemia accompanies the reaction in the moderately enlarged spleen. In chronic venous congestion, there is diffuse enlargement of the spleen.

The venous congestion may be of systemic origin, caused by intrahepatic obstruction to portal venous drainage or by obstructive venous disorders in the portal or splenic veins. Systemic venous congestion is found in cardiac decompensation involving the right side of the heart. It is particularly severe in tricuspid or pulmonary valvular disease and in chronic cor pulmonale.

The most common causes of striking congestive splenomegaly are the various forms of cirrhosis of the liver. It is also caused by obstruction to the extrahepatic portal or splenic vein (e.g., spontaneous portal vein thrombosis).

Hypersplenism

Hypersplenism is a symptom complex characterized by congestive splenomegaly, leukopenia, and anemia. It was referred to as *Bonti's disease* and was considered a primary hematologic disorder with secondary involvement of the spleen. Currently splenic involvement is believed to be primary.

The hypersplenic syndrome has been divided into primary and secondary types. In primary hypersplenism, there is increased splenic activity and size of unknown cause. Secondary hypersplenism may occur in patients whose splenomegaly has a known origin, such as leukemia or lymphoma. In both forms the spleen is almost always enlarged.

Infarcts

Splenic infarcts are comparatively common lesions caused by occlusion of the major splenic artery or any of its branches (Fig. 10-11). They are almost always the result of emboli that arise in the heart, produced either from mural thrombi or from vegetations on the valves of the left side of the heart.

FOCAL DISEASE

Focal disease of the spleen may be single or multiple and may be found in normal or enlarged spleens. The major nontraumatic causes of focal splenic defects include tumors (benign and malignant), infarction, abscesses, and cysts. Splenic defects may be discovered incidentally, as in another imaging study, or specific, as in the case of a splenic infarct or abscess.

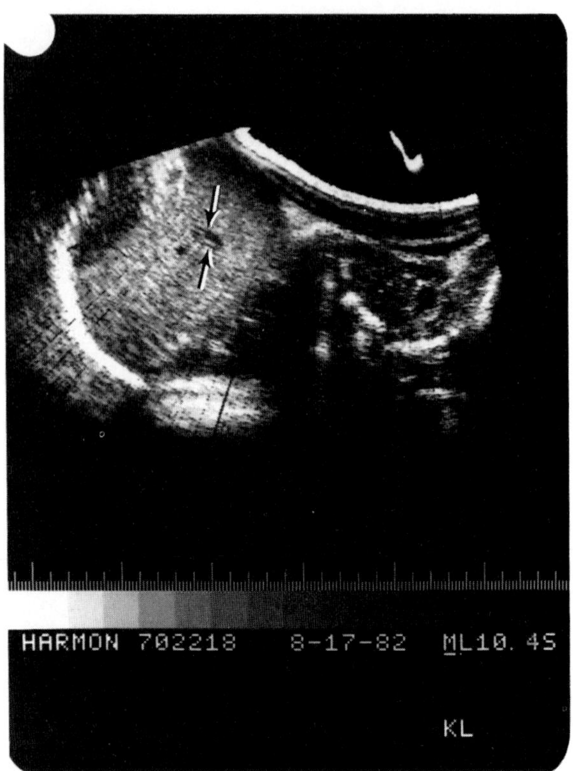

FIG. 10-11 Sagittal scan of the left upper quadrant shows a small collection within the spleen, which was representative of an infarct *(arrows)*.

DIFFUSE DISEASE

Erythropoietic Abnormalities

Erythropoietic abnormalities include the following: sickle cell, hereditary spherocytosis, hemolytic anemia, chronic anemia, polycythemia vera, thalassemia, and myeloproliferative disorders. On ultrasound, they tend to produce an isoechoic pattern.

Sickle Cell Anemia. In the earlier stage of sickle cell anemia, as seen in infants and children, the spleen is enlarged with marked congestion of the red pulp. Later the spleen undergoes progressive infarction and fibrosis and decreases in size until, in adults, only a small mass of fibrous tissue may be found (autosplenectomy). It is generally believed that these changes result when sickled cells plug the vasculature of the splenic substance, effectively producing ischemic destruction of the spleen.

Hereditary or Congenital Spherocytosis. In hereditary or congenital spherocytosis the spleen may be enlarged. An intrinsic abnormality of the red cells gives rise to erythrocytes that are small and spheroid rather than the normal, flattened, biconcave disks. The two results of this disease are the production by the bone marrow of spherocytic erythrocytes and the increased destruction of these cells in the spleen. The spleen destroys spherocytes selectively.

Hemolytic Anemia. *Hemolytic anemia* is the general term applied to anemia referable to decreased life of the erythrocytes. When the rate of destruction is greater than the bone marrow can compensate for, then anemia results.

Autoimmune Hemolytic Anemia. Autoimmune anemia can occur in its primary form without underlying disease, or it may be seen as a secondary disorder in patients already suffering from some disorder of the reticuloendothelial or hematopoietic systems, such as lymphoma, leukemia, or infectious mononucleosis. In the secondary form the splenic changes are dominated by the underlying disease; in the primary form the spleen is variably enlarged.

Polycythemia Vera. In polycythemia vera the spleen is variably enlarged, rather firm, and blue-red. Infarcts and thrombosis are common in polycythemia vera.

Thalassemia. The spleen is severely involved in thalassemia. This hemoglobinopathy differs from the others in that an abnormal molecular form of hemoglobin is not present. Instead, there is a suppression of synthesis of beta or alpha polypeptide chains, resulting in deficient synthesis of normal hemoglobin. The erythrocytes are not only deficient in normal hemoglobin but also abnormal in shape; many are target cells, whereas others vary considerably in size and shape. Their life span is short because they are destroyed by the spleen in large numbers.

The disease ranges from mild to severe. The changes in the spleen are greatest in the severe form, called *thalassemia major* (Fig. 10-12). The spleen is very large, often seeming to fill the entire abdominal cavity.

Myeloproliferative Disorders. Myeloproliferative disorders include acute and chronic myelogenous leukemias, polycythemia vera, myelofibrosis, megakarocytic leukemia, and erythroleukemia (Fig. 10-13). An isoechoic ultrasound pattern is seen because the parenchyma is hypoechoic compared with the liver.

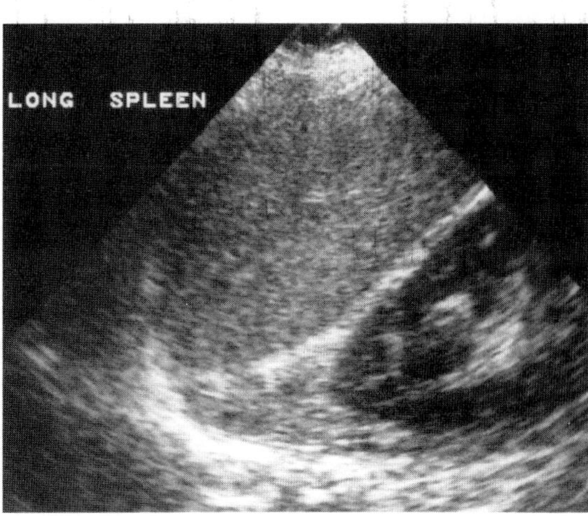

FIG. 10-12 A middle-aged, oriental patient with thalassemia major. The spleen can become very large, filling most of the abdominal cavity on the left.

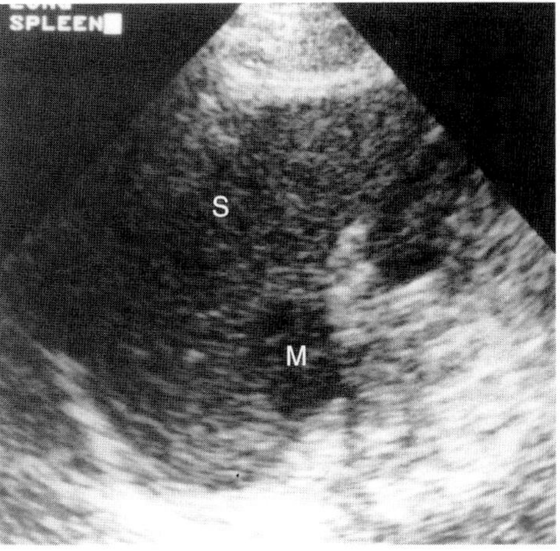

FIG. 10-13 Longitudinal scan in a patient with acute myelogenous leukemia. An isoechoic pattern is seen as the splenic parenchyma is hypoechoic, as compared with the liver. Spleen, *S;* mass, *m*.

Lymphopoietic Abnormalities

Lymphopoietic abnormalities include lymphocytic leukemias, lymphoma, and Hodgkin's disease. Ultrasound shows a diffusely hypoechoic splenic pattern with focal lesions. Patients with non-Hodgkin's lymphoma have been reported as having an isoechoic echo pattern.

Leukemia. Chronic myelogenous leukemia may be responsible for more extreme splenomegaly than any other disease. Chronic lymphocytic leukemia produces less severe splenomegaly.

Granulocytopoietic Abnormalities

Granulocytopoietic abnormalities include cases of reactive hyperplasia resulting from acute or chronic infection (i.e., splenitis sarcoid, tuberculosis). On ultrasound, splenomegaly is seen with a diffusely hypoechoic pattern (less dense than the liver).

Patients who have had a previous granulomatous infection present with bright echogenic lesions on ultrasound, with or without shadowing. Histoplasmosis and tuberculosis are the most common; sarcoidosis is rare. The sonographer may also find calcium in the splenic artery (Figs. 10-14 and 10-15).

Reticuloendotheliosis

Diseases characterized by reticuloendothelial hyperactivity and varying degrees of lipid storage in phagocytes are included in the category of reticuloendotheliosis. On ultrasound the spleen appears isoechoic.

Gaucher's Disease. All age groups can be affected by Gaucher's disease. About 50% of patients are under 8 years of age and 17% are under 1 year of age. Clinical features follow a chronic course, with bone pain and changes in skin pigmentation. On ultrasound there is splenomegaly, diffuse inhomogeneity, and multiple splenic nodules (well-defined hypoechoic lesions). These nodules may be irregular, hy-

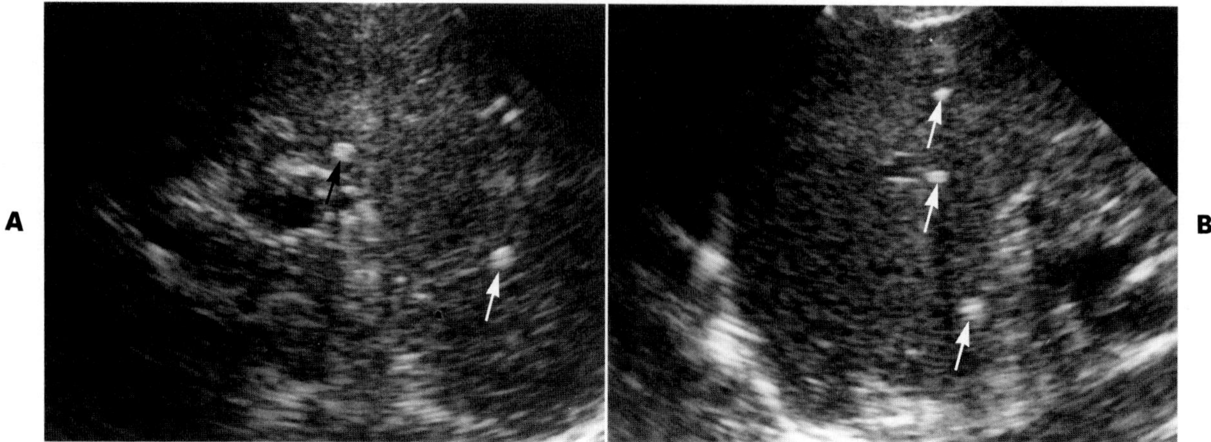

FIG. 10-14 **A,** Transverse, and **B,** longitudinal scans of a patient with granulomatous infection. The bright echogenic lesions are seen within the splenic parenchyma *(arrows)*.

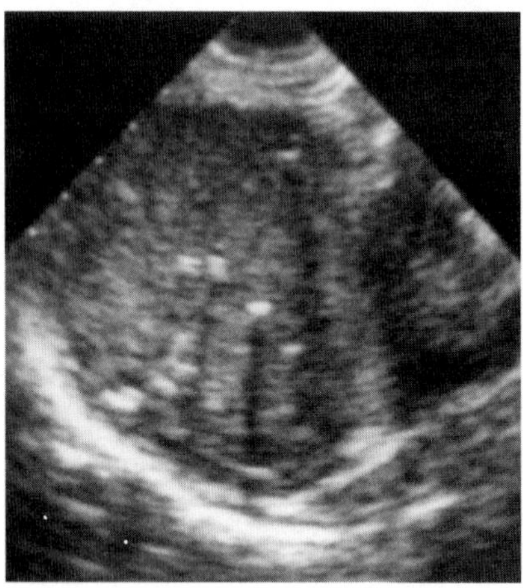

FIG. 10-15 Splenic calcifications are seen in this young Hispanic female with tuberculosis.

perechoic, or mixed. They represent focal areas of Gaucher's cells associated with fibrosis and infarction.

Niemann-Pick Disease. Niemann-Pick disease is a rapidly fatal disease that predominantly affects female infants. The clinical features consist of hepatomegaly, digestive disturbances, and lymphadenopathy.

Letterer-Siwe Disease. In Letterer-Siwe disease, sometimes called *nonlipid reticuloendotheliosis,* there is proliferation of reticuloendothelial cells in all tissues but particularly in the splenic lymph nodes and bone marrow. Usually the spleen is only moderately enlarged, although the change may be more severe in affected older infants. This disease is generally found in children below the age of 2 years. Clinical features are hepatosplenomegaly, fever, and pulmonary involvement. It is rapidly fatal.

Hand-Schüller-Christian Disease. Hand-Schüller-Christian disease is benign and chronic in spite of many features similar to those of Letterer-Siwe disease. It usually affects children over 2 years of age. The clinical features are a chronic course, diabetes, and moderate hepatosplenomegaly.

Abscess and Splenic Infection

Splenic Abscess. Splenic abscesses are uncommon, probably because of the phagocytic activity of the spleen's efficient reticuloendothelial system and leukocytes. The system may be infected by the following: subacute bacterial endocarditis, septicemia, decreased immunologic states, or drug abuse. In the majority of patients the infection is spread from distant foci in the abdomen, or an inflammatory process extends directly from adjacent organs. Extrinsic processes (i.e., perinephric or subphrenic abscess, perforated gastric or colonic lesions, or pancreatic abscess) may invade.

Clinical findings may be subtle with fever, left upper quadrant tenderness, abdominal pain, left shoulder and flank pain, and splenomegaly.

Ultrasound Findings. Sonography shows a mixed echo pattern (Fig. 10-16). The lesion may be hypoechoic, often with a hyperechoic foci that represents debris or gas. Other findings include the following: thick or shaggy walls, anechoic (without echoes within a mass), poor definition of the lesion, and increased to decreased transmission (depending on the presence of gas). An abscess may be difficult to distinguish from an infarct, neoplasm, or hematoma, and clinical correlation is necessary.

Splenic Infection. Many infections can affect the spleen. The most prominent feature is splenomegaly. Many immunocompromised patients also have multiple nodules within the spleen.

Patients with hepatosplenic candidiasis may show irregular masses within the spleen, the "wheels-within-wheels" pattern, with the outer wheel representing the ring of fibrosis surrounding the inner echogenic wheel of inflammatory cells and a central hypoechoic area. Other patterns found are bull's eye (hypoechoic rim with a echogenic central core), hypoechoic nodule, or hyperechoic nodule.

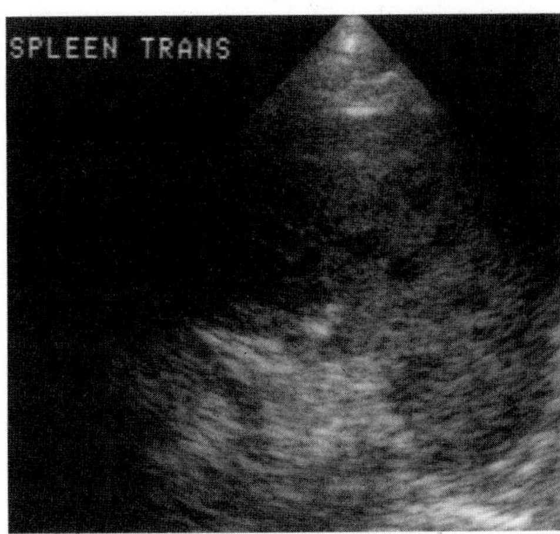

FIG. 10-16 Multiple hypoechoic lesions are seen within this transverse view of the splenic parenchyma. This patient was a drug addict who presented with fever and left shoulder and flank pain. Multiple splenic abscess collections were suspected when blood cultures returned position for subbacterial endocarditis.

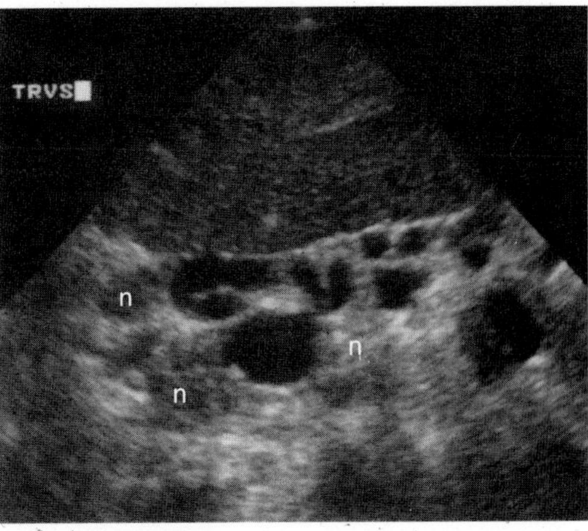

FIG. 10-17 Young, human immunodeficiency virus (HIV)—positive patient presented with tenderness in the upper abdomen. Multiple nodes are seen along the splenic hilum with prominent splenic vacular structures.

Patients with mycobacterial infections show tiny echogenic foci diffusely throughout the spleen. Active tuberculosis shows echo-poor or cystic masses representing small abscess lesions.

Acquired Immune Deficiency Syndrome. In acquired immune deficiency syndrome patients the most common finding is splenomegaly. These patients may have multiorgan involvement (i.e., liver, spleen, kidneys) (Figs. 10-17 and 10-18). The focal lesions include candida, pneumocystis, mycobacterium, disseminated pneumocystis, Kaposi's sarcoma, and lymphoma.

Splenic Infarction

Splenic infarction is the most common cause of focal splenic lesions. An infarction of the spleen occurs because of septic emboli and local thrombosis in patients with pancreatitis, subacute bacterial endocarditis, leukemia, lymphomatous disorders, sickle cell anemia, sarcoidosis, or polyarteritis nodosa.

Ultrasound may show a localized hypoechoic area, depending on the time of onset. Fresh hemorrhage has a hypoechoic appearance; healed infarctions appear as echogenic peripheral wedge-shaped lesions with their base toward the subcapsular surface of the spleen. The infarction may become nodular or hyperechoic with time.

Trauma

The spleen is most commonly injured as the result of blunt abdominal trauma. If the patient has severe left upper quadrant pain secondary to trauma, a splenic hematoma or subcapsular hematoma should be considered. The tear may result in linear or stellate lacerations or capsular tears, puncture wounds from foreign bodies or rib fractures or subcapsular hematomas.

Blunt trauma has two outcomes. If the capsule is intact the outcome may be intraparenchymal or subcapsular hematoma; if the capsule ruptures, a focal or free intraperitoneal hematoma may form. In delayed ruptures, a subcapsular hematoma may develop with subsequent rupture.

Clinical Findings. The patient typically presents with left upper quadrant pain, left shoulder pain, left flank pain, or dizziness. On clinical evaluation the patient may have tenderness over the left upper quadrant, hypotension, and decreased hemoglobin, indicating a bleed.

Ultrasound Findings. The most prominent finding is splenomegaly, with progressive enlargement as the bleed continues. In addition, an irregular splenic border, hematoma, contusion (splenic inhomogeneity), subcapsular and pericapsular fluid collections, free intraperitoneal blood, or left pleural effusion may be present.

Focal hematomas may have intrasplenic fluid collections. Perisplenic fluid is seen in patients with subcapsular hematomas. The sonographer should be aware that blood exhibits various echo patterns, depending on the time that has passed since the trauma. Fresh hemorrhage may appear hypoechoic and be difficult to distinguish from normal splenic tissue—look for a double-contour sign depicting the hematoma as separate from the spleen. As the protein and cells reabsorb the hematoma, it becomes organized and the fluid becomes hyperechoic and similar to splenic tissue. In focal areas, tiny splenic lacerations give rise to small collections of blood interspersed with disrupted splenic pulp (contusion). With time, the hematoma becomes more fluid or lucent-appearing.

The echo-free, intraperitoneal fluid is probably blood mixed with peritoneal transudate. Healing of the lesion takes time, often extending into months. The free fluid disappears quicker because the fluid is moved across the pleural and peritoneal membranes rapidly (2 to 4 weeks). Intrasplenic hematomas and contusions take longer because the

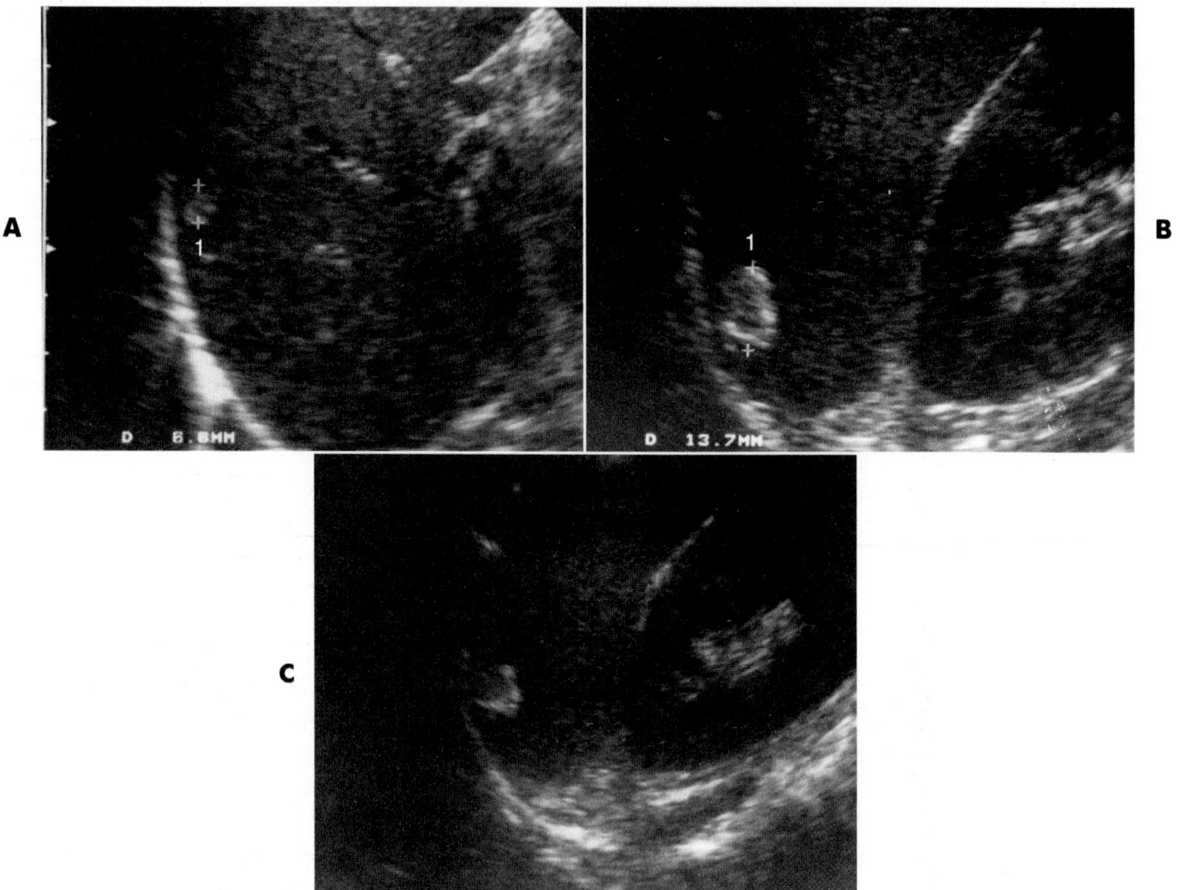

FIG. 10-18 A to **C.** The most common finding in acquired immunodeficiency syndrome patients is splenomegaly. These patients have multiple-organ involvement. This patient had two bright echogenic foci along the lateral margin of the spleen.

fluid, protein, and necrotic debris must be resorbed from within a solid organ in which the blood supply has already been focally disrupted. When the spleen returns to normal, small irregular foci may remain—or the parenchyma may be normal.

Splenic Cysts

Splenic cysts may be classified as parasitic or nonparasitic in origin. *Echinococcus* is the only parasite that forms splenic cysts; it is uncommon in the United States. Parasitic cysts appear as anechoic lesions with possible daughter cysts and calcification, or as solid masses with fine internal echoes and poor distal enhancement. Nonparasitic cysts of the spleen have been categorized as either primary or true.

Primary, or epidermoid, cysts contain an epithelial lining and are considered to be of congenital origin. False or secondary cysts lack a cellular lining, probably developing as a result of prior trauma to the spleen and account for 80% of nonparasitic splenic cysts. True cysts are usually solitary and unilocular and rarely contain calcification. The internal surface of the cyst may be smooth or trabeculated. The fluid may be clear or turbid, and may contain protein, iron, bilirubin, fat, and cholesterol crystals. Primary cysts occur more frequently in females; 50% occur in patients under 15 years of age. Clinically they present with an asymptomatic left upper quadrant mass.

Ultrasound Findings. Ultrasound shows a hypoechoic or anechoic foci with well-defined walls and increased through-transmission (Fig. 10-19). Primary cysts can have internal echoes at increased gain. Hemorrhage within the cyst may produce a fluid level.

Primary Tumors of the Spleen

Generally speaking, primary tumors of the spleen are rare. The tumors may be divided into two groups, benign or malignant. With the benign primary tumors, splenomegaly is the first indication of an abnormality. Most of these tumors appear isoechoic compared with the normal splenic parenchyma. Benign primary tumors include hamartoma, cavernous hemangioma, and cystic lymphangioma.

Malignant tumors of the spleen are also uncommon. Primary tumors found in the spleen may be lymphoma, Hodgkin's tumor, or hemangiosarcoma.

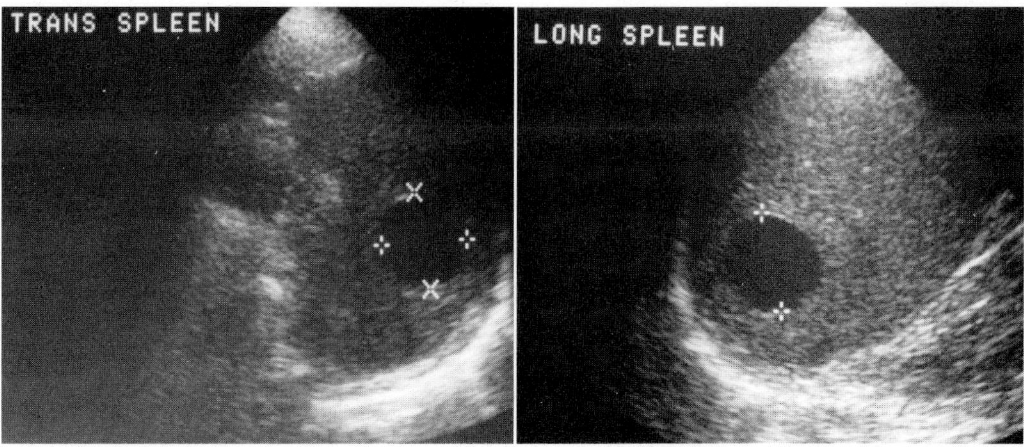

FIG. 10-19 Young patient with right upper quadrant pain had an incidental finding of a splenic cyst. The borders are well defined and the mass is anechoic.

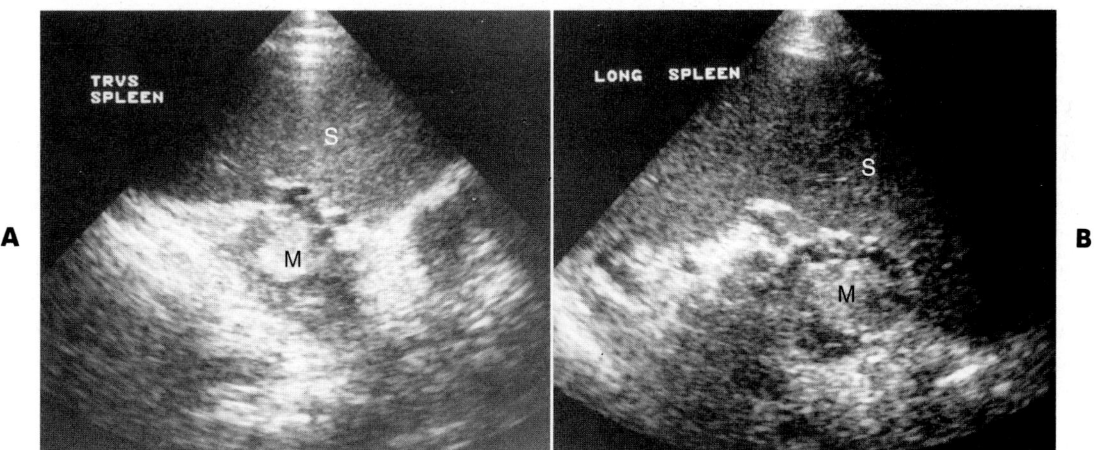

FIG. 10-20 A, and **B,** 43 year old, human immunodeficiency virus (HIV)—positive with alcoholic pancreatitis and pseudocyst in the tail of the pancreas. He presented to the emergency room with abdominal pain and fever. Ultrasound findings revealed a complex mass in the area of the previous pseudocyst. This may represent an infected pseudocyst with purulent fluid, hemorrhage within the pseudocyst, or fatty deposition. This patient had multiple nodes along the head of the pancreas (not shown).

Benign Primary Neoplasms

Hamartoma. Hamartoma has both solid and cystic components and is generally hyperechoic on ultrasound. The patient is a symptomatic. The tumor may be solitary or multiple and is considered well-defined but not encapsulated. The hamartoma is composed of lymphoid tissue or a combination of sinuses and structures equivalent to pulp cords of normal splenic tissue.

Cavernous Hemangioma. Cavernous hemangioma is a large inhomogeneous echogenic mass with multiple small hypoechoic areas. The patient presents with no symptoms and only becomes symptomatic when the size of the spleen increases and compresses other organs. Complications occur when the tumor increases in size to cause a splenic rupture with peritoneal symptoms. The ultrasound appearance is a complex pattern; infarction with coagulated blood or fibrin in the cavities may be seen but is unspecific. Hydatid cyst, abscess, dermoid cyst, and metastases should be considered in the differential diagnosis.

Cystic Lymphangioma. Cystic lymphangioma is a benign malformation of lymphatics, composed of endothelium-lined cystic spaces. It appears as a mass with extensive cystic replacement of splenic parenchyma. Lymphangiomatosis affects predominately the somatic soft tissue (found in the neck, axilla, mediastinum, retroperitoneum, and soft tissues of the extremities). It may involve multiple organ systems or be confined to solitary organs, such as the liver, spleen, kidney, or colon. Splenic involvement is rare, but when it occurs a multicystic appearance is characteristic.

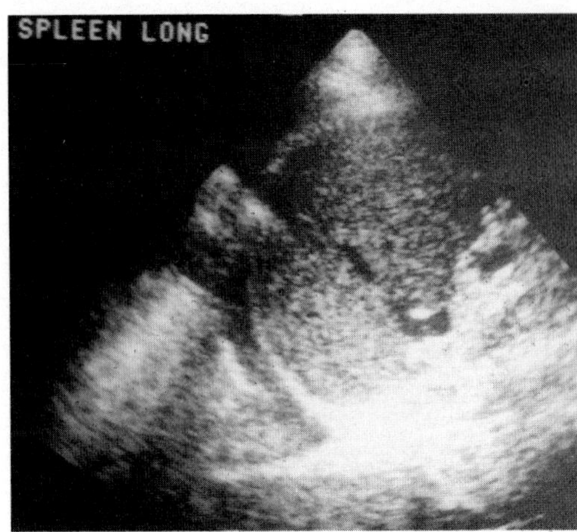

FIG. 10-21 Metastases is the result of a hematogenous spread from another primary site. The spleen is the tenth most common site of tumors spread from the breast, lung, ovary, stomach, melanoma, and prostate. This patient present with secondary signs of metastases—malignant ascites.

Malignant Primary Neoplasm

Hemangiosarcoma is a rare malignant neoplasm arising from the vascular endothelium of the spleen. The mixed cystic ultrasound pattern resembles that of a cavernous hemangioma, but it can also be hyperechoic.

Lymphoma. The spleen is commonly involved in lymphoma. It may be difficult to detect splenic lymphoma by ultrasound. When it is seen, however, it appears to be typically hypoechoic; some focal areas are also seen.

Metastases. Metastases are the result of a hematogenous spread from another primary site. The spleen is the tenth most common site of metastases, which may originate from the breast, lung, ovary, stomach, or prostate, or from melanoma (Figs. 10-20 and 10-21). The metastatic tumors may be microscopic, causing no symptoms. The splenic parenchyma should be carefully evaluated by the sonographer to detect the abnormalities of the splenic parenchyma.

Melanoma deposits appear hypoechoic but are of higher echo amplitude than lymphoma; some are echodense.

REVIEW QUESTIONS

1. Is the spleen intraperitoneal or extraperitoneal?
2. What is an accessory spleen? What problems may arise in the accessory spleen?
3. Define the *wandering spleen*.
4. What is the significance of splenic agenesis?
5. What organs are part of the reticuloendothelial system?
6. How big is the normal spleen?
7. Describe the echogenic pattern of the spleen.
8. Name five conditions that can cause splenomegaly.
9. What would the sonographer see on ultrasound in a patient with a sickle-cell crisis?
10. What is the appearance of lymphomatous involvement of the spleen?
11. Describe some conditions that can cause a splenic abscess.
12. What is the appearance of a splenic infarct on ultrasound?
13. Describe subcapsular hematoma and its ultrasound appearance.
14. Name three common benign primary tumors of the spleen.

REFERENCES

1. Hicken P, Sauerbrei EE, and Cooperberg PL: Ultrasonic coronal scanning of left upper quadrant, J Can Assoc Radiol 32:107, 1981.

BIBLIOGRAPHY

Al-Moyaya S, Al-Awami M, Vaidya MP, et al: Hydatid cyst of the spleen, Am J Trop Med Hyg 35:995, 1986.

Balcar I, Seltzer SE, Davis S, and Geller S: Computed tomography patterns of splenic infarction: a clinical and experimental study, Radiology 151:723, 1984.

Bhimji SD, Cooperberg PL, and Naiman S: Ultrasound diagnosis of splenic cysts, Radiology 122:787, 1977.

Costello P, Kane RA, Oster J, et al: Focal splenic disease demonstrated by ultrasound and computed tomography, J Can Assoc Radiol 36:22, 1985.

Delamarre J, Capron JP, Drouard F, et al: Splenosis: ultrasound and computed tomography findings in a case complicated by an intraperitoneal implant traumatic hematoma, Gastrointest Radiol 13:275, 1988.

Duddy MJ and Calder CJ: Cystic hemangioma of the spleen: findings on ultrasound and computed tomography, Br J Radiol 62:180, 1989.

Franquet T, Montes M, Lecumberri FJ, et al: Hydatid disease of the spleen: imaging findings in nine patients, Am J Roentgenol 154:525, 1990.

Hill SC, Reinig JW, Barranger JA, et al: Gaucher's disease: sonographic appearance of spleen, Radiology 160:631, 1986.

Lupien C and Sauerbrie EE: Healing in the traumatized spleen: sonographic investigation, Radiology 150:181, 1984.

Manor A, Starinsky R, Gorfinkel D, et al: Ultrasound features of a symptomatic splenic hemangioma, J Clin Ultrasound 12:95, 1984.

Maresca G, Mirk P, DeGaetano AM, et al: Sonographic patterns in splenic infarction, J Clin Ultrasound 14:23, 1986.

Mostbeck G, Sommer G, Haller J, et al: Accessory spleen: presentation as a large abdominal mass in an asymptomatic young woman, Gastrointest Radiol 12:337, 1987.

Muller H, Schneider H, Ruckauer K, et al: Accessory spleen torsion: clinical picture, sonographic diagnosis and differential diagnosis, Klin Pediatr 200:419, 1988.

Nishitani H, Hayashi T, Onitsuka H, et al: Computed tomography of accessory spleens, Radiat Med 2:222, 1984.

Pastakia B, Shawker TH, Thalar M, et al: Hepatosplenic candidiasis: wheels within wheels, Radiology 166:417, 1988.

Plaja Ramon P, Also Puertolas C, and Sanchis Solera L: Wandering spleen: discussion apropos of a case, An Esp Pediatr 26:69, 1987.

Stevens PG, Kumari-Subaiya SS, and Kahn LB: Splenic involvement in Gaucher's disease: sonographic findings, J Clin Ultrasound 15:397, 1987.

Turk CO, Lipson SB, and Brandt TD: Splenosis mimicking a renal mass, Urology 31:248, 1988.

Vyborny CJ, Merrill TN, Reda J, et al: Subacute subcapsular hematoma of the spleen complicating pancreatitis: successful percutaneous drainage, Radiology 169:161, 1989.

Wilson LS, Robinson DE, Griffiths KA, et al: Evaluation of ultrasonic attenuation in diffuse diseases of spleen and liver, Ultrasound Imaging 9:236, 1987.

Yee JM, Raghavendra BN, Horii SC, et al: Abdominal sonography in AIDS: a review, J Ultrasound Med 8:705, 1989.

CHAPTER

11

The Retroperitoneum

Sandra L. Hagen-Ansert

The retroperitoneal space is the area between the posterior portion of the parietal peritoneum and the posterior abdominal wall muscles (Fig. 11-1). It extends from the diaphragm to the pelvis. Laterally the boundaries extend to the extraperitoneal fat planes within the confines of the transversalis fascia, and medially the space encloses the great vessels. It is subdivided into the following three categories: anterior pararenal space, perirenal space, and posterior pararenal space.

The perirenal space surrounds the kidney, adrenal, and perirenal fat. The anterior pararenal space includes the duodenum, pancreas, and ascending and transverse colon. The posterior pararenal space includes the iliopsoas muscle, ureter, and branches of the inferior vena cava and aorta, and their lymphatics.

The retroperitoneum is protected by the spine, ribs, pelvis, and musculature and has been a difficult area to assess clinically by ultrasound. Computerized tomography imaging is better to outline the retroperitoneal cavity. Occasionally, however, the sonographer is asked to rule out fluid collection, hematoma, urinoma, or ascitic fluid in the retroperitoneal space.

NORMAL RETROPERITONEAL ANATOMY

The retroperitoneum is delineated anteriorly by the posterior peritoneum, posteriorly by the transversalis fascia, and laterally by the lateral borders of the quadratus lumborum muscles and peritoneal leaves of the mesentery. As one proceeds from a superior to inferior direction, the retroperitoneum extends from the diaphragm to the pelvic brim. Superior to the pelvic brim, the retroperitoneum can be partitioned into the lumbar and iliac fossae. The pararenal and perirenal spaces are included in the lumbar fossa.

Pathologic processes can stretch from the anterior abdominal wall to the subdiaphragmatic space, mediastinum, and subcutaneous tissues of the back and flank. The retrofascial space, which includes the psoas, quadratus lumborum, and iliacus muscles (muscles posterior to the transversalis fascia), is often the site of extension of retroperitoneal pathologic processes.

Ultrasound of the Retroperitoneum

There is no specific preparation to image the retroperitoneal cavity, although 6 to 8 hours of fasting may help to eliminate bowel gas. To image the retroperitoneum, scans should be made in the longitudinal and transverse plane from the diaphragm to the iliac crest with the patient in a supine or prone position and from the crest to the symphysis in a supine position with the patient having a full bladder. The upper abdomen may also be scanned with the patient in a decubitus position. All scans should include the kidneys and retroperitoneal muscles.

Anterior Pararenal Space

The anterior pararenal space is bound anteriorly by the posterior parietal peritoneum and posteriorly by the anterior renal fascia. It is bound laterally by the lateroconal fascia formed by the fusion of the anterior and posterior leaves of the renal fascia. (This space merges with the bare area of the liver by the coronary ligament.) The pancreas, duodenal sweep, and ascending and transverse colon are the organs included in the anterior pararenal space (Fig. 11-2).

Perirenal Space

The perirenal space is surrounded by the anterior and posterior layers of the renal fascia (Gerota's fascia), attaching to the diaphragm superiorly. They are united loosely at their inferior margin at the iliac crest level or superior border of the false pelvis. Collections in the perinephric space can communicate within the iliac fossa of the retroperitoneum (Fig. 11-3).

The lateroconal fascia (the lateral fusion of the renal fascia) proceeds anteriorly as the posterior peritoneum. The posterior renal fasciae fuse medially with the psoas or quadratus lumborum fascia (Fig. 11-4). The anterior renal fascia fuses medially with connective tissue surrounding the great vessels. (This space contains the adrenal gland, kidney, and ureter; the great vessels, also within this space, are largely isolated within their connective tissue sheaths.) The perirenal space contains the adrenal gland and kidney (in a variable amount of echogenic perinephric fat, the thickest portion posterior and lateral to the kidney's lower pole). The kidney is anterolateral to the psoas muscle, an-

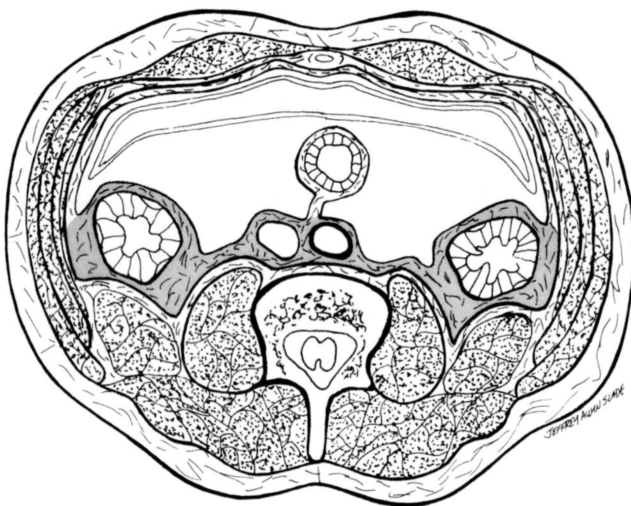

FIG. 11-1 Schematic transverse section of the abdominal cavity at the level of the fourth lumbar vertebra. The retroperitoneal space is outlined in gray.

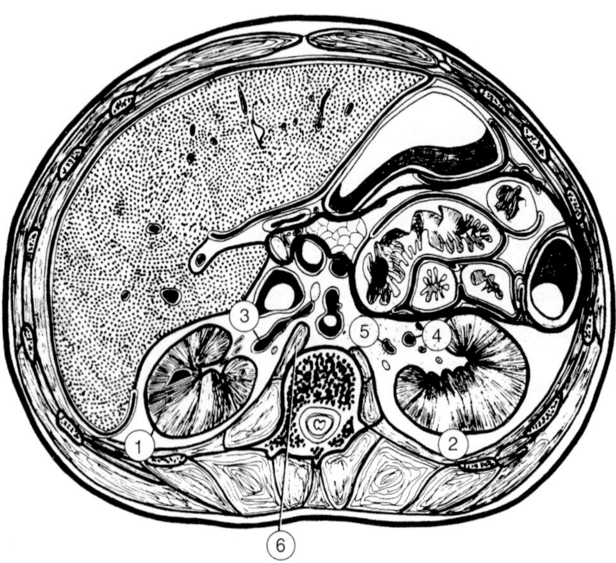

FIG. 11-2 Transverse line drawing of the anterior pararenal space. Right kidney, *1;* left kidney, *2;* right renal artery, *3;* left renal vein, *4;* left renal artery, *5;* and crus of the diaphragm, *6.* This space is bound anteriorly by the posterior parietal peritoneum and the anterior renal fascia. It is bound laterally by the lateroconal fascia formed by the fusion of the anterior and posterior leaves of the renal fascia. The pancreas, duodenal sweep, and the ascending and transverse colon are included in the anterior pararenal space. (From Hagen-Ansert SL: The anatomy workbook. Philadelphia, 1986, JB Lippincott)

terior to the quadratus lumborum muscle, and posteromedial to the ascending and descending colon.

The second portion of the duodenum is anterior to the kidney hilum on the right. On the left the kidney is bounded by the stomach anterosuperiorly, the pancreas anteriorly, and the spleen anterolaterally.

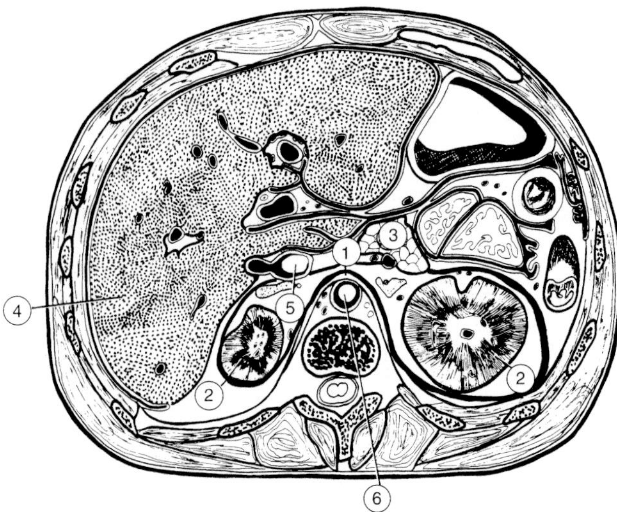

FIG. 11-3 Transverse line drawing of the perirenal space. Crus, *1;* kidneys, *2;* pancreas, *3;* right lobe of the liver, *4;* inferior vena cava, *5;* and aorta, *6.* This is surrounded by the anterior and posterior layers of the renal fascia. These layers join and attach to the diaphragm superiorly, but they are united only loosely at their inferior margin at the level of the iliac crest. (From Hagen-Ansert SL: The anatomy workbook. Philadelphia, 1986, JB Lippincott)

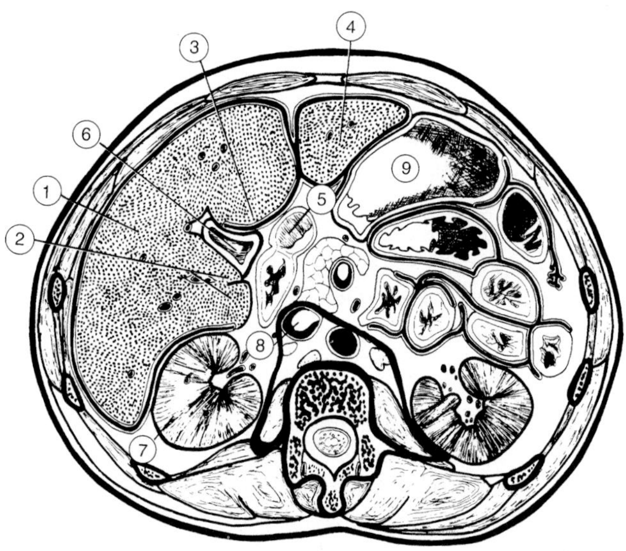

FIG. 11-4 Transverse line drawing of the posterior pararenal space. Right lobe, *1;* caudate lobe, *2;* left lobe (medial), *3;* left lobe (lateral), *4;* duodenum, *5;* gallbladder, *6;* right kidney, *7;* inferior vena cava, *8;* and stomach, *9.* This space is located between the posterior renal fascia and the transversalis fascia. It communicates with the periotneal fat, lateral to the lateroconal fascia. The space merges inferiorly with the anterior pararenal space and retroperitoneal tissues of the iliac fossa. (From Hagen-Ansert SL: The anatomy workbook. Philadelphia, 1986, JB Lippincott)

Adrenal Glands

In the adult patient the adrenal glands are anterior, medial, and superior to the kidneys (Fig. 11-5). The right adrenal is more superior to the kidney, whereas the left adrenal is more medial to the kidney. The medial portion of

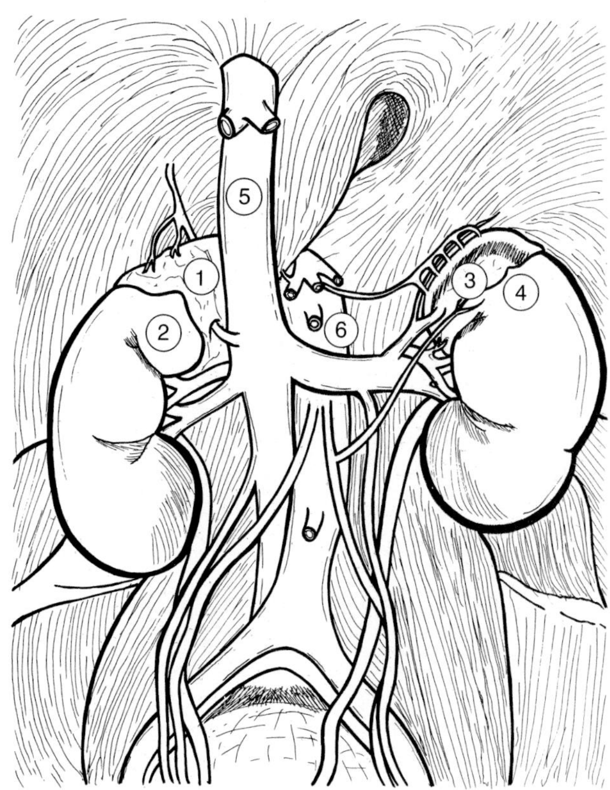

FIG. 11-5 The adrenal glands are retroperitoneal organs that lie on the upper pole of each kidney. Right adrenal gland, *1;* upper pole of the right kidney, *2;* left adrenal gland, *3;* upper pole of the left kidney, *4;* inferior vena cava, *5;* and the aorta, *6.* They are surrounded by perinephric fascia and are separated from the kidneys by perinephric fat. The right adrenal gland is triangular and caps the upper pole of the right kidney. It extends medially behind the inferior vena cava, and rests posteriorly on the diaphragm. The left adrenal gland is semilunar and extends along the medial borders of the left kidney. It lies posterior to the pancreas, the lesser sac, and the stomach, and rests posteriorly on the diaphragm. (From Hagen-Ansert SL: The anatomy workbook. Philadelphia, 1986, JB Lippincott)

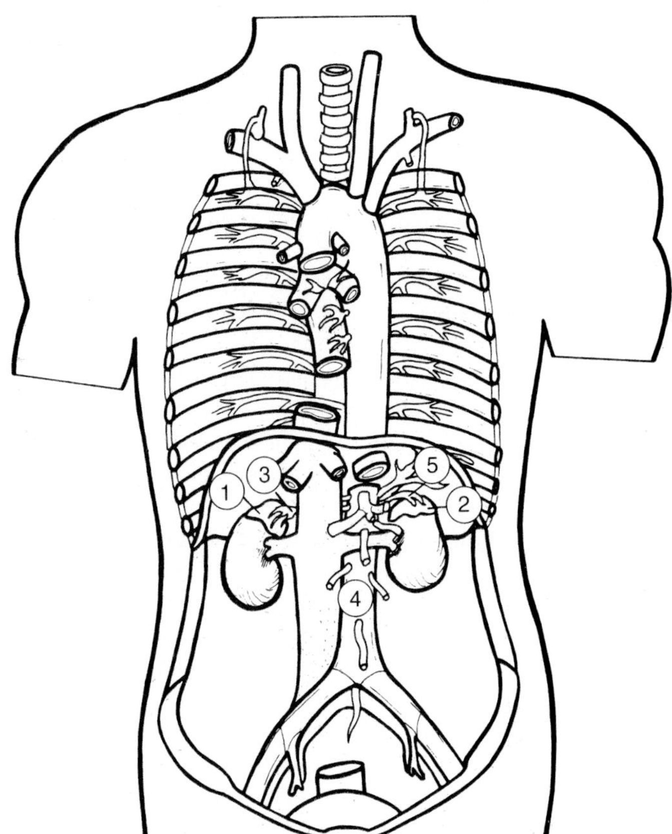

FIG. 11-6 There are three arteries supplying each gland—the suprarenal branch of the inferior phrenic artery, the suprarenal branch of the aorta, and the suprarenal branch of the renal artery. A single vein arises from the hilum of each gland and drains into the inferior vena cava on the right and into the renal vein on the left. Left adrenal gland, *1;* right adrenal gland, *2;* suprarenal arteries, *3* and *5*; abdominal aorta, *4.* (From Hagen-Ansert SL: The anatomy workbook. Philadelphia, 1986, JB Lippincott)

the right adrenal gland is immediately posterior to the inferior vena cava (above the level of the portal vein and lateral to the crus). The lateral portion of the gland is posterior and medial to the right lobe of the liver and posterior to the duodenum.

The left adrenal gland is lateral or slightly posterolateral to the aorta and lateral to the crus of the diaphragm. The superior portion is posterior to the lesser omental space and posterior to the stomach. The inferior portion is posterior to the pancreas. The splenic vein and artery pass between the pancreas and the left adrenal gland.

The adrenal glands vary in size, shape, and configuration; the right adrenal is triangular in shape and caps the upper pole of the right kidney. The left adrenal is semilunar in shape and extends along the medial border of the left kidney from the upper pole to the hilus. The internal texture is medium in consistency; the cortex and medulla are not distinguished.

The adrenal gland is a distinct hypoechoic structure; sometimes highly echogenic fat is seen surrounding the gland. The size is usually smaller than 3 cm (3 to 6 cm long, 3 to 6 mm thick, 2 to 4 cm wide).

Neonatal Adrenal

The neonatal adrenal glands are characterized by a thin echogenic core surrounded by a thick transonic zone. This thick rim of transonicity represents the hypertrophied adrenal cortex, whereas the echogenic core is the adrenal medulla. The infant adrenal is proportionally larger than the adult (one third the size of the kidney; in adults it is one thirteenth the size).

Vascular Supply of the Adrenal Glands

Three arteries supply each adrenal gland: the suprarenal branch of the inferior phrenic, the suprarenal branch of the aorta, and the suprarenal branch of the renal artery (Fig. 11-6). A single vein from the hilum of each gland drains into the inferior vena cava on the right and on the left the vein drains into the left renal vein.

Physiology

Each adrenal gland is comprised of two endocrine glands. The cortex, or outer part, secretes a range of steroid hormones; the medulla, or core, secretes epinephrine and norepinephrine.

Cortex

The steroids secreted by the adrenal cortex fall into the following three main categories:

1. Mineralocorticoids—regulate electrolyte metabolism. Aldosterone is the principal mineralocorticoid. It has a regulatory effect on the relative concentrations of mineral ions in the body fluids and therefore on the water content of tissues. An insufficiency of this steroid leads to increased excretion of sodium and chloride ions and water into the urine. This is accompanied by a fall in sodium, chloride, and bicarbonate concentrations in the blood, resulting in a lowered pH or acidosis.
2. Glucocorticoids—play a principal role in carbohydrate metabolism. They promote deposition of liver glycogen from proteins and inhibit use of glucose by the cells, thus increasing blood sugar level. Cortisone and hydrocortisone are the primary glucocorticoids. They diminish allergic response, especially the more serious inflammatory types (rheumatoid arthritis and rheumatic fever).
3. Sex hormones—androgens (male) and estrogens (female). The adrenal gland secretes both types of hormones regardless of the patient's gender. Normally these are secreted in minute quantities and have almost insignificant effects. With oversecretion, however, a marked effect is seen. Adrenal tumors in women can promote aggressive homosexuality and secondary masculine characteristics. Hypersecretion of the hormone in prepubertal boys accelerates adult masculine development and the growth of pubic hair. The adrenal cortex is controlled by adrenocorticotropic hormone (ACTH) from the pituitary. A diminished glucocorticoid blood concentration stimulates the secretion of ACTH. Consequent increase in adrenal cortex activity inhibits further ACTH secretion.

Hypofunction of the adrenal cortex in humans is called *Addison's disease*. Symptoms and signs include hypotension, general weakness, loss of appetite and weight, and a characteristic bronzing of the skin.

Oversecretion of the adrenal cortex may be caused by an overproduction of ACTH resulting from a pituitary tumor or a tumor in the cortex itself. Cushing's disease is one type of oversecretion disease of the adrenal cortex. Symptoms include increased sodium retention—which leads to tissue edema, increased plasma volume, and a mild alkalosis. Muscle and bone weakness is common. Secretion of androgens is increased and causes masculinizing effects in women.

Medulla[1]

The adrenal medulla makes up the core of the gland, in which groups of irregular cells are located amid veins that collect blood from the sinusoids. This gland produces epinephrine and norepinephrine. Both of these hormones are amines, sometimes referred to as *catecholamines*. They elevate the blood pressure, the former working as an accelerator of the heart rate and the latter as a vasoconstrictor. The two hormones together promote glycogenolysis, the breakdown of liver glycogen to glucose, which causes an increase in blood sugar concentration.

The adrenal medulla is not essential for life and can be removed surgically without causing untreatable damage.

Ultrasound of the Adrenal Glands

Although sonography has proven useful in evaluating soft tissue structures within the abdominal cavity, visualization of the adrenal glands has been difficult because of its small size, medial location, and the surrounding perirenal fat. If the adrenal gland becomes enlarged secondary to disease, it is easier to image and separate it from the upper pole of the kidney.

Visualization of the adrenal area depends on several factors: the size of the patient and the amount of perirenal fat surrounding the adrenal area, the presence of bowel gas, and the ability to change the patient into multiple positions.

With the patient in the decubitus position the sonographer should attempt to align the kidney and ipsilateral paravertebral vessels (inferior vena cava or aorta). The right adrenal gland has a "comma" or triangular shape in the transaxial plane. The best visualization is obtained by a transverse scan with the patient in a left lateral decubitus position. As the patient assumes this position, the inferior vena cava moves forward and the aorta rolls over the crus of the diaphragm to offer a good window to image the upper pole of the right kidney and adrenal. If the patient is obese, it may be difficult to recognize the triangular- or crescent-shaped adrenal gland. The adrenal should not appear rounded; if it does, the finding suggests a pathologic process.

The longitudinal scan is made through the right lobe of the liver, perpendicular to the linear right crus of the diaphragm. The retroperitoneal fat must be recognized as separate from the liver, crus of the diaphragm, adrenal gland, and great vessel (Fig. 11-7).

The left adrenal gland is closely related to the left crus of the diaphragm and the anterior-superior-medial aspect of the upper pole of the left kidney. It may be more difficult to image the left adrenal because of the stomach gas interference. The patient should be placed in a right lateral decubitus position and transverse scans made in an attempt to align the left kidney and the aorta. The left adrenal is seen by scanning along the posterior axillary line. The patient should be in deep inspiration in an effort to bring the adrenal and renal area into better view (Fig. 11-8).

Ultrasound pitfalls[5]

1. Right crus of the diaphragm
2. Second portion of the duodenum
3. Esophagogastric junction (cephalad to the left adrenal gland)[2]

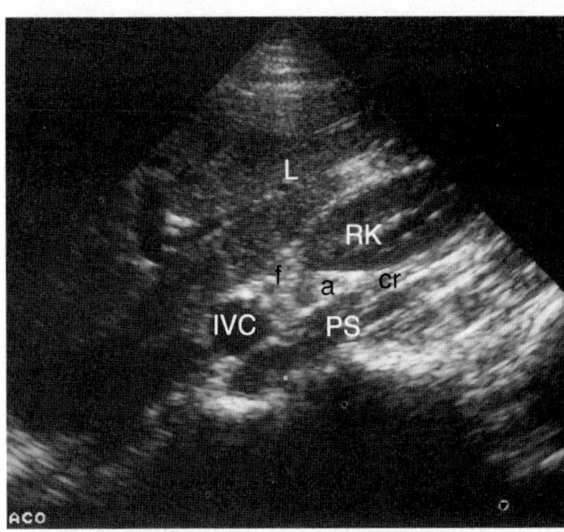

FIG. 11-7 The longitudinal scan of the right adrenal gland is made through the right lobe of the liver, perpendicular to the right crus of the diaphragm. The retroperitoneal fat, *f*, should be recognized as separate from the liver, *L*, crus, *cr*, adrenal gland, *a*, psoas, *Ps*, and upper pole of the right kidney, *RK*.

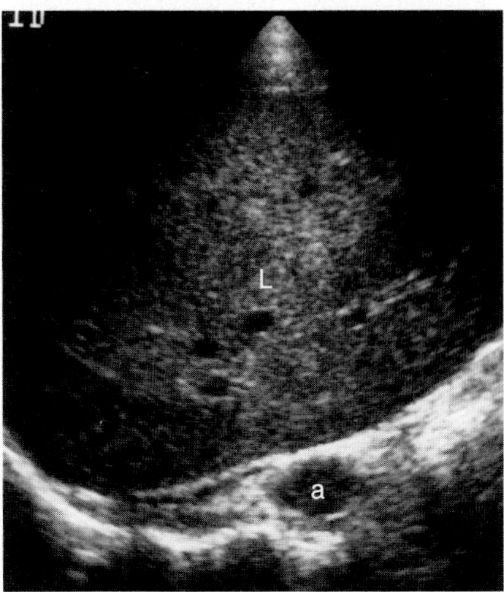

FIG. 11-9 Adrenal cysts, *a*, may become calcified, which gives them the ultrasound appearance of a "solid" mass with decreased transmission.

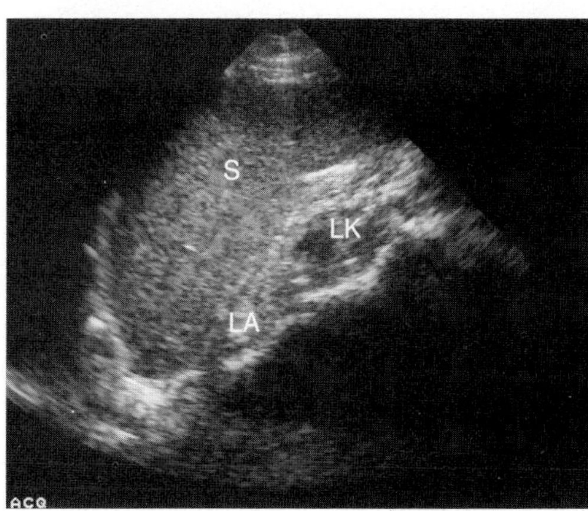

FIG. 11-8 The left adrenal gland, *LA*, is closely related to the left crus of the diaphragm and the anterior-superior-medial aspect of the upper pole of the left kidney, *LK*, and spleen, *S*.

4. Medial lobulations of the spleen[7]
5. Splenic vasculature
6. Body-tail region of the pancreas
7. Fourth portion of the duodenum

Sample[3] states the normal right adrenal gland can be visualized in over 90% of patients, whereas the left is seen in 80% of patients.[4]

Pathology

Sonographically, adrenal cysts present a typical cystic pattern, as seen in other organs of the body, having a strong back wall, no internal echoes, and good through-transmission. Adrenal cysts have the tendency to become calcified, which gives them the ultrasound appearance of a somewhat solid mass with no internal echoes (a sharp posterior border with poor through-transmission) (Figs. 11-9 and 11-10). The cyst may have hemorrhaged, and then it appears as a complex mass with multiple internal echoes and good through-transmission (Fig. 11-11).

Further pathology of the adrenal glands is related to the tumors arising within them and their hyposecretion or hypersecretion of hormones. Endocrine deficiencies may be produced when the glands are destroyed by hemorrhage, infarction, or tumor.[8] Pituitary dysfunction may also play a role in the function of the adrenals and their control of hormones.

There are several cortical syndromes that the sonographer may encounter while scanning for an adrenal mass[8]:

1. Addison's disease. This may be of adrenal or pituitary origin and is the chronic result of adrenal hypofunction. The deficiency may result from a primary adrenal tumor or metastases.
2. Adrenogenital syndrome. This is the result of excessive secretion of the sex hormones.
3. Conn's syndrome. This is caused by excessive secretion of aldosterone, usually because of a cortical adenoma.
4. Cushing's syndrome. This is produced by excessive secretion of glucocorticoids resulting from hyperplasia, a benign tumor, or carcinoma. The syndrome can also be caused by an anterior pituitary tumor.
5. Waterhouse-Friderichsen syndrome. This commonly results from bilateral hemorrhage into the adrenal glands.

The pheochromocytes of the adrenal medulla may produce a tumor called a *pheochromocytoma* that secretes epinephrine and norepinephrine in excessive quantities. These patients present with intermittent hypertension. The tumor has a homogeneous pattern that can be differentiated from a cyst by its weak posterior wall and poor through-transmission (Fig. 11-12). Pheochromocytomas may be large bulky tumors with a variety of sonographic patterns including cystic, solid, and calcified components.[6]

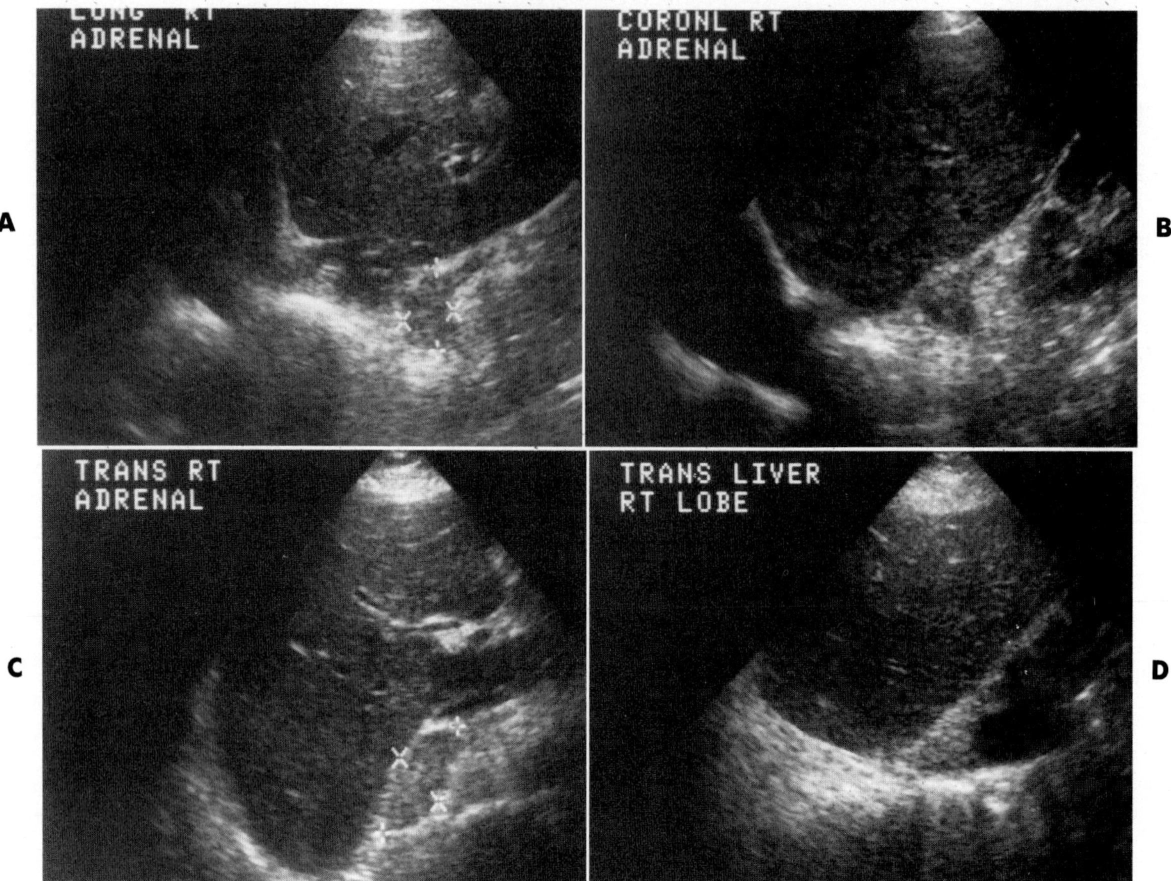

FIG. 11-10 The normal adrenal gland is quite difficult to image consistently in the adult patient. When it becomes enlarged, hyperplasia, hemorrhage, or tumor formation should be considered. **A,** Longitudinal right adrenal. **B,** Coronal right adrenal. **C,** Transverse right adrenal. **D,** Transverse oblique right adrenal.

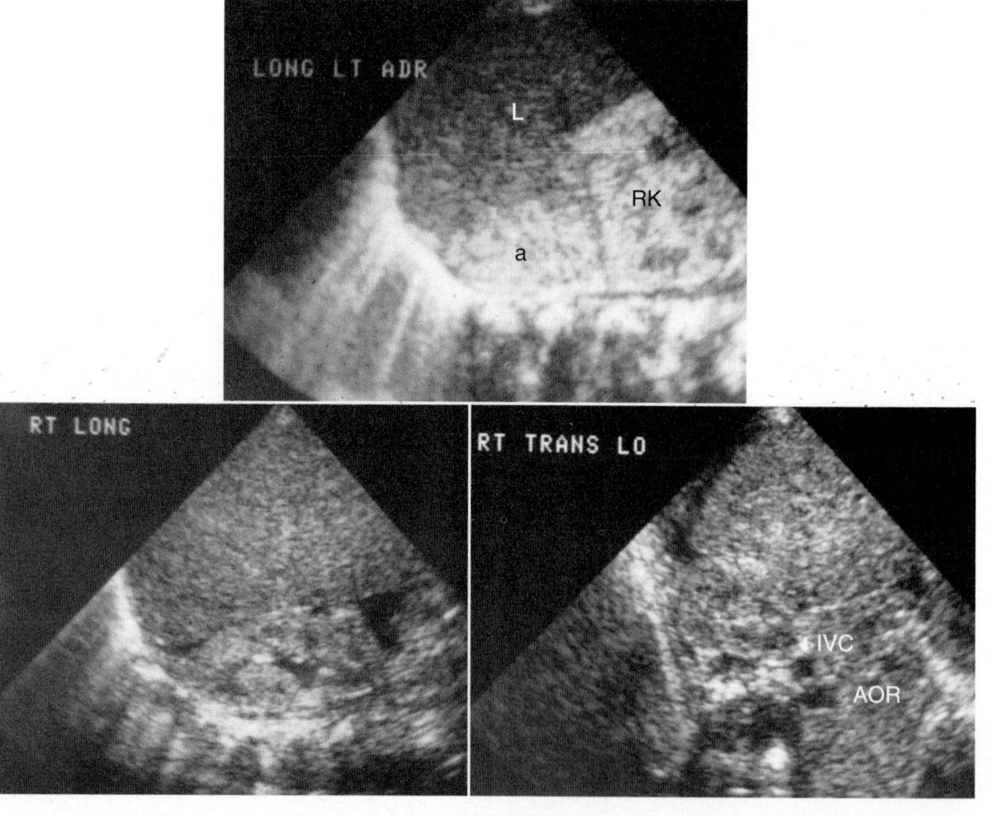

FIG. 11-11 Adrenal hemorrhage in a 1-month-old neonate. The mass appears as a complex lesion with multiple internal echoes and generalized enlargement of the gland.

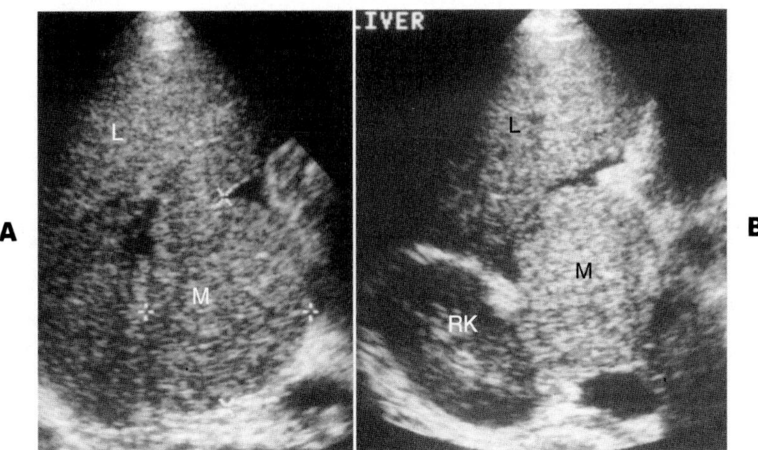

FIG. 11-12 The pheochromocytoma is a homogeneous tumor that has a weak posterior wall and decreased through-transmission. This tumor can grow quite large. **A,** Longitudinal: liver, *L*, mass, *m*. **B,** Transverse: liver, *L*, right kidney, *RK*, inferior vena cava, *IVC*, and mass, *m*.

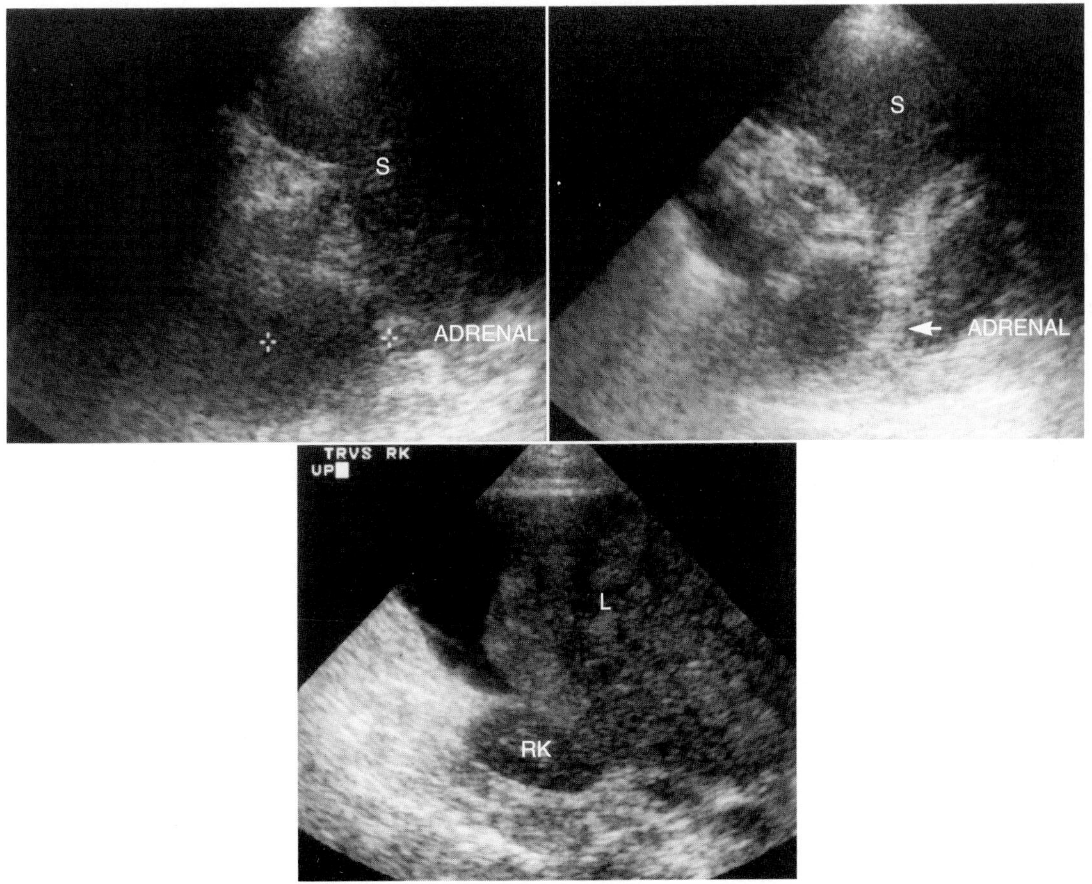

FIG. 11-13 Ill-defined mass in the area of the adrenal gland in a patient with metastatic liver disease. Liver, *L*, spleen, *S*.

Most adrenal carcinomas are not functional, but they may account for Cushing's syndrome or hyperaldosteronemia.[6] The origin of the tumor should be clearly defined. Metastases to the adrenals vary in size and echogenicity (Figs. 11-13 to 11-15). Often central necrosis causes areas of sonolucency within the tumor.

The adrenal neuroblastoma is the most common malignancy of the adrenal glands in childhood and the most common tumor of infancy. Generally it arises within the adrenal medulla. Although children are usually asymptomatic, some do present with a palpable abdominal mass that must be differentiated from a neonatal hemorrhage and hydrone-

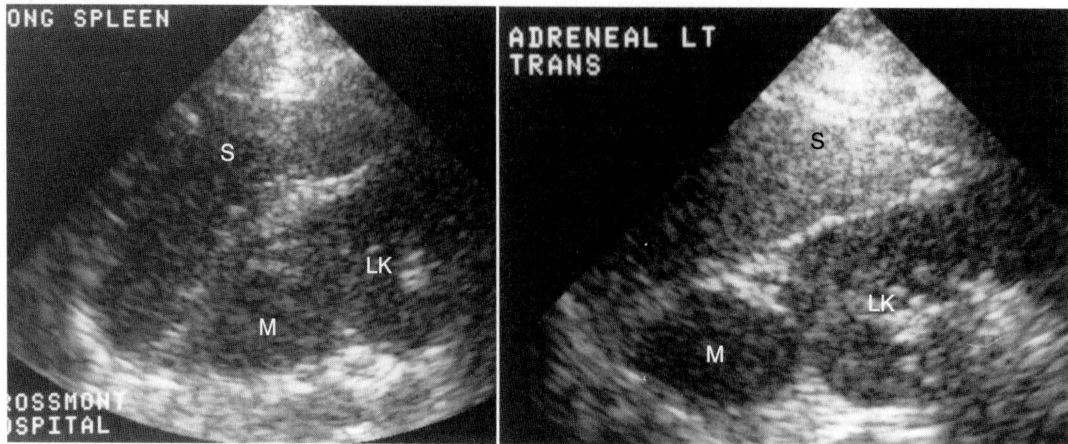

FIG. 11-14 Patient with a large mass in the left adrenal gland representing metastases. Spleen, *S*, left kidney, *LK*, adrenal mass, *m*.

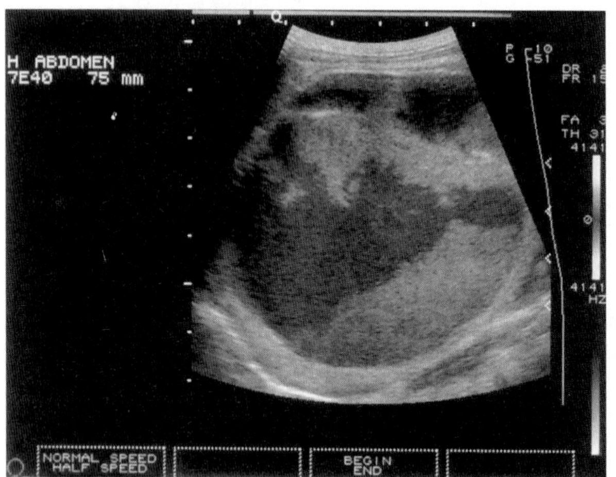

FIG. 11-15 Huge complex right adrenal mass. The sonographer would have to demonstrate this mass as separate from the right kidney, liver, and retroperitoneum.

phrosis.[6] Sonographically the tumor appears as an echogenic mass. It may be large, and evaluation of the surrounding retroperitoneum and liver should be made to rule out metastases.

Aorta

The aorta enters the abdomen posterior to the diaphragm at the level of L1 and passes posterior to the left lobe of the liver. The aorta has a straight course to the level of L4, where it bifurcates into the iliac arteries. A slight anterior curve of the aorta is the result of lumbar lordosis.

Inferior Vena Cava

The inferior vena cava extends from the junction of the two common iliac veins to the right of L5 and travels cephalad through the liver. Unlike the aorta, it curves anterior toward its termination into the right atrial cavity.

Diaphragmatic Crura

The diaphragmatic crura begin as tendinous fibers from the lumbar vertebral bodies, disks, and transverse processes of L3 on the right and L1 on the left (Fig. 11-16). The right crus is longer, larger, and more lobular and is associated with the anterior aspect of the lumbar vertebral ligament. The right renal artery crosses anterior to the crus and posterior to the inferior vena cava at the level of the right kidney. The right crus is bounded by the inferior vena cava anterolaterally and the right adrenal and right lobe of liver posterolaterally.

The left crus courses along the anterior lumbar vertebral bodies in a superior direction and inserts into the central tendon of the diaphragm.

Ultrasound of the Crus of the Diaphragm

The crus of the diaphragm may be imaged in the transverse or longitudinal coronal plane. The right crus is seen in a plane that passes through the right lobe of the liver, kidney, and adrenal gland (Fig. 11-17). The left crus is seen using the spleen and left kidney as a window with the crus to the left of the aorta.

Lymph Nodes

There are two major lymph node–bearing areas in the retroperitoneal cavity: the iliac and hypogastric nodes within the pelvis, and the paraortic group in the upper retroperitoneum. The lymphatic chain follows the course of the thoracic aorta, abdominal aorta, and iliac arteries (Fig. 11-18). Common sites are the paraortic and paracaval areas near the great vessels, peripancreatic, renal hilar area, and mesenteric. Normal nodes are smaller than the tip of a finger, less than 1 cm, and are not imaged with ultrasound. However, if these nodes enlarge because of infection or tumor, they can be seen with ultrasound.

Ultrasound Evaluation of Paraortic Nodes

Ultrasound patterns associated with nodes include rounded, focal echo-poor lesions 1 to 3 cm in size, and

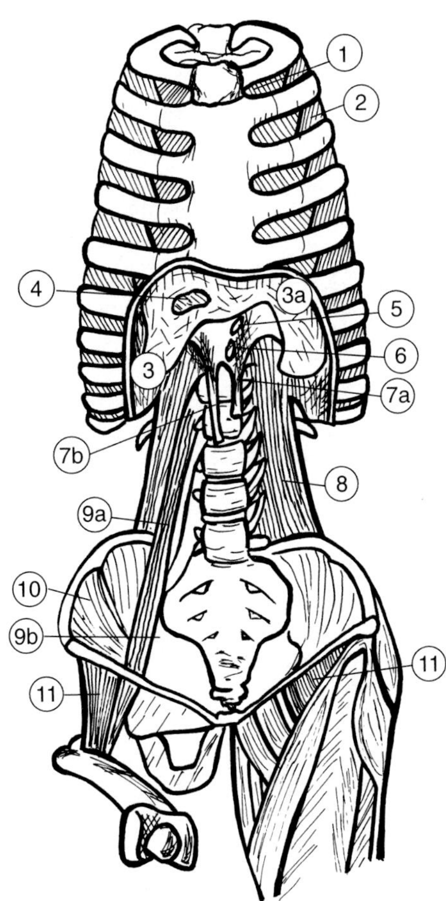

FIG. 11-16 The crura of the diaphragm begins as tendinous fibers from the lumar vertebral bodies, disks, and transverse processes of L3 on the right and L1 on the left. Internal intercostal muscle, *1;* external intercostal muscle, *2;* diaphragm, *3;* central tendon, *3a;* inferior vena cava, *4;* esophagus, *5;* aorta, *6;* left crus, *7a;* right crus, *7b;* quadratus lumborum muscle, *8;* psoas major muscle, *9a;* psoas minor muscle, *9b;* iliacus muscle, *10;* iliopsoas muscle, *11*. (From Hagen-Ansert SL: The anatomy workbook. Philadelphia, 1986, JB Lippincott)

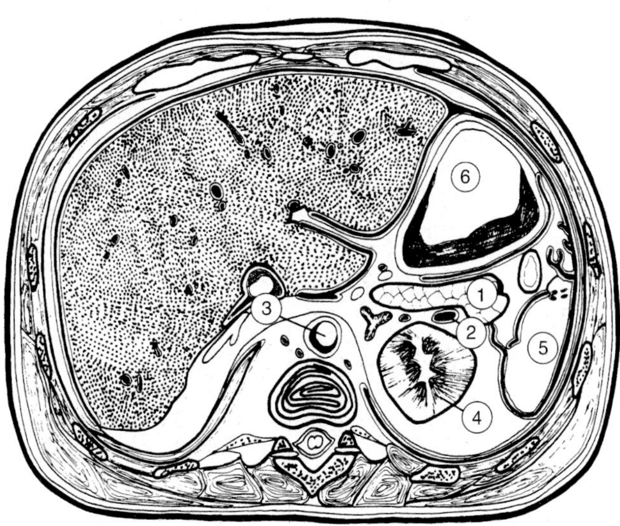

FIG. 11-17 The right crus of the diaphragm passes posterior to the inferior vena cava, whereas the left crus passes anterior to the aorta. Pancreas (tail), *1;* splenic vein, *2;* aorta, *3;* left kidney, *4;* spleen, *5;* stomach, *6*. (From Hagen-Ansert SL: The anatomy workbook, Philadelphia, 1986, JB Lippincott)

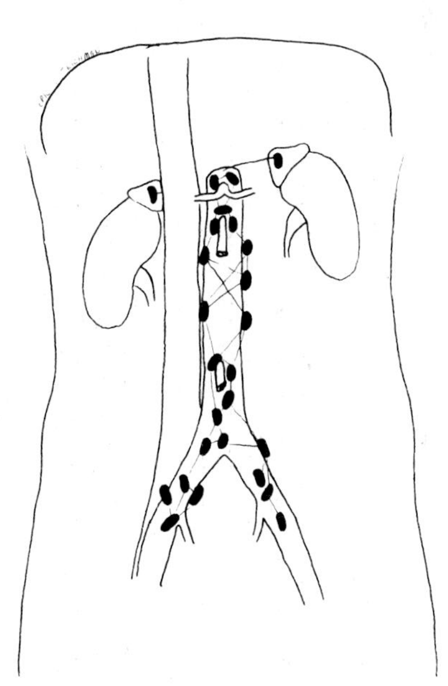

FIG. 11-18 Lymphatic chain along the aorta and iliac artery.

larger, confluent, echo-poor masses, which often displace the kidney laterally. The sonographer may also detect a "mantle" of nodes in the paraspinal location, a "floating" or anterior displaced aorta secondary to the enlarged nodes, or the mesenteric "sandwich" sign representing the anterior and posterior node masses surrounding mesenteric vessels (Figs. 11-19 to 11-22).

The lymph nodes lie along the lateral and anterior margins of the aorta and inferior vena cava; thus, the best scanning is done with the patient in the supine or decubitus position. It is always important to examine the patient in two planes, since the enlarged nodes may mimic an aortic aneurysm or tumor in only one plane.

Longitudinal scans may be made first to outline the aorta and to search for enlarged lymph nodes. The aorta provides an excellent background for the hypoechoic nodes. Scans should begin at the midline, and the transducer should be angled both to the left and right at small angles to image the anterior and lateral borders of the aorta and inferior vena cava.

Transverse scans are made from the level of the xyphoid to the symphysis. Careful identification of the great vessels, organ structures, and muscles is important. Patterns of a fluid-filled duodenum or bowel may make it difficult to outline the great vessels or may cause confusion in diagnosing lymphadenopathy.

Scans below the umbilicus are more difficult because of interference from the small bowel. Careful attention should be given to the psoas and iliacus muscles within the pelvis as the iliac arteries run along their medial border. Both mus-

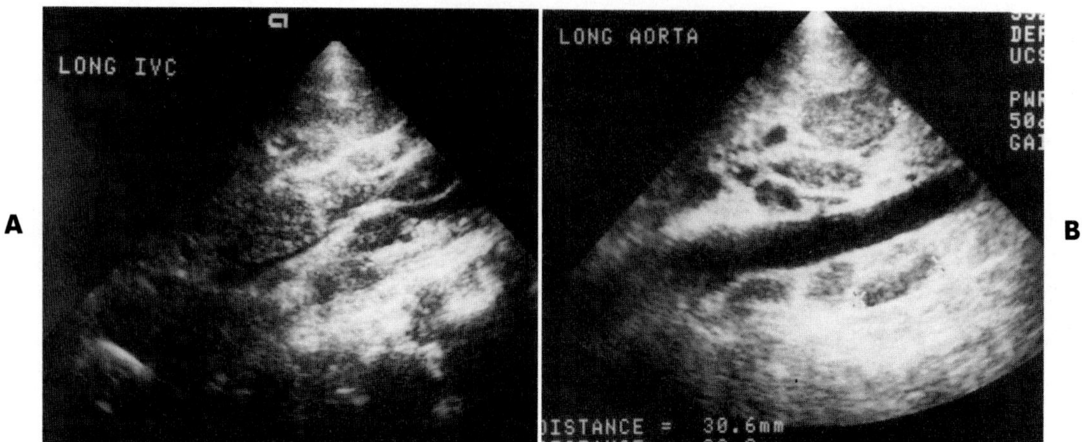

FIG. 11-19 A, Longitudinal scans over the inferior vena cava and **B,** aorta show multiple nodes elevating the inferior vena cava and surrounding the aorta.

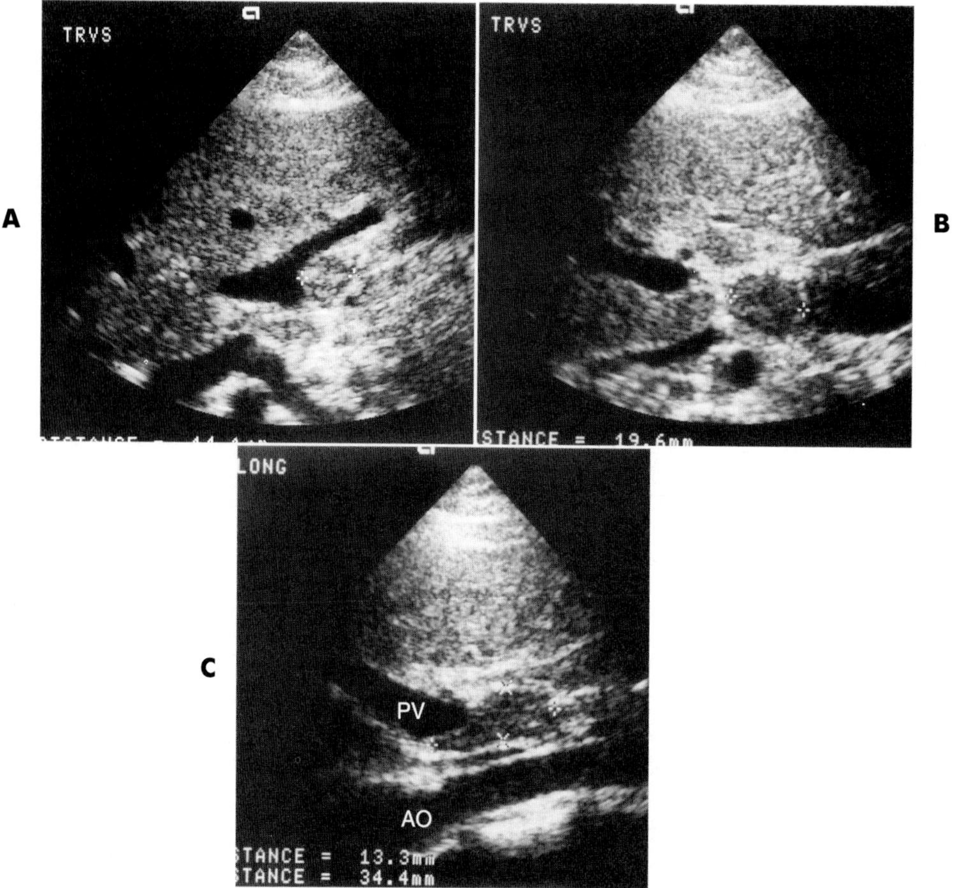

FIG. 11-20 A to **C,** A 32-year-old female with right upper quadrant pain and fever. Two paracaval nodes *(crossbars)* were seen anterior to the aorta and inferior to the portal vein.

cles serve as a hypoechoic marker along the pelvic side wall. Enlarged lymph nodes can be identified anterior and medial to these margins. A smooth sharp border of the muscle indicates no nodal involvement. The bladder should be filled to help push the small bowel out of the pelvis and to serve as an acoustic window to better image the vascular structures. Color Doppler may also be used to help delineate the vascular structures.

Splenomegaly should also be evaluated in patients with lymphadenopathy. As the sonographer moves caudal from

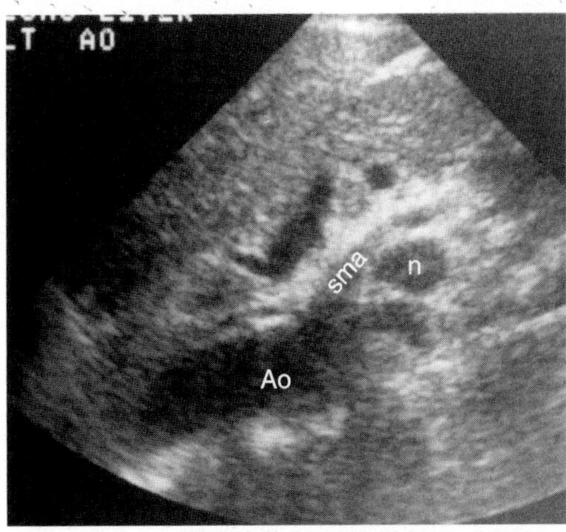

FIG. 11-21 Longitudinal view of the aorta with the superior mesenteric artery. If the angle of the SMA exceeds 15 degrees, lymphadenopathy should be considered, *n*.

the xyphoid, attention should be on the splenic size and great vessel area to detect nodal involvement near the hilus of the spleen (Figs. 11-23 and 11-24).

In our experience, lymph nodes remain as consistent patterns, whereas bowel and the duodenum present with changing peristaltic patterns when imaged with ultrasound. As gentle pressure is applied with the transducer in an effort to displace the bowel, the lymph nodes remain constant in shape. The echo pattern posterior to each structure is different. Lymph nodes are homogeneous and thus transmit sound easily; the bowel presents a more complex pattern with dense central echoes from its mucosal pattern. Often the duodenum has some air within its walls, causing a shadow posteriorly. Enlarged lymph nodes should be reproducible on ultrasound. After the abdomen is completely scanned, repeat sections over the enlarged nodes should demonstrate the same pattern as before.

POSTERIOR PARARENAL SPACE AND ILIAC FOSSA

The posterior pararenal space is located between the posterior renal fascia and the transversalis fascia. It communi-

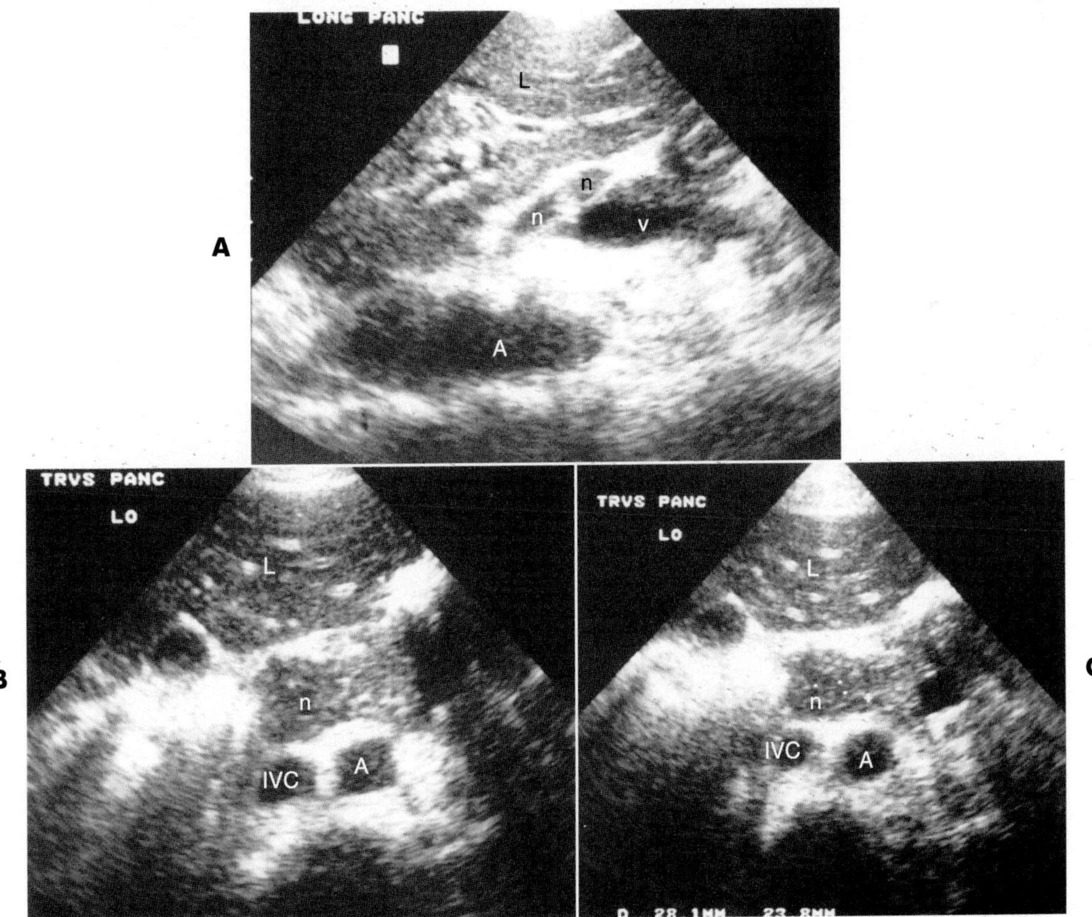

FIG. 11-22 A 46-year-old male with a history of AIDS. Liver function tests were abnormal. Hepatosplenomegaly was present. Adjacent to the pancreas are numerous small nodal masses, the largest measuring 2 cm. **A,** Longitudinal: aorta, *A;* superior mesenteric vein, *v;* nodes, *n*. **B** and **C,** Transverse: aorta, *A;* inferior vena cava, *IVC;* nodes, *n;* liver, *L*.

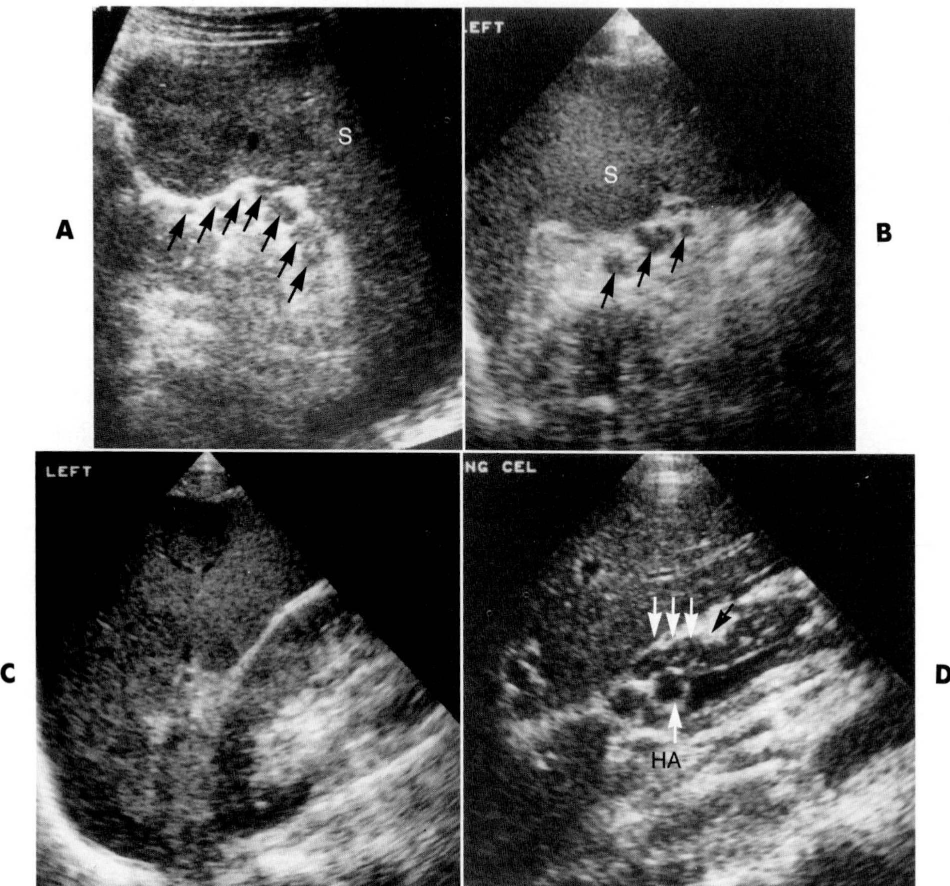

FIG. 11-23 **A** to **D**, Splenomegaly should be evaluated in patients with lymphadenopathy. Enlarged nodes *(arrows)* are seen in the area of the hilus of the spleen, *S*. This patient also has a metastatic lesion near the periphery of the spleen.

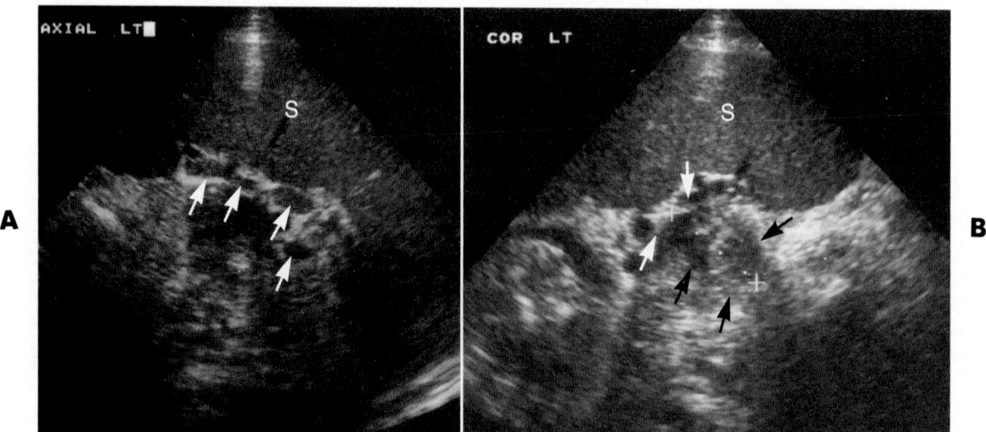

FIG. 11-24 **A** and **B**, Axial and coronal scans of a patient with splenomegaly and enlarged nodes in the area of the splenic hilus. Color flow should be used to document that the lesions are nodes and not dilated vascular structures. Spleen, *S;* nodes *(arrows)*.

cates with the peritoneal fat, lateral to the lateroconal fascia. The posterior pararenal space merges inferiorly with the anterior pararenal space and retroperitoneal tissues of the iliac fossa (see Fig. 11-4).

The psoas muscle, the fascia of which merges with the posterior transversalis fascia, makes up the medial border of this posterior space. This space is open laterally and inferiorly. The blood and lymph nodes embedded in fat may be found in the posterior pararenal space.

Iliac Fossa

The iliac fossa is the region extending between the internal surface of the iliac wings from the crest to the iliopectineal line. This area is known as the *false pelvis* and contains the ureter and major branches of the distal great vessels and their lymphatics. The transversalis fascia extends into the iliac fossa as the iliac fascia.

Retrofascial Space

The retrofascial space is comprised of the posterior abdominal wall, muscles, nerves, lymphatics, and areolar tissue behind the transversalis fascia. It is divided into the following three compartments: (1) psoas, (2) lumbar (quadratus lumborum), and (3) iliac, by the leaves of the transversalis fascia.

Quadratus Lumborum

The quadratus lumborum originates from the iliolumbar ligament, the adjacent iliac crest, and the superior borders of the transverse process of L3 and L4, and inserts into the margin of the twelfth rib (Fig. 11-25). It is adjoining and posterior to the colon, kidney, and psoas muscle.

Psoas

The psoas muscle spans from the mediastinum to the thigh (Fig. 11-26). The fascia attaches to the pelvic brim.

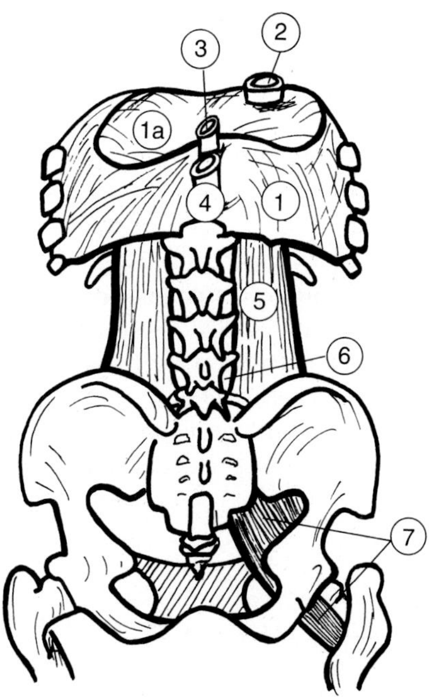

FIG. 11-25 The quadratus lumborum muscle originates from the iliolumar ligament, the adjacent iliac crest, and the superior borders of the transverse process of L3, L4, and inserts into the margins of the twelth rib. Diaphragm, *1;* central tendon, *1a;* inferior vena cava, *2;* esophagus, *3;* aorta, *4;* quadratus lumborum muscle, *5;* psoas major muscle, *6;* iliopsoas muscle, *7.* (From Hagen-Ansert SL: The anatomy workbook, Philadelphia, 1986, JB Lippincott)

Iliacus

The iliacus makes up the iliac space and extends the length of the iliac fossa. The psoas passes through the iliac fossa medial to the iliacus and posterior to the iliac fascia (Fig. 11-27). These two muscles merge together as they extend into the true pelvis. The iliopsoas takes on a more anterior location caudally to lie along the lateral pelvic side wall.

PELVIC RETROPERITONEUM

The pelvic retroperitoneum lies between the sacrum and pubis from back to front, between the pelvic peritoneal reflection above and pelvic diaphragm (coccygeus and levator ani muscles) below, and between the obturator internus and piriformis muscles. There are four subdivisions: (1) prevesical, (2) rectovesical, (3) presacral, and (4) bilateral pararectal (and paravesical) spaces.

Prevesical Space

The prevesical space spans from the pubis to the anterior margin of the bladder. It is bordered laterally by the obturator fascia. The connective tissue covering the bladder, seminal vesicles, and prostate is continuous with the fascial lamina within this space. The space is an extension of the retroperitoneal space of the anterior abdominal wall deep to the rectus sheath, which is continuous with the transversalis fascia. The space between the bladder and rectum is the rectovesical space (Fig. 11-28).

Presacral Space

The presacral space lies between the rectum and fascia covering the sacrum and posterior pelvic floor musculature.

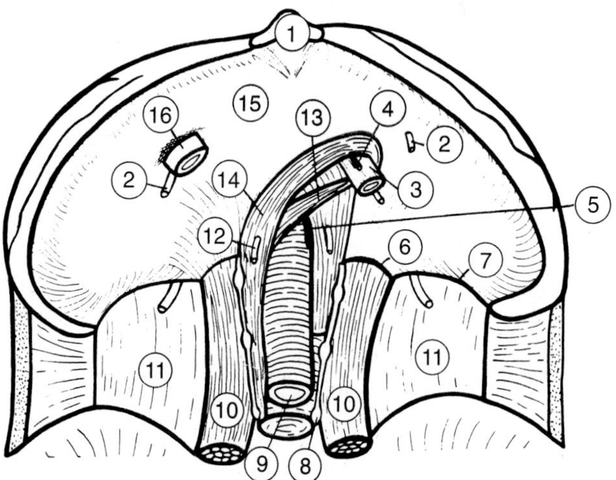

FIG. 11-26 The psoas muscle extends from the mediastinum to the thigh. Xyphoid process, *1;* right and left phrenic nerves, *2;* esophagus, *3;* vagi, *4;* median arcuate ligament, *5;* medial arcuate ligament, *6;* lateral arcuate ligament, *7;* sympathetic trunk, *8;* aorta, *9;* psoas muscle, *10;* quadrate lumborum muscle, *11;* splanchnic nerves, *12;* left crus, *13;* right crus, *14;* central tendon, *15;* inferior vena cava, *16.* (From Hagen-Ansert SL: The anatomy workbook, Philadelphia, 1986, JB Lippincott)

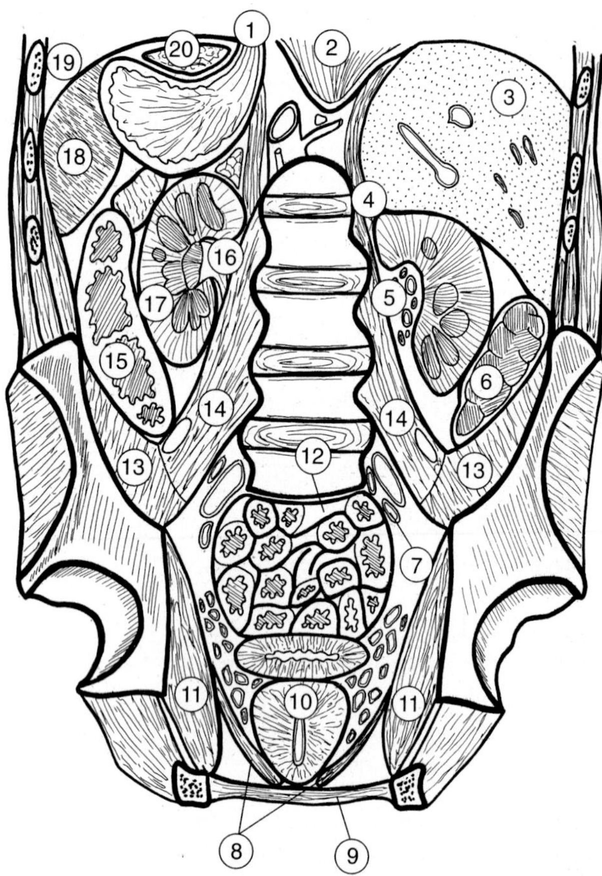

FIG. 11-27 The iliacus muscle extends the length of the iliac fossa. The psoas muscle passes through the iliac fossa medial to the iliacus. The psoas and iliacus muscles merge as they extend into the true pelvis. The iliopsoas muscle takes on a more anterior location caudally to lie along the lateral pelvic sidewall. Cardiac orifice of the stomach, *1;* diaphragm, *2;* right lobe of the liver, *3;* right suprarenal gland, *4;* renal sinus, *5;* ascending colon, *6;* iliac artery and vein, *7;* levator ani muscle, *8;* transverse perineal muscle, *9;* prostrate, *10;* obturator internus muscle, *11;* ileum, *12;* iliacus muscle, *13;* psoas major muscle, *14;* descending colon, *15;* renal pelvis, *16;* renal capsule, *17;* spleen, *18;* costodiaphragmatic recess, *19;* left lobe of the liver, *20.* (From Hagen-Ansert SL: The anatomy workbook, Philadelphia, 1986, JB Lippincott)

Bilateral Pararectal Space

The pararectal space is bounded laterally by the piriformis and levator ani fascia and medially by the rectum. It extends anteriorly from the bladder, medially to the obturator internus, and laterally to the external iliac vessels (Figs. 11-29 and 11-30).

The paravesical and pararectal spaces are traversed by the two ureters. The pelvic wall muscles, iliac vessels, ureter, bladder, prostate, seminal vesicles, and cervix are retroperitoneal structures within the true pelvis. The obturator internus muscle lines the lateral aspect of the pelvis. Posteriorly, the piriformis muscle is seen extending anterolaterally from the region of the sacrum.

Retroperitoneal Fat

The lesions in the liver or in Morison's pouch displace the echoes posterior and inferior, whereas renal and adrenal lesions cause anterior displacement of structures. An extrahepatic mass may shift the inferior vena cava anteromedially (anterior displacement of right kidney).

Primary Retroperitoneal Tumors

A primary retroperitoneal tumor is one that originates independently within the retroperitoneal space. The tumors can arise anywhere, and most are malignant. Like other tumors, they may exhibit a variety of sonography patterns from homogeneous to solid to a mixture of complex tissue masses.

Neurogenic tumors are usually encountered in the paravertebral region, where they arise from nerve roots or sympathetic chain ganglia. Sonographically their pattern is quite variable.

Leiomyosarcomas are prone to undergo necrosis and cystic degeneration. Their sonographic pattern is complex. Liposarcomas produce a highly reflective sonographic pattern because of their fat interface.

Fibrosarcomas and rhabdomyosarcomas may be quite invasive and may infiltrate widely into muscles and adjoining soft tissues. They often present with extension across the midline and appear very similar to lymphomas. Sonographically they are highly reflective tumors.

Teratomatous tumors may arise within the upper retroperitoneum and the pelvis. They may contain calcified echoes from bones, cartilage, and teeth, as well as soft tissue elements.

Tumors of uniform cell type generally have a homogeneous appearance unless there is hemorrhage or necrosis. Often the presence of necrosis depends on the size and growth of the mass.

Secondary Retroperitoneal Tumors

Secondary retroperitoneal tumors are primarily recurrences from previously resected tumors. Recurrent masses from previous renal carcinoma are frequent. Ascitic fluid along with a retroperitoneal tumor usually indicates seeding or invasion of the peritoneal surface. Evaluation of the paraaortic region should be made for extension to the lymph nodes. The liver should also be evaluated for metastatic involvement.

RETROPERITONEAL FLUID COLLECTIONS

Urinoma

A urinoma is a walled-off collection of extravasated urine that develops spontaneously after trauma, surgery, or a subacute or chronic urinary obstruction. Urinomas usually collect about the kidney or upper ureter in the perinephric space. Occasionally urinomas dissect into the pelvis and compress the bladder. Generally their sonographic pattern is sonolucent unless they become infected.

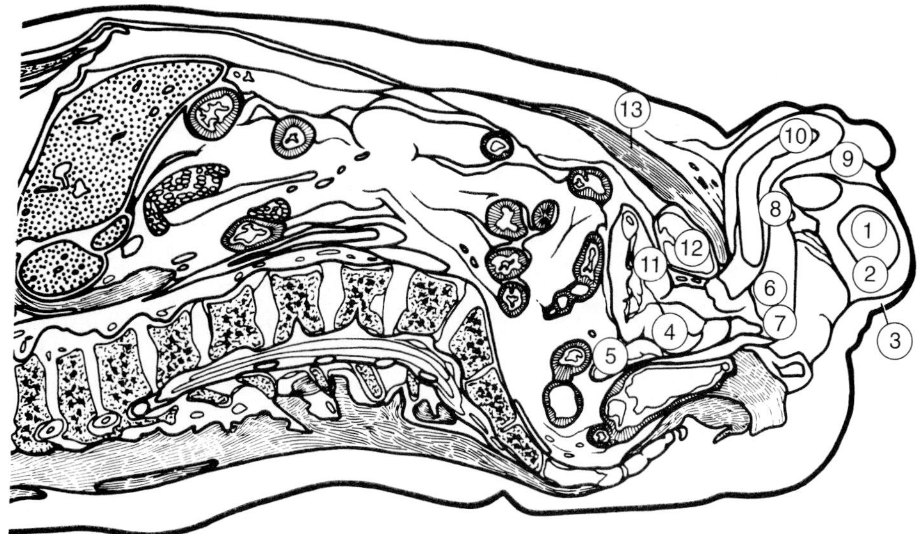

FIG. 11-28 The prevesical space extends from the pubis to the anterior margin of the bladder. It is bordered by the obturator fascia on its lateral margins. The space between the bladder and rectum is the rectovesical space. Testis, *1;* epididymis, *2;* scrotum, *3;* prostrate, *4;* seminal vesicles, *5;* bulb of the penis, *6;* bulbospongiousus muscle, *7;* corpus spongiosum penis, *8;* glans penis, *9;* corpus cavernosum penis, *10;* rectum, *11;* symphysis pubis, *12;* pyramidalis muscle, *13*. (From Hagen-Ansert SL: The anatomy workbook, Philadelphia, 1986, JB Lippincott)

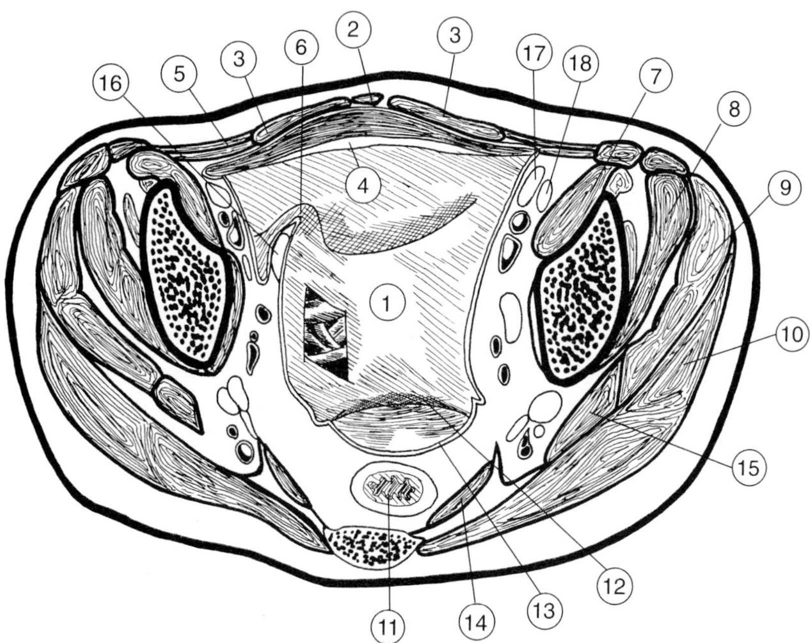

FIG. 11-29 The pararectal space is bounded laterally by the piriformis and levator and fascia and medially by the rectum. Uterus, *1;* pyramidalis muscle, *2;* rectus abdominis muscle, *3;* peritoneal cavity, *4;* obturator internus muscle, *5;* fallopian tube, *6;* iliopsoas muscle, *7;* gluteus minimus muscle, *8;* gluteus medius muscle, *9;* gluteus maximus muscle, *10;* rectum, *11;* pouch of douglas, *12;* peritoneum, *13;* coccygeus muscle, *14;* piriformis muscle, *15;* ovary, *16;* external iliac vein, *17;* external iliac artery, *18*. (From Hagen-Ansert SL: The anatomy workbook, Philadelphia, 1986, JB Lippincott)

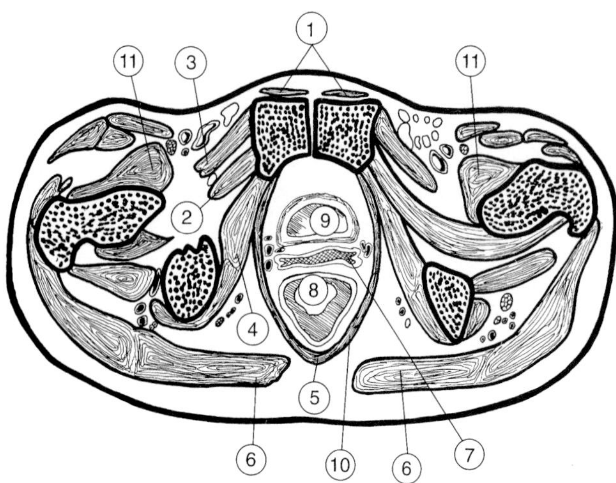

FIG. 11-30 The pararectal space extends anteriorly from the bladder, medially to the obturator internus and laterally to the external iliac vessels. Pyramidalis muscle, *1;* obturator externus muscle, *2;* pectineus muscle, *3;* obturator internus muscle, *4;* fascia of the pelvic diaphragm, *5;* gluteus maximus muscle; *6;* vagina, *7;* rectum, *8;* bladder, *9;* levator ani muscle, *10;* iliopsoas muscle, *11*. (From Hagen-Ansert SL: The anatomy workbook, Philadelphia, 1986, JB Lippincott.)

Hemorrhage

A retroperitoneal hemorrhage may occur in a variety of conditions, including trauma, vasculitis, bleeding diathesis, leaking aortic aneurysm, or bleeding neoplasm. Sonographically it may be well localized and produce displacement of other organs, or it may present as a poorly defined infiltrative process.

Fresh hematomas present as sonolucent areas whereas organized thrombus and clot formation show echo densities within the mass. Calcification may be seen in longstanding hematomas.

Abscess

Abscess formation may result from surgery, trauma, or perforations of the bowel or duodenum. Sonographically the abscess usually has a more complex pattern with debris. Gas within the abscess is reflective and casts an acoustic shadow. One should be careful not to misdiagnose a gas-containing abscess for "bowel" patterns. The radiograph should be evaluated in this case. The abscess frequently extends along or within the muscle planes, is of an irregular shape, and lies in the most dependent portion of the retroperitoneal space.

RETROPERITONEAL FIBROSIS

Retroperitoneal fibrosis is a disease of unknown etiology characterized by thick sheets of fibrous tissue in the retroperitoneal space. The disease may occur in association with abdominal aortic aneurysms. It may encase and obstruct the ureters and vena cava, with resultant hydronephrosis. A discrete mass of abnormal tissue lying anterior and lateral to the great vessels has been described by Sanders et al.[2] It may mimic lymphoma and thus must be further delineated for benignity or malignancy.

REVIEW QUESTIONS

1. Define the retroperitoneal space, anterior pararenal space, perirenal space, and posterior pararenal space.
2. Describe the appearance of the neonatal adrenal gland.
3. Describe the function of the adrenal cortex and medulla.
4. What is the best ultrasound window to record the adrenal glands?
5. List four pitfalls the sonographer should be aware of in evaluating the adrenal gland.
6. Describe the diaphragmatic crura and their significance in sonography.
7. Describe the path of the lymph nodes and their size and sonographic appearance.
8. Define these signs: mantle, floating, and sandwich.
9. What is the difference between the true and false pelvis?
10. Which muscles comprise the pelvic diaphragm?
11. What is the rectovesical space?
12. Name three primary retroperitoneal tumors.
13. What is an urinoma and how does it appear on ultrasound?

REFERENCES

Adrenal Glands

1. Anderson PD: Clinical anatomy and physiology for allied health sciences, Philadelphia, 1976, WB Saunders.
2. Rao AKR and Silver TM: Normal pancreas and splenic variants simulating suprarenal and renal tumors, Am J Roentgenol 126:530, 1976.
3. Sample WF: A new technique for the evaluation of the adrenal gland with gray scale ultrasonography, Radiology 124:463, 1977.
4. Sample WF: Adrenal ultrasonography, Radiology 127:461, 1978.
5. Sample WF: Ultrasonography of the adrenal gland. In Resnick MI and Sanders RC, editors: Ultrasound in urology, Baltimore, 1979, Williams & Wilkins.
6. Sample WF: Renal, adrenal, retroperitoneal, and scrotal ultrasonography. In Sarti DA and Sample WF, editors: Diagnostic ultrasound: text and cases, Boston, 1980, GK Hall.
7. Sample WF and Sarti DA: Computed tomography and gray scale ultrasonography of the adrenal gland: a comparative study, Radiology 128:377, 1978.
8. Talmont CA: Adrenal glands. In Taylor KJW et al, editors: Manual of ultrasonography, New York, 1980, Churchill Livingstone.

BIBLIOGRAPHY

Antonious A, Spetseropoulos J, Vlahos L, et al: The sonographic appearance of adrenal involvement in non-Hodgkin's lymphoma, J Ultrasound Med 2:235, 1983.

Belville JS, Morgentaler A, Loughlin KR, et al: Spontaneous perinephric and subcapsular renal hemorrhage: evaluation with computed tomography, ultrasound and angiography, Radiology 172:733, 1989.

Bitter DA and Ross DS: Incidentally discovered adrenal masses, Am J Surg 158:159, 1989.

Bowerman RA, Silver TM, Jaffe MH, et al: Sonography of adrenal pheochromocytomas, Am J Roentgenol 137:1227, 1981.

Callen PW, filly RA, and Marks WM: The quadratus lumborum muscle: a possible source of confusion in sonographic evaluation of the retroperitoneum, J Clin Ultrasound 7:3459, 1979.

Callen PW, Filly RA, Sarti DA, et al: Ultrasonography of the diaphragmatic crura, Radiology 130;721, 1979.

Chesbrough RM, Burkhard TK, Martinez AT, et al: Gerota versus Zuckerkandl: the renal fascia revisited, Radiology 173:845, 1989.

Creed L, Reger K, Pond GD, et al: Potential pitfall in computed tomography and sonographic evaluation of suspected lymphoma, Am J Roentgenol 139:606, 1982.

Cunningham JJ: Ultrasonic findings in "primary" lymphoma of the adrenal area, J Ultrasound Med 2:467, 1983.

Davidson AJ and Hartman DS: Lymphangioma of the retroperitoneum: computed tomography and sonographic characteristics, Radiology 175:507, 1990.

Davidson AJ, Hartman DS, and Goldman SM: Mature teratoma of the retroperitoneum: radiologic, pathologic, and clinical correlation, Radiology 172:421, 1989.

Davies RP and Lam AH: Adrenocortical neoplasm in children: ultrasound appearance, J Ultrasound Med 6;325, 1987.

DeLange EE, Black WC, and Mills SE: Radiologic features of retroperitoneal cystic hamartoma, Gastrointest Radiol 13:266, 1988.

Derchi LE, Rizzatto G, Banderali A, et al: Sonographic appearance of primary retroperitoneal cysts, J Ultrasound Med 8:381, 1989.

Dodds WJ, Darweesh RMA, Lawson TL, et al: The retroperitoneal spaces revisited, Am J Roentgenol 147:1155, 1989.

Ebisuno S, Yamauchi T, Fukatani T, et al: Retroperitoneal Castleman's disease: a case report and brief review of tumors of the pararenal area, Urol Int 44:169, 1989.

Fagan CJ, Amparo EG, and Davis M: Retroperitoneal fibrosis, Semin Ultrasound 3:123, 1982.

Glazer HS, Weyman PJ, Sagel SS, et al: Nonfunctioning adrenal masses: incidental discovery on computed tomography, Am J Roentgenol 139:81, 1982.

Glynn TP, Kreipke DL, and Irons JM: Amyloidosis: diffuse involvement of the retroperitoneum, Radiology 170:726, 1989.

Gore RM, Callen PW, and Filly RA: Displaced retroperitoneal fat: sonographic guide to right upper quadrant mass localization, Radiology 142:701, 1982.

Graif M, Manor A, and Itzchak Y: Sonographic differentiation of extra- and intrahepatic masses, Am J Roentgenol 141:553, 1983.

Graif M, Martinovitz U, Strauss S, et al: Sonographic localization of hematomas in hemophiliac patients with positive iliopsoas sign, Am J Roentgenol 148:121, 1987.

Grizzle WE: Pathology of the adrenal gland, Semin Roentgenol 23:323, 1988.

Gunther RW, Kelbel C, and Lenner V: Real-time ultrasound of normal adrenal glands and small tumors, J Clin Ultrasound 12:211, 1984.

Hamper UM, Fishman EK, Hartma DS, et al: Primary adrenocortical carcinoma: sonographic evaluation with clinical and pathologic correlation in 26 patients, Am J Roentgenol 148:915, 1987.

Hubbard MM, Husami TW, and Abumrad NN: Nonfunctioning adrenal tumors: dilemmas in management, Am J Surg 5:516, 1989.

Jing B: Diagnostic imaging of abdominal and pelvic lymph nodes in lymphoma. In Libshitz HI, editor: Imaging the lymphomas. Radiol Clin North Am 801, 1990.

Lang EK: Renal, perirenal, and pararenal abscesses: percutaneous drainage, Radiology 174:109, 1990.

Magill HL, Tonkin ILD, Bada H, et al: Advantages of coronal ultrasonography in evaluating the neonatal retroperitoneum, J Ultrasound Med 2:289, 1983.

Marchal G, Gelin J, Verbeken E, et al: High-resolution real-time sonography of the adrenal glands: a routine examination? J Ultrasound Med 5:65, 1986.

Morehouse HT, Weiner SN, and Hoffman-Treatin JC: Inflammatory disease of the kidney, Semin Ultrasound, CT, MR 7:246, 1986.

Piccirillo M, Rigsby CM, and Rosenfield AT: Sonography of renal inflammatory disease, Urol Radiol 9:66, 1987.

Ritchey ML, Kinard R, and Novicki DE: Adrenal tumors: involvement of the inferior vena cava, J Urol 138:1134, 1987.

Rubenstein WA and Whalen JP: Extraperitoneal spaces. Am J Roentgenol 147:1162, 1986.

Sacks D, Banner MP, Meranze SG, et al: Renal and related retroperitoneal abscesses: percutaneous drainage, Radiology 167:447, 1988.

Sanders RC, Duff T, McLoughlin MG, et al: Sonography in the diagnosis of retroperitoneal fibrosis, J Urol 118:944, 1977.

Savader SJ, Otero RR, and Savader BL: Puerperal ovarian vein thrombosis: evaluation with computed tomography, ultrasound and magnetic resonance, Radiology 167:637, 1988.

Shirkhoda A: Computed tomography of perirenal metastases, J Comput Assist Tomogr 10:435, 1986.

Shirkhoda A, Mann MA, Staab EV, et al: Soft-tissue hemorrhage in hemophiliac patients: computed tomography and ultrasound study, Radiology 147:811, 1983.

Silverman ML and Lee AK: Anatomy and pathology of the adrenal glands, Urol Clin North Am 16:417, 1989.

Soffer M, Abecassis J, and Bonnin A: Percutaneous drainage of retroperitoneal abscesses, Radiology 170:280, 1989.

Solla JA and Reed K: Primary retroperitoneal sarcomas, Am J Surg 152:496, 1986.

Subramanyam BR, Balthazar EJ, and Horii SC: Sonography of the accessory spleen, Am J Roentgenol 143:47, 1984.

Suesada Y, Nakao N, Miura K, et al: Pseudolymphoma of the retroperitoneum, Eur J Radiol 6:144, 1987.

Yeh H: Ultrasonography of the adrenals, Semin Roentgenol 23:250, 1988.

CHAPTER 12

Peritoneal Cavity and Abdominal Wall

Sandra Hagen-Ansert

Peritoneal Cavity

DETERMINATION OF INTRAPERITONEAL LOCATION

Pleural versus Subdiaphragmatic

Because of the coronary ligament attachments, collections in the right posterior subphrenic space cannot extend between the bare area of the liver and the diaphragm. The right pleural space extends medially to the attachment of the right superior coronary ligament, therefore pleural collections may appear opposed to the bare area of the liver (Fig. 12-1). The pleural fluid tends to distribute posteromedially in the chest.

Subcapsular Versus Intraperitoneal

Subcapsular liver and splenic collections are seen when they are inferior to the diaphragmatic echocomplex unilaterally and they conform to the shape of an organ capsule. They may extend medially to the attachment of the superior coronary ligament.

Retroperitoneal Versus Intraperitoneal

A mass is confirmed to be within the retroperitoneal cavity when anterior renal displacement or anterior displacement of the dilated ureters can be documented. The mass interposed anteriorly or superiorly to kidneys can be located either intraperitoneally or retroperitoneally (Fig. 12-2).

Fatty and collagenous connective tissues in the perirenal or anterior pararenal space produce echoes that are best demonstrated on sagittal scans. Retroperitoneal lesions displace echoes ventrally and cranially; hepatic and subhepatic lesions produce inferior and posterior displacement (Fig. 12-3).

The anterior displacement of the superior mesenteric vessels, splenic vein, renal vein, and inferior vena cava excludes an intraperitoneal location. A large right-sided retroperitoneal mass rotates the intrahepatic portal veins to the left. This causes the left portal vein to show reversed flow.

Right posterior hepatic masses of similar dimensions may produce minor displacement of the intrahepatic portal vein. Primary liver masses should move simultaneously with the liver.

Extraperitoneal Versus Intraperitoneal

An undisrupted peritoneal line distinguishes extraperitoneal from intraperitoneal locations. The demonstration of posterior or lateral bladder displacement suggests an extraperitoneal or retroperitoneal location.

SONOGRAPHIC IDENTIFICATION OF INTRAPERITONEAL COMPARTMENTS

Perihepatic and Upper Abdominal Compartments

Ligaments on the right side of the liver form the subphrenic and subhepatic spaces (Fig. 12-4). The falciform ligament divides the subphrenic space into right and left components. The ligamentum teres hepatis ascends from the umbilicus to the umbilical notch of the liver within the free margin of the falciform ligament before coursing within the liver.

The bare area is delineated by the right superior and inferior coronary ligaments, (Fig. 12-5), which separate the posterior subphrenic space from the right superior subhepatic space (Morison's pouch). Lateral to the bare area and right triangular ligament, the posterior subphrenic and subhepatic spaces are continuous.

A single large and irregular perihepatic space surrounds the superior and lateral aspects of the left lobe of the liver with the left coronary ligaments anatomically separating the subphrenic space into anterior and posterior compartments.

The left subhepatic space is divided into an anterior compartment (the gastrohepatic recess) and a posterior compartment (the lesser sac) by the lesser omentum and stomach (Fig. 12-6)). The lesser sac lies anterior to the pancreas and posterior to the stomach.

With fluid in the lesser and greater omental cavities, the lesser omentum may be seen as a linear, undulating echodensity extending from the stomach to the porta hepatis.

Gastrosplenic Ligament

The gastrosplenic ligament is the left lateral extension of the greater omentum that connects the gastric greater curvature to the superior splenic hilum and forms a portion of the left lateral border of the lesser sac (see Fig. 12-6).

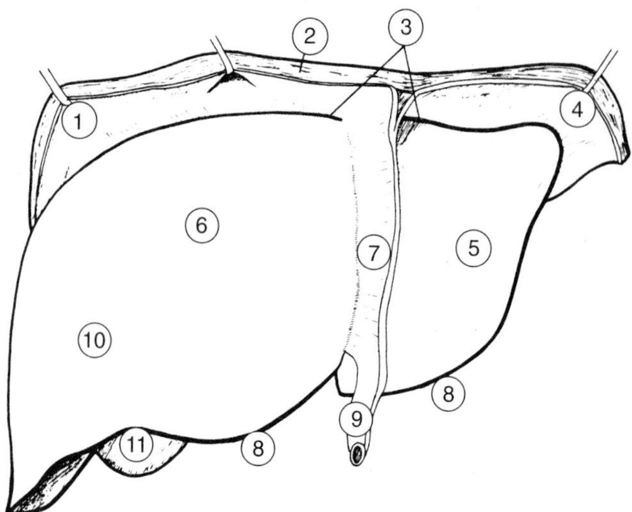

FIG. 12-1 The right pleural space extends medially to the attachment of the right superior coronary ligament. Therefore pleural collections may appear opposed to the bare area of the liver. Right triangular ligament, *1;* diaphragm (pulled up), *2;* coronary ligament, *3;* left triangular ligament, *4;* left lobe, *5;* right lobe, *6;* falciform ligament, *7;* inferior margin, *8;* ligamentum teres, *8;* ligamentum teres, *9;* costal impression, *10;* gallbladder, *11.* (From Hagen-Ansert SL: The anatomy workbook, Philadelphia, 1986, JB Lippincott.)

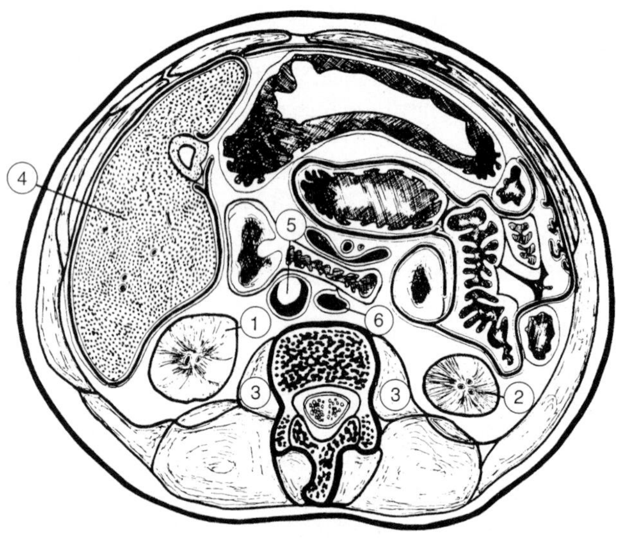

FIG. 12-2 A mass is confirmed to be within the retroperitoneal cavity when there is anterior renal displacement or anterior displacement of the dilated ureters. Right kidney, *1;* left kidney, *2;* psoas muscle, *3;* right lobe of the liver, *4;* inferior vena cava, *5;* aorta, *6.* (From Hagen-Ansert SL: The anatomy workbook, Philadelphia, 1986, JB Lippincott.)

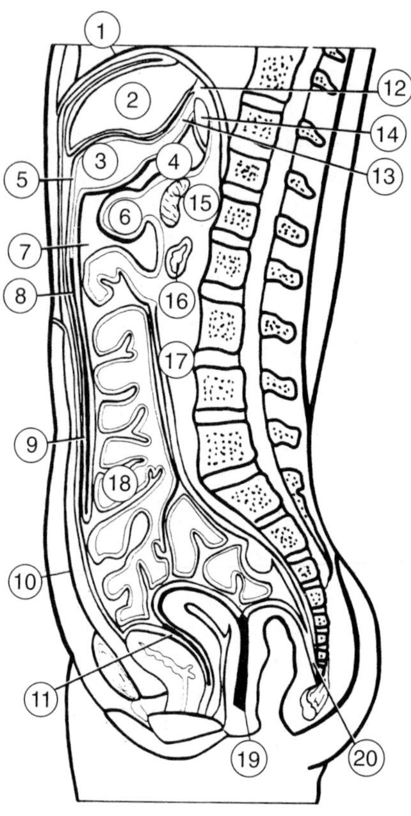

FIG. 12-3 The parietal peritoneum along the anterior abdominal wall may be traced from the falciform ligament to the diaphragm. The visceral peritoneum covers the anterior and inferior surfaces of the liver to the porta hepatis. At this point, it passes to the lesser curvature of the stomach as the anterior layer of the lesser omentum. It covers the anterior surface of the stomach to form the greater omentum. The peritoneum folds upward and forms the posterior layer of the transverse mesocolon. The peritoneum passes over the anterior border of the pancreas and runs downward, anterior to the third part of the duodenum. The peritoneum leaves the posterior abdominal wall as the anterior layer of the mesentery of the small intestine. The visceral peritoneum covers the jejunum and forms the posterior layer of the mesentery. The peritoneum returns to the posterior abdominal wall into the pelvis to cover the anterior rectum. In the female, it reflects onto the posterior vagina to form the rectouterine pouch, or pouch of Douglas. It passes over the vagina to its anterior surface to the upper surface of the bladder to the anterior abdominal wall. In the male, it reflects off of the bladder and seminal vesicles to form the rectovesical pouch. Diaphragm, *1;* liver, *2;* stomach, *3;* omental bursa, *4;* gastric ligament, *5;* transverse colon, *6;* peritoneal cavity, *7;* greater omentum, *8;* parietal peritoneum, *9;* linea alba, *10;* vesicouterine pouch, *11;* subphrenic space, *12;* lesser omentum, *13;* caudate lobe of the liver, *14;* pancreas, *15;* duodenum, *16;* retroperitoneum, *17;* intestine, *18;* rectouterine pouch, *19;* anococcygeus ligament, *20.* (From Hagen-Ansert SL: The anatomy workbook, Philadelphia, 1986, JB Lippincott.)

Splenorenal Ligament

The splenorenal ligament is formed by the posterior reflection of the peritoneum of the spleen and passes inferiorly to overlie the left kidney (Fig. 12-7). It forms the posterior portion of the left lateral border of the lesser sac and separates the lesser sac from the renosplenic recess.

The Lesser Omental Bursa

The lesser omental bursa is subdivided into a larger lateroinferior and a smaller mediosuperior recess by the gastropancreatic folds, which are produced by the left gastric and hepatic arteries. The lesser sac extends to the diaphragm. The superior recess of the bursa surrounds the an-

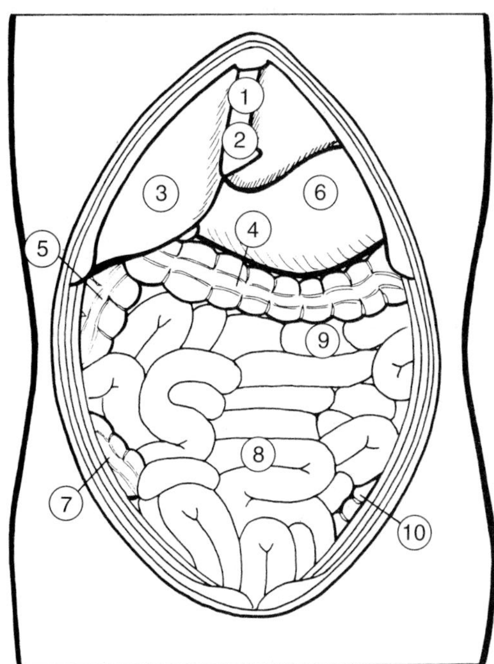

FIG. 12-4 The falciform ligament divides the subphrenic space into right and left components. The ligamentum teres ascends from the umbilicus to the umbilical notch of the liver within the free margin of the falciform ligament prior to coursing within the liver. Falciform ligament, *1;* ligamentum teres, *2;* right lobe of the liver, *3;* transverse colon, *4;* ascending colon, *5;* stomach, *6;* cecum, *7;* ileum, *8;* jejunum, *9;* descending colon, *10*. (From Hagen-Ansert SL: The anatomy workbook, Philadelphia, 1986, JB Lippincott.)

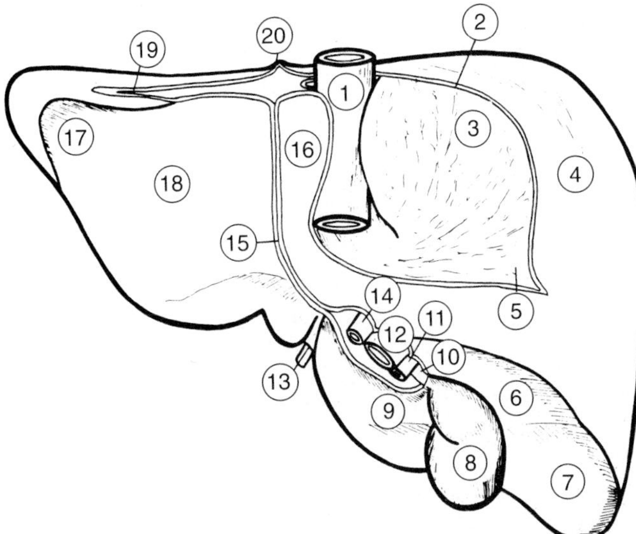

FIG. 12-5 Posterior view of the diaphragmatic surface of the liver. The bare area of the liver is delineated by the right superior and inferior coronary ligaments, which separate the posterior subphrenic space from the right superior subhepatic space known as Morison's Pouch. Inferior vena cava, *1;* coronary ligaments, *2;* bare area, *3;* right lobe, *4;* right triangular ligament, *5;* renal impression, *6;* colic impression, *7;* gallbladder, *8;* quadrate lobe, *9;* cystic duct, *10;* hepatic duct, *11;* portal vein, *12;* ligamentum teres, *13;* hepatic artery, *14;* attachment of the lesser omentum, *15;* caudate lobe, *16;* gastric impression, *17;* left lobe, *18;* left triangular ligament, *19;* falciform ligament, *20*. (From Hagen-Ansert SL: The anatomy workbook, Philadelphia, 1986, JB Lippincott.)

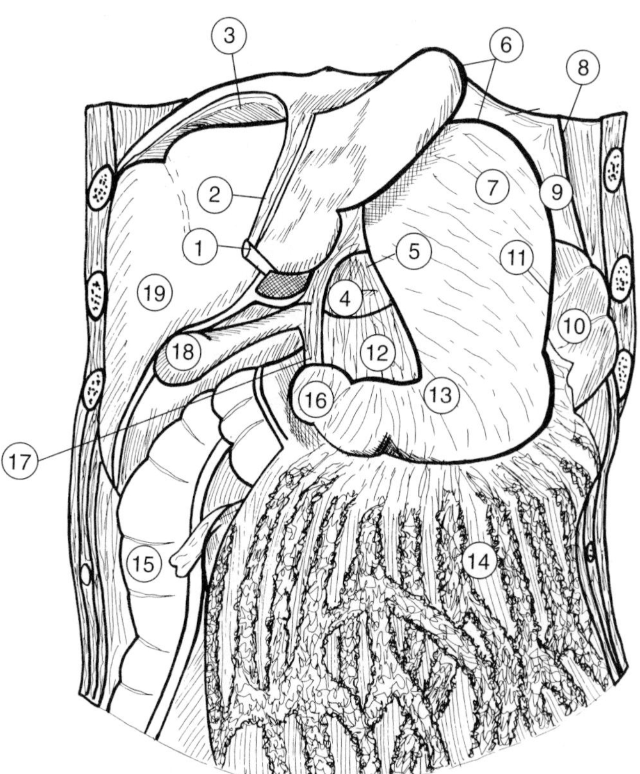

FIG. 12-6 The left subhepatic space is divided into an anterior compartment (gastrohepatic recess) and a posterior compartment (lesser sac) by the lesser omentum and stomach. The gastrosplenic ligament is the left lateral extension of the greater omentum that connects the gastric greater curvature to the superior splenic hilum and forms a portion of the left lateral border of the lesser sac. Ligamentum teres, *1;* falciform ligament, *2;* hepatic coronary ligament, *3;* caudate lobe of the liver, *4;* hepatogastric ligament, *5;* cardiac ligament, *6;* fundus of the stomach, *7;* diaphragm, *8;* parietal peritoneum, *9;* spleen, *10;* gastrosplenic ligament, *11;* lesser omentum, *12;* lesser curvature of the stomach, *13;* greater omentum, *14;* ascending colon, *15;* pylorus, *16;* epiploic foramen, *17;* gallbladder, *18;* liver, *19*. (From Hagen-Ansert SL: The anatomy workbook, Philadelphia, 1986, JB Lippincott.)

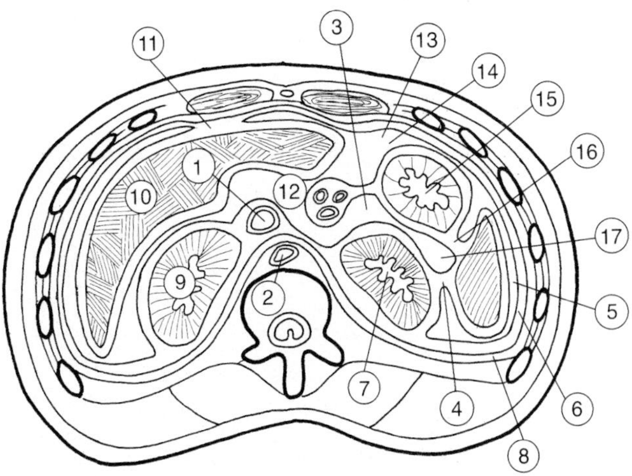

FIG. 12-7 The splenorenal ligament is formed by the posterior reflection of the peritoneum of the spleen and passes inferiorly to overlie the left kidney. Inferior vena cava, *1;* aorta, *2;* lesser sac, *3;* lienorenal ligament, *4;* peritoneum, *5;* subserous fascia, *6;* left kidney, *7;* diaphragm, *8;* right kidney, *9;* liver, *10,* falciform ligament, *11;* epiploic foramen, *12;* greater sac, *13;* lesser omentum, *14;* stomach, *15;* gastrolienal ligament, *16;* spleen, *17*. (From Hagen-Ansert SL: The anatomy workbook, Philadelphia, 1986, JB Lippincott.)

terior, medial, and posterior surfaces of the caudate lobe, making the caudate a lesser sac structure. The lesser sac collections may extend a considerable distance below the plane of the pancreas by inferiorly displacing the transverse mesocolon or extending into the inferior recess of the greater omentum.

Lower Abdominal and Pelvic Compartments

The supravesical space and the medial and lateral inguinal fossae represent intraperitoneal paravesical spaces formed by indentation of the anterior parietal peritoneum by the bladder, obliterated umbilical arteries, and inferior epigastric vessels.

The retrovesical space is divided by the uterus into an anterior vesicouterine recess and a posterior rectouterine sac (pouch of Douglas).

The peritoneal reflection over the dome of the bladder may have an inferior recess extending anterior to the bladder. Ascites displaces the distended urinary bladder inferiorly but not posteriorly. Intraperitoneal fluid compresses the bladder from its lateral aspect in cases of loculation. Fluid in the extraperitoneal prevesical space has a "yoke-over-bell" configuration, displacing the bladder posteriorly and compressing it from the sides along its entire length.

Ascites

Serous ascites appears as echo-free fluid regions indented and shaped by the organs and viscera it surrounds or between which it is interposed. The amount of intraperitoneal fluid depends on the location, volume, and patient position. Fluid may accumulate from several sources, namely peritoneal pressure, an area from which fluid originates, rapidity of accumulation, presence or absence of adhesions, density of fluid with respect to other abdominal organs, and bladder fullness.

The fluid first fills the pouch of Douglas, then the lateral paravesical recesses, before it ascends to both paracolic gutters. The major flow from the pelvis is via the right paracolic gutter.

In patients with concomitant hiatal hernia, ascites may involve the chest, from the abdomen into the posterior mediastinum and through the esophageal hiatus (Fig. 12-8). Small volumes of fluid in the supine patient first appear around the inferior tip of the right lobe in the superior portion of the right flank and in the pelvic cul-de-sac, then in

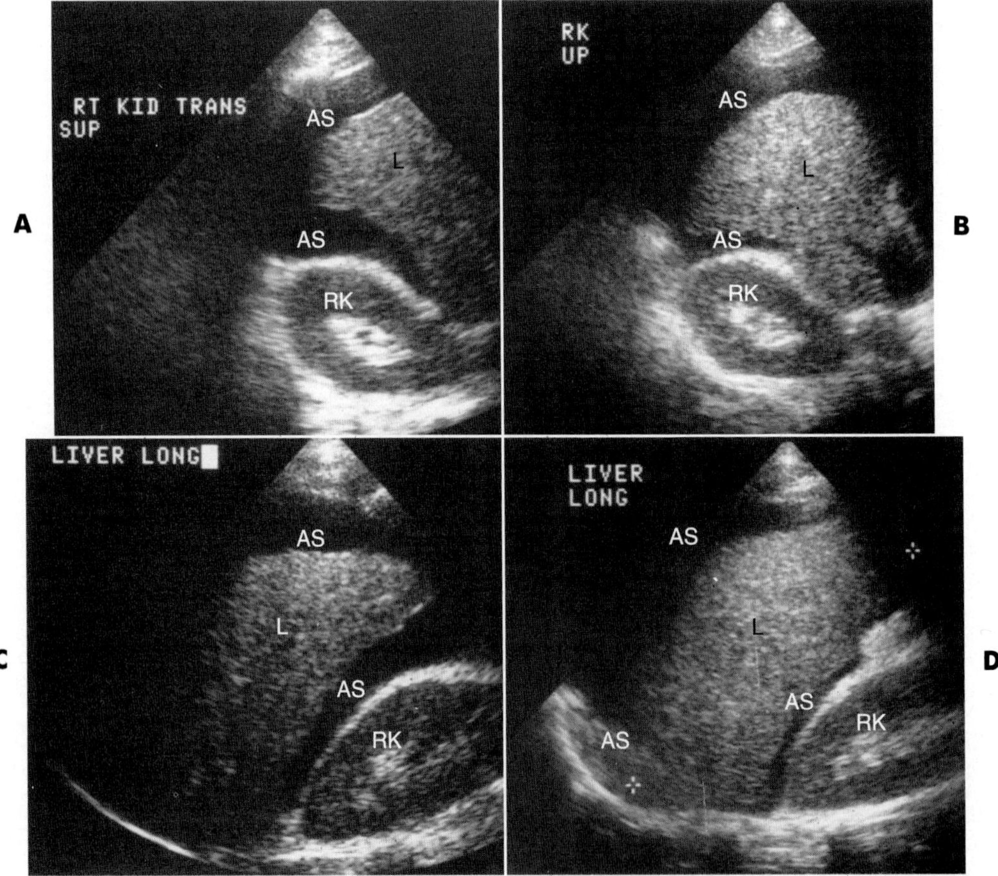

FIG. 12-8 Ascites may fill the peritoneal cavity. Small volumes of fluid in the supine position first appear around the inferior tip of the right lobe of the superior portion of the right flank. **A,** Transverse: liver, *L;* right kidney, *RK;* ascites, *As.* **B,** Transverse. **C,** Longitudinal with fluid in Morison's pouch. **D,** Longitudinal.

the paracolic gutters, before moving lateral and anterior to the liver.

The small bowel loops sink or float in the surrounding ascitic fluid, depending on relative gas content and amount of fat in the mesentery. The middle portion of the transverse colon usually floats on top of fluid because of its gas content, whereas the ascending portions of colon, which are fixed retroperitoneally, remain in their normal location with or without gas.

Floating loops of small bowel, anchored posteriorly by mesentery and with fluid between the mesenteric folds, have a characteristic anterior convex fan shape or arcuate appearance. An overdistended bladder may mask small quantities of fluid.

Inflammatory or Malignant Ascites

In searching for inflammatory or malignant ascites the sonographer should look for fine or coarse internal echoes: loculation; unusual distribution, matting, or clumping of bowel loops; and thickening of interfaces between the fluid and neighboring structures (Fig. 12-9).

Hepatorenal Recess

Generalized ascites, inflammatory fluid from acute cholecystitis, fluid resulting from pancreatic autolysis, or blood from a ruptured hepatic neoplasm or ectopic gestation may contribute to the formation of hepatorenal fluid collections. (Figs. 12-10 to 12-12). Abdominal fluid collections do not persist 1 week after abdominal surgery as a normal part of the healing process.

Loculated ascites tends to be more irregular in outline, shows less mass effect, and may change shape slightly with positional variation.

Abscess Formation and Pockets in the Abdomen and Pelvis

An abscess is a cavity formed by necrosis within a solid tissue or a circumscribed collection of purulent material.

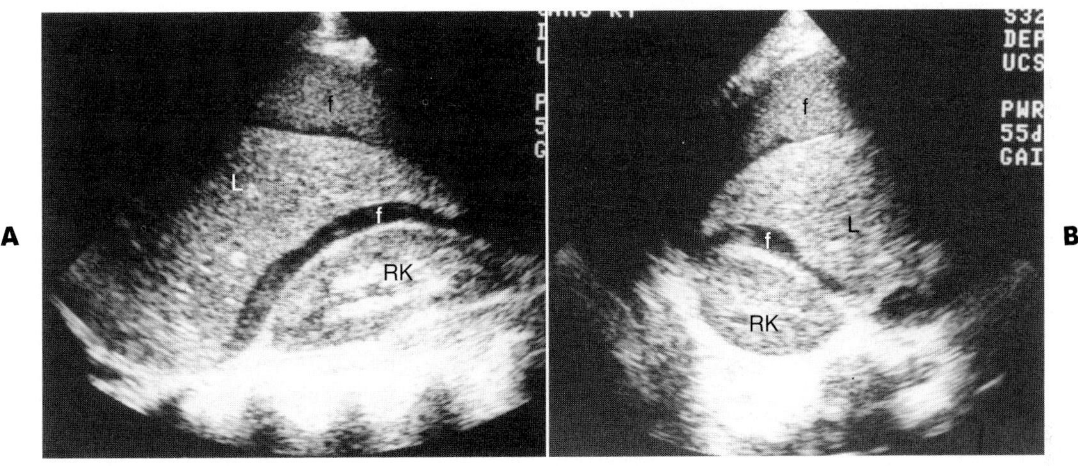

FIG. 12-9 Fine echoes within the ascitic fluid may represent debris, hemorrhage, bacteria, or tumor infiltration. **A,** Longitudinal: liver, *L;* right kidney, *RK;* fluid *f.* **B,** Transverse.

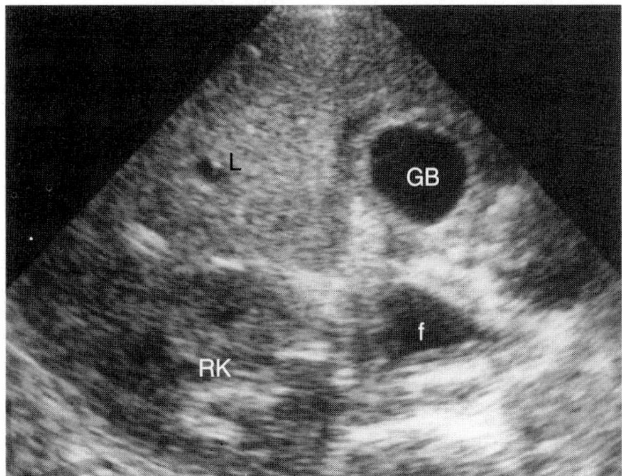

FIG. 12-10 Fluid collection in Morison's pouch in a patient with acute cholecystitis. Liver, *L;* right kidney, *RK;* fluid, *f;* gallbladder, *GB*.

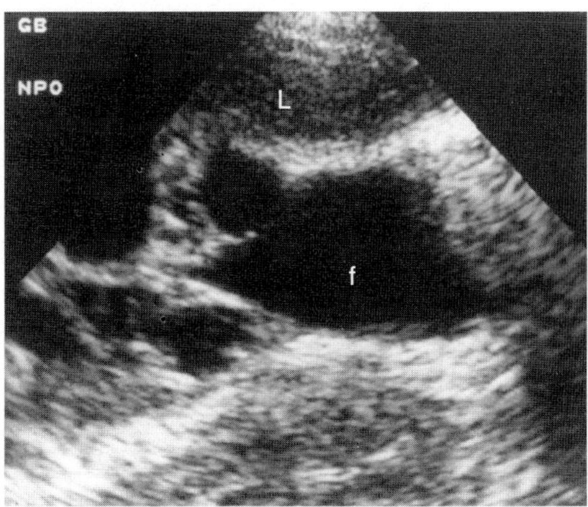

FIG. 12-11 A 45-year-old male after cholecystectomy with spiking temperatures and right upper quadrant tenderness. Fluid collection, *f,* is seen in the area of Morison's pouch.

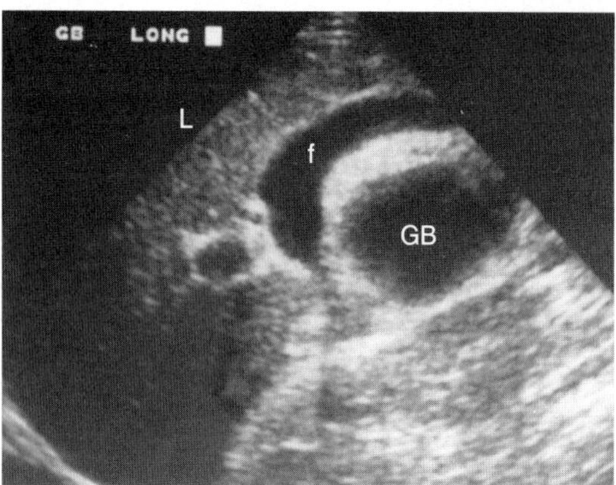

FIG. 12-12 Crescent-shaped fluid collection anterior to the gallbladder. The gallbladder wall is thickened, measuring more than 2 mm.

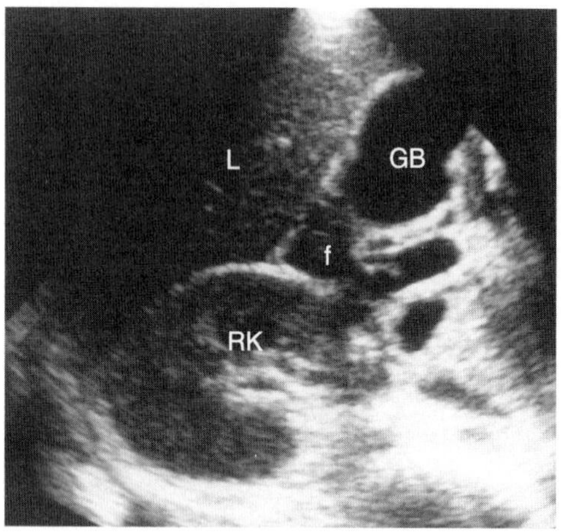

FIG. 12-13 Abscess collections appear with varied echogenicity, shape, and borders. This scan was from a 36-year-old febrile patient in acute right upper quadrant pain. Rupture of the gallbladder wall is seen, *f*.

The sonographer is frequently asked to evaluate a patient to rule out an abscess formation. The patient may present with a fever of unknown origin or with tenderness and swelling from a postoperative procedure. Other clinical signs include chills, weakness, malaise, and pain at the localized site of infection. Laboratory findings include normal liver function values, increased white blood cell count, generalized sepsis, and bacterial cultures (if superficial).

General Sonographic Appearance

Abscess collections can appear quite varied in their texture depending on the length of time the abscess has been forming and the space available for the abscess to localize. Therefore many collections appear predominantly fluid-filled with irregular borders; they can also be complex with debris floating within the cystic mass, or they may show a more solid pattern (Fig. 12-13). If the collection is in the pelvis, careful analysis of bowel patterns and peristalsis should be made in an attempt to separate the bowel from the abscess collection.

Classically an abscess appears as an elliptical sonolucent mass with thick and irregular margins. The margins tend to be under tension and displace surrounding structures. A septated appearance may result from previous or developing adhesions. Necrotic debris produces low-level internal echoes that may be seen to "float" within the abscess. Fluid levels are secondary to layering, probably because of the settling of debris.

Gas-containing Abscess

Gas-containing abscesses present with varying echo patterns. Generally they appear as a densely echogenic mass with or without acoustic shadowing and otherwise increased through-transmission (Fig. 12-14). A teratoma may mimic the pattern of a gas-containing abscess, but clinical history and x rays exclude this tumor from the diagnosis. A gas-containing abscess may be confused with a solid lesion be-

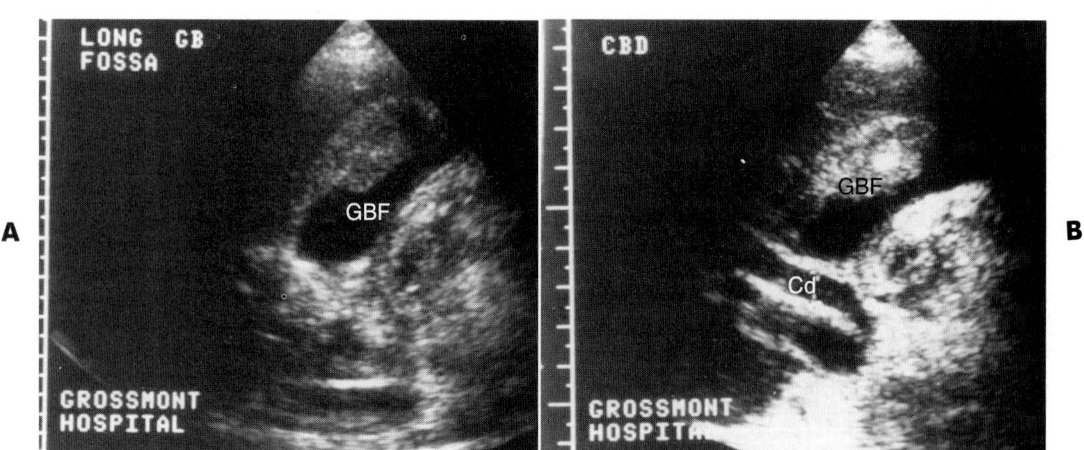

FIG. 12-14 A 57-year-old male after cholecystectomy presents with fever and tenderness over the right upper quadrant. **A,** A large pocket of fluid was seen in the gallbladder fossa, *GBf,* with multiple areas of shadowing representing gas within the abscess collection. **B,** The common duct, *cd,* is still dilated after surgery.

cause it can be difficult to determine the presence of through-transmission.

Peritonitis

Peritonitis and the resultant abscess formation may be a generalized or localized process. Multiloculated abscesses or multiple collections should be documented and their size determined as accurately as possible to help plan drainage and improve accuracy in follow-up studies.

Lesser-sac Abscess

The small slitlike epiploic foramen usually seals off the lesser sac from inflammatory processes extrinsic to it. If the process begins within the lesser sac, such as with a pancreatic abscess, the sac may be involved along with other secondarily affected peritoneal and retroperitoneal spaces. Differential diagnosis should include pseudocyst, pancreatic abscess, gastric outlet obstruction, and fluid-filled stomach.

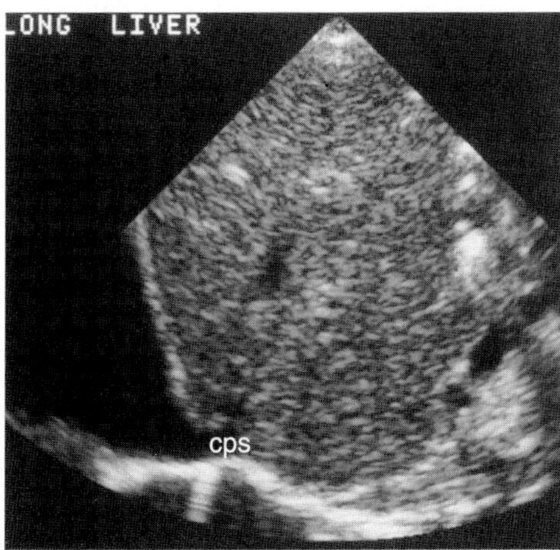

FIG. 12-15 Large right pleural effusion superior to the dome of the liver. The fluid fills the costophrenic sulcus, *cps*.

Subphrenic Abscess

The left upper quadrant may be difficult to examine because of the air interference. The sonographer may alter the patient's position to a right lateral decubitus and scan along the coronal plane of the body or prone to use the spleen as a window.

A sonographer must be careful of pleural effusions that appear above the diaphragm. The sonographer may scan the patient upright to better demonstrate the pleural and subdiaphragmatic areas (Figs. 12-15 and 12-16).

Subcapsular Collections

Subcapsular collections of fluid within the liver can mimic loculated subphrenic fluid. Intraabdominal fluid may be differentiated by its smooth border and its tendency to conform to the contour of the liver. It displaces the liver medially, rather than indenting the border locally, as subcapsular fluid might. A tense subphrenic abscess can displace the liver.

It may be difficult to distinguish a subphrenic abscess from ascites. To do so, the sonographer can look at the margins of the fluid collection or look for other collections of fluid (in pelvis) to distinguish ascites from fluid. Preperitoneal fat anterior to the liver may mimic a localized fluid collection.

An abscess collects in the most dependent area of the body, so all the "gutters" should be evaluated, including the "pockets" and "pouches" and the spaces above and around the various organs.

If an abscess is suspected (e.g., the patient has a fever of unknown origin), the sonographer should evaluate the following areas:

- Subdiaphragmatic area (liver and spleen)
- Splenic recess and borders
- Hepatic recess and borders
- Liver and right kidney
- Pericolic gutters

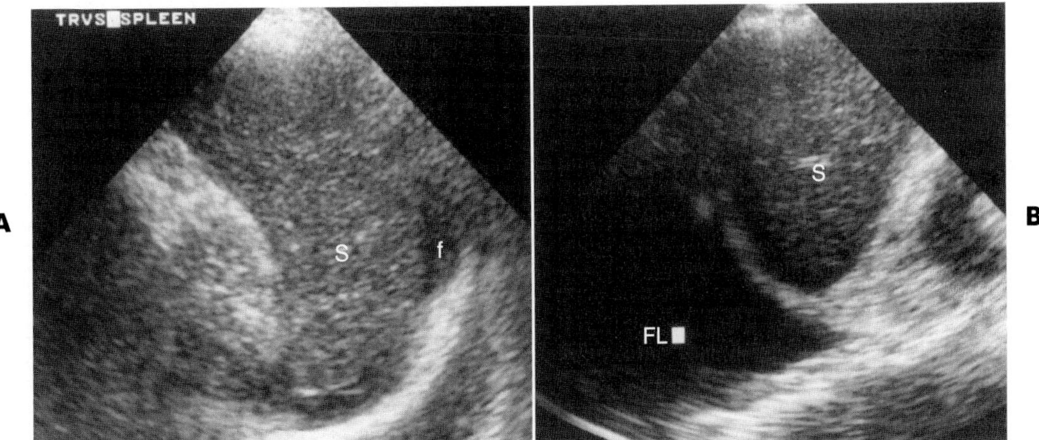

FIG. 12-16 Pleural effusion in the left pleural cavity seen superior to the spleen and diaphragm. If this area cannot be adequately scanned in the supine position, the patient may sit upright for scans along the posterior pleural surface. **A,** Transverse: spleen, *S;* fluid, *FL*. **B,** Longitudinal: spleen, *S;* fluid, *FL*.

- Lesser omentum
- Transverse mesocolon
- Morison's pouch
- Gastrocolic ligament
- Phrenicosplenic ligament
- Recesses between intestinal loops and colon
- Extrahepatic falciform ligament
- Pouch of Douglas
- Broad ligaments (female)
- The area anterior to the urinary bladder

Liver

There are five major pathways through which bacteria can enter the liver and cause abscess formation:

1. Through the portal system
2. By way of ascending cholangitis of the common bile duct (this is the most common cause in the United States)
3. Via the hepatic artery secondary to bacteremia
4. By direct extension from an infection
5. By implantation of bacteria after trauma to the abdominal wall

Kidney

Renal abscesses are classified according to their locations. A renal carbuncle is an abscess that forms within the renal parenchyma. Clinical symptoms vary from none to fever, leukocytosis, and flank pain (Fig. 12-17). Sonography may show a discrete mass within the kidney, which may be cystic, cystic with debris, or solid.

A perinephric abscess is usually the result of a perforated renal abscess that leaks purulent material into the tissues adjacent to the kidney. Sonographic findings include a fluid collection around the kidney or an adjacent mass, which can vary from a cystic to a more solid appearance.

Generalized Abdominal Abscess

A high percentage of abdominal and pelvic abscesses appear after surgery or trauma. The hepatic recesses and perihepatic spaces are the most common sites for abscess formation. The pelvis is another common site (free fluid below the transverse mesocolon often flows into the pouch of Douglas and perivesical spaces).

An abscess may form in the right subhepatic space. The fluid ascends the right pericolic gutter into Morison's pouch. When the fluid fills Morison's pouch, it spreads past the coronary ligament over the dome of the liver. The presence of a right subhepatic abscess generally implies previous contamination of the right subhepatic space.

Appendiceal Abscess

Acute appendicitis is the most common abdominal pathologic process that requires immediate surgery. The cause of obstruction of the appendix is a fecolith at its origin in the cecum. The appendix becomes distended rapidly after obstruction.

Clinical symptoms include fever and severe pain near McBurney's point in the right lower quadrant (to locate this point, draw a straight line between the umbilicus and the anterior superior iliac spine and then move 2 inches along the line from the iliac spine). Laboratory findings show an increased white blood cell count. The differential diagnosis includes pelvic inflammatory disease, twisted or ruptured ovarian cyst, acute gastroenteritis, and mesenteric lymphadenitis.

Sonogram findings. On sonography, a complex mass is found in the right lower quadrant (Fig. 12-18). The sonographer should also examine other gutters to rule out differentials.

Abdominal Wall Masses

An abscess in the abdominal wall may occur after surgery. The sonogram may show cystic, complex, or solid characteristics. Generally the masses are very superficial and are easy to locate and tap if necessary. A high-

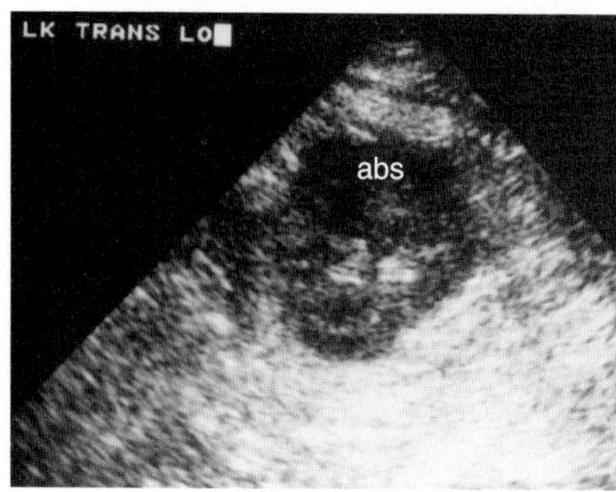

FIG. 12-17 A 26-year-old female with left flank pain and increased white blood count. A large, irregular area was seen in the lower pole of the left kidney representing a renal abscess, *abs*.

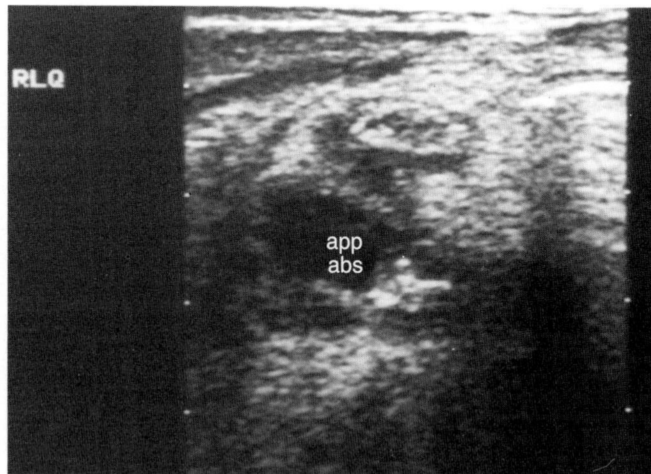

FIG. 12-18 A 22-year-old male with right lower quadrant pain near McBurney's point. White blood cell count was increased. A complex mass represents an appendiceal abscess, *app abs*.

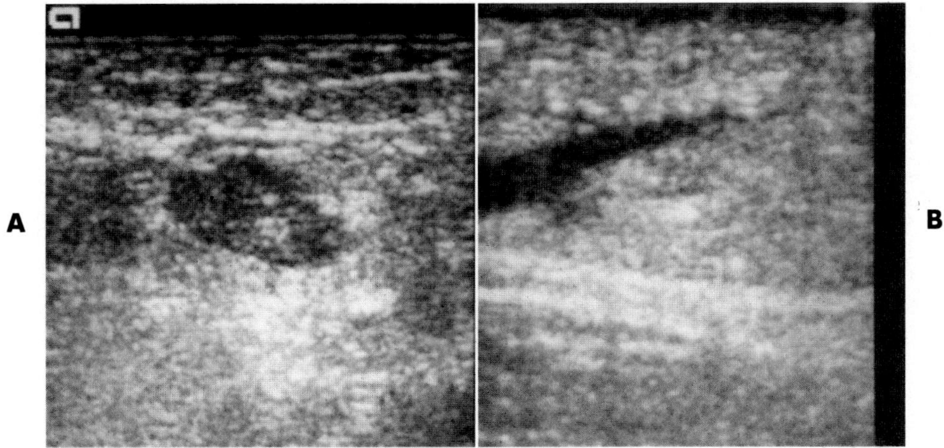

FIG. 12-19 A and **B,** Hematomas may occur anywhere in the abdomen, superficial muscular area, groin, or extremities. New bleeds are primarily cystic with some debris along the posterior border. As the blood organizes, the blood clots form, and thus the mass becomes more complex. This patient recently had a cardiac catheterization and developed a hematoma after catheterization.

frequency, linear-array transducer should be used to image the superficial area.

Hematoma

Hematomas are caused by surgical injury to tissue or by blunt trauma to the abdomen. Laboratory values may show a decrease in hematocrit and red blood cell count; the patient may go into shock. The sonographic appearance depends on the stage of the bleed (Fig. 12-19). New bleeds are primarily cystic with some debris and blood clots; as the blood begins to organize, the mass becomes more "solid" in appearance. New clots may be very homogeneous.

Hematomas can become infected and at any stage may be sonographically indistinguishable from abscesses. They may mimic subphrenic fluid.

Lymphoceles

Lymphoceles generally look like loculated, simple fluid collections, although they may have a more complex, usually septated, morphology. Differentiation from loculated ascites is usually possible because the mass effect of a lymphocele that is under tension displaces the surrounding organs. Differentiation from other fluid collections is mainly made by aspiration.

Peritoneum

The peritoneal lining is not seen as a distinct structure during sonography unless it is thickened. This is usually secondary to metastatic implants or to direct extension of tumor from the viscera or mesentery. Primary mesotheliomas occur rarely.

Biloma

Bilomas are extrahepatic loculated collections of bile that may develop because of iatrogenic, traumatic, or spontaneous rupture of the biliary tree. On ultrasound, they may appear cystic with weak internal echoes or a fluid-fluid level if clots or debris are not present. They usually have sharp margins. The extrahepatic bilomas are usually crescentic, surrounding and compressing structures with which they come in contact.

Cystic Lesions of the Mesentery, Omentum, and Peritoneum

Abdominal cysts may have (1) embryologic, (2) traumatic or acquired, (3) neoplastic, or (4) infective and degenerative sources. Mesenteric and omental cysts are uniloculated or multiloculated with smooth walls and thin internal septations. The internal echoes are correlated with fat globules, debris, superimposed hemorrhage, or infection. They may follow the contour of underlying bowel and conform to the anterior abdominal wall rather than produce distention.

Hemorrhage into the omental or mesenteric cysts may cause rapid distention and clinically mimic ascites. Peritoneal inclusion cysts are considered in the differential diagnosis when large adnexal cystic structures are identified in a young woman. Fungal infections present as peritoneal cystic lesions.

Urinoma

A urinoma, an encapsulated collection of urine, may result from a closed renal injury or surgical intervention or may arise spontaneously secondary to an obstructing lesion. The extraperitoneal extravasation may be subcapsular or perirenal: the latter collections are sometimes termed *uriniferous pseudocysts*. The extravasation may leak around the ureter, where the perinephric fascia is weakest, or into adjoining fascial planes and peritoneal cavity.

Cystic masses are most often oriented inferomedially with upward and lateral displacement of the lower pole of

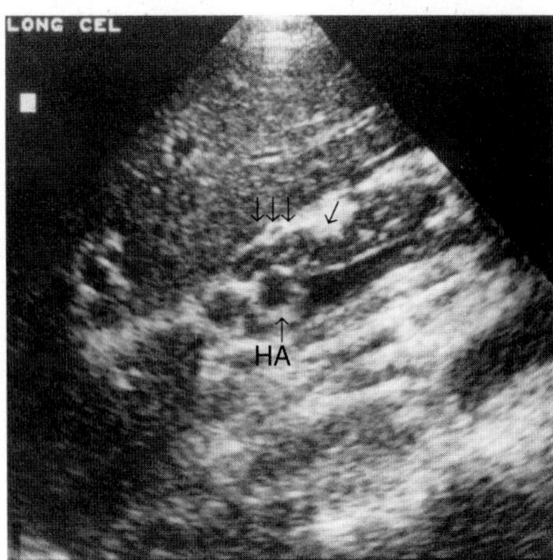

FIG. 12-20 Nodes in the superior mesenteric/celiac axis area may cause the vessels to be compressed or elevated from their origin from the abdominal aorta. Multiple small nodes *(arrows)* are seen to encompass the hepatic artery, *HA*.

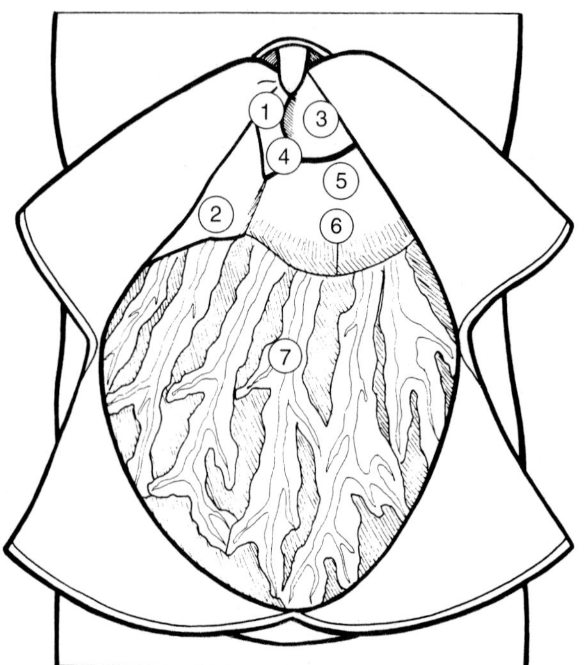

FIG. 12-21 Tumor may infiltrate the greater omentum and can coat the abdominal cavity to envelop and matt together in the abdominal viscera. Falciform, *1;* right lobe of the liver, *2;* left lobe of the liver, *3;* ligamentum teres, *4;* stomach, *5;* greater curvature of the stomach, *6;* greater omentum, *7*. (From Hagen-Ansert SL: The anatomy workbook, Philadelphia, 1986, JB Lippincott.)

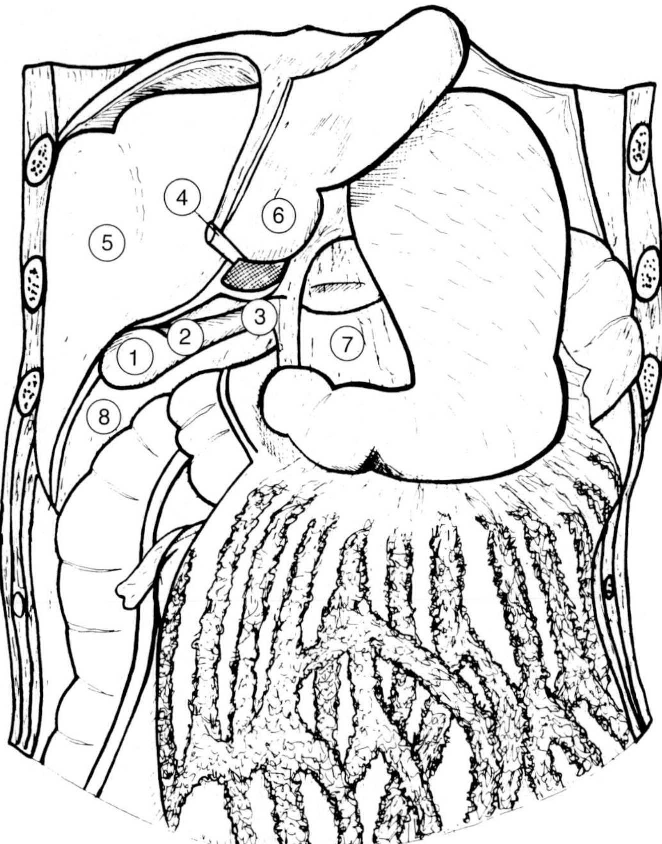

FIG. 12-22 The omentum can send tumor cells to the level of the diaphragm, liver, and splenic hilum. Fundus of the gallbladder, *1;* body of the gallbladder, *2;* neck of the gallbladder, *3;* ligamentum teres, *4;* right lobe of the liver, *5;* caudate lobe of the liver, *6;* lesser sac, *7;* duodenum, *8*. (From Hagen-Ansert SL: The anatomy workbook, Philadelphia, 1986, JB Lippincott.)

the kidney along with medial displacement of the ureter. They usually present on ultrasound as anechoic or contain low-level echoes.

Urachal Cyst

A urachal cyst is an incomplete regression of the urachus during development. On ultrasound the sonographer may see a cystic mass between the umbilicus and the bladder. The mass may be small or giant multiseptated, extending into the upper abdomen.

Peritoneal Metastases

The peritoneal metastases develop from cellular implantation across the peritoneal cavity. The most common primary sites are the ovaries, stomach, and colon. Other less common sites are the pancreas, biliary tract, kidneys, testicles, and uterus. Metastases may arise from tumors such as sarcomas, melanomas, teratomas, or embryonic tumors. The metastases form a nodular, sheetlike irregular configuration. Multiple small nodules are seen along the peritoneal line. The larger masses obliterate the line and cause adhesion to bowel loops.

Lymphoma of Omentum and Mesentery

Lymphoma presents as a uniformly thick, hypoechoic, band-shaped structure that follows the convexity of the anterior and lateral abdominal wall, creating the omental band. On ultrasound, they present as a lobulated confluent hypoechoic mass surrounding a centrally positioned echogenic area. The "sandwich sign" represents a mass infiltrating the mesenteric leaves and encasing the superior mesenteric artery (Fig. 12-20).

Tumors of Peritoneum, Omentum, and Mesentery

Secondary tumors and lymphoma are neoplasms that most commonly involve the peritoneum and mesentery.

Peritoneal and Omental Mesothelioma

Peritoneal and omental mesothelioma most often occur in middle-aged men as the result of exposure to asbestos. The common symptoms are abdominal pain, weight loss, and ascites. The tumor may present as a large mass with discrete smaller nodes scattered over large areas of the visceral and parietal peritoneum, or it may present as diffuse nodes and plaques that coat the abdominal cavity and envelope and mat together in the abdominal viscera (Figs. 12-21 and 12-22).

Abdominal Wall

NORMAL ANATOMY

The paired rectus abdominis muscles are delineated medially in the midline of the body by the linea alba. Laterally the aponeuroses of external oblique, internal oblique, and transversus abdominis muscles unite to form a bandlike vertical fibrous groove called the *linea semilunaris* or *spigelian fascia* (Fig. 12-23). The sheath of the three anterolateral abdominal muscles invests the rectus both anteriorly and posteriorly. Midway between the umbilicus and symphysis pubis the aponeurotic sheath passes anteriorly to the rectus (Fig. 12-24).

Below the line the rectus muscle is separated from the intraabdominal contents only by the transversalis fascia and the peritoneum (Fig. 12-25). The rectus muscles are seen as a biconvex muscle group delineated by the linea alba and linea semilunaris. The peritoneal line is seen as a discrete linear echogenicity in the deepest layer of the abdominal wall.

PATHOLOGY

Extraperitoneal Hematoma

Extraperitoneal rectus sheath hematomas are acute or chronic collections of blood lying either within the rectus muscle or between the muscle and its sheath. They arise as the result of direct trauma, pregnancy, cardiovascular and degenerative muscle diseases, surgical injury, anticoagulation therapy, steroids, or extreme exercise.

Clinically the patient may present with acute, sharp, persistent nonradiating pain. On ultrasound the sonographer notices an asymmetry between the rectus sheath muscles. The hematoma may present as an anechoic mass with scattered internal echoes.

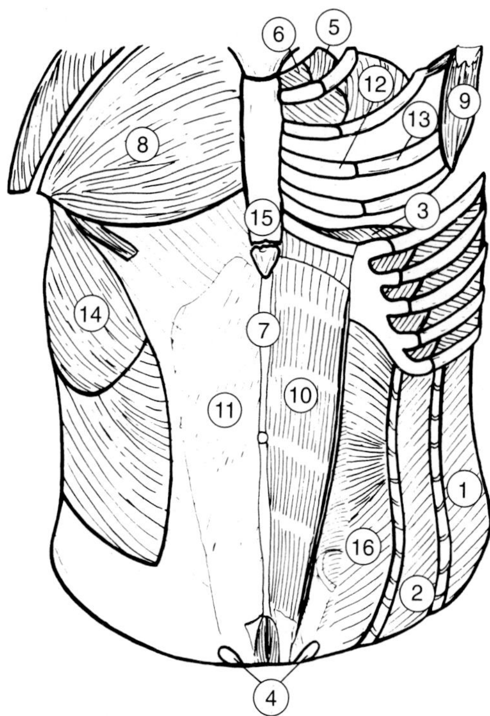

FIG. 12-23 The muscles of the anterior and lateral abdominal walls include the external oblique, the internal oblique, the transversus, the rectus abdominis, and the pyramidalis. External oblique muscle, *1;* internal oblique muscle, *2;* diaphragm, *3;* external inguinal ring, *4;* external intercostal muscle, *5;* internal intercostal muscle, *6;* linea alba, *7;* pectoralis major muscle, *8;* pectoralis minor muscle, *9;* rectus abdominis muscle, *10;* rectus sheath, *11;* costal cartilage, *12;* rib, *13;* serratus anterior muscle, *14;* sternum, *15;* transverse abdominis muscle, *16.* (From Hagen-Ansert SL: The anatomy workbook, Philadelphia, 1986, JB Lippincott.)

Bladder-Flap Hematoma

A bladder-flap hematoma is a collection of blood between the bladder and lower-uterine segment, resulting from a lower-uterine transverse cesarean section and bleeding from the uterine vessels.

Subfascial Hematoma

A subfascial hematoma is found in the prevesical space and is caused by a disruption of the inferior epigastric vessels or their branches during a cesarean section.

Inflammatory Lesion

Abdominal Wall Abscess

On ultrasound an abdominal wall abscess presents as an anechoic or echoic mass with internal echoes from debris. The mass usually has irregular margins and shape. It may have gas bubbles within that show shadowing on the ultrasound image.

Neoplasm

Neoplasms of the abdominal wall include lipomas, desmoid tumors, or metastases. The tumor may present as hypoechoic to cystic (except lipomas). The desmoid tumor is

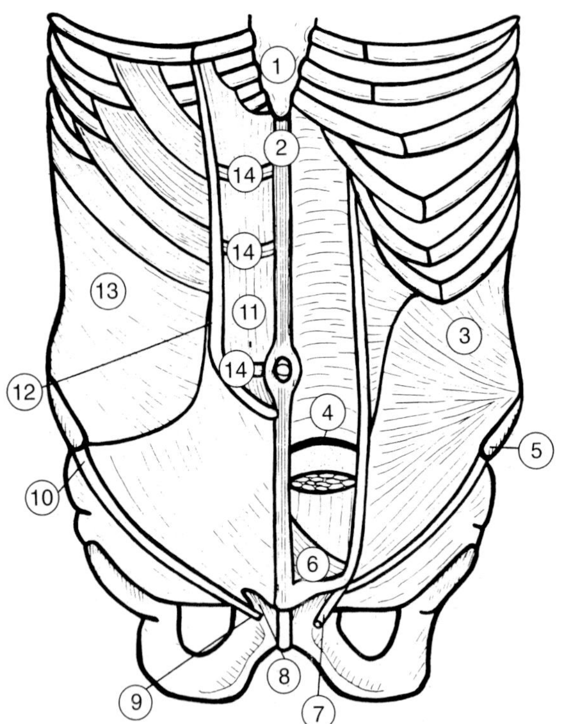

FIG. 12-24 The rectus abdominis muscle arises from the front of the symphysis pubis and the pubic crest. Upon contraction, its lateral margin forms a palpable curved surface, termed the linea semilunaris, that extends from the ninth costal cartilage to the pubic tubercle. The anterior surface of the rectus muscle is crossed by three tendinous intersections that are firmly attached to the anterior wall of the rectus sheath. The pyramidalis muscle arises by its base from the anterior surface of the pubis and inserts into the linea alba. It lies anterior to the lower part of the rectus abdominis muscle. Xyphoid process, *1;* linea alba, *2;* internal oblique muscle, *3;* arcuate line, *4;* anterior superior iliac spine, *5;* pyramidalis muscle, *6;* spermatic cord, *7;* superficial inguinal ring, *8;* pubic tubercle, *9;* inguinal ligament, *10;* rectus muscle, *11;* linea semilunaris, *12;* external oblique muscle, *13;* tendinous intersections, *14*. (From Hagen-Ansert SL: The anatomy workbook. Philadelphia: JB Lippincott.)

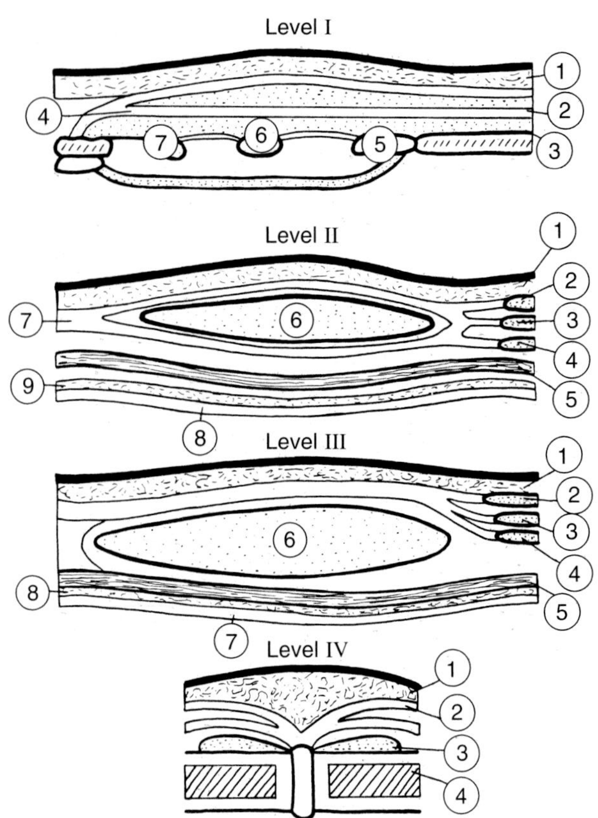

FIG. 12-25 Level 1 (above the costal margin). Superficial fascia, *1;* pectoralis major muscle, *2;* rectus muscle, *3;* aponeurosis of the external oblique muscle, *4;* external oblique muscle, *5;* internal oblique muscle, *6;* transversus muscle, *7*. Level II (between the costal margin and the level of the anterior superior iliac spine). Superficial fascia, *1;* external oblique muscle, *2;* internal oblique muscle, *3;* transverse muscle, *4;* fascia transversalis, *5;* rectus muscle, *6;* linea alba, *7;* peritoneum, *8;* extraperitoneal fat, *9*. Level III (below the level of the anterior superior iliac spine and above the pelvis). Superficial fascia, *1;* external oblique muscle, *2;* internal oblique muscle, *3;* transverse muscle, *4;* fascia transversalis, *5;* rectus muscle, *6;* peritoneum, *7;* extraperitoneal fat, *8*. Level 4 (at the level of the pubis). Superficial fascia, *1*; aponeurosis of the external oblique muscle, *2*; rectus muscle, *3*; pubis, *4*. (From Hagen-Ansert SL: The anatomy workbook. Philadelphia, 1986, JB Lippincott.)

a benign fibrous neoplasm of aponeurotic structures. It most commonly arises in relation to the rectus abdominis and its sheath. On ultrasound, it presents as anechoic to hypoechoic with smooth and sharply defined walls.

Hernia

If a hernia is suspected, the sonographer should look for peristalsing bowel within the mass, although the peristalsis may be absent with incarceration. The hernia may involve the omentum only or it may mimic other masses. The hernia commonly originates near the junction of the linea semilunaris and arcuate line. The hernia penetrates both the transversus abdominis and internal oblique muscles, expanding laterally in the space between the two oblique muscles. The sonographer should scan obliquely between the anterior superior iliac spine and pubic crest, along the course of the inguinal ligament.

The femoral artery and vein are seen anterior to the iliopubic junction. The psoas muscle and lymphatic channels occupy a space between the anterior superior iliac spine and iliopubic junction. Masses arising in relation to the femoral vessels and beneath the inguinal ligament include the femoral hernias, lipomas, soft-tissue sarcomas, and lymph nodes. Abnormalities arising superior to the femoral vessels and inguinal ligament include direct and indirect inguinal hernias, ectopic testicles, and extension of femoral hernias.

REVIEW QUESTIONS

1. How do the coronary ligaments help the sonographer determine if the fluid is pleural rather than subdiaphragmatic?

2. How can the sonographer determine if the mass is retroperitoneal or intraperitoneal?
3. What is the significance of anterior displacement of the superior mesenteric vessels?
4. What divides the subphrenic space into right and left components?
5. Describe the bare area of the liver and where it is located.
6. Describe the lesser sac boundaries.
7. What is the retrovesical space? What is the posterior rectouterine sac called?
8. How does serous ascites appear on ultrasound? Where does the fluid accumulate first?
9. How would malignant ascites appear on ultrasound?
10. What is the sonographic appearance of an abscess on ultrasound?
11. Describe the clinical findings for a patient with an abdominal abscess.
12. What are some causes of a lesser-sac abscess?
13. How can the sonographer differentiate a subcapsular hematoma from ascites?
14. Name at least five areas the sonographer should investigate in the search for an abscess collection.
15. Describe the five pathways by which bacteria can enter the liver and cause abscess formation.
16. What is a renal carbuncle and how would it present on ultrasound?
17. Describe McBurney's point and its significance to the sonographer.
18. Define a biloma.
19. What is the source of abdominal cysts?
20. Define a urinoma. How is it caused and how it would appear on ultrasound?
21. Describe the appearance of lymphoma on ultrasound.
22. What is the normal composition of the anterior abdominal wall?
23. How can the sonographer differentiate a rectus sheath hematoma from an abscess collection?
24. Name three forms of abdominal wall tumors.
25. How can the sonographer determine if a mass is a hernia or an abscess or cystic collection?

BIBLIOGRAPHY

Abu-Yusef MM, Wiese JA, and Shamma AR: Case report. The "to-and-for" sign: duplex Doppler evidence of femoral artery pseudoaneurysm, Am J Roentgenol 150:632, 1988.

Archer A, Choyke PL, O'Brien W, et al: Scrotal enlargement following inguinal herniorrhaphy: ultrasound evaluation, Urol Radiol 9:249, 1988.

Baron RL and Lee JK: Mesenteric desmoid tumours, Radiology 140:777, 1981.

Behan M and Kazam E: The echogenic characteristics of fatty tissues and tumors, Radiology 129:143, 1978.

Benaceraff BK, Adzick NS: Fetal diaphragmatic hernia: ultrasound diagnosis and clinical outcome in 19 cases, Am J Obstet Gynecol 156:573, 1987.

Black D, Vora J, Hayward M, et al: Measurement of subcutaneous fat thickness with high frequency pulsed ultrasound: comparison with a caliper and a radiographic technique, Clin Phys Physiol Measurement 9:57, 1988.

Brugman SM, Bjelland JJ, Thomasson JE, et al: Sonographic findings with radiographic correlation in meconium peritonitis, J Clin Ultrasound 7:305, 1979.

Bruneton JN, Caramella E, Hery M, et al: Axillary lymph node metastasis in breast cancer: preoperative detection with US, Radiology 158:325, 1986.

Bruneton JN and Normand F: Cervical lymph nodes: In Bruneton JN, editor: Ultrasonography of the neck, Berlin, 1987, Springer, pp. 81-92.

Bruneton JN, Normand F, Balu-Maestro C, et al: Lymphomatous superficial lymph nodes: US detection, Radiology 165:233, 1987.

Bruneton JN, Roux P, Caramella E, et al: ear, nose, and throat cancer: ultrasound diagnosis of metastasis to cervical lymph nodes, Radiology 142:771, 1984.

Comstock CH: The antenatal diagnosis of diaphragmatic anomalies, J Ultrasound Med 5:391, 1986.

Coughlin BF and Paushter DM: Peripheral pseudoaneurysms: evaluation with duplex US, Radiology 168:339, 1988.

Diakoumakis EE, Weinberg B, and Seife B: Unusual case studies of anterior wall mass as diagnosed by ultrasonography, J Clin Ultrasound 12:351, 1984.

Diament MJ, Boerhat MI, and Kangarloo H: Real-time sector ultrasound in the evaluation of suspected abnormalities of diaphragmatic motion, J Clin Ultrasound 13:539, 1985.

Engel JM and Deitch EE: Sonography of the anterior abdominal wall, Am J Roentgenol 137:73, 1981.

Fischer JD and Turner FW: Abdominal incisional hernias—a 10 year review, Can J Surg 17:202, 1974.

Golding RH, Li DKB, and Cooperberg PL: Sonographic demonstration of air-fluid levels in abdominal abscesses, J Ultrasound Med 1:151, 1982.

Gooding GAW and Cummings SR: Sonographic detection of ascites in liver disease, J Ultrasound Med 3:169, 1984.

Gooding GAW, Effeney DJ, and Goldstone J: The aortofemoral graft: detection and identification of healing complications by ultrasonography, Surgery 89:949, 1981.

Haber K, Asher WM and Freimann AK: Echographic evaluation of diaphragmatic motion in intra-abdominal disease, Radiology 114:141, 1975.

Halvorsen RA, Jones MA, Rice RP, and Thompson WM: Anterior left subphrenic abscesses: characteristic plain film and CT appearance, Am J Roentgenol 139:283, 1982.

Hillman BJ and Haber K: Echographic characteristics of malignant lymph nodes, JCU 8:213, 1980.

Jones PR, Davies PS and Norgan NG: Ultrasonic measurements of subcutaneous adipose tissue in man, Am J Phys Anthropology 73:359, 1986.

Kaftori JK, Rosenberger A, Pollack S, Fish JH: Rectus sheath hematoma: ultrasonographic diagnosis, Am J Roentgenol 128:283, 1977.

Kordan B and Payne SD: Fat necrosis simulating a primary tumor of the mesentery: sonographic diagnosis, J Ultrasound Med 7:345, 1988.

Landay MJ, Setiawan H, Hirsch G, et al: Hepatic and thoracic amebiasis Am J Roentgenol 135:449, 1980.

Lee PWR, Bark M, Macfie J, and Pratt D: The ultrasound diagnosis of rectus sheath haematoma, Br J Surg 64:633, 1977.

Lessner AM, Lempert N, Pietrocola DM, et al: Diagnosis and treatment of pelvic lymphoceles in the renal transplant patient, NY State J Med 84:491, 1984.

Levitt RG, Kohler RE, Sagel SS, et al: Metastatic disease of the mesentery and omentum, Radiol Clin North Am 20:501, 1982.

Lundstedt C, Hederström E, Holmin T, et al: Radiological diagnosis in proven intra-abdominal abscesses formation: a comparison between plain films of the abdomen, ultrasonography and computed tomography, Gastroinest Radiol 8:261, 1983.

Marchal G, Oyen R, Verschakelen J, et al: Sonographic appearance of normal lymph nodes, J Ultrasound Med 4:417, 1985.

Marshak RH, Lindner AE, Maklansky D, et al: Mesenteric fat necrosis simulating a carcinoma of the cecum, Am J Gastroenterol 5:459, 1980.

Meyers MA: Distribution of intra-abdominal malignant seeding: dependency on dynamics of flow and ascitic fluid, Am J Roentgenol 119:198, 1973.

Meyers MA: Metastatic disease along the small bowel mesentery: roentgen features, Am J Roentgenol 123:67, 1975.

Meyers MA and McSweeney J: Secondary neoplasms of the bowel, Radiology 133:419, 1979.

Middleton WD, Erickson S, and Melson GL: Perivascular color artifact: pathologic significance and appearance on color Doppler US images, Radiology 171:647, 1989.

Mitchell DG, Needleman L, Bezzi M, et al: Femoral artery pseudoaneurysm: diagnosis with conventional duplex and color Doppler US, Radiology 164:687, 1987.

Mittelstaedt C: Ultrasonic diagnosis of omental cysts, Radiology 114:673, 1975.

Morton MJ, Charboneau JW, and Banks PM: Inguinal lymphadenopathy simulating a false aneurysm on color-flow Doppler sonography, Am J Roentgenol 151:115, 1988.

Müeller PR, Ferrucci JT Jr, Harbin WP, et al: Appearance of lymphomatous involvement of the mesentery by ultrasonography and body computed tomography: the "sandwich sign," Radiology 134:467, 1980.

Müeller PR and Simeone JF: Intra-abdominal abscess: diagnosis by sonography and computed tomography, Radiol Clin North Am 21:425, 1983.

Nicolet V, Gagnon A, Filiatrault D, and Biosvert J: Sonographic appearance of an abdominal cystic lymphangioma, J Ultrasound Med 3:85, 1984.

O'Neil JD, Ros PR, Storm BL, et al: Cystic mesothelioma of the peritoneum, Radiology 170:333, 1989.

Proto AV, Lane EJ, and Marangola JA: A new concept of ascitic fluid distribution, Am J Roentgenol 126:974, 1976.

Sacks D, Robinson MD, and Perlmutter GS: Femoral arterial injury following catheterization duplex evaluation, J Ultrasound Med 8:241, 1989.

Sandler MA, Alpern MB, Madrazo BL, et al: Inflammatory lesions of the groin: ultrasonic evaluation, Radiology 151:747, 1984.

Savage PE, Joseph AEA, and Adam EJ: Massive abdominal wall hematoma: real-time ultrasound localization of bleeding, J Ultrasound Med 4:157, 1985.

Schneider JA and Zelnick EJ: Benign cystic peritoneal mesothelioma, J Clin Ultrasound 13:190, 1985.

Shafir R, Itzchak Y, Heymen Z, et al: Preoperative ultrasonic measurements of the thickness of cutaneous malignant melanoma, J Ultrasound Med 3:205, 1984.

Spangen L: Ultrasound as a diagnostic aid in ventral abdominal hernia, JCU 3:211, 1975.

Spring DB, Schroeder D, Babu S, et al: Ultrasonic evaluation of lymphocele formation after staging lymphadenectomy for prostatic cancer, Radiology 141:479, 1981.

Subramanyam BR, Balthazar EJ, Raghavendra BN, et al: Sonographic diagnosis of scrotal hernia, Am J Roentgenol 139:535, 1982.

Tromans A, Campbell N, and Sykes P: Rectus sheath haematoma. Diagnosis by ultrasound, Br J Surg 68:518, 1981.

van Sonnenberg E, Müeller PR, and Ferrucci JT: Percutaneous drainage of 250 abdominal abscesses and fluid collections. Part I: results, failures and complications, Radiology 151:337, 1984.

Wu C-C, Chow K-S, Lü T-N and Huang F-T: Sonographic features of tuberculous omental cakes in peritoneal tuberculosis, J Clin Ultrasound 16:195, 1988.

Yeh H-C, Halton KP, and Gray CE: Anatomic variations and abnormalities in the diaphragm seen with ultrasound, Radiographics 10:1019, 1990.

• PART TWO •

Superficial Structures

CHAPTER 13
Breast

Sandra L. Hagen-Ansert

One out of eleven American women will develop breast cancer. It is the leading cause of death for the middle-aged woman. Early detection of the tumor is vital, since the disease can spread rapidly. Delays in early detection and treatment can be particularly tragic because the 5-year survival rate for localized breast cancer adequately treated is 98% after 5 years and 95% after 10 years.[7] Metastatic cancer shows survival rates of only 30% to 50% after 10 years.

The clinical diagnosis of breast cancer may fall under several categories, depending on the age of the patient, whether the lesion is palpable, the risk factors of the patient, and previous medical history. The practice of self-examination is an important issue in the detection of early lesions or subtle changes in the breast parenchyma that one may notice only from a regular routine examination.

The purpose of this chapter is to present an overview of breast lesions with particular reference to the aspects with which a sonographer is concerned either directly or indirectly, and its primary emphasis is on the technique of sonography.

As early as 1951 the first paper on ultrasound of the breast was published by John Wild using A-mode techniques. The following year, Wild used the B-mode with a water bag technique to image the breast parenchyma. Several years later, in 1956, the Japanese used an overhead water bag method with a 2 MHz transducer and noted that malignancies returned strong echoes. In 1967 the Australians developed a similar overhead water bag technique with a 2 MHz transducer and noticed the breast was greatly compressed by this attempt. Contrary to previous work reported, the group at the Ultrasonics Institute discovered that malignancies returned low-level echoes, whereas stronger echoes were obtained from the surrounding fibrous connective tissue.

The following year Elizabeth Kelly-Fry developed an overhead water bag method with an open drape allowing the breast to protrude from a hole, held firm by adhesive tape and a plastic drape. In 1969 grey-scale instrumentation was developed by the Ultrasonics Institute and had a significant impact on tissue differentiation seen on ultrasound images. In 1974 the Australians modified their instrumentation so the patient would lie in a prone position with her breast immersed in a warm water bath. A single 4.5 MHz transducer was used to provide the high resolution necessary to image the breast tissue.

Most clinical laboratories today use the high-resolution real time scanner to visualize palpable breast lesions. The high-frequency 5, 7.5, and 10 MHz transducers have the short-to-medium focus necessary to obtain high-quality images of the breast parenchyma.

ANATOMY

The function of the female breast is to secrete milk during lactation. The breast is a differentiated apocrine sweat gland. Its parenchymal elements are the lobes, ducts, lobules, and acini. Because the mammary gland is a skin derivative, the stromal elements include dense connective tissue, loose connective tissue, and fat. Sonographically fat is the least echogenic tissue within the breast. The interface between fat and loose connective tissue is less echogenic than that between fat and dense connective tissue. The position of these interfaces in relation to the beam determines their reflectivity. The age and functional state of the breast dictate the amount and arrangement of various parenchymal and stromal elements. There may be variation of these elements in women of the same age group, in breasts of similar functioning states, and from region to region in the same breast.

The breast is composed of 15 to 20 lobes. Each lobe contains the parenchymal elements of the breast. Ducts extend from the lobes through the breast parenchyma to converge in a single papilla, the nipple, which is surrounded by the areola (Fig. 13-1). The ducts are covered with a connective tissue layer that varies in thickness and density from breast to breast. The normal duct usually measures about 2 mm in diameter. The patient who is nursing may have a lactating duct that measures as much as 8 mm.

The entire breast is enveloped in a duplication of superficial pectoral fascia. The posterior part of the fascia is connected to the pectoral musculature; the anterior part is connected to the skin by thin connective septa (Fig. 13-2). The anterior and posterior fascial planes are connected by curvilinear connective tissue septa known as *Cooper's ligaments*.[4] These ligaments are the supporting structures of the breast and provide the shape and consistency of its paren-

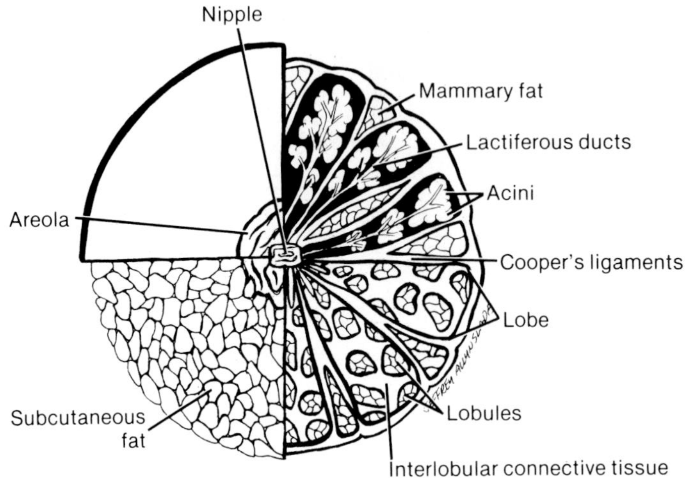

FIG. 13-1 Anatomy of the breast. (Modified from Townsend CM: Clin Symp 32:1, 1980.)

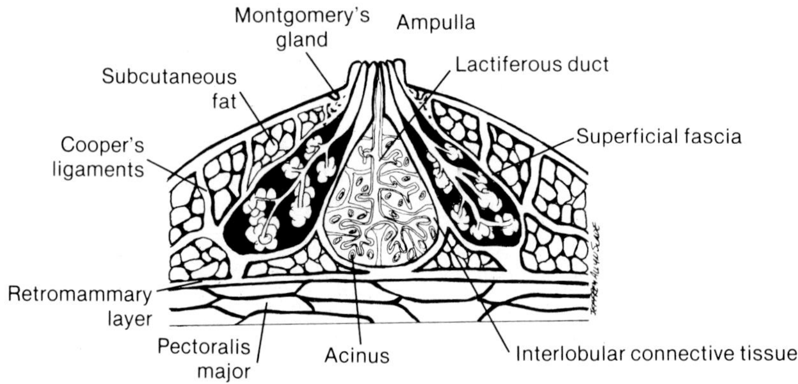

FIG. 13-2 Anatomy of the breast. (Modified from Townsend CM: Clin Symp 32:1, 1980.)

chyma. The connective tissue septa envelop the lobules and lobes of the breast and become the interlobular and interlobar connective tissues that surround the fat lobules and parenchyma of the breast.

There are three well-defined layers in the breast: subcutaneous, mammary, and retromammary (Fig. 13-3). The subcutaneous layer is bounded superficially by the dermis and deeply by the superficial connective tissue plane.[2] The principal component of this layer is fat lobules enclosed by connective tissue septa. The mammary layer is composed of breast parenchyma and is found between the superficial and deep connective tissue layers. Fat is seen to be interspersed in a lobular fashion throughout the entire breast parenchyma. The sonographic pattern within this layer shows the greatest variation with the patient's age and functional state of the breast.[2] The retromammary layer consists of fat lobules that are separated anteriorly from the mammary layer by the deep connective tissue plane and posteriorly by the fascia over the pectoralis major.

During pregnancy the ducts and parenchymal elements of the breast expand to such a degree that the mammary layer takes up the entire breast. The subcutaneous fat layer and the retromammary layer are so squeezed that they appear very narrow on the sonogram. The interfaces in the pregnant breast are less echogenic.

The major portion of the breast contained within the superficial fascia of the anterior thoracic wall is situated between the second or third rib superiorly, the sixth or seventh costal cartilage inferiorly, the anterior axillary line laterally, and the sternal border medially.[9] The greatest amount of glandular tissue is located in the upper outer quadrant of the breast, which explains why tumors are more frequently found here.

The major pectoral muscle lies posterior to the retromammary layer. The minor pectoral muscle lies superolaterally posterior to it. The pectoralis minor courses from its rib cage origin to the point where it inserts into the coracoid process. The lower border of the pectoralis major forms the anterior border of the axilla. Breast tissue can extend into this region and is referred to as the *axillary tail* or *tail of Spence* (Fig. 13-4).

Vascular Supply and Lymph Drainage

The principal blood supply to the breast is from branches of the internal mammary and the lateral thoracic arteries. The intercostal artery plays a subordinant role. Venous

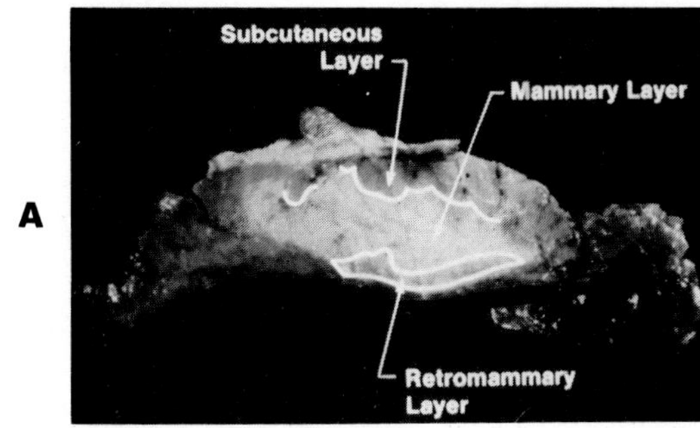

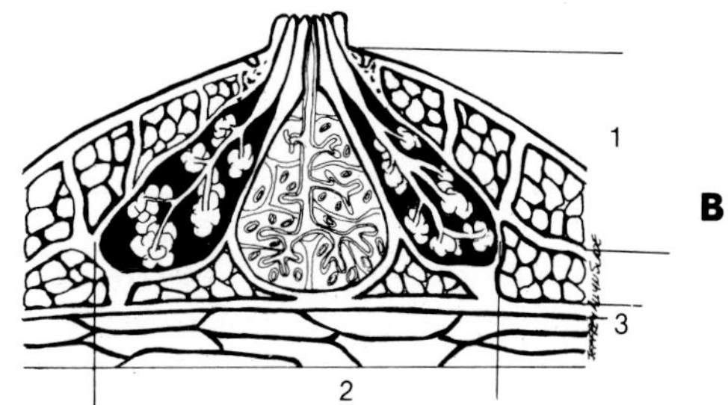

FIG. 13-3 Three layers of breast tissue. **A,** Anatomic section. **B,** Diagram. *1,* Subcutaneous fatty layer; *2,* mammary layer; *3,* retromammary layer. (Modified from Townsend CM: Clin Symp 32:1, 1980.)

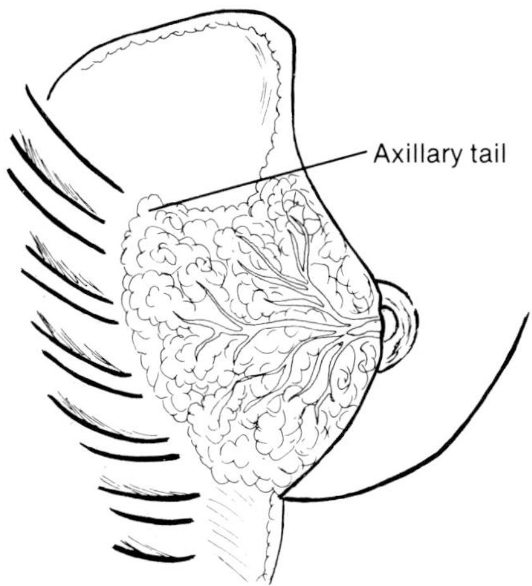

FIG. 13-4 A projection of tissue, called the *axillary tail* or *tail of Spence,* usually extends from the upper outer quadrant into the axilla.

drainage is through superficial and deep veins. The superficial veins are usually arranged in a transverse or longitudinal pattern and can be seen on the sonogram. The deep veins are not visible. In the axilla the axillary vein is sonographically visible, with the axillary artery located superior and a bit posterior to it.

The lymphatics of the breast originate in the lymph capillaries of the mammary connective tissue grid. The lymph capillaries are similar to blood capillaries and are abundant in the breast tissue. They have valves to assure flow in the direction of the venous system (away from the tissues). The lymph vessels empty into lymph nodes; thus when cancer cells invade the lymphatic system, they reach the lymph nodes, which act as a filter and retain the malignant cells. These then grow at the expense of the node and gradually destroy it.

The axillary lymph nodes are closely related to the axillary vein. The majority of the lymph drainage passes to this group of nodes. Other drainage pathways are along the inferior margin of the pectoralis major. Flow may also be directed to groups of lymph nodes around the third, fourth, and fifth prongs of the serratus anterior, as well as toward the intercostal and mediastinal node group. Lymph drainage is also routed to the subdiaphragmatic lymph nodes. Medial lymph drainage eventually reaches the parasternal and anterior mediastinal lymph nodes. In addition, there are abundant lymphatic connections to the opposite breast.

Variations in Parenchymal Patterns

The first pattern, and the one most difficult to image by sonography, is the fatty breast. Fatty replacement of the parenchymal elements of the breast occurs with each pregnancy. With the onset of menopause there is atrophy of the ducts. As a result, all three layers appear fatty. Generally radiography images this type of breast quite adequately.

The second pattern is still largely fat. Histologically there is some periductal connective tissue, which sonographically presents as bright reflectors. The breast basically appears fatty.

The next pattern is complex. It consists of progressing degrees of fibrosis. Sonographically degrees of coalescence of the dense connective tissue and a scalloped effect of the superficial connective tissue plane can often be seen. There is still some residual fat present in this pattern.

The last pattern shows no residual fat in the mammary layer. The fat is replaced by dense connective tissue.

PHYSIOLOGY

The breast is an endocrine gland and is affected in its physical and microscopic state by changing hormonal levels. The growth of the breast begins before the onset of menstruation. At puberty the combined influences of the hypothalamus and anterior pituitary, and later the ovaries, cause growth of the breast. Although these are the primary endocrine sources responsible for breast growth, complete development also requires normal levels of insulin and thyroid hormone secretions.[5]

During the first year or two of menstruation, ovulation does not occur and there is an increased output of estrogen. This causes the mammary ducts to elongate. Their epithelial lining reduplicates and proliferates as the ends of the mammary tubules form sprouts of future lobules. Estrogen stimulates the vascularity of the breast tissue, increases the volume and elasticity of the connective tissues, and induces fat deposition in the breast.

With the onset of maturity (i.e., when ovulation occurs and the progesterone-secreting corpora lutea are formed), the second stage of mammary development occurs.[8] This is the formation of the lobules and acinar structures and gives the mammary gland the characteristic lobular structure found during childbearing years. Further acinar development continues in proportion to the intensity of the hormonal stimuli during each menstrual cycle.

During pregnancy, changes occur that make milk production possible. In addition to estrogen and progesterone, hormones such as placental lactogen, prolactin, and chorionic gonadotropin are required for complete gestational development of the breast.[11] At delivery there is a loss of estrogen and progesterone. Prolactin then predominates and the alveolar cells actively synthesize and secrete milk. During the 3 months after cessation of lactation, involution of the breast occurs. The breast remains larger because of the fatty tissue replacement. Post-lactation involution is a decrease in the size of the lobular-alveolar components as compared to their enlargement during pregnancy.

EVALUATION OF THE PATIENT WITH A BREAST MASS

Medical History

A complete medical history is very important in assessing the patient with a breast mass. The following pertinent questions may aid the clinician in the final diagnosis:

- Age (the greater the age the higher the risk, especially over 35 years of age)
- Previous cancer of the breast (up to 16% will develop cancer in the other breast)
- Family history (40% chance of developing cancer if mother had cancer)
- Late first pregnancy (28 years of age or over)
- Nulliparous women
- Late menopause (54 years of age or older)
- Previous biopsy for benign disease
- Exposure to radiation at an early age
- Mammographic appearance of a prominent duct pattern or marked dysplasia
- Obesity
- Suppression of emotions (especially anger)

The age of the patient is important since malignancy is rarely found in women under 25 years of age and the incidence steadily increases with age. If the patient or the clinician detects a breast mass, symptoms such as pain, tenderness, or nipple discharge should be noted. The patient is questioned about whether these symptoms occur cyclically, during pregnancy, or in relation to trauma or previous breast disease. Patients with a previous biopsy-proved breast lesion or who have had breast cancer are at an increased risk for cancer. The incidence of cancer is greater in a patient whose mother or sister has had breast cancer. Early menarche and late menopause have also been associated with an increased risk of breast cancer.[8]

Diagnostic Techniques

A complete physical examination of the patient's breasts should be performed after the medical history has been taken. It is essential that the size, location, consistency, and mobility of the mass be noted, as well as the site of biopsy scars, asymmetry between the breasts, skin changes or discoloration, and the presence of skin dimpling.

One of the most reliable methods for detecting breast masses is palpation, which may be done by either the physician or the patient. Premenopausal women should examine their breasts at the same time of the month, preferably 5 to 7 days after cessation of menses, so that subtle changes can be detected.

Most breast lumps are benign, with only 20% to 25% of those surgically removed revealing malignancy. More than 90% of the lumps are found by breast self-examination.

Mammography

The most accurate noninvasive method for the detection of breast lesions is mammography. With dedicated mammographic equipment, the diagnosis of cancer can be made if the examination is optimally performed and interpreted.

The mammographic diagnosis of breast cancer depends on the demonstration of a mass having poorly defined stellate or knobby margins or a cluster of tiny rod-shaped calcifications. The benign lesions are known to have sharply defined margins and smooth contours. If calcifications are present in the benign lesion, they are round or oval shape. To better visualize these small areas of calcification, fine detail is critical. The development of mammographic magnification offers improved detail and sharpness for the interpreter to determine if the lesion is benign or malignant.

The American Cancer Society recommends that all women between the ages of 35 and 40 have a baseline mammogram performed, followed by an annual or biennial mammogram screening until the age of 50. Women beyond 50 years of age, should have a mammogram yearly. With the development of high-resolution and low-radiation techniques, this recommendation is actively being promoted across the nation in an effort to reduce the mortality figures from breast cancer.

Technologic advances in combining mammography with ultrasound have produced an even higher diagnostic accuracy. Although mammography is the most sensitive technique for detecting cancer in the fatty breast, tissue, ultrasound is more useful in women under 35 years of age and in women with dense, fibrous, glandular breasts. Ultrasound also gives information about tissue characteristics that mammography does not provide.

Ultrasound

Ultrasound has been found clinically useful in the following conditions: patients with radiographic dense breasts (any age), younger patients, patients with an equivocal mammographic finding, symptomatic patients who are pregnant or lactating, and patients with breast prostheses. It is also of great value in distinguishing a cystic from a solid lesion in a patient with a known breast mass.

Real Time Technique. Patients who present with a palpable breast lesion are examined with high-resolution real time ultrasound. The patient may be examined in a supine-oblique position, as she is rolled about 35 degrees toward the side opposite the breast to be examined. A sponge or folded towel is placed under her hips and shoulders to support her position. Her arm (on the side of the breast to be examined) is placed behind her head to help provide a stable scanning surface.

A high-frequency, 5.0 or 7.5 MHz, small-diameter transducer is used to image the breast parenchyma. The time gain compensation is adjusted to balance the skin echo, subcutaneous fat, dense breast core or mammary layer, retromammary layer, and pectoral muscles. The sensitivity of the equipment is adjusted to visualize the low-level subcutaneous layer, the echogenic mammary layer, and bright reflection from the retromammary layer, and the medium-level reflection from the pectoral muscles.

The mass is localized and its boundaries noted with a marking pen. The area surrounding the mass in a 3 cm square is then marked off with the marking pen. Scans are made in the transverse direction beginning at the inferior margin and moving cephalad by the smallest intervals possible. Subsequent scans are made in the sagittal direction beginning at the medial border of the square and moving laterally by small intervals. Extreme care should be taken to scan very lightly over the breast area so as not to distort the architecture. If the mass is very mobile, you may need to isolate it between two fingers. This will secure the lesion so it will not slip from under the transducer as you are scanning. The following characteristics of the mass should be noted: shape, size, definition of borders, amount of transmission or attenuation, presence or absence of internal echoes, and degree of reflection from the anterior or posterior wall. Because the mass must be evaluated carefully, it is important to assess these characteristics when the beam is directly over the major part of the lesion. Small lesions, under 1 cm, may not be easily visualized by this technique because of the wide beam width, which fails to visualize a mass smaller than the transducer diameter.

Ultrasonic Description of the Normal Breast

There are many variations in the normal breast, and these must be fully appreciated to interpret the sonographic image and differentiate normal patterns from pathologic processes. The breast of a premenopausal patient is discussed in detail.

The boundaries of the breast are the skin line, nipple, and retromammary layer. These generally give strong, bright echo reflections. The areolar area may be recognized by the slightly lower echo reflection as compared with the nipple and skin. The internal nipple may show low to bright reflections and is quite variable (Fig. 13-5).

Subcutaneous fat displays areas of generally low reflectivity intermixed with bright reflections from Cooper's ligaments and other connective tissue (Fig. 13-6). Cooper's ligaments are seen if the beam strikes them at a perpendicular angle. Often compression of the breast allows even more ligaments to be visualized.

The mammary layer, often referred to as the *breast core* or *active glandular breast tissue,* is generally displayed as a somewhat cone-shaped or triangular area beneath the subcutaneous fat layer and anterior to the retromammary layer. It is shown to converge toward the nipple (Fig. 13-7). The fatty tissue interspersed throughout the mammary layer dictates the amount of intensity reflected from the breast parenchyma. If little fat is present, there is a uniform architecture with a strong echogenic pattern (because of colla-

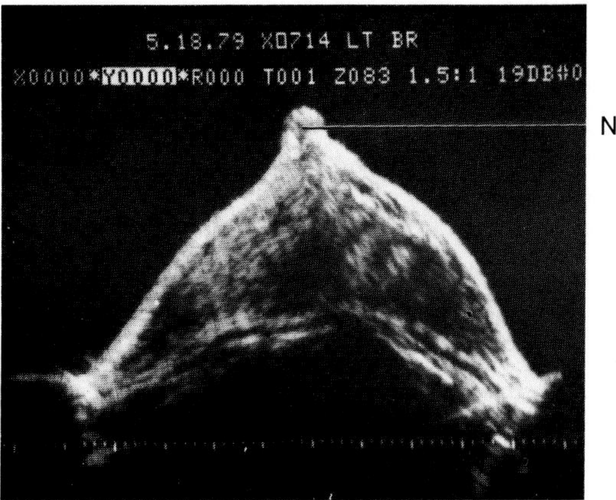

FIG. 13-5 Transverse scan of a noncompressed breast nipple, *N*.

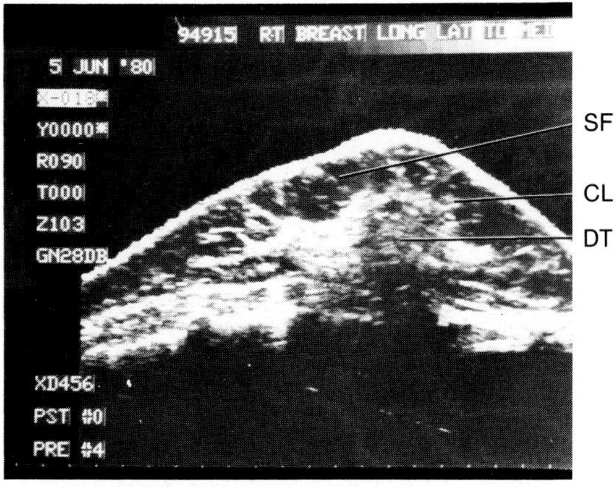

FIG. 13-6 Subcutaneous fat, *SF*, displays areas of low reflectivity interspersed with bright reflectors from Cooper's ligament, *CL*. Dense tissue, *DT*.

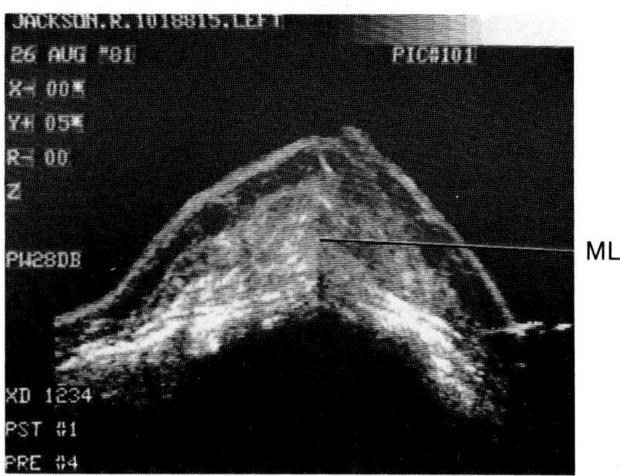

FIG. 13-7 Transverse scan of the mammary layer of the breast, *ML*.

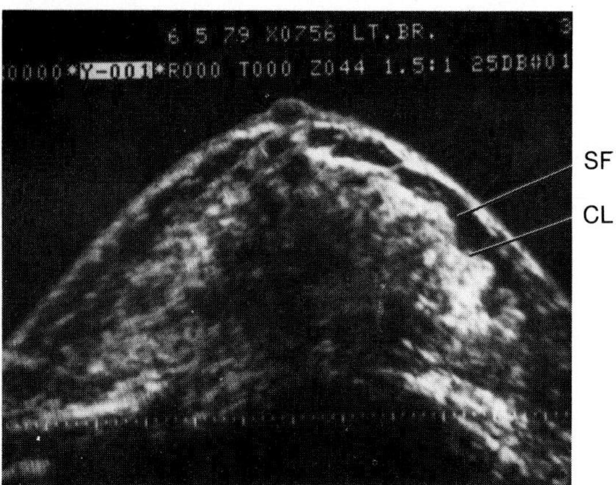

FIG. 13-8 Dense breast. Subcutaneous fat; *SF*. Cooper's ligament, *CL*.

gen and fibrotic tissue) throughout the mammary layer. When fatty tissue is present, areas of low-level echoes become intertwined with areas of strong echoes from the active breast tissue. The analysis of this pattern becomes critical to the final diagnosis, and one must be able to separate lobules of fat from a marginated lesion.

The retromammary layer is similar in texture to the subcutaneous layer, although the boundary echoes resemble skin reflections. The pectoral muscles are shown as low-level echo areas posterior to the retromammary layer. Ribs and intercostal margins are seen as bright and anechoic areas posterior to the pectoral muscles.

The echo appearance of the breast does change with age: the younger the patient, the greater the volume of the mammary layer, the denser the breast, and the more effective sonography is over mammography (Fig. 13-8). The older patient has more fatty tissue, and it is more difficult to distinguish disruptions in architecture than in the younger denser breast (Fig. 13-9).

Many breast lesions occur diffusely within the breast parenchyma (i.e., fibrous infiltration and fibrocystic disease). The recognition of these processes involves assessing the magnitude, texture, and distribution of echoes throughout the breast core.

Changes associated with a diffuse breast lesion may be characterized by the following:

1. Increase in fibrotic tissue (more echogenic)
2. Increase in amplitude of echoes
3. Increase in fatty tissue (less echogenic)

Usually fatty infiltrations are not well circumscribed. Diffuse conditions lack the uniformity and texture seen in normal breast tissue.

Localized lesions may exhibit cystic or solid appearances depending on their particular characteristics. The lesions should be observed using the following criteria:

1. Boundary echoes
2. Attenuation or transmission characteristics
3. Shape and position of the lesion
4. Disruption of normal architecture

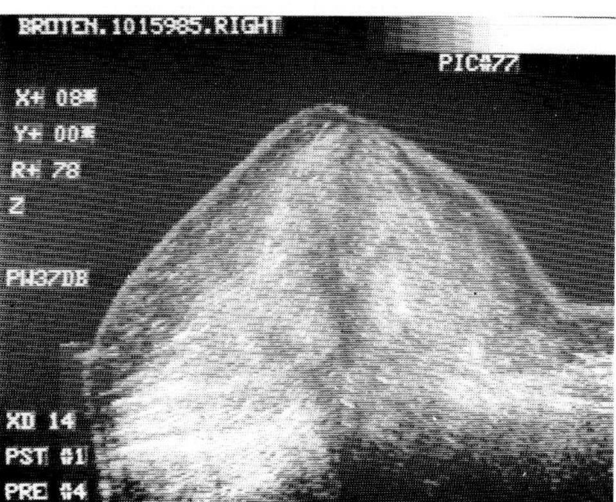

FIG. 13-9 Fatty replaced breast.

5. Nature of surrounding tissues
6. Homogeneity
7. Presence of calcifications
8. Skin changes

Each of these changes is discussed in the next section as they relate to cystic versus solid lesions and the distinction between benign and malignant breast lesions.

PATHOLOGY OF BREAST MASSES

The most common pathologic lesions of the female breast are, in order of decreasing frequency, fibrocystic disease, carcinoma, fibroadenoma, intraductal papilloma, and duct ectasia.[11] Benign lesions are the most common breast lesions, occurring in 70% of proved lesions biopsied or removed. Several parameters must be considered when a dominant mass has been palpated: patient's age, physical characteristics of the mass, and previous medical history. Lesions more common to younger women are fibrocystic disease and fibroadenomas. Older or postmenopausal women are more likely to have intraductal papillomas, duct ectasia, and cancer.

The benign and malignant masses are discussed with their clinical findings and symptoms, mammographic findings,[4] and ultrasound findings.

CHARACTERISTIC SIGNS OF BREAST MASSES[4]

Contour or margin
- Smooth
- Irregular
- Spiculated

Shape
- Round
- Oval
- Tubular
- Lobulated

Internal echo pattern
- Anechoic (homogeneous)
  - Strong
  - Intermediate
  - Weak
  - Mixed

Boundary echoes
- Anterior and/or posterior
  - Strong
  - Weak
  - Absent

Attenuation effects
- Acoustic enhancement
- Acoustic shadowing
  - Central
  - Bilateral
  - Unilateral

Distal echoes
- Strong
- Intermediate
- Weak
- Absent

Disruption of architecture

Differential Diagnosis of Breast Masses

Symptoms of breast masses include pain, a palpable mass, spontaneous or induced nipple discharge, skin dimpling, ulceration, or nipple retraction. The benign process is usually associated with pain, tumor, and nipple discharge. Skin dimpling or ulceration and nipple retraction nearly always result from cancer. Solid tumors are rubbery, mobile, and well delineated (as seen in a fibroadenoma) or stone hard and irregular (as in a carcinoma). Soft tumors usually represent a lipoma (fat tissue). Cystic masses are like a balloon of water, well delineated but not as mobile as fibroadenomas because they form part of the breast parenchyma, whereas a fibroadenoma has a capsule.

BENIGN DISEASE

Cystic Disease

Cystic disease is commonly seen in women 35 to 55 years of age. Symptoms include history of a changing menstrual cycle, pain (especially when the cyst is growing rapidly), recent lump, and tenderness. The disease may be microcystic or macrocystic. The small cyst may regress incompletely during the premenstrual phase. In the microcystic form the cysts are multiple with some pain and tenderness of the breast. The macrocystic form has three-dimensional lesions, which are well-delineated and slightly mobile (Fig. 13-10). These cysts may be aspirated for analysis of the fluid.

Mammographic Findings

1. Usually smooth walled with sharp borders
2. A cyst and noncalcified fibroadenoma are hard to differentiate
3. Lucent rim of fat around cyst

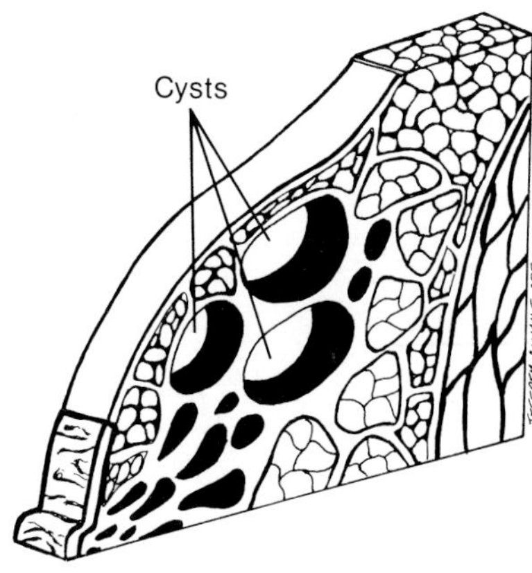

FIG. 13-10 Schema of multiple cysts in a breast. (Modified from Townsend CM: Clin Symp 32:1, 1980.)

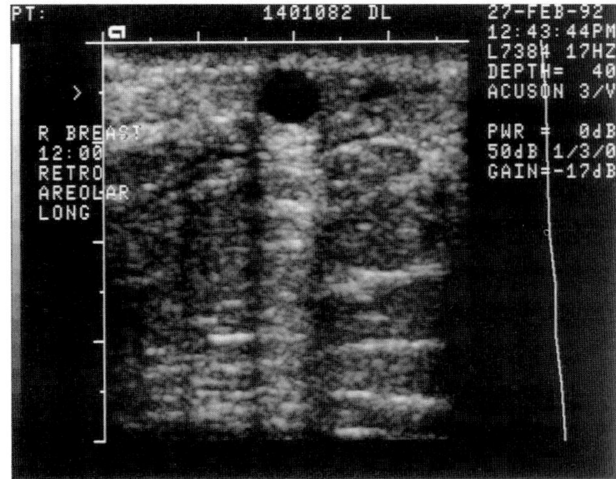

FIG. 13-11 Transverse scan of the right breast. The cystic lesion is noted at the 12 o'clock position. The borders are smooth and well defined, the through-transmission is good, and there are no internal echoes within the mass. The shadowing seen along either side of the cyst is from the beam divergence as it strikes the curved lateral borders.

Ultrasound Findings[5]

1. Smooth, sharp, well-defined borders (Figs. 13-11 through 13-15)
2. Lateral edge shadowing (arises from the low-energy loss as the beam passes normally through the distal cyst wall, leaving sufficient energy to cause multireflections between the distal cyst wall and the chest wall[6])
3. Anechoic
4. Posterior enhancement

Fibrocystic Disease

Fibrocystic disease produces histologic changes in the terminal ducts and lobules of the breast in both the epithelial and the connective tissue. It is usually accompanied by pain in the breast.

Its etiology is thought to be a disturbance in the estrogen-progesterone balance, since it does not occur during pu-

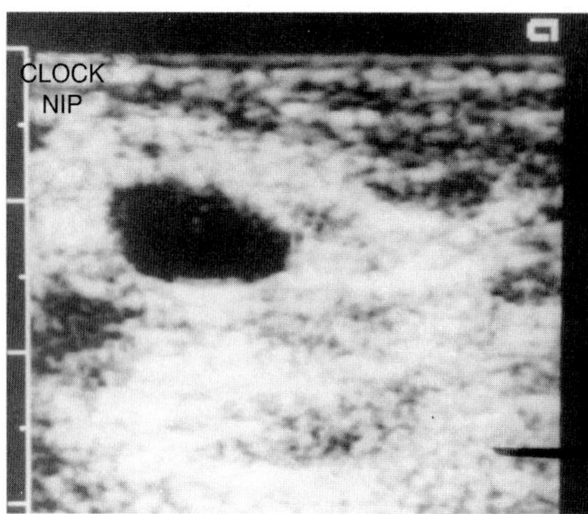

FIG. 13-12 Transverse scan of the small cyst in the breast. This scan shows the gain increased too high, causing the borders to become somewhat irregular.

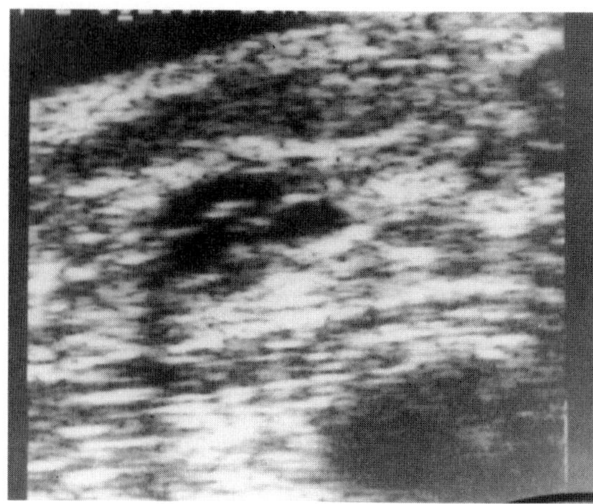

FIG. 13-14 Transverse scans along the right upper quadrant show three small cystic structures clustered together. The increased transmission is not apparent until you look beyond the posterior border.

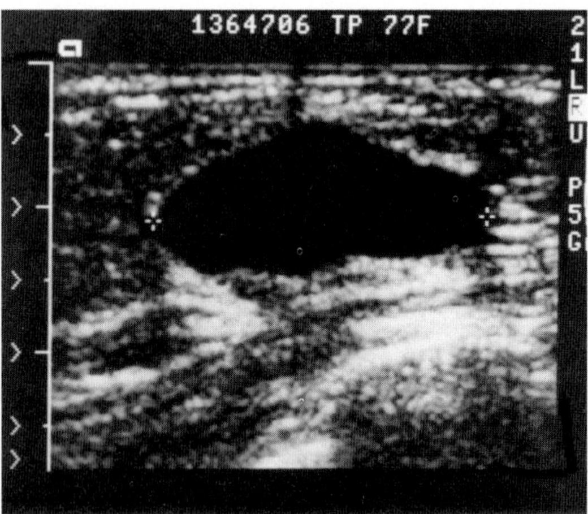

FIG. 13-13 This breast mass was seen in a 77-year-old female. It fulfills all of the qualifications of a cystic lesion except for the increased through-transmission. There is not increased transmission because the mass is lying next to the pectoralis major muscle group (this muscle absorbs some of the sound transmission).

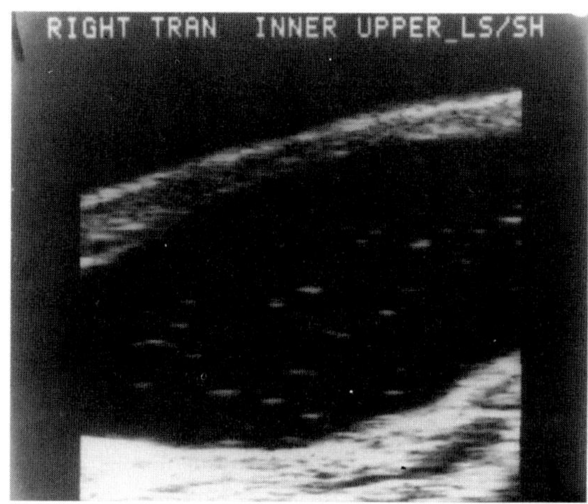

FIG. 13-15 The cystic mass developed low-level echoes within secondary to hemorrhage after biopsy.

berty. It is a cyclic dysplasia, with signs and symptoms that vary according to the menstrual cycle. (Other diseases, such as mammary dysplasia, fibroadenoma, cystosarcoma phylloides, and papillomas, do not change with the menstrual cycle.)

The changes in fibrocystic disease occur in the breast parenchyma according to the patient's age. General symptoms are pain, nodularity, a dominant mass, cysts, and occasional nipple discharge.

There are three distinct stages. Stage 1, mazoplasia or mastodynia, is characterized by increased proliferation of the stroma and by the small number of lobules or acini.[10] Stage 2, adenosis, entails hyperplasia and proliferation for the epithelial component of the ducts.[10] Stage 3, cystic disease, involves the involution of the lobules and hyperplasia of the surrounding stroma, leading to the formation of cysts [10] (Fig. 13-13).

Another facet of fibrocystic disease is the dilation of the ducts, known as *comedomastitis*. This is seen in middle-aged women and is characterized by the dilation of ducts filled with a secretion produced by desquamated cells from the duct wall. The secretion is manifested clinically by a multicolored and sticky nipple discharge. It often is accompanied by a retroareolar or periareolar redness and burning pain and itching. If untreated, the terminal ducts dilate and thicken. If the process is chronic, the ducts become tortuous (varicocele of Bloodgood) and may cause nipple retraction that simulates cancer.

Fibrocystic disease is a benign condition, although a patient with duct hyperplasia and atypia has a five-times greater risk of developing breast cancer.[10]

Apocrine metaplasia with atypia carries a slightly decreased risk. The condition has been termed *precancerous mastopathy* by Haagensen.[3]

Gross cystic disease and breast cancer occur in the same

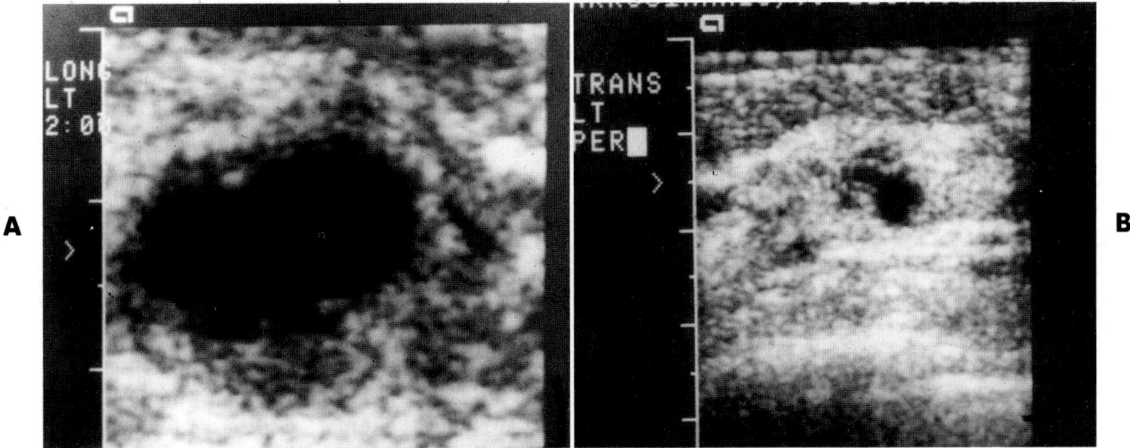

FIG. 13-16 A, This middle-aged female presented with cyclic breast tenderness. Both breasts demonstrated multiple cystic lesions throughout the mammary glandular tissue representative of fibrocystic disease. This image shows one large cyst, with a smaller cyst along its lateral border. **B,** This image shows the somewhat irregular cyst compressed by two smaller cysts. This pattern was present throughout the breast.

age group of patients, 40 to 50 years. Thus the method for diagnosis and treatment must be specific, to rule out a benign process versus a malignant one.

In the stage of mastodynia or mazoplasia the breasts are very painful, especially in the premenstrual period. The upper outer quadrants seem to be the most sensitive. This process is commonly seen in young women. Since it is a benign condition, it may subside spontaneously with time, medication, or pregnancy.

Stage 2, adenosis, is commonly seen in women 25 to 40 years of age. The pain is premenstrual and less severe. The patient may also have nipple discharge. (To be clinically significant, the discharge must be spontaneous and unprovoked.) The breast parenchyma is more pronounced and irregular because of nodularity. The nodules are usually of small size; they are considered more dominant as they reach 1 cm.

If the hyperplasia is surrounded by an intense proliferation of fibrous tissue, these areas may form a dominant mass that may be mistaken clinically for cancer. It is helpful to distinguish a tumor, which has three dimensions (height, width, and depth) and occupies space, whereas a mass has only two dimensions (height and width) and represents thickening.

Mammographic Findings

1. Scattered fine, coarse, round, or lobulated densities and masses in combination with proliferation of parenchyma and linear strands of fibrous (stromal) tissue

Ultrasound Findings (Fig. 13-16)

1. Average amount of subcutaneous fat
2. Areas of fibrous stroma that appear brighter than the parenchyma
3. Small cysts scattered throughout the breast (cystic stage)
4. Large cysts may also be present

Fibroadenoma

Fibroadenoma is one of the most common benign breast tumors, the most common in childhood, and occurs primarily in young adult women. It may be found in one breast only or bilaterally.

The growth of the fibroadenoma is stimulated by the administration of estrogen. Under normal circumstances hormonal influences on the breast (estrogen) result in the proliferation of epithelial cells in lactiferous ducts and in stromal tissue during the first half of the menstrual cycle. During the second half this condition regresses, allowing breast tissue to return to its normal resting state. In certain disturbances of this hormonal mechanism the regression fails to occur and results in the development of fibrous and epithelial nodules that become fibroadenomas, fibromas, or adenomas, depending on the predominant cell type. They may also be related to pregnancy and lactation.

Clinically the fibroadenoma is firm, rubbery, freely mobile, and clearly delineated from the surrounding breast tissue (Fig. 13-17). It is round or ovoid, smooth or lobulated, and usually does not cause loss of contour of the breast unless it develops to a large size. It rarely causes mastodynia, and it does not change size during the menstrual cycle. It grows very slowly. A sudden increase in size with acute pain may be a result of hemorrhage within the tumor. Calcification may follow hemorrhage or infarction, and thus the tumor may mimic a carcinoma.

Mammographic Findings

1. Smooth contour
2. Difficult to differentiate from a cyst (except when lobulated)
3. May contain calcium deposits, which make differential diagnosis easier; as degeneration of tumor progresses, size and number of deposits increase

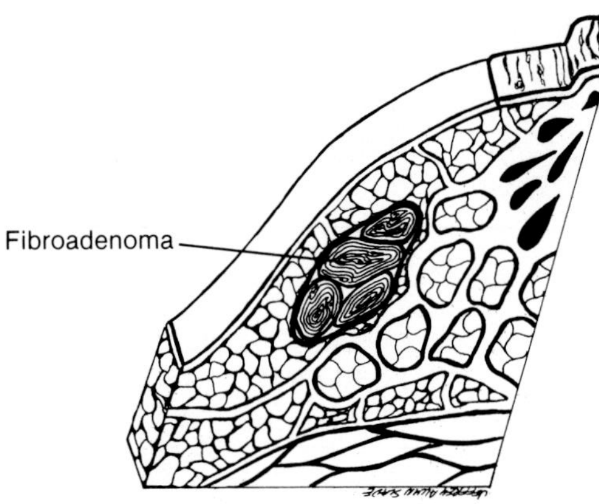

FIG. 13-17 Schema of a fibroadenoma. The lesion is palpated as a solitary, smooth, firm, well-demarcated nodule. (Modified from Townsend CM: Clin Symp 32:1, 1980.)

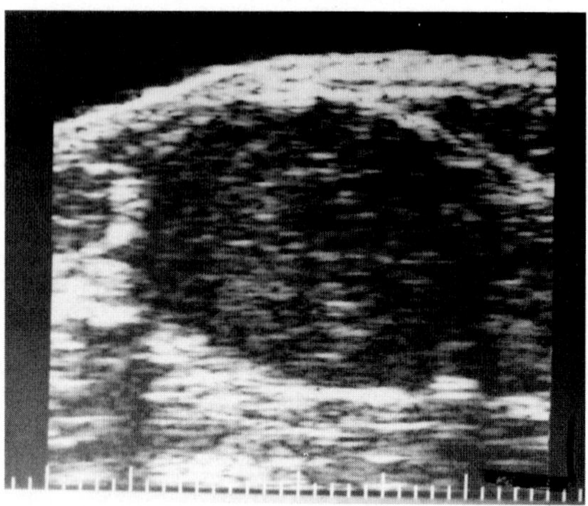

FIG. 13-18 Transverse view of a large fibroadenoma. The mass has smooth borders, uniform low-level echoes, and decreased through-transmission.

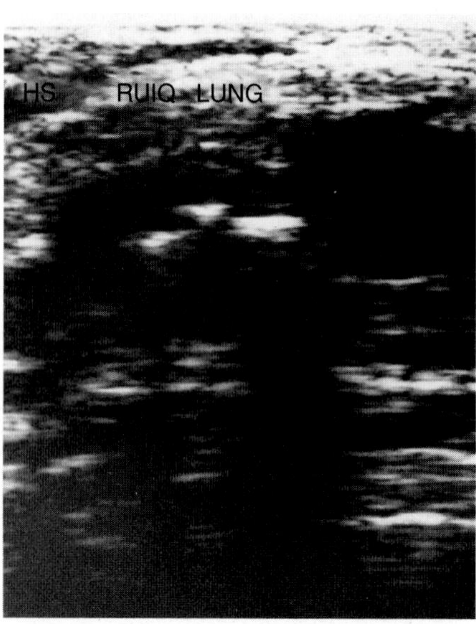

FIG. 13-19 Another characteristic finding in a fibroadenoma is the presence of calcifications, as shown in this image. The dense shadows are seen posterior to the bright calcifications.

Ultrasound Findings[2]

1. Smooth or lobulated borders (Figs. 13-18 and 13-19)
2. Strong anterior wall
3. Intermediate posterior enhancement
4. Low-level homogeneous internal echoes (sometimes strong)

Lipoma

A pure lipoma is entirely composed of fatty tissue. Other forms of lipoma consist of fat with fibrous and glandular elements interspersed (fibroadenolipoma). The lipoma may assume a large size before it is clinically detected. It is usually found in middle-aged or menopausal women.

Clinically, on palpation a large, soft, poorly demarcated mass is felt that cannot be clearly separated from the surrounding parenchyma. There is no thinning or fixation of the overlying skin.

Mammographic Findings

1. Sharply defined capsule
2. Radiolucent (fat cells)
3. No calcification; appears benign and homogeneous
4. May extend to beneath the skin and displace the subcutaneous fat

Ultrasound Findings

1. Difficult or impossible to detect in the fatty breast
2. Internal low-level echo content similar to that of fat
3. Posterior enhancement
4. Smooth walls

Fat Necrosis

Fat necrosis may be caused by trauma to the breast or plasma cell mastitis, or it may be related to an involutional process or other disease present in the breast, such as cancer. It is more frequently found in older women.

Clinical palpation reveals a spherical nodule that is generally superficial under a layer of calcified necrosis. A deep-lying focus of necrosis may cause scarring with skin retraction and thus mimic carcinoma.

Mammographic Findings

1. Area of nodular fibrosis or typical linear cystlike calcifications

Ultrasound Findings

1. Irregular complex mass with low-level echoes
2. May mimic a malignant lesion
3. May appear as fat but is separate and different from the rest of the breast parenchyma

Acute Mastitis

Acute mastitis may result from infection, trauma, mechanical obstruction in the breast ducts, or other reasons. It often occurs during lactation, beginning in the lactiferous ducts and spreading via the lymphatics or blood. Acute mastitis is often confined to one area of the breast.

Diffuse mastitis results from the infection being carried via the blood or breast lymphatics and thus affecting the entire breast.

Mammographic Findings
1. Increased density, ill-defined
2. Difficult to diagnose in the dense lactating breast unless sufficient fat is interspersed to provide differences in density
3. Skin thickening resulting from edema

Chronic Mastitis

An inflammation of the glandular tissue is considered to be chronic mastitis. It is very difficult to differentiate by ultrasound; the echo pattern is mixed and diffuse with sound absorption. It usually is found in elderly women. There is a thickening of the connective tissue that results in narrowing of the lumina of the milk ducts. The cause is inspissated intraductal secretions, which are forced into the periductal connective tissue.

Clinically the patient usually has a nipple discharge, and frequently the nipple has retracted over a period of years. Palpation reveals some subareolar thickening but no dominant mass.

Mammographic Findings
1. Coarse road type of calcifications
2. Skin thickening
3. Nipple retraction (may or may not be present)

Abscess

An abscess may be single or multiple. Acute abscesses have a poorly defined border, whereas mature abscesses are well encapsulated with sharp borders. A definite diagnosis cannot be made from the mammogram alone. Aspiration is needed.

Clinical findings show pain, swelling, and reddening of the overlying skin. The patient may be febrile, and swollen painful axillary nodes may be present.

Ultrasound Findings (Figs. 13-20 and 13-21)
1. Diffuse mottled appearance of the breast
2. Dense breast
3. Irregular borders (some may be smooth)
4. Posterior enhancement
5. May have low-level internal echoes

Cystosarcoma Phyllodes

Cystosarcoma phyllodes is an uncommon breast neoplasm, yet it is the most frequent sarcoma of the breast. It is more commonly found in women in their fifties and usually is unilateral. It may arise from a fibroadenoma, as well as de novo. Many patients may notice a small breast mass that has been present for a long time suddenly begin to grow rapidly. At least 27% of these tumors are malignant; 12% metastasize.

When the tumor is small, it is well delineated, firm, and mobile, much like a fibroadenoma. As it enlarges, the surface may become irregular and lobulated. Skin changes can develop from increasing pressure. Edema may produce a skin change. As pressure increases, it causes tropic changes and eventual skin ulcerations. Infection and abscess formation may be a secondary complication. The tumor never adheres to the adjacent soft tissue or underlying pectoral muscle; therefore dimpling of the skin or fixation of the tumor is not observed.[10]

Mammographic Findings
1. May be solitary and extremely large or a conglomerate of several masses
2. Borders smooth and sharp

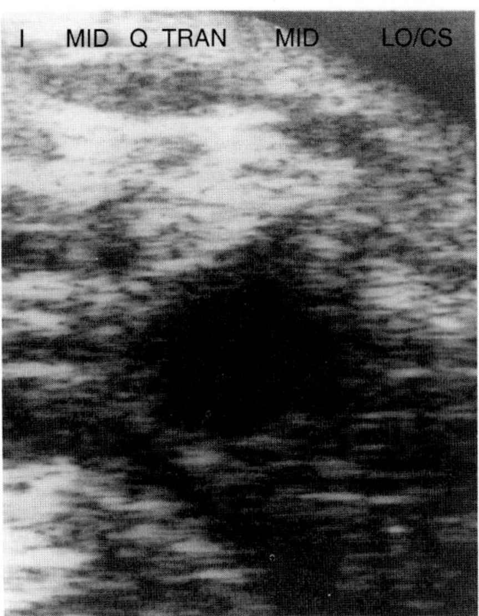

FIG. 13-20 Ill-defined abscess appears with a variety of patterns, depending on the consistency of the abscess. This lesion has irregular borders and decreased through-transmission. The patient had a biopsy performed 2 days earlier and presented with a red, swollen, tender breast.

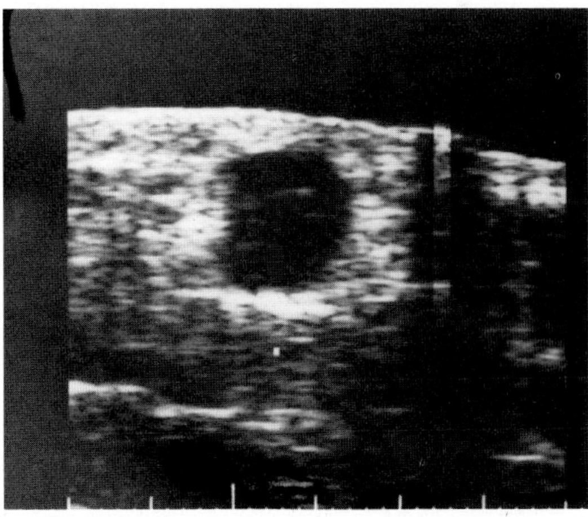

FIG. 13-21 This patient had a biopsy of her breast cyst 1 week earlier. A well-defined mass with low-level internal echoes is seen in the area of the biopsy.

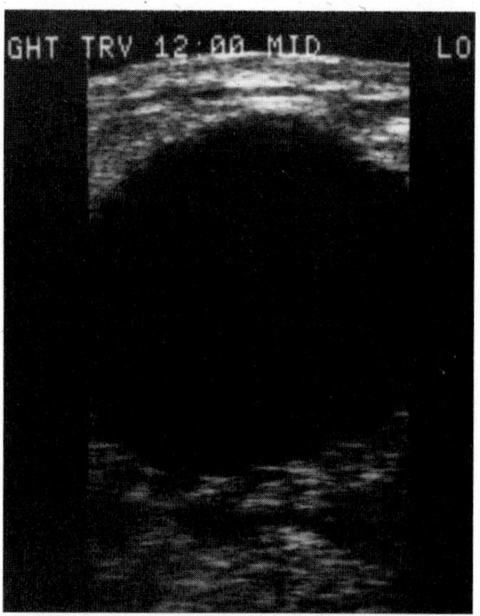

FIG. 13-22 A cystosarcoma phyllode appears as a mass with low-level or anechoic internal echoes, a weak posterior margin, and associated architectural disruption. This lesion generally presents as a very large mass in the breast.

3. Calcifications not usually seen as with fibroadenomas
4. Overlying skin thickened and stretched
5. More difficult to recognize in the young dense breast, where tumor occupies most of the breast

Ultrasound Findings (Fig. 13-22)

1. Borders somewhat irregular
2. Anechoic or low level
3. Usually very large
4. Weak posterior margin
5. Architectural disruption

Intraductual Papilloma

Intraductal papilloma occurs most frequently in women 40 to 50 years of age. The predominant symptom is spontaneous nipple discharge arising from a single duct. When the discharge is copious, it is usually preceded by a sensation of fullness or pain in the areola or nipple area and is relieved as the fluid is expelled.

Papillomas are usually small, multiple, and multicentric. They consist of simple proliferations of duct epithelium projecting outward into a dilated lumen from one or more focal points (Fig. 13-23), each supported by a vascular stalk from which it receives the blood supply. Trauma may rupture the stalk, filling the duct with blood or serum. Papillomas may also grow to a large size and thus become palpable lesions. They are somewhat linear, resembling the terminal duct, and are usually benign.

MALIGNANT DISEASE

Malignant disease generally develops over a long period. It is not unusual for several years to pass from the first appearance of atypical hyperplasia to the final diagnosis of in situ cancer.

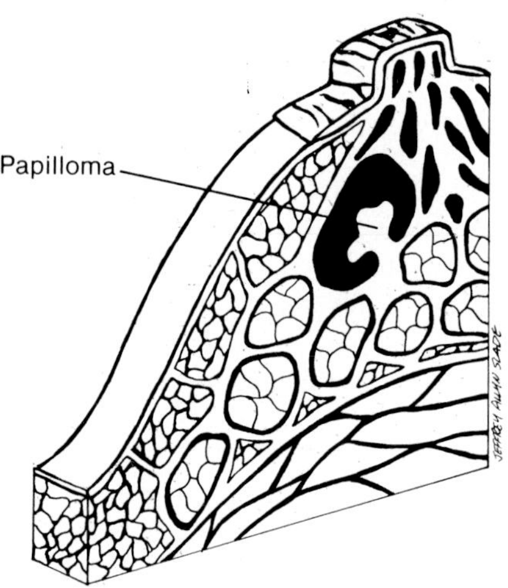

FIG. 13-23 Solitary intraductal papilloma. (Modified from Townsend CM: Clin Symp 32:1, 1980.)

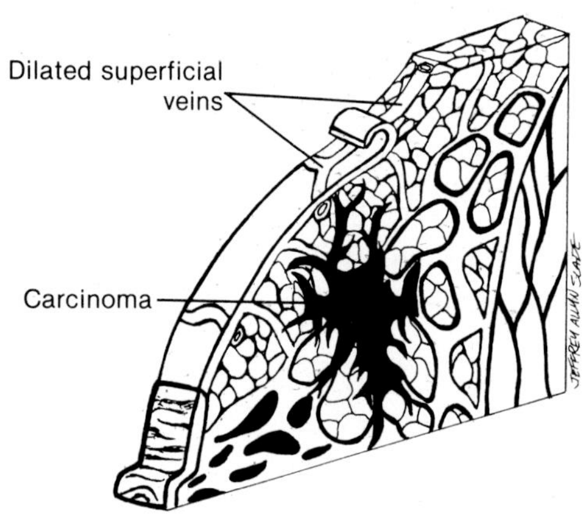

FIG. 13-24 Vascular signs of malignant disease. (Modified from Townsend CM: Clin Symp 32:1, 1980.)

Malignant cells grow along a line of least resistance, such as in fatty tissue. In fibrotic tissue, most cancer growth occurs along the borders. Lymphatics and blood vessels are frequently used as pathways for new tumor development (Fig. 13-24). If the tumor is encapsulated, it continues to grow in one area, compressing and distorting the surrounding architecture. When the carcinoma is contained and has not invaded the basal membrane structure, it is considered in situ. Most cancer originates in the ducts, whereas a smaller percentage originates in the glandular tissue.

Cancer of the breast is of two types: sarcoma and carcinoma. *Sarcoma* refers to breast tumors that arise from the supportive or connective tissues. Sarcoma is the usual type, growing rapidly and invading fibrous tissue. *Carcinoma* refers to breast tumors that arise from the epithelium, in the ductal and glandular tissue, and usually has tentacles. Other malignant diseases affecting the breast are a result of systemic neoplasms, such as leukemia or lymphoma.

Cancer is further classified as infiltrating and noninfiltrating. Infiltrating carcinoma has infiltrated the tissue beyond the basement membrane and into adjacent tissue. Chances of metastases are enhanced with the time and type of growth present. Infiltrating carcinomas are histologically designated into several types. Some produce more fibrosis and therefore are categorized as infiltrating ductal carcinoma with productive fibrosis. Others, such as medullary carcinoma, have little associated fibrosis. Colloid carcinoma is a type of cancer in which mucin production occurs and the fibrotic reaction may be variable. Over 80% of carcinomas fall into the category of infiltrating ductal carcinoma with productive fibrosis. Noninfiltrating carcinoma is carcinoma of the lactiferous ducts that has not infiltrated the basement membrane but is proliferating within the confines of the ducts and their branches. There is no danger of metastases under these circumstances. This also may be referred to as *carcinoma in situ*. Most in situ lesions develop from longstanding epithelial hyperplasia of ducts and lobules.

The more favorable cancers, which remain localized to the breast longer and have a 75% survival rate after 10 years, represent only 10% to 12% of all breast cancer.[1] This group includes medullary, intracystic papillary, papillary, colloid, adenoid cystic, and tubular carcinoma.

Malignant cystosarcoma phyllodes and stromal sarcomas rarely metastasize to regional nodes and have a better than average prognosis after treatment. Occasional spread to distant areas of the body has been reported with these tumors.

The exact type of tumor can be determined only by a histologic diagnosis, not by other noninvasive means. It is the role of mammography and ultrasound to clarify whether a mass is present and whether it has cystic or solid characteristics; then a differential can be made as to its benign or malignant probabilities.

The characteristics most often seen by ultrasound in a malignant mass are as follows:

1. Irregular spiculated contour or margin
2. Round or lobulated
3. Weak nonuniform internal echoes
4. Intermediate anterior and absent or weak posterior boundary echoes
5. Great attenuation effects

The exception to this list of criteria is medullary carcinoma. Because of its cellularity and occasional encapsulation, it may present more like a fibroadenoma. Its characteristics are smooth borders and round uniform to absent internal echoes.

Intraductal Solid Carcinoma (Comedocarcinoma)

In intraductal solid carcinoma, macroscopically the lactiferous ducts are filled with a yellow pastelike material that looks like small plugs (comedones) when sectioned. Histologically the ducts are filled with plugs of epithelial tumor that have a central necrosis, giving rise to the pastelike material. Both invasive and noninvasive forms exist.

The clinical picture depends on the stage of the disease.

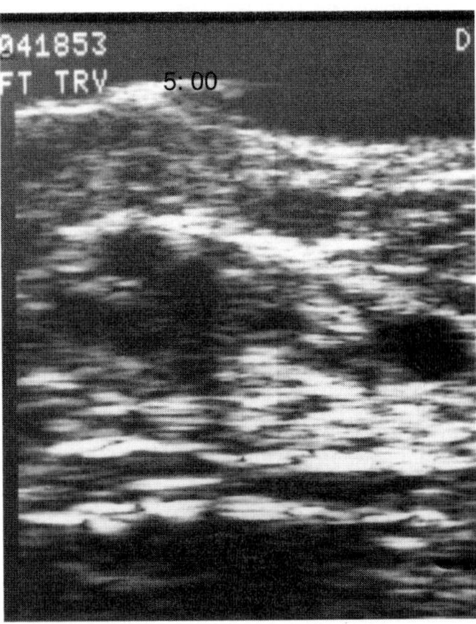

FIG. 13-25 Intraductal carcinoma appears as a mass with irregular borders, diffuse internal echoes, and attenuation with shadowing.

Noninvasive forms may lack any clinical or palpatory findings. If there is a nipple discharge, it is more frequently clear than bloody (unlike papillary carcinoma, in which bloody discharge is typical). The patient may complain of pain or the sensation of insects crawling on the breast. With early invasion, minimal thickening of the surrounding breast tissue may be palpated. In the advanced stage the clinical signs are nipple retraction, dominant mass, and fixation.

Mammographic Findings

1. Microcalcifications

Ultrasound Findings

1. Irregular border (Fig. 13-25)
2. Diffuse internal echo pattern
3. Attenuation with shadowing

Juvenile Breast Cancer

Juvenile breast cancer is similar to the intraductal carcinoma and infiltrating ductal carcinoma found in adults. Generally it occurs in young females, between 8 and 15 years of age, and has a good prognosis when treated.

Papillary Carcinoma

Papillary carcinoma is a tumor that initially arises as an intraductal mass. It may also take the form of an intracystic tumor, but that is rare.

The early stage of papillary carcinoma is noninfiltrating. The tumor occasionally arises from a benign ductal papilloma. It is associated with little fibrotic reaction.

Both intraductal and intracystic forms exist, and these represent 1% to 2% of all breast carcinomas. The earliest clinical sign of intraductal papillary carcinoma is bloody nipple discharge. Occasionally a mass can be palpated as a small, firm, well-circumscribed area; this may be mistaken for a fibroadenoma. There may be nodules of blue or red discoloration under the skin with central ulceration. A diffusely nodular appearance overlying the skin is a special variant of multiple intraductal papillary carcinoma. Intracystic papillary carcinoma is clinically indistinguishable in its early stages from a cyst or fibroadenoma. When the tumor has invaded through the cyst wall, it is palpable as a poorly circumscribed mass.

Mammographic Findings

1. Intraductal—not often diagnosed in early stages
2. Intracystic—recognized when invasion beyond the wall of the cyst occurs; the sharp contours of the cyst are lost because of surrounding edema and infiltration

Ultrasound Findings

1. Irregular borders
2. Heterogeneous internal echo pattern
3. Attenuation with acoustic shadowing

Paget's Disease

Paget's disease arises in the superficial subareolar or deeper lactiferous ducts and grows in the direction of the nipple, spreading into the intraepidermal region of the nipple and areola. It may be confused with a melanoma.

The disease induces changes of the nipple and areola. Any ulceration, enlargement, or deformity of the nipple and areola should suggest Paget's disease. This is a relatively rare tumor, accounting for 2.5% of all breast cancers. It occurs in older women, over 50 years of age. Differential diagnosis includes benign inflammatory eczematous condition of the nipple, since palpatory findings are frequently not present. The primary duct cancer may be quite deep or embedded in fibrotic tissue.

Mammographic Findings

1. Thickened areolar tissue resulting from eczema or tumor infiltration
2. Solid tumor mass occasionally
3. Microcalcifications (if seen in either a punctate or a linear display, strongly suggestive of duct carcinoma)

Ultrasound Findings

1. Irregular borders
2. Heterogeneous internal echoes
3. Attenuation with posterior shadow
4. Subareolar solid mass
5. Skin echo thin and deformed, suggesting infiltration

Scirrhous Carcinoma

Scirrhous carcinoma is a type of duct tumor with extensive fibrous tissue proliferation (productive fibrosis). Focal calcification may also be present. Histologically the cells are found in narrow files or strands, clusters, or columns and may form lumina with varying frequency.

Scirrhous is the most common form of breast cancer. The classical clinical signs are a firm, nodular, frequently nonmovable mass often with fixation, as well as flattening of overlying skin and nipple retraction. The retraction is a result of an infiltrative shortening of Cooper's ligaments because of productive fibrosis (Fig. 13-26). Fixation and retraction of the nipple may be the result of a subareolar carcinoma but may also be caused by benign fibrosis of the breast. It is important to note that some patients normally have inverted nipples. The size of the cancer may vary from a few millimeters to involvement of nearly the entire breast. The deep-lying scirrhous carcinoma may grow into and become fixed to the thoracic wall. A sanguineous discharge is rare in this tumor.

Mammographic Findings

1. Central mass with lobular and ill-defined contour from which numerous fibrous strands extend into surrounding breast tissue
2. Diagnosis easier in the fatty breast than in the dense breast
3. Microcalcification present in 35%

Ultrasound Findings

1. Irregular mass with ill-defined borders
2. Attenuation with posterior shadow
3. Disruption of architecture

Medullary Carcinoma

Medullary carcinoma is a densely cellular tumor containing large, round, or oval tumor cells. It usually is a well-circumscribed mass whose center is frequently necrotic, as well as hemorrhagic and cystic.

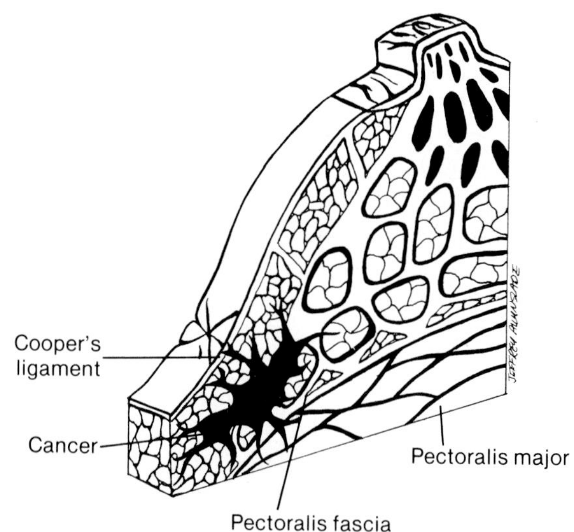

FIG. 13-26 Skin dimpling. (Modified from Townsend CM: Clin Symp 32:1, 1980.)

Medullary carcinomas are relatively rare, comprising less than 5% of breast cancers. The age of occurrence is slightly lower than for the average breast cancer. The skin fixation over the mass is an infrequent finding. It will occasionally reach large proportions and may have a diameter up to 10 cm. Discoloration of the overlying skin is often seen. Bilateral occurrence is more frequent than in other cancers.

Mammographic Findings

1. Round, oval, or lobulated mass
2. Margins appear to be smooth but with nonuniformity and adjacent edema
3. Connective tissue strands occasionally
4. In larger tumors, secondary signs of subcutaneous fatty tissue infiltration, skin thickening, and increased vascularity

Ultrasound Findings

1. May resemble fibroadenoma (Fig. 13-27; see color image.)
2. Well-defined border
3. Homogeneous internal echoes
4. Posterior enhancement

Colloid Carcinoma

Colloid carcinoma (mucinous) is also a type of duct carcinoma. The cells of the tumor produce secretions that fill lactiferous ducts or the stromal tissues that the tumor cells are invading.

Clinically it presents as a smooth not particularly firm mass at palpation. Because of its smooth, nonfibrosing nature, plateauing or fixation is not seen, as with scirrhous carcinoma.

Mammographic Findings

1. Smoothly contoured mass resembling a benign tumor

Ultrasound Findings

1. Similar to a fibroadenoma
2. Well-defined borders
3. Posterior enhancement

Lobular Carcinoma

Lobular carcinoma originates in the ductules of the lobules. When the basement membrane is not invaded and there are no signs of infiltration, the disease is called *lobular carcinoma in situ*. Secondary involvement of adjacent terminal ductules and neighboring lobules may occur. Multiple foci of lobular carcinoma throughout the breast are not rare.

It most commonly is found in women between the ages of 40 and 50. Frequently it is found in the upper outer quadrants, perhaps because in the involuted breast the residual breast tissue remains in the upper outer quadrants, whereas the other areas are replaced by fat. There are no typical clinical symptoms that indicate lobular carcinoma in situ. The indication for biopsy depends on abnormal palpatory findings. It commonly occurs bilaterally; thus prophylactic biopsy and mammography of the opposite breast are recommended.

Mammographic Findings

1. Microcalcifications (Some clinicians believe that the tumor is adjacent to the calcifications. However, it is not certain whether the calcifications occur as a result of the

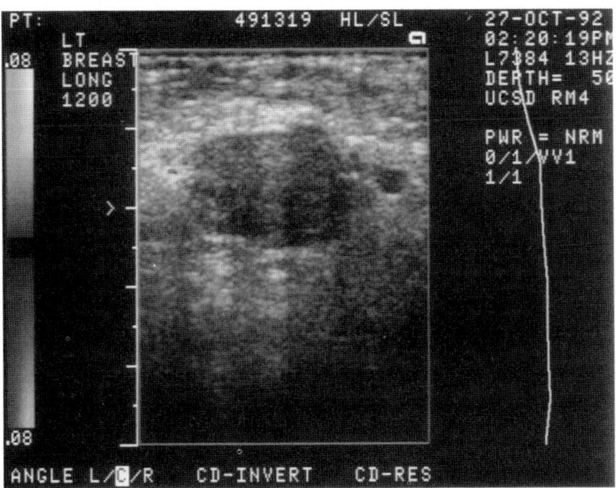

FIG. 13-27 Medullary carcinoma may resemble a fibroadenoma. The borders are well-defined, there are homogeneous internal echoes, and posterior enhancement may be present (see color image).

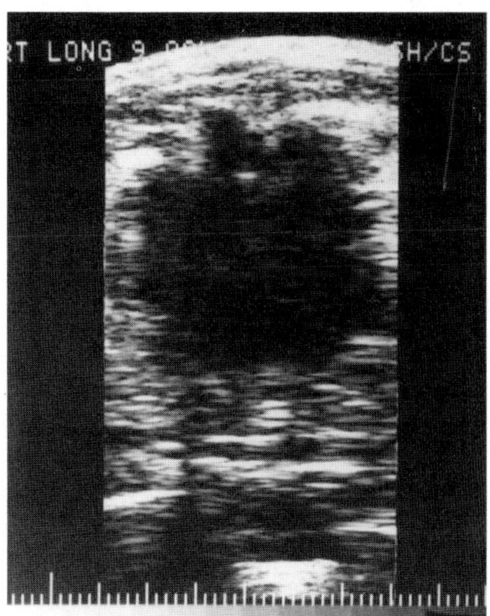

FIG. 13-28 Lobular carcinoma presents with weak internal echoes with irregular distribution; the anterior and lateral wall echoes may be irregular and disrupted. The posterior wall is weak to absent.

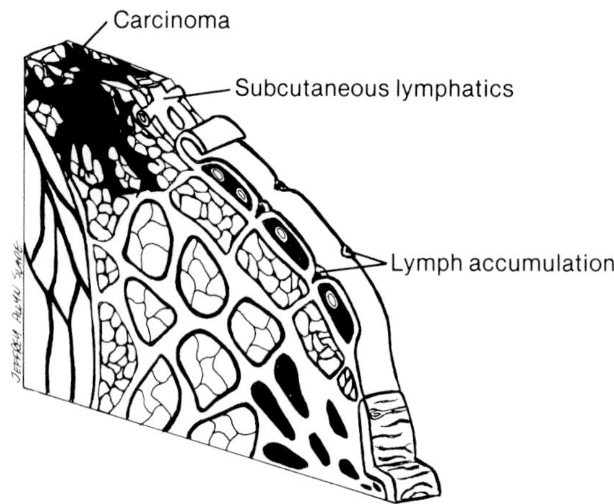

FIG. 13-29 Skin edema. (Modified from Townsend CM: Clin Symp 32:1, 1980.)

lobular carcinoma itself or whether the two processes have an increased tendency to occur together.)

Ultrasound Findings (Fig. 13-28)
1. Weak internal echo pattern, irregular distribution
2. Intermediate anterior and lateral wall echoes
3. Absent posterior wall
4. Irregular central shadow present
5. Tumor surrounded by bright punctate echoes of breast stroma, especially in the mammary layer

Diffuse Carcinoma

Diffuse carcinoma (inflammatory carcinoma) presents with all infiltrative types of breast carcinoma (e.g., scirrhous, medullary, colloid). Characteristically there is a diffuse spread of disease throughout the breast because of capillary invasion and involvement of lymphatics of the skin (Fig. 13-29).

It usually is found in middle-aged to older women. The breast is often very large, the progression of inflammatory carcinoma very rapid, and the course very short. The skin shows an erythematous blotchy pattern, and the nipple may be retracted. There is diffuse skin thickening.

Mammographic Findings
1. Generalized skin thickening
2. Parenchyma not as cloudy as with inflammatory mastitis, but proliferation of abnormal tissue of increased density
3. Occasionally a dominant mass from which the carcinoma originates
4. Sometimes malignant calcifications in linear or intraductal forms

Ultrasound Findings
1. If dominant mass present, borders irregular with high attenuation by shadow
2. Skin thickening in comparison with the normal breast

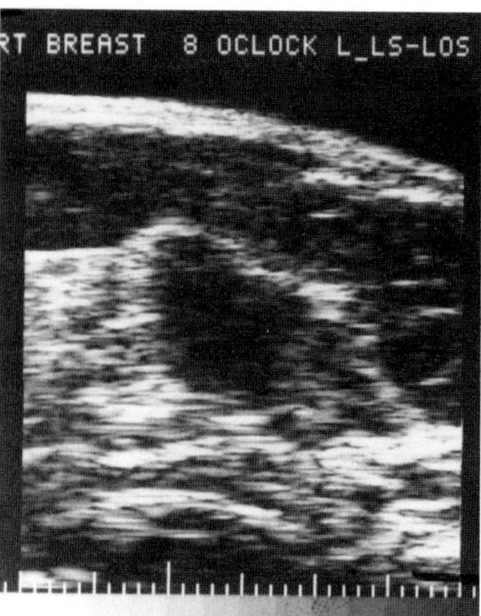

FIG. 13-30 The patient who presents with a breast mass that does not fulfill a simple cyst may elect to have a biopsy performed. Ultrasound can help the clinician define the boundaries of the lesion, describe how deep the lesion lies beneath the skin surface, and define the internal echo consistency of the lesion.

BIOPSY TECHNIQUES FOR BREAST TUMORS

Three events have occurred that affect the number and type of invasive diagnostic procedures used on women with breast masses (Fig. 13-30).

First, women are becoming more informed about their diagnostic choices. They are asking their physicians to order an ultrasound examination to determine whether the mass is cystic or solid before subjecting themselves to an excisional biopsy.

Second, as physicians have ultrasound available, they are more confident in its use and are more willing to perform a needle aspiration of a cystic area rather than the more invasive excisional biopsy. This judgment depends on the physical characteristics of the breast mass, the age of the patient, and the associated risk factors determined from the patient's history.

Third, needle biopsy is more acceptable to both patients and physicians. Although it is not as accurate as the open biopsy, it has become a useful diagnostic tool in breast lesions suspected of being carcinomatous. The advantages of the technique are that it is an office procedure, it is cost effective, it is simple to perform, and it is relatively atraumatic. Needle biopsy or excisional biopsy is the only reliable method for determining the exact malignancy of a breast mass.

REVIEW QUESTIONS

1. What is the incidence of breast cancer in the female population?
2. Describe the function of the female breast.
3. Name the three layers of the breast.

4. Describe the ligaments and inner structure of the normal breast.
5. Describe the four parenchymal patterns of the breast.
6. Name at least five risk factors associated with breast cancer.
7. How is ultrasound effective in imaging the breast? For what type of patients should ultrasound be requested?
8. Name the boundaries of the breast.
9. What is the ultrasound appearance of the subcutaneous fatty layer and Cooper's ligaments in the breast?
10. Describe the ultrasound appearance of the mammary layer.
11. Describe the changes associated with a diffuse breast lesion.
12. What criteria are used in determining the nature of the breast lesion?
13. Discuss the characteristic signs of breast masses and their significance in simple cyst, abscess or mastitis, benign lesions, and solid lesions.
14. Describe fibrocystic disease.

REFERENCES

1. Calderson D, Vilkomerson D, Mezrich R, et al: Differences in the attenuation of ultrasound by normal, benign, and malignant breast tissue, J Clin Ultrasound 4:249, 1976.
2. Cole-Beuglet CM, Goldberg BB, Patchefsky AS, et al: Atlas of breast ultrasound; correlation of anatomy, pathology, mammography, and ultrasonography, Denver, 1980, Technicare.
3. Haagensen ED: Diseases of the breast, ed 2, Philadelphia, 1971, WB Saunders.
4. Hoeffken W and Lanyi M: Mammography, Philadelphia, 1977, WB Saunders.
5. Jellins J, Kossoff G, and Reeve TS: Detection and classification of liquid filled masses in the breast by grey scale echography, Radiology 125:205, 1977.
6. Kobayashi T: Clinical ultrasound of the breast, New York, 1978, Plenum.
7. Laing FC: Ultrasonographic evaluation of breast masses, J Assoc Can Radiol 27:278, 1976.
8. Netter F: Reproductive system. In Ciba collection of medical illustrations, vol 2, Summit, NJ, 1965, Ciba Pharmaceutical.
9. Omni Education: Breast examination (module), New York, 1974, Ortho Pharmaceutical.
10. Pilnik S: Clinical diagnosis of benign breast diseases, J Reprod Med 22:277, 1979.
11. Townsend CM: Breast lumps, Clin Symp 32:1, 1980.

BIBLIOGRAPHY

Harper P, et al: Ultrasound visualization of the breast symptomatic patients, Radiology 137:1980.

Kelly-Frye E: Breast imaging. In Sabbagha RE: Diagnostic ultrasound applied to obstetrics and gynecology, New York, 1980, Harper & Row.

Kelly-Fry E, Fry FJ, and Gardner GW: Recommendations for widespread application of ultrasound visualization techniques for examination of the female breast. In White D and Brown RE, editors: Ultrasound in medicine, vol 3A, New York, 1977, Plenum.

Kelly-Fry E, Fry FJ, Sanghvi NT, et al: A combined clinical and research approach to the problem of ultrasound visualization of breast. In White D, editor: Ultrasound in medicine, vol 1, New York, 1975, Plenum.

Kobayashi T: Gray-scale echography for breast cancer, Radiology 122:207, 1977.

Kossoff G, Kelly-Fry E, and Jellins J: Average velocity of ultrasound in the human female breast, J Acoust Soc Am 53:1730, 1973.

Pilnik S and Leis HP Jr: Clinical diagnosis of breast lesions. In Gallager HS et al: The breast, St Louis, 1978, Mosby.

Pilnik S and Leis HP Jr: Nipple discharge. In Gallager HS et al, editors: The breast, St Louis, 1978, Mosby.

Rubin CS, Kurtz AB, Goldberg BB, et al: Ultrasound mammographic parenchymal patterns: a preliminary report, Radiology 130:515, 1979.

CHAPTER 14

Thyroid

Traci Parker

Ultrasound is used to evaluate normal thyroid anatomy and pathologic conditions. The thyroid lies superficially in the neck and is well visualized with high-frequency real time ultrasound. Sonography is safe; no radiation is used. The test is simple and very well tolerated by patients.

Thyroid ultrasound is used to determine the nature of a nodule. It can determine whether the mass is:

- Single or multiple.
- Solid or cystic.
- Complex or calcified.

The size and location of lesions and any adjacent adenopathy can be noted. Ultrasound is used to define the anatomy of the thyroid gland rather than the function of the gland. The functional state is determined by scintigraphy, which is a nuclear medicine test.

ANATOMY AND PHYSIOLOGY

The thyroid is located in the anterior neck at the level of the hyoid cartilage. The thyroid gland consists of right and left lobes, which are connected across the midline by the thyroid isthmus. The thyroid straddles the trachea anteriorly, and the lobes extend on either side and are bounded laterally by the carotid arteries and jugular veins. The lobes are equal in size and are 5 to 6 cm in length and 2 cm in the anterioposterior measurement. The isthmus, which lies anterior to the trachea, is variable in size. A pyramidal lobe that extends superiorly from the isthmus is present in 15% to 30% of thyroid glands (Fig. 14-1). Normal thyroid parenchyma appears sonographically as a homogeneous gland of medium- to high-level echoes.

Along the anterior surface of the thyroid gland lie the strap muscles, including the sternothyroideus, the omohyoideus, and the sternohyoideus, which are seen as thin sonolucent bands. The longus colli muscle is posterior and lateral to each thyroid lobe and appears as a hypoechoic triangular structure adjacent to the cervical vertebrae (Fig. 14-2).

Blood is supplied to the thyroid by four arteries. Two superior thyroid arteries arise from the external carotids and descend to the upper poles. Two inferior thyroid arteries arise from the thyrocervical trunk of the subclavian artery and ascend to the lower poles. Corresponding veins drain into the internal jugular veins (see Fig. 14-1).

The role of the thyroid, an endocrine gland, is to maintain normal body metabolism, growth, and development by the synthesis, storage, and secretion of thyroid hormones. The mechanism for producing thyroid hormones is iodine metabolism. The thyroid gland traps iodine from the blood and, through a series of chemical reactions, produces the thyroid hormones triiodothyronine (T_3) and thyroxine (T_4). These are stored in the colloid of the gland. When thyroid hormone is needed by the body, it is released into the bloodstream by the action of thyrotropin or thyroid-stimulating hormone (TSH), which is produced by the pituitary gland. The secretion of TSH is regulated by thyrotropin-releasing factor, which is produced by the hypothalmus (located in the brain). The level of thyrotropin-releasing factor is controlled by the basal metabolic rate. A decrease in the basal metabolic rate, a result of a low concentration of thyroid hormones, causes an increase in thyrotropin-releasing factor. This causes increased secretion of TSH and a subsequent increase in the release of thyroid hormones. When the blood level of hormones is returned to normal, the basal metabolic rate returns to normal and TSH secretion stops.

ULTRASOUND TECHNIQUE

Before beginning the scan, obtain a good history about the patient's general health, thyroid medications, imaging studies already performed (scintigraphy, for example), family history of hyperparathyroidism or thyroid cancer, and any previous neck irradiation or surgery.

The patient should be in the supine position with the neck hyperextended. To accomplish this, put a pillow under both of the patient's shoulders. In this position the lower lobes are more readily visualized.

A high-resolution linear 7.5- to 10-MHz transducer should be used. Each lobe requires careful scanning in both the longitudinal and transverse planes. The lateral, middle, and medial parts of each lobe are examined in the longitudinal plane (Fig. 14-3) and so labeled. The upper, middle, and lower portions are examined and labeled in the transverse plane (Fig. 14-4). The patient's turning the head to

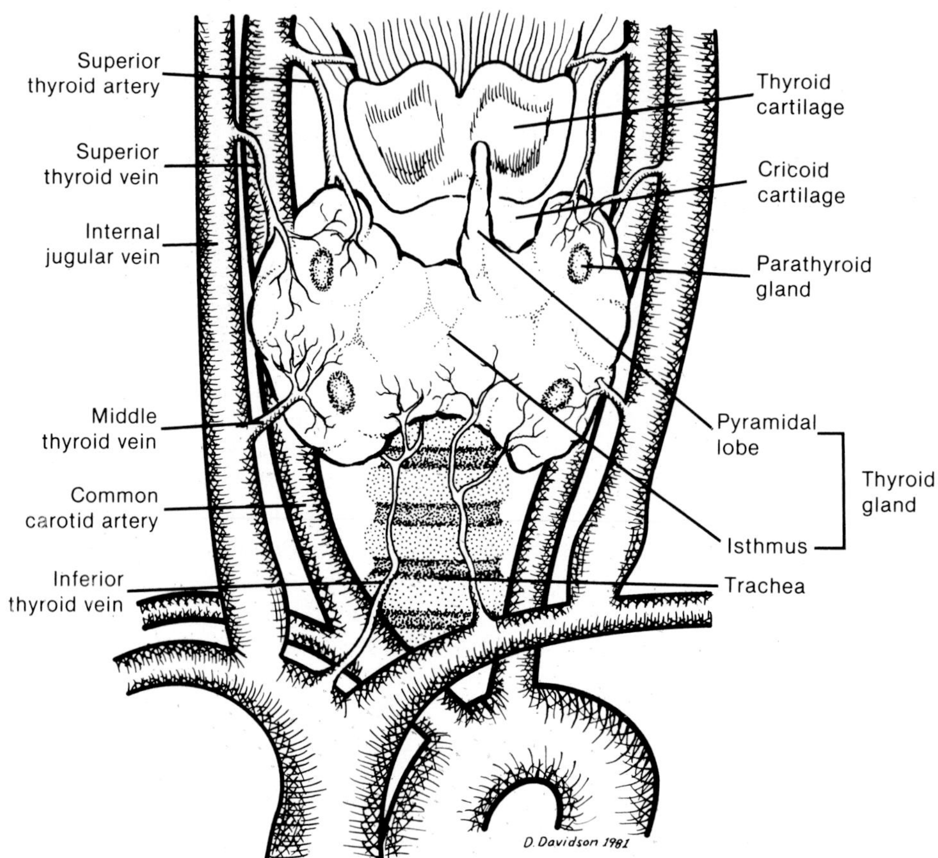

FIG. 14-1 Anterior view of the thyroid and parathyroid regions. (Modified from Forsham PH: Endocrine system and selected metabolic diseases, ed 3, Summit, NJ, 1974, Ciba Pharmaceutical)

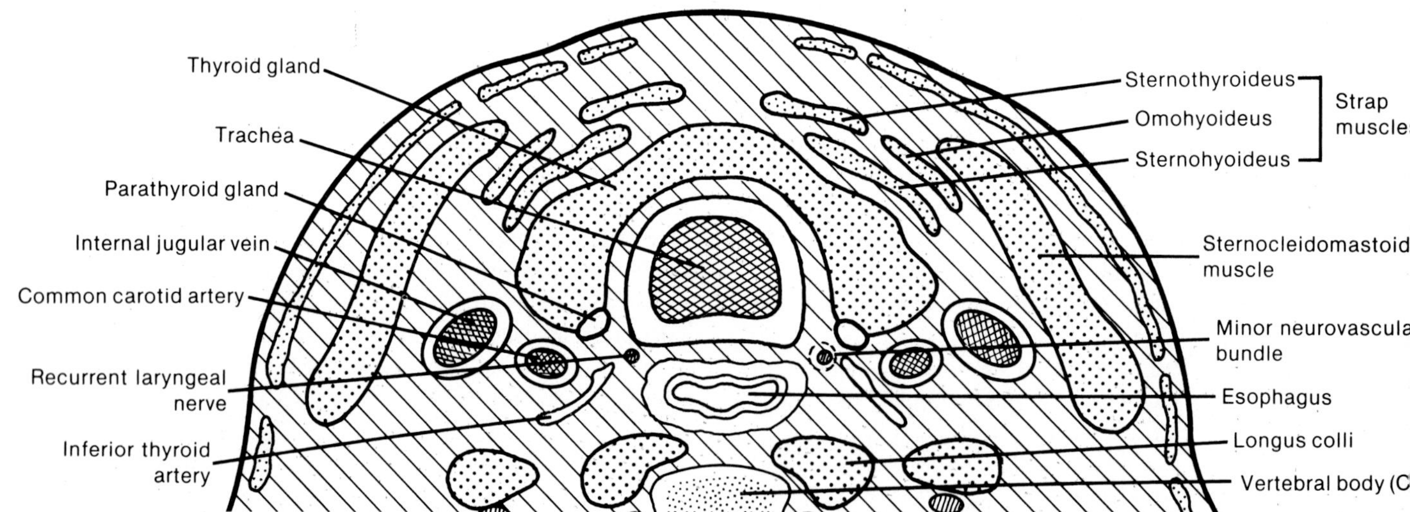

FIG. 14-2 Cross-section of the thyroid region showing organ, vessel, and muscle relationships. (Modified from Forsham PH: Endocrine system and selected metabolic diseases, ed 3, Summit, NJ, 1974, Ciba Pharmaceutical)

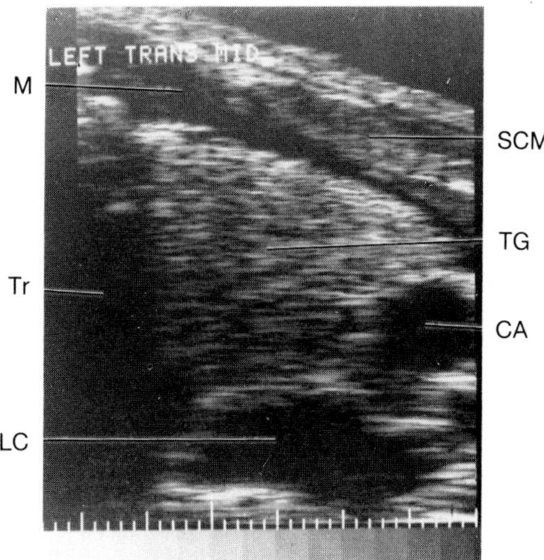

FIG. 14-3 Transverse scan of the left lobe of the normal thyroid gland, *TG,* demonstrating the relationships of the carotid artery, *CA,* trachea, *Tr,* and muscles. Note the homogeneous texture of the gland.

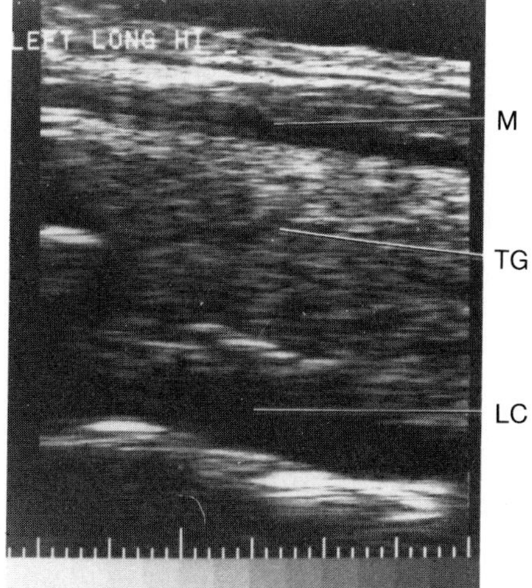

FIG. 14-4 Longitudinal scan of the upper pole of the normal thyroid, *TG.* Strap muscles, *M,* border the gland anteriorly and the longus colli, *LC,* borders posteriorly. *SCM,* sternocleidomastoid muscle.

the opposite side of the side being scanned enables the sonographer to better visualize each individual lobe. Transverse and longitudinal images of the isthmus must also be obtained (Fig. 14-5). The examination should also extend laterally to include the region of the carotid artery and jugular vein to identify enlarged cervical lymph nodes.

If an abnormality is encountered, all characteristics (i.e., cystic areas, calcification, or a halo) should be demonstrated. It is not uncommon for sonography to demonstrate multiple nodules in a gland previously suspected of having only a solitary lesion.

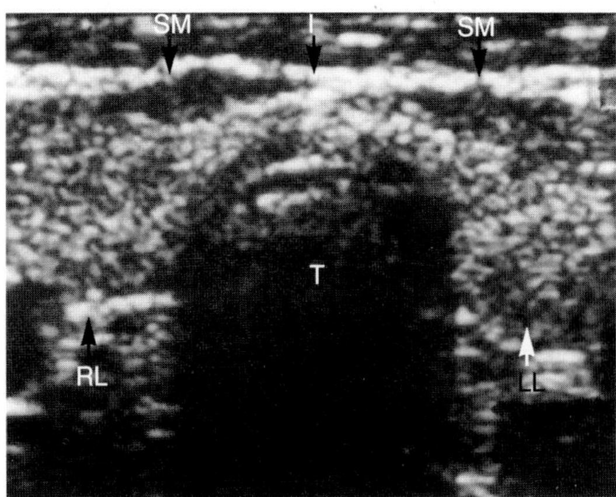

FIG. 14-5 Transverse scan of the normal isthmus of the thyroid. *T,* Trachea; *Sm,* strap muscle; *I,* isthmus; *RL,* right lobe; *LL,* left lobe.

PATHOLOGY

The most common cause of thyroid disorders worldwide is iodine deficiency, leading to goiter formation and hypothyroidism. In areas not deficient in iodine, autoimmune processes are believed to be the basis for most cases of thyroid disease, which ranges from hyperthyroidism to hypothyroidism.[5] Enlargement of the thyroid gland is termed *goiter. Nodular hyperplasia, multinodular goiter,* and *adenomatous hyperplasia* are some of the terms used to describe goiter, which is the most common thyroid abnormality.[4] Goiters can be diffuse and symmetric or irregular and nodular. Sonography shows that the goiterous gland is usually enlarged, nodular, and sometimes inhomogeneous.

Goiters may result from hyperplasia, neoplasia, or an inflammatory process. Normal thyroid function, hyperfunction, or hypofunction can also cause enlargement of the gland.

Hyperthyroidism

Hyperthyroidism is a hypermetabolic state in which increased amounts of thyroid hormones are produced. Patients present with weight loss, nervousness, and an increased heart rate. Exopthalmos may develop when the condition is severe. Hyperthyroidism associated with a diffuse hyperplastic goiter is termed *Graves' disease*. The overactivity of Graves' disease is manifested sonographically by increased vascularity on color Doppler.[3]

Hypothyroidism

Hypothyroidism is a hypometabolic state resulting from inadequate secretion of thyroid hormones. Lethargy, sluggish reactions, and a deep, husky voice are manifestations.

Benign Lesions

Cysts

Cysts are thought to represent cystic degeneration of a follicular adenoma. Approximately 20% of solitary nodules

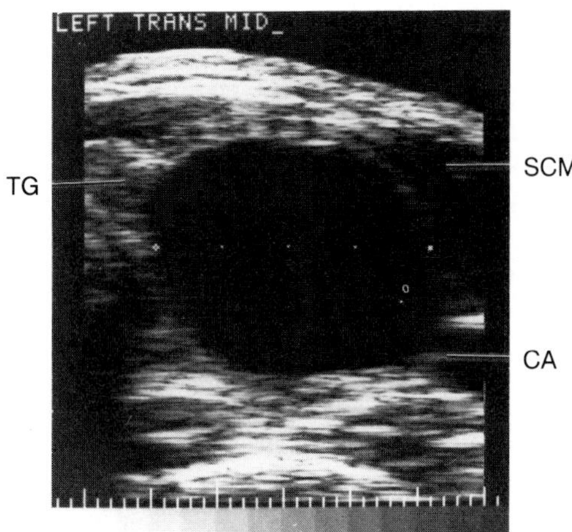

FIG. 14-6 A 2-cm thyroid cyst occupies most of the left lobe on this transverse scan. *TG,* thyroid gland, isthmus; *CA,* carotid artery; *SCM,* sternocleidomastoid muscle.

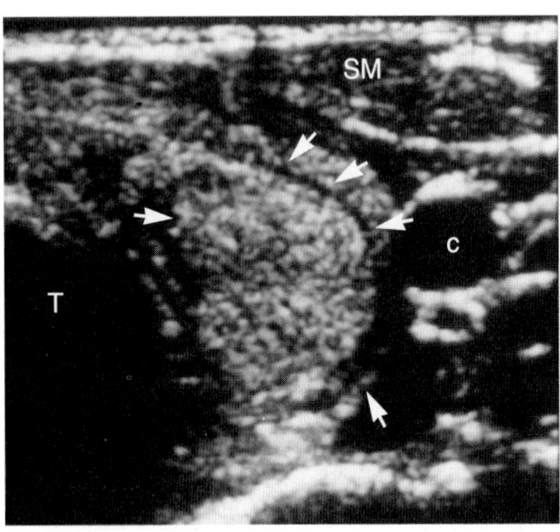

FIG. 14-7 Transverse scan of a large thyroid adenoma demonstrating a peripheral halo. *Sm,* Strap muscle; *C,* carotid; *T,* trachea; *Arrows,* halo appearance.

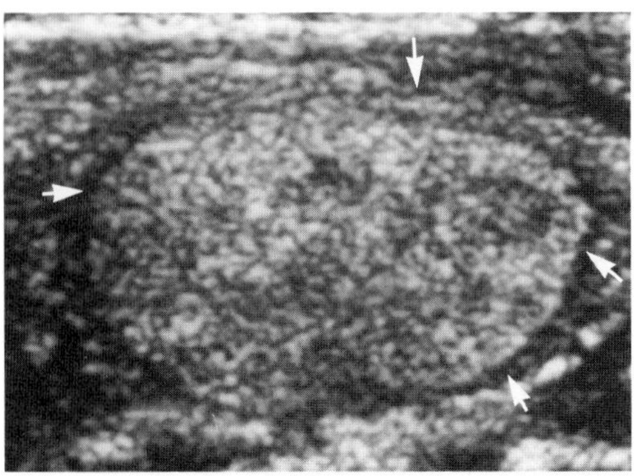

FIG. 14-8 Heterogeneous appearance within an adenoma with discrete borders. Also demonstrates a halo. *Arrows,* halo appearance.

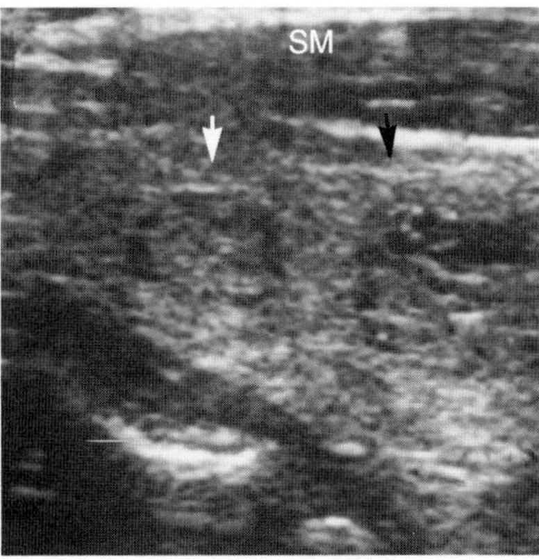

FIG. 14-9 Multiple adenomas, with hypoechoic cystic degeneration within each. *Arrows,* Adenoma; *Sm,* strap muscle.

are cystic. Blood or debris may be present within them. As with all simple cysts, the sonographic appearance of a simple thyroid cyst must be anechoic and have sharp, well-defined walls and distal acoustic enhancement (Fig. 14-6).

Adenoma

An adenoma is a benign thyroid neoplasm characterized by complete fibrous encapsulation. Adenomas have a broad spectrum of ultrasound appearances. They range from echolucent (no echoes) to completely echo-dense and commonly have a peripheral halo. The halo, or thin echolucent rim surrounding the lesion, may represent edema of the compressed normal thyroid tissue or the capsule of the adenoma (Figs. 14-7 and 14-8). In a few instances, it may be blood around the lesion. Although the halo is a relatively consistent finding in adenomas, additional statistical information is necessary to establish its specificity.

Adenomas that contain echolucent areas are a result of cystic degeneration (probably from hemorrhage) (Fig. 14-9 and 14-10) and usually lack a well-rounded margin. This lack of a discrete cystic margin is helpful in differentiation from a simple cyst. Calcification, characteristically rimlike, can also be associated with adenomas. Its acoustic shadow may preclude visualization posteriorly (Figs. 14-11 and 14-12).[3]

Diffuse Nontoxic Goiter

Diffuse nontoxic goiter (colloid goiter) occurs as a compensatory enlargement of the thyroid gland resulting from thyroid hormone deficiency. The gland becomes diffusely and uniformly enlarged. In the first stage hyperplasia occurs; in the second stage, colloid involution. Progression of this process leads to an asymmetric and multinodular gland (Fig. 14-13).

Adenomatous Hyperplasia

Adenomatous hyperplasia (multinodular goiter) is one of the most common forms of thyroid disease. Nodularity of the gland can be the end stage of diffuse nontoxic goiter. This can be followed by focal scarring, focal areas of ische-

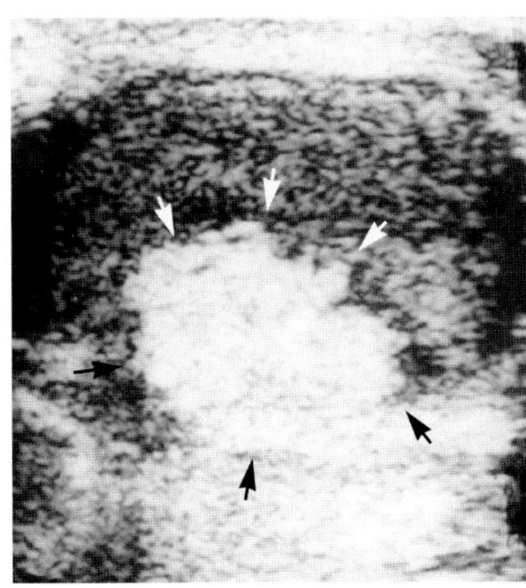

FIG. 14-10 Longitudinal scan demonstrating an echogenic hemorrhagic adenoma. *Arrows,* Adenoma.

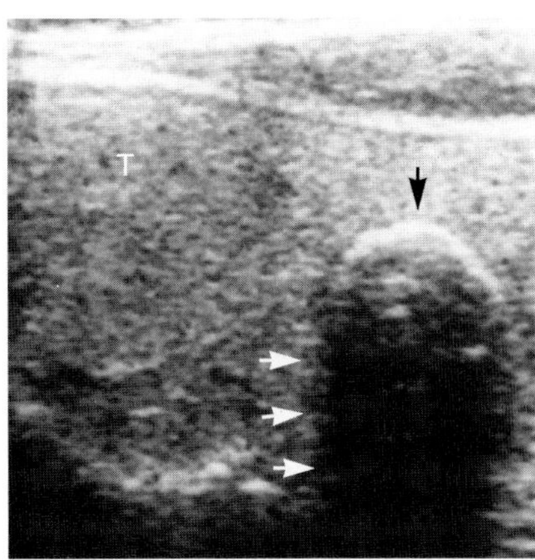

FIG. 14-12 Longitudinal scan demonstrating a calcified adenoma. *T,* Normal thyroid tissue; *T,* calcified adenoma; *white arrow,* shadowing from the calcification.

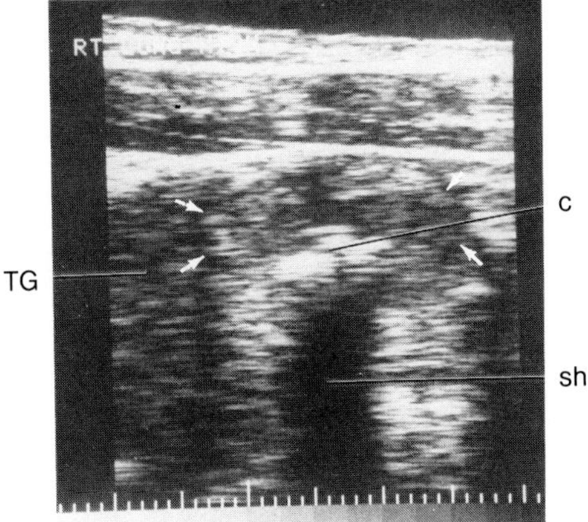

FIG. 14-11 Longitudinal scan of a thyroid adenoma demonstrating a halo *(arrows)* and a large central calcification, *c,* with shadow, *sh. TG,* thyroid gland.

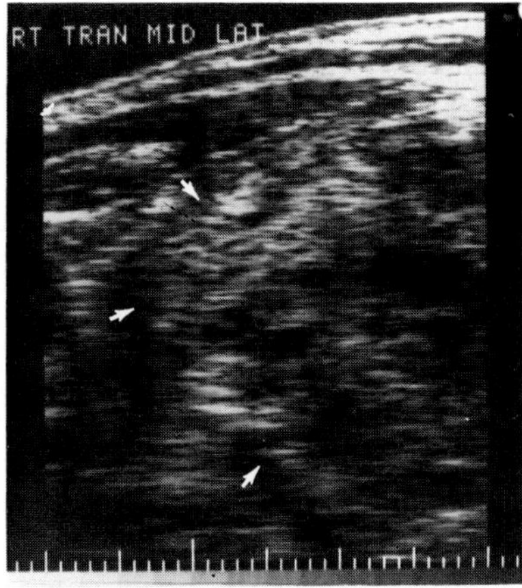

FIG. 14-13 Areas of cystic degeneration and a poorly defined halo *(arrowheads)* can be identified on this transverse scan of a multinodular goiter. Discrete nodule margins are difficult to perceive.

mia, and necrosis and cyst formation (Fig. 14-14). Fibrosis or calcifications may also manifest. Some of the nodules are poorly circumscribed; others appear to be encapsulated. Enlargement can involve one lobe to a greater extent than the other and sometimes causes difficulty in breathing and swallowing.

Lesions in multinodular goiter have many features of true adenomas. The multiple nodules of adenomatous hyperplasia may demonstrate halos and may have clear or nondiscrete borders.

The solid portion of the lesions may have the same echotexture as the normal thyroid tissue. Calcifications and cystic areas may be present within the nodules.

Thyroiditis

Thyroiditis causes swelling and tenderness of the thyroid. Thyroiditis is caused by infection or can be related to autoimmune abnormalities. By sonography, the gland appears as enlarged and hypoechoic. There are many forms of thyroiditis. The common goiterous form of autoimmune thyroiditis is called *Hashimoto's thyroiditis.* The thyroid in Hashimoto's thyroiditis is always diffusely abnormal on ultrasound, with decreased and inhomogeneous echogenicity. The gland may be normal or increased in size and may have an irregular surface.

Malignant Lesions

Carcinoma of the thyroid is rare. A solitary nodule may be malignant in 10% to 25% of cases, but the risk of malignancy decreases with the presence of multiple nodules. A solitary thyroid nodule in the presence of cervical adenopathy on the same side suggests malignancy.[1]

The ultrasound appearance of thyroid cancer is highly variable. The neoplasm can be of any size, single or multiple, and can appear as a solid, partially cystic, or largely cystic mass. Occasionally, thyroid cancer presents as a

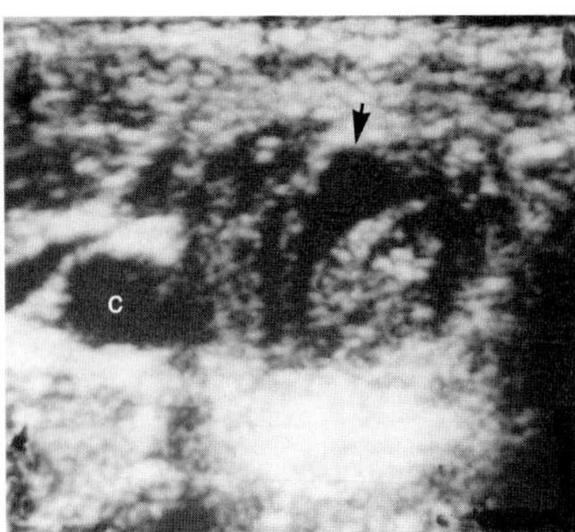

FIG. 14-14 Multinodular goiter demonstrating focal areas of ischemia and cystic areas. *C*, Carotid; *arrow*, cystic areas.

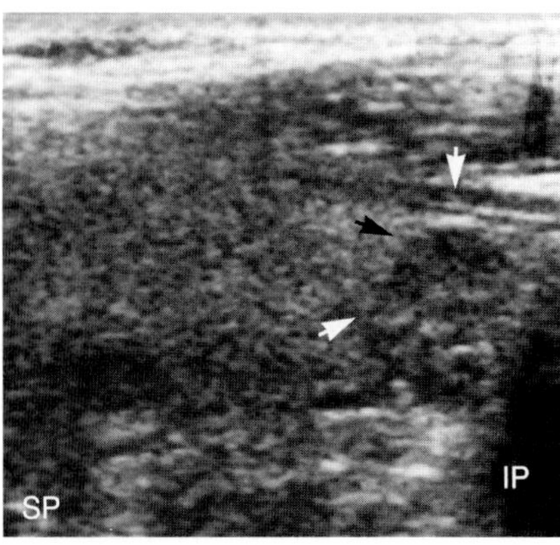

FIG. 14-16 Longitudinal scan of medullary carcinoma causing enlargement of the inferior pole of the right lobe of the thyroid. *Sp*, Superior pole; *Ip*, inferior pole; *Arrows*, medullary carcinoma lesion.

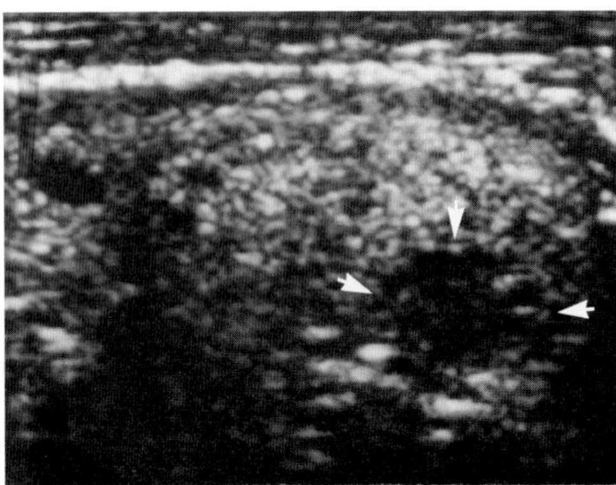

FIG. 14-15 Solitary lesion representing papillary carcinoma upon biopsy. In addition, this patient had cervical lymph adenopathy. *Arrows*, Papillary carcinoma lesion.

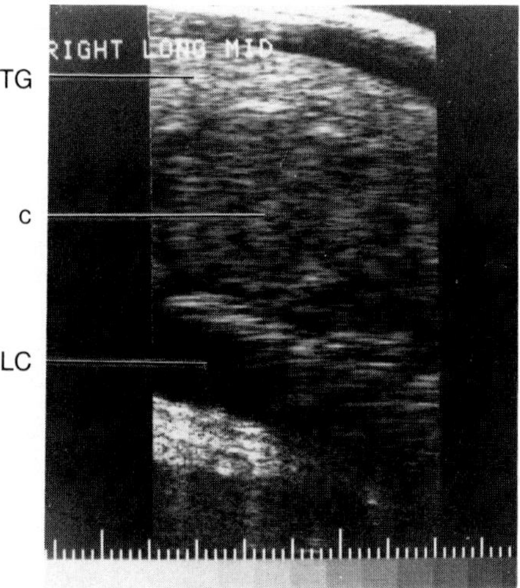

FIG. 14-17 Longitudinal section revealing the 3-cm thyroid carcinoma, *c*, to be less echogenic than the normal thyroid, *TG*. Longus colli, *LC*.

small solid nodule (Fig. 14-15). Thyroid cancer is usually hypoechoic relative to normal thyroid, but thyroid carcinomas with the same echo texture as normal thyroid have been reported. Calcifications are present in 50% to 80% of all types of thyroid carcinoma.

Papillary thyroid cancer is the most common of the thyroid malignancies and is the predominant cause of thyroid cancer in children. Approximately 20% of patients with papillary thyroid cancer have metastatic cervical adenopathy.

Follicular Carcinoma

Follicular carcinoma of the thyroid is usually a solitary mass of the thyroid. An irregular, firm, nodular enlargement is characteristic. This type of thyroid cancer is more aggressive than papillary cancer.

Medullary Carcinoma

Medullary carcinoma accounts for 10% of thyroid cancers. It presents as a hard, bulky mass that causes enlargement of a small portion of the gland (Fig. 14-16) and can involve the entire gland.

In patients with medullary thyroid carcinoma, thyroid lesions appear as punctuated, bright echogenic foci within solid masses.[2] These correspond pathologically to deposits of calcium surrounded by amyloid. Ultrasound is highly sensitive in detecting metastatic lymphadenopathy in these patients; thus, careful evaluation of the entire neck area surrounding the thyroid is important.

Anaplastic Carcinoma

Anaplastic (undifferentiated) carcinoma is rare and accounts for less than 10% of thyroid cancers. It usually occurs after 50 years of age. This lesion presents as a hard, fixed mass with rapid growth. Its growth is locally invasive into surrounding neck structures, and it usually causes death by compression and asphyxiation because of invasion of the trachea (Fig. 14-17).

Thyroid cancer is commonly isoechoic or hypoechoic by ultrasound. The interfaces of the lesion are often poorly defined and a halo is rarely present. Cystic degeneration, if present, is minimal. Specks of calcium may also be noted but are seldom peripheral as with adenomas.

PARATHYROID

Anatomy

The parathyroid glands are normally located on the posterior medial surface of the thyroid gland. Most people have four parathyroid glands but to have three to five parathyroid glands is not uncommon. Parathyroid glands have been found in different places such as in the neck and mediastinum. The four parathyroid glands are paired. Two lie posterior to each superior pole of the thyroid, and the other two lie posterior to the inferior pole.

Each gland is flat and disc-shaped. The echo texture is similar to that of the overlying thyroid gland. For this reason, the normal sized glands (<4 mm) are usually not seen by ultrasound, but occasionally a single one may be imaged and appear as a flat hypoechoic structure posterior to the thyroid and adjacent to it. Enlarged glands (>5 mm) have a decreased echo texture and appear sonographically as elongated masses between the posterior longus coli muscle and the anterior thyroid lobe.

Physiology

The parathyroid glands are the calcium-sensing organs in the body. They produce parathormone (PTH) and monitor the serum calcium feedback mechanism.

The stimulus to PTH secretion is a decrease in the level of blood calcium. When the serum calcium level decreases, the parathyroid glands are stimulated to release PTH. When the serum calcium level increases, parathyroid activity decreases. PTH acts on bone, kidney, and intestine to enhance calcium absorption. Patients with unexplained hypercalcemia detected on routine blood chemistry screening are the most common referrals for parathyroid echography. Symptomatic renal stones, ulcers, and bone pain are other indications.

Ultrasound Technique

For successful sonographic detection of parathyroid abnormalities, a high-resolution (7.5- to 10-MHz) transducer must be used. The patient is placed supine with the neck slightly hyperextended. From the upper neck, just under the jaw, to the sternal notch, transverse and longitudinal planes must be examined and recorded. To detect any inferiorly located parathyroid glands, the patient is asked to swallow to elevate the thyroid gland during real time scanning. Normal parathyroid glands are seldom identified.

Pathology

Primary Hyperparathyroidism

Primary hyperparathyroidism is a state of increased function of the parathyroid glands. Women have primary hyperparathyroidism two to three times more frequently than men; it is particularly common after menopause. Primary hyperparathyroidism is characterized by hypercalcemia, hypercalciuria, and low serum levels of phosphate.

Most patients are asymptomatic at the time of diagnosis and have no manifestations of hyperparathyroidism, such as nephrolithiasis and osteopenia. Primary hyperparathyroidism occurs when increased amounts of PTH are produced by an adenoma, primary hyperplasia, or, rarely, carcinoma located in the parathyroid gland.

Adenoma

Adenoma is the most common cause of primary hyperparathyroidism (80% of cases). A solitary adenoma may involve any one of the four glands with equal frequency. Adenomas are benign and are usually less than 3 cm. The most common shape of a parathyroid adenoma is oval. Parathyroid adenomas are hypoechoic (Figs. 14-18 and 14-19), and the vast majority are solid. Adenomas are encapsulated and have a discrete border. Differentiation of adenomas and hyperplasia is difficult on histologic and morphologic grounds.

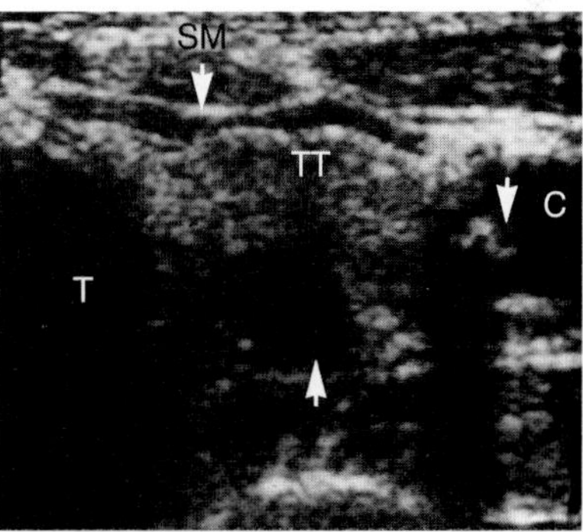

FIG. 14-18 Transverse scan of enlarged parathyroid gland. *Sm,* Strap muscles; *TT,* thyroid tissue; *T,* trachea; *Arrow,* parathyroid gland; *C,* carotid; *right arrow,* coincidental plaque in carotid.

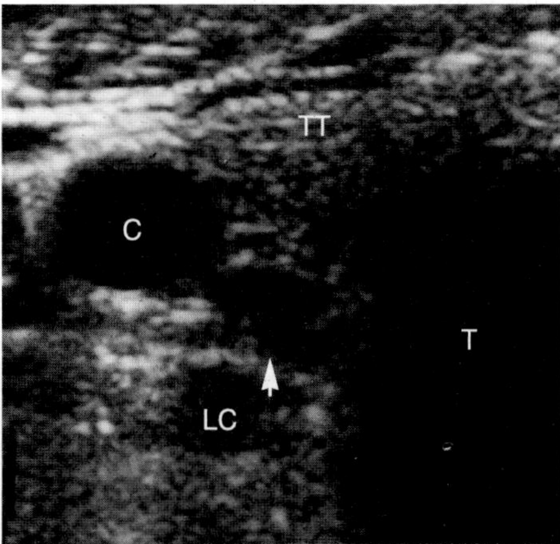

FIG. 14-19 Transverse scan of enlarge parathyroid gland. *C,* Carotid; *TT,* thyroid tissue; *LC,* longus colli; *Arrow,* parathyroid; *T,* tractea.

Primary Hyperplasia

Primary hyperplasia is defined as hyperfunction of all parathyroid glands with no apparent cause. Only one gland may significantly enlarge with the remaining glands only mildly affected, or all glands may be enlarged. In any case, they rarely reach more than 1 cm in size.

Carcinoma

Histologic differentiation of adenoma and carcinoma is very difficult. Metastases to regional nodes or distant organs, capsular invasion, or local recurrence must be present for cancer to be diagnosed.

Most cancers of the parathyroid glands are small, irregular, and rather firm masses. They sometimes adhere to surrounding structures. If death results, it is more likely to be caused by hyperparathyroid complications than by the malignancy itself.

Secondary Hyperparathyroidism

Secondary hyperparathyroidism is a chronic hypocalcemia, caused by renal failure, vitamin D deficiency (rickets), or malabsorption syndromes. These abnormalities induce PTH secretion, which leads to secondary hyperparathyroidism. The hyperfunction of the parathyroids is apparently a compensatory reaction; renal insufficiency and intestinal malabsorption cause hypocalcemia, which leads to stimulation of PTH. All four glands are usually affected.

Ultrasound Appearances

Normal

With high-resolution scanners, it is possible to resolve the parathyroid glands. The anatomic relationship (i.e., the parathyroids are closely attached to or embedded in the thyroid gland and lack acoustical differences) makes the resolution of parathyroid glands difficult.

In many cases a prominent longus colli (see Fig. 14-19) appears as a discrete area posterior to the thyroid; it is important not to confuse this normal anatomy with a mass. Longitudinal sections can usually solve the problem. A linear appearance of the muscle is evident in this plane. The minor neurovascular bundle, composed of the inferior thyroid artery and recurrent laryngeal nerve, may also be a source of confusion. Longitudinal scans can often eliminate this confusion by identifying its tubular appearance.

MISCELLANEOUS NECK MASSES

The role of ultrasound in evaluating palpable neck masses is to determine site of origin and assess lesion texture.

Developmental Cysts

Thyroglossal Duct Cysts

Thyroglossal duct cysts are congenital anomalies that present in the midline of the neck anterior to the trachea (Fig. 14-20). They are fusiform or spherical masses rarely larger than 2 or 3 cm.

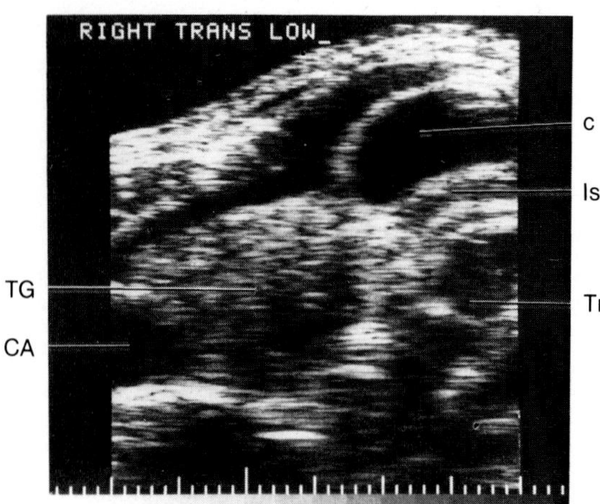

FIG. 14-20 Transverse scan at the level of the thyroid gland, *TG*, demonstrating a thyroglossal duct cyst, *c*, in the midline anterior to the trachea, *Tr*. Carotid artery, *CA;* isthmus of thyroid gland, *Is*.

A remnant of the tubular development of the thyroid gland may persist between the base of the tongue and the hyoid bone. This narrow hollow tract, which connects the thyroid lobes to the floor of the pharynx, normally atrophies in the adult. Failure to atrophy creates the potential for cystic masses to form anywhere along it.

Branchial Cleft Cysts

Branchial cleft cysts are cystic formations usually located laterally. During embryonic development the branchial cleft is a slender tract extending from the pharyngeal cavity to an opening near the auricle or into the neck. A diverticulum may extend either laterally from the pharynx or medially from the neck.

Although primarily cystic in appearance, these lesions may present with solid components, usually of low-level echogenicity, particularly if they have become infected.

Cystic Hygroma

Cystic hygroma of the neck results from congenital modification of the lymphatics. It presents from the posterior occiput and is most frequently seen as a large cystic mass on the lateral aspect of the neck. It can be multiseptated and multilocular.

Abscess

Abscess can arise in any location in the neck. The sonographic appearance ranges from primarily fluid-filled to completely echogenic. Most commonly, it is a mass of low-level echogenicity with rather irregular walls. Chronic abscess may be particularly difficult to demonstrate, since the indistinct margins blend with surrounding tissue.

The role of ultrasound in evaluating abscess is localization for percutaneous needle aspiration and follow-up examination during and after treatment.

Adenopathy

Low-level echogenicity of well-circumscribed masses is the classical sonographic appearance of enlarged lymph nodes. However, in some cases they appear echo-free. Inflammatory processes may also exhibit a cystic nature.

Differentiation of inflammation from neoplastic processes is not always possible by sonographic criteria alone. To confirm a neoplastic process, biopsy is performed.

REVIEW QUESTIONS

1. Describe the anatomic landmarks used to locate the thyroid gland.
2. Name the muscles adjacent to the thyroid gland.
3. Describe the ultrasound technique used to image the thyroid gland.
4. What is a goiter? Describe its sonographic appearance.
5. How is Graves' disease detected by ultrasound?
6. What is an adenoma of the thyroid gland?
7. Name the most common forms of thyroid disease.
8. Name the forms of thyroiditis.
9. Describe the appearance of carcinoma of the thyroid.
10. Describe the location of the parathyroid glands.
11. Name the disease state that causes increased function of the parathyroid gland.
12. What is the most common cause of primary hyperparathyroidism?
13. What is a thyroglossal duct cyst?
14. Describe the ultrasound appearance of a cystic hygroma.

REFERENCES

1. Gooding G: Thyroid and parathyroid. In Mittlestaedt C, editor: General ultrasound pp. 105-139, New York, 1992, Churchill Livingstone.
2. Gorman B, Charboneau JW, and James EM: Medullary thyroid carcinoma: role of high-resolution ultrasound, Radiology 162:147, 1987.
3. Ralls PW, Mayekawa DS, and Lee K: Color flow Doppler sonography in Graves' disease, Am J Roentgenol 150:781, 1988.
4. Rosai J: Thyroid gland. In Ackerman's surgical pathology, ed 7, p. 391, St. Louis, 1989, Mosby.
5. Turnbridge WM and Caldwell G: The epidemiology of thyroid diseases, pp. 530, 578, Philadelphia, 1991, J.B. Lippincott.

CHAPTER 15

The Scrotum and Other Superficial Structures

Traci Parker

Scrotum

Ultrasound is an excellent tool for evaluating the scrotum and its contents. The anatomic structures as well as the vascular physiology can be investigated with ultrasound. The clinical diagnosis of abnormalities can be confirmed and differentiated.

Sonography is useful for the following:

- Evaluating testicular size
- Differentiating intratesticular or extratesticular abnormalities causing scrotal enlargement or a palpable mass
- Finding an occult (concealed) neoplasm
- Evaluating the condition of the testicle in cases of trauma or infection
- Differentiating the causes of acute scrotum
- Determining the presence or absence of a varicocele in an infertility work-up
- Locating an undescended testis

NORMAL ANATOMY

The scrotum is a pendent sac divided into two lateral compartments by a septum called the *median raphe*. Each compartment contains a testicle, an epididymis, a vas deferens, and a spermatic cord. The scrotal sac is lined internally by the parietal layer of the tunica vaginalis. The visceral layer of the tunica vaginalis surrounds the testicle, except for a small area posteriorly, which is termed the *bare area*. At this site, the testicle is against the scrotal wall, preventing torsion. Blood vessels, lymphatics, nerves, and spermatic ducts travel through the bare area.[1]

The testes are the male reproductive glands. Each testicle is ovoid in shape and measures approximately 2 to 3 cm in diameter and 3 to 5 cm long. The testicular parenchyma is encased within a thick fibrous capsule known as the *tunica albuginea*. The tunica albuginea is surrounded by the parietal layer of the tunica vaginalis. The tunica albuginea inserts into the posterior aspect of the testicle, where the efferent ductules and blood vessels enter to form a vertical septum called the *mediastinum*.

Each testicle is made up of several hundred lobules. Each lobule is made up of one or several very tortuous tubules called *seminiferous tubules*. In the normal seminiferous tubule, mitosis and spermatogenesis take place (Figs. 15-1 and 15-2).

The seminiferous tubules converge at the mediastinum and form the rete testis. The mediastinum appears as an echogenic line going through the testicle (Fig. 15-3). The tubules of the rete testis then empty into the efferent ducts. The efferent ducts continue on to empty into the epididymis.

The epididymis lies along the posterolateral aspect of the testis and is made up of a head, body, and tail. Its overall size is 6 to 7 cm, and it contains more than 6 m of coiled tubule. The epididymal head (also called the *globus major*) is located over the upper pole of the testicle. It is round or triangular in shape and measures approximately 6 to 15 mm in width. A small protuberance may arise from the epididymal head, known as the *appendix of the epididymis* (Fig. 15-4). This is present in approximately 33% of males.[5] The body courses along the posterolateral surface of the testicle to the tail, which is located under the lower pole of the testicle.

Beginning with the body and ending at the tail of the epididymis, the vas deferens is formed from these structures. The vas deferens ascends medially and cephalad and carries semen. The vas deferens continues cephalad until reaching an ampulla just proximal to the prostate and adjacent to the seminal vesicles.

The majority of the blood supplied to the testis comes from the testicular artery, which arises directly from the aorta. The vas deferens and epididymis receive blood from the deferential artery (a branch of the vesical [bladder] artery). The peritesticular tissue is supplied by the cremasteric artery, which is a branch of the inferior epigastric artery.[4] Both the deferential and cremasteric arteries anastomose with the testicular artery.[6]

The testicle is drained by a network of veins that arise from the mediastinum to form the pampiniform plexus, which is located within the spermatic cord. The pampini-

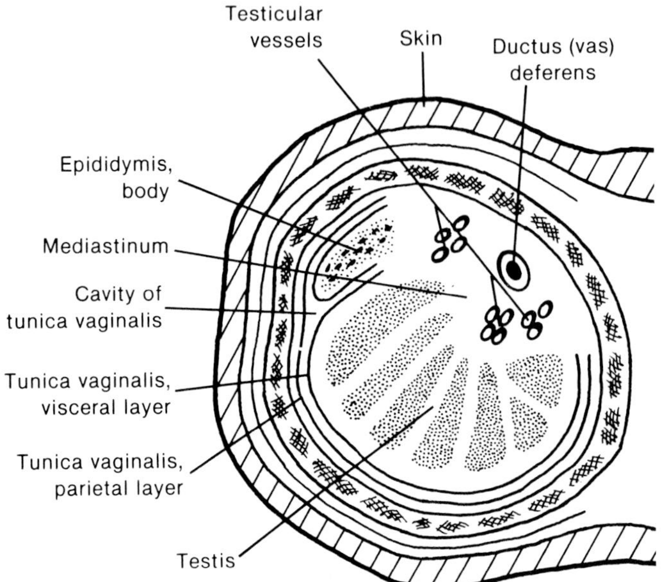

FIG. 15-1 Cross-section through the midpoint of the scrotum and right testis. (Redrawn from Anson BJ: Morris' human anatomy, ed 12, New York, 1966, McGraw-Hill Book.)

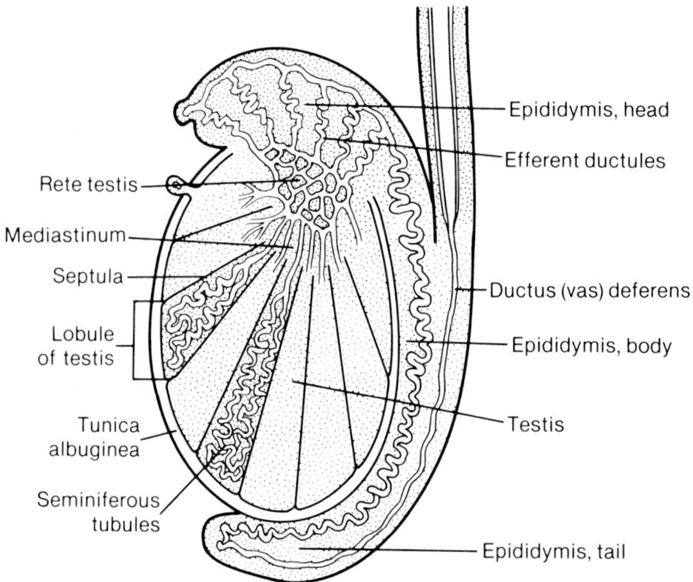

FIG. 15-2 Longitudinal section of the testis and epididymis. (The size of the seminiferous tubules is exaggerated). (Redrawn from Anson BJ: Morris' human anatomy, ed 12, New York, 1966, McGraw-Hill Book.)

form plexus converges into three veins, the testicular, deferential, and cremasteric. The right testicular vein drains directly into the vena cava and the left drains into the left renal vein.

TECHNIQUE

To optimally visualize the scrotum, a high-resolution, real time 7.5- to 10-MHz linear transducer should be used. Instrumentation capable of demonstrating flow with color and spectral Doppler is extremely helpful to demonstrate flow in normal and abnormal conditions. The Doppler settings should be set for low-volume, low-velocity flow to optimize the visualization of the small testicular arteries. Color Doppler is also helpful in finding a vessel for further evaluation by pulsed Doppler.

To prepare for the scan the patient should be placed in the supine position. Avoid a cold room to reduce testicular retraction and skin thickening. The penis should be gently drawn up toward the patient's lower abdomen and covered

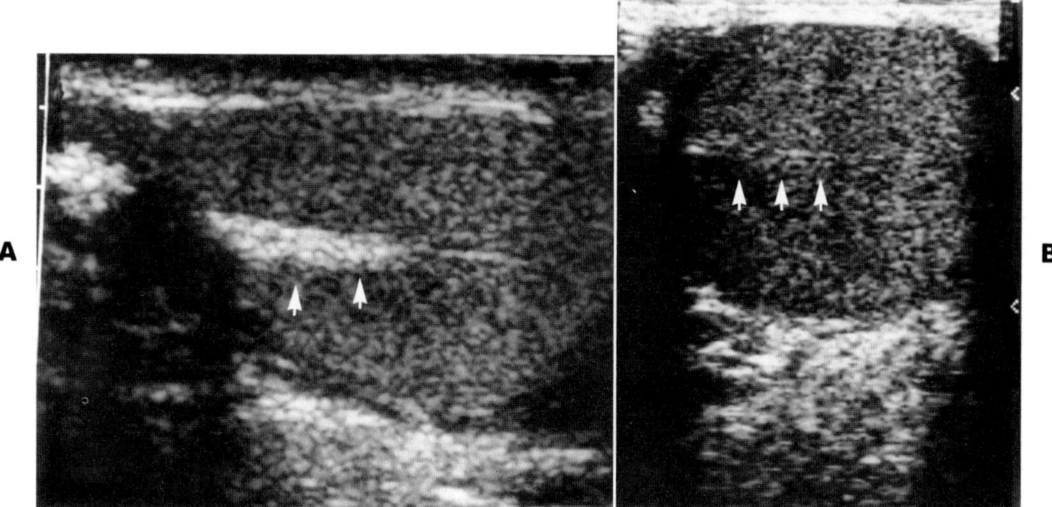

FIG. 15-3 A, Longitudinal scan demonstrating the echogenic mediastinum *(arrows)*. **B**, Transverse scan demonstrating the echogenic mediastinum *(arrows)*.

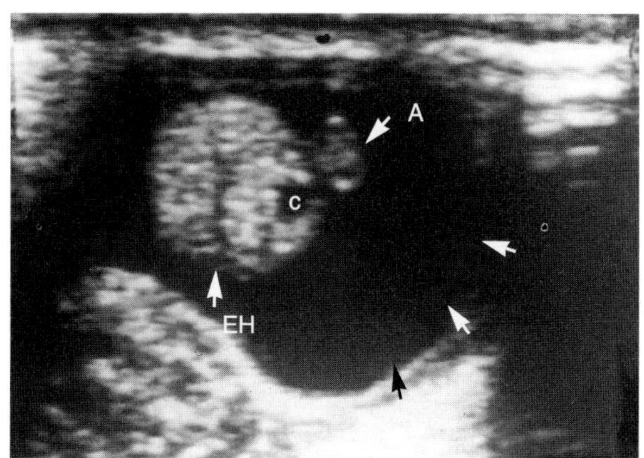

FIG. 15-4 Transverse scan of the epididymal head with a small epididymal cyst and protruding appendix of the epididymis. Hydrocele, *Arrows;* appendix, *A;* epididymal cyst, *C;* epididymal head, *EH*.

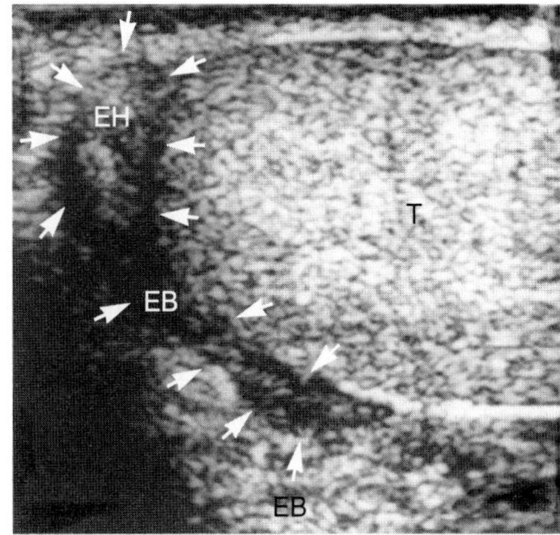

FIG. 15-5 Longitudinal scan demonstrating the normal relationship and echotexture of the epididymal head and testicle. Epididymal body, *EB;* epididymal head, *EH;* normal testicular texture, *T*.

with a towel. A second towel can then be placed under the scrotum for support during imaging. An alternative method for support is to cradle the scrotum in the examiner's gloved hand.

Both testicles should be scanned completely, in both the longitudinal and transverse planes. The longitudinal plane should indicate the lateral, middle, and medial portions of the testicle. A separate image of the epididymal head in relation to the superior portion of the testicle should be obtained (Fig. 15-5). Upper, middle, and lower transverse planes should be evaluated as well. An image comparing the echogenicity and size of both testes should be included in the examination (Fig. 15-6).

The epididymal head and body, as well as the tail, if possible, should be evaluated. The tail is small and therefore

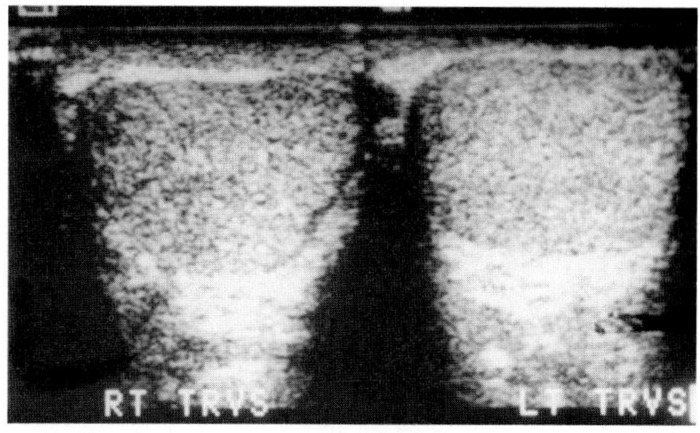

FIG. 15-6 Transverse sonogram of both testicles showing symmetry in size and echotexture.

difficult to distinguish. The spermatic cord area should be scanned from the inguinal canal to the scrotum.

CONGENITAL ANOMALIES

Undescended Testicle

The testes are formed in the retroperitoneum of a male fetus. The testes then descend into the scrotum via the inguinal canal shortly before birth or early in the neonatal period. A deficiency of gonadotropin hormonal stimulation or physical factors such as adhesions or anatomical maldevelopments can interrupt the descent of the testes.[2]

Approximately 80% of undescended testes are found in the inguinal canal, but they are occasionally found intraabdominally or in the femoral area.[5] Undescended testes in the inguinal canal can be demonstrated with ultrasound. The undescended testicle is ovoid in shape and smaller and more hypoechoic than a normal testicle.

Surgical treatment of an undescended testicle by freeing it and implanting it into the scrotum is known as *orchiopexy*. If orchiopexy is not performed at an early age, the testis becomes atrophic and is at a high risk for cancer.[1]

MALIGNANT TESTICULAR TUMORS

Primary Testicular Cancer

Primary testicular cancer occurs in young men ages 15 to 34, in which 10% to 50% present with acute scrotal pain. About 95% of primary testicular neoplasms are of germ-cell origin.[3] Ultrasound is very sensitive in detecting testicular masses. Sonography can determine if a mass is intratesticular or extratesticular. This is important because most intratesticular masses are malignant and most extratesticular masses are benign.[1] Although testicular masses can be well described and differentiated using ultrasound, the ultrasound examination cannot confirm absolutely that a mass is malignant. The sonographic features of a mass may suggest a certain type of tumor, however. In general, testicular tumors are divided into germ-cell and sex-cord stromal tumors. Approximately 95% of all testicular tumors are of germ-cell type.

Seminoma is the most common germinal tumor and peaks in the fourth decade. Seminomas spread via the lymphatics and are very radiosensitive. Seminomas have the best prognosis (Fig. 15-7).

Embryonal cell tumors are less common, but are much more aggressive and lethal than seminomas. The 20-to 30-year age group is the most susceptible. Embryonal cell tumors spread through the blood and via the lymph nodes (Fig. 15-8).

Malignant testicular tumors appear on ultrasound as well-defined masses and are hypoechoic, although they can be heterogeneous. Seminomas tend to be more homogeneous and hypoechoic than other germ-cell tumors.

Yolk sac tumors are the most common germ-cell testicular tumors of infancy and childhood.

Choriocarcinoma is a rare primary malignancy of the testicle. Choriocarcinoma presents itself only as a small nodule, often with no testicular enlargement. The mass may have cystic areas as a result of hemorrhage and necrosis.

Germ-cell tumors are associated with an elevated HCG and AFP. Tumors larger than 1.5 cm are usually hypervascular and tend to have disorganized blood flow. Color Doppler cannot distinguish benign tumors from malignant tumors. Tumors of the sex-cord stroma include Leydig cell tumors and Sertoli cell tumors. These masses occur less commonly than germ-cell tumors and appear sonographically as an inhomogeneous testis.

BENIGN TESTICULAR LESIONS

Benign intratesticular lesions are rare. Testicular cysts presenting with well-rounded borders, anechoic with pos-

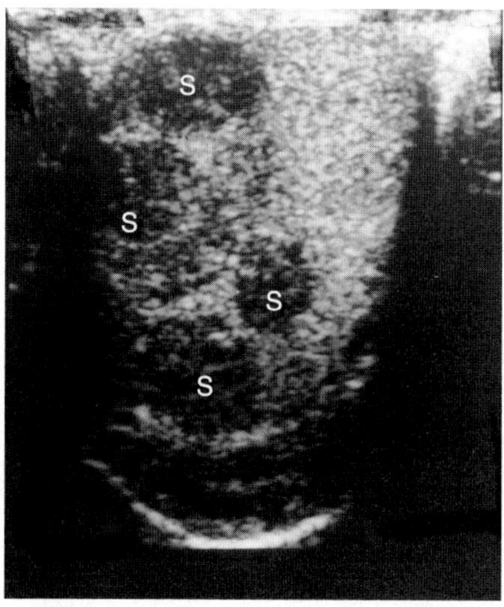

FIG. 15-7 Sonogram of the testicle containing multiple well-defined tumors with decreased echogenicity, demonstrating seminoma. (Courtesy Alvarado Hospital Ultrasound Department, San Diego, CA.)

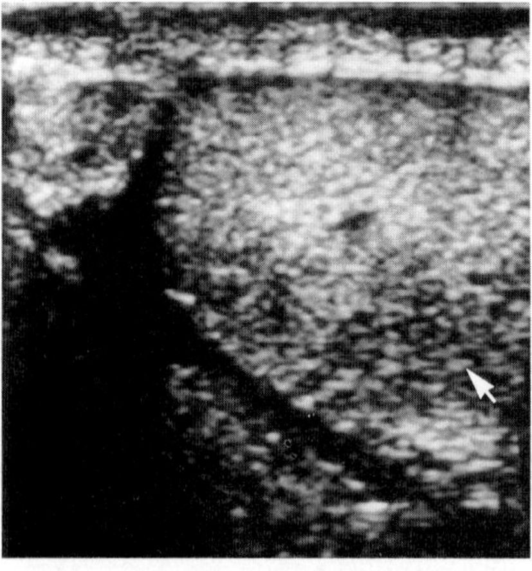

FIG. 15-8 Longitudinal scan of a large mass in the testicle; biopsy confirmed embryonal cell carcinoma.

terior enhancement, are also rare, although more common than once thought because of the use of high-frequency, real time ultrasound.[3] An echo-poor or complex abnormality within the testis could be an abscess, orchitis, torsion, or benign or malignant tumor.

Two or three calcifications in the testicle are common, although multiple tiny calcifications throughout the testes have been found; this is termed *microlithiasis*. Microlithiasis has been seen in normal patients, but it is associated with tumors, sterility, and cryptorchidism. Sonographically, microlithiasis appears as multiple echogenic nonshadowing areas throughout the testis, and these calcifications obscure other pathology (Fig. 15-9).

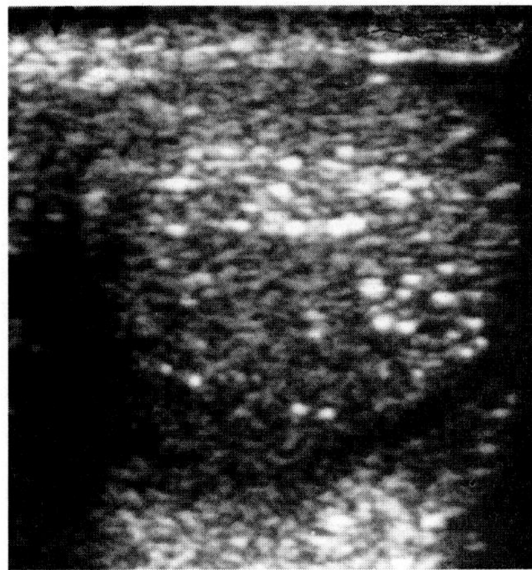

FIG. 15-9 Transverse sonogram of the testicle containing multiple bright echoes resulting from tiny calcifications demonstrating microlithiasis. (Courtesy Alvarado Hospital Ultrasound Department, San Diego, CA.)

EXTRATESTICULAR PROCESSES

The testicle is attached to the scrotum at the bare area. If the bare area is small, a small remnant stalk of tunica vaginalis allows the testicle to be mobile. Torsion occurs when the testicle revolves one or more times on this short stalk, which obstructs blood flow to the testicle and results in severe pain. Torsion is more common in males less than 25 years of age, with a peak incidence at 13 years of age.

Once torsion occurs, the testicle becomes congested and edematous because of the veins in the twisted cord. Pressure within the testicle begins to build because of arterial obstruction, which leads to testicular ischemia. It is important to correctly diagnose this abnormality early because necrosis of the torsed testicle occurs within 24 hours.

The ultrasound image is normal in the first 4 hours of torsion. Although the real time appearance of the testes is normal at this time, color and pulsed Doppler are abnormal. There is absence of flow in the testicle and the epididymis.

After 4 hours, the torsed testicle appears enlarged and hypoechoic (Fig. 15-10, *A*). The testicle may have some inhomogeneity resulting from hemorrhage. Other findings include enlargement of the epididymis (Fig. 15-10, *B*), a reactive hydrocele, and scrotal wall thickening. As in the early phase of torsion, Doppler demonstrates absence of flow within the testicle and epididymis.

INFECTIONS

With epididymitis, the scrotum becomes swollen and tender. In most cases, it is unilateral. The patient presents with a fever and painful urination. Infection usually begins in the epididymis and spreads to the testicle. Severe infection can lead to the development of an abscess in the epididymis or testicle.

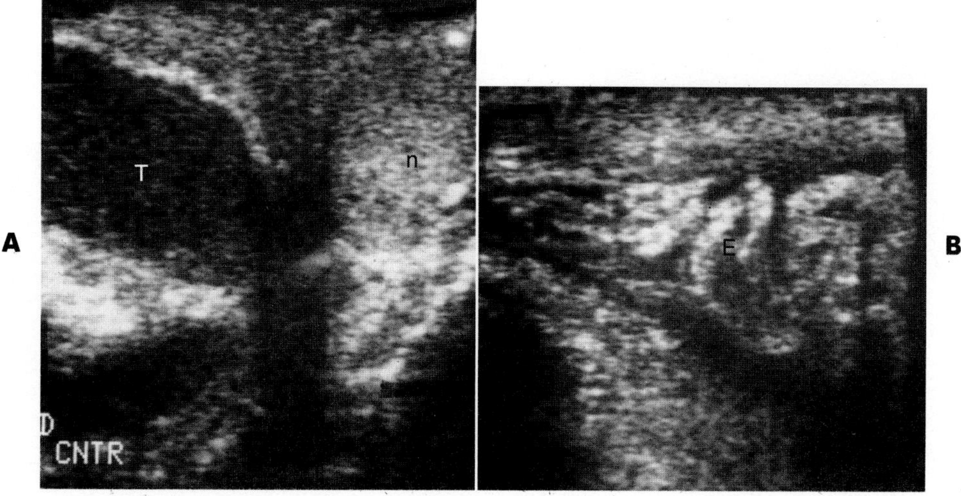

FIG. 15-10 A, Transverse sonogram of both testicles showing asymmetry of echogenicity and size. The torsed testicle *(T)* is hypoechoic and enlarged. Normal testicle, *N;* torsed testicle, *T.* **B,** Longitudinal scan of the enlarged epididymis in a torsed testicle. Epididymis, *E.*

Sonographically, acute epididymitis usually shows enlargement of the epididymal head, with decreased echogenicity secondary to edema. A reactive hydrocele may be present (Fig. 15-11). Color Doppler findings include an increased amount of flow in and around the epididymis. If an abscess has formed, complex cystic areas may be identified in the epididymis.

Infection that has spread to the testicle is termed *orchitis*. With orchitis, the testicle may appear normal or enlarged in size. The echogenicity may be decreased or heterogeneous (Fig. 15-12). Reactive hydroceles and skin thickening are associated with orchitis. With color Doppler, the testicle has increased blood flow (Fig. 15-13; see color image). The ultrasound appearance of chronic orchitis appears as layers of heterogeneous testicular parenchyma (Fig. 15-14).

Focal orchitis occurs without involvement of the epididymis and has the same appearance as a neoplasm. Focal orchitis cannot be distinguished from a neoplasm, although clinical symptoms, such as fever and an increased white blood count, strongly suggest an infectious process.

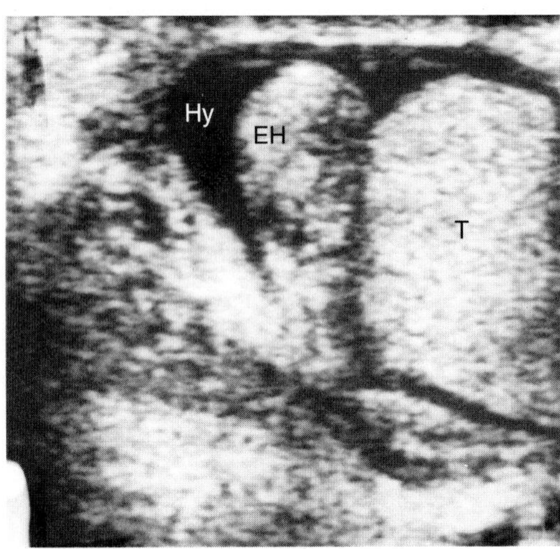

FIG. 15-11 Longitudinal sonogram of epididymitis, demonstrating an enlarged epididymis with a reactive hydrocele. Epididymal head, *EH;* hydrocele, *Hy;* testicle, *T*.

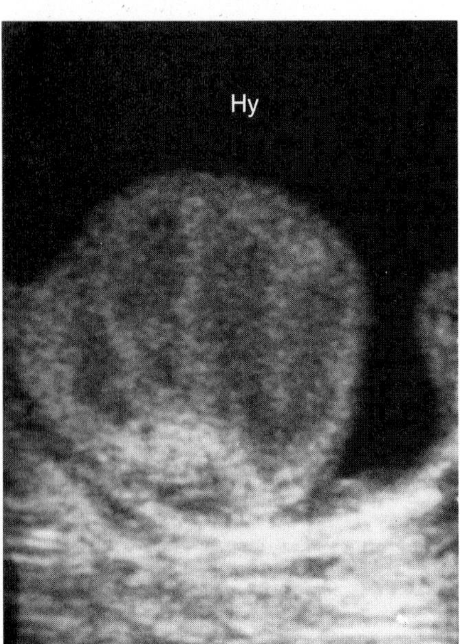

FIG. 15-12 Transverse scan of a testicle demonstrating areas of heterogeneous testicular tissue secondary to orchitis. Reactive hydrocele, *Hy*.

VARICOCELE

A varicocele is the abnormal dilation and tortuosity of the veins in the pampiniform plexus of the spermatic cord. Varicoceles are more common on the left but can occur bilaterally. The right internal spermatic vein drains directly into the inferior vena cava, whereas the left internal spermatic vein drains into the left renal vein at a 90-degree angle. This angle prevents the formation of a valve. As a result, 99% of varicoceles are left-sided and only 1% are bilateral.[6]

Varicoceles may cause infertility because they are associated with low sperm counts and decreased motility.[1] Varicoceles appear sonographically as an extratesticular collection of tortuous tubular structures (Fig. 15-15). Having the patient perform the Valsalva maneuver or stand may increase the size of the varicoceles, making them more obvious. Blood flow is present and can even be reversed but failure to detect flow cannot exclude diagnosis of a varicocele.

HYDROCELE

A hydrocele is a collection of fluid between the visceral and parietal layers of the tunica vaginalis. Hydroceles can

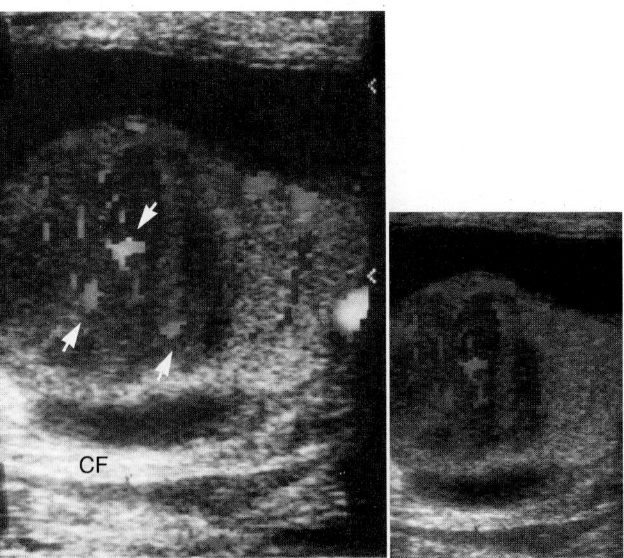

FIG. 15-13 Color Doppler scan demonstrating an increase in vascularity related to orchitis. Color flow, *CF* (see color flow image).

be congenital, idiopathic, or acquired. The size of hydroceles varies from just a few cubic centimeters to as much as a liter. Acquired hydroceles are a result of infarction, inflammation, neoplasm, or trauma. Hydroceles appear on ultrasound as anechoic fluid in the scrotum surrounding the testicle and epididymis. Occasionally, small particles and septations are seen in the fluid (Fig. 15-16).

EPIDIDYMAL CYSTS

Spermatoceles are benign cysts consisting of nonviable sperm. They are commonly located in the head of the epididymis, but have been found in the body and tail. Septations have been seen and spermatoceles can be singular or multiple. On ultrasound a spermatocele appears as an anechoic cyst, with posterior enhancement and rounded well-defined walls (Fig. 15-17).

A spermatocele cannot be differentiated from a simple epididymal cyst. Epididymal cysts are composed of clear serous fluid, not sperm. They are much less common than spermatoceles.[1]

HERNIA

Scrotal hernia occurs when a section of bowel herniates through a patent processus vaginalis into the scrotum. A patient presents with scrotal enlargement. Ultrasound can be used to diagnose hernia by demonstrating peristalsing loops of bowel in the scrotum (Fig. 15-18).

TRAUMA

In cases of scrotal trauma, ultrasound can be helpful in evaluating the extent of the injury. Testicular parenchymal injury or hemorrhage can alter the normal homogeneous appearance of the testicle (Fig. 15-19). Hematomas in the epididymis or scrotal wall have variable sonographic appearances. Like hematomas in other parts of the body, the

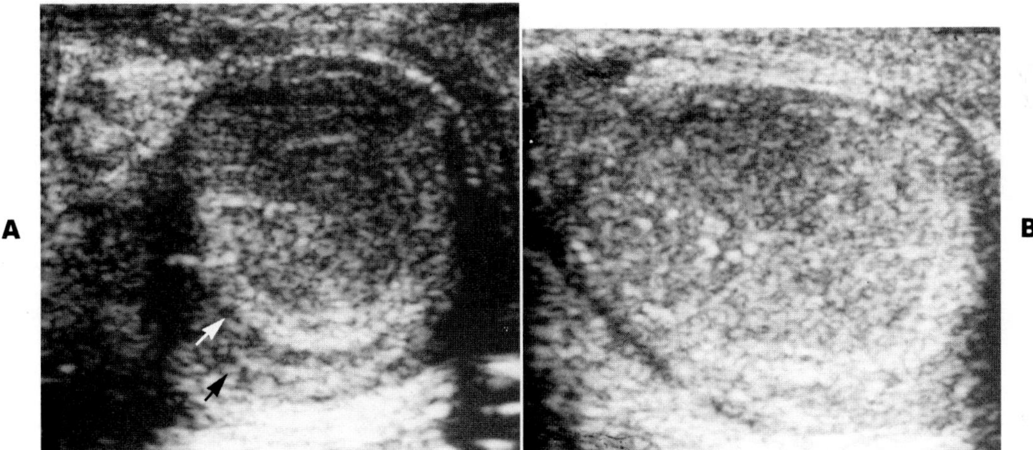

FIG. 15-14 A, Chronic orchitis. Transverse scan demonstrates the layering effect of a chronic condition of orchitis. **B,** Longitudinal scan of chronic orchitis. (Courtesy Alvarado Hospital Ultrasound Department, San Diego, CA.)

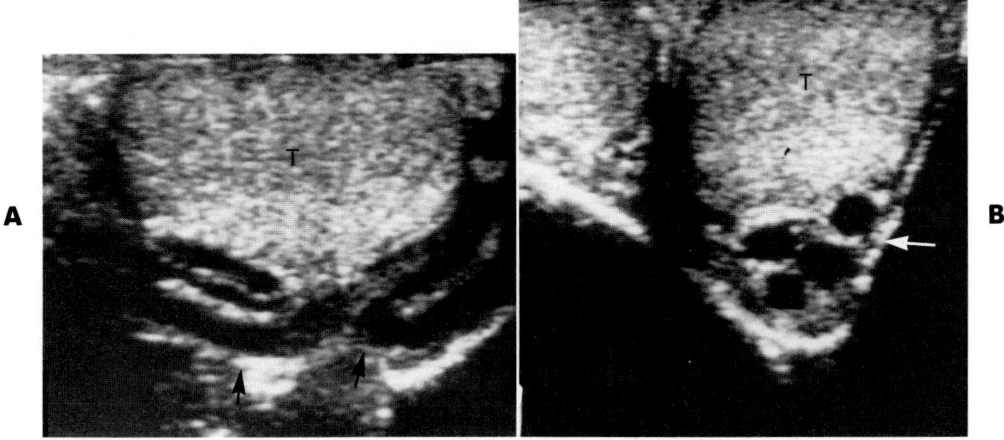

FIG. 15-15 A, Longitudinal scan of dilated veins of left pampiniform plexus representing a varicocele. Testicle, *T*. **B,** Transverse scan of dilated veins in a varicocele. Testicle, *T*.

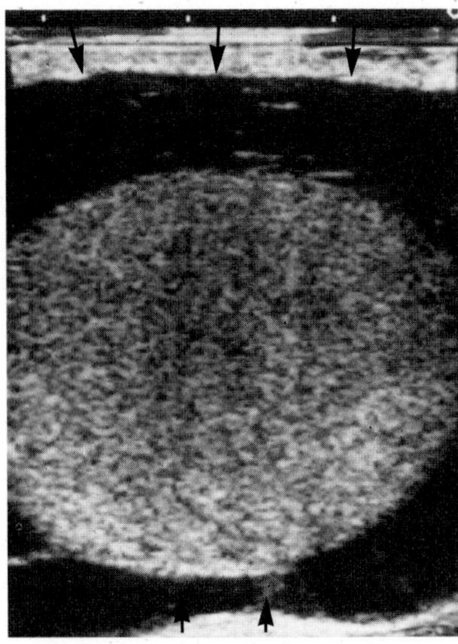

FIG. 15-16 Hydrocele with septations.

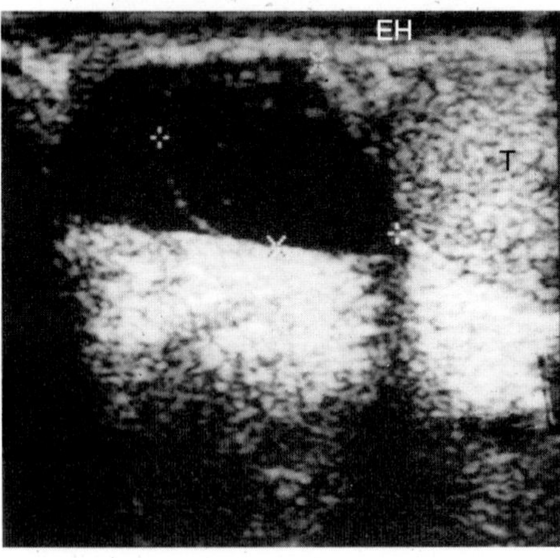

FIG. 15-17 Large spermatocele. Epididymal head, *EH;* testicle, *T*.

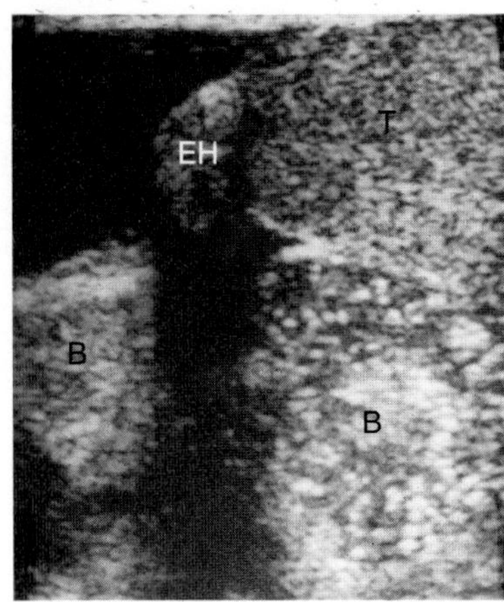

FIG. 15-18 A, Scrotal hernia. Epididymal head, *EH;* testicle, *T;* peristalsing bowel, *B*.

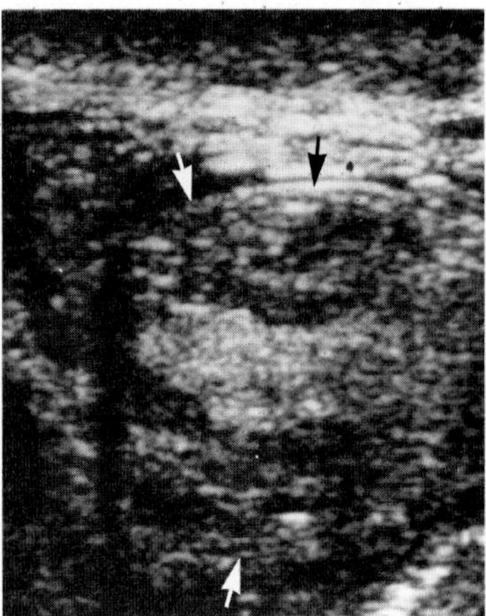

FIG. 15-19 Heterogeneous appearance of the testicle secondary to trauma. Hypoechoic areas represent hemorrhage resulting from testicular parenchymal injury.

appearance is different depending on the age of the hematoma. The first appearance of a hematoma is hypoechoic. As the hematoma ages, its appearance becomes more echogenic.

Other Superficial Structures

VASCULAR ACCESS FOR HEMODIALYSIS

Approximately 40,000 patients in the United States are undergoing chronic hemodialysis for end-stage renal disease. These are patients whose severely damaged kidneys are not capable of removing toxic products from the blood. Dialysis removes these substances and maintains electrolyte hemostasis by passing the patient's blood through a dialyzing solution.

Anatomy and Physiology

Circulatory access for hemodialysis depends on the creation of an easily accessible high-flow vascular system. This is accomplished by some form of surgical connection between an artery and vein. After anastomosis the veins frequently enlarge because of increased flow of arterialized blood through them. Needles can then be inserted into the arterialized veins to provide adequate flow for dialysis.

Creation of a successful arteriovenous (AV) anastomosis requires a situation in which adequate arteries and veins can be joined without stress and without jeopardy to circulation of the extremity involved. The forearm and thigh are the usual locations, with common hookups being radial artery to cephalic vein, brachial artery to antecubital vein, and femoral artery to saphenous vein. The anastomosis can be of the side-to-side, end-to-end, or end-to-side design. This description refers to the respective arterial-venous or graft-venous relationship.

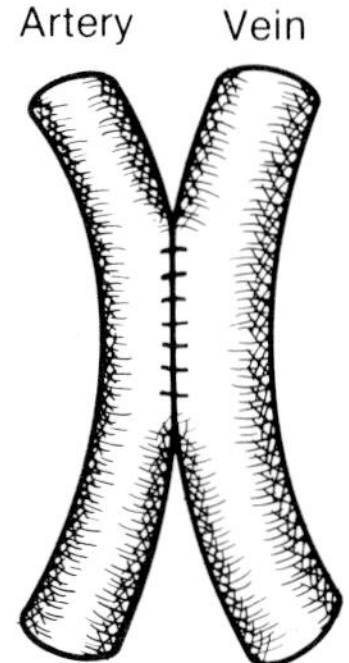

FIG. 15-20 Typical side-to-side arrangement for an arteriovenous fistula. (Redrawn from Massry S and Sellers A: Clinical aspects of uremia and dialysis, Springfield, Ill, 1976, Charles C Thomas.)

Vascular access systems are of two types. One is a direct AV fistula using the patient's own vessels; the other involves the use of tubes, either heterologous (usually bovine) or synthetic materials.

Arteriovenous Fistula

The AV fistula proved to be a major advance over the previously used external Silastic (Scribner) shunts in terms of complications and failures. It is usually the arrangement of choice for initial vascular access.

A side-to-side anastomosis between an artery and the largest available adjacent vein is made (Fig. 15-20). Increased blood flow created by fistula formation causes the subcutaneous veins to become progressively dilated, thereby providing sufficient blood flow for hemodialysis.

Bovine Heterograft

Bovine heterografts made from processed carotid arteries of cows are usually reserved for patients whose vessels will not permit establishment of an AV fistula or whose fistula has failed.

The anastomosis is frequently the end-to-side type (Fig. 15-21). A loop fistula between the radial or ulnar artery and the antecubital or a deep vein in the forearm is also common. The thigh is usually reserved as a last resort because of an increased incidence of graft complications in this location.

Synthetic Graft

Polytetrafluoroethylene (Gore-Tex) has become a popular material for use in vascular access. Grafts of synthetic material are easier to handle and easier to reoperate on, and they have a better rate of patency than do bovine heterografts.

Straight or U-shaped anastomoses are used with preference for the proximal radial artery and a medial vein at or above the elbow joint (Fig. 15-22).

Pathology

A number of complications can lead to failure of the access. AV fistulas and bovine heterografts have higher complication rates in patients with proved arterial disease. The most likely cause is low blood flow.

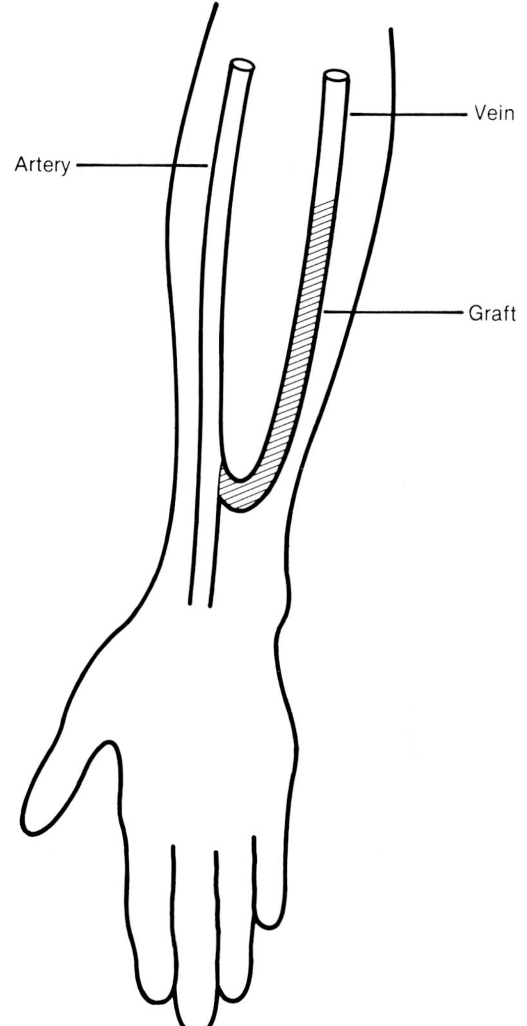

FIG. 15-21 Schema of a bovine heterograft. (Courtesy Christine Skram, RDMS, University of California Medical Center, San Diego.)

Thrombosis

The most common complication to cause access failure is thrombosis. It develops because of low blood flow, which is a result of inadequate arterial inflow or high venous resistance (outflow obstruction). Common sites of thrombosis are anastomotic and puncture sites. Occlusion can develop as a result of thrombus accumulation. Thrombectomy or reconstruction can be performed in an attempt to salvage the access.

Infection

Early detection of infection is crucial in vascular accesses, since graft replacement is often required in inadequately treated cases. Infection can result from repeated venipunctures or after operation. Bovine heterografts are es-

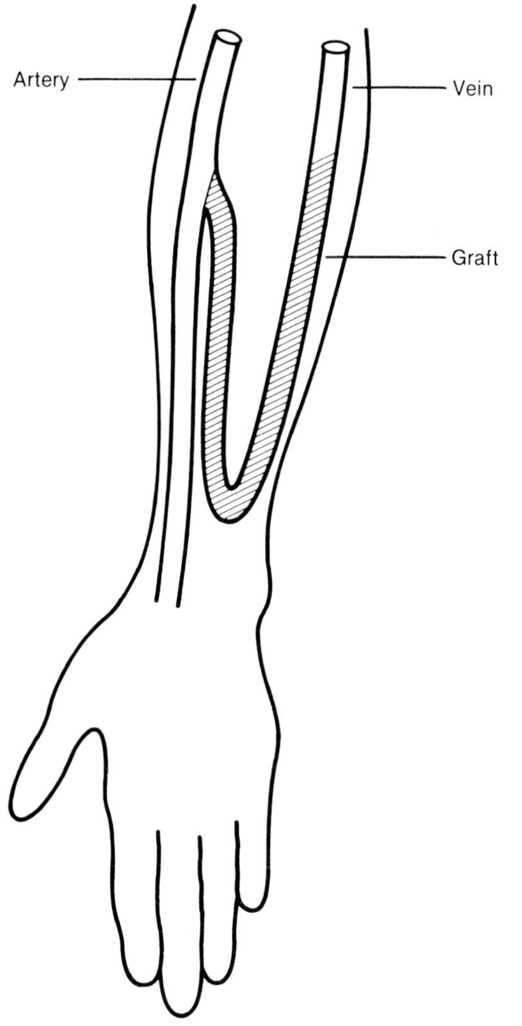

FIG. 15-22 Schema of a synthetic graft. (Courtesy Christine Skram, RDMS, University of California Medical Center, San Diego.)

pecially susceptible to infection, but this is not a significant problem with radiocephalic AV fistulas. Treatment with systemic and/or topical antibiotics is effective. Localized abscesses can be drained, but if they are grossly infected, the graft must be removed.

Aneurysm

An aneurysm is the result of weakness of the venous wall resulting from high venous pressure or repeated dialysis trauma. Thrombus can develop within the aneurysm. More ominously, graft degeneration with hemorrhage or infection may occur.

Pseudoaneurysm

A false aneurysm, which probably results from extravasation, may develop as a result of trauma or infection. It is usually found at the site of anastomosis (usually arterial) or at a needle puncture tear.

Ultrasound Evaluation

Scanning Technique

To evaluate arm fistulas the patient is placed recumbent, primarily for purposes of stability and support of the arm. The arm of interest is closest to the operator and is extended (hand up) and supported on the bed beside the patient. If the arm cannot be positioned as described, a firm flat device for support from shoulder to hand may be used. The patient's arm is abducted approximately 45 degrees with the support device positioned under it and the shoulder. If necessary, the examination may be performed with the patient in a wheelchair. Support of the extended arm can be obtained with the device stabilized on the arm of the wheelchair.

For evaluation of leg fistulas the patient is supine on a bed with the leg of interest closest to the operator. A slight frogleg position facilitates transducer access.

A preliminary review of the patient's surgical anatomy (and pathosis if present) should be undertaken before image recording.

Since the vein is usually of larger caliber and easier to identify, it is located first and the survey is begun longitudinally near the elbow. With an AV fistula the vein is traced toward the wrist to the anastomosis. After examination of the anastomosis the artery is then traced back to the elbow. A graft is evaluated similarly: scanning is performed toward the wrist through the vein, venous anastomosis, and graft. The arterial anastomosis and artery are then identified, and the sonographer continues to scan back toward the elbow.

After preliminary exploration, scanning is repeated with image documentation of the vein, venous anastomosis, graft, arterial anastomosis, artery, and any pathologic condition that may be present. Transverse scanning is performed using this routine. The flexibility of real time allows the vasculature to be delineated with relative ease.

Ultrasound Appearances

Arteriovenous Fistula. Since existing vasculature is used in creation of an AV fistula, the artery and vein are seen as anechoic tubular channels. With survey through the vessels the anastomosis, usually side-to-side, can be identified where the vein becomes contiguous with the artery (Fig. 15-23). The vascular thrill detected on palpation is helpful in localizing the anastomosis.

Bovine Heterograft. The appearance of a normal bovine heterograft is of an anechoic tubular channel whose walls are smooth and regular. It has essentially the same echographic appearance as a patient's normal blood vessels. The anastomoses can be difficult to identify because of the echographic similarity of the heterograft and the native vessel; however, a slight wall irregularity is often evident at the suture site. The end-to-side arterial anastomosis can be identified by tracing the heterograft to its insertion into the side of the artery.

Synthetic Graft. The synthetic graft appears as a very

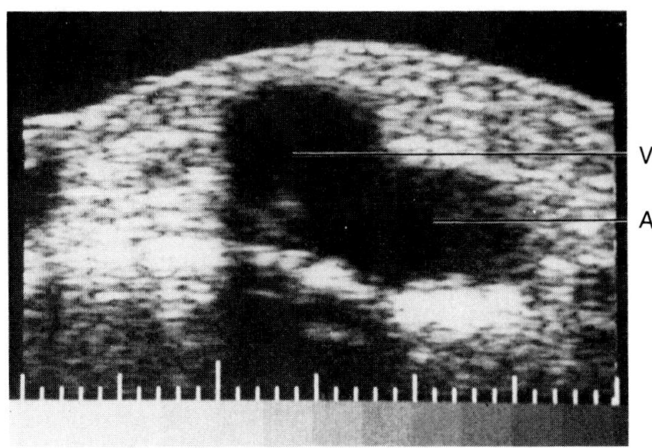

FIG. 15-23 Transverse section through arterial, *A*, to venous, *V*, anastomosis of a normal arteriovenous fistula.

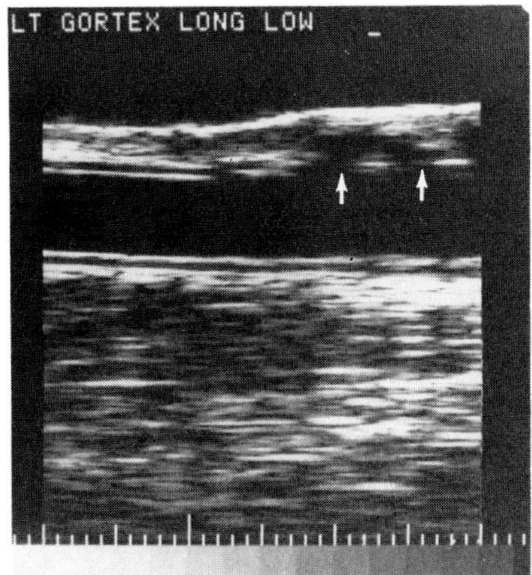

FIG. 15-24 Longitudinal sonogram of a synthetic graft. Note the smooth walls of the graft interrupted at the needle puncture sites *(arrows)*.

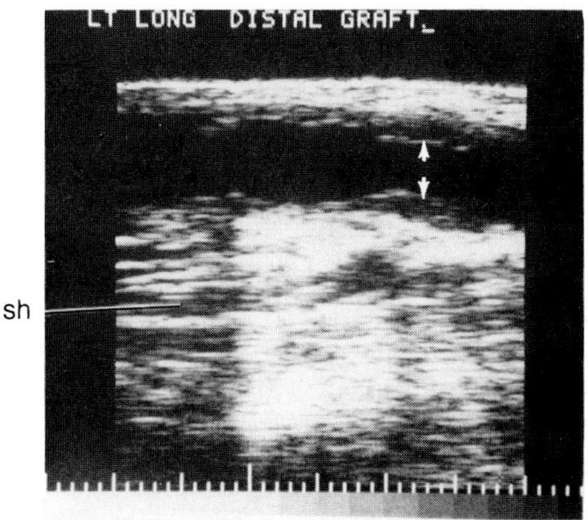

FIG. 15-25 Scan of synthetic graft anastomosis. The junction between the graft and the host vein can be identified by the shadowing, *sh*, deep to the graft. Minimal stenosis *(between arrowheads)* is also present within the vein.

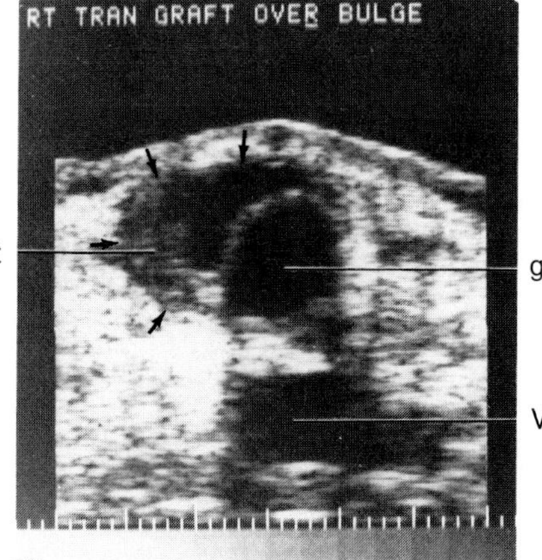

FIG. 15-26 Transverse scan of a synthetic graft, *g*, demonstrating a pseudoaneurysm *(arrows)* partially filled with thrombus, *t*. Native vessel, *V*.

discrete anechoic channel (Fig. 15-24). Because of its acoustic properties, synthetic graft material demonstrates a greater beam attenuation than do native vessels. The anastomosis can be clearly identified by the sharp difference in echo attenuation between the graft and the host vessel (Fig. 15-25).

Complications. A number of complications have been reported.

Thrombosis of a vascular access appears as an irregular echo reflection within the otherwise anechoic lumen of the vessel and may create an acoustic shadow. The amount and extent of resultant stenosis can be demonstrated. Special note should be made of wall irregularities from needle puncture, since they may be sites of thrombus deposition.

On rare occasions, soft or early thrombus may not create sufficient acoustic impedance to be sonographically evident. Doppler sonography may be useful in these instances.

Infection can appear as a sonolucent or complex mass around the graft or as vegetations within the graft appearing as echoes projecting from the wall of the lumen. Vegetations may flap with pulsations that can be documented by real time. Special attention should be paid to repeated venipuncture sites since they are potential abscess formation sites.

A palpable mass of vascular grafts is frequently an aneurysm. A localized increase in the normal caliber of the vein is characteristic. Thrombus may occur within the aneurysm, which is an area of relative stasis.

A pseudoaneurysm occurs most commonly at the anastomotic site or at a needle-puncture site. A thrombus may totally fill the pseudoaneurysm (Fig. 15-26).

REVIEW QUESTIONS

1. Name five uses of ultrasound diagnosis of the scrotum.
2. Describe the anatomy of the scrotum.
3. Define the anatomic location of the epididymis.

4. What ultrasound technique is used to image the scrotum?
5. Which transducer should be used to image the scrotum?
6. Where are the testes formed? What is the abnormality called if their migration is incomplete?
7. What are the clinical signs of primary testicular cancer?
8. Why is it important to know if the mass is intratesticular or extratesticular?
9. What are the categories of testicular tumors?
10. Which tumor type has the best prognosis?
11. What is the significance of microlithiasis?
12. Describe the development of testicular torsion and its significance.
13. What is the ultrasound appearance of torsion?
14. Describe the sonographic appearance of acute epididymitis.
15. What is orchitis? Describe the ultrasound findings.
16. What is a varicocele? How does the Valsalva maneuver help the sonographer determine if a varicocele is present?
17. Name the cause of the development of a hydrocele.
18. How can the sonographer determine if a hernia is present?
19. Describe the complications of an anastomosis between the artery and vein in a dialysis patient.
20. How is color flow useful in the diagnosis of a pseudoaneurysm?

REFERENCES

1. Benson C and Doubilet P: Scrotum. In Mittlestaedt C, editor: General ultrasound, pp. 1134-1145, New York, 1992, Churchill Livingston.
2. Garnick MB, Prout GR, and Canellos GP: Germinal tumors of the testis. In Holland JF and Frei E, editors: Cancer medicine, Philadelphia, 1982, Lea & Febiger.
3. Gooding GAW, Leonhart W, and Stein R: Testicular cysts: ultrasound findings, Radiology 163:537, 1987.
4. Harrison R: The distribution of the vasal and cremasteric arteries to the testis and their functional importance, J Anat 82:267, 1989.
5. Krone KD and Carroll BA: Scrotal ultrasound, Radiol Clin North Am 23:121, 1985.
6. Netter F: Scrotum: reproductive system, p. 73, West Caldwell, 1989, CIBA 1965.

• PART THREE •

Pediatric Applications

CHAPTER

16

Neonatal Echoencephalography

Sandra Hagen-Ansert • Raul Bejar

Brain damage is common in premature infants. Intraventricular and subependymal hemorrhages occur in 40% to 70% of premature neonates under 34 weeks gestation. Multifocal necrosis of the white matter or periventricular leukomalacia can develop in 12% to 20% of infants weighing less than 2000 g. These lesions are associated with increased mortality and an abnormal neurologic outcome.

With advancements in ultrasound, computerized tomography, and magnetic imaging, the last decade has brought increased understanding of the intracranial lesions of premature babies. For many reasons, echoencephalography continues to be the technique of choice to visualize the neonatal brain. This technique continues to be available at the bedside, is nonionizing and noninvasive, and is tolerated by even the sickest infants.

Real time technology has allowed the sonographer to image the neonatal skull through high-resolution gray scale with retained spatial relationships. Real time also allows the sonographer to follow the continuity of structures within the brain. This feature is important when following structures such as the choroid plexus in the lateral ventricles. The purpose of this chapter is to present our approach to imaging the normal and abnormal neonatal brain. First we review fetal brain anatomy. A discussion of the techniques of sonographic evaluation then leads the reader into the visualization of both the normal and the abnormal brain. Finally, we review many different parameters that may help interpret the images.

EMBRYOLOGIC DEVELOPMENT OF THE NEONATAL BRAIN

Development of the brain begins early in the embryo and continues until birth. At approximately 18 days of embryonic life the neural plate begins to develop. From this neural plate, the neural tube forms, eventually differentiating into the central nervous system (brain and spinal cord). The cranial end of the neural tube, which forms the brain, differentiates and grows the fastest.[32] At approximately the fourth week of development the expanding neural folds fuse to form the following three primary brain vesicles: the forebrain or prosencephalon, the midbrain or mesencephalon, and the hindbrain or rhombencephalon (Fig. 16-1). From these three primary vesicles arise all the anatomic landmarks necessary for neonatal brain evaluation. An understanding of this development helps the sonographer understand the anatomy encountered during the ultrasound examination. The following discussion is a concise summary of embryologic development to help the sonographer understand the development of the fetal brain.

As the neural tube folds, forming the primary brain vesicles, there is some associated flexing ventrally. The rapid growth of the brain causes this bending; the midbrain and the cervical flexures result. Later another flexure forms, which is caused by uneven growth; this is the pontine flexure (Fig. 16-2). The pontine flexure, midbrain flexure, and cervical flexure all shape the evolving brain for the final stages of development.

The pontine flexure divides the hindbrain into caudal (myelencephalon) and rostral (metencephalon) parts. The myelencephalon becomes the medulla oblongata, and the metencephalon gives rise to the pons and cerebellum (Fig. 16-3). The fourth ventricle arises from the cavity of the hindbrain.

The midbrain (mesencephalon) undergoes relatively few changes. The third and fourth ventricles are joined by the cerebral aqueduct as the neural canal narrows (Fig. 16-4). Just rostral to the developing cerebellum the cerebral peduncles are formed of fibers growing down from the cerebrum. The cerebral peduncles become more prominent as more descending fibers pass through the developing midbrain on their way to the brain stem.

The forebrain or prosencephalon has a central part called the *diencephalon* and lateral expansions called the *telencephalon*. The walls of the diencephalon become the thalami, and the cavity forms the third ventricle (Fig. 16-5). The thalamus on each side develops rapidly and bulges into the cavity of the third ventricle. This pressure on the third ventricle reduces it to a narrow slit, which explains why the third ventricle is so difficult to see in the normal state with ultrasound. In approximately 70% of fetal heads the thalami meet and fuse in the midline.[32] This forms a bridge of gray matter across the third ventricle, called the *mass*

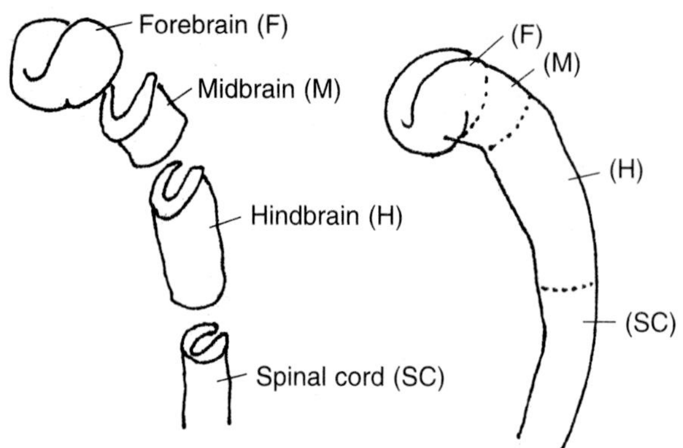

FIG. 16-1 Early development of the brain in the fourth week of development shows the neural folds as they fuse to form three primary brain vesicles—the forebrain, *F*, or prosencephalon, the midbrain, *M*, or mesenencephalon, and the hindbrain, *H*, or rhombencephalon.

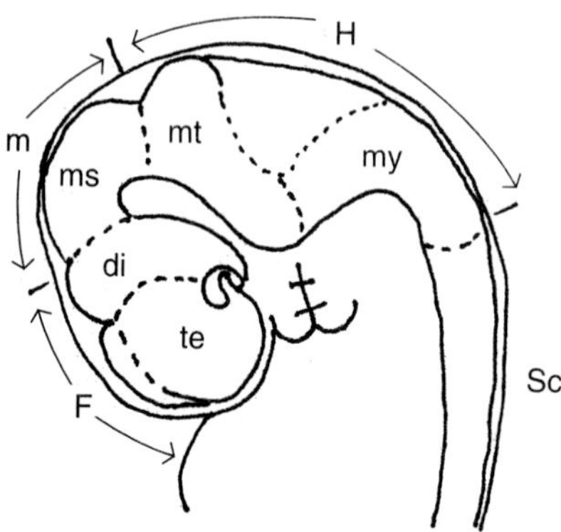

FIG. 16-2 As the neural tube folds, forming the primary brain vesicles, there is some associated flexing ventrally. The midbrain and the cervical flexures both bend forward. Forebrain, *F;* telencephalon, *te,* diencephalon, *di;* midbrain, *M;* mesenceaphlon, *ms;* hindbrain, *H;* metencephalon, *mt;* myelencephalon, *my;* spinal cord, *sc.*

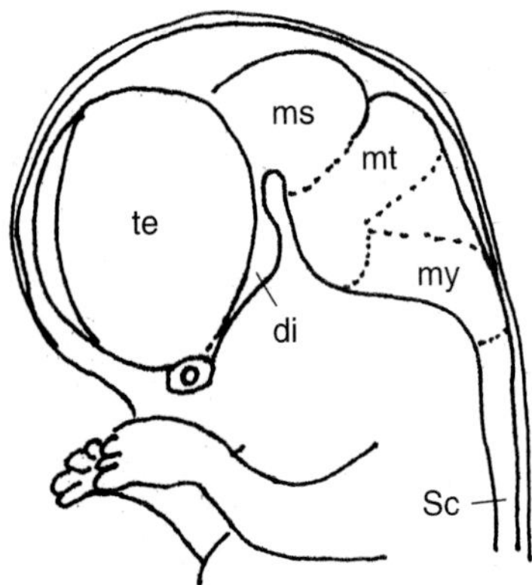

FIG. 16-3 The pontine flexure divides the hindbrain into caudal, myelencephalon, *my,* rostral, metencephalon, *mt,* parts. The myelencephalon becomes the medulla oblongata, and the metencephalon gives rise to the pons and cerebellum. Telencephalon, *te;* mesencephalon, *ms;* diencephalon, *di;* spinal cord, *sc.*

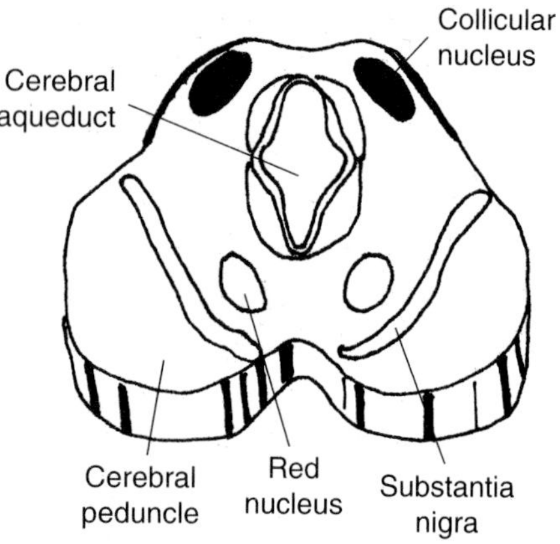

FIG. 16-4 The third and fourth ventricles are joined by the cerebral aqueduct as the neural canal narrows.

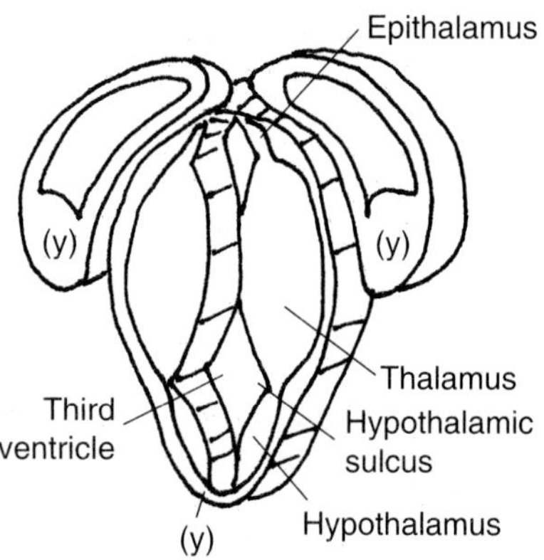

FIG. 16-5 The forebrain has a central part called the *diencephalon* and lateral expansions called the *telencephalon.* The walls of the diencephalon become the thalami, and the cavity forms the third ventricle.

intermedia, which can be seen by ultrasound only in the abnormal state.

The cavity of the telencephalon forms the lateral ventricles and the extreme anterior part of the third ventricle. At first the lateral ventricles (at this early stage called the *cerebral vesicles*) are in wide communication with the third ventricle through the interventricular foramina. As the cerebral hemispheres expand, they cover the diencephalon, midbrain, and hindbrain. Eventually the hemispheres meet at the midline, flattening their medial surfaces. This decreases the size of the interventricular foramina and forms the longitudinal fissure between them, called the *falx cerebri.* As the hemispheres grow, they assume a C shape. This differential growth and curvature also affects the shape of the developing lateral ventricles. The ventricles likewise assume a C shape, with frontal, posterior, and temporal horns forming. As the cerebral cortex differentiates, fibers passing to and from it divide into the caudate and lentiform nuclei. The caudate nucleus becomes elongated and C shaped, conforming to the outline of the lateral ventricle (Fig. 16-

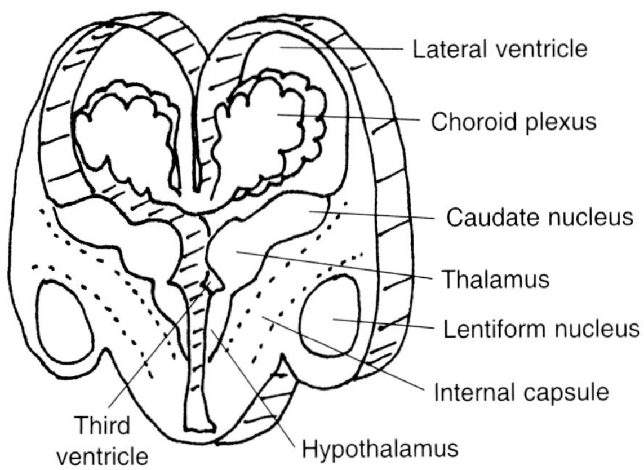

FIG. 16-6 As the cerebral cortex differentiates, fibers passing to and from it divide into the caudate and lentiform nuclei. The caudate nucleus becomes elongated and C-shaped, conforming to the outline of the lateral ventricle.

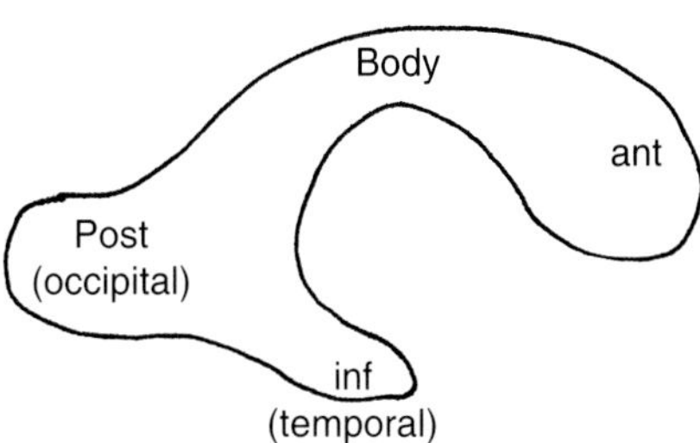

FIG. 16-7 Sagittal section of the lateral ventricle divided into anterior, body, posterior (occipital), and inferior (temporal) horns.

6). Its head and body lie in the floor of the anterior horn and body of the lateral ventricle. Its tail makes a U-shaped turn, winding up on the roof of the temporal horn of the lateral ventricle.

As the ventricles and cerebrum are developing and taking shape, changes are occurring that will produce the choroid plexus. All four ventricles are lined by an ependymal membrane. This ependymal lining, covered externally by vascular pia mater, forms the tela choroidea. The very active proliferation of the vascular pia mater causes the tela choroidea to invaginate into the ventricular cavity. There is further differentiation until the tufted choroid plexuses form. This process takes place at the roof of the third and fourth ventricles and posteromedial walls of the lateral ventricles to form the choroid plexus. When formed, the choroid plexuses are responsible for the secretion and absorption of cerebrospinal fluid.

The rate of growth varies in the various parts of the brain. The ventricles grow slower than the cerebral hemispheres. This explains the high ventricular-to-hemispheric ratio at 15 weeks (40% to 70%) compared with the low ventricular-to-hemispheric ratio at term (23% to 33%).[25] The growth and development of the different parts of the brain are also very complicated in the early stages. Fortunately most of the complicated differential growth occurs before the intracranial structures in the neonate are evaluated by ultrasound. After 20 to 35 weeks the brain is essentially developed and is just increasing in size and maturing.[32]

ANATOMY OF THE NEONATAL BRAIN

The sonographer must be familiar with specific anatomic structures within the brain to perform a complete ultrasound examination of the neonatal head. The cranial cavity contains the brain and its surrounding meninges and portions of the cranial nerves, arteries, veins, and venous sinuses.

Ventricular System

The lateral ventricles are the largest of the cerebral spinal fluid cavities located within the cerebral hemispheres. They communicate with the third ventricle through the interventricular foramen. There are two lateral ventricles, located on either side of the brain. The lateral ventricles are divided into the following four segments: frontal horn, body, and occipital and temporal horns (Fig. 16-7). The atrium or trigone is the site where the anterior, occipital, and temporal horns join together.

The body of the lateral ventricle extends from the foramen of Monro to the trigone. The corpus callosum forms the roof and the septum pellucidum forms the medial wall. The thalamus touches the inferior lateral ventricular wall and the body of the caudate nucleus borders the superior wall.

The temporal horn extends anteriorly from the trigone through the temporal lobe. The roof is formed by the white matter of the temporal lobe and by the tail of the caudate nucleus. The hippocampus forms the medial wall.

The occipital horn extends posteriorly from the trigone. The occipital cortex and white matter form the medial wall. The corpus callosum forms the proximal roof and lateral wall.

The frontal horn is divided posteriorly by the foramen of Monro near the body of the ventricle. The roof is formed by the corpus callosum. The septum pellucidum forms the medial wall and the head of the caudate nucleus forms the lateral wall.

The third ventricle is connected by the foramen of Monro to the lateral ventricles. The aqueduct of Sylvius connects the third and fourth ventricles. The medulla oblongata forms the floor of the ventricle. The roof is formed by the cerebellar vermis and posterior medullary vellum. The massa intermedia is a soft-tissue structure visualized with ventricular dilation.

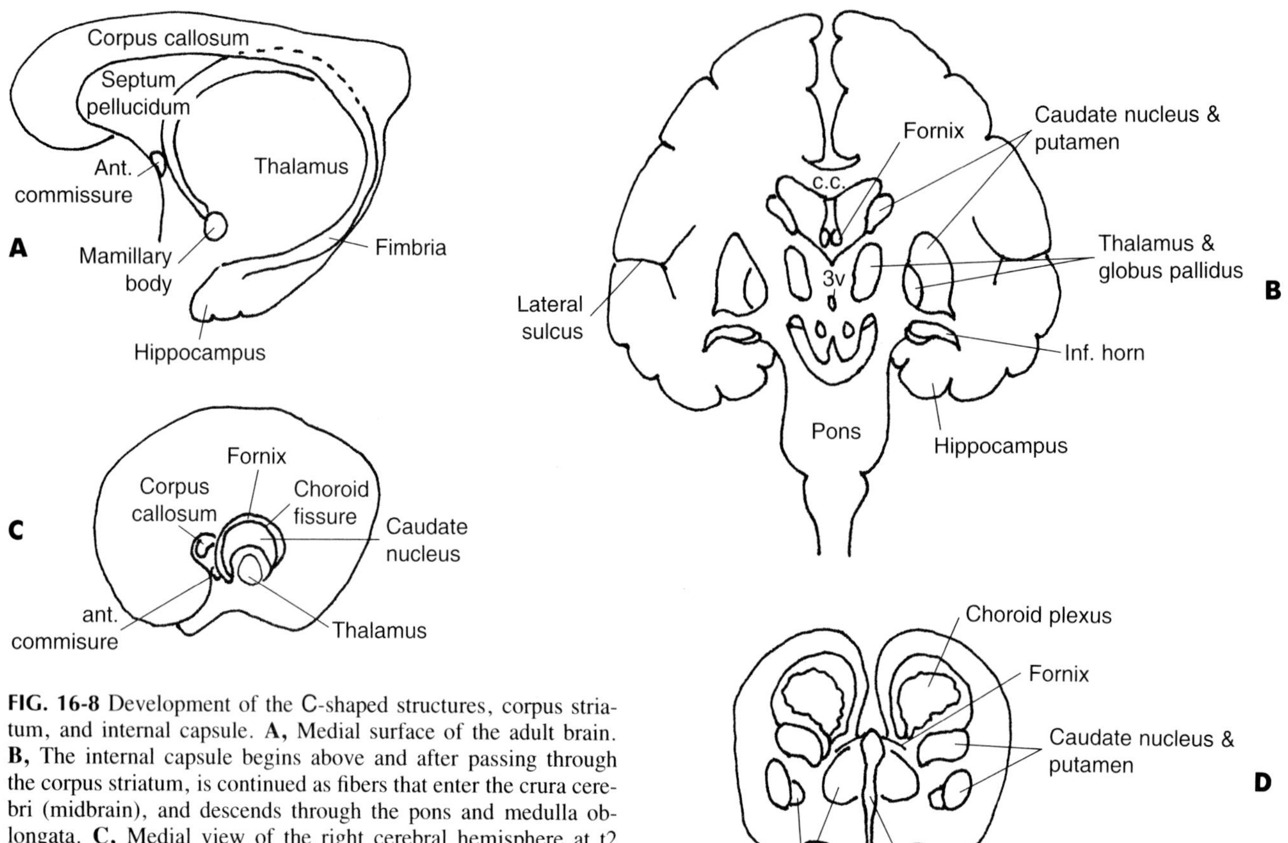

FIG. 16-8 Development of the C-shaped structures, corpus striatum, and internal capsule. **A,** Medial surface of the adult brain. **B,** The internal capsule begins above and after passing through the corpus striatum, is continued as fibers that enter the crura cerebri (midbrain), and descends through the pons and medulla oblongata. **C,** Medial view of the right cerebral hemisphere at t2 weeks. The fornix and choroid fissure have begun their C-shaped course, but the corpus callosum has not yet grown backward. **D,** The longitudinal fissure between the cerebral hemispheres leads directly onto the roof of the third ventricle.

The fourth ventricle is a cavity of the hindbrain. The fourth ventricle is connected to the third by the cerebral aqueduct. This aqueduct of Sylvius is seen with massive ventricular enlargement. Below, the fourth ventricle is continuous with the central canal of the spinal cord.

Cavum Septum Pellucidum. The cavum septum pellucidum is a thin triangular hole filled with cerebrospinal fluid, which lies between the anterior horn of the lateral ventricles. The cavum vergae is found at the posterior tip of the cavum septum pellucidi. It closes at 24 weeks of gestation (Fig. 16-8, *A*).

Brain Stem. The brain stem is the part of the brain connecting the forebrain and the spinal cord. It consists of the midbrain, pons, and medulla oblongata.

Cerebellum/Vermis. The cerebellum/vermis is the portion of the brain that lies posterior to the pons and medulla oblongata and below the tentorium. It lies in the posterior cranial fossa under the tentorium cerebelli. The two hemispheres are connected by the vermis. It is connected to the midbrain by the cerebellar peduncles. The middle cerebellar peduncles connect the cerebellum to the pons and the inferior cerebellar penduncles connect the cerebellum to the medulla.

Pons. The pons is found on the anterior surface of the cerebellum below the midbrain and above the medulla oblongata (Fig. 16-8, *B*).

Tentorium. The tentorium is a V-shaped echogenic structure separating the cerebrum and the cerebellum; it is an extension of the falx cerebri.

Falx Cerebri. The falx is a fibrous structure separating the two cerebral hemispheres.

Cisterna Magna. The cisterna magna is located in the posterior fossa of the brain. It is an enclosed space serving as a reservoir for cerebral spinal fluid.

Caudate Nucleus. The caudate nucleus is the portion of the brain that forms the lateral borders of the frontal horns of the lateral ventricles and lies anterior to the thalamus. It is further divided into the head, body, and tail. The head of the caudate nucleus is a common site for hemorrhage (Fig. 16-8, *C*).

Corpus Collosum. The corpus collosum is a mass of white matter that connects the two cerebral hemispheres. This structure forms the roof of the lateral ventricles. The corpus collosum sits on top of the cavum septum vellucidum (see Fig. 16-8, *C*).

Cerebral Hemispheres. There are two cerebral hemispheres connected by the corpus callosum. They extend from the frontal to the occipital bones, above the anterior and middle cranial fossae. Posteriorly they extend above the tentorium cerebelli. They are separated by a longitudinal fissure into which projects the falx cerebri.

Thalamus. The thalamus consists of two ovoid, egg-shaped brain structures situated on either side of the third ventricle superior to the brain stem (Fig. 16-8, *A* and *D*).

Cavum Septi-pellucidum. The cavum septi-pellucidum is a thin, triangular hole filled with cerebral spinal fluid that lies between the anterior horns of the lateral ventricles.

Choroid Plexus. The choroid plexus is a mass of special cells located in the atrium of the lateral ventricles. These cells regulate the intraventricular pressure by secretion or absorption of cerebral spinal fluid. The glomus is the tail of the choroid plexus and is a major site for bleeds (see Fig. 16-8, *D*).

Germinal Matrix. The germinal matrix includes periventricular tissue and the caudate nucleus. It is located 1 cm above the caudate nucleus in the floor of the lateral ventricle. It sweeps from the frontal horn posteriorly into the temporal horn.

Midbrain. The midbrain portion of the brain is narrow and connects the forebrain to the hindbrain. It consists of two halves called the *cerebral penduncles*. The cerebral aqueduct is a narrow cavity of the midbrain that connects the third and fourth ventricles. The tectum is part of the tegmentum located behind the cerebral aqueduct. It has four small surface swellings called the *superior* and *inferior colliculi*.

Meninges. The meninges are the brain coverings and spinal cord coverings. There are dura mater, arachnoid, and pia mater membranes.

Ependyma. The ependyma is a membrane lining the cerebral ventricles. The subependyma is the area immediately beneath the ependyma.

Fontanelle. Fontanelles are the spaces between the bones of the skull. In the neonate the fontanelles have not closed completely. The transducer is placed carefully on the fontanelle to record multiple images of the brain in the coronal, axial, and sagittal planes.

Fissures. The interhemispheric fissure is the area in which the falx cerebri sits and separates the two cerebral hemispheres. The sylvian fissure is bilateral and is the area where the middle cerebral artery is located. The quadramgemia fissure is located posterior and inferior from the cavum vergae. The vein of Galen is posterior, so the sonographer must be aware that Doppler should be performed to make sure it is a fissure and not an enlarged vein of Galen.

Gyrus and Sulcus. The gyri are convolutions on the surface of the brain caused by infolding of the cortex. The sulcus is a groove or depression on the surface of the brain separating the gyri. The sulci further divide the hemispheres into frontal, parietal, occipital, and temporal lobes.

METHODS OF EVALUATION

In preparing the ultrasound room for the neonatal examination a number of considerations must be taken into account. First, even though the neonate may be well enough to come to the laboratory, he or she is still fragile and susceptible to any environmental changes. Consequently blankets, radiant heaters, oxygen hookups, and heating pads are all essential to making the environment in the laboratory suitable. Second, if there are any problems with the child, a crash cart and life support systems must be immediately available. A neonatal nurse specialist will probably accompany the neonate to the laboratory. However, the ultrasound equipment may be easily transported to the neonatal intensive care unit for initial evaluation and follow-up.

Sonographic Evaluation of the Neonatal Brain

Ultrasound Techniques. Phased array or linear sector transducers are the equipment of choice to perform echoencephalography studies. The small transducer makes it possible to obtain excellent contact with the skull through the fontanelles and sutures and to avoid the curvature of the calvarium. Consequently, the brain is visualized well even in infants with small fontanelles.[3,36] A 7.5- to 10-MHz transducer should be used with the premature infant. In larger babies the studies can be obtained with a 7.5-MHz transducer for structures located close to the fontanelles and a 5-MHz transducer for visualization of the anatomy in areas situated farther away from the transducer.

Multiple planes and views are used to study the supratentorial and infratentorial compartments.[9,10,12] Supratentorial studies show both cerebral hemispheres, the basal ganglia, the lateral and third ventricles, the interhemispheric fissure, and the subarachnoid space surrounding the hemispheres. Infratentorial studies visualize the cerebellum, the brain stem, the fourth ventricle, and the basal cisterns.

Both compartments are studied in the coronal, modified coronal, sagittal, and parasagittal planes. The sagittal, parasagittal, and modified coronal planes are imaged from the anterior fontanelle (Fig. 16-9). Since the structures in the infratentorial compartment are located relatively far from the transducer, a medium or long focal distance transducer is recommended, particularly in older infants. The coronal views for the infratentorial compartment are obtained from the mastoid fontanelle and the occipitotemporal suture (Fig. 16-10).

At this point, we examine the cross-sectional relationship of structures within the brain so correlation can be made with ultrasound. There are many ways to divide the brain in cross-section. We deal only with the three planes that are commonly used in ultrasound: axial, coronal, and sagittal.

A recommended protocol used in our department is provided.

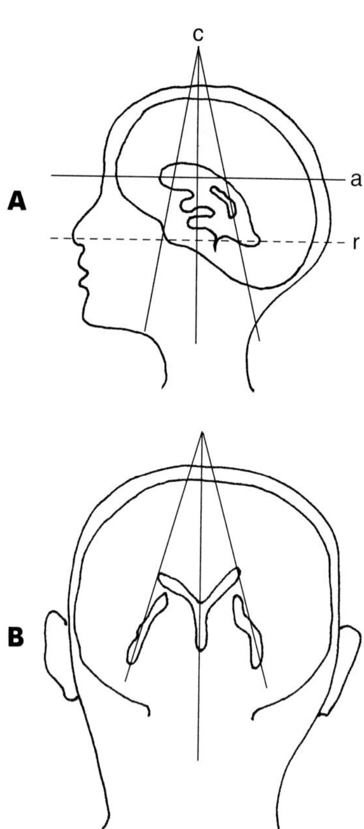

FIG. 16-9 **A,** Coronal views of the neonatal head are made through the anterior fontanelle, *c*. The transducer is angled from the anterior skull to the posterior skull to record various parts of the neonatal brain anatomy. Axial plane of view, *a;* reid's baseline, *r*. **B,** Sagittal views of the neonatal head are made through the sagittal suture.

NEONATAL HEAD EXAMINATION PROTOCOL

Transducer

- 5.0 MHz for over 34 weeks or macrocephaly
- 7.0 MHz for under 34 weeks
- 10.0 MHz for 24 to 26 weeks

Coronal*

1. Anterior: orbits
2. Anterior: anterior horns and lateral ventricles
3. Anterior: anterior horns and lateral ventricles
4. Middle: lateral ventricles, cavum septum pellucidum, third ventricle, and corpus callosum
5. Middle: same
6. Middle: same

1. Post: ambient wings and cisterna magnum
2. Post: tentorium and cisterna magnum
3. Post: choroid
4. Post: glomus of choroids
5. Post: far posterior brain (occipital)
6. Post: all the way back to the posterior of the brain

*This protocol assumes a 6:1 multiformat disk or a camera is used.

Sagittal

The steps should be done separately for each side.

1. Very lateral at sylvian fissure (middle cerebral artery)
2. Lateral ventricle: anterior, body, and occipital (temporal if hydrocephalic)
   a. Caudothalamic groove (notch)
   b. Thalamus
3. Lateral ventricle: same
4. Lateral ventricle: same
5. Lateral ventricle: same
6. Midline: cavum septum pellucidum, corpus callosum, third ventricle, and foramen of Monro
   a. Aqueduct of Sylvius
   b. Fourth ventricle
   c. Cerebellum (tentorium)
   d. Cisterna magna

Axial

Measure lateral ventricles from lateral wall to lateral wall. This view is very important for hydrocephalus and follow-up studies to determine increase in the ventricular size. It is also good to show the bleed in or out of the ventricle to determine the grade of the bleed.

You may want to use the linear 5-MHz transducer for the initial baseline study to better delineate the subarachnoid fluid and interhemispheric fissure.

Coronal

1. Three anterior images.
2. Three posterior images.

If the fontanelle is difficult to image because of overlapping bones, you may want to place the transducer in the posterior fontanelle to image the choroid plexus and lateral ventricles.

Coronal and Modified Coronal Plane. Coronal sections are obtained by making slices approximately 90 degrees from the axial sections. Technically a coronal view is 90 degrees to Reid's baseline. However, a number of different angles to Reid's baseline are used in performing the examination. When looking at the sections, the vertex of the skull is at the top and the left side of the brain is to the right of the image. To perform these studies the transducer is placed on the anterior fontanelle with the scanning plane following the coronal suture (Fig. 16-11). The middle of the crystal must be centered in the coronal suture to reduce bone interference and to procure the most extensive image of the brain. Symmetrical images must be obtained. This is accomplished using the skull bones and the middle cerebral arteries at the Sylvian fissure as landmarks (Fig. 16-12). The skull bones and the arteries should be the same size bilaterally. After a symmetric view is obtained, the transducer is angled anteriorly and posteriorly to enable complete visualization of the lateral and third ventricles, the deep subcortical white matter, and the basal ganglia.

When the transducer is angled anteriorly, the frontal horns of the lateral ventricles appear as nonechogenic slit-

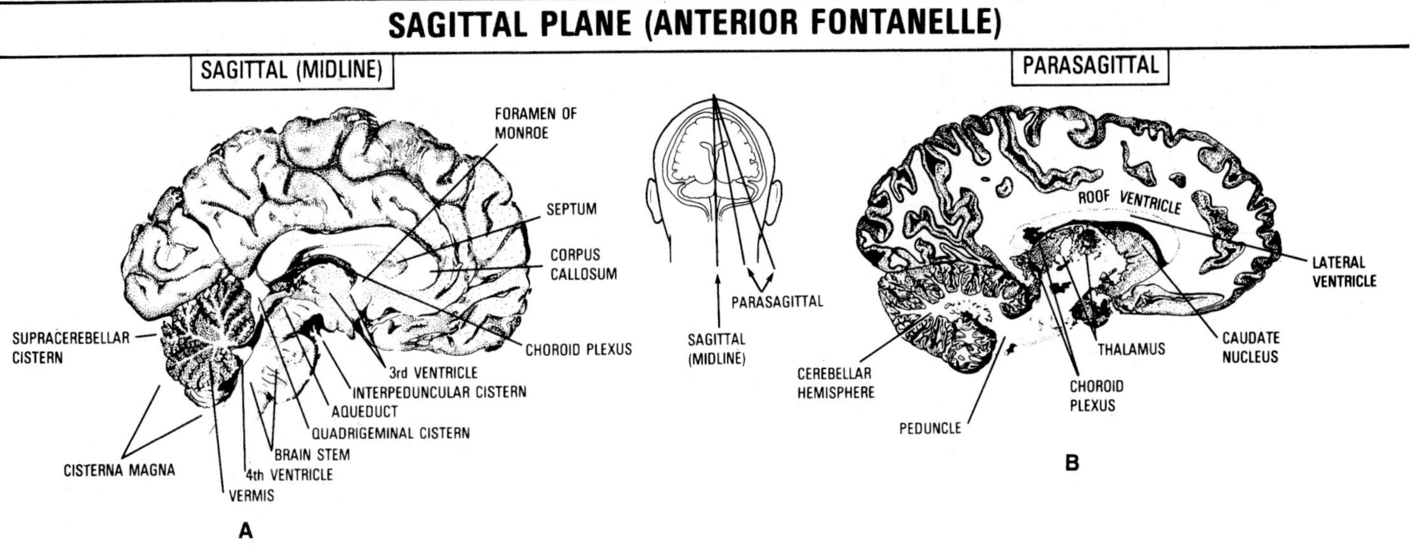

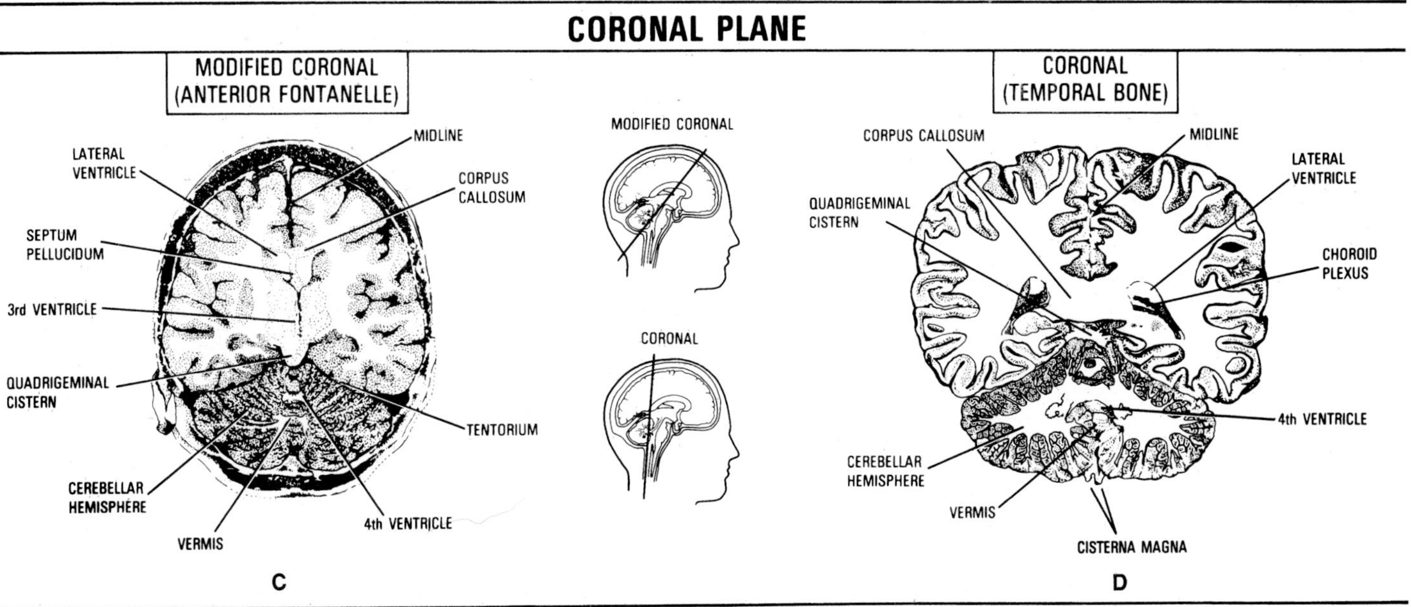

FIG. 16-10 Schema of the structures of the infratentorial compartment. **A** and **B,** Sagittal and parasagittal planes respectively. **C,** Modified coronal plane (through the anterior fontanelle). **D,** Coronal plane of the posterior fossa (through the temporal suture). Note the distance existing from the place where the transducer is positioned and the structures of the posterior fossa (cerebellum, cisterna magna, fourth ventricle, etc.).

like cystic formations. As the transducer is angled posteriorly, the ventricles acquire a commalike shape, and their width increases from 2 mm at the frontal lobes to a maximum of 3 to 6 mm at the region of the choroid plexus (bodies of the lateral ventricles) (Fig. 16-13).

The choroid plexus is an intraventricular structure lying in the floor of the lateral ventricles and extending from the temporal horn into the atrium and body of the lateral ventricles (Fig. 16-14). At the foramen of Monro the plexus enters into the third ventricle. Consequently the frontal (anterior) and the occipital (posterior) horns are devoid of choroid plexus. The choroid plexus becomes enlarged at the level of the atria (glomus of the choroid plexus). At the atria the plexus can almost entirely fill the ventricular cavity. Echoencephalography shows the choroid plexus as a very echogenic structure inside the ventricular cavities surrounding the thalamic nuclei. The size of the choroid plexus depends on the gestational age of the infants. The plexus is very large in very immature infants (less than 25 weeks), and it should not be mistaken for intraventricular hemor-

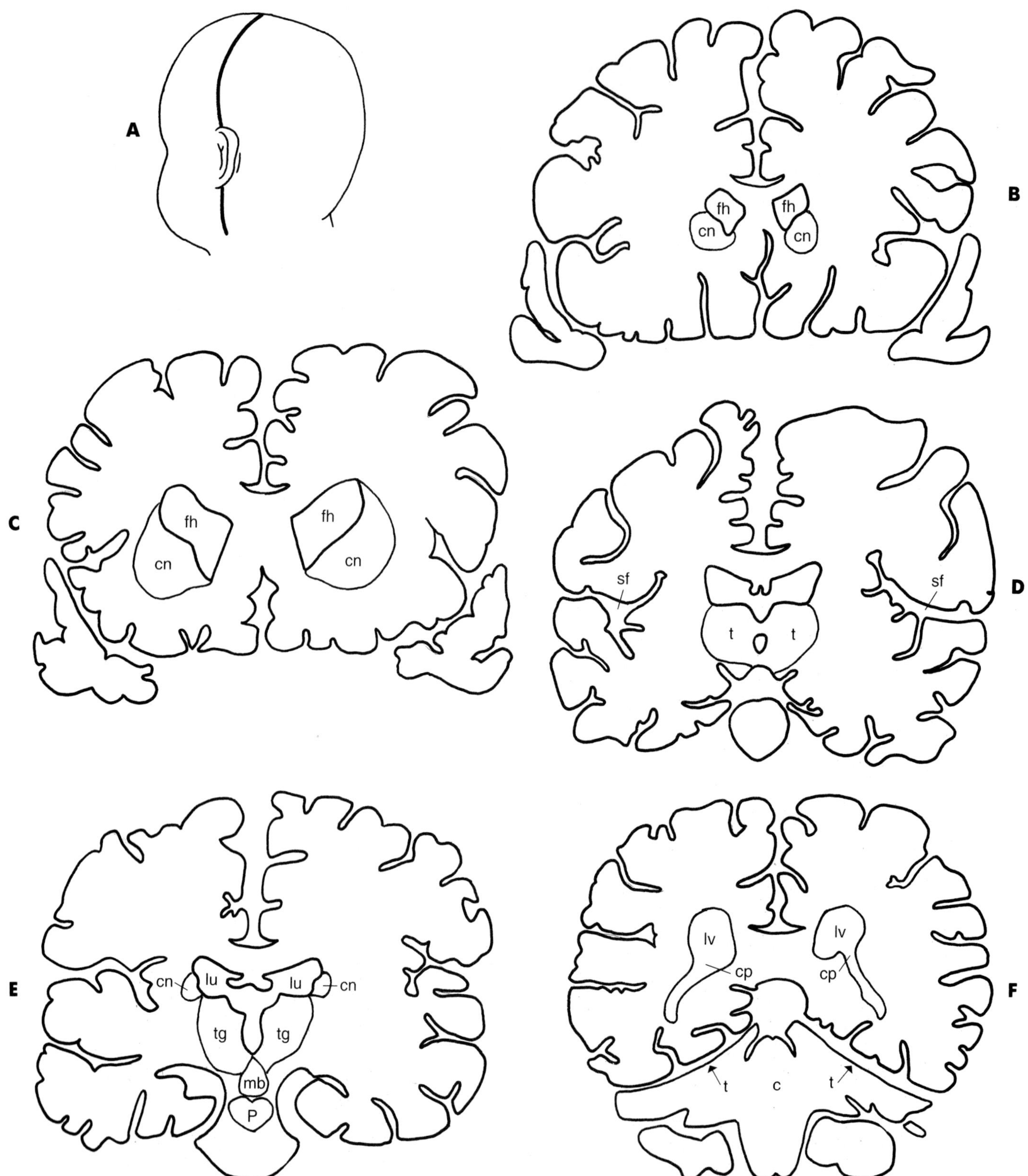

FIG. 16-11 A, A coronal view is 90 degrees from Reid's baseline. **B,** The anterior section of the brian shows the relationship of the frontal horns, *fh,* of the lateral ventricles to the caudate nuclei, *cn*. The caudate nuclei lie posterolateral to the frontal horns. The interhemispheric fissure is shown, *if*. **C,** The cavum septi pellucidi, *sp,* is seen between the frontal horns, *fh*. Caudate nuclei, *cn*. **D,** The thalami, *t,* and third ventricle, *3V* are more posterior. The foramen of Monroe is also seen, *fm*. The sylvian fissures, *sf,* are seen along the lateral walls of the brain. **E,** The pons, *p,* and hippocampal gyrus, *hg,* are shown posterior to the bodies of the lateral ventricles, *lv,* and caudate nuclei, *cn*. Trigonum, t; midbrain, mb. **F,** The trigonum of the lateral ventricle, *lv,* and the choroid plexus, *cp,* is shown as it lies anterior to the cerebellum, *c,* and tentorium, *tn*.

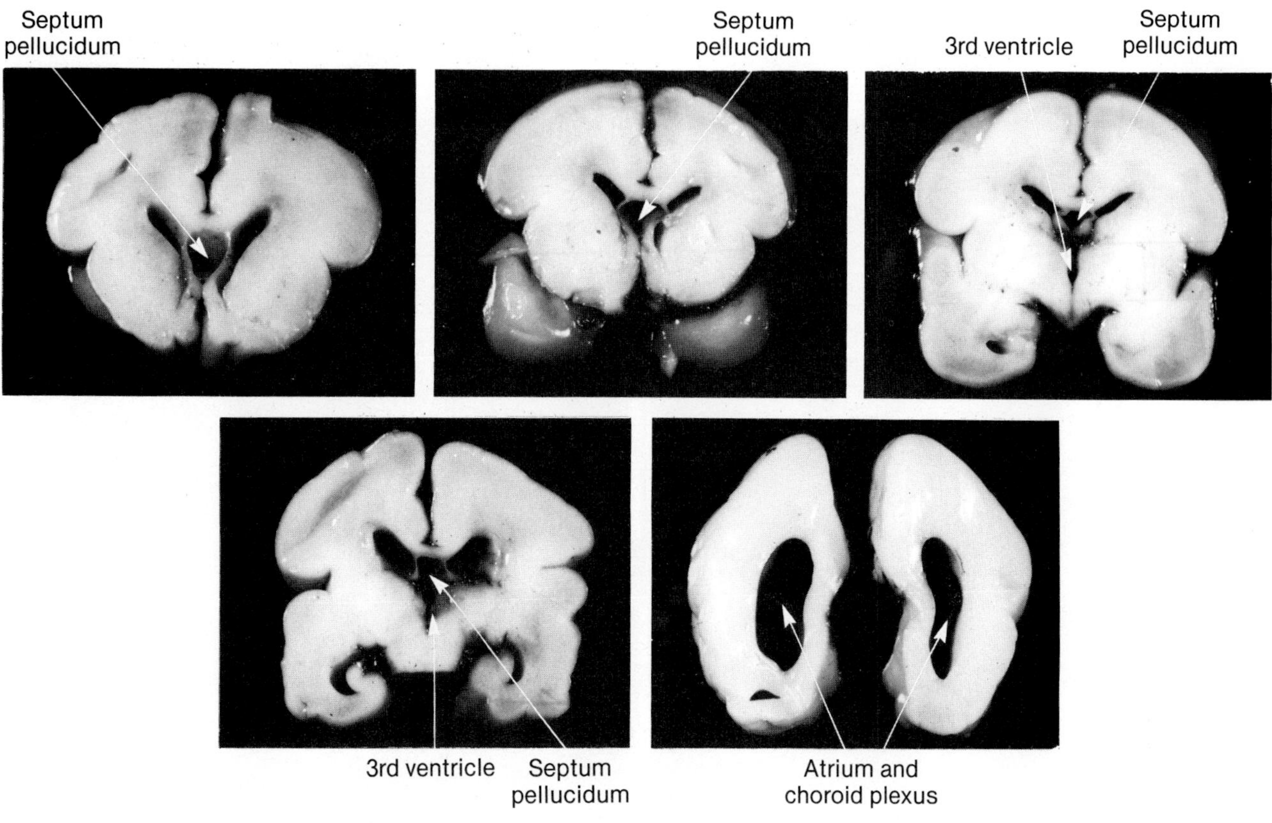

FIG. 16-12 Anatomic slices of a premature brain in the coronal plane.

rhages. The plexus becomes smaller with increasing gestational age. Between 30 weeks of gestation and term, the size is approximately 2 to 3 mm at the body of the lateral ventricles and 4 to 5 mm at the atria (glomus of the choroid plexus).

The third ventricle is not visualized in normal conditions in the coronal or modified coronal studies. Occasionally a thin and very echogenic formation can be seen in the midline immediately below the septum pellucidum. This echogenic image corresponds to the choroid plexus extending into the third ventricle. The septum pellucidum appears as a midline cystic structure separating the bodies and frontal horns of the lateral ventricles. The septum constitutes the internal wall of the bodies and posterior part of the frontal horns.

Coronal and modified coronal views also visualize the basal ganglia and the white matter. The caudate nuclei constitute the inferior and lateral walls of the ventricles at the bodies and posterior part of the frontal horns (Fig 16-15). In very small infants the caudate nuclei may have higher echogenicity than the rest of the brain parenchyma. In these infants the nuclei should not be mistaken for subependymal hemorrhages. The thalamic ganglia are located laterally to the third ventricle, and they are visualized as areas of low echogenicity. The white matter is situated between the lateral ventricles and the cortex. The white matter has low echogenicity with thin echogenic streaks that correspond to small vessels.

Modified Coronal Studies. The modified coronal plane demonstrates the body of the lateral ventricles, the third ventricle, and the posterior fossa. To obtain this view the transducer is positioned over the anterior fontanelle with an angle of approximately 30 to 40 degrees between the scanning plane and the surface of the fontanelle. In this view the tentorium, the cerebellar vermis, the fourth ventricle, the cerebellar hemispheres, and the cisterna magna can be seen in the infratentorial compartment. The vermis is a very echogenic structure in the midline. The fourth ventricle appears in the midline as a small anechoic space approximately 2 to 3 mm wide, located anteriorly to the vermis. The cerebellar hemispheres have low echogenicity and are contiguous with the echogenic vermis. The cisterna magna corresponds to a nonechogenic space between the vermis, the cerebellar hemispheres, and the occipital bone (Fig. 16-16).

Coronal Studies. A straight coronal view of the posterior fossa is obtained by placing the transducer on the mastoid fontanelle or the occipitotemporal suture, immediately behind the ear. The scanning plane should be kept perpendicular to the canthomeatal line. The tentorium, cerebellar hemispheres, cisterna magna, and supracerebellar cistern are visualized (see Fig. 16-16). Angling the transducer an-

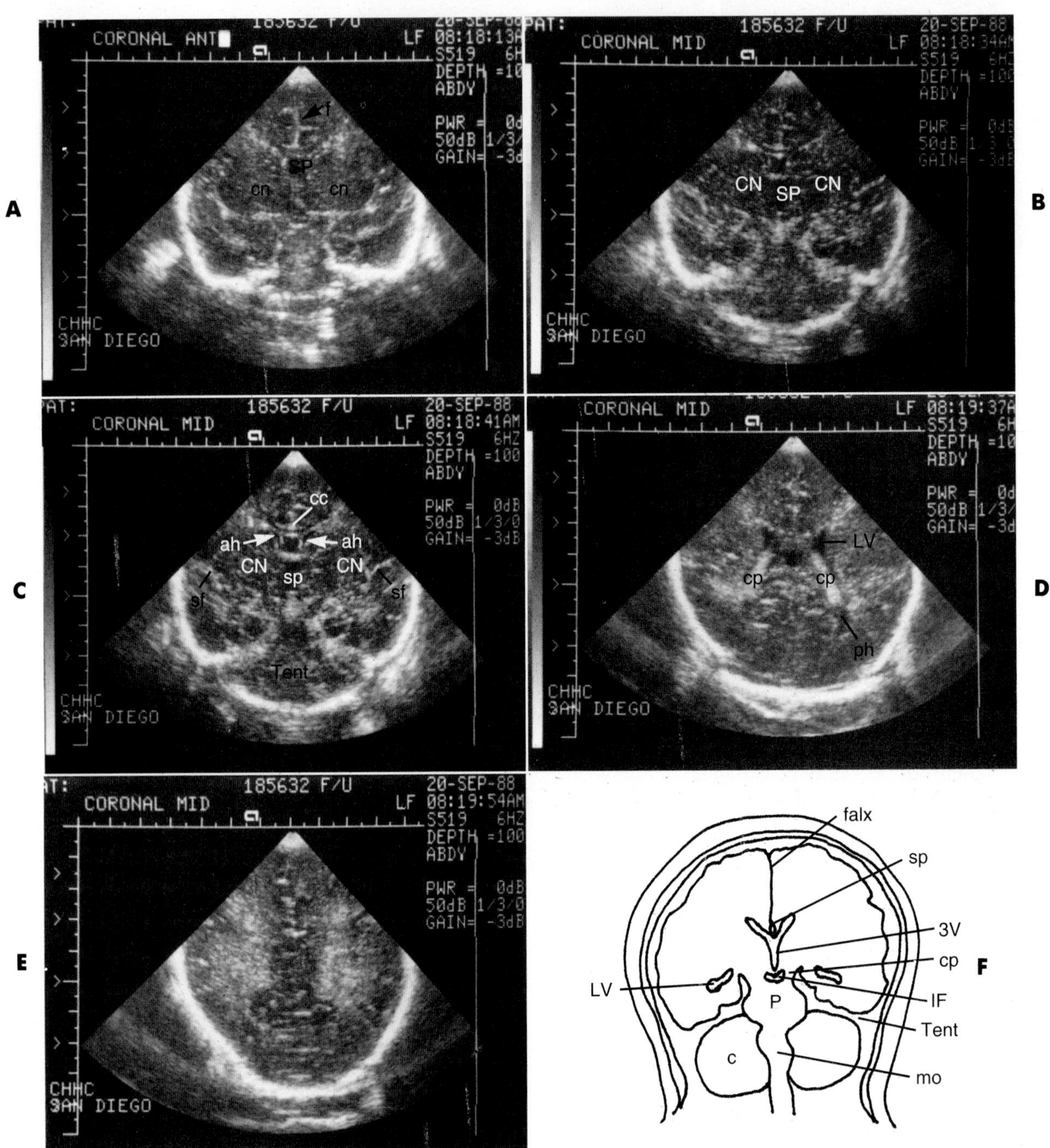

FIG. 16-13 A, Anterior coronal view. Falx, *f,* septum pellucidum, *sp,* caudate nucleus, *cn.* **B,** Midcoronal view. Caudate nucleus, *cn,* septum pellucidum, *sp.* **C,** Midcoronal view. Corpus collosum, *cc;* anterior horn *ah;* caudate nucleus, *cn;* septum pellucidum, *sp;* sylvian fissure, *sf;* tentorium, *tent.* **D,** Midcoronal view. Lateral ventricle, *LV;* choroid plexus *cp;* posterior horn, *ph.* **E,** Midposterior view of the brain parenchyma. **F,** Modified coronal view. Septum pellucidum, *sp;* Third ventricle, *3V;* choroid plexus, interpeduncular fossa, *If;* tentorium cerebelli, *Tent;* medulla oblongata, *MO;* pons, *P;* cerebellar hemisphere, *C;* lateral ventricle, *LV.*

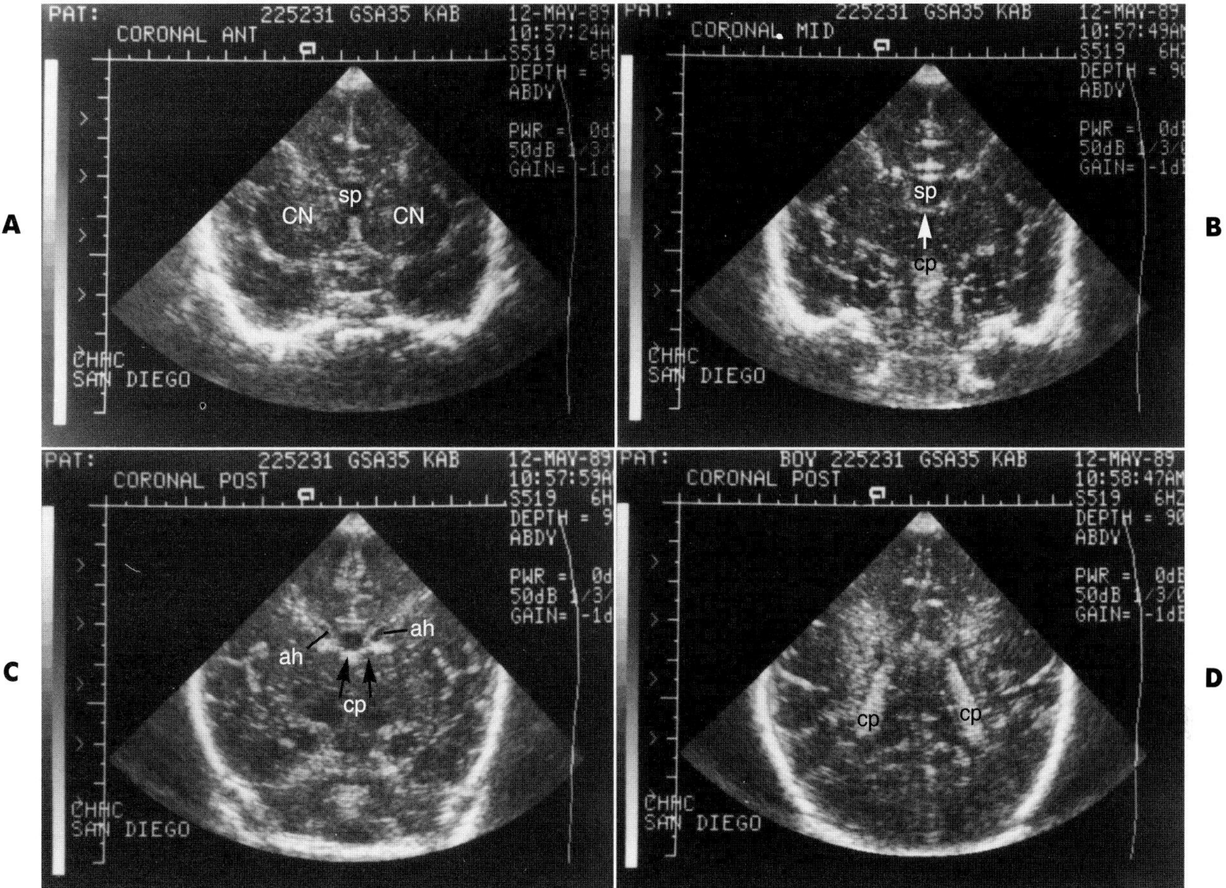

FIG. 16-14 The choroid plexus is an intraventricular structure lying in the floor of the lateral ventricles and extending from the temporal horn into the atrium and body of the lateral ventricles. **A,** Anterior coronal view. Caudate nucleus, *cn,* septum pellucidum, *sp.* **B,** Midcoronal view. Septum pellucidum, *sp,* choroid plexus, *cp.* **C,** Postcoronal view. Anterior horn, *ah,* choroid plexus, *cp.* **D,** Postcoronal view. Choroid plexus, *cp.*

teriorly brings the fourth ventricle and the brain stem into view. The fourth ventricle appears as a triangle inside the cerebellum, and the most ventral aspect of the supracerebellar cistern is also seen.

Sagittal and Parasagittal Plane. Sagittal sections are made by rotating the coronal plane approximately 30 degrees. These sections are viewed with the anterior brain to the left and the occipital portion of the brain to the right. To obtain these studies the transducer is positioned over the anterior fontanelle with the scanning plane following the sagittal suture (Fig. 16-17). Sagittal studies provide the most extensive visualization of the brain.

The straight sagittal study (the only view strictly in the sagittal plane) shows the midline structures in the supratentorial and infratentorial compartments. The straight midline view should be obtained before performing the right and left parasagittal studies. This view is a guide to determine if a parasagittal study corresponds to the right or left side (Fig. 16-18).

The supratentorial structures shown by the sagittal studies are the corpus callosum, septum pellucidum, and third ventricle (see Fig. 16-18). The corpus callosum appears as two thin parallel lines separated by a thin nonechogenic space. The septum pellucidum appears as an anechoic (cystic) structure immediately below the corpus callosum. The third ventricle is normally anechoic and is located inferiorly to the septum. The echogenic choroid plexus appears to enter the top of the third ventricle through the foramen of Monro. The supraoptic recess of the third ventricle is shown as a triangular nonechogenic structure extending inferiorly and anteriorly toward the suprasellar region.

In the straight sagittal plane the infratentorial structures visualized are the cerebellar vermis, the fourth ventricle, the cisterna magna, the supracerebellar and quadrigeminal cisterns, and the brain stem (Fig. 16-19). The vermis of the cerebellum appears as a very echo-dense formation, separated from the occipital bone by an anechoic space that corresponds to the cisterna magna. The other cisterns also are anechoic spaces located above and behind the cerebellar vermis. The fourth ventricle appears as a small V with

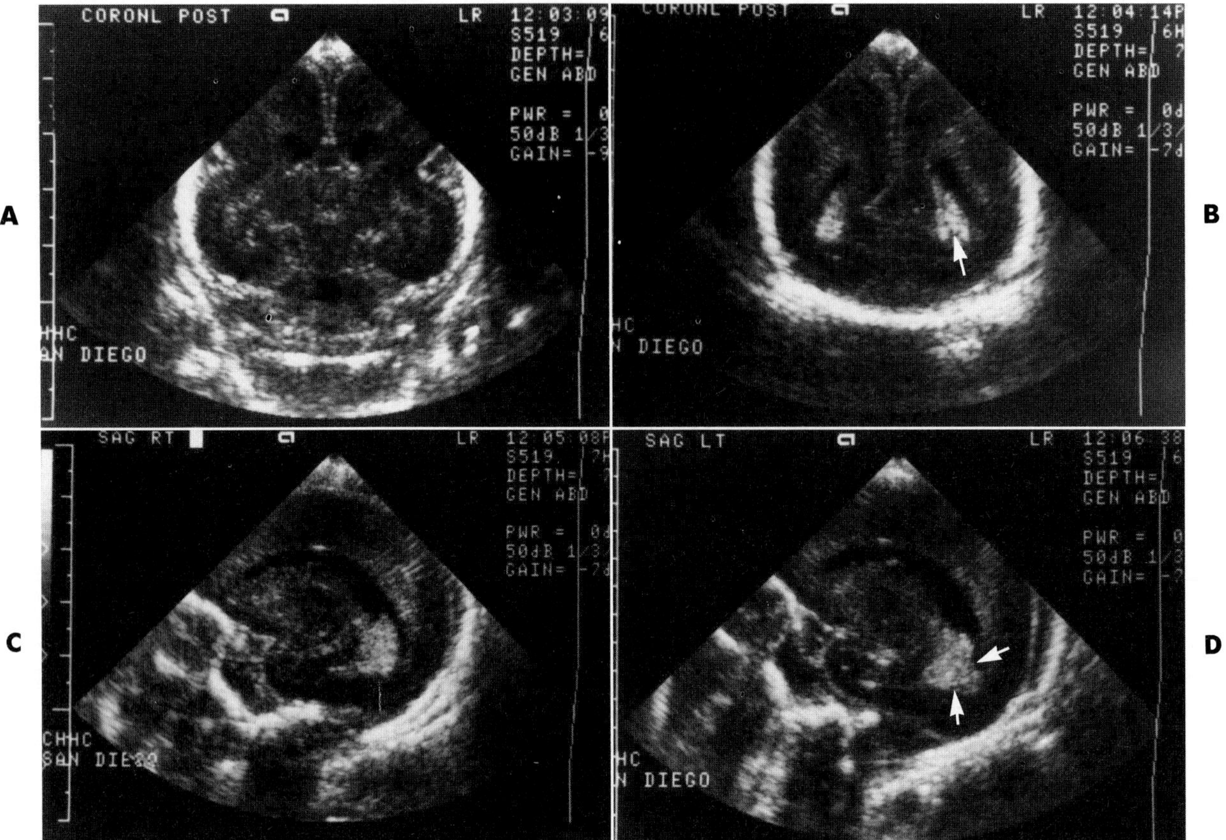

FIG. 16-15 Neonatal head in a 23-week premature infant shows the echogenic choroid plexus in the ventricles. **A,** The left ventricle looks slightly more echogenic than the right **(B)**; the sagittal views of the right, **C,** and left ventricle, **D,** shows an irregular border of the choroid plexus, indicating a small grade I bleed *(D—arrows)*.

the vertex oriented posteriorly inside the echogenic vermis. The fourth ventricle is limited anteriorly by the brain stem. The brain stem has low echogenicity, with an echo-dense anterior border demarcated by the basilar artery.

Parasagittal Studies. After having studied the midline, the transducer is moved/angled slightly to the left and right sides to visualize the cerebellar hemispheres in the parasagittal plane. The cerebellar hemispheres appear as round, low echogenic formations with moderately hyperechoic surfaces.

The parasagittal views are obtained by angling the transducer to the right or left side of the skull (Fig. 16-20). Three parasagittal studies should be performed. The first parasagittal image should be close to the midline to visualize the caudate nuclei in detail, since subependymal hemorrhages begin in the germinal matrix that is located at the level of these ganglia. These views image the frontal horn and body of the lateral ventricles, the thalamus, the head of the caudate nucleus, and the choroid plexus. The frontal horns and bodies of the lateral ventricles appear as narrow nonechogenic cavities. The height of the bodies of the ventricles normally is less than 7 mm at the level of the midthalamus. The floor of lateral ventricles is determined by the boundary between the very echogenic choroid plexus and the less echogenic thalamus. The choroid plexus appears as a small (2 to 3 mm height), very echogenic structure lying against the thalamus. The plexus appears to end at the thalamic-caudate groove, which is the most frequent location of subependymal hemorrhages. The floor of the ventricles ventral to the groove is formed by the head of the caudate nucleus, which in very small infants has higher echogenicity than the surrounding tissues.

The second parasagittal image is made slightly lateral to the first image and includes the entire ventricular cavity. Since the ventricular cavity is not entirely parallel to the midline (i.e., the posterior horns are more lateral or external than the anterior horns), the transducer must be rotated slightly counterclockwise to form an acute angle with the sagittal suture anteriorly. These views show the entire ventricular horns, the choroid plexus including the glomus, the thalami, the caudate nuclei, and the white matter superior and anterior to the lateral ventricles.

The third parasagittal view images the white matter located lateral (externally) to the lateral ventricles. This view is useful in studying intraparenchymal hemorrhages, porencephaly, and periventricular leukomalacia.

NORMAL RTE OF PRETERM INFANTS

MODIFIED CORONAL PLANE
INTERHEMISPHERE FISSURE
SEPTUM PELLUCIDUM
LATERAL VENTRICLE
MIDDLE CEREBRAL ARTERY IN THE SYLVIAN FISSURE
CHOROID PLEXUS
3rd VENTRICLE
THALAMUS
TENTORIUM
CHOROIDAL FISSURE
CEREBELLAR HEMISPHERES
TENTORIUM
4th VENTRICLE
VERMIS
CISTERNA MAGNA
QUADRIGEMINAL CISTERN

CORONAL PLANE (Post)
SUPERIOR
MIDLINE
PARIETAL BONE
ATRIUM & CHOROID PLEXUS
QUADRIGEMINAL CISTERN
TENTORIUM
TEMPORAL BONE
CEREBELLAR HEMISPHERE
CISTERNA MAGNA

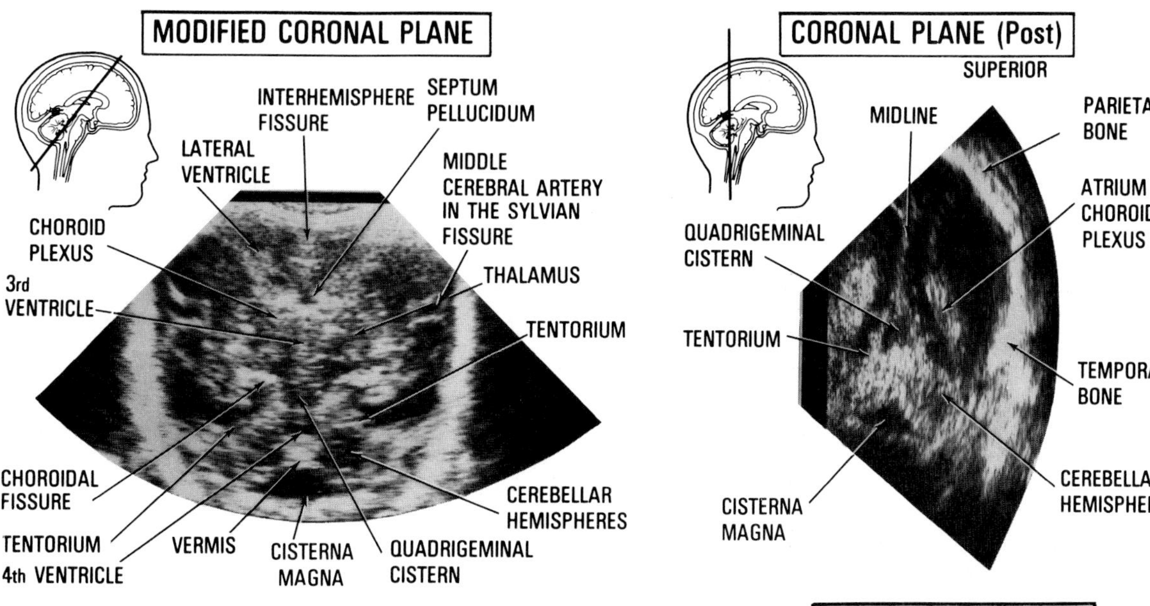

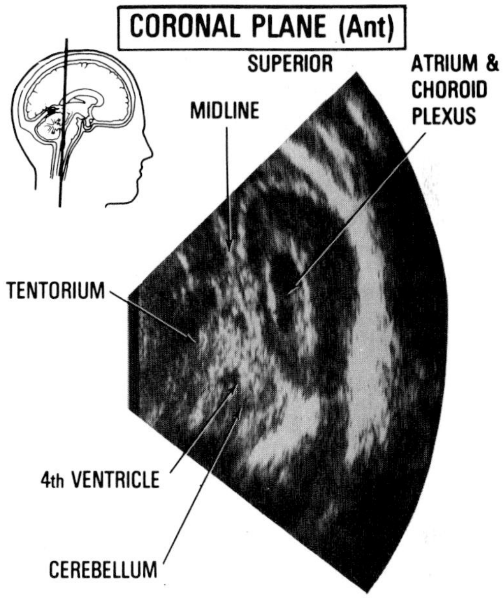

CORONAL PLANE (Ant)
SUPERIOR
ATRIUM & CHOROID PLEXUS
MIDLINE
TENTORIUM
4th VENTRICLE
CEREBELLUM

FIG. 16-16 Normal ultrasound studies focused in the infratentorial compartment. In the parasagittal study, note the normal ultrasonographic characteristics of the cerebellar hemispheres. See text for more descriptions.

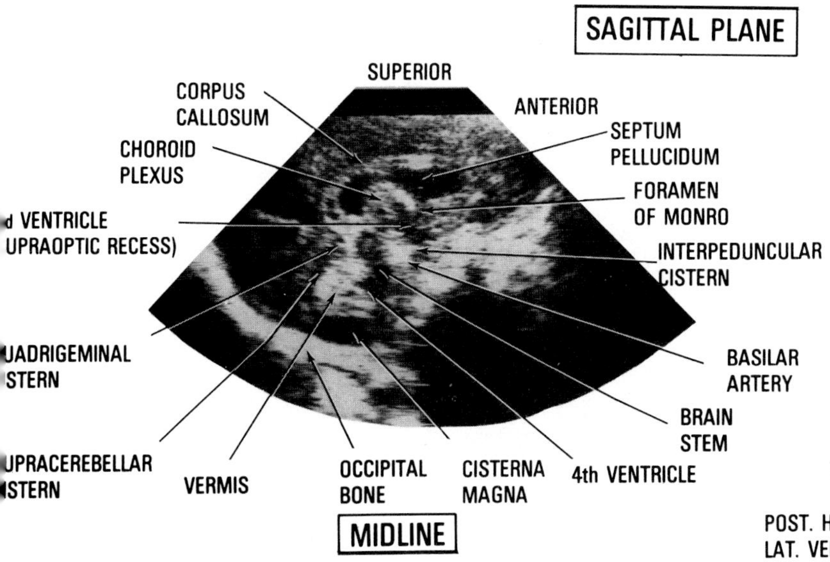

SAGITTAL PLANE
SUPERIOR
CORPUS CALLOSUM
ANTERIOR
SEPTUM PELLUCIDUM
CHOROID PLEXUS
FORAMEN OF MONRO
d VENTRICLE
UPRAOPTIC RECESS)
INTERPEDUNCULAR CISTERN
UADRIGEMINAL
STERN
BASILAR ARTERY
BRAIN STEM
UPRACEREBELLAR
ISTERN
VERMIS
OCCIPITAL BONE
CISTERNA MAGNA
4th VENTRICLE
MIDLINE

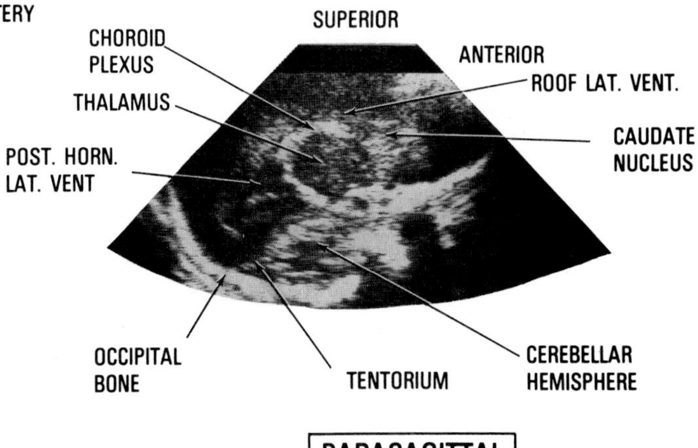

SUPERIOR
CHOROID PLEXUS
ANTERIOR
ROOF LAT. VENT.
THALAMUS
CAUDATE NUCLEUS
POST. HORN. LAT. VENT
OCCIPITAL BONE
TENTORIUM
CEREBELLAR HEMISPHERE
PARASAGITTAL

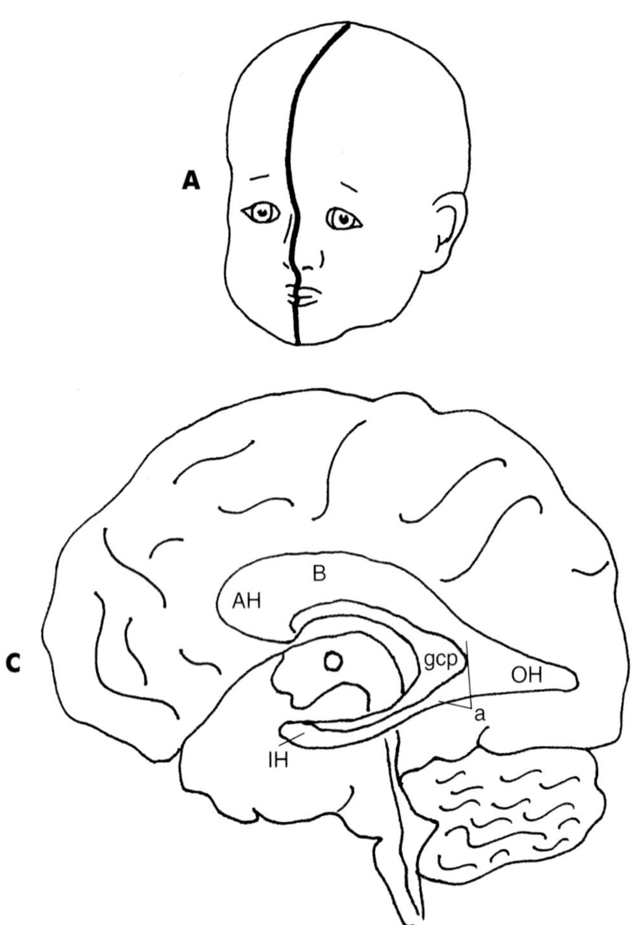

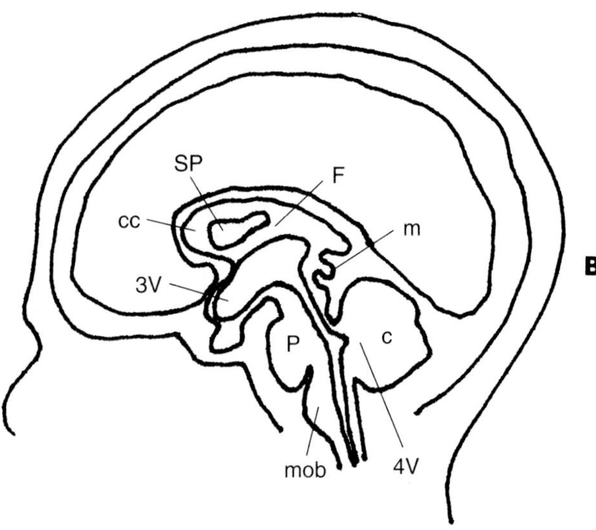

FIG. 16-17 A, Sagittal suture through the neonatal skull. **B,** Midline sagittal view. Third ventricle, *3V;* corpus callosum, *cc;* septum pellucidum, *sp;* fornix, *f;* mesencephlic tectum, *m;* cerebellum, *c;* medulla oblongata, *mob;* pons, *p;* fourth ventricle, *4V.* **C,** Parasagittal view. Anterior horn, *ah;* body, *b;* occipital horn, *oh;* inferior horn, *Ih;* glomus choroid plexus, *gcp;* atrium, *a.*

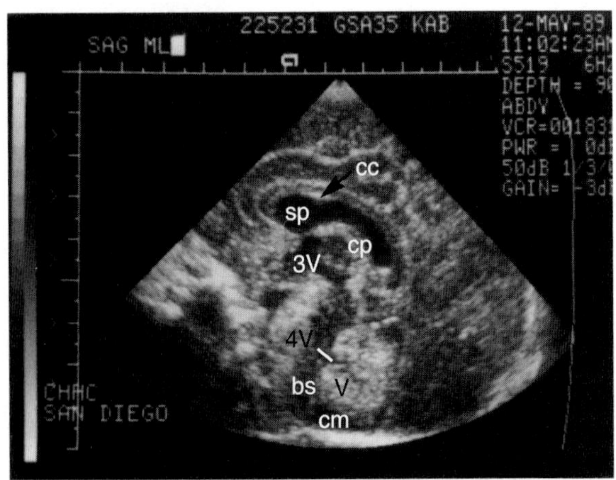

FIG. 16-18 "Straight" sagittal view of the midline structures. Supratentorial structures: corpus callosum, *cc;* septum pellucidum, *sp;* choroid plexus, *cp;* third ventricle, (3V). Infratentorial structures: cerebellar vermis, *v;* fourth ventricle, *4V;* cisterna magna, *cm;* brain stem, *bs.*

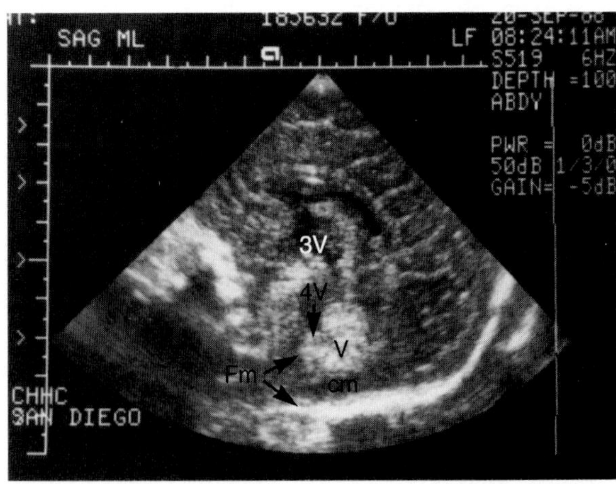

FIG. 16-19 Slight parasagittal view of the third ventricle, *3V,* fourth ventricle, *4V,* vermis, *v,* foramen magnum, *fm,* and cisterna magna, *cm.*

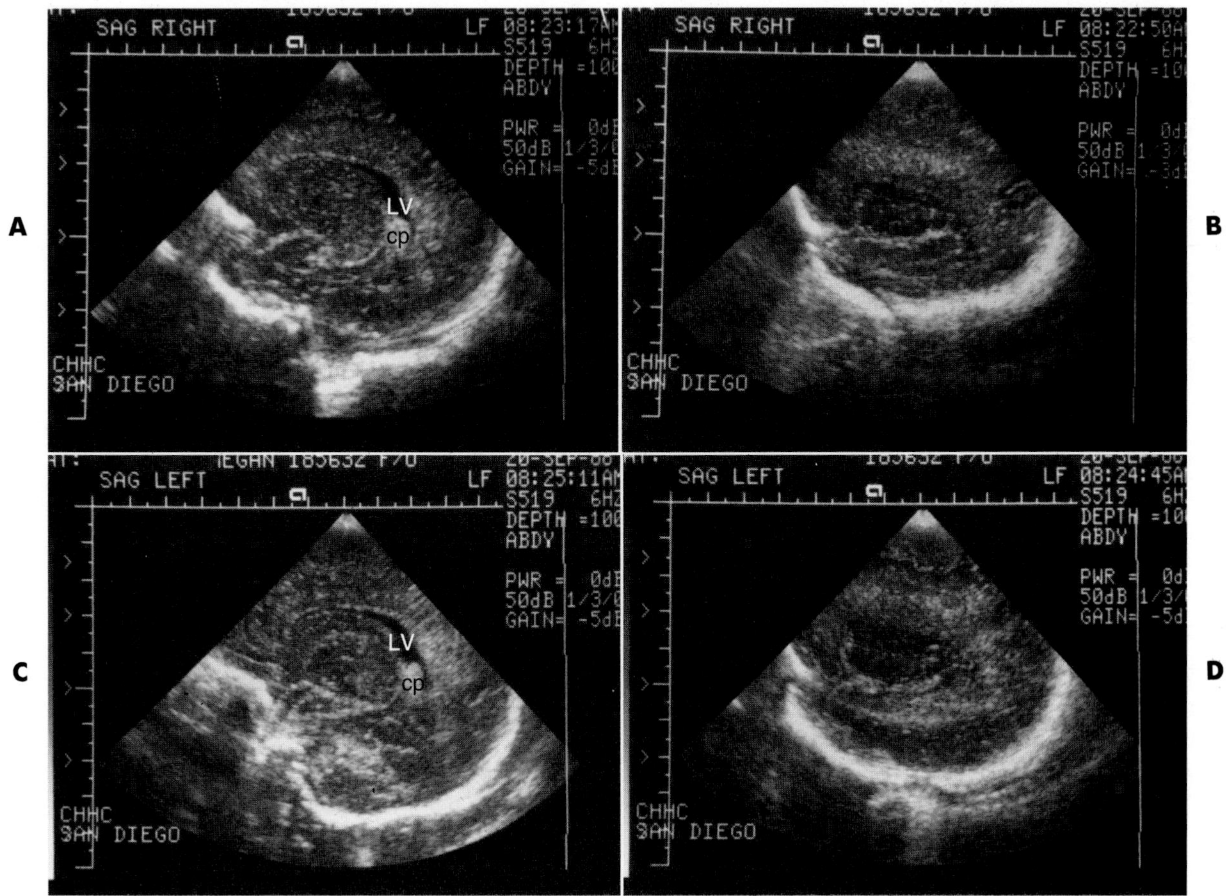

FIG. 16-20 Parasagittal views to the right and left of the midline show the lateral ventricles, *LV*, choroid plexus, *cp*, in images **A** and **C.** The far parasagittal images angled away from the ventricles show the brain parenchyma, **D.**

Axial Plane. An axial section of the brain is one in which the brain is sliced from one lateral side to the other, parallel with the canthomeatal line. The axial view is obtained by scanning the brain through either the mastoid or the posterior fontanelle (Fig. 16-21). Through the mastoid fontanelle the posterior horn, atrium, and glomus of the choroid plexus can be visualized. The echogenic choroid plexus almost fills the ventricular cavity at the atrium but it rarely extends into the occipital horns. The axial image is useful in following the size of the atria and occipital horns in patients with hydrocephalus. Using the choroid plexus as a reference, it is possible to obtain consistent serial measurements of the ventricular size in the same anatomical position (Fig. 16-22).

In the level just above the external auditory meatus, many anatomic landmarks are seen that are important for ultrasound evaluation. Posteriorly the cerebellum can be seen with the tentorium separating it from the cerebrum. Moving anteriorly on this section, the cerebral peduncles can be seen with the fourth ventricle just behind. In front of the peduncles the suprasellar cistern can be found; it contains the cerebrovascular circle of Willis. Moving the transducer approximately 5 mm above the external auditory meatus reveals the ambient cisterns between the hippocampal gyrus and the cerebral peduncles and inferior colliculi. More anteriorly and laterally are the bilateral sylvian fissures, which contain the middle cerebral arteries. Another image slightly higher displays the thalami as two symmetric areas on each side of the midline.

The third ventricle lies between the thalami. Anterior to the thalami are the frontal horns of the lateral ventricles. Posterolateral to each frontal horn is the region of the caudate nucleus. In premature infants the germinal matrix lies in the subependymal layer along the caudate nuclei. This is of critical anatomic importance, since it is the most common site of intracranial hemorrhage in premature infants. Posterior to the thalami are the occipital horns of the lateral ventricles. Between the occipital horns and frontal horns is the area of the interhemispheric fissure.

As the transducer is angled higher, the bodies of the lateral ventricles are imaged. The corpus callosum is seen between the lateral ventricles. At this level the caudate nuclei lie in the lateral walls of the lateral ventricles. The choroid plexus can also be seen within the lateral ventricles. At the

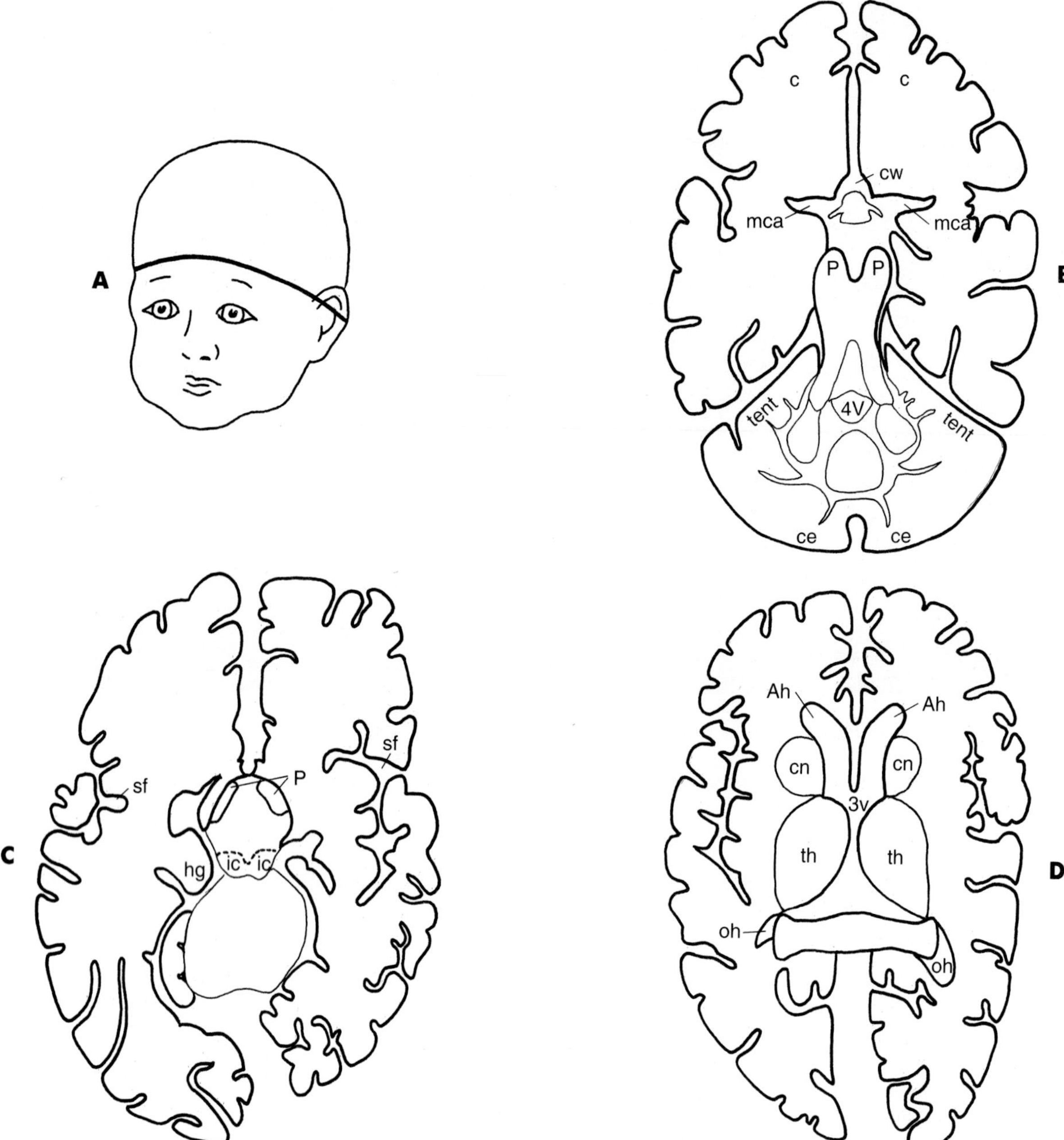

FIG. 16-21 A, The axial plane is made parallel with the canthomeatal line. **B,** Axial section of the brian at the level of the external auditory meatus. Cerebellum, *ce;* tentorium, *tent;* cerebrum, *c;* fourth ventricle, *4V;* cerebral peduncle, *p;* circle of Willia, *cw;* middle cerebral artery, *mca.* **C,** Axial section of the brain 5 mm above the external auditory meatus. Hippocampal gyrus, *hg;* cerebral peduncle, *p;* inferior colliculus, *ic;* sylvian fissure, *sf.* **D,** Axial section of the brain 10 mm above the external auditory meatus. Anterior horn, *ah;* caudate nucleus, *cn;* thalamus, *th;* third ventricle, *3V;* occipital horn, *oh.* **E,** Axial section of the brain 15 to 20 mm above the external auditory meatus. Lateral ventricle, *LV;* choroid plexus, *cp;* caudate nucleus, *cn;* corpus callosum, *cc.* **F,** Axial section of the brain 20 to 25 mm above the canthomeatal line. Lateral ventricle, *LV.*

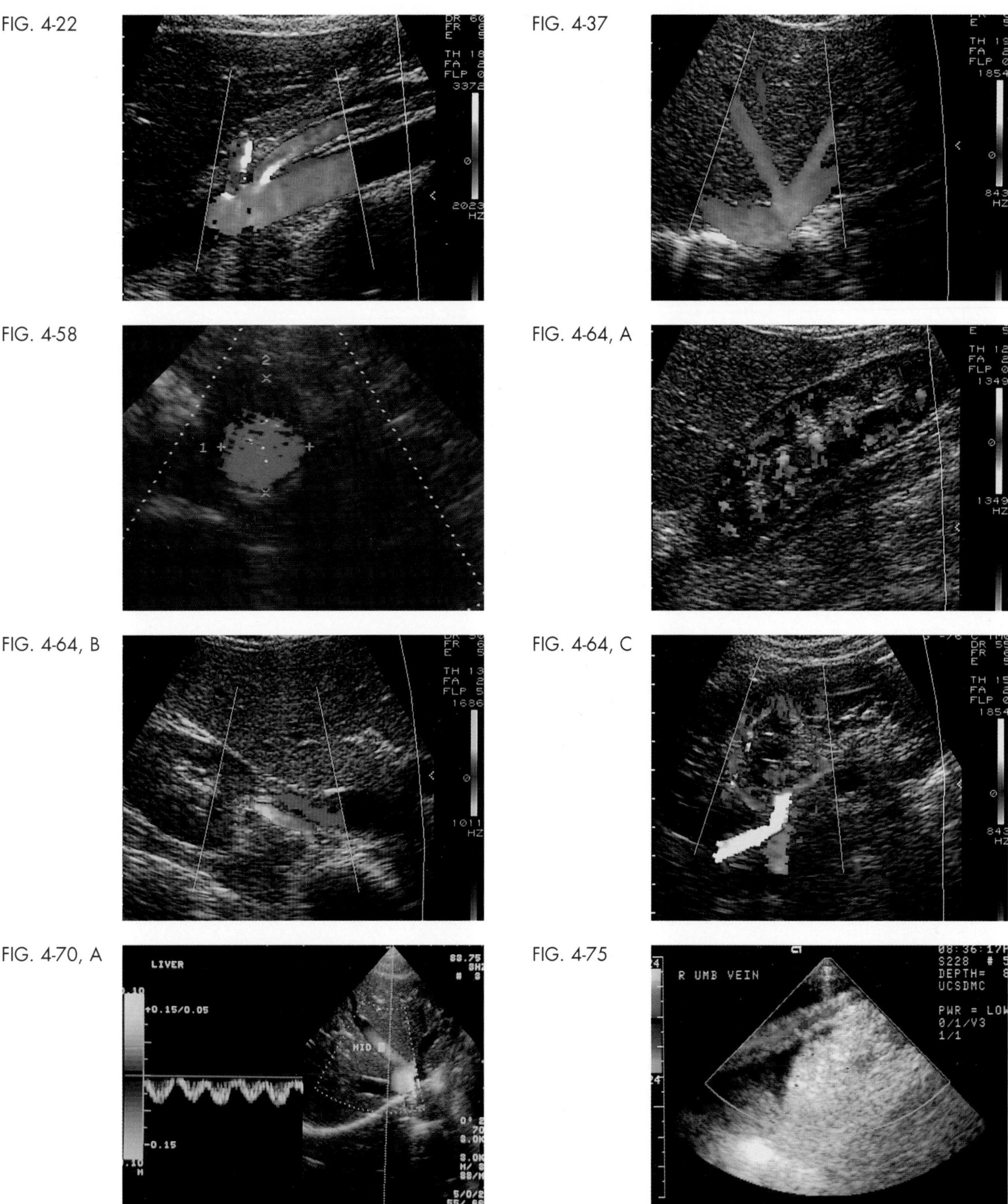

FIG. 4-22 Color flow of the image highlighting the arterial vessels. **FIG. 4-37** Normal color flow showing the flow of the hepatic veins into the inferior vena cava. **FIG. 4-58** Color helps determine the presence of false channels (dissection) and the amount of lumen that remains open secondary to clot formation. **FIG. 4-64 A,** Sagittal. **B,** Transverse of the right kidney shows flow in the renal artery *(red)* and vein *(blue).* **C,** Sagittal view of the main renal artery *(red),* renal vein *(blue),* and interlobar and arcuate arteries and veins. **FIG. 4-70 A,** Transverse scan of the middle hepatic vein shows normal flow patterns. **FIG. 4-75** Color-flow sagittal scans in a patient with a recanalized umbilical vein *(red).*

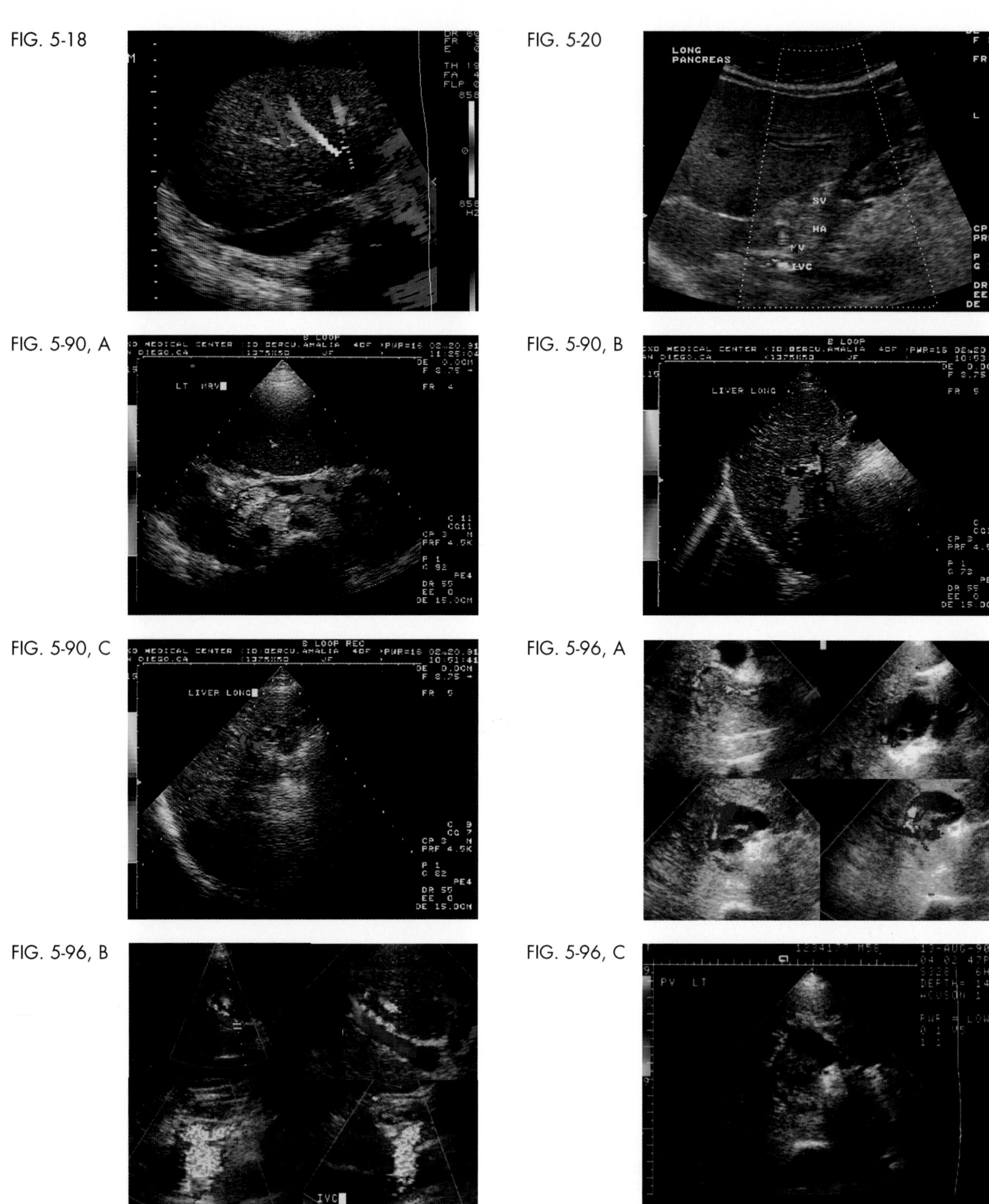

FIG. 5-18 Color flow of the intrahepatic vascular vessels shows the hepatic veins *(blue)* as they flow into the inferior vena cava. The portal veins *(red)* flow into the liver parenchyma. **FIG. 5-20** Color Doppler in the longitudinal plane shows the hepatic arterial flow, *HA,* anterior to the portal vein, *PV,* and inferior vena cava, *IVC.* **FIG. 5-90 A-C,** Cavernous transformation of the portal vein is identified, with multiple small periportal collaterals seen on color-flow imaging. Multiple collateral channels and varices are also identified on the surface of the left lobe of the liver. **FIG. 5-96 A-C,** The portacaval shunt was patent with turbulent flow. The portal vein flow was hepatofugal. There was hepatopedal flow in the superior mesenteric vein and splenic vein.

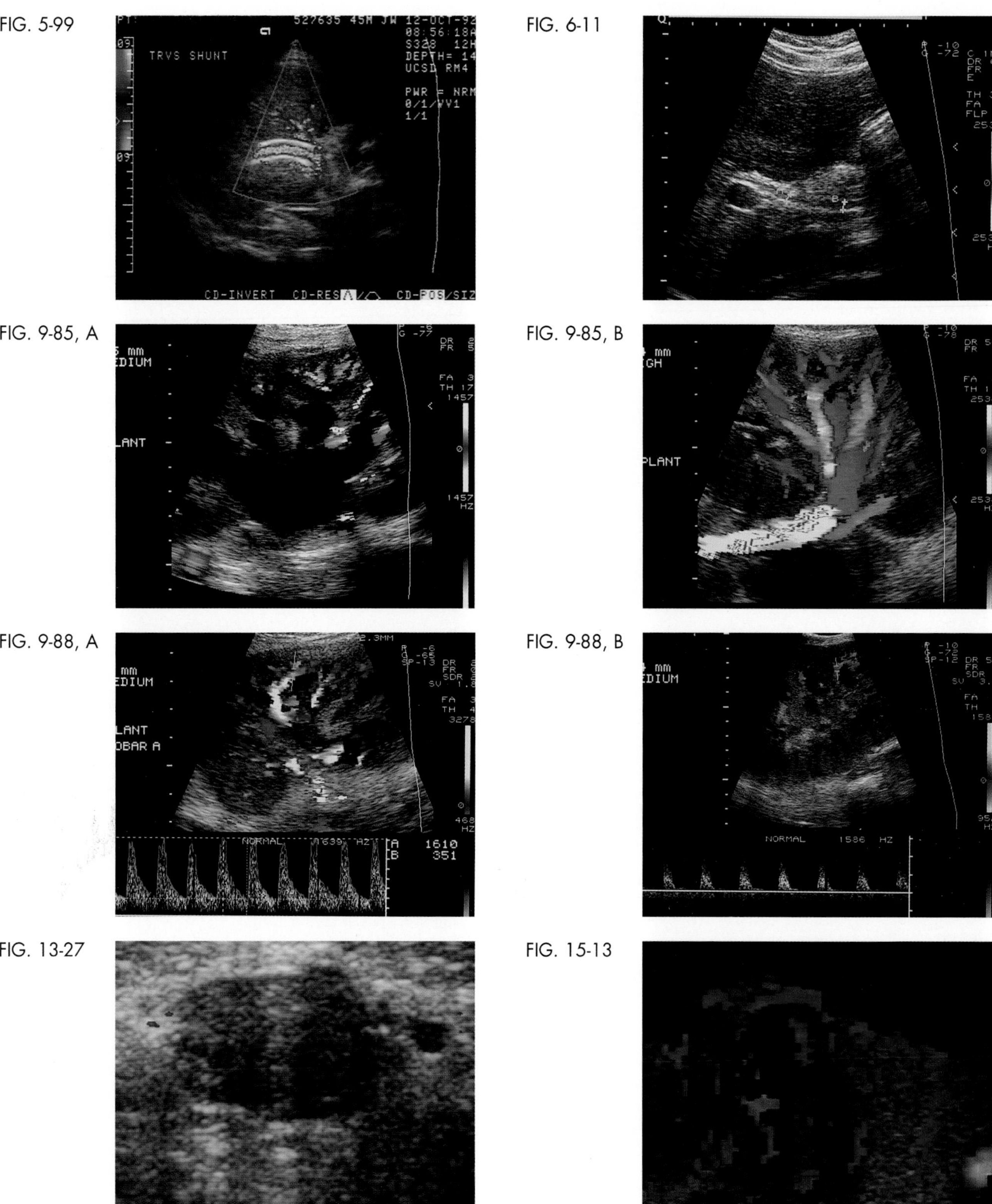

FIG. 5-99 This patient showed turbulence within the patent shunt. The jugular vessels were evaluated as well. **FIG. 6-11** Longitudinal oblique scans of the common bile duct as it lies anterior to the color-filled portal vein. The ductal structures will not fill with color, thus helping the sonographer to separate distended ducts from vascular structures. **FIG. 9-85 A** and **B,** Images of the distended renal transplant with hydronephrosis versus a normal renal transplant. **FIG. 9-88 A** and **B,** Color flow and Doppler images of a normal flow pattern with good perfusion versus an abnormal flow pattern with no diastolic flow, as seen in a patient with rejection. **FIG. 13-27** Medullary carcinoma may resemble a fibroadenoma. **FIG. 15-13** Color Doppler scan demonstrating an increase in vascularity related to orchitis. Color flow, *CF.*

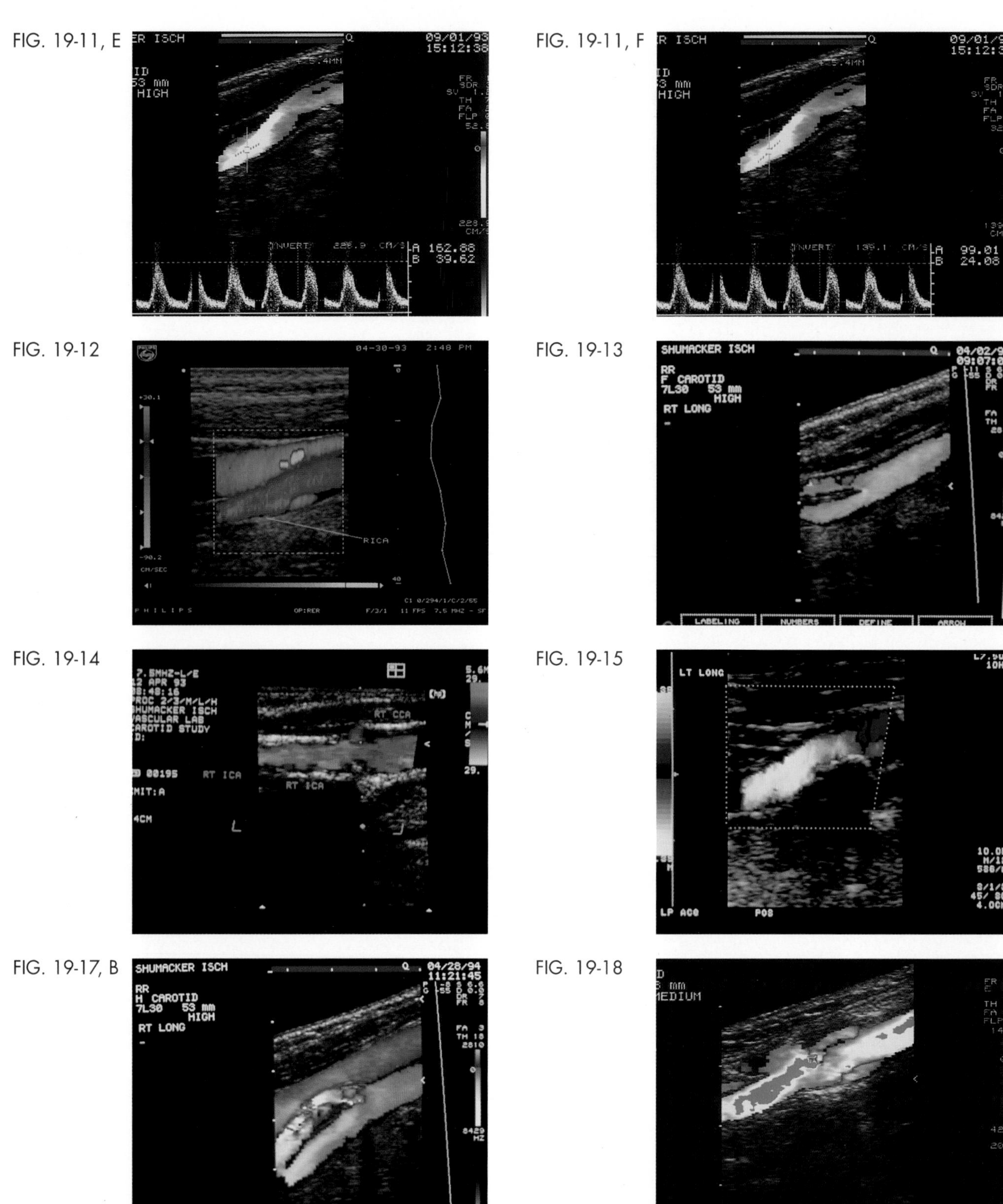

FIG. 19-11 E, With color flow on, the streamline is visible, the vector line does not align with it, and the velocity readings are artifactually elevated and could be interpreted as abnormal. **F,** Correcting the angle to parallel the streamline brings the velocities into a correct and more normal range. **FIG. 19-12** An area of normal flow reversal appears as the blue area within the otherwise red internal carotid artery; this represents an area of flow separation. **FIG. 19-13** An example image from a system that uses a standoff wedge. **FIG. 19-14** An example image from a system that uses beam-steering. **FIG. 19-15** An example image from a beam-steered system that makes use of a color box or flow window. **FIG. 19-17 B,** Extensive plaque is obscured when color flow is turned on. **FIG. 19-18** All frequencies above 2019 Hz are tagged using a green color to distinguish them from slower velocities within the vessel.

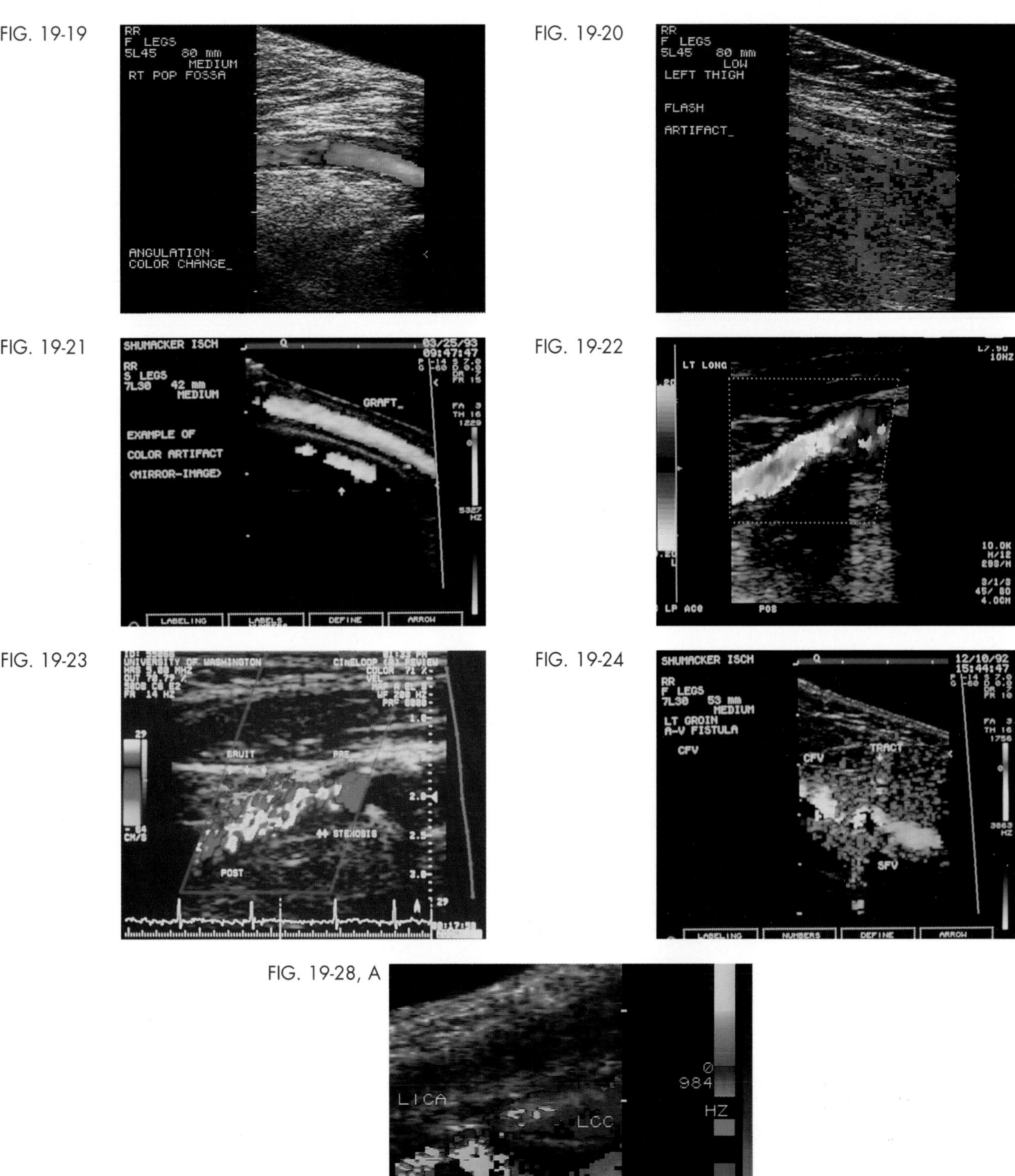

FIG. 19-19 If tortuous vasculature is present or if curvatures cause flow to move toward the transducer elements in one segment and away from the elements in another, both red and blue flow patterns may appear within the same vascular structure. **FIG. 19-20** Flash artifact. **FIG. 19-21** Mirror-image color-flow artifact. **FIG. 19-22** Color aliasing. Normal flow away from the transducer should be coded as shades of red in this vessel; the velocity threshold is too low and higher forward velocities "wrap around" to the reverse, or blue, side of the color bar, as evidenced by the shades of blue in the center streamline area. **FIG. 19-23** A bruit from a stenosis may generate color disturbances around the vessel that are centered at the area of turbulence. **FIG. 19-24** An arteriovenous fistula or extremely turbulent vessel generates a mixed color pattern. **FIG. 19-28 A,** A severe internal carotid stenosis identified by duplex.

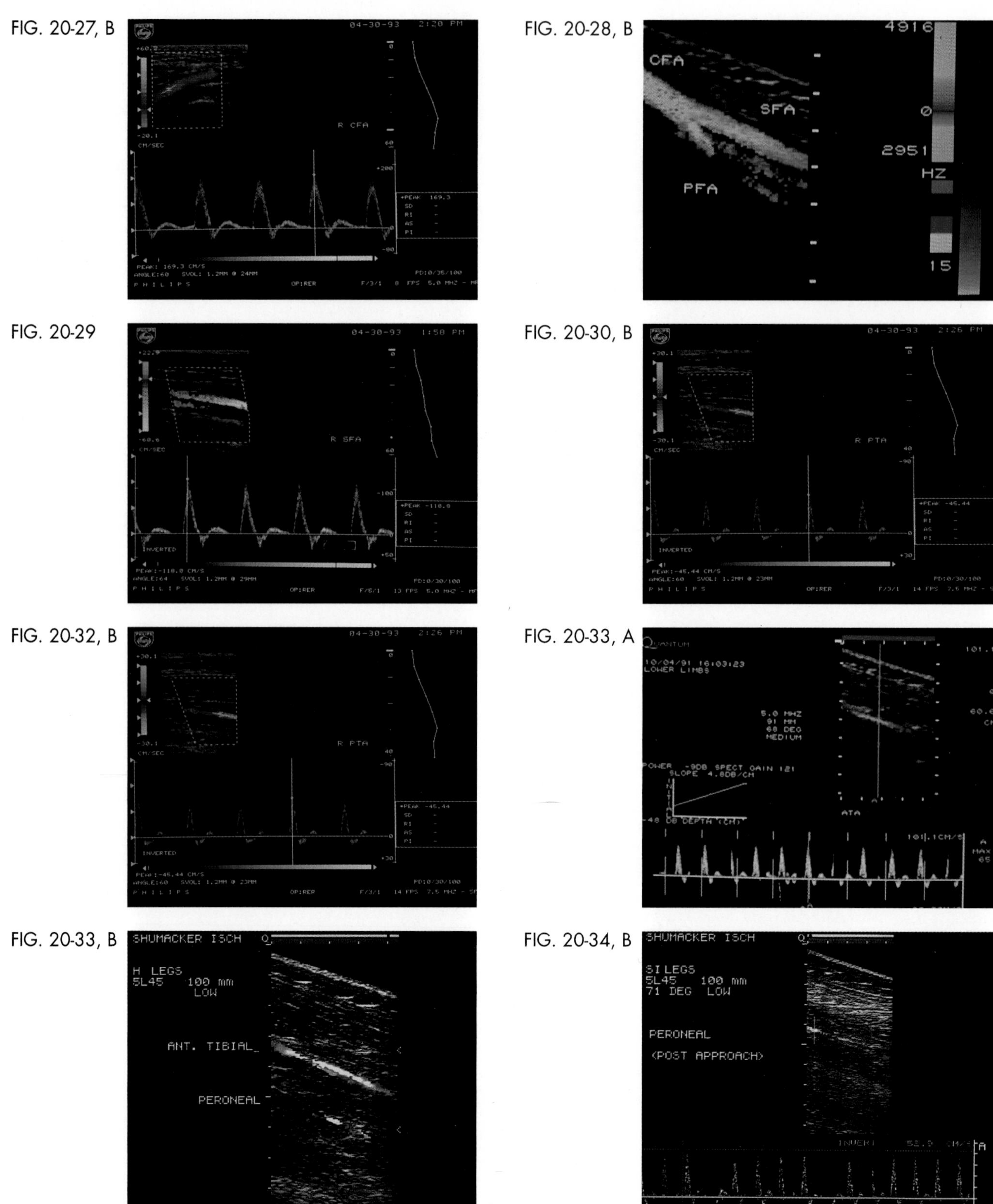

FIG. 20-27 B, Distal external iliac-common femoral artery with normal duplex spectral Doppler waveform. **FIG. 20-28 B,** Superficial femoral artery common-profunda femoris artery bifurcation off the common femoral artery. **FIG. 20-29** Superficial femoral artery with normal duplex spectral Doppler waveform. **FIG. 20-30 B,** Popliteal artery with normal duplex spectral Doppler waveform. **FIG. 20-32 B,** Posterior tibial artery with normal duplex spectral Doppler waveform. **FIG. 20-33 A,** Anterior tibial artery with normal duplex spectral Doppler waveform. **B,** Anterior tibial artery showing the peroneal artery deep to it in the anterior scanning position. **FIG. 20-34 B,** Peroneal artery with normal duplex spectral Doppler waveform.

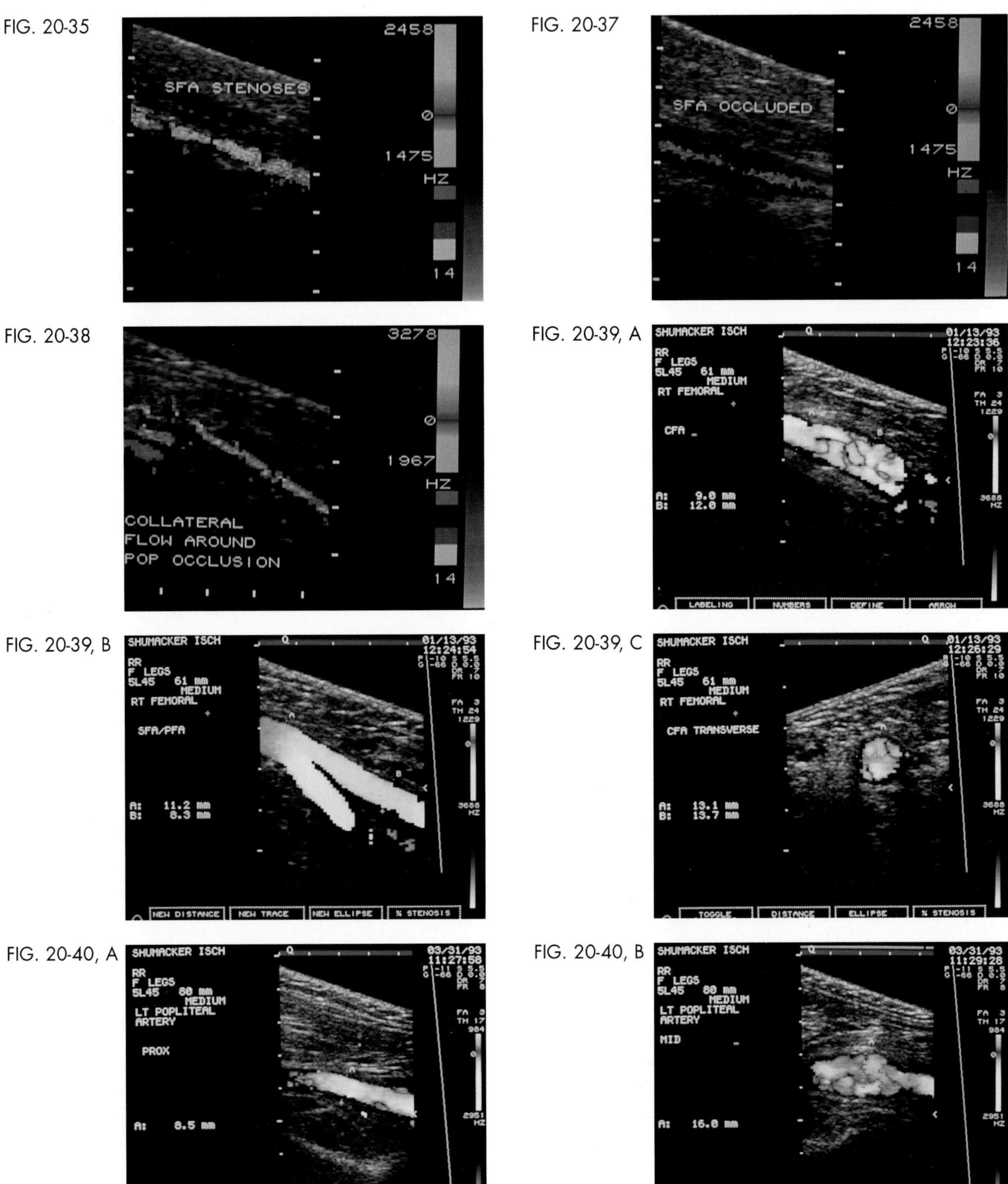

FIG. 20-35 A longitudinal image of a superficial femoral artery showing multiple irregular stenoses within the segment. Note the acceleration of the color-flow streamlines and the presence of flow disturbances. **FIG. 20-37** Occluded superficial femoral artery (note patent superficial femoral vein deep to the artery with normal blue venous color flow). **FIG. 20-38** Example showing collaterals directing flow from a patent proximal popliteal artery around an occluded distal segment. **FIG. 20-39 A-C,** Common femoral ectasia. **FIG. 20-40** Popliteal aneurysm. This popliteal artery measures 8.5 mm in a straight segment proximal to the popliteal fossa. **A,** Just distal to this, the artery has an aneurysmal segment that measures 16 mm in anteroposterior diameter. **B,** The vessel assumes a normal diameter distal to the aneurysm (right side of **B**).

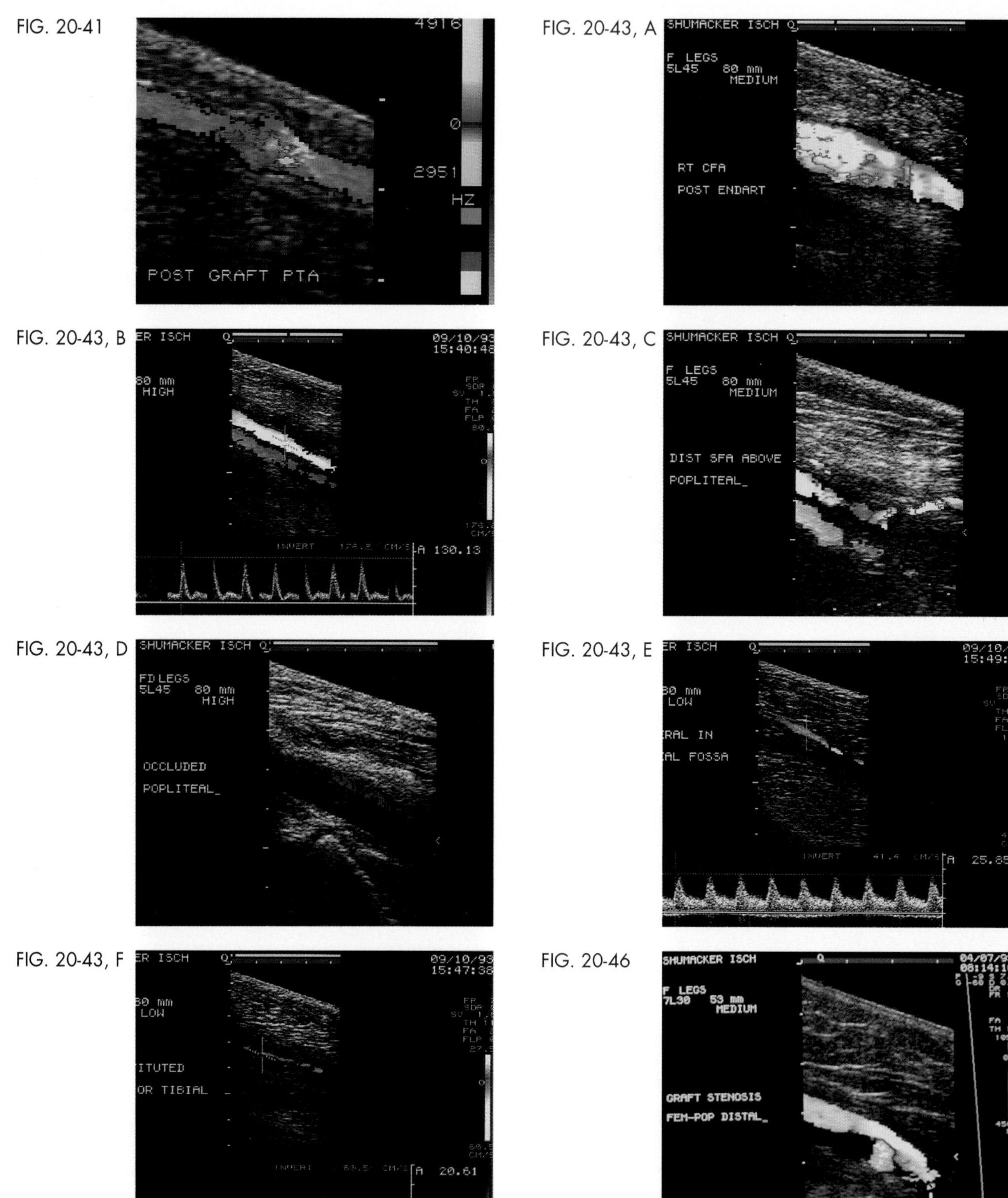

FIG. 20-41 This arterial in situ graft segment received a percutaneous transluminal balloon angioplasty for a focal stenosis, causing normal postangioplasty dilation of the artery. **FIG. 20-43** CFA endarterectomy and popliteal occlusion. **A,** Common femoral artery. **B,** Superficial femoral artery and corresponding Doppler spectral waveform. **C,** Distal superficial femoral artery. **D,** Occluded popliteal artery. **E,** Popliteal collateral and corresponding Doppler spectral waveform. **F,** Posterior tibial artery and corresponding Doppler spectral waveform. **FIG. 20-46** This stenotic area in a vein bypass graft is occurring at a valve sinus, with thrombotic material lodged in a residual valve cusp. Note the hemodynamic flow streamline, and the area of flow separation on the distal side of the stenosis.

FIG. 20-50

FIG. 20-54, A

FIG. 20-54, B

FIG. 20-55, A

FIG. 20-55, B

FIG. 20-55, C

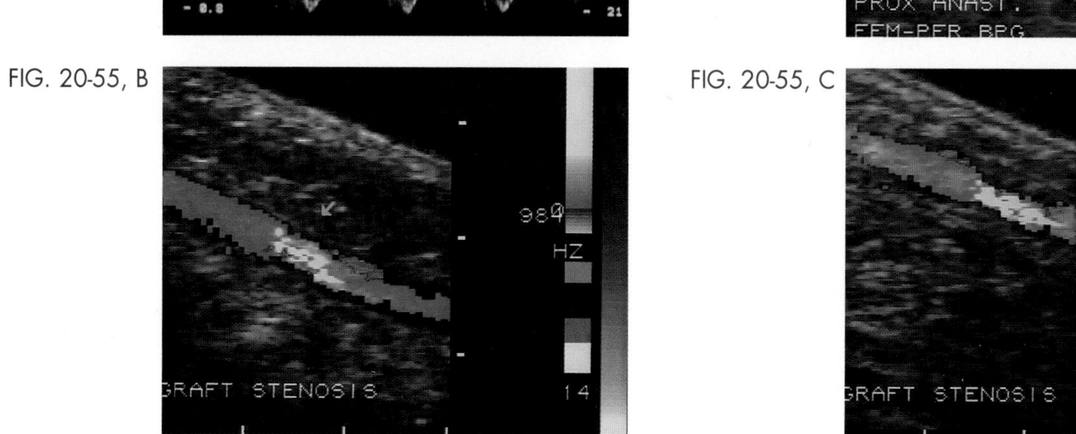

FIG. 20-55, D

FIG. 20-55, E

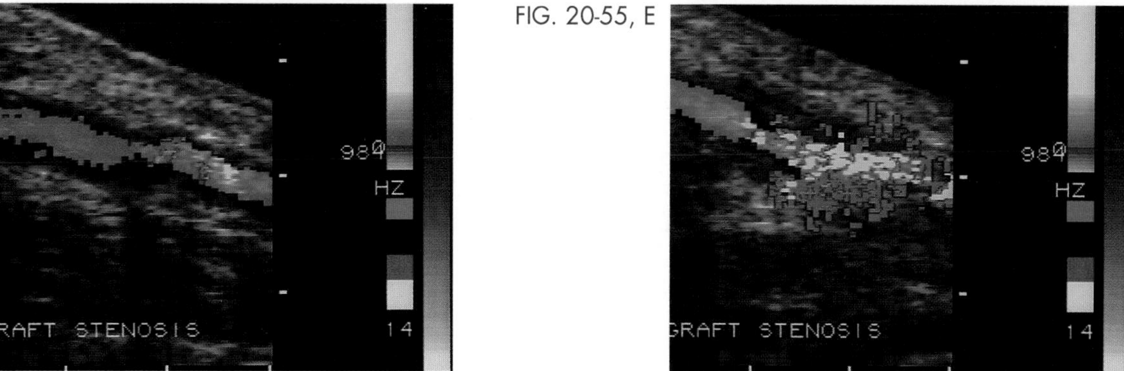

FIG. 20-50 Appearance of an occluded Gore-Tex bypass graft. Note absence of color flow within and the bright walls of the synthetic material. **FIG. 20-54 A,** Normal femoropopliteal graft, proximal segment. **B,** Normal femoropopliteal graft, distal segment. **FIG. 20-55 A,** Proximal graft anastomosis. **B,** Above-knee graft stenosis. **C,** Below-knee graft stenosis. **D,** Midcalf level graft stenosis (see text). **E,** Graft stenosis above distal anastomosis.

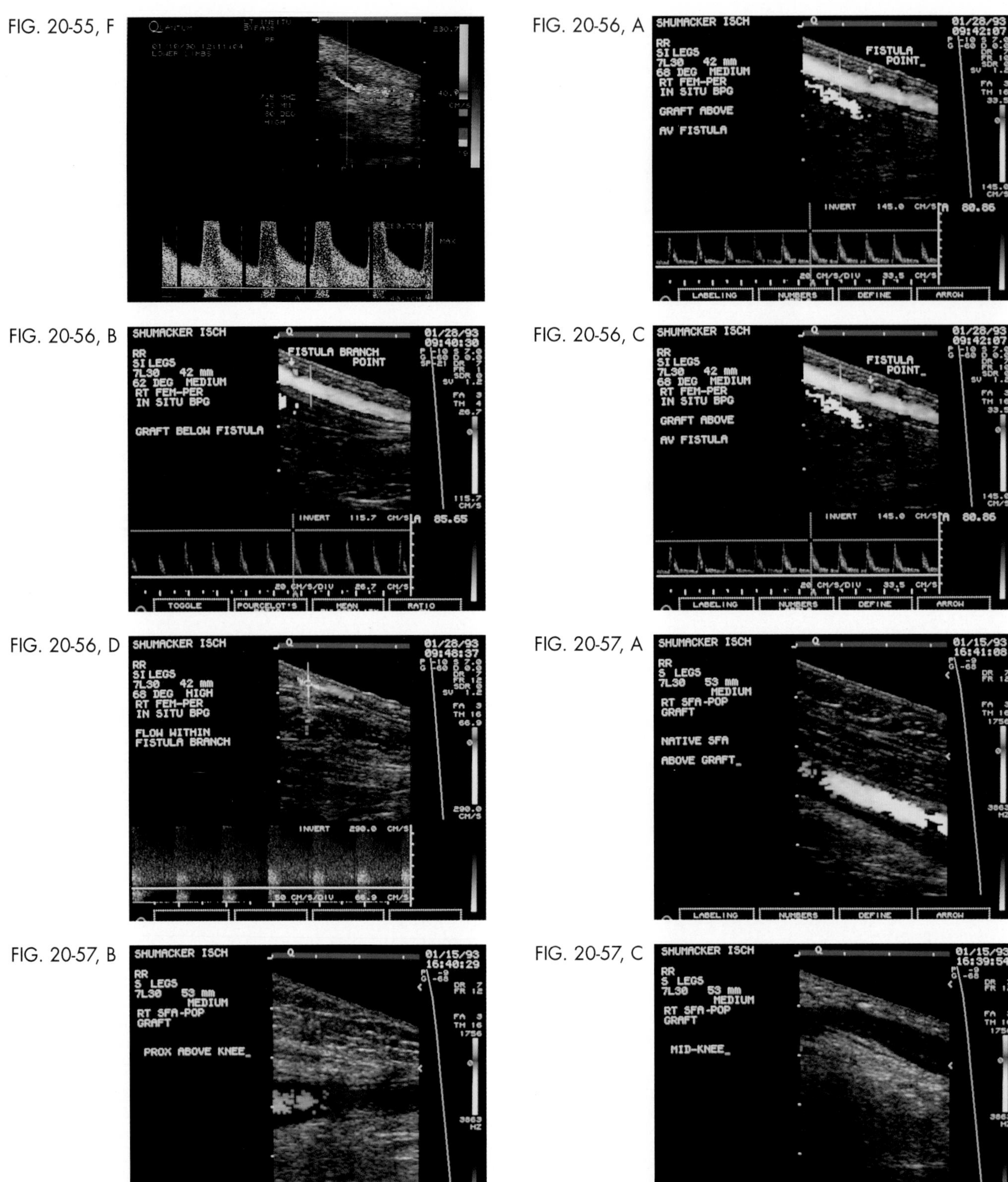

FIG. 20-55 F, Doppler spectral waveforms at distal stenosis shown in **E. FIG. 20-56 A,** In situ graft with waveforms and velocity proximal to arteriovenous fistula takeoff. **B,** Distal to arteriovenous fistula takeoff. **C,** Waveform in the proximal segment of the arteriovenous fistula. Note the elevated velocity scale. **D,** Distal segment of the arteriovenous fistula. **FIG. 20-57** Occluded superficial graft. **A,** Native SFA. **B,** Proximal anastomosis. **C,** Center graft.

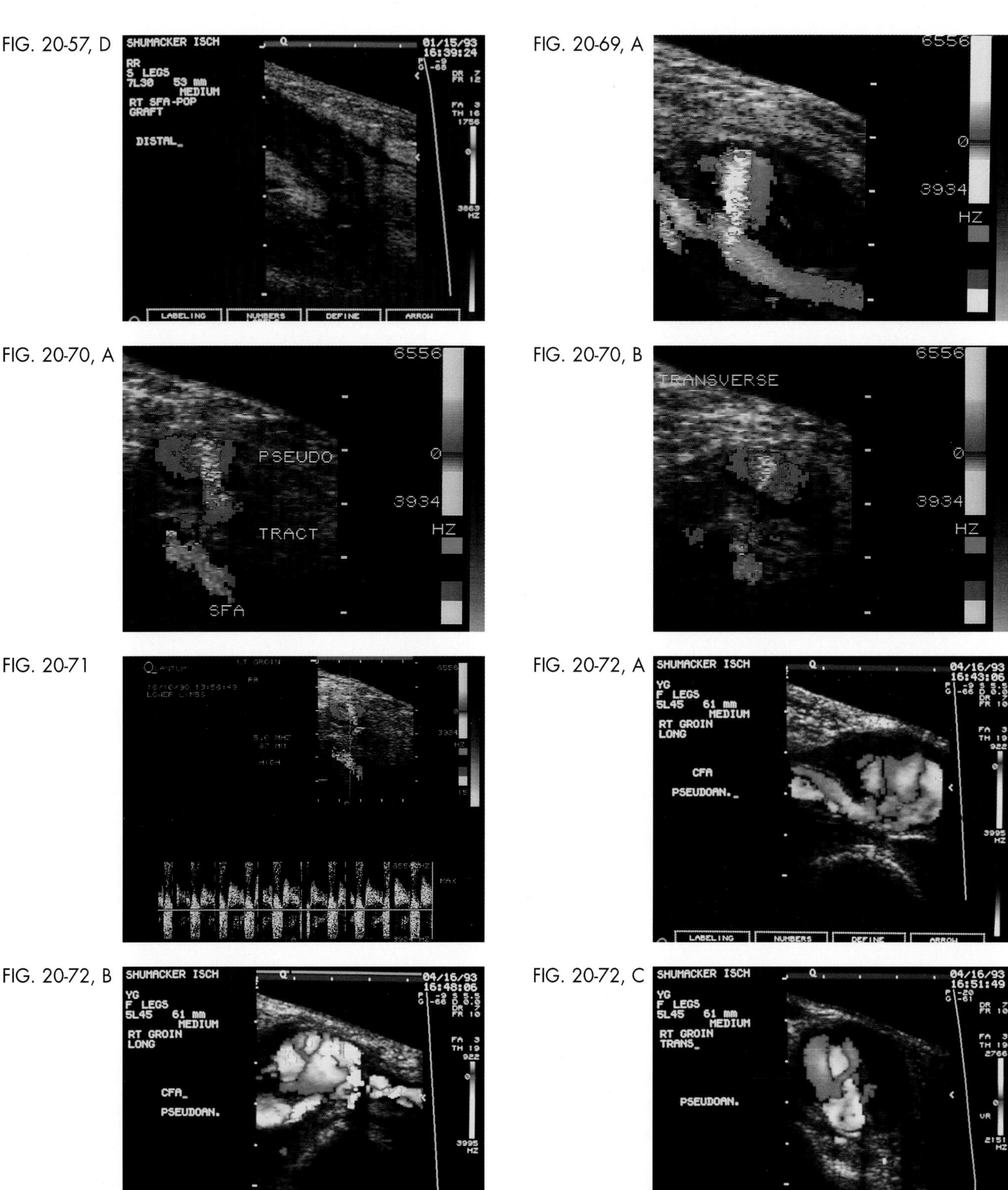

FIG. 20-57 D, Distal anastomosis. **FIG. 20-69** "Swirling" color-flow patterns in a pseudoaneurysm. **A,** An axial jet from the tract is directed toward the transducer (which appears as blue color flow). **FIG. 20-70** This superficial femoral artery pseudoaneurysm has a clearly defined tract that can be identified in both the **A,** longitudinal and **B,** transverse planes. **FIG. 20-71** Characteristic bidirectional to-and-fro flow pattern in the tract of the pseudoaneurysm shown in Fig. 20-70. **FIG. 20-72 A,** Right anastomotic pseudoaneurysm, long axis, proximal. **B,** Long axis, distal. **C,** Transverse.

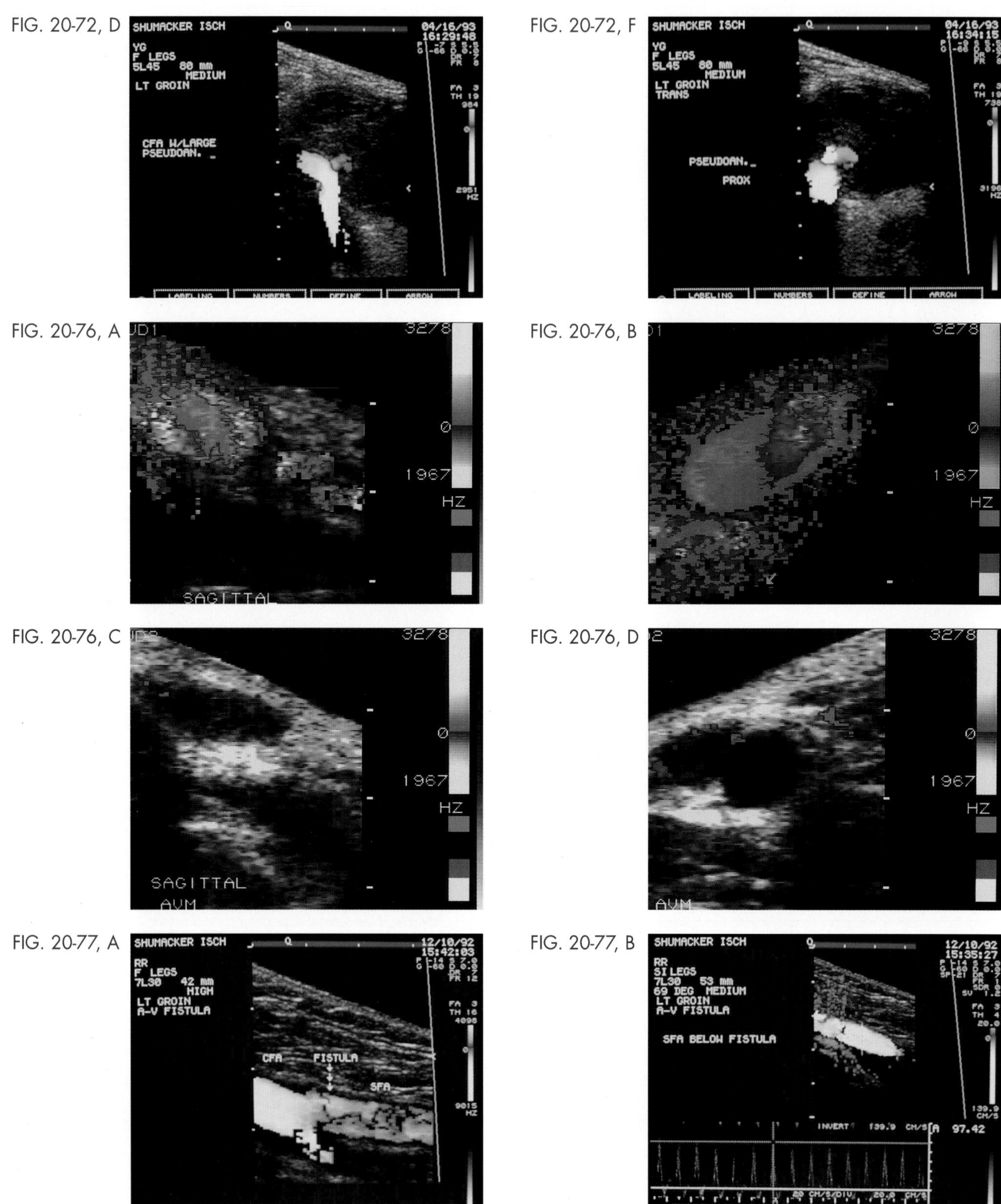

FIG. 20-72 D, Left anastomotic pseudoaneurysm, long axis, proximal. **F,** Transverse, proximal. **FIG. 20-76 A,** Upper-extremity arteriovenous fistula, aneurysmal fistula and branches, sagittal plane. **B,** Transverse plane (see text). **C,** Sagittal plane, postembolization. **D,** Transverse plane, postembolization. **FIG. 20-77** Arteriovenous fistula. **A,** Native SFA. **B,** Doppler spectral waveforms at SFA distal to fistula origin.

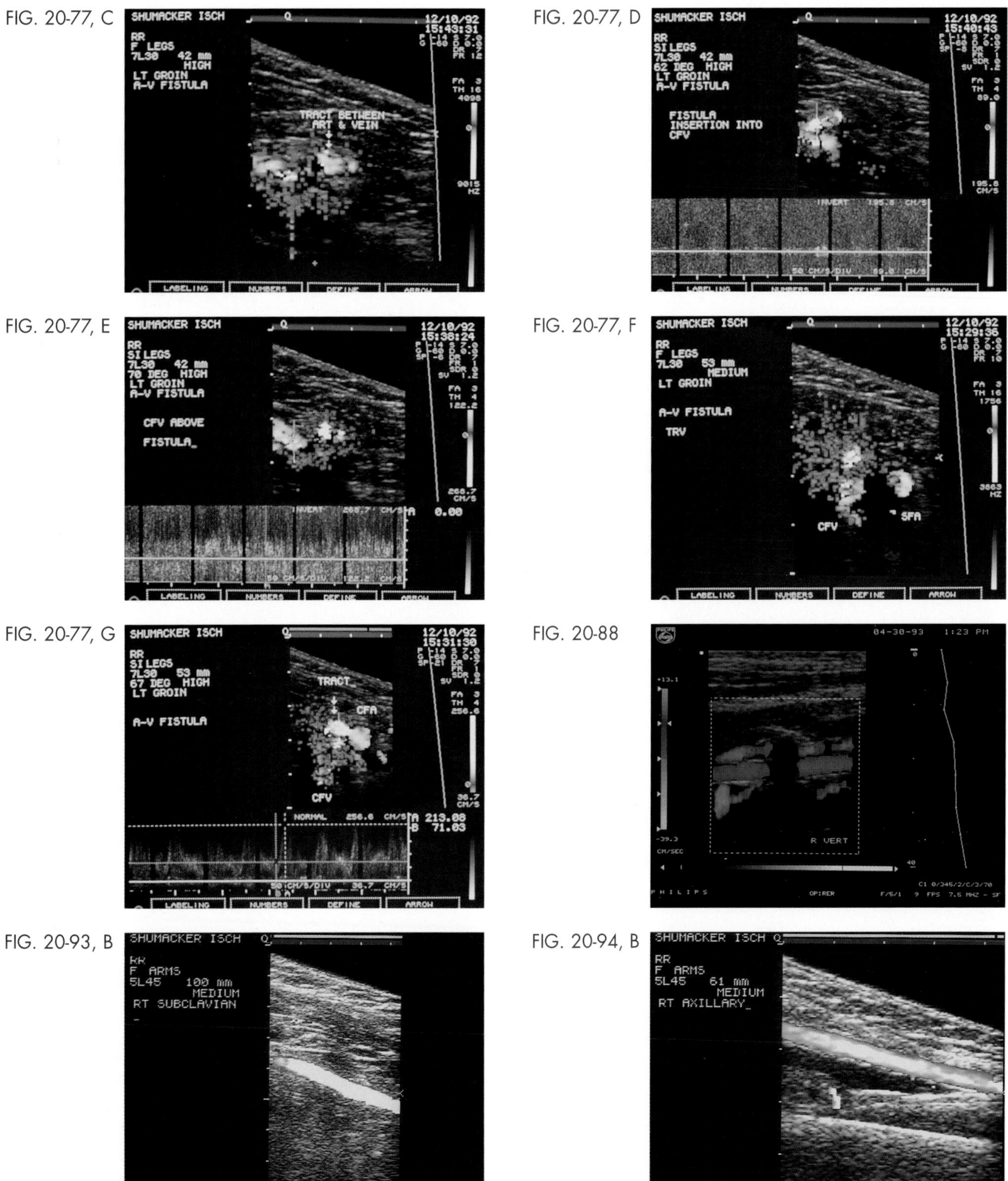

FIG. 20-77 C, Long-axis localization of fistula tract. **D,** Doppler spectral waveforms in fistula tract at insertion into CFV. **E,** Doppler spectral waveforms in CFV proximal to fistula tract insertion. **F,** Transverse plane view of fistula tract in relationship to SFA and CFV. **G,** Doppler spectral waveforms within fistula tract, transverse plane (see text). **FIG. 20-88** Normal color-flow appearance of the antegrade vertebral artery (red) and vertebral veins (blue). Note the shadow from the transverse vertebral process. **FIG. 20-93 B,** Normal subclavian artery. **FIG. 20-94 B,** Normal axillary artery.

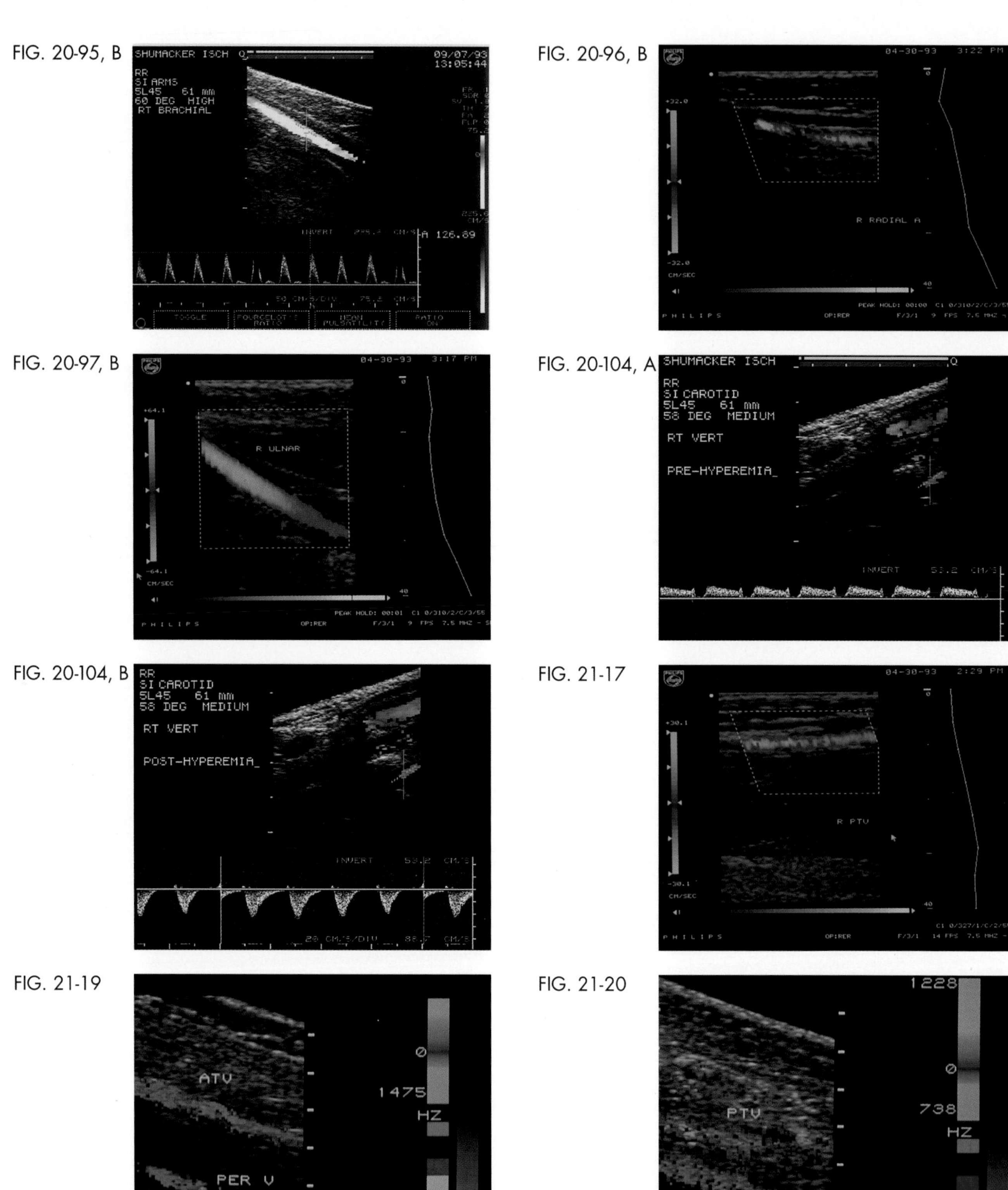

FIG. 20-95 B, Normal brachial artery with spectral waveform. **FIG. 20-96 B,** Normal radial artery. **FIG. 20-97 B,** Normal ulnar artery. **FIG. 20-104** Subclavian steal hyperemia test. The transient vertebral signal in **A** reverses in systole but does not go below the baseline. After 3 minutes of brachial occlusion with a pressure cuff and release, reactive hyperemia in the arm causes the signal to fully reverse below the baseline in systole and diastole, **B. FIG. 21-17** Normal posterior tibial vein. **FIG. 21-19** Normal proximal anterior tibial vein (note the relationship of the peroneal vein visualized deep to it). **FIG. 21-20** Longitudinal relationship of the peroneal vein deep to the posterior tibial vein in the mediolateral scan plane.

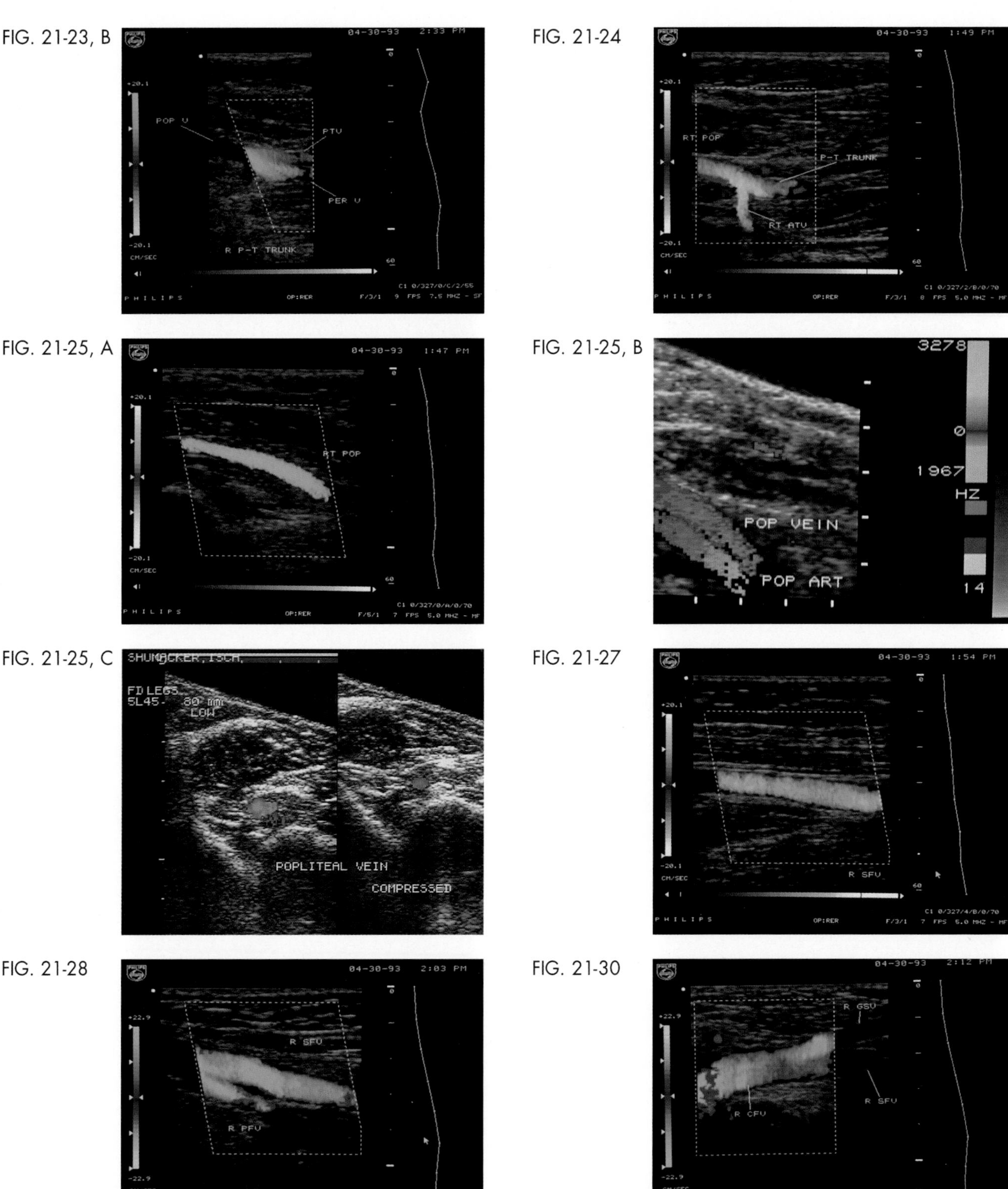

FIG. 21-23 B, Normal peroneal-tibial junction with the distal popliteal vein. **FIG. 21-24** Normal distal popliteal vein, showing the insertion of the anterior tibial vein. **FIG. 21-25 A,** Longitudinal of the normal popliteal vein across the central popliteal fossa. **B,** Longitudinal of the popliteal vein and popliteal artery in the posterior imaging plane. **C,** Transverse view of a normal popliteal vein showing the uncompressed vein on the left image and the vein compressed on the right image. Note that the walls coapt easily. **FIG. 21-27** Normal superficial femoral vein. **FIG. 21-28** Superficial femoral–deep femoral junction with the common femoral vein. **FIG. 21-30** Normal common femoral vein (note the saphenofemoral junction to the right).

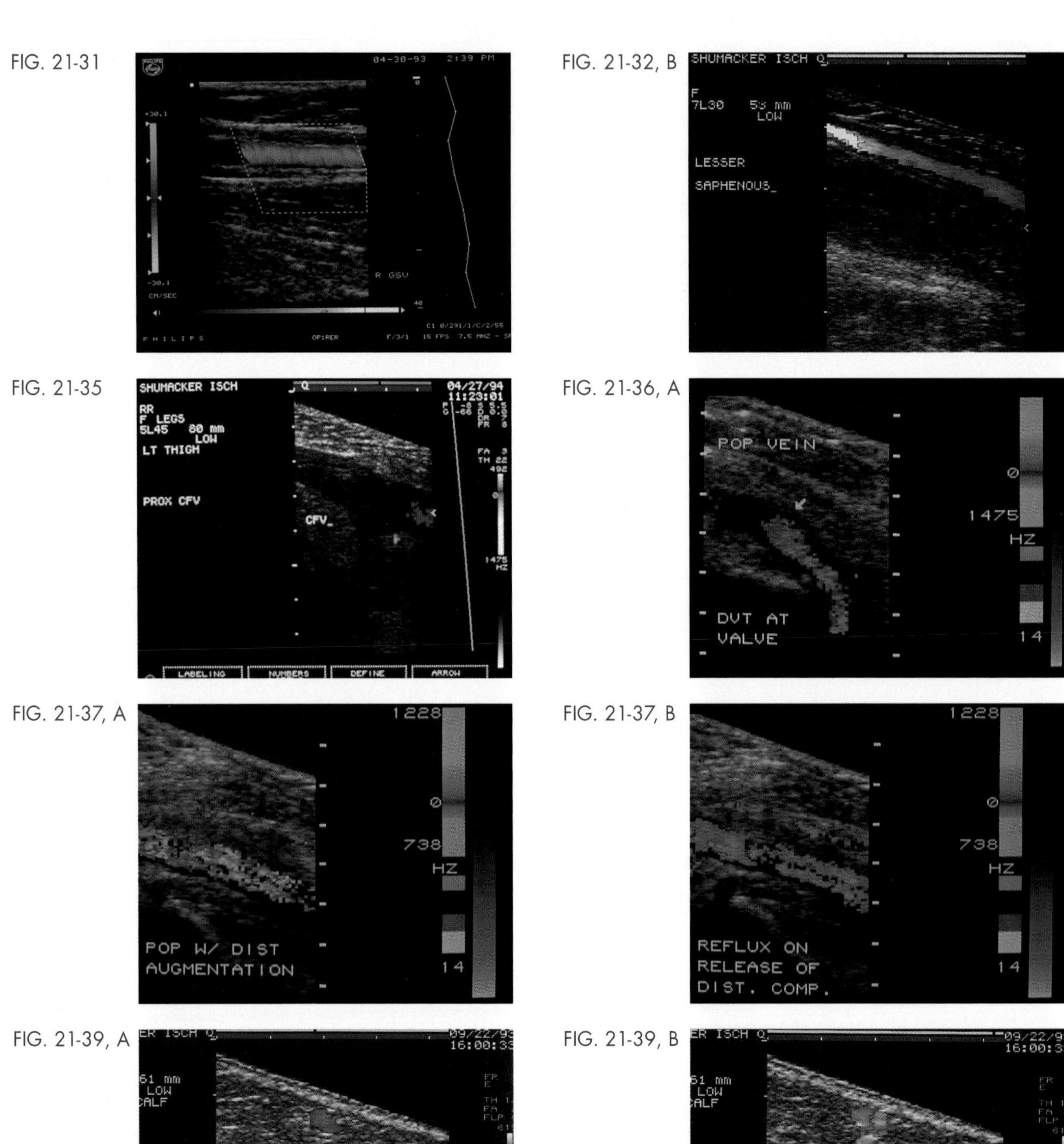

FIG. 21-31 Great saphenous vein. **FIG. 21-32 B,** Color-flow duplex of the lesser saphenous vein distal to the saphenopopliteal junction. **FIG. 21-35** The proximal portion of common femoral vein filled with echogenic homogeneous thrombus. **FIG. 21-36 A,** A popliteal vein has thrombus concentrating near a valve *(arrow)*. **FIG. 21-37 A,** Color-flow appearance of reflux. Distal calf augmentation shows normal blue antegrade flow through this chronically recanalized popliteal vein. **B,** On release of calf compression, strong red retrograde flow is seen rushing back through the venous segment. **FIG. 21-39 A,** With distal compression of the foot, flow travels normally through the perforator from the superficial vein to the deep vein (flow is away from the transducer, thus is coded red—see scale to the right). **B,** On release of distal compression, flow becomes retrograde in the perforator (flowing back toward the transducer and thus coded blue), flowing back into the superficial vein.

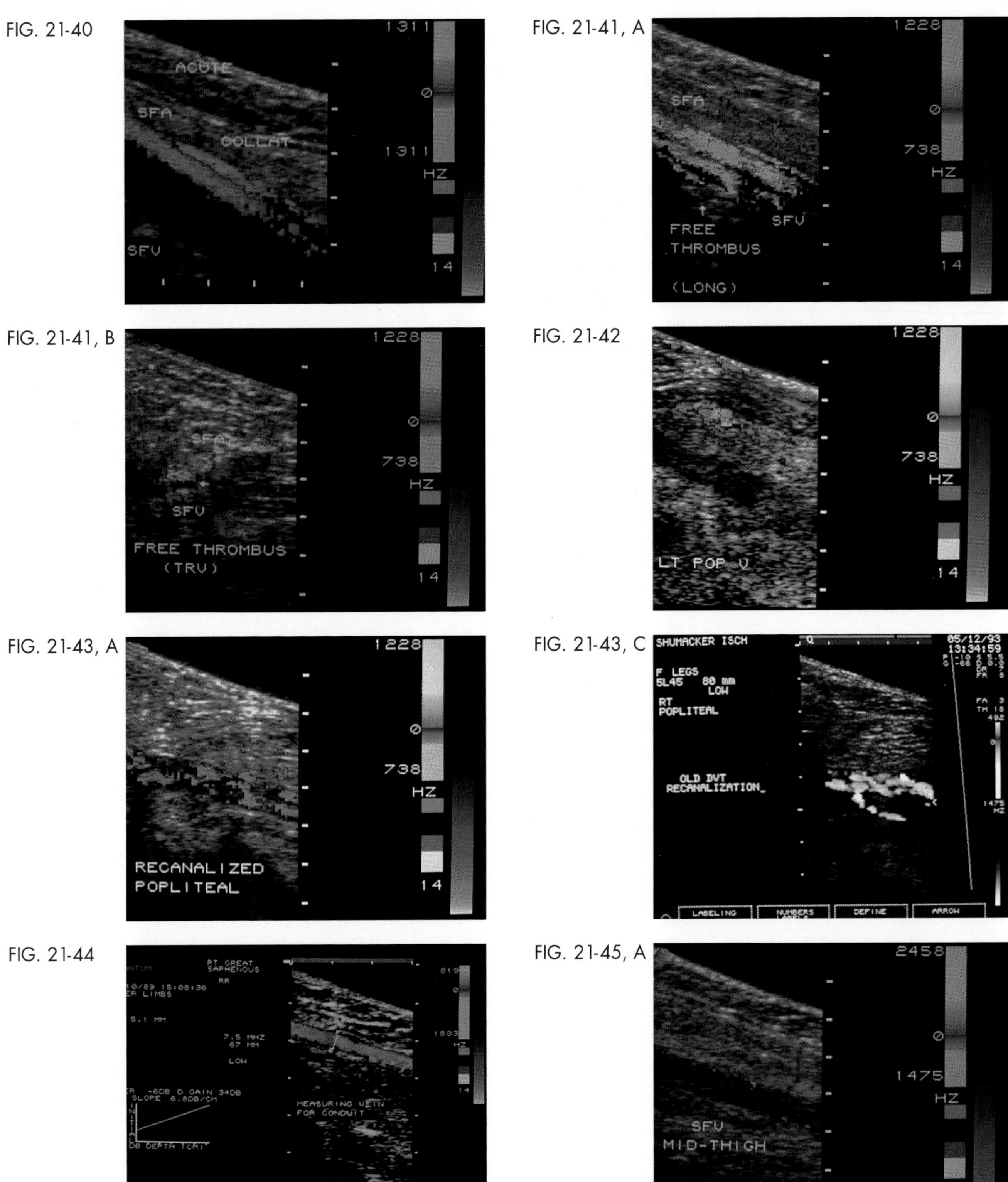

FIG. 21-40 Acute thrombus. **FIG. 21-41** Adherent or free thrombus. **A,** In longitudinal section, note the "tongue" of thrombus in the superficial femoral vein, which is adherent to the wall proximally but appears to "float" within the color-flow pattern, almost giving a double-lumen appearance. **B,** The true nature of the thrombus becomes more apparent in the transverse plane, where it is surrounded on three sides by color flow and adheres to the lateral wall (to the right). **FIG. 21-42** Chronic thrombus. **FIG. 21-43** Recanalized thrombus. **A,** The popliteal vein in this segment has old chronic thrombus through which numerous pathways have developed. **C,** This popliteal vein has recanalized almost completely from an old thrombosis. **FIG. 21-44** Measuring the size of the great saphenous vein to determine suitability for bypass conduit. **FIG. 21-45** Recurrent deep-vein thrombosis. **A,** The superficial femoral vein is completely thrombosed.

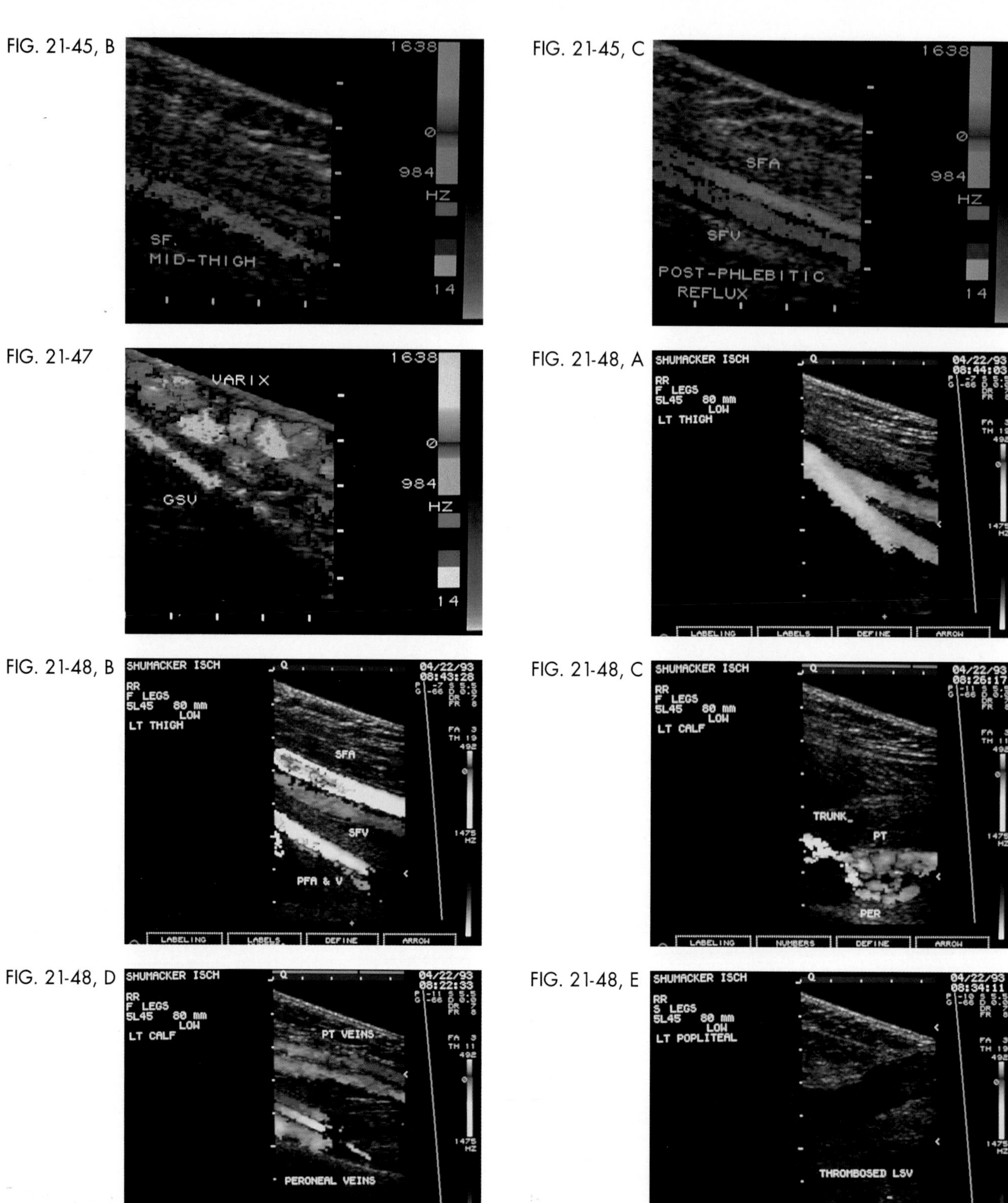

FIG. 21-45 Recurrent deep-vein thrombosis. **B,** In a follow-up examination 6 months after anticoagulation therapy the same segment is now patent with some residual irregularity, although post-phlebitic reflux is present, **C. FIG. 21-47** This large dilated varicosity appeared on external physical examination to involve the great saphenous vein; duplex sonography shows the varix to be an entirely separate, and thus focally treatable, venous branch (note the normal saphenous vein deep to the varix). **FIG. 21-48 A,** Normal lower-extremity deep system—junction of the common femoral vein, superficial femoral vein, and profunda femoris vein. **B,** Superficial femoral vein, profunda femoris vein. **C,** Peroneal-tibial junction. **D,** Posterior tibial and peroneal veins. **E,** Thrombosed saphenopopliteal junction and proximal lesser saphenous vein.

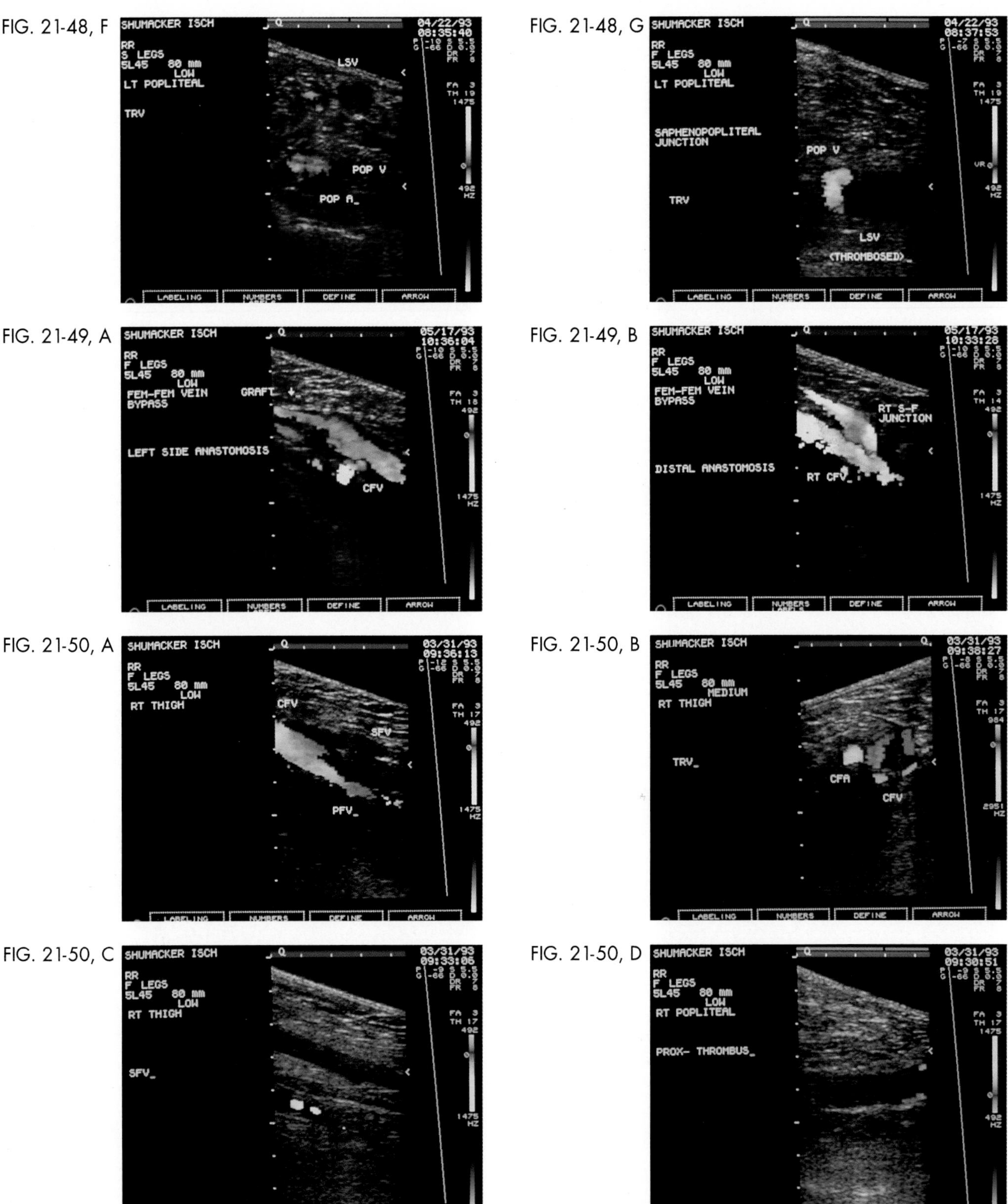

FIG. 21-48 F, Transverse view—patent popliteal vein and thrombosed lesser saphenous vein (proximal calf). **G,** Transverse view—saphenopopliteal junction, patent popliteal vein. **FIG. 21-49 A,** Femorofemoral venous bypass—left anastomosis, left common femoral vein (see text). **B,** Femorofemoral venous bypass—right saphenofemoral junction, right common femoral vein (see text). **FIG. 21-50 A,** Partial distal common femoral vein thrombosis, superficial femoral vein thrombosis—longitudinal view. **B,** Transverse view. **C,** Thrombosed superficial femoral vein, midthigh. **D,** Thrombosed proximal popliteal vein.

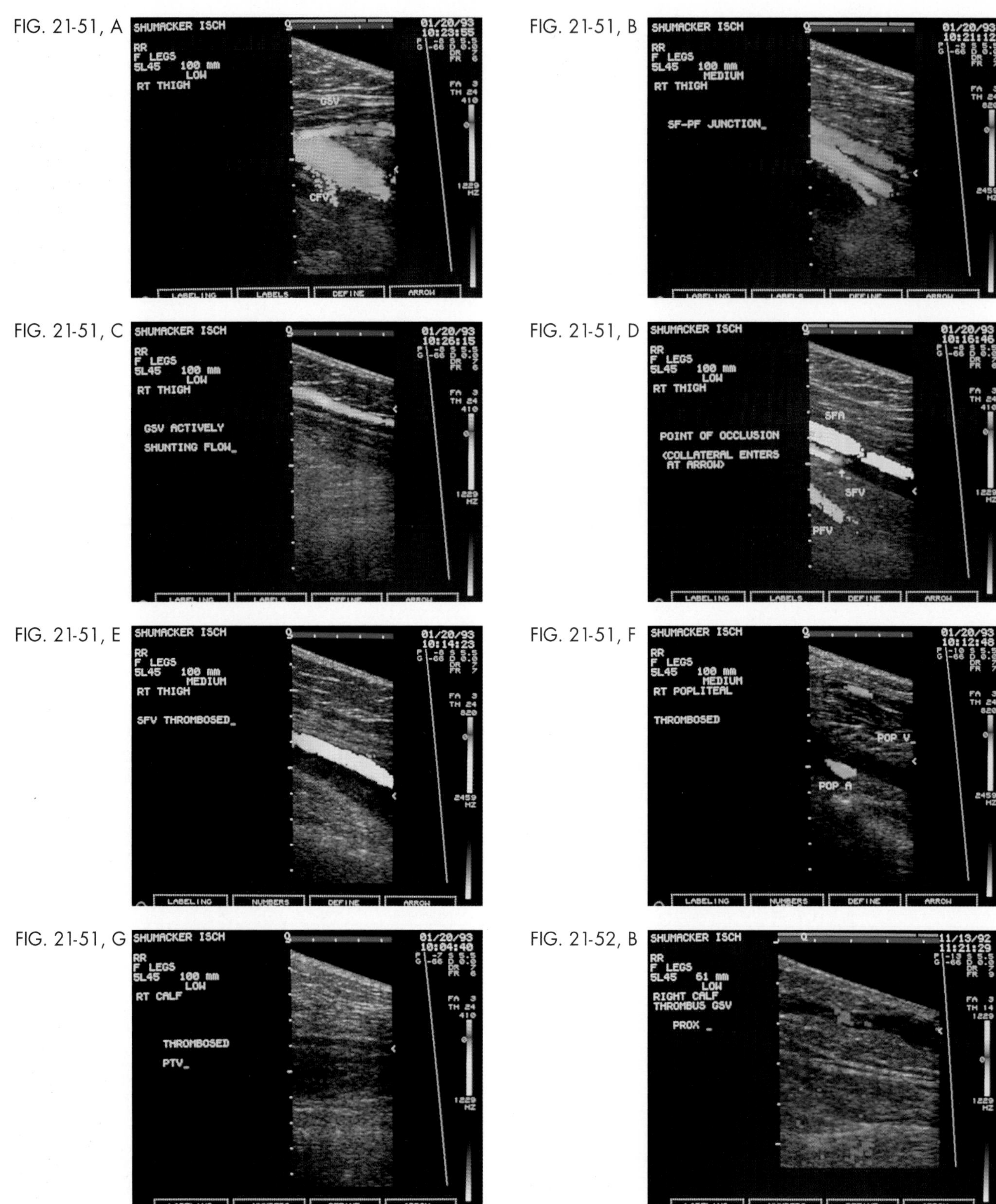

FIG. 21-51 A, Patent common femoral vein and saphenofemoral junction. **B,** Patent junction of common femoral vein, profunda femoris vein, and superficial femoral vein. **C,** Great saphenous vein with high-velocity continuous flow. **D,** Proximal extent of superficial femoral vein occlusion with collateral inflow. **E,** Thrombosed superficial femoral vein, middistal level (see text). **F,** Thrombosed popliteal vein. **G,** Thrombosed posterior tibial vein. **FIG. 21-52 B,** Thrombus in the great saphenous vein just below the knee.

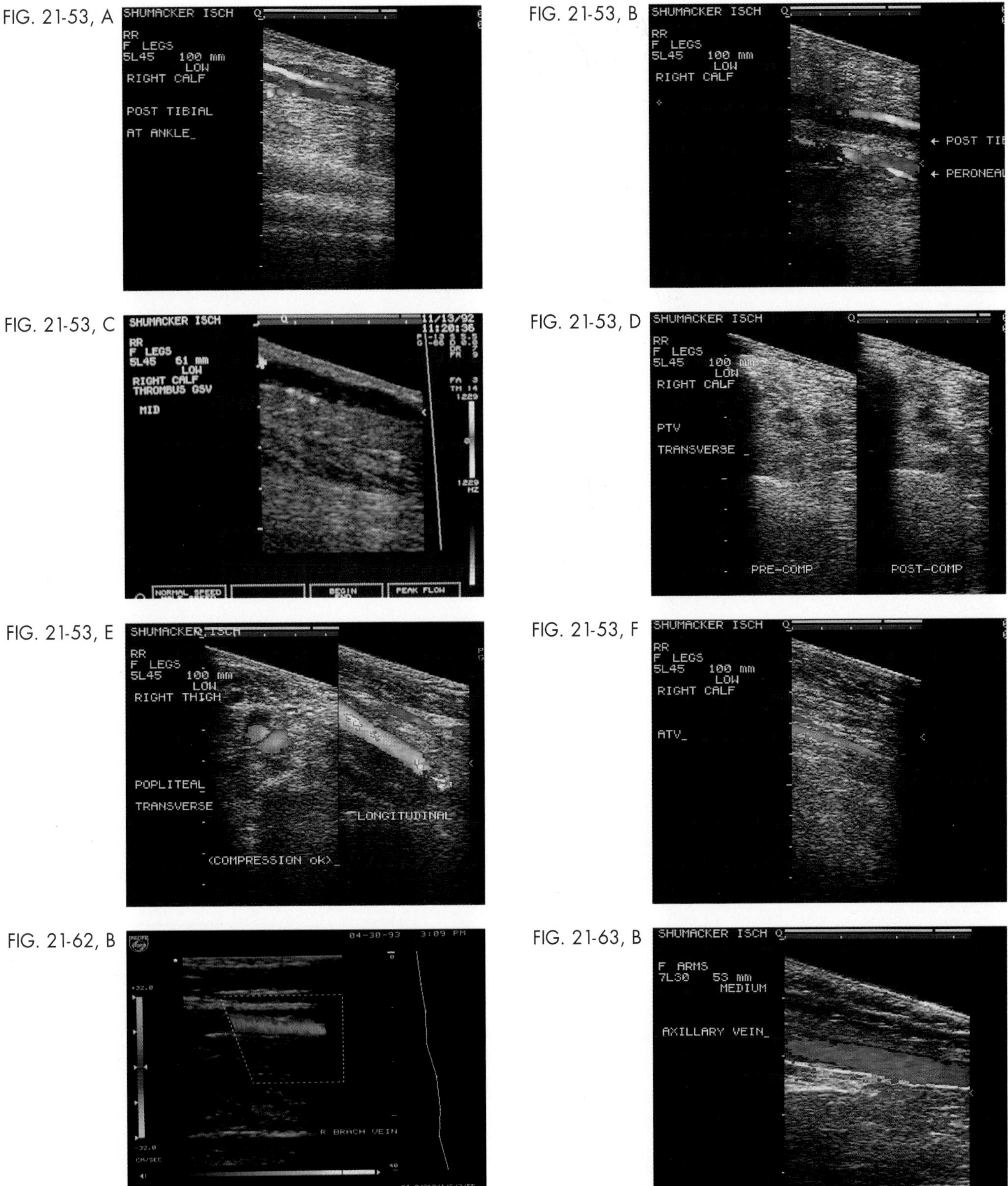

FIG. 21-53 A, Patent distal posterior tibial veins. **B,** Thrombosed posterior tibial veins, patent peroneal veins. **C,** Thrombus in the great saphenous vein along the midcalf segment. **D,** Thrombosed posterior tibial vein, midcalf level, transverse plane, with and without transducer compression. **E,** Patent popliteal vein (longitudinal and transverse planes). **F,** Patent anterior tibial vein. **FIG. 21-62 B,** Color-flow duplex appearance of a normal brachial vein. **FIG. 21-63 B,** Normal axillary vein.

FIG. 21-64

FIG. 21-65, B

FIG. 21-65, C

FIG. 21-67, A

FIG. 21-67, B

FIG. 21-68, A

FIG. 21-68, B

FIG. 21-68, C

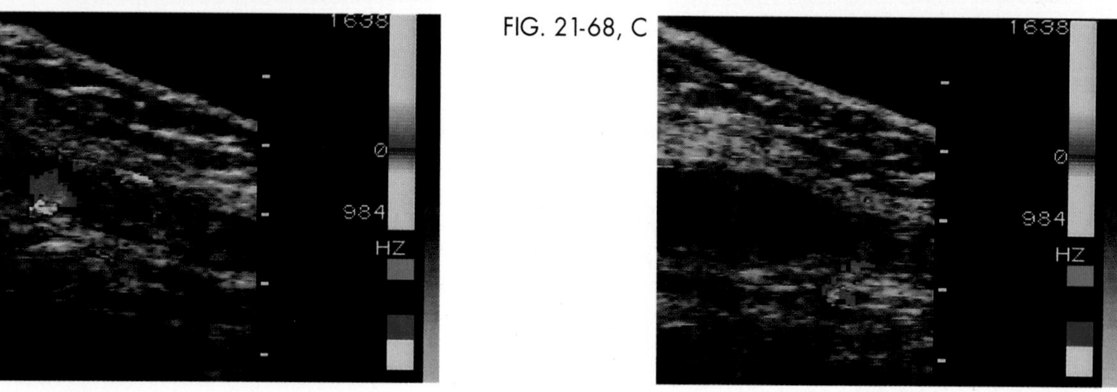

FIG. 21-64 Brachial-basilic vein junction with the normal axillary vein. **FIG. 21-65 B,** Normal subclavian vein in the longitudinal plane. **C,** Normal subclavian vein in the transverse plane. **FIG. 21-67 A,** Normal internal jugular vein with the internal carotid artery and carotid bulb seen deep to it in the longitudinal plane. **B,** Transverse view of the same internal jugular vein, taken somewhat more proximally with the common carotid deep and medial to it. **FIG. 21-68 A,** Poorly augmenting patent distal brachial vein. Note edge of thrombus to left. **B,** Thrombosed proximal brachial vein with collaterals. **C,** Thrombosed axillary vein.

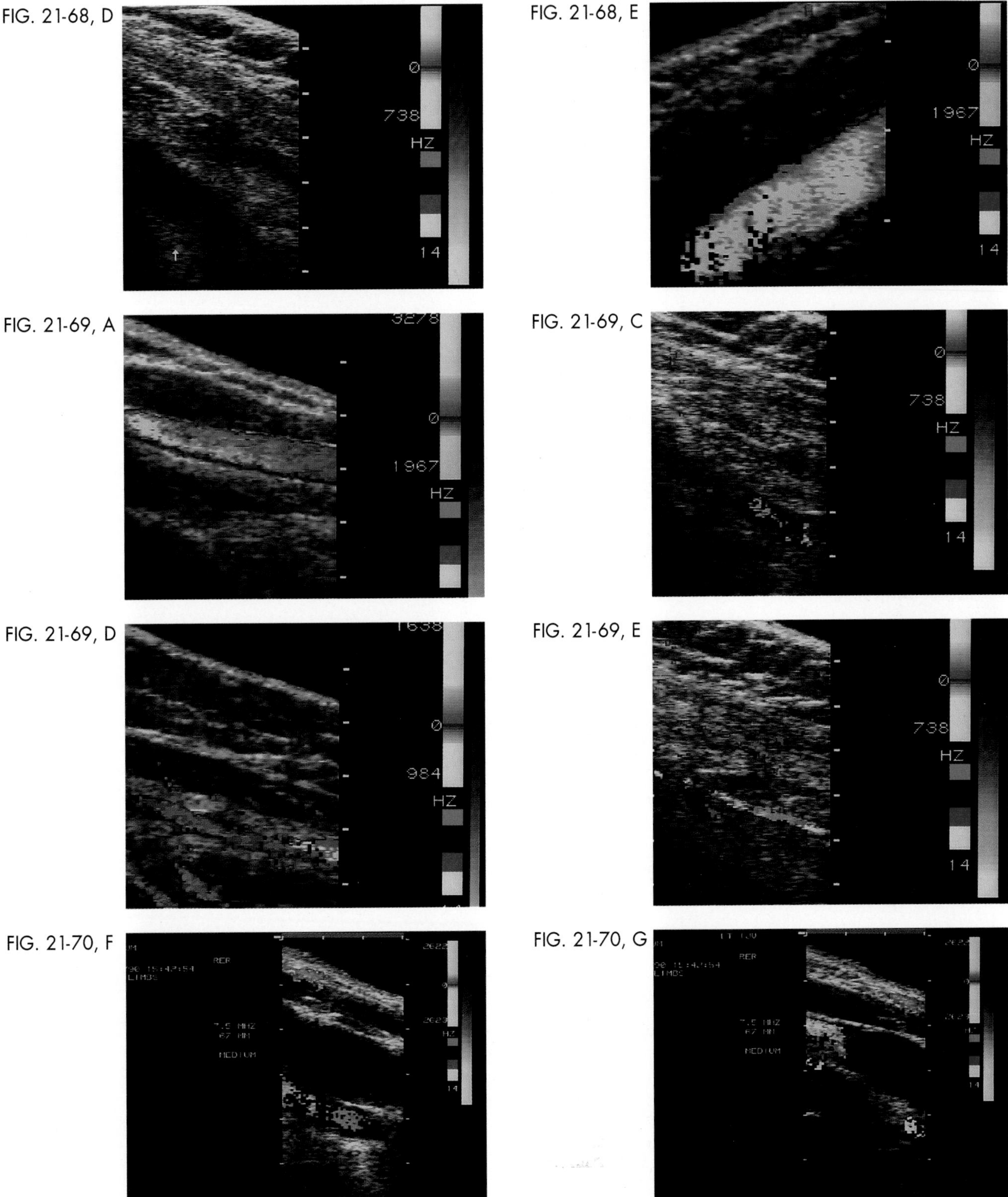

FIG. 21-68 D, Thrombosed subclavian vein. **E,** Patent internal jugular vein. **FIG. 21-69 A,** Patent distal brachial vein. **C,** Thrombosed and partly recanalized subclavian vein. **D,** Active collaterals in axilla (note thrombosed axillary vein above collaterals). **E,** Patent active collateral paralleling subclavian vein. **FIG. 21-70 F,** Acutely thrombosed proximal internal jugular vein (head to left). Note the common carotid deep to the vein. **G,** Middistal segment of the thrombosed internal jugular vein above; note the border of the thrombus and the patent segment to the left of the image.

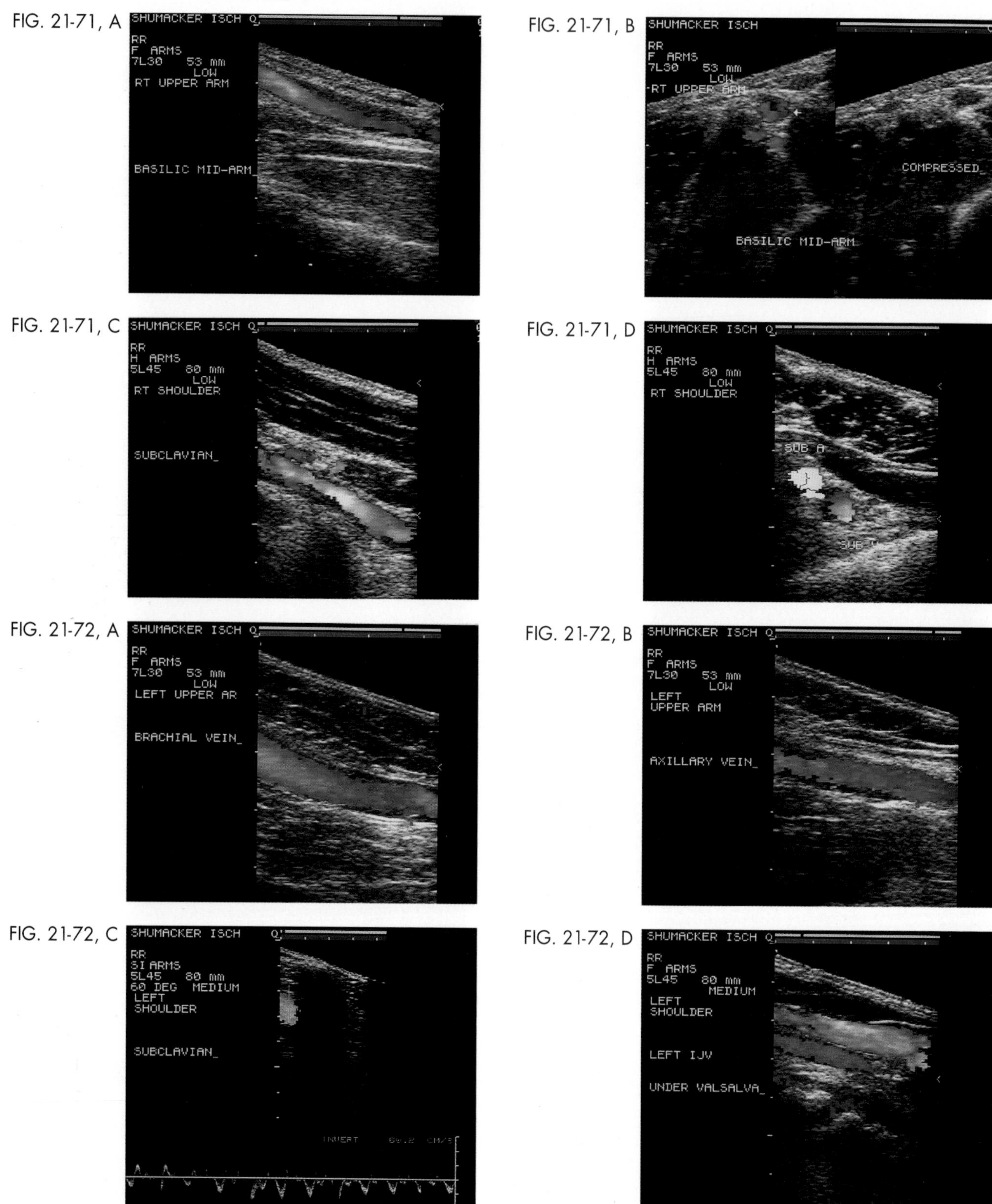

FIG. 21-71 A, Longitudinal view of basilic vein with nonobstructive partial thrombus on superficial wall. **B,** Transverse views of the above partially thrombosed basilic vein *(arrow),* before *(left),* and after *(right)* transducer compression. Note that the vein does not flatten because of the presence of the thrombus. **C,** Subclavian vein with nonobstructive partial thrombus on deep wall. **D,** Transverse view of the subclavian vein in **C**. Note the relationship of the subclavian artery (head is to left of image). **FIG. 21-72 A,** Normal, patent brachial vein. **B,** Normal, patent axillary vein. **C,** Normal, patent subclavian vein (partly obscured by clavicle), showing a normal slightly pulsatile subclavian venous signal. **D,** Normal, patent internal jugular vein.

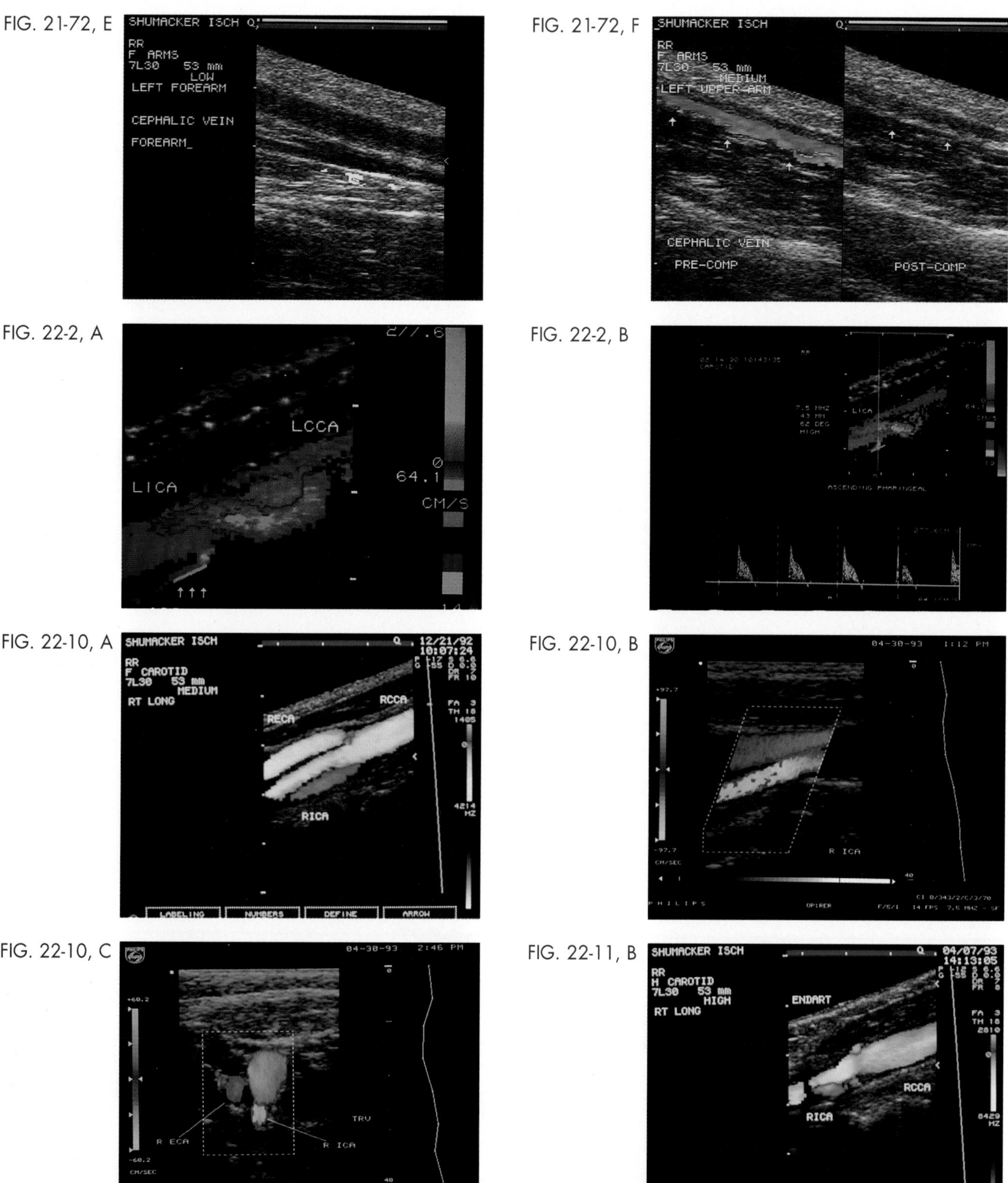

FIG. 21-72 E, Thrombosed cephalic vein in forearm. **F,** Partially thrombosed cephalic vein in upper arm, showing incomplete compressibility. **FIG. 22-2 A,** Ascending pharyngeal artery arising from a normal internal carotid origin. **B,** A Doppler shows a high-resistance flow pattern typical of a branch artery. **FIG. 22-10** Normal carotid system. **A,** Longitudinal view of the carotid bifurcation, showing normal color-flow filling in the ICA (with an area of normal color-flow separation), ECA, and distal CCA. **B,** Longitudinal view of the internal carotid artery, with the internal jugular vein shown superficially to it, showing normal color-flow filling. **C,** Transverse image showing the relationships of the internal jugular vein, internal carotid artery, and external carotid artery. **FIG. 22-11 B,** Internal carotid artery with plaque shows increased streamline and blue flow separation on the distal side of the stenotic plaque.

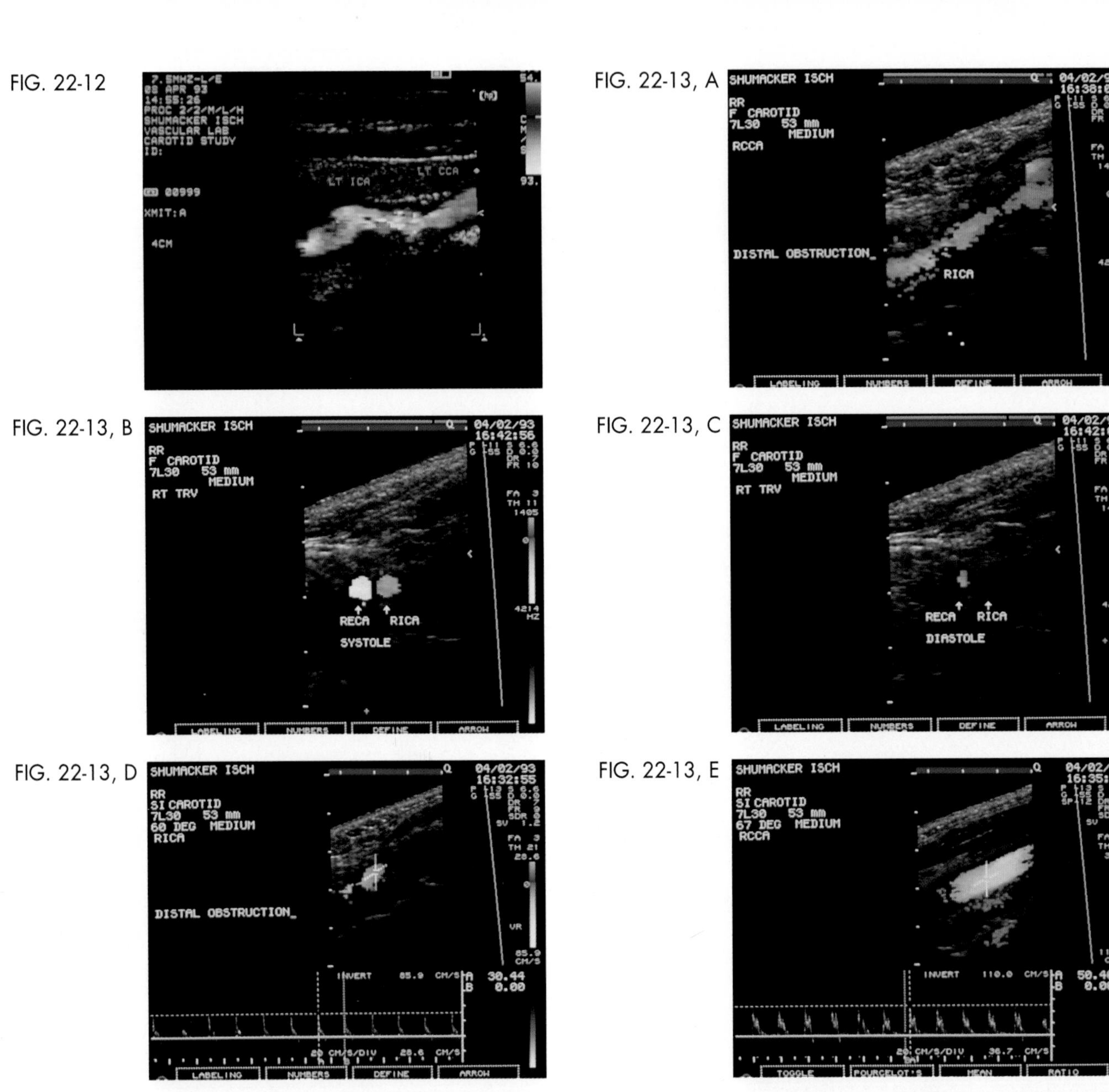

FIG. 22-12 Carotid bifurcation showing blue flow eddies along the surface of an irregular plaque. **FIG. 22-13** High distal ICA obstruction. **A,** Slightly stenosed but patent-appearing internal carotid artery, longitudinal view, with color in systole. **B,** Patent-appearing ICA and ECA in the transverse view, with color in systole. **C,** Same as *B* in diastole. Note absence of color flow in the ICA. **D,** Doppler in the ICA, showing abrupt systolic peak and absence of diastolic flow. **E,** Doppler in the CCA, showing the typical appearance of a preocclusion common carotid waveform with a complete absence of diastolic flow. **FIG. 22-14 B,** Internal carotid artery origin showing axial and tangential flow jets caused by the weblike plaque. **FIG. 22-22** A longitudinal view of the vertebral artery in the central cervical section of the neck, imaged between the transverse processes of the cervical vertebrae (shadow).

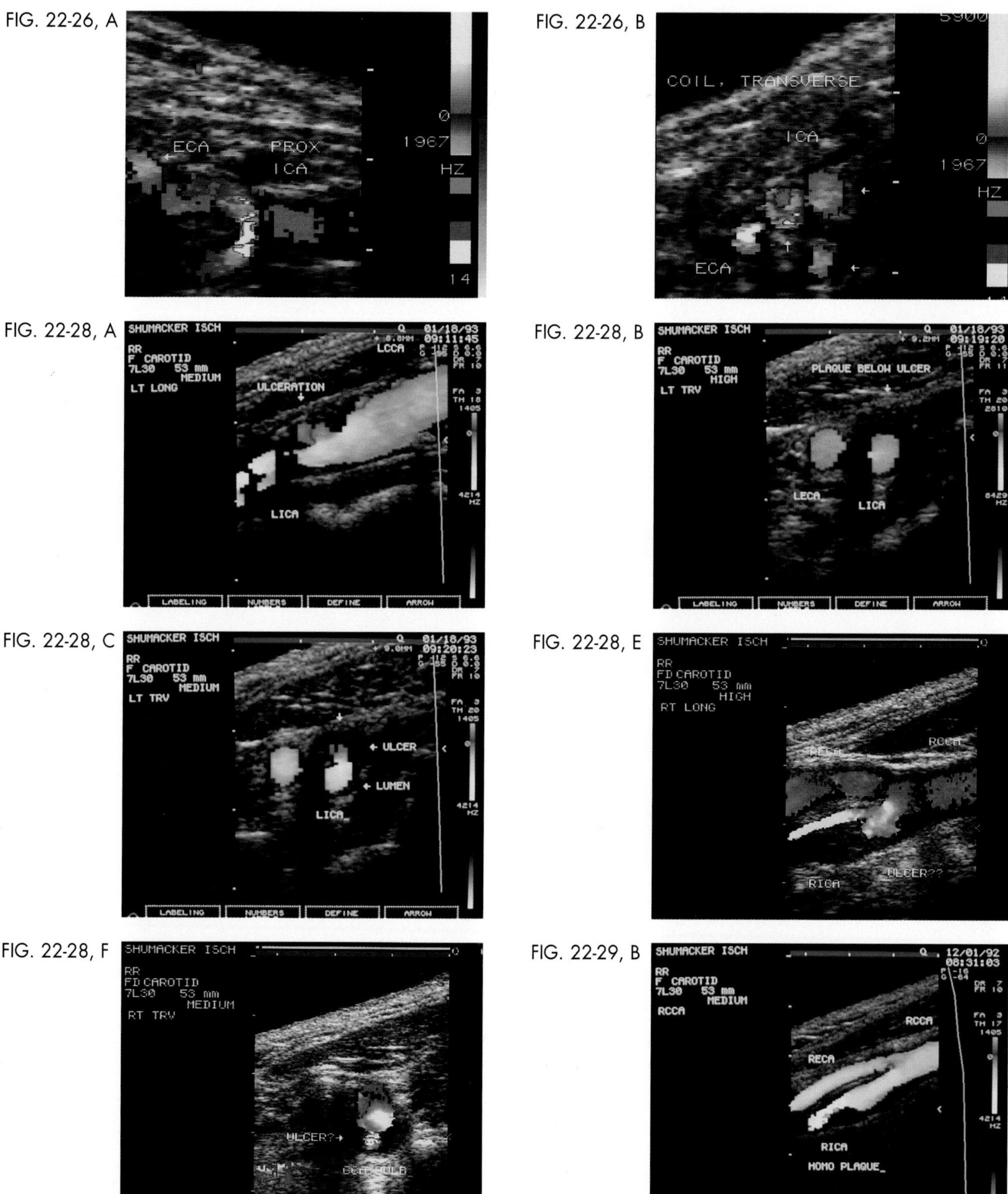

FIG. 22-26 Internal carotid artery coil. **A,** Longitudinal showing loop in ICA. **B,** Transverse. Note the false appearance of three lumens, all part of the same ICA *(arrows);* color helps delineate the flow direction in the visualized segments that make up the coil. **FIG. 22-28** Ulcerated plaque. **A,** Longitudinal image showing a distinct ulceration in a heterogeneous plaque on the superficial wall of the ICA origin. Note the blue color-flow reversal within the ulceration. **B,** Transverse image showing the proximal portion of the plaque below the ulceration. **C,** Transverse image across the ICA and plaque at the level of the ulceration. **E,** Longitudinal image showing the flow patterns into the ulceration and the jet of flow across the smooth distal taper of the plaque. **F,** Transverse image across the ECA and the ICA at the level of the ulceration. **FIG. 22-29 B,** Longitudinal view of a hemodynamically significant fatty (homogeneous) plaque in the distal ICA.

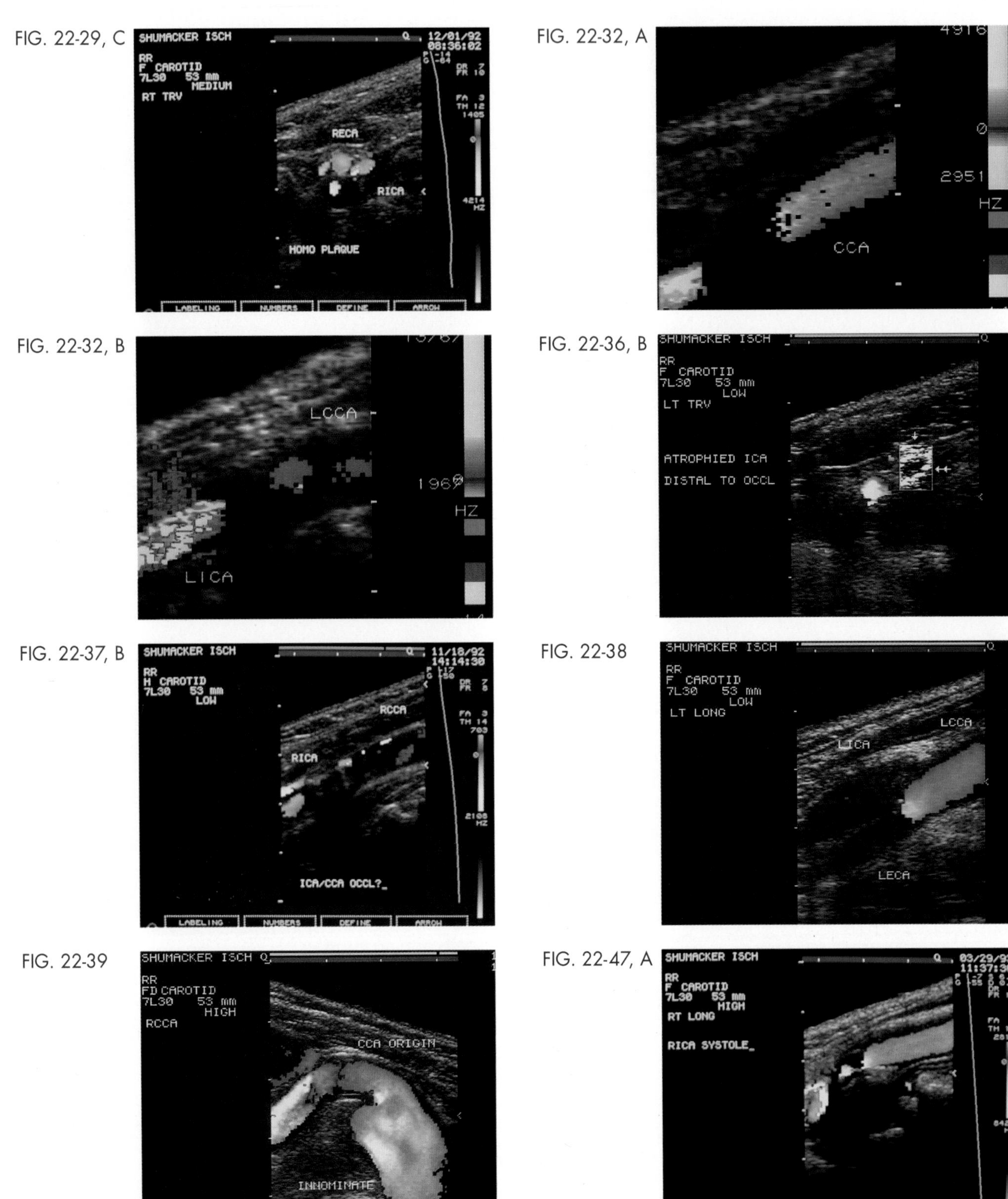

FIG. 22-29 C, Transverse view plaque in the ICA. **FIG. 22-32 A,** The color-flow patterns distal to the calcific shadow are uniform with no turbulence and a normal streamline, implying a hemodynamically insignificant stenosis. **B,** A jet streamline along the superficial wall distal to the calcific shadow with marked flow separation and a visualized bruit. **FIG. 22-36 B,** Transverse view of the atrophied occluded internal carotid artery. **FIG. 22-37** Complete proximal occlusion with reconstituted ICA and ECA. **B,** Longitudinal view. **FIG. 22-38** Longitudinal image showing a completely occluded ICA and ECA with a patent CCA. **FIG. 22-39** Longitudinal image demonstrating a superficial, supraclavicularly positioned, tortuous origin of the CCA. **FIG. 22-47 A,** Longitudinal image showing a severe stenosis with a tight streamline *(left)* distal to the stenosis and an area of flow separation beneath the jet in systole.

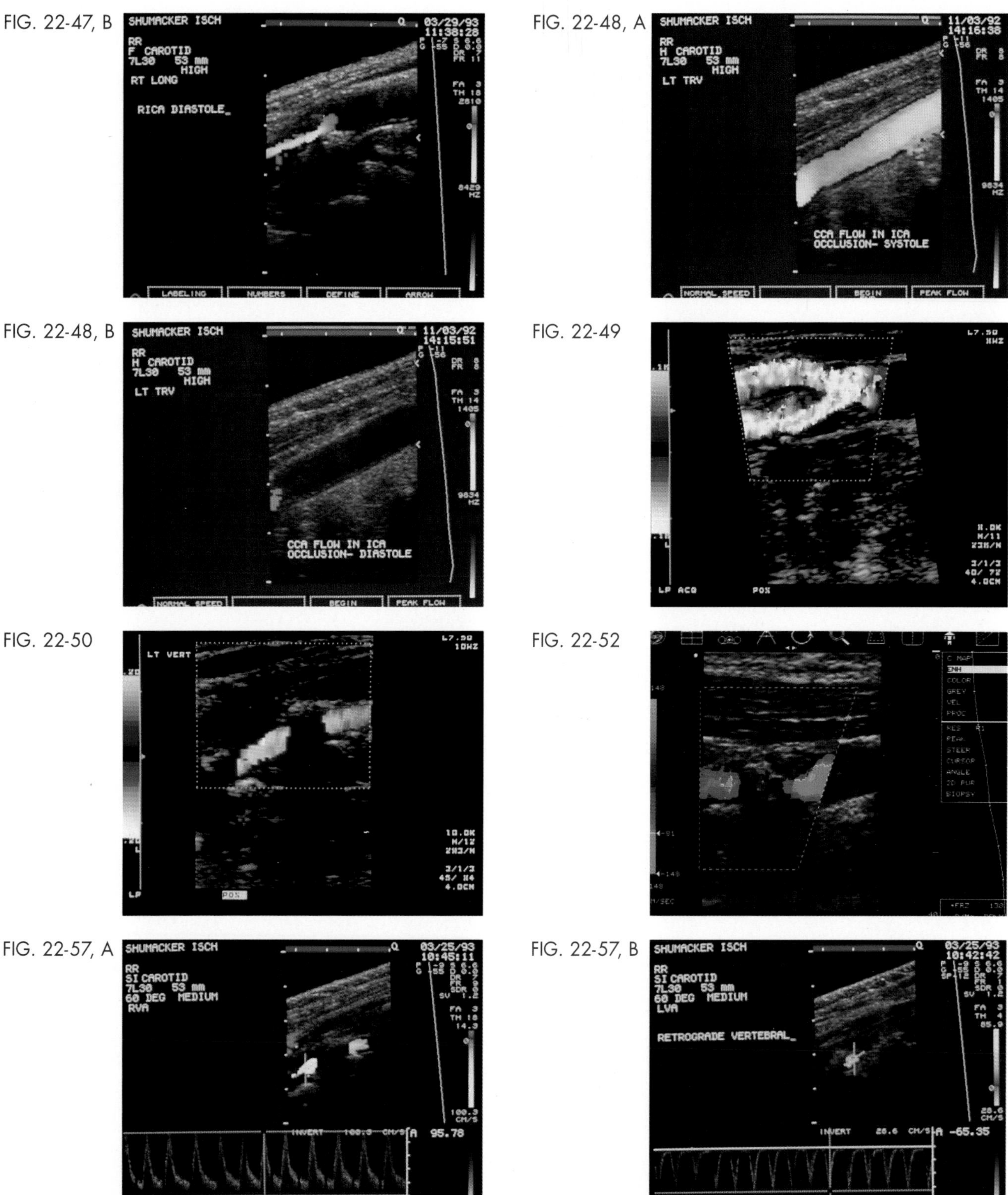

FIG. 22-47 B, The same image as in **A,** taken during the diastolic portion of the cardiac cycle, shows the streamline persisting with continued elevated velocities within it. **FIG. 22-48** Common carotid in complete distal occlusion, demonstrating the on-off pattern. **A,** Common carotid pattern in systole. **B,** Common carotid pattern in diastole. **FIG. 22-49** Color-flow pattern lacks uniformity because of stenosis and luminal irregularity; numerous areas of mixed red and blue are seen from disturbed flow (some aliasing is occurring in the central streamline). **FIG. 22-50** Retrograde (blue) color-flow pattern in a vertebral artery, seen in complete subclavian steal. **FIG. 22-52** Image of an internal carotid stenosis, showing velocity green tagging; velocities greater than 81 cm/sec are colored green. **FIG. 22-57** Vertebral arteries in left subclavian steal. **A,** Antegrade Doppler flow signal in the right vertebral artery. **B,** Fully retrograde Doppler flow signal in the left vertebral artery.

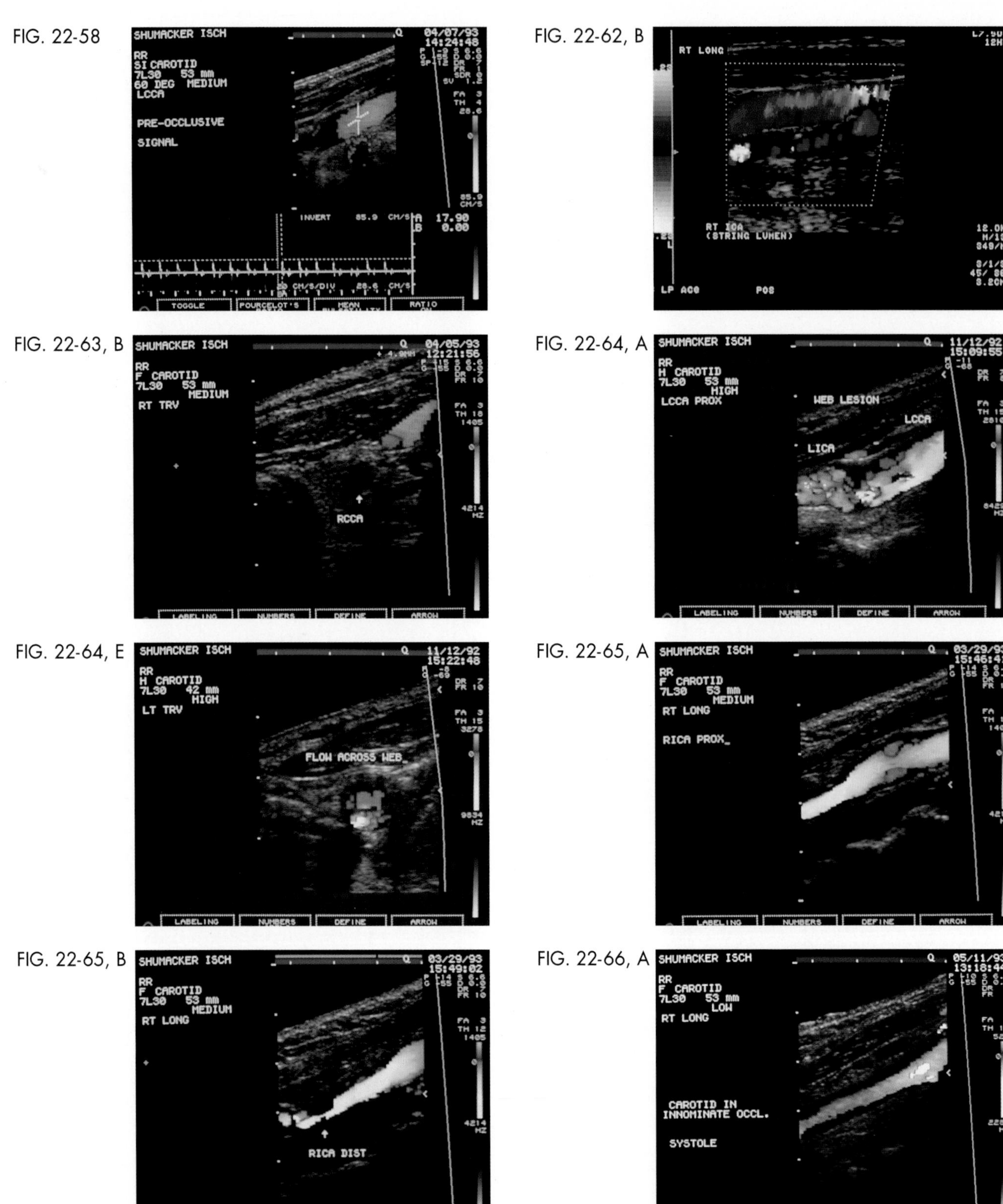

FIG. 22-58 Example of a high-resistance, low-velocity Doppler spectral waveform proximal to a complete ICA occlusion. Note that there is no diastolic flow. **FIG. 22-62 B,** A greater than 95% ICA stenosis, showing a narrow patent lumen. **FIG. 22-63** Total occlusion of the CCA, ICA, and ECA. **B,** Transverse image of the occluded CCA, showing a patent internal jugular vein for comparison. **FIG. 22-64** Weblike lesion, left CCA. **A,** Distal CCA and proximal ICA, longitudinal plane. **E,** Mid-CCA across septate lesion, transverse plane. **FIG. 22-65** Distal ICA stenosis. **A,** Proximal ICA and bifurcation, longitudinal plane. **B,** Distal ICA, longitudinal plane. **FIG. 22-66** ECA dominant early carotid steal. **A,** Right CCA, systole.

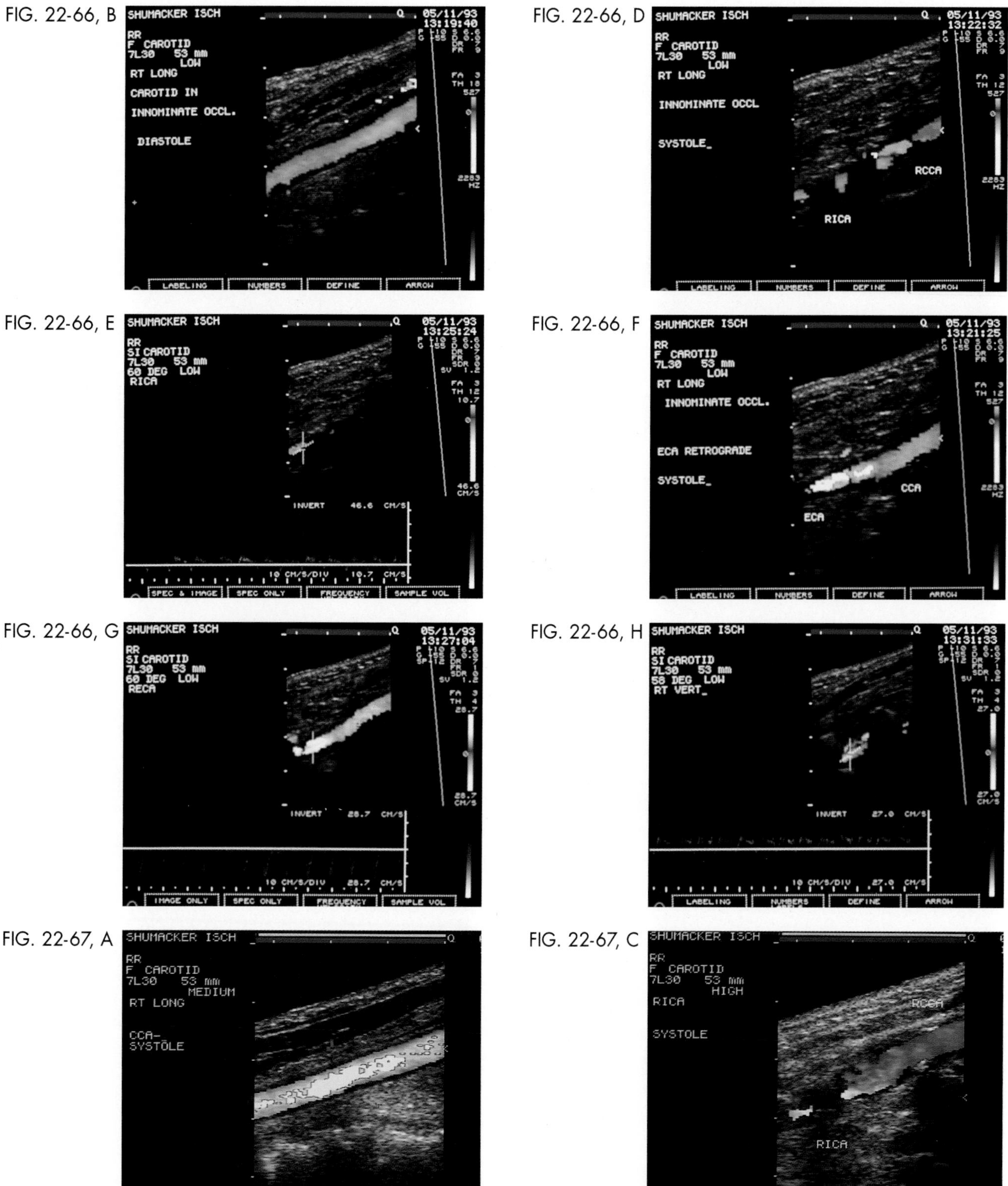

FIG. 22-66 ECA dominant early carotid steal. **B,** Right CCA, diastole. **D,** Right ICA and CCA at bifurcation with transient ICA flow in systole. **E,** Low-velocity transient flow, right ICA. **F,** Right ECA and CCA at bifurcation with retrograde ECA flow in systole. **G,** Retrograde flow in right ECA. **H,** Right vertebral artery, showing antegrade but early transitional systolic retrograde flow. **FIG. 22-67** ICA and vertebral dominant early carotid steal. **A,** Right CCA, systole. **C,** Right ICA and CCA at bifurcation in systole.

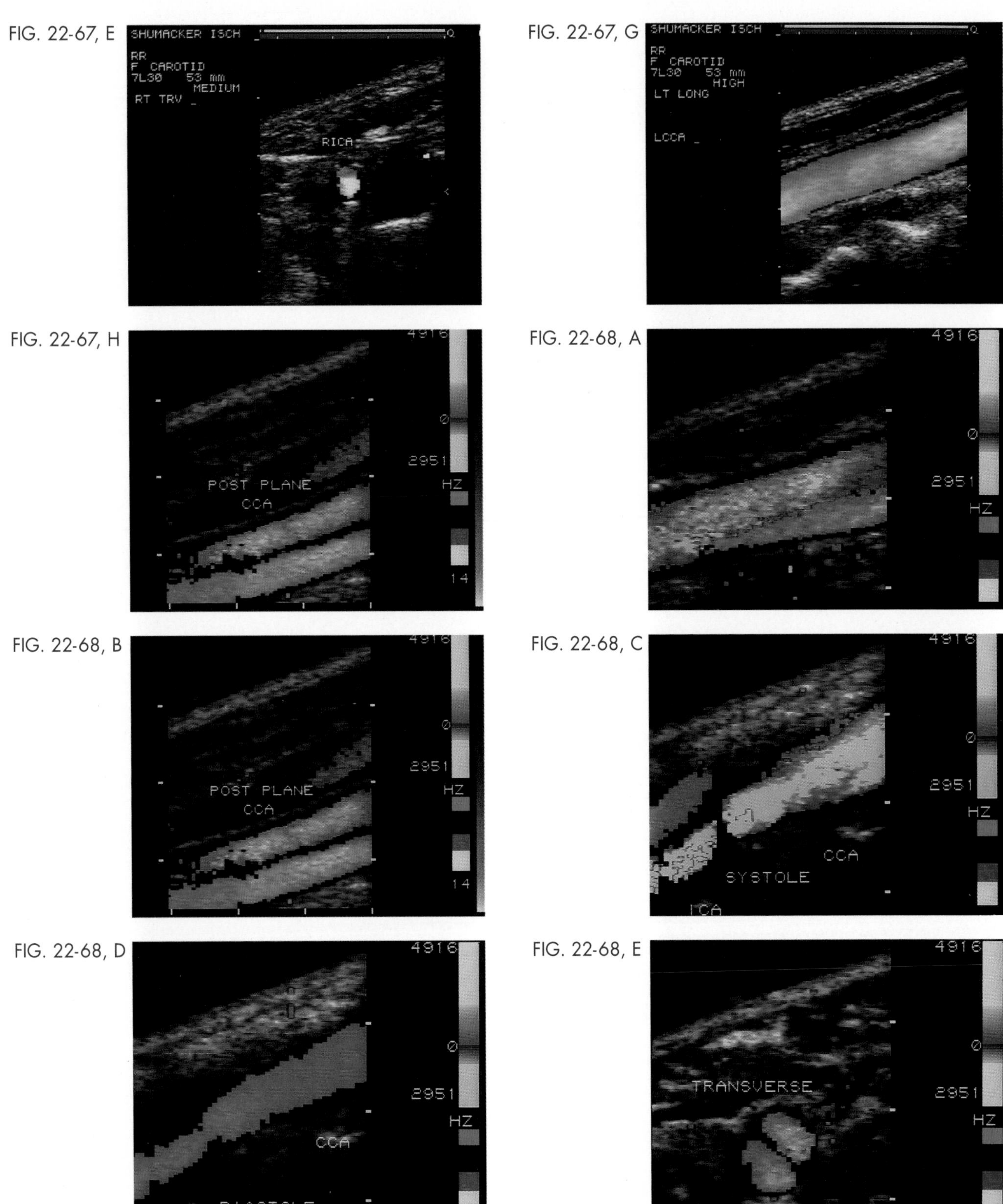

FIG. 22-67 ICA and vertebral dominant early carotid steal. **E,** Right ICA, transverse plane, in systole. **G,** Left CCA, systole. **H,** Left ICA, ECA, and CCA at bifurcation in systole. **FIG. 22-68** Carotid dissection. **A,** CCA, longitudinal. **B,** CCA, longitudinal from posterior scanning plane, showing double lumen. **C,** ICA and CCA at bifurcation in systole. **D,** ICA and CCA at bifurcation in diastole. **E,** CCA, transverse plane.

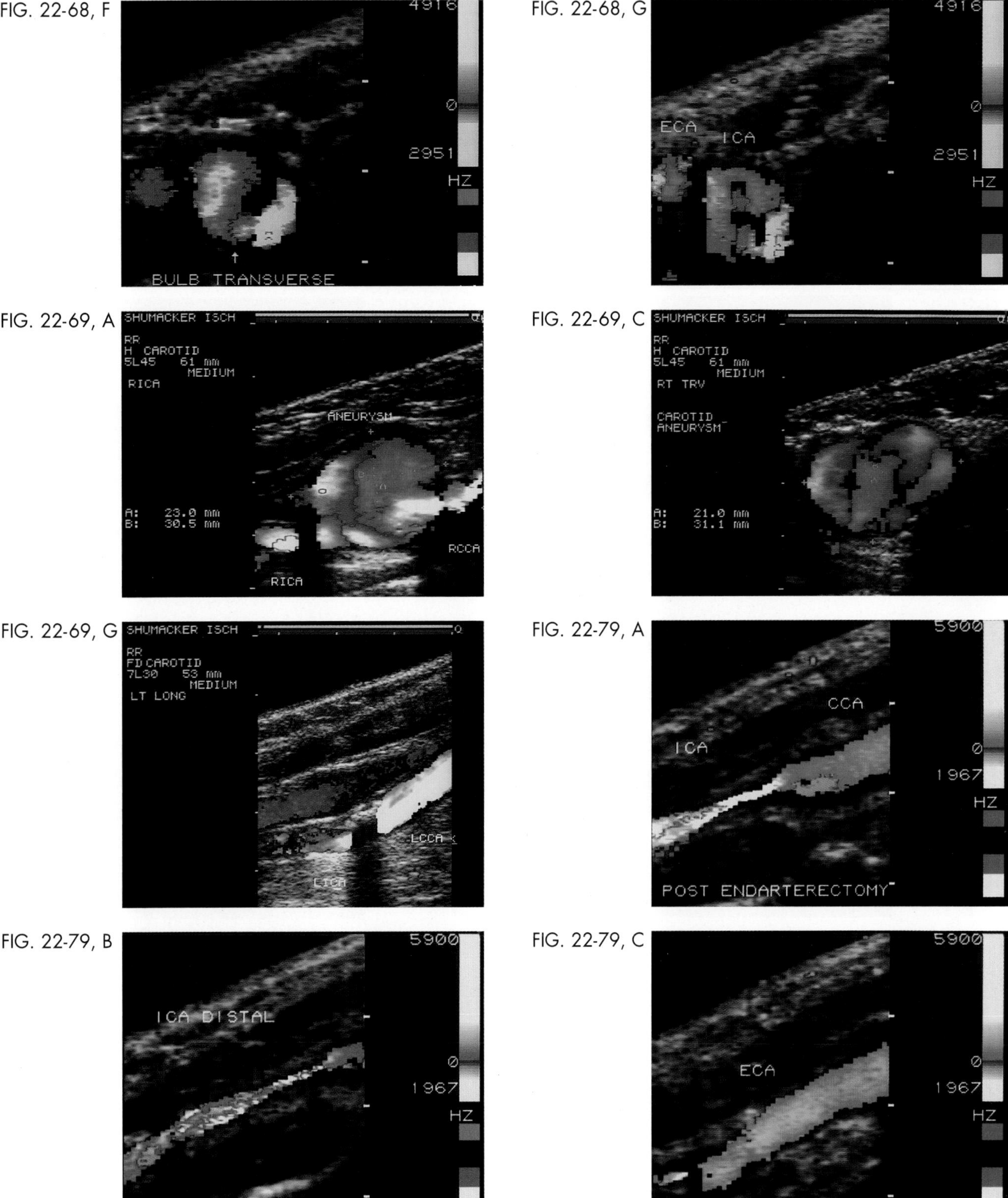

FIG. 22-68 Carotid dissection. **F,** Bulb area, transverse plane. **G,** ECA and ICA, transverse plane. **FIG. 22-69** Right carotid aneurysm and 20% to 59% left ICA stenosis. **A,** Right bifurcation in the longitudinal plane, showing the aneurysm and its relationship to the ICA and CCA. **C,** Transverse color-flow image of the aneurysm. **G,** Left ICA and CCA at bifurcation, longitudinal plane. **FIG. 22-79** Fibrointimal hyperplasia, after endarterectomy. **A,** Longitudinal image of the bifurcation, showing a physically narrowed proximal ICA with a high-velocity flow jet. **B,** Longitudinal image of the distal ICA, showing flow disturbance distal to the jet. **C,** Longitudinal normal image of the ECA. Compare its size with that of the hyperplastic ICA.

FIG. 22-79, D

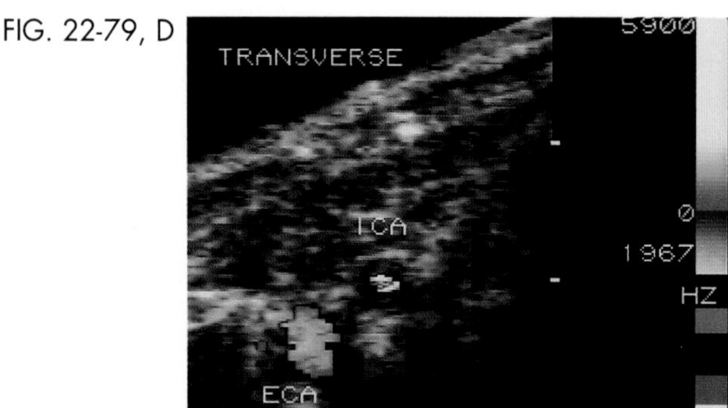

FIG. 22-79, E

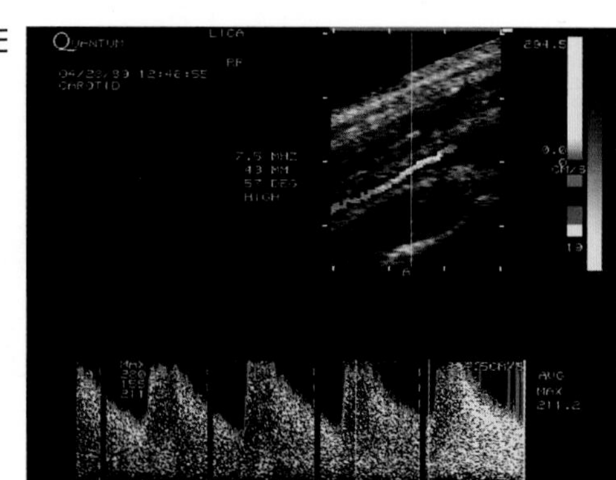

FIG. 22-79, F

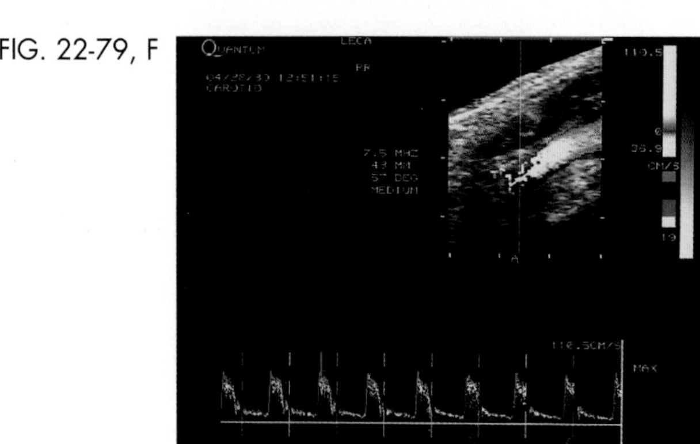

FIG. 22-80, A

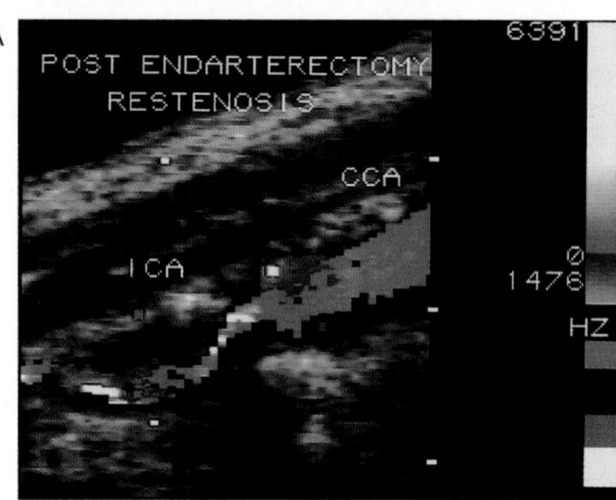

FIG. 22-79 Fibrointimal hyperplasia, after endarterectomy. **D,** Transverse view of the ICA and ECA. Note the small ICA lumen. **E,** High-velocity abnormal Doppler spectral waveform from the hyperplastic ICA. **F,** Normal Doppler spectral waveform from the ECA. **FIG. 22-80** Recurrent stenosis, after endarterectomy. **A,** Longitudinal view of an ICA after endarterectomy, showing the presence of a severe stenosis from recurrent atheroma.

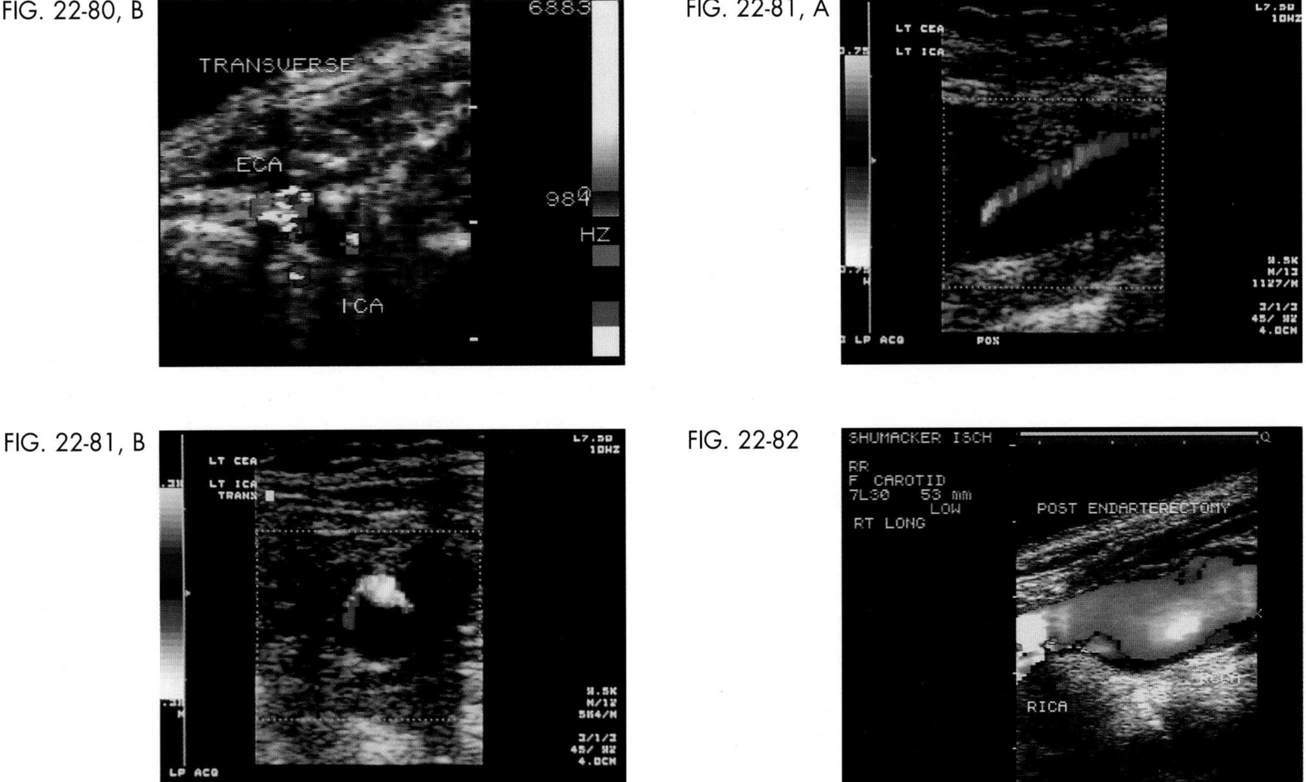

FIG. 22-80 Recurrent stenosis, after endarterectomy. **B,** Transverse view of the stenosed ICA and ECA, showing the residual lumen. **FIG. 22-81** Thrombus formation, after endarterectomy. **A,** Longitudinal view of an ICA after endarterectomy, showing the presence of homogeneous thrombus along the deep wall. **B,** Transverse view of the same ICA, showing that the thrombus is hemodynamically nonobstructive. **FIG. 22-82** Normal appearance in a patched carotid artery after endarterectomy.

FIG. 22-83

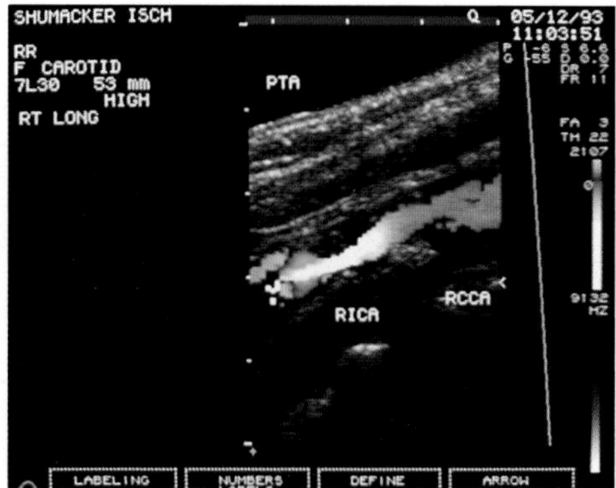

FIG. 22-86, A

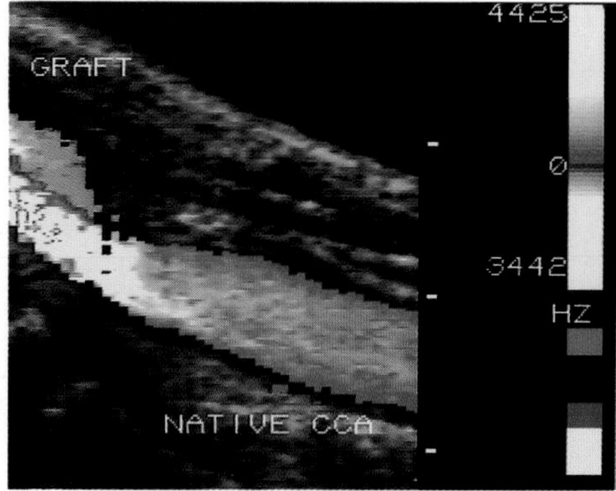

FIG. 22-86, B

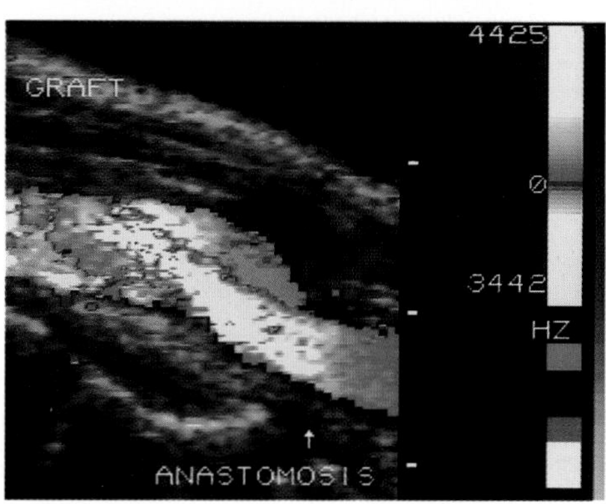

FIG. 22-86, C

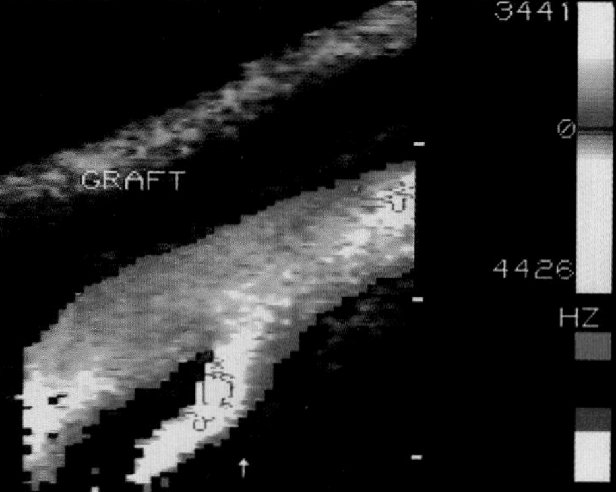

FIG. 22-83 Image of an internal carotid artery stenosis after percutaneous transluminal angioplasty. Residual stenotic material remains along the superficial wall. **FIG. 22-86** CCA to ICA saphenous vein interposition graft. **A,** Longitudinal image of the proximal native CCA. The proximal anastomosis with the graft is to the left. **B,** Longitudinal image of the proximal graft, showing normal flow separation from diameter change. **C,** Image of the new "bifurcation" with the ECA implanted into the graft.

FIG. 22-86, D

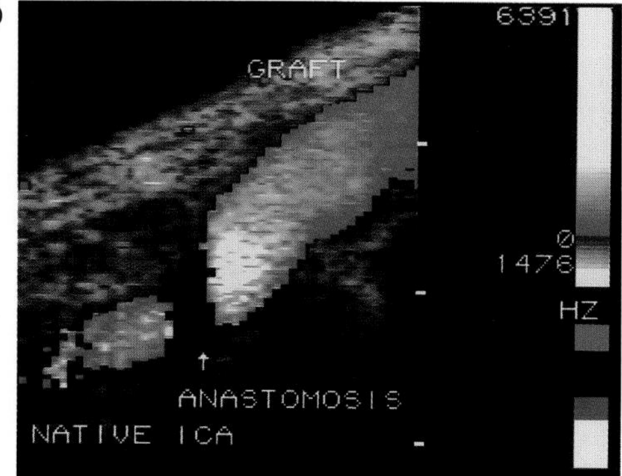

FIG. 22-86, E

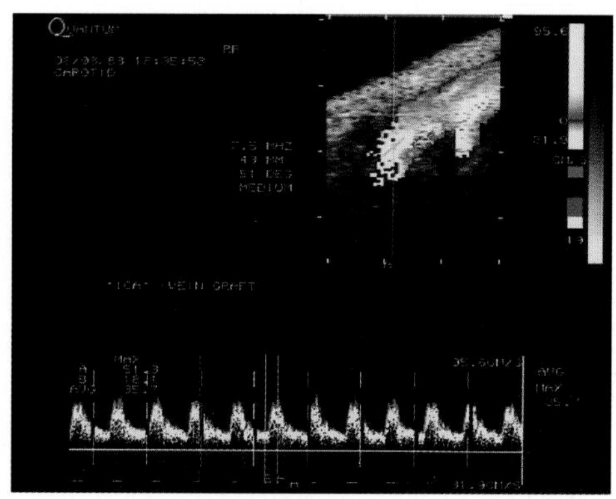

FIG. 22-86, F

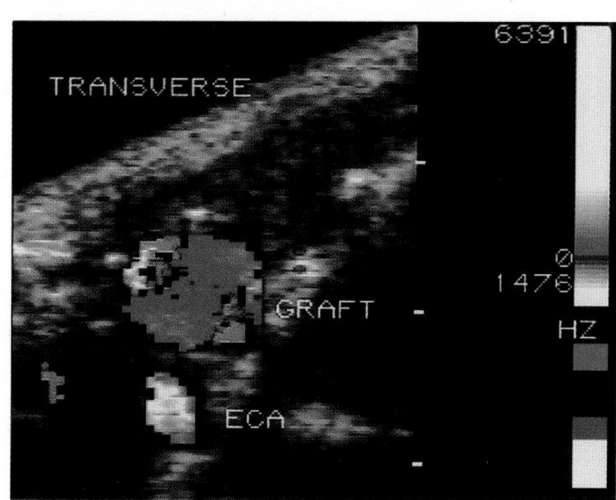

FIG. 22-87, A

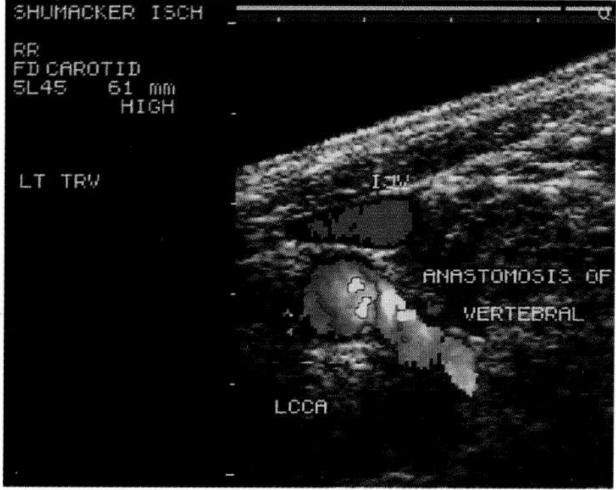

FIG. 22-86 CCA to ICA saphenous vein interposition graft. **D,** Longitudinal image of the distal graft anastomosis with the native ICA. **E,** Normal Doppler spectral waveform in the "ICA" portion of the distal graft. **F,** Transverse view above the "bifurcation," showing the graft (which resembles an endarterectomized ICA) and the ECA. **FIG. 22-87** Reimplantation, vertebral to CCA. **A,** Transverse view of a CCA with a reimplanted vertebral artery.

FIG. 22-88

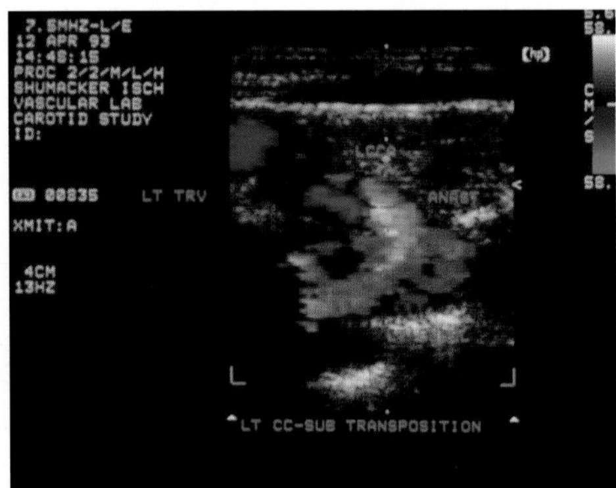

FIG. 22-89

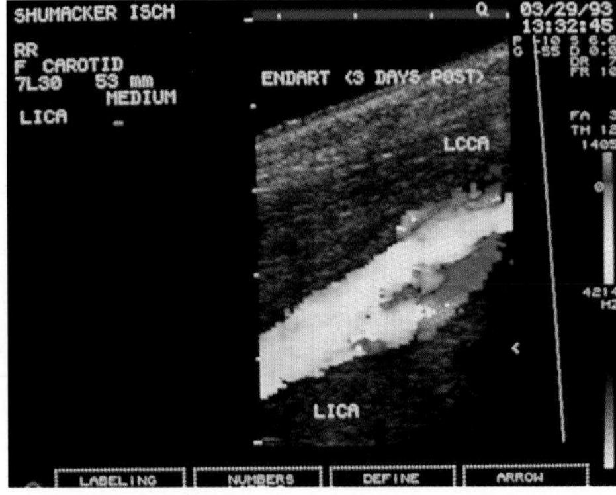

FIG. 22-104

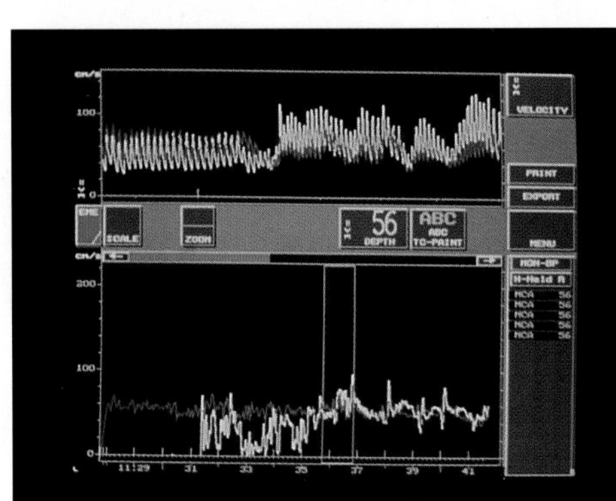

FIG. 22-108, A

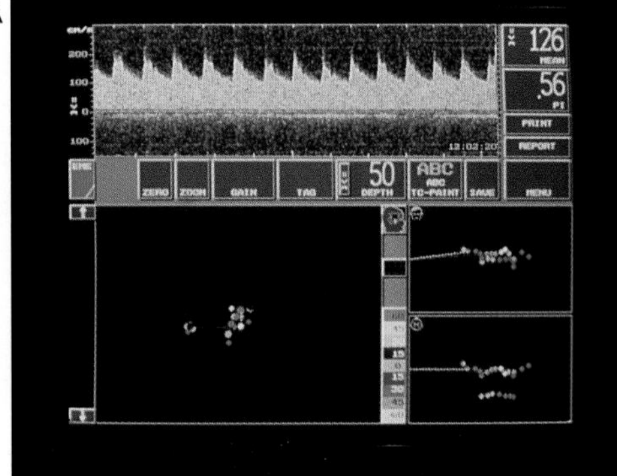

FIG. 22-88 Image of a CCA-to-subclavian-artery transposition. **FIG. 22-89** Image of an ICA, 3 days after endarterectomy and patch angioplasty. **FIG. 22-104** Long-term monitoring TCD tracing during carotid surgery; the spectral envelope *(white line)* is monitored together with the blood pressure *(red line)*. The upper waveform display is an enlarged section from the lower compressed long-term display. **FIG. 22-108** The upper third of the display shows the spectral waveform at the current sample site. The spatial maps *(bottom images)* are arranged to show a side view (lateral—*bottom left*), AP frontal view (coronal—*upper right*), and top-down view (horizontal—*lower right*) of the vessels in **A.** Flow direction toward (red hues) or away from (blue hues) the transducer in the vessels is shown by the plotted sample points. **A,** Abnormal, elevated middle cerebral artery Doppler waveform with a mean velocity of 126 cm/sec *(top),* taken from the left MCA.

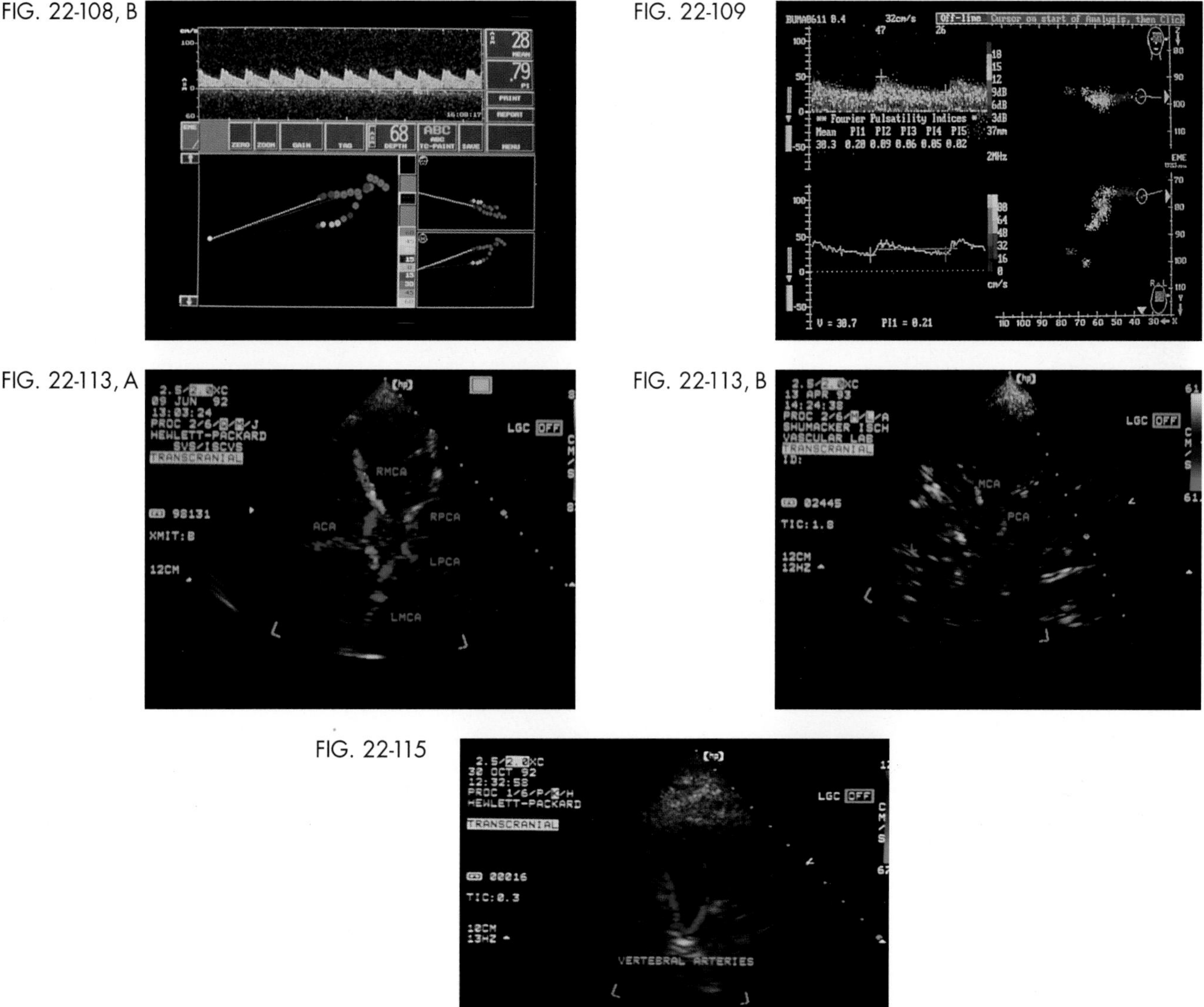

FIG. 22-108 B, This image shows a normal vertebral signal *(top),* and the vertebral and basilar arteries in a top-down view (bottom—*left and lower right*) and AP frontal view (bottom—*upper right*). (Courtesy EME/Nicolet.) **FIG. 22-109** Three-dimensional image from a patient with a traumatic ICA dissection; the left MCA has reduced pulsatility *(top left),* the left carotid siphon and ACA are not detected, and velocities and dot brightness are increased in the collateralizing left PCoA. (From Ries F, Bernstein EF: Vascular Diagnosis, ed 4, St. Louis: Mosby, 1993.) **FIG. 22-113 A,** Transtemporal axial scan showing an exceptional complete view of the circle of Willis. **B,** A more typical view of the right MCA and PCA and left ACA, seen in a 64-year-old man. **FIG. 22-115** Transoccipital color-flow scan showing both distal vertebral arteries.

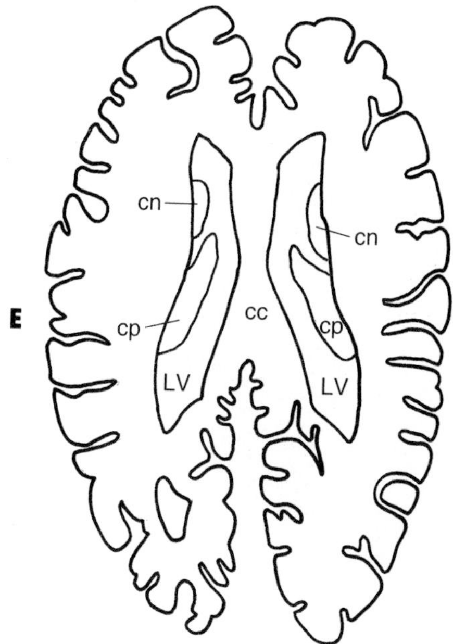

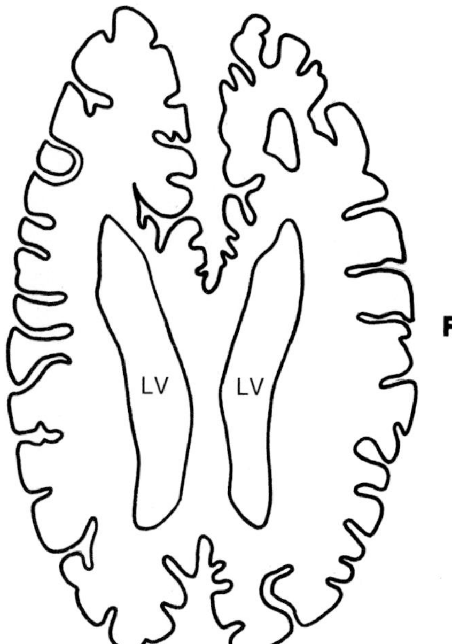

Fig. 16-21, cont'd. For legend see opposite page.

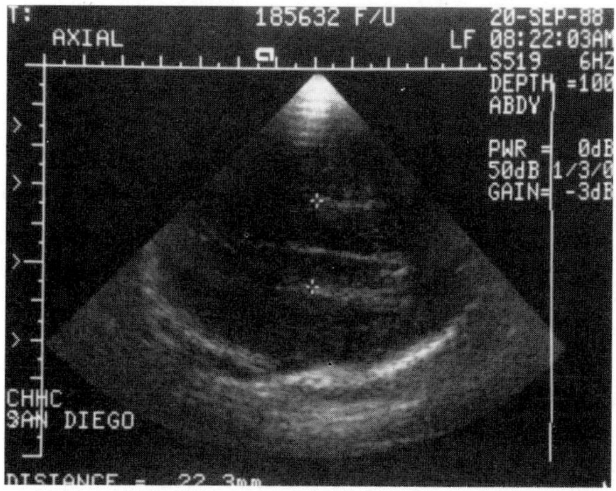

FIG. 16-22 Axial section through the lateral ventricles show the ventricular measurement made at the widest point. Normal ventricular measurement is 10 mm (or 20 mm for both ventricles.)

next higher level, only the lateral ventricles can be seen. This level, where there is no choroid plexus showing, is the correct level for measuring ventricular size.

Through the posterior fontanelle, the occipital horns appear as small, triangular cystic structures with the vertex oriented posteriorly. At the base of the triangle appears the highly echogenic glomus of the choroid plexus. To obtain symmetric images, the frontal bones must be used as a reference.

In the axial plane the posterior horns are closer to the transducer than in studies from the anterior fontanelle; thus the occipital horns and the occipital and temporal lobes are within the focal zone of the transducer. Consequently, axial studies increase the sensitivity and precision of the technique for studying the structures located far from the anterior fontanelle. This is important for detecting small amounts of blood in the occipital horns as well as small ischemic lesions in the white matter of the occipital and temporal lobes.

Studies from the Cervical Spinal Column. Pathology in the posterior fossa and in the spinal cord can be studied through the neck using a high-definition, short-focused transducer. The transducer is placed at the posterior part of the neck just below the occipital bone, with the scanning plane in the same direction as the spinal cord (sagittal plane) (Fig. 16-23, *A*). Then the transducer is rotated up to visualize the medulla and the cervical spinal cord surrounded by the anechoic subarachnoid space. At the top of this view the cisterna magna and the inferior part of the vermis can easily be identified (Fig. 16-23, *B*). Since the structures of the posterior fossa are distant from the transducer when they are scanned from the anterior fontanelle, studying the posterior fossa in the coronal plane from the mastoid fonticullus and in the sagittal plane through the neck enables more precise identification of subarachnoid and intracerebellar hemorrhages.

DEVELOPMENTAL PROBLEMS OF THE BRAIN

Chromosome Abnormalities. Two thirds of children and fetuses with chromosomal anomalies showed no pathologic changes in the brain. The overall appearance of the brain was small in size with a variety of minor morphologic abnormalities.

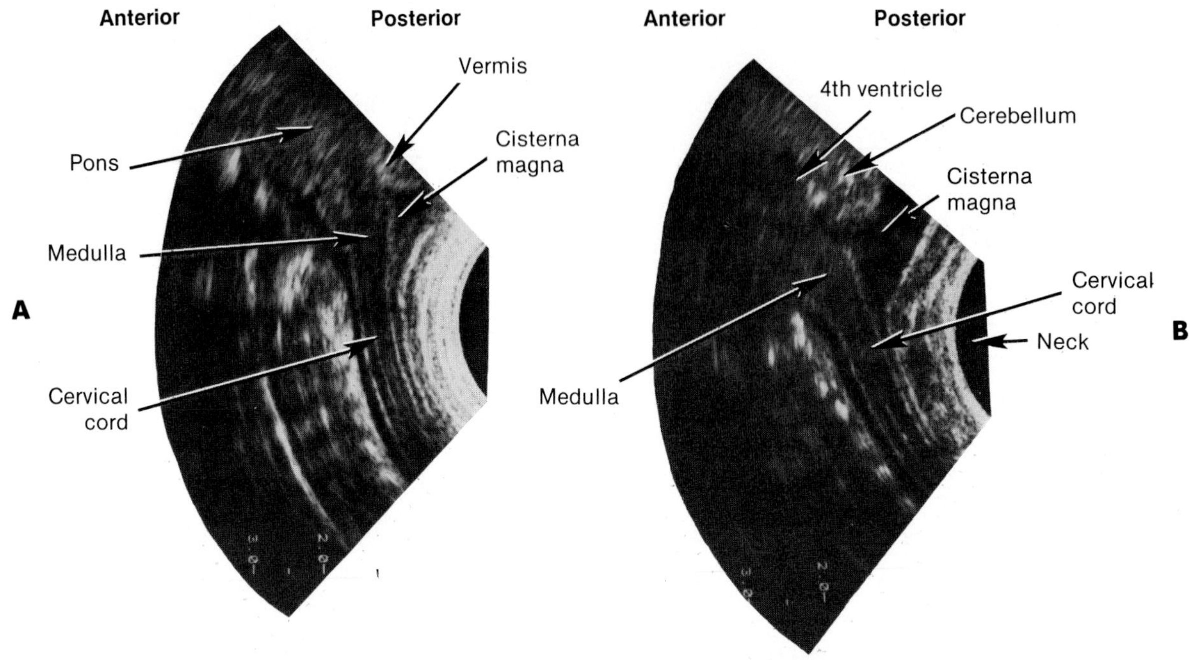

FIG. 16-23 Sagittal visualization of the posterior fossa from the cervical column (nuchal view). To obtain a view similar to **A,** the transducer should be applied to the middle of the cervical column with the scanning plane oriented in the sagittal plane. The cervical cord, the brain stem, the cisterna magna, and the inferior part of the cerebellum may be seen. After obtaining view **A,** the transducer should be oriented upward to visualize the cisterna magna, the cerebellum, and the brain stem in more detail, **B.** Note the normal echogenicity of the spinal cord compared with the subarachnoid space and the vermis of the cerebellum.

Patients with trisomy 21 have a small brain with a small frontal lobe and reduced distance in the A-P diameter. Trisomy 13 shows an abnormality of the forebrain. The overall appearance of the brain is small but normal. One third of the patients show holoprosencephaly with or without cyclopia, various degrees of semilobar and lobar holoprosencephaly, or isolated absence of olfactory bulbs and tracts. Cerebellar heterotopias are present; they may be large.

Patients with trisomy 18 have gyral abnormalities and dysplasia of the hippocampus and inferior olive. Cerebellar heterotopias are found, and the corpus callosum is absent. Various neural tube defects are associated with this chromosome anomaly, including holoprosencephaly.

Teratogens. Patients with maternal diabetes may deliver a neonate with holoprosencephaly and caudal regression syndrome. Fetal alcohol syndrome may cause microencephaly, hydrocephaly, cerebral and cerebellar dysrhaphia, agenesis of the corpus callosum, and other anomalies.

NEURAL TUBE DEFECTS

A number of different anomalies may occur in fetal brain development. These anomalies, such as anencephaly, meningomyelocele, meningocele, and encephalocele, are discussed in more detail in Chapter 29, in the ultrasound and high-risk pregnancy chapter. The following list briefly describes the anomaly and the affected area of the brain:

- ARNOLD-CHIARI MALFORMATION. An Arnold-Chiari malformation is a congenital anomaly associated with spina bifida in which the cerebellum and brain stem are pulled toward the spinal cord and secondary hydrocephalus develops.
- HOLOPROSENCEPHALY. Holoprosencephaly is characterized by a grossly abnormal brain in which there is a common large central ventricle.
- DANDY-WALKER SYNDROME. Dandy-Walker syndrome is a congenital anomaly in which a huge fourth ventricle cyst occupies the area where the cerebellum usually lies, with secondary dilation of the third and lateral ventricles. The Dandy-Walker malformation of the cerebellum is the result of a disturbance of the growth of the roof of the fourth ventricle. The vermis is absent in 25% of the population. The fourth ventricle is enlarged. The posterior fossa is enlarged with the sinuses displaced upward. It may be associated with the following malformations: hydrocephalus, agenesis of the corpus callosum, infundibular hamartomas, or brain-stem lipomas.
- AGENESIS OF THE CORPUS CALLOSUM. Agenesis of the corpus callosum is a condition in which the fibers of the corpus callosum cross from side to side on a glial sling; agenesis may occur as an isolated anomaly without any clinical effect. The corpus callosum is absent in severe holoprosencephaly. Agenesis of the corpus callosum may be associated with Arnold-Chiari malformation

and hydrocephalus. In neonates with this anomaly the cerebral hemispheres have ventricles with pointed upper corners (bat-wing appearance).

- ARTERIO-MALFORMATION OF THE VEIN OF GALEN. Arterio-malformation of the vein of Galen is an anomaly that presents with cardiac failure as the shunt of blood travels through the venous malformation. The underlying cerebral parenchyma may be infarcted secondary to the shunt.
- CHOROID PLEXUS CYSTS. The appearance of these small cysts within the choroid plexus has no clinical significance without other cerebral or visceral anomalies.
- HYDROCEPHALUS. Hydrocephalus is caused by the obstruction of cerebral spinal fluid. The earlier it occurs, the greater the enlargement of the head. This dilation results in widely separated sutures and huge, bulging fontanelles. The sonographer should look for the blunting of the lateral angles of the lateral ventricles.

Arnold-Chiari Malformation

Arnold-Chiari malformation is characterized by the following:

- Displacement of the fourth ventricle and upper medulla into the cervical canal
- Displacement of the inferior part of the cerebellum through the foramen magnum
- Defects in the calvarium and spinal column

Arnold-Chiari malformation is frequently associated with myelomeningocele, hydrocephalus, dilation of the third ventricle, and absence of the septum pellucidum. About 80% to 90% of infants with myelomeningocele have Arnold-Chiari malformations. Hydrocephalus is usually caused by obstruction of the CSF pathway at the fourth ventricle or in the posterior fossa, or secondary to aqueductal stenosis, which is present in 40% to 75% of infants with Arnold-Chiari malformations.[8,23,44,45]

Arnold-Chiari malformation can be correctly diagnosed with ECHO. Sagittal studies from the anterior fontanelle show a small cerebellum, absence of the cisterna magna, low position of the fourth ventricle, and displacement of the cerebellum through the foramen magnum associated with hydrocephalus, absence of the septum pellucidum, and widening of the third ventricle (Fig. 16-24).

Holoprosencephaly

Holoprosencephaly is caused by disturbances in the process of ventral induction very early in life. The neuropathologic features include a single cerebrum with single ventricular cavity, absence of the corpus callosum and frontal horns, and a thin membrane arising from the roof of the third ventricle, which may extend posteriorly forming a supratentorial cyst[6,23,44,45] (Fig. 16-25).

After the ventral induction has occurred, ischemic lesions in the midline may induce malformations of the telencephalon similar to holoprosencephaly. As in holoprosencephaly, there is a single ventricular cavity and absence of the corpus callosum. However, the presence of two frontal horns helps differentiate these malformations caused by ischemic lesions from true holoprosencephaly. When holoprosencephaly is suspected, it is important to obtain modified coronal studies of the whole frontal lobes to determine whether two frontal horns are present.

Dandy-Walker Malformation

The typical Dandy-Walker malformation is characterized by absence of the cerebellar vermis, cystic changes in the fourth ventricle with the development of a large cyst in the posterior fossa (Dandy-Walker cyst), and hydrocephalus (Fig. 16-26). The hydrocephalus is caused by the atresia of the foramina of Luschka and Magendie (congenital obstructive hydrocephalus). When the vermis is absent, the fourth ventricle communicates directly with the cyst.[24,35,37] A Dandy-Walker variant is present when there is an enlarged cisterna magna communicating with the fourth ventricle in the presence of a normal or hypoplastic cerebellar vermis (Fig. 16-27).

Agenesis of the Corpus Callosum

The corpus callosum is the great commissure connecting the brain hemispheres. Hypoplasia or agenesis of the corpus callosum may occur during the processes of ventral induction or cellular migration. Agenesis of the corpus callosum is often combined with migrational disorders such as heterotopias and polymicrogyria.[24,44,45] Absence of the corpus callosum may also be induced by ischemic lesions in the midline or by intrauterine encephalomalacia (Fig. 16-27). Other defects associated with this defect are porencephaly, hydrocephalus, microgyria, and fusion of the hemispheres.

Complete absence of the corpus callosum is distinguished by narrow frontal horns, as well as marked separation of the anterior horns and bodies of the lateral ventricles associated with widening of the occipital horns and the third ventricle. The ventricular cavities acquire the distinctive appearance of "vampire wings." These characteristics are easily identified by ECHO (Fig. 16-28).

Congenital Hydrocephalus

Hydrocephalus refers to any condition in which enlargement of the ventricular system is caused by an imbalance between production and reabsorption of cerebrospinal fluid (CSF). When this instability ensues in the fetus, the widening of the ventricular system is present at birth. Infants born with ventricular enlargement are considered to have congenital hydrocephalus. Hydrocephalus is infrequently caused by over production of fluid. Excessive fluid production may occur in infants with papilloma of the choroid plexus, a tumor that actively secretes CSF.[31,44]

Two anatomic types of hydrocephalus are distinguished.

Obstructive Hydrocephalus. Obstructive hydrocephalus is characterized by interference in the circulation of CSF within the ventricular system itself, causing subsequent en-

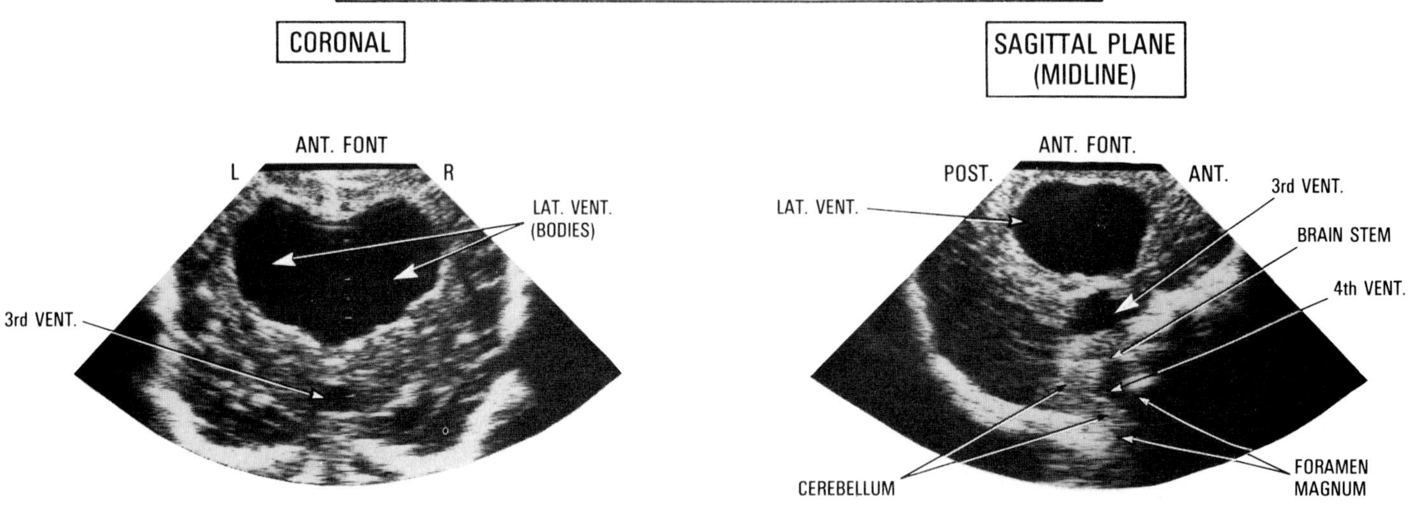

FIG 16-24 Arnold-Chiari malformation. Note the low position of the fourth ventricle, the absence of the cisterna magna, and the extension of the inferior part of the cerebellum into the foramen magnum.

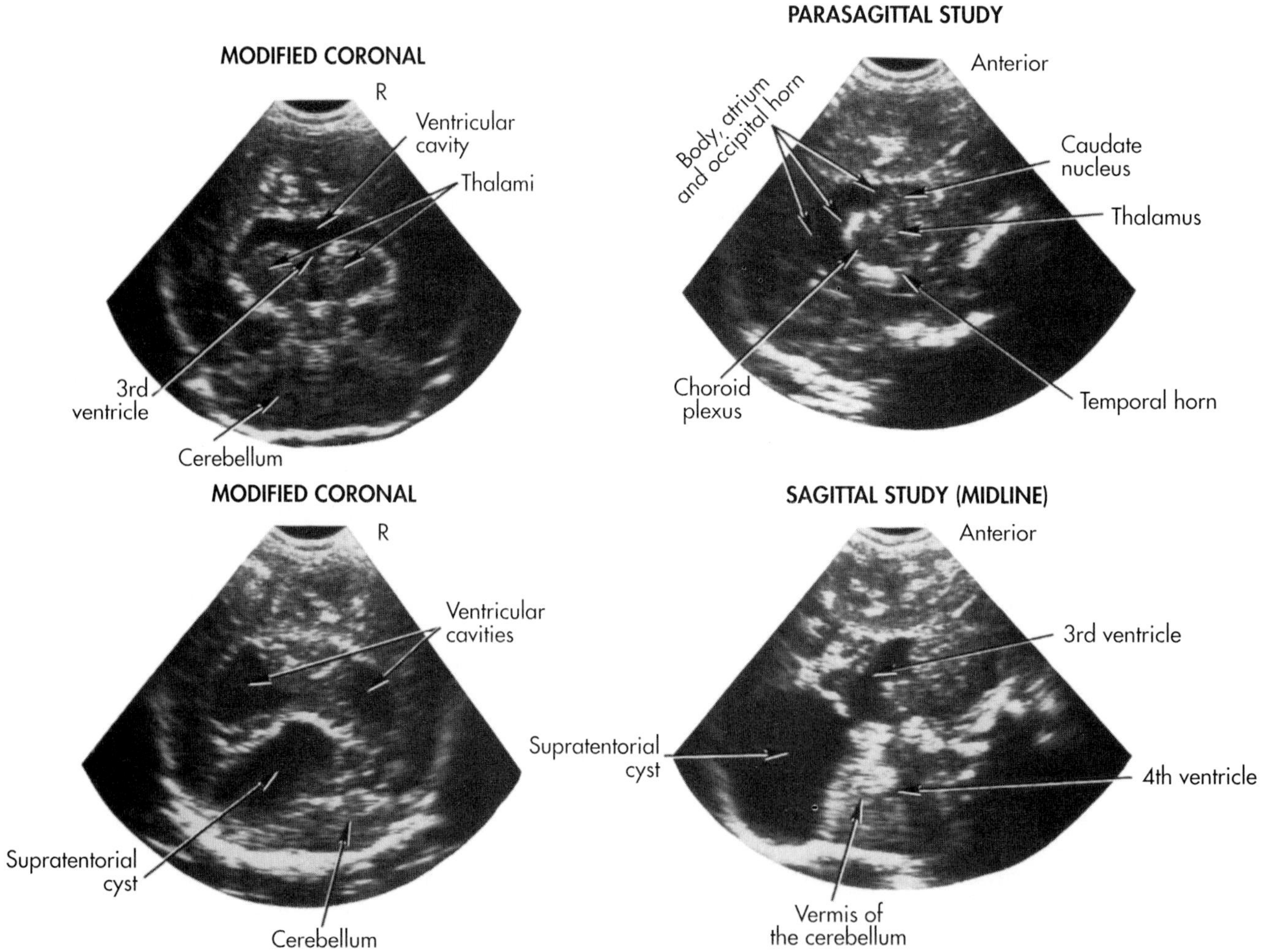

MODIFIED CORONAL

R

Ventricular cavity

Thalami

3rd ventricle

Cerebellum

PARASAGITTAL STUDY

Anterior

Body, atrium and occipital horn

Caudate nucleus

Thalamus

Choroid plexus

Temporal horn

MODIFIED CORONAL

R

Ventricular cavities

Supratentorial cyst

Cerebellum

SAGITTAL STUDY (MIDLINE)

Anterior

3rd ventricle

Supratentorial cyst

4th ventricle

Vermis of the cerebellum

FIG. 16-25 Holoprosencephaly. Note the crescent shape of the central cavity extending into the third ventricle, the absence of corpus callosum, septum pellucidum, and frontal horns (parasagittal studies), and the large supratentorial cyst protruding from the third ventricle.

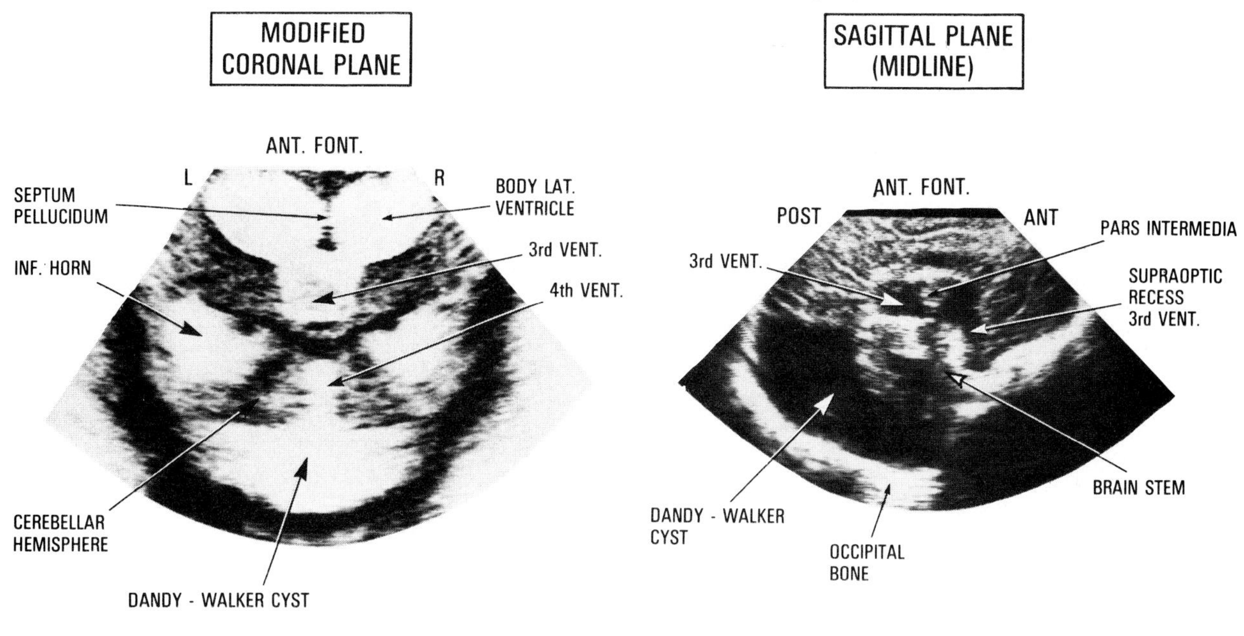

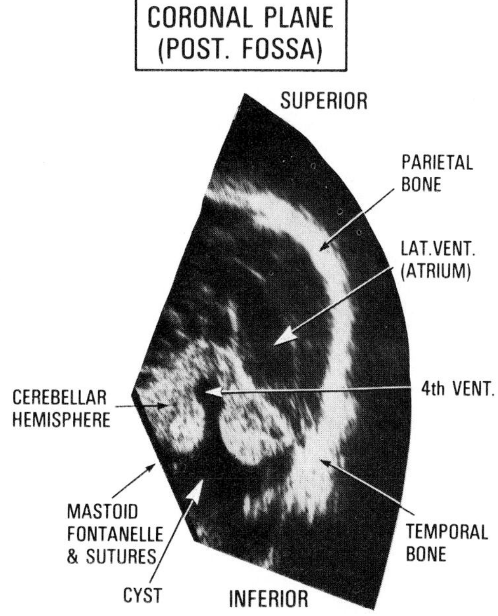

FIG. 16-26 Echoencephalograms in Dandy-Walker malformation. Note the posterior fossa cyst in the modified coronal and sagittal planes. The coronal studies show that the vermis was absent and that there was an open communication between the fourth ventricle and the cyst.

largement of the ventricular cavities proximal to the obstruction.[44,45]

Communicant Hydrocephalus. In communicant hydrocephalus the CSF pathways are open within the ventricular system but there is decreased absorption of CSF. Absorption of CSF can be impeded by occlusion of the subarachnoid cisterns in the posterior fossa or the obliteration of the subarachnoid spaces over the convexities of the brain. The entire ventricular system becomes uniformly distended.[44,45]

The most common cause of congenital hydrocephalus is aqueductal stenosis. The aqueduct of Sylvius is narrowed or replaced by multiple small channels with blind ends. Occasionally aqueductal stenosis may be caused by extrinsic lesions posterior to the brain stem such as congenital aneurysm of the vein of Galen. Aqueductal stenosis can be diagnosed with ECHO when an infant is born with widening of the lateral and third ventricles and a normal-size fourth ventricle. If the hydrocephalus is very large, the posterior fossa is smaller than usual, and the cerebellum is displaced toward the occipital bone with the disappearance of the cis-

ABSENCE OF THE CORPUS CALLOSUM AND DANCY WALKER MALFORMATION

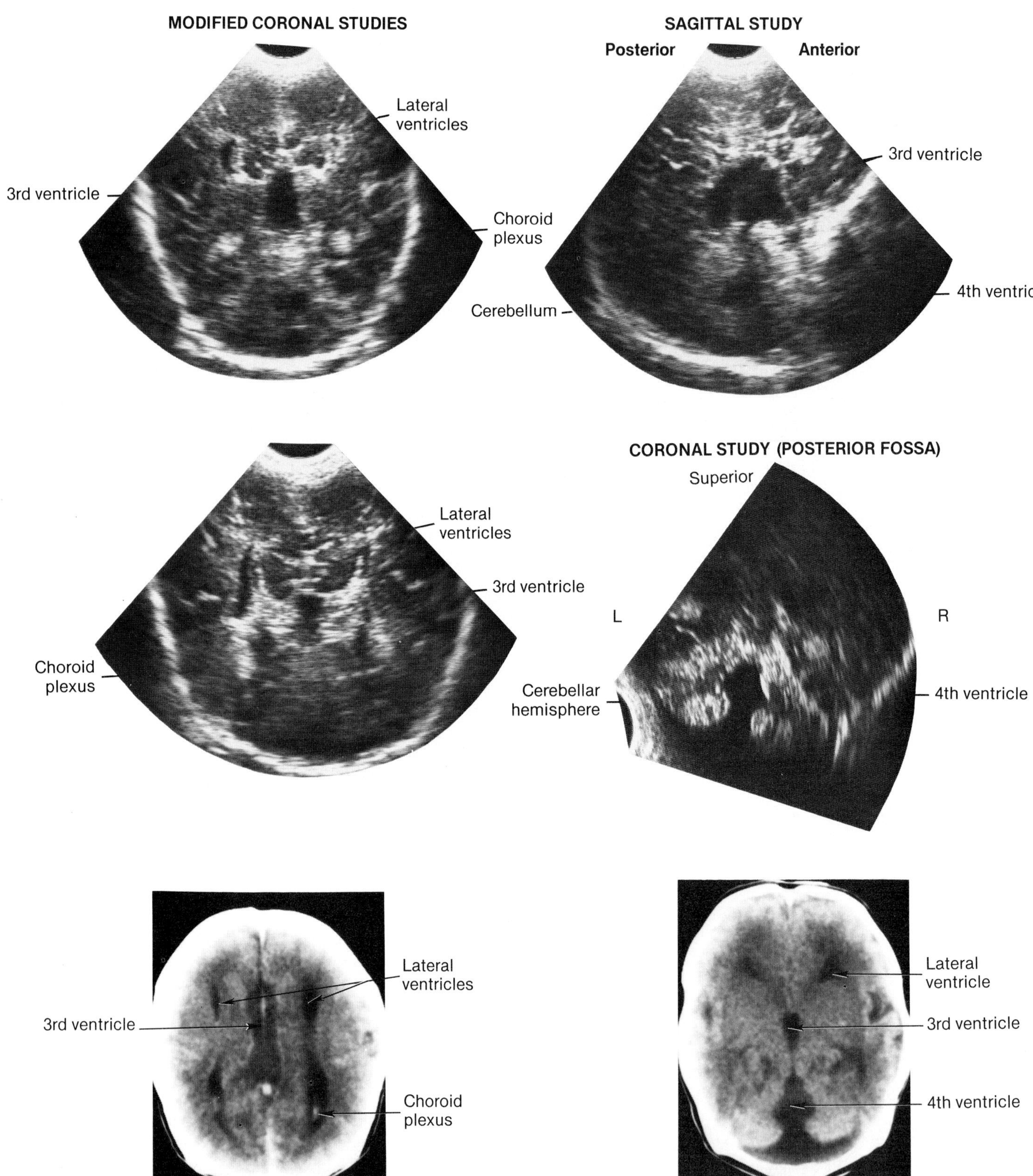

FIG. 16-27 Agenesis of the corpus callosum associated with Dandy-Walker malformation. Complex malformation showing anomalies characteristic of agenesis of the corpus callosum (compare with Fig. 19-39). The lateral ventricles are parallel to the midline, there is a very large third ventricle displaced upward, and the frontal horns have the typical shape of vampire wings. The posterior fossa shows anomalies distinctive of Dandy-Walker malformation (absence of the vermis, enlarged fourth ventricle, and large cisterna magna).

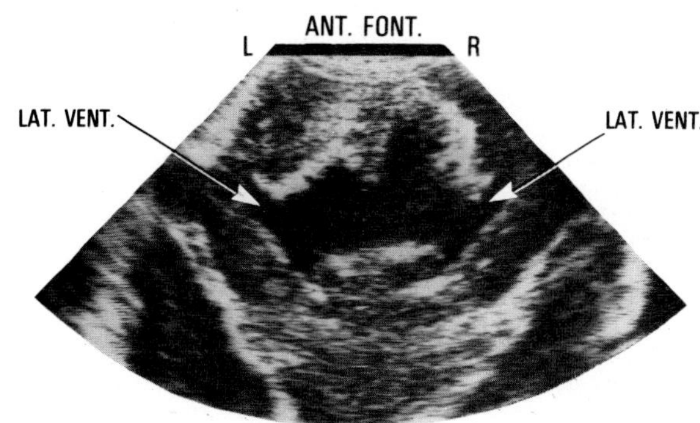

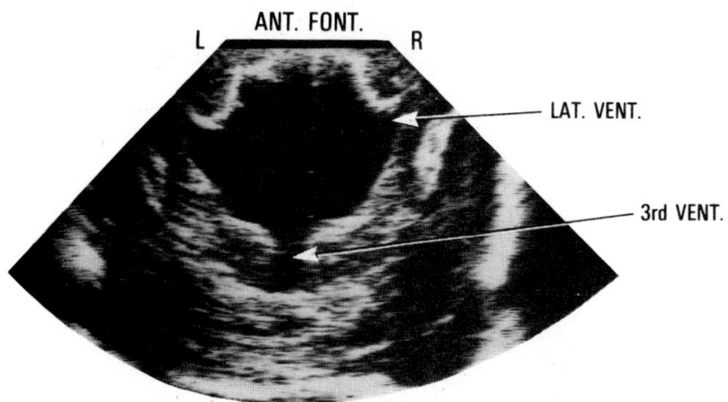

FIG. 16-28 Absence of the corpus callosum caused by a large midline infarction. Note the areas of increased echogenicity in the frontal lobes close to the midline. These echodense zones are associated with destruction of the corpus callosum and a large porencephalic cavity communicating with the lateral ventricles.

terna magna. However, the cerebellum is not dislodged into foramen magnum, thus differentiating aqueductal stenosis from the Arnold-Chiari malformation (Fig. 16-29).

Arnold-Chiari and Dandy-Walker malformations, other important causes of congenital hydrocephalus, already have been described.

Subarachnoid Cysts

Subarachnoid cysts are lined by arachnoid tissue and contain cerebrospinal fluid.[35] The following three major etiologies are postulated to explain the formation of these cysts:

- Localized entrapment of fluid during embryogenesis
- Residual subdural hematoma
- Fluid extravasation secondary to leptomeningeal tear or ventricular rupture

The cysts may be located in the infratentorial or supratentorial compartments. Subarachnoid cysts in the posterior fossa are associated with a normal vermis and a normal fourth ventricle, which differentiates subarachnoid cysts from the Dandy-Walker malformation. In a supratentorial compartment, these cysts usually arise from the suprasellar or quadrigeminal plate cisterns. The most frequent locations are the interhemispheric fissure, the suprasellar region, and the cerebral convexities. These cysts may be symptomatic secondary to cerebral compression or hydrocephalus, or they may be totally asymptomatic.[2,23,35]

Subarachnoid cysts usually appear in ECHO studies as nonechogenic cystic structures arising from the quadrigeminal plate cistern or the suprasellar region. Sagittal studies are useful to determine the location and size of these cysts. Sequential studies should be obtained in infants with this complication, since the cysts may have progressive growth and may need to be drained by ventriculoperitoneal shunts (Fig. 16-30).

ECHOENCEPHALOGRAPHIC DIAGNOSIS OF NEONATAL BRAIN LESIONS

Real time echoencephalography is ideal for timing the onset and sequentially following the evolution of a large number of brain lesions in newborn infants.

Hemorrhagic Pathology (see box on p. 398)

Subependymal-intraventricular Hemorrhages. Subependymal-intraventricular hemorrhages (SEHs-IVHs) are the most common hemorrhagic lesions in preterm newborn infants. These lesions affect 30% to 50% of infants less than 34 weeks of gestation.[45] SEHs-IVHs are a developmental disease, since they originate in the subependymal germinal matrix.[20] The germinal matrix is the tissue where neurons and glial cells develop before migrating from the subventricular (subependymal) region to the cortex. The germinal matrix is highly cellular, has poor connective supporting tissue, and is richly vascularized with very thin capillaries. This increased capillary fragility may explain the high frequency of these hemorrhages in tiny infants. Furthermore, the germinal matrix has a high fibrinolytic activity that may be important for the extension of the capillary hemorrhages that originate in this tissue.[20] By 24 weeks of gestation most of the neuronal and glial migration has occurred. However, pockets of germinal matrix remain until 40 weeks of gestation in the subependymal area at the head of the caudate nuclei. This may explain why subependymal hemorrhages are less frequent in term infants and why the majority of the intraventricular hemorrhages in these infants originate in the choroid plexus.[27,45]

Subependymal hemorrhages (SEHs) are caused by capillary bleeding in the germinal matrix. The most frequent location is at the thalamic-caudate groove. If bleeding continues, the hemorrhage enlarges, pushing the ependyma into the ventricular cavity, which can then become completely occluded by the subependymal hemorrhage. Eventually large SEHs rupture through the ependyma into the ventricular cavity, forming an intraventricular hemorrhage (IVH).

IVHs and SEHs are easily detected with real time echoencephalography as very echo-dense structures, since fluid and clotted blood have higher acoustic impedance than the

SAGITTAL PLANE (MIDLINE)

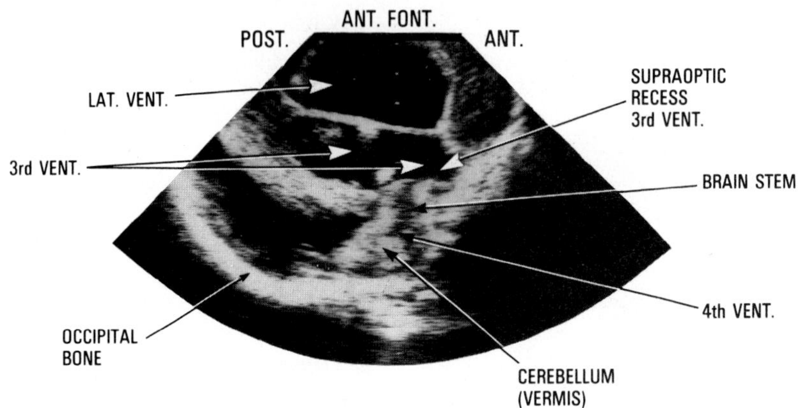

MODIFIED CORONAL PLANE

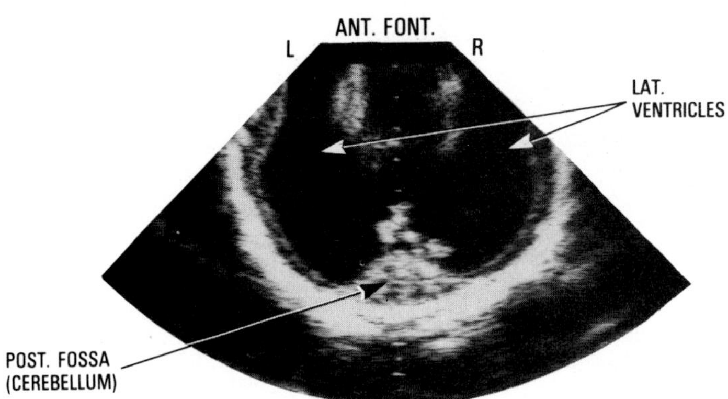

FIG. 16-29 Stenosis of the aqueduct causing congenital hydrocephalus. Note that the third ventricle is very enlarged and that the fourth ventricle is normal in size. The cerebellum appears displaced toward the occipital bone, but the cerebellum does not protrude into the foramen magnum. Compare with Fig. 16-24 (Arnold-Chiari malformation).

SEH-IVH HEMORRHAGE

- Grade I: SEH or IVH without ventricular enlargement
- Grade II: SEH or IVH with minimal ventricular enlargement
- Grade III: SEH or IVH with moderate or large ventricular enlargement
- Grade IV: SEH or IVH with intraparenchymal hemorrhage

brain parenchyma and the CSF. Overall, ECHO is more sensitive for detecting IVHs-SEHs than computerized tomography (CT). Hemoglobin concentrations greater than 5 to 6 mg/dl are required to detect blood in the ventricular cavities with CT, whereas ECHO can visualize blood when the concentration of red blood cells in the CSF is only 1 to 2 mg/dl (Fig. 16-31).[7]

SEHs-IVHs can be studied in the coronal, modified coronal, sagittal, parasagittal, and axial planes. A subependymal hemorrhage is usually seen at the thalamic-caudate notch as a very echo-dense lesion pushing up the floor and external wall of the lateral ventricle with partial obliteration of the ventricular cavity. The SEH can extend by continuous bleeding and perforate the ventricular wall with partial or total flooding of the ventricular system (intraventricular hemorrhage, IVH). IVHs appear as echo-dense structures inside the anechoic ventricular cavities. Depending on the amount of blood, the ventricle can become full and dilated. Subsequently the SEH may obstruct the circulation and absorption of the cerebrospinal fluid, causing the ventricles to dilate further with CSF and ultimately resulting in posthemorrhagic hydrocephalus.

Studies from the anterior fontanelle may not detect small

SAGITTAL PLANE (MIDLINE)

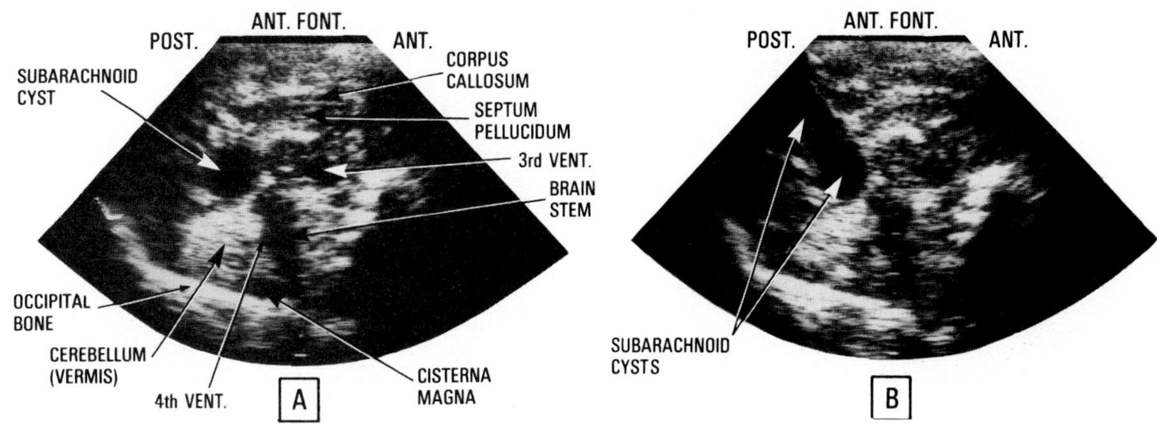

MODIFIED CORONAL PLANE

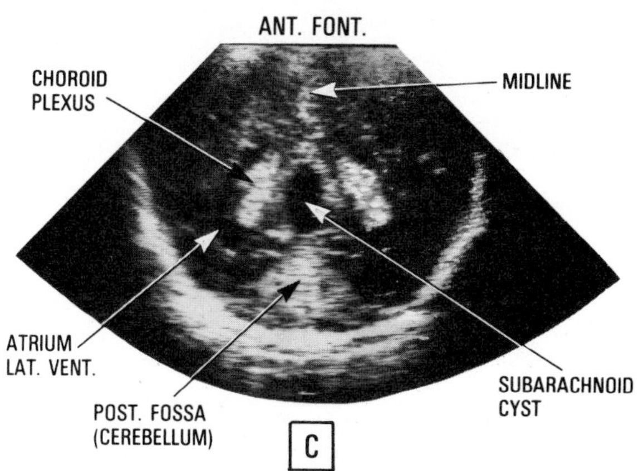

FIG. 16-30 Subarachnoid cyst. Large cystic structure in the midline. The cyst appears to emerge from the quadrigeminal plate and extends upward in the midline. **D,** Posterior coronal view of the lateral ventricles with the choroid plexus. Small cystic structures are seen within the choroid plexus representing a choroid cyst. **E,** Sagittal view of the left ventricle showing the small choroid cysts *(arrow)*.

D

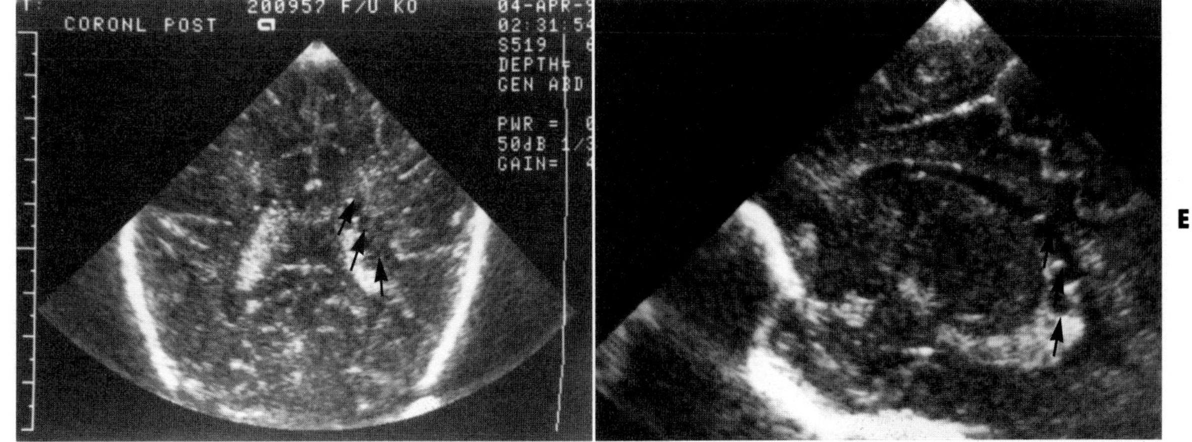

E

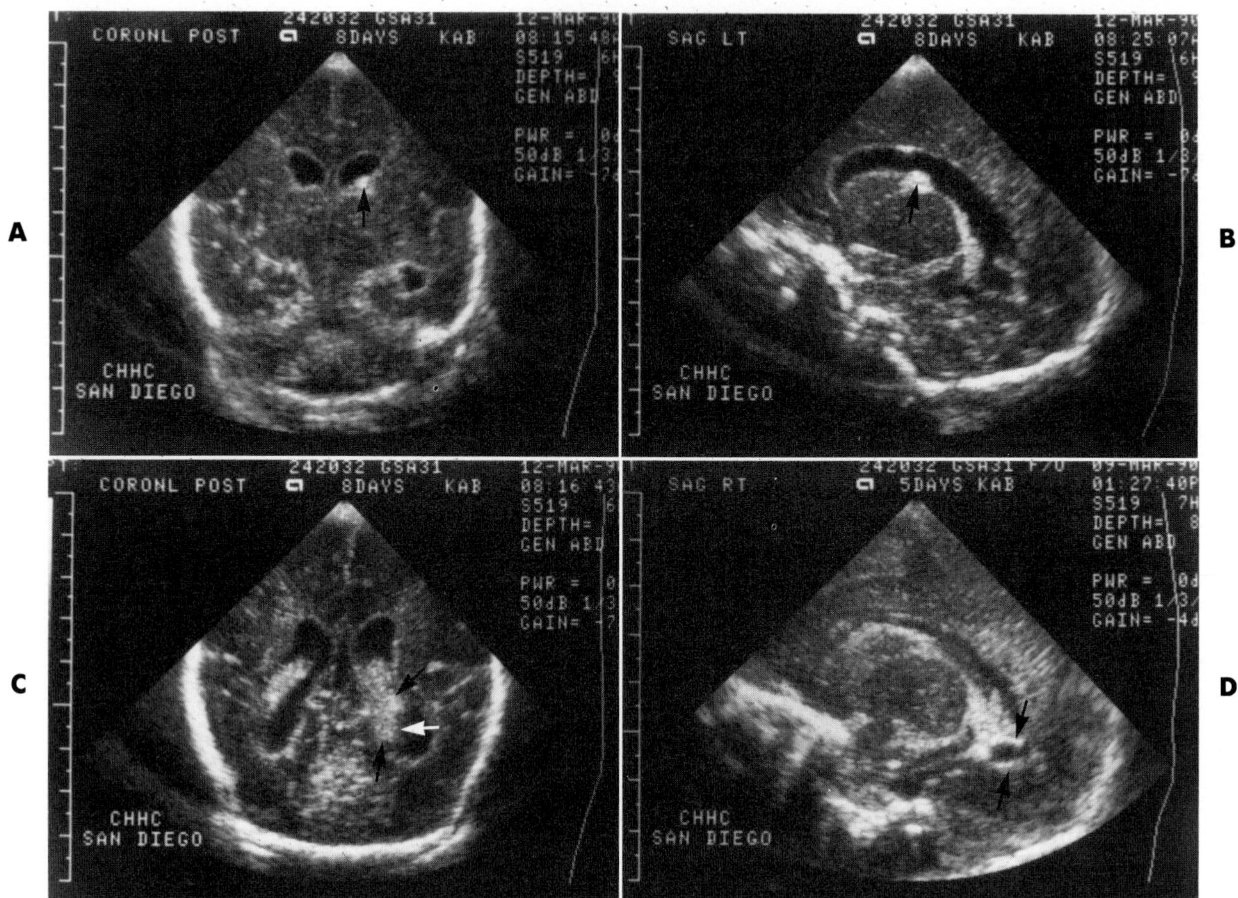

FIG 16-31 **A,** Posterior coronal view of a 8-day-old premature infant with a bilateral grade III bleed. The ventricles are slightly dilated with a subependymal bleed that extends into the ventricular cavity. **B,** Sagittal view of the left ventricle shows the subependymal bleed. **C,** Posterior coronal view of the full choroid plexus secondary to the hemorrhage. **D,** Sagittal view of the premie at 5 days shows fullness at the base of the occipital horn with a necrotic hemorrhage.

IVHs, since intraventricular blood tends to "settle out" in the posterior horns. These small IVHs can be diagnosed when the occipital horns are visualized in the axial plane from the mastoid or from the posterior fontanelles. Since these fontanelles are closer to the occipital horns than the anterior fontanelle, the occipital horns are within the focal range of the transducer, and a greater amount of ultrasonic energy can reach the sedimented red blood cells.

IVHs-SEHs are not a sudden event; they usually expand slowly (Fig. 16-32). This phenomenon is probably secondary to the high fibrinolytic activity of the germinal matrix. However, in some infants the IVHs-SEHs extend very fast; sudden flooding and distension of the ventricles by hemorrhage is associated with the clinical symptoms of shock, seizures, hypoxemia, and a sudden decrease in the hematocrit. Typically, when a small IVH-SEH progresses to a large IVH-SEH (usually during the first 4 postpartum days), the IVHs-SEHs are asymptomatic. Since approximately 70% of hemorrhages are asymptomatic, it is necessary to have a technique, such as ECHO, to routinely scan all the infants at risk for these lesions.

Classification of SEH-IVH hemorrhage is based on the extension of the hemorrhage and the resultant changes in the ventricular size.

Only ventricular enlargement produced by the intraventricular hemorrhage should be considered. Small SEHs-IVHs may occlude the foramen of Monro or the aqueduct of Sylvius and thereby produce moderate to large dilation of the lateral ventricles by CSF.

The ventricular size is measured in the sagittal plane (height of the body of the ventricles at the midthalamus) and in the axial plane (width of the atrium at the level of the choroid plexus). Based on these measurements, ventricular dilation may be classified as follows:

- **Mild dilation:** Ventricular size measuring 8 to 10 mm
- **Moderate dilation:** Ventricular size measuring 11 to 14 mm
- **Large dilation:** Ventricular size greater than 14 mm

After the hemorrhage has occurred, the blood spreads following the CSF pathways, reaching the fourth ventricle and eventually the cisterns in the posterior fossa, with the development of subarachnoid hemorrhages (SAH) (Fig. 16-

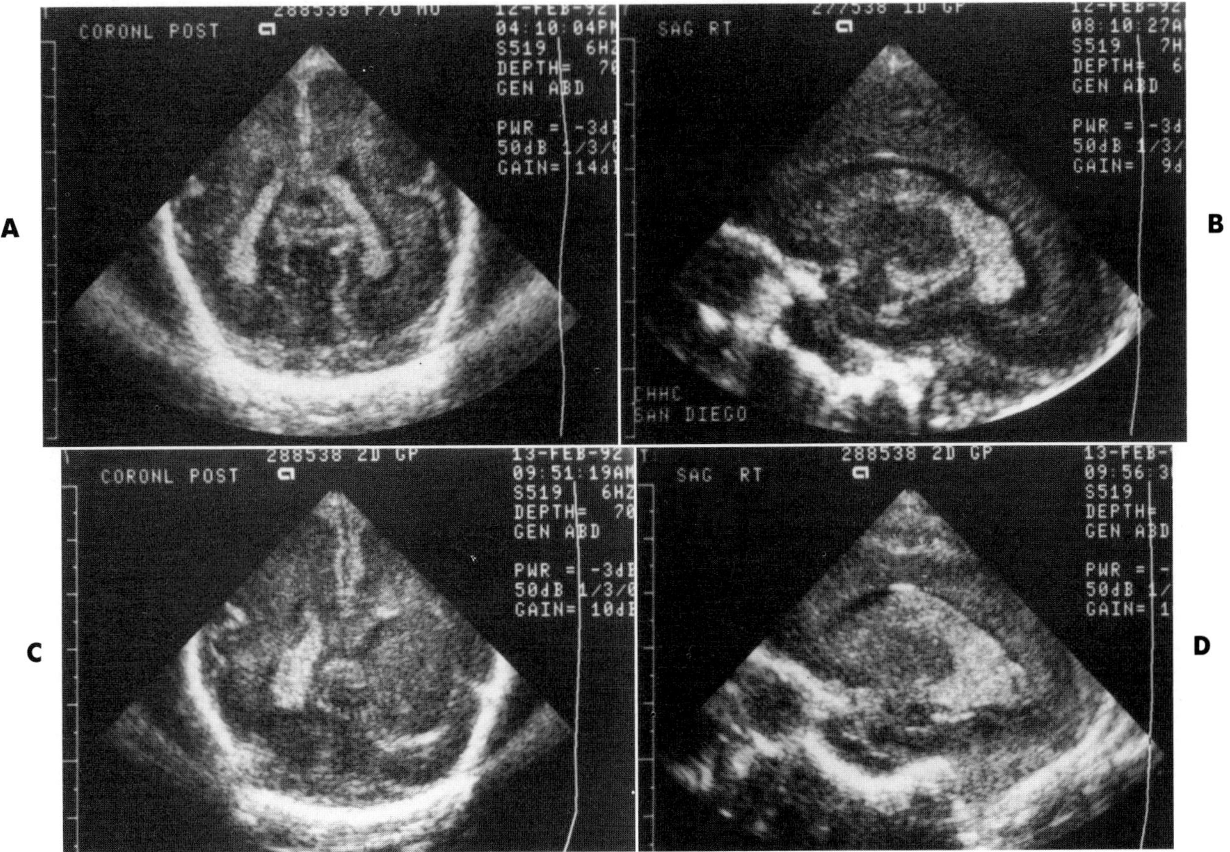

FIG. 16-32 A and **B,** Coronal and sagittal images of a premature twin with a grade II bleed shortly after birth that progressed to a grade III bleed in 1 day (**C** and **D**).

33). Subsequently, obstruction of the CSF pathways and obliterans arachnoiditis occurs, causing imbalance between production and reabsorption of CSF. Posthemorrhagic ventricular dilation develops as a consequence of this imbalance.[45] If the ventricular dilation is progressive, the patient is considered to have posthemorrhagic hydrocephalus (Fig. 16-34). This complication occurs in approximately 35% of infants with large hemorrhages. Usually mild to moderate ventricular dilation resolves spontaneously. However, placement of a ventriculoperitoneal shunt may be necessary for severely dilated ventricles (Fig. 16-35).

Posthemorrhagic hydrocephalus may be silent, since the white matter of newborn infants is very compliant and easily compressed as the ventricles widen.[45] This factor explains why initial ventricular dilation occurs without changes in the head circumference. The head circumference starts to enlarge only after significant compression of the white matter has developed.[45] Sequential studies are required in infants with SEHs-IVHs to diagnose posthemorrhagic ventricular dilation in the silent phase.

ECHO is the most reliable technique to diagnose and follow changes in the ventricular size and in the intraventricular clots. IVHs-SEHs resolve in several days or weeks, depending on the size of the bleed and on the individual patient. Although intraventricular clots are easily detected by CT, they resolve as the concentration of hemoglobin decreases, and they are not seen after 10 to 14 days in CT studies.[3,21,35,36]

Intraventricular clots undergo characteristic changes with time. Initially they are very echogenic, then low echogenic areas appear. Eventually they become completely cystic with visualization of the choroid plexus inside the cystic ventricular cast. Large cystic intraventricular clots may cause persistent ventricular dilation despite drainage of the CSF by a ventriculoperitoneal shunt.

Intraparenchymal Hemorrhages. Intraparenchymal hemorrhages (IPHs) complicate SEHs-IVHs in approximately 15% to 25% of the infants.[30b,45] IPHs are a severe complication, since they indicate that the brain parenchyma has been destroyed. Although IPHs originally were considered an extension of SEHs-IVHs, recent evidence suggests that this lesion may actually be a primary infarction of the periventricular and subcortical white matter with destruction of the lateral wall of the ventricle. When the necrotic tissue liquefies, the IVH extends into the necrotic areas.

Intraparenchymal hemorrhages appear as very echogenic zones in the white matter adjacent to the lateral ventricles.

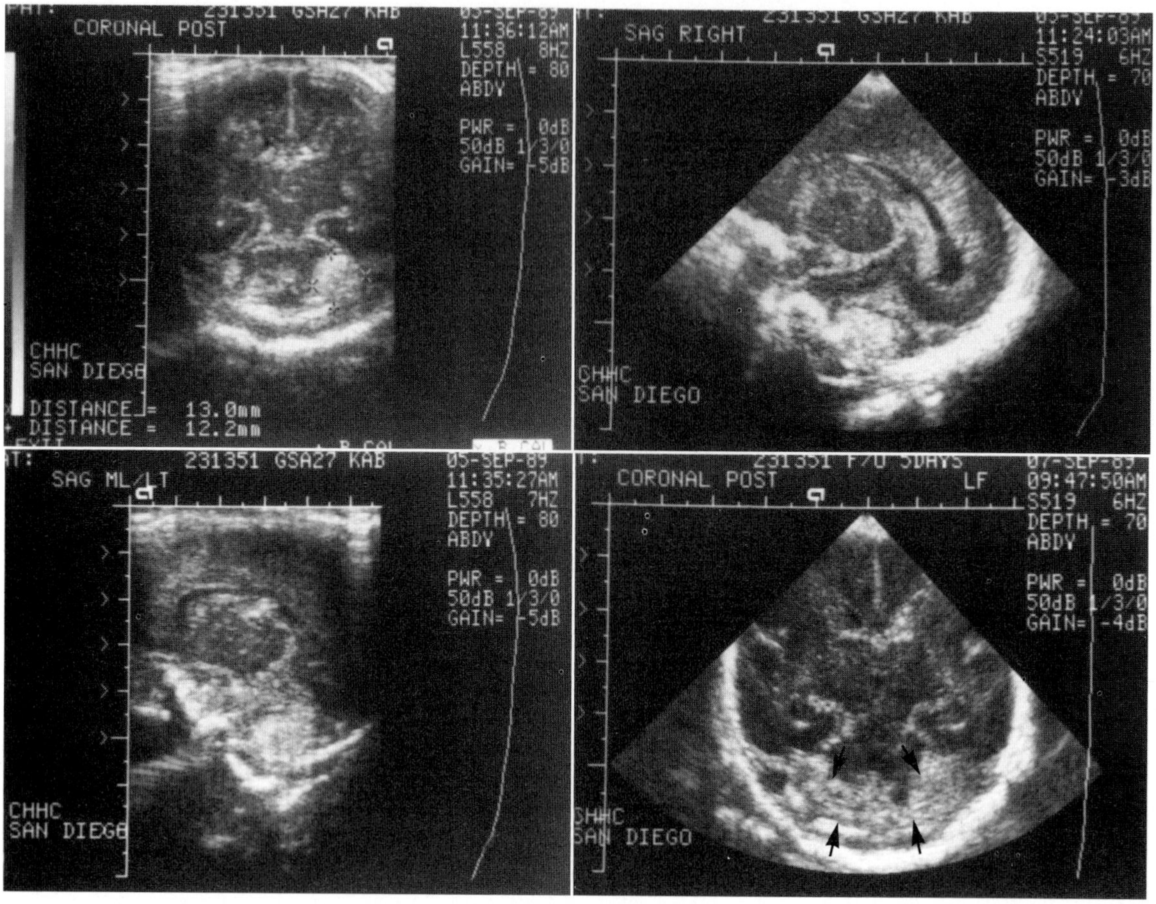

FIG. 16-33 **A** to **D**, Multiple coronal and sagittal images in a 27-week premature infant with a large cerebellar bleed. In 5 days the bleed had progressed throughout the cerebellar compartment.

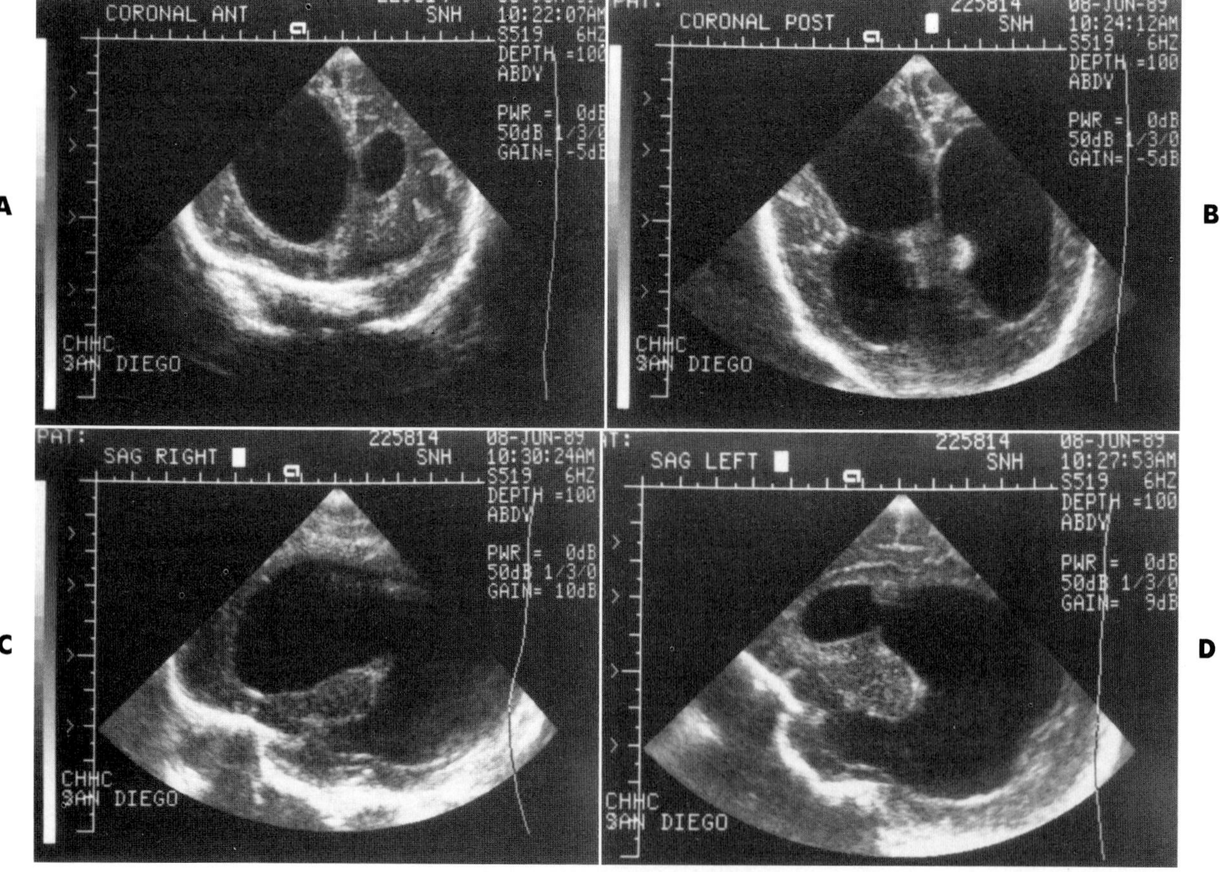

FIG. 16-34 **A** to **D**, A 4-month-old infant with hydrocephalus shows dilation of the lateral ventricles.

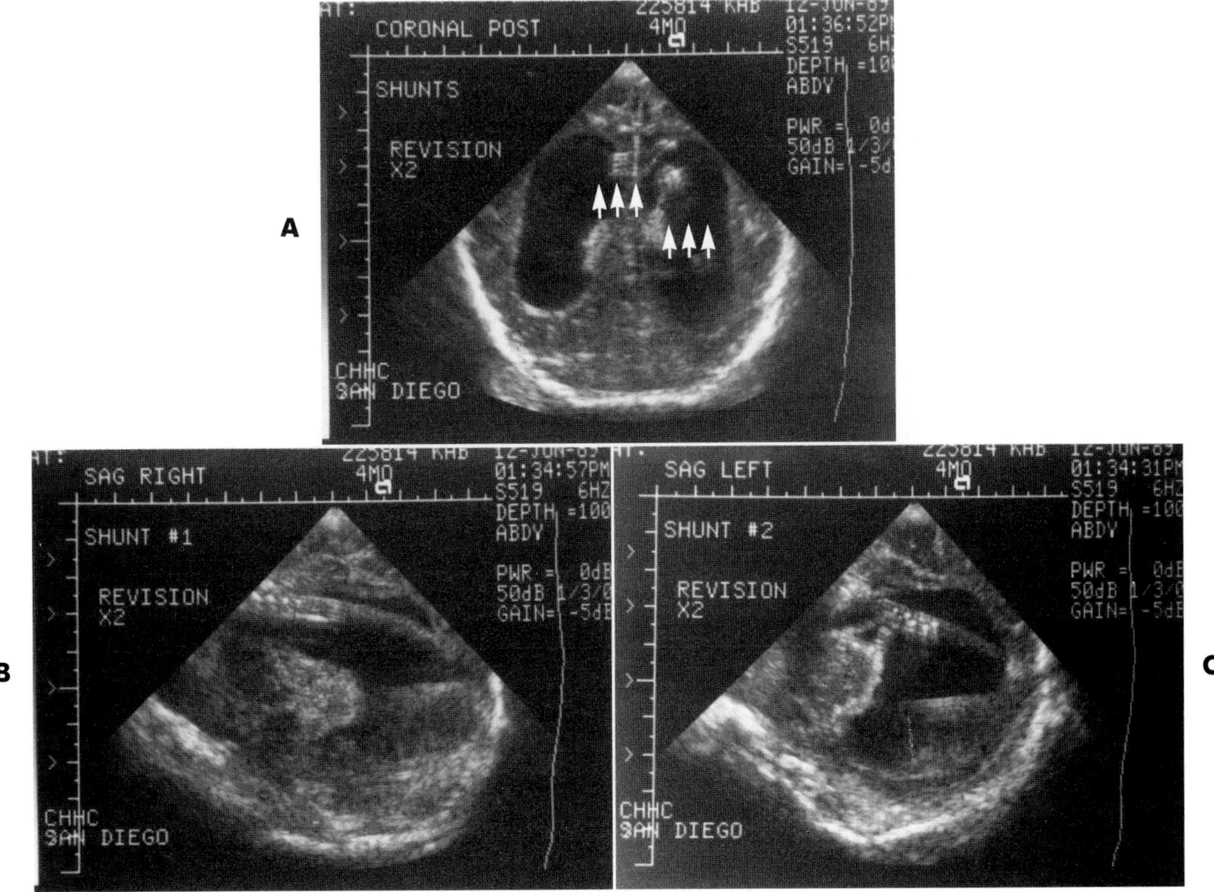

FIG. 16-35 A to **C,** Follow-up study of the infant in fig. 16-34 shows the shunt tubing in place for drainage of the hydrocephalus. Ultrasound is very useful in following the shunt placement, as well as monitoring the drainage of the dilated ventricle.

Echogenic areas in the white matter may correspond to IPHs or to hemorrhagic infarctions or extensive periventricular leukomalacia. In the classic grade IV IPH, there is a clot extending from the white matter into the ventricular cavity (Fig. 16-36). Intraparenchymal clots follow the same evolution as intraventricular clots. A few days after the acute bleeding the clots become cystic and are reabsorbed completely in 3 or 4 weeks, leaving a cavity communicating with the lateral ventricle (porencephalic cyst).

When SEHs-IVHs associated with IPH evolve to posthemorrhagic hydrocephalus, the increased intraventricular pressure is transmitted to the porencephalic cyst. Hydrocephalus after hemorrhage associated with porencephaly is an indication for early ventriculoperitoneal shunt placement to minimize the deleterious effects of progressive compression and ischemia of the brain parenchyma (Fig. 16-37).

Subarachnoid Hemorrhages. Subarachnoid hemorrhages may be isolated or secondary to IVHs-SEHs. The etiology of isolated SAH is not clearly understood. Birth trauma and hypoxia or asphyxia have been considered the most probable causes.[45] In the case of IVHs-SEHs, blood coming from the germinal matrix or the choroid plexus collects in the infratentorial subarachnoid cisterns (cisterna magna and supracerebellar cistern). The blood may extend to the subarachnoid space surrounding the convexity of the cerebral hemispheres. The diagnosis of SAHs is important, inasmuch as obstruction of the CSF pathways may occur with subsequent development of hydrocephalus or transitory ventricular dilation.

Subarachnoid hemorrhages are characterized by strong echoes in the anechoic subarachnoid space.[18] Increased echogenicity in the Sylvian fissure has been considered diagnostic of SAH. However, this criterion is associated with a high incidence of false-negative and false-positive diagnoses. SAHs can be diagnosed easily if the cisterns in the posterior fossa are studied. Scanning the posterior fossa in the coronal, modified coronal, and sagittal planes, and from the neck enables unequivocal diagnosis of SAHs (Fig. 16-38). Blood coming from the ventricles may obstruct the aqueduct of Sylvius and the foramina of Luschka and Magendie. Bicompartmental hydrocephalus may develop, since the fourth ventricle has choroid plexus. This process may lead to gigantic dilation of the fourth ventricle with

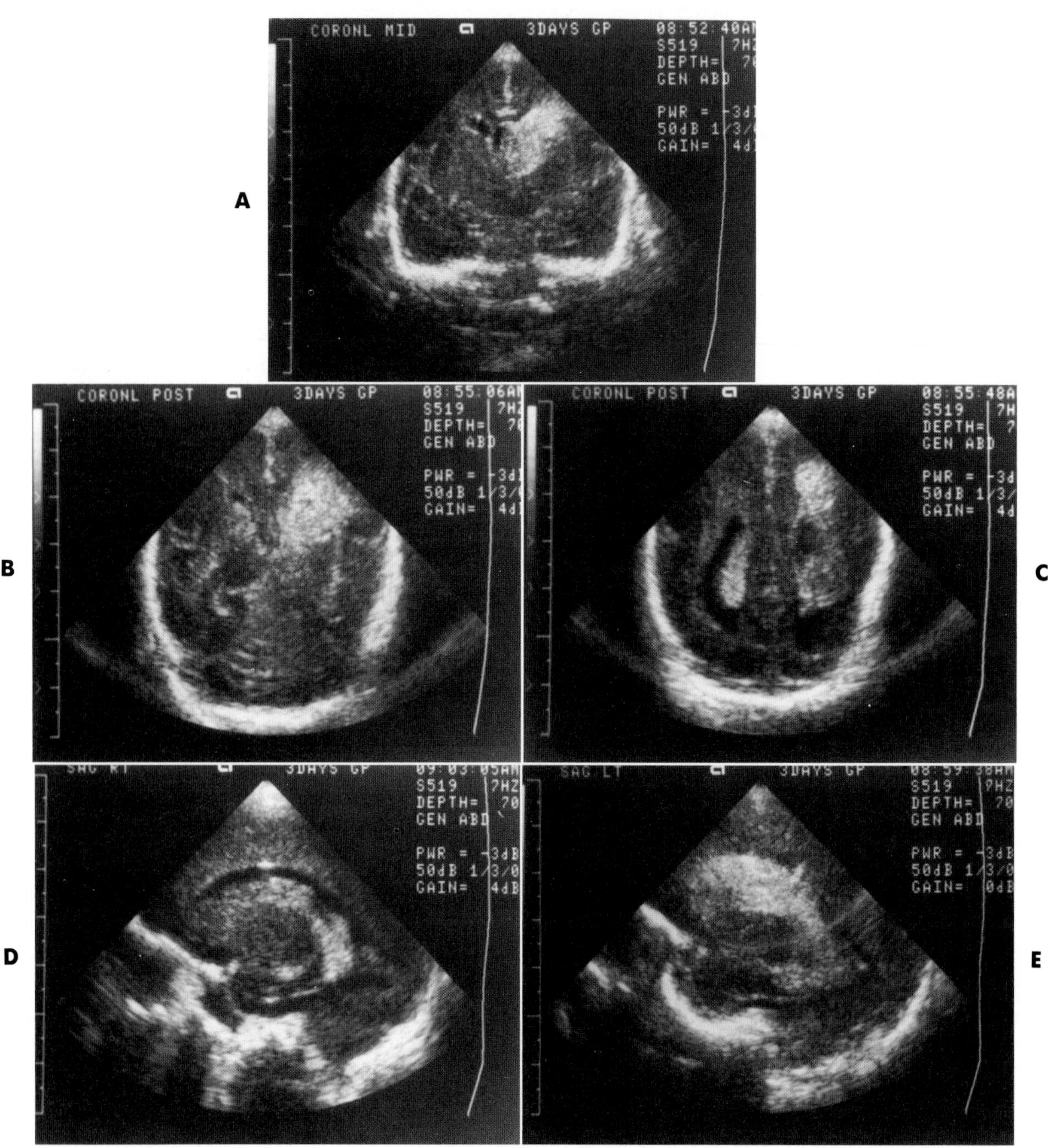

FIG. 16-36 A to **E,** A 3-day-old premature infant presents with a grade III bleed on the right and grade IV bleed on the left with extension into the brain parenchyma.

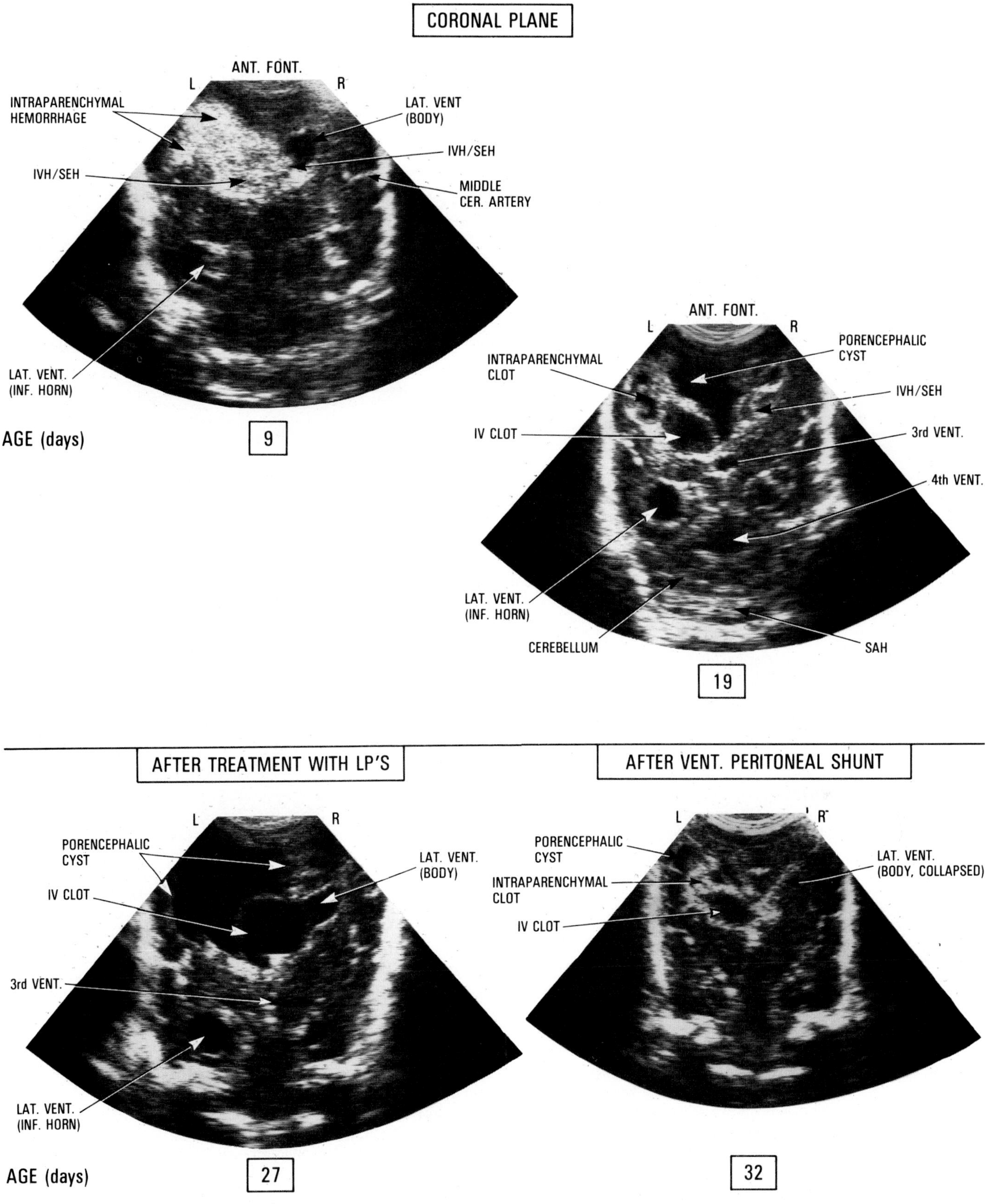

CORONAL PLANE
ANT. FONT.
L
R
INTRAPARENCHYMAL HEMORRHAGE
LAT. VENT (BODY)
IVH/SEH
IVH/SEH
MIDDLE CER. ARTERY
LAT. VENT. (INF. HORN)
AGE (days)
9
ANT. FONT.
L
R
PORENCEPHALIC CYST
INTRAPARENCHYMAL CLOT
IVH/SEH
IV CLOT
3rd VENT.
4th VENT.
LAT. VENT. (INF. HORN)
CEREBELLUM
SAH
19
AFTER TREATMENT WITH LP'S
AFTER VENT. PERITONEAL SHUNT
L
R
PORENCEPHALIC CYST
LAT. VENT. (BODY)
IV CLOT
3rd VENT.
LAT. VENT. (INF. HORN)
L
R
PORENCEPHALIC CYST
INTRAPARENCHYMAL CLOT
IV CLOT
LAT. VENT. (BODY, COLLAPSED)
AGE (days)
27
32

FIG. 16-37 Coronal, sagittal, parasagittal, and axial studies in a preterm infant with large IVH/SEH, extensive IPH, posthemorrhagic hydrocephalus, and porencephaly. Note the unique clot extending from the ventricle into the brain parenchyma and the changes in the intraparenchymal clot with the development of a large porencephalic cyst. The cyst communicates with the body of the left lateral ventricle. The parasagittal studies through the lateral wall of the ventricle and the axial views were useful to define precisely the extension of the IPH and the porencephalic cyst. A VPS produced significant reduction of the ventricular size and the porencephalic cyst.

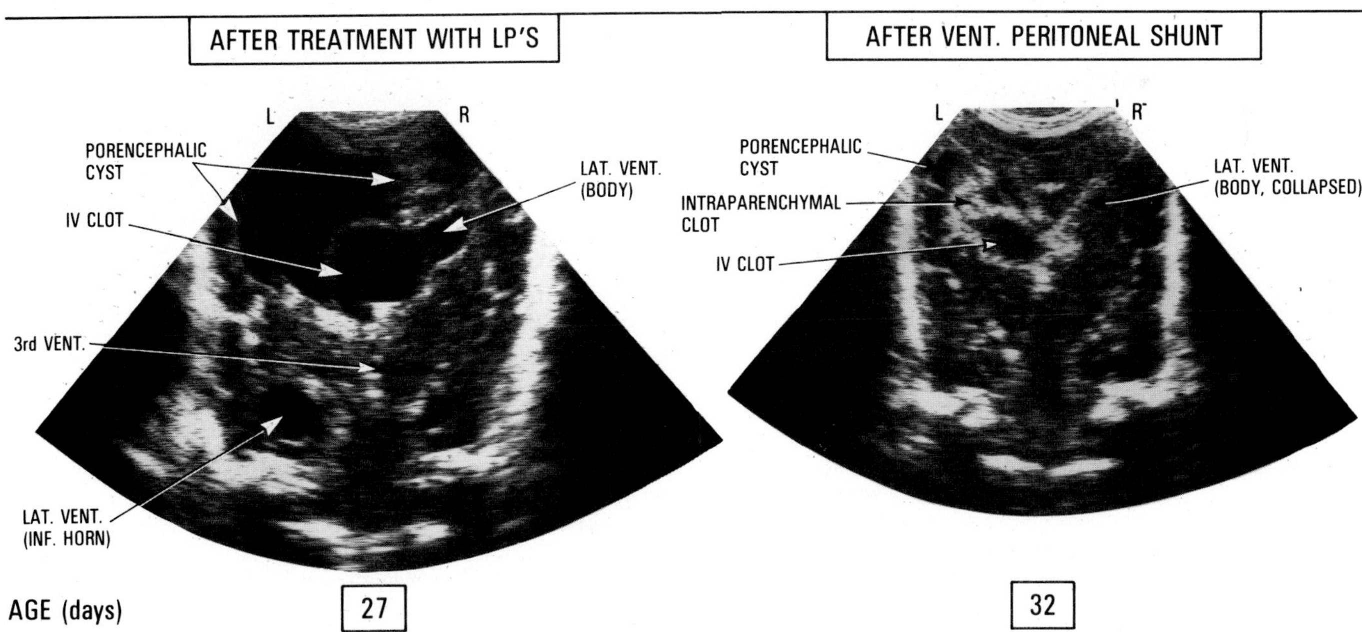

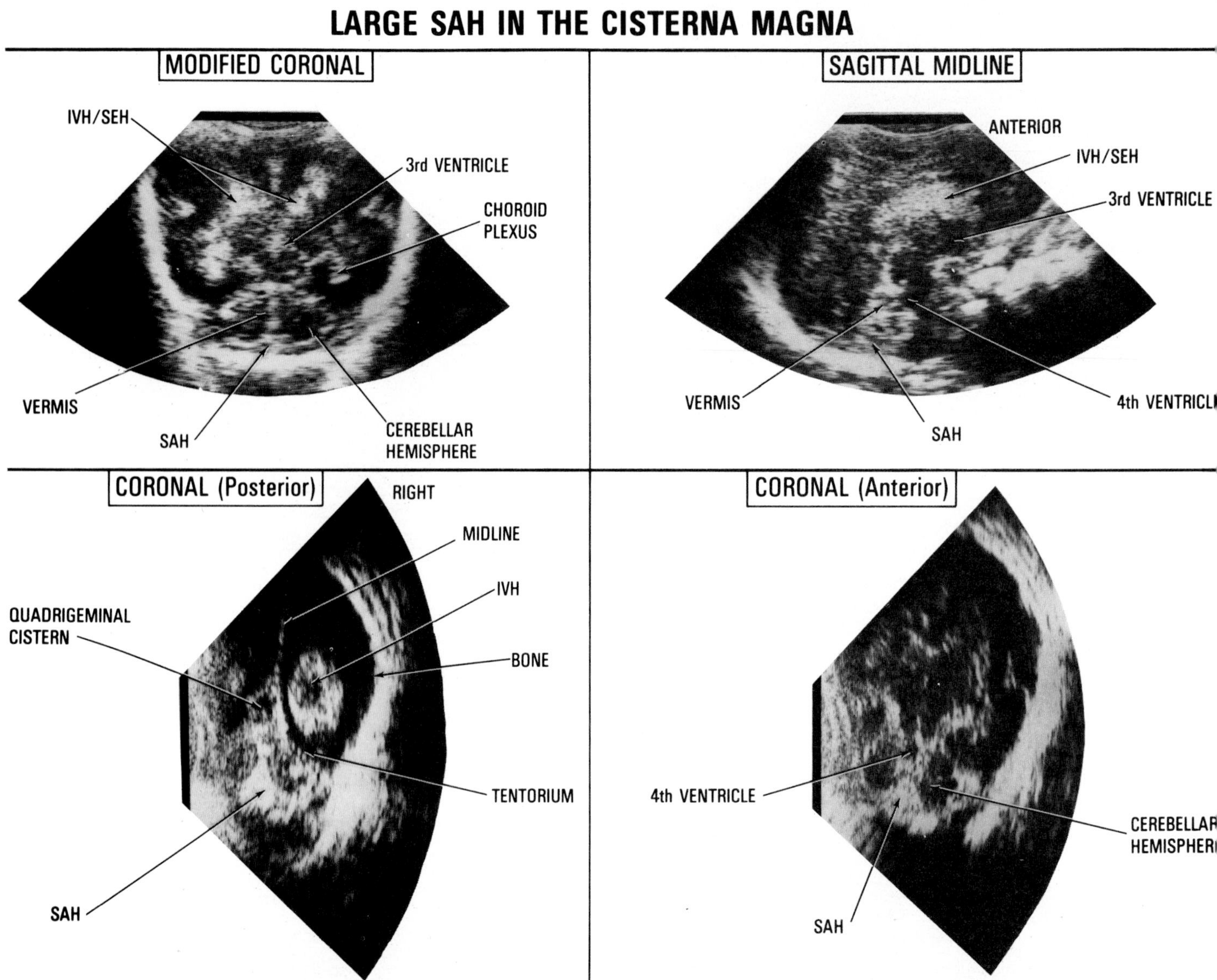

FIG. 16-38 Large SAHs in the posterior fossa in two premature infants with IVHs-SEHs. The coronal studies of the posterior fossa through the mastoid fontanelle were useful to diagnose SAH in the first patient. Note the increased echogenicity in the cisterna magna and in the supracerebellar cistern. In the second patient the fourth ventricle enlarged acutely. Lumbar punctures decompressed transiently the fourth ventricle without significant change in the size of the lateral ventricles. By 19 days the fourth ventricle was gigantic, displacing the brain stem anteriorly. A ventriculoperitoneal shunt corrected the hydrocephalus but failed to reduce the size of the fourth ventricle, indicating bicompartmental hydrocephalus.

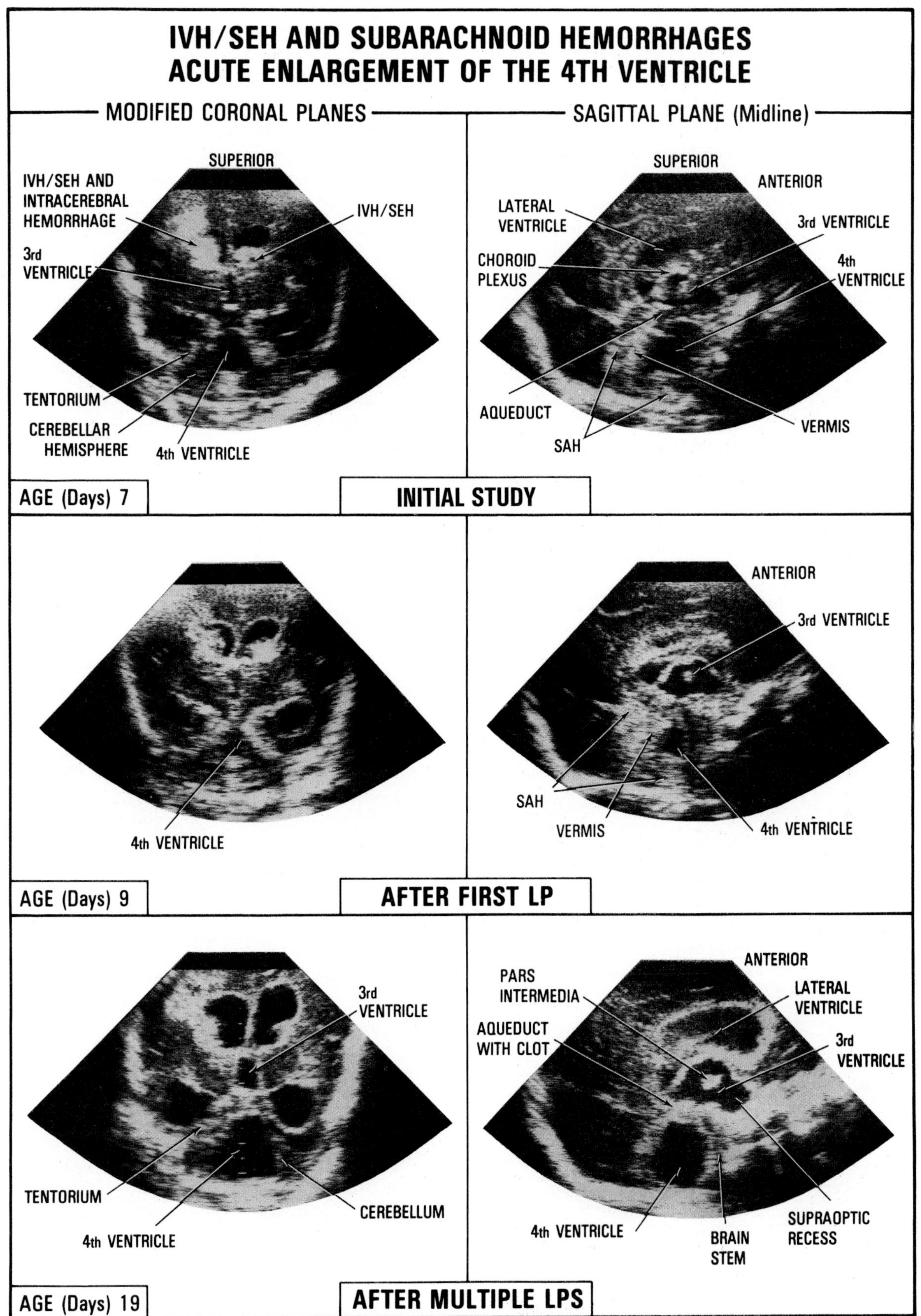

FIG. 16-39 See legend for Fig. 16-38.

displacement and compression of the brain stem (Fig. 16-39).

Intracerebellar Hemorrhages. Four categories of intracerebellar hemorrhage are described as follows:

- Primary intracerebellar hemorrhage
- Venous infarction
- Traumatic laceration resulting from occipital diastasis
- Extension to the cerebellum of a large SEH-IVH

In premature neonates, there are areas of germinal matrix located around the fourth ventricle in the cerebellar hemispheres. The cerebellar germinal matrix has the same vulnerability to hemorrhage as the telencephalic germinal matrix. Intracerebellar hemorrhages have been reported in approximately 5% to 10% of postmortem studies of neonatal populations.[45] The incidence in live infants is significantly lower. This discrepancy is probably a result of the difficulties in diagnosing these hemorrhages.

Using modified coronal, sagittal, and parasagittal views of the posterior fossa (infratentorial compartment), it is possible to diagnose unequivocally intracerebellar hemorrhages.[9] These hemorrhages appear as very echogenic structures inside the less echogenic cerebellar parenchyma. Coronal views through the mastoid fontanelle may be essential to differentiate intracerebellar hemorrhages from large SAHs in the cisterna magna, the supracerebellar cistern, or both. Intracerebellar hemorrhages become cystic with time, leaving cavitary lesions in the cerebellar hemispheres. These characteristic sequential changes are useful in making a positive diagnosis of intracerebellar hemorrhages.

Epidural Hemorrhages and Subdural Collections. Epidural hemorrhages and subdural fluid collections are better diagnosed by CT. Since these lesions are located peripherally along the surface of the brain, they are often not adequately visualized by ECHO. Subdural collections appear as nonechogenic spaces between the echogenic calvarium and the cortex. Epidural hemorrhages are seen as echogenic formations located immediately underneath the calvarium (Fig. 16-40).

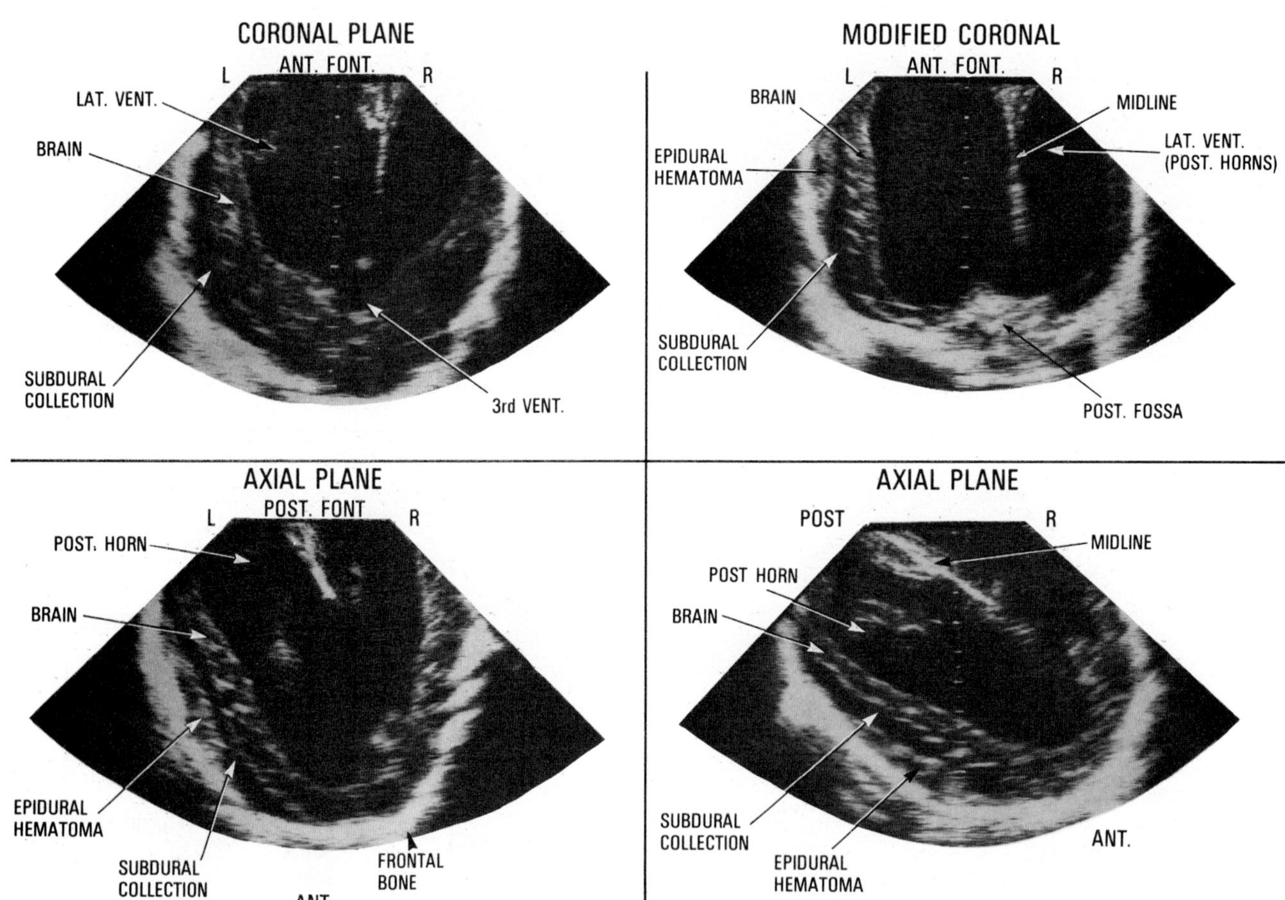

FIG. 16-40 Subdural collection and epidural hemorrhage in a premature infant with congenital hydrocephalus. The epidural hemorrhage is characterized by an area of increased echogenicity immediately underneath the skull. The subdural collection has the same echogenicity as the CSF.

Ischemic-hypoxic Lesions

Ischemic-hypoxic cerebral injury is a frequent complication of sick newborn infants. These lesions are usually associated with abnormal neurologic outcome.[7,45] Five major types of neonatal hypoxic-ischemic brain injury have been described[45]:

- Selective neuronal necrosis
- Status marmoratus
- Parasagittal cerebral injury
- Periventricular leukomalacia or white-matter necrosis
- Focal brain necrosis

ECHO is not a very precise technique to diagnose necrotic ischemic lesions. In ischemic-hypoxic encephalopathy, ECHO may show areas of increased echogenicity in the subcortical and deep white matter and in the basal ganglia* (Figs. 16-41 to 16-46). The increased echogenicity is caused by congestion and microhemorrhages, which are characteristically present in the acute stage of ischemic injuries.[7] However, echodensities are not pathognomonic of ischemic necrosis, inasmuch as they have been observed in

*References 7, 9, 12, 14, 22, 26, 28, 42.

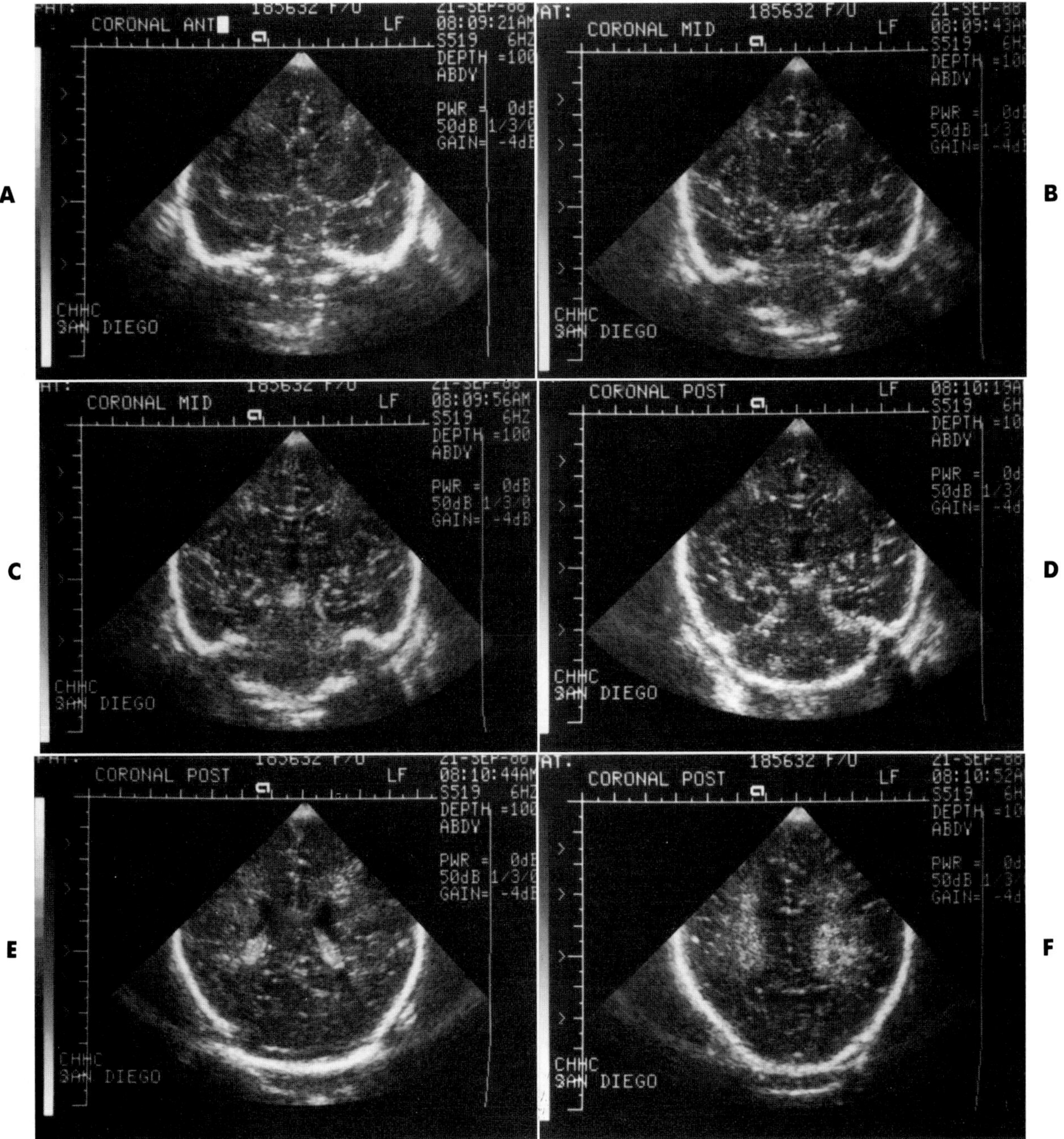

FIG. 16-41 A to **F,** Coronal images of a premature infant with PVL in the posterior parenchyma (**F**).

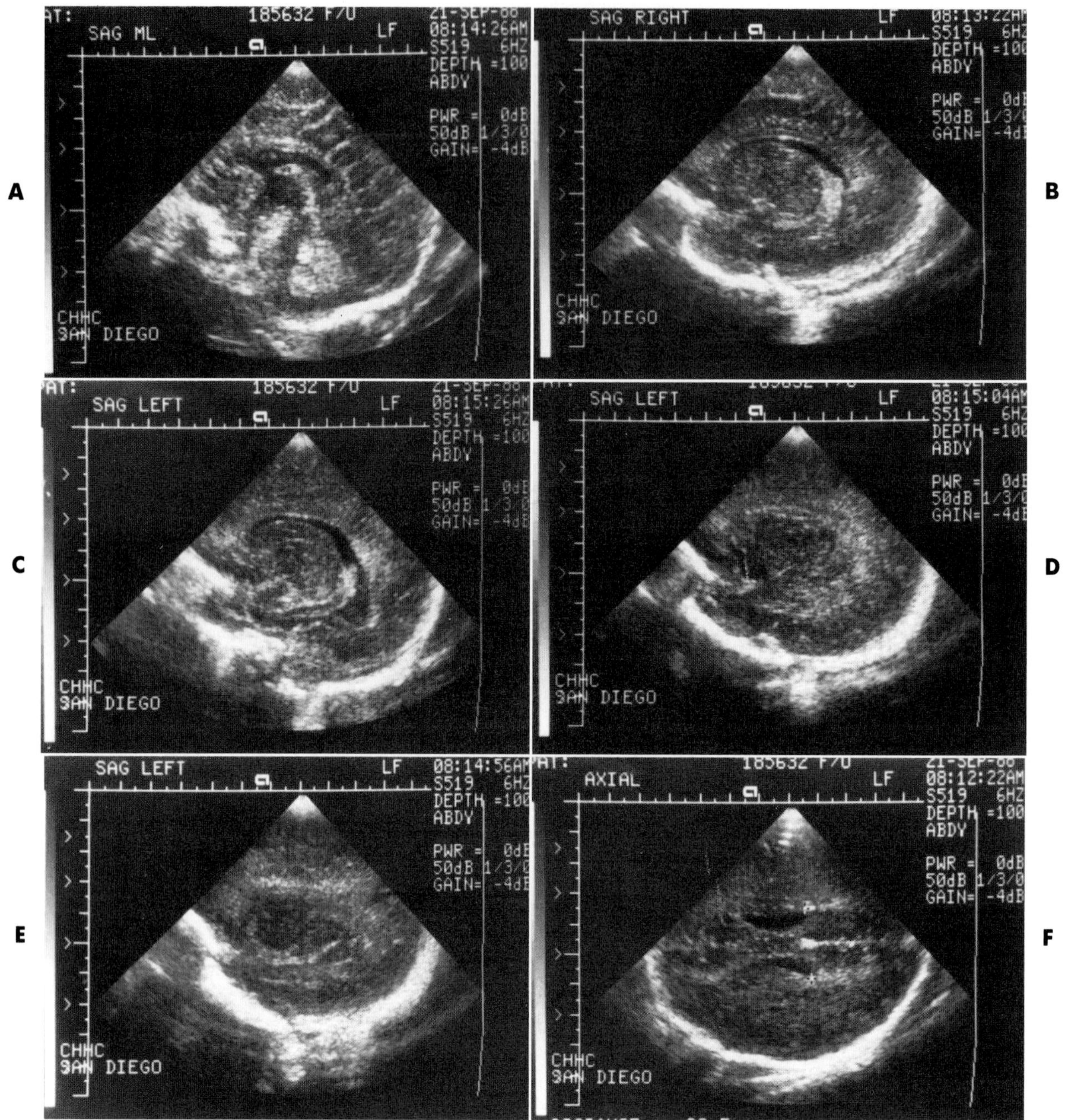

FIG. 16-42 A to **E,** Sagittal scans and F axial scans of the patient in Fig. 16-41. Increased white matter necrosis is seen in the left parenchymal hemisphere.

infants having only congestion and microhemorrhages without necrosis.[7] If necrosis is present in the echogenic areas, cavitary lesions appear 2 or more weeks after the ischemic insult. Echolucencies or cysts are the landmark for the diagnosis of ischemic brain injury in newborn infants.[7]

ECHO appears useful in diagnosing multifocal white matter necrosis (periventricular leukomalacia) and focal ischemic lesions.

Periventricular Leukomalacia or Multifocal White Matter Necrosis. Multifocal white matter necrosis (WMN) or periventricular leukomalacia is the most frequent ischemic lesion in the immature brain. This lesion is associated with anomalous myelination of the immature brain, as well as abnormal neurologic development including cerebral palsy.* WMN is probably the most important cause of abnormal neurodevelopmental sequelae in preterm infants.

WMN is found in 20% to 80% of neonatal autopsies.[6,64] Pathologists describe an acute phase characterized by multiple foci or coagulation necrosis in deep and periventricular white matter, and a chronic phase depicted by cavita-

*References 1, 7, 10-12, 29, 46

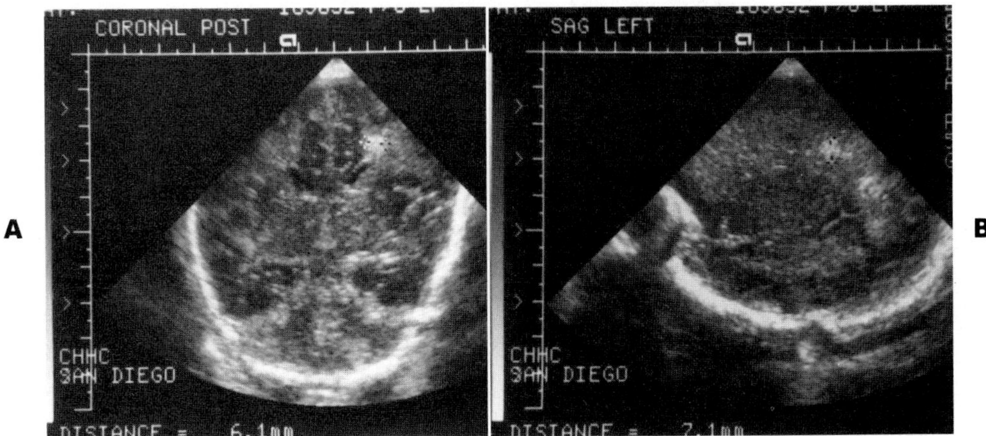

FIG. 16-43 A to **B,** Progression of the PVL in the patient shown in Fig. 16-41.

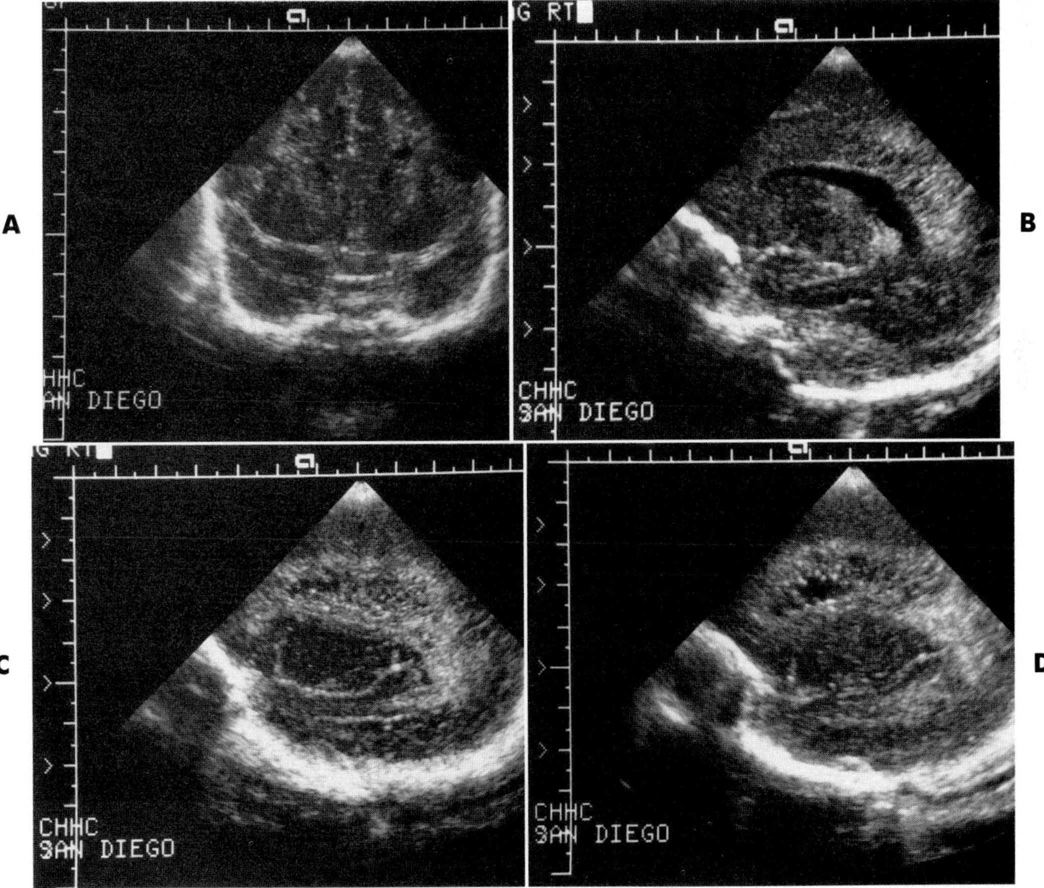

FIG. 16-44 A to **D,** The same patient with subsequent progression of the PVL bilaterally as seen 2 weeks later.

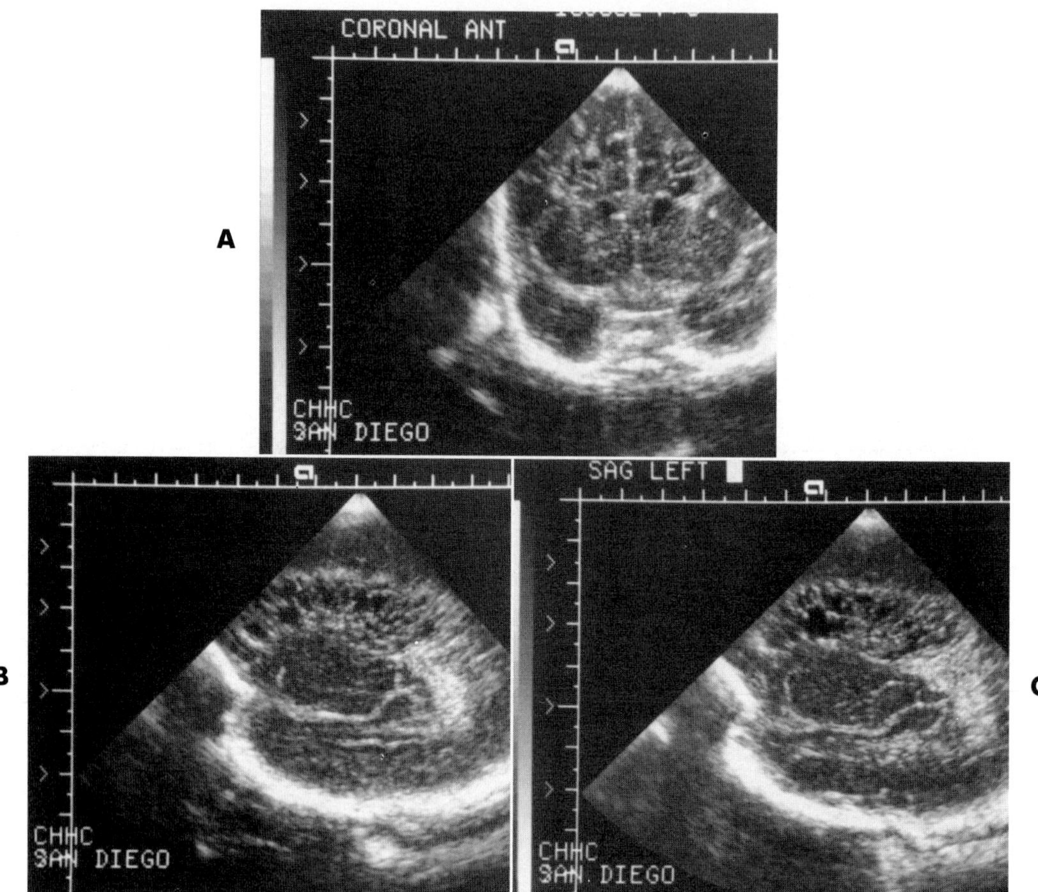

FIG. 16-45 A to **C,** The same patient 3 weeks later has multiple anechoic areas throughout the right and left hemispheres secondary to the PVL.

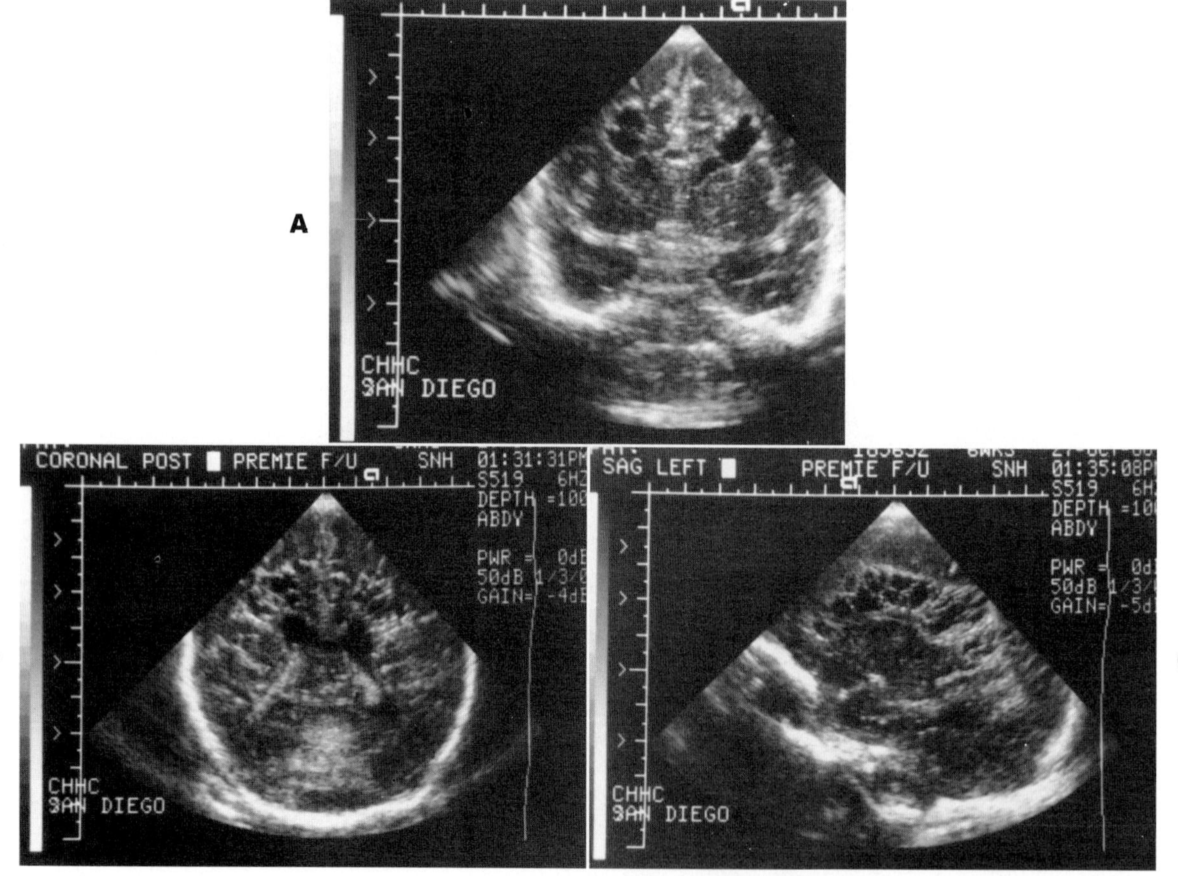

FIG. 16-46 A to **C,** The smaller anechoic areas develop into large anechoic areas throughout the brain parenchyma 6 weeks later.

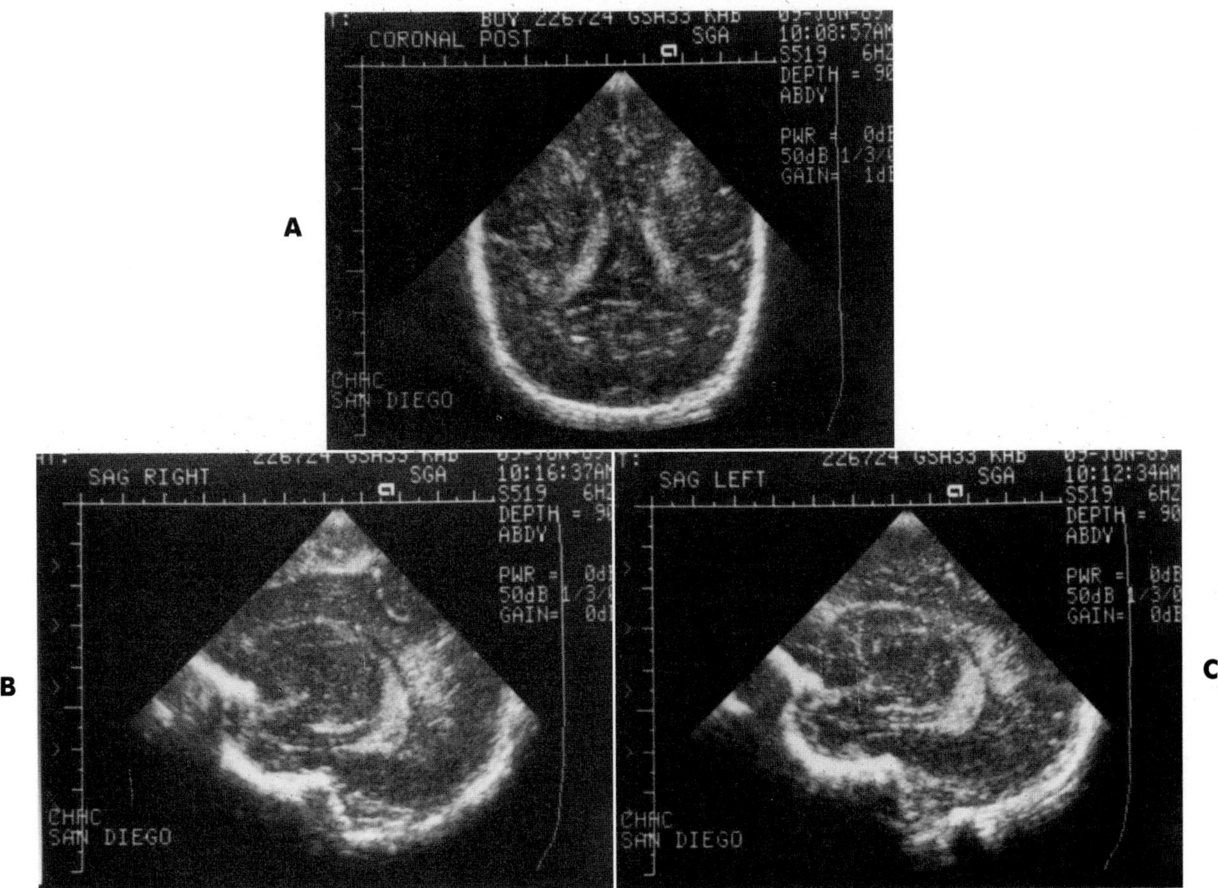

FIG. 16-47 **A,** Coronal posterior. **B** and **C,** Sagittal scans of a 33-week premature infant with white matter necrosis along the lateral ventricular borders. Follow-up studies show if this congestion develops into a hemorrhage or clears up completely.

tion and scarring appearing one or more weeks after the cerebral insult.[1,3,7] Early in the chronic stage multiple cavities develop in the necrotic white matter adjacent to the lateral walls of the frontal horns, body, atria, and occipital horns of the lateral ventricles.[11,29] These lesions are frequently located in the lateral wall of the atria and occipital horns, causing damage to the optic radiations.[6] Eventually the cavities resolve, leaving gliotic scars and diffuse cerebral atrophy.[40] Necrotic lesions with only microscopic cavities may also lead to cerebral atrophy.[15]

Until recently, white-matter necrosis was diagnosed only at autopsy. Consequently the etiology, incidence, natural evolution, and neurologic consequences of WMN have not been precisely identified. Brain ischemia caused by systemic hypotension and endotoxemia are considered the putative agents of WMN. Both proposed etiologies are supported by experimental and clinical studies. Endotoxin may be the mediator between infection and white-matter pathology. Gilles et al.[16,17] first produced WMN in newborn kittens by intraperitoneal injection of endotoxin from *Escherichia coli*. Young et al.[47] showed that hypotension secondary to hemorrhage or endotoxemia produced brain ischemia and necrosis of the cerebral white matter in newborn puppies. Leviton et al.[29] showed that 85% of infants who died with white-matter lesions had terminal gram-negative bacteremia. Data from the National Perinatal Collaborative Project also has shown that amniotic fluid and maternal urinary tract infections are associated with psychomotor dysfunction and cerebral palsy. Nelson and Ellenberg[34] cited the importance of prenatal factors associated with cerebral palsy. They showed that chorioamnionitis, prolonged rupture of membranes, and congenital malformations were the major predictors of cerebral palsy. Sims et al.[41] found that brain lesions of prenatal onset were associated with amnionitis and acute intrauterine infection. In addition, Naeye[33] noted a significant increase in neurodevelopmental handicaps in infants with amniotic fluid infections.

Currently, WMN may be diagnosed in infants with echoencephalography.* Several authors have reported an incidence of WMN in preterm infants between 5% and 25%.† Real time ultrasound appears very accurate in diagnosing WMN.[43] The acute stage of WMN is characterized by highly echogenic areas in the cerebral white matter supe-

*References 7, 9, 10, 12, 13, 19, 22, 28, 36, 42, 44, 45
†References 11, 12, 22, 28, 37, 38, 42

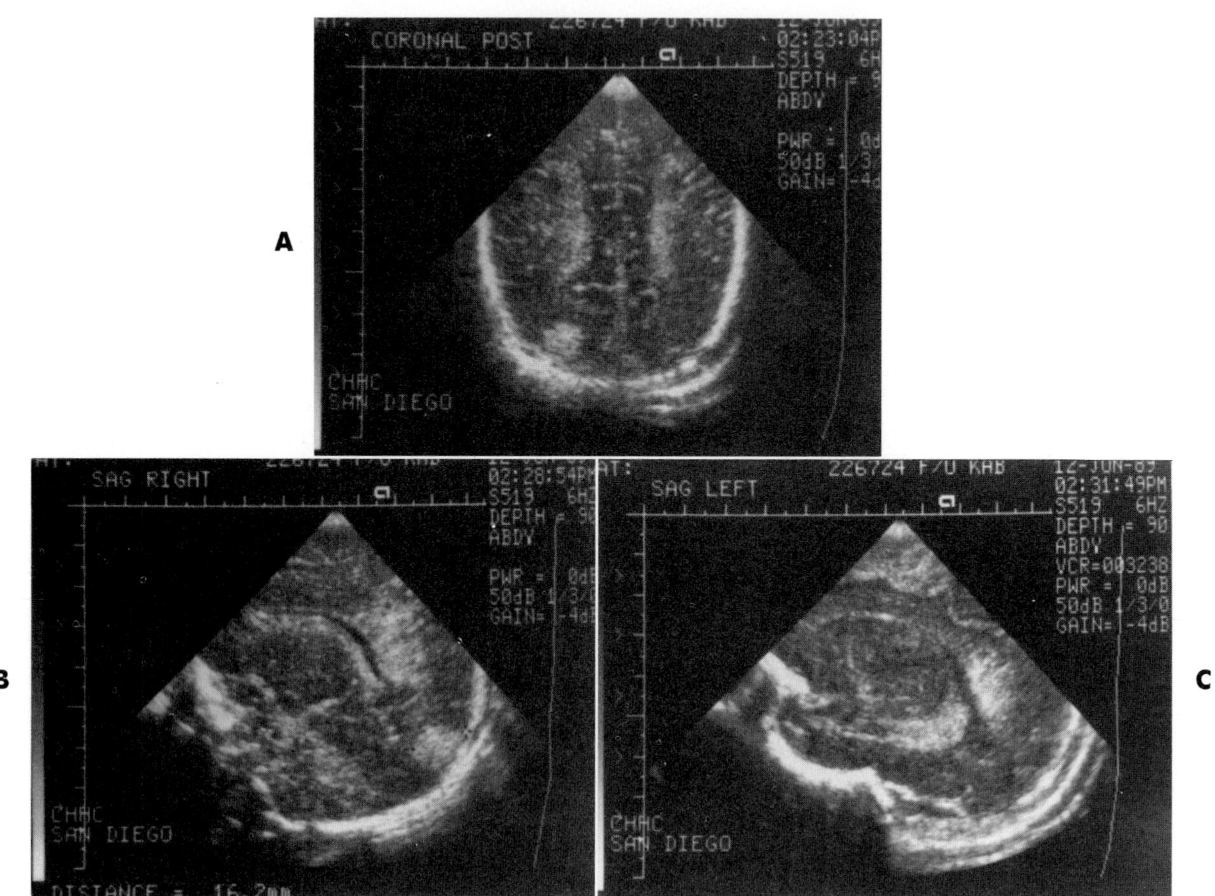

FIG. 16-48 A to **C**, Follow-up study of the patient in Fig. 16-47 shows small cystic changes within the congested parenchyma representing PVL. This patient had a history of nephrotic syndrome and a cerebellar bleed in the right.

rior and lateral to the frontal horns, bodies, atria, and occipital horns of the lateral ventricles (Figs. 16-47 to 16-49). Echodense areas are present during the first week after delivery and usually resolve in the following weeks.‡ Microscopically, the echodensities consist of congestion, microhemorrhages, and foci of necrosis.[7] However, echodensities may be associated only with congestion and microhemorrhages without necrosis.[7]

The chronic stage of WMN is identified with ultrasound when echolucencies develop in the echogenic white matter (Figs. 16-50 to 16-52). Pathologic studies have confirmed that echolucent lesions correspond to cavitary lesions in the white matter.[7] The presence of echolucencies is prima facie evidence that necrotic injury exists in the cerebral white matter. Echodensities alone suggest, but do not prove, that the echodense white matter is necrotic. The absence of cystic lesions in the echoencephalogram precludes definitive diagnosis of WMN. Since very echogenic white matter can be simply congestion without coagulation, and in fact not necessarily white matter necrosis at all, careful sequential observations must be performed to identify cavitary lesions developing in the echo-dense white matter. Cystic lesions in WMN may be microscopic or smaller than the resolution of the ultrasound scanners. Consequently WMN may exist in the absence of cavitary lesions in the sonograms.

Both neuropathologic and echoencephalographic studies have shown that a period of 1 to 6 weeks ensues between the acute stage of WMN and the development of cystic lesions. Echogenic areas and cysts decrease in size and eventually disappear 2 to 5 months after the diagnosis of acute necrosis. If the necrosis was extensive, brain atrophy may be the only indication that WMN occurred during the perinatal period. ECHO is also useful to diagnose the atrophic phase of the chronic stage. This phase is identified by an enlarged subarachnoid space, widened interhemispheric fissure, and persistent ventricular dilation in an infant with a normal or small head circumference (Fig. 16-53).

Focal Brain Necrosis. These necrotic lesions occur within the distribution of large arteries. This complication is present in term and preterm infants, but it is infrequent under 30 weeks gestational age.[5,45] Vascular maldevelopment, asphyxia or hypoxia, embolism from the placenta,

‡References 4, 21, 30b, 35, 45

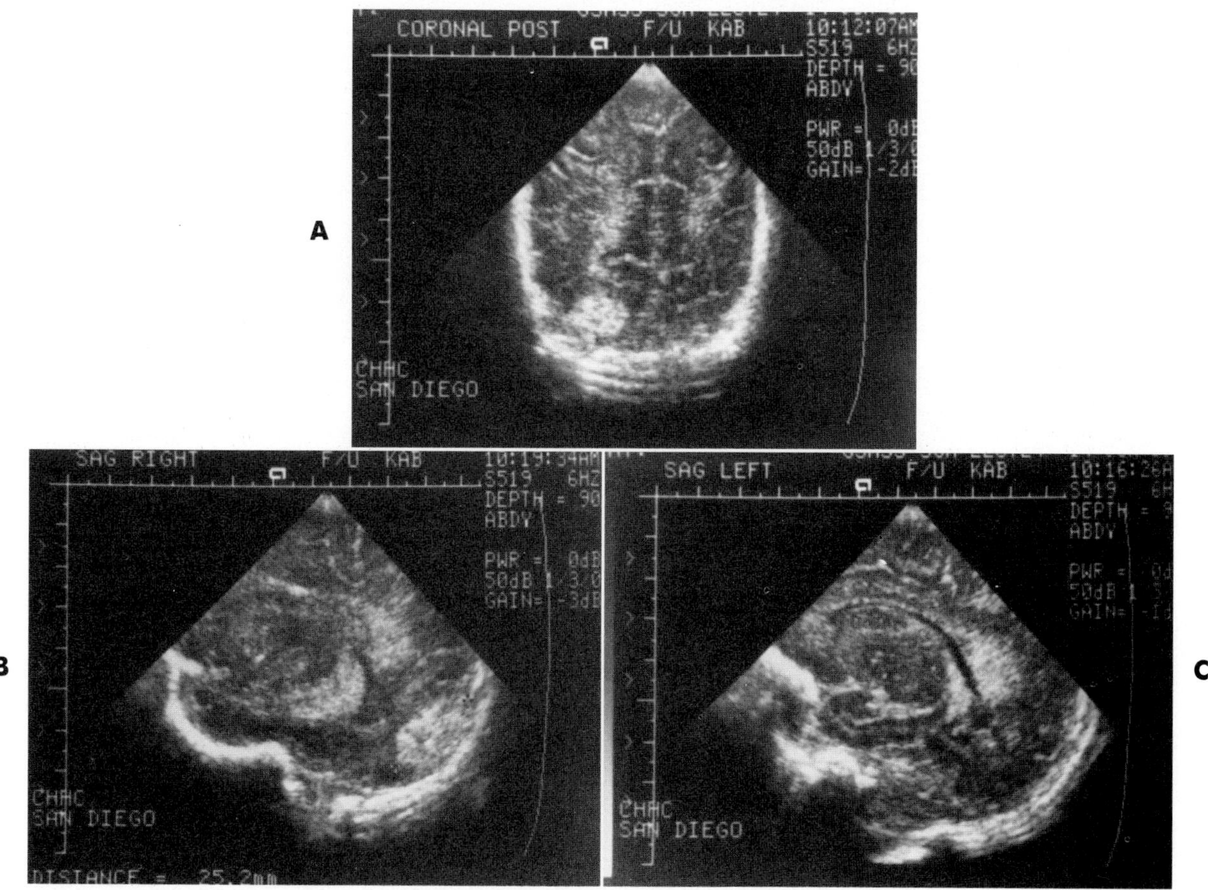

FIG. 16-49 A and **B,** Follow-up study 1-week later of the same patient in Fig. 16-47 and 48 shows the brightly echogenic bleed in the cerebellar area on the right along with congestion and small cystic changes in the parenchyma.

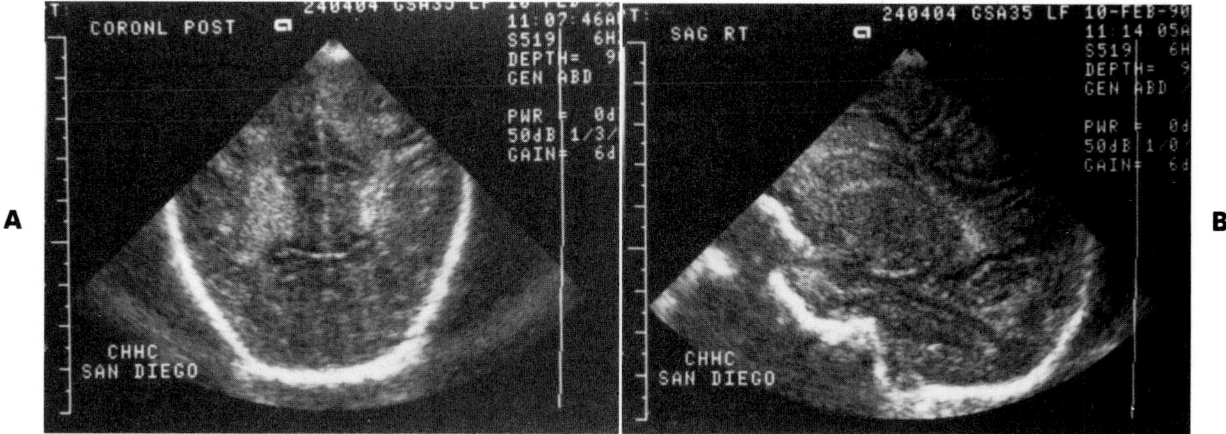

FIG. 16-50 A and **B,** A 35-week-old premature infant with meningitis and PVL.

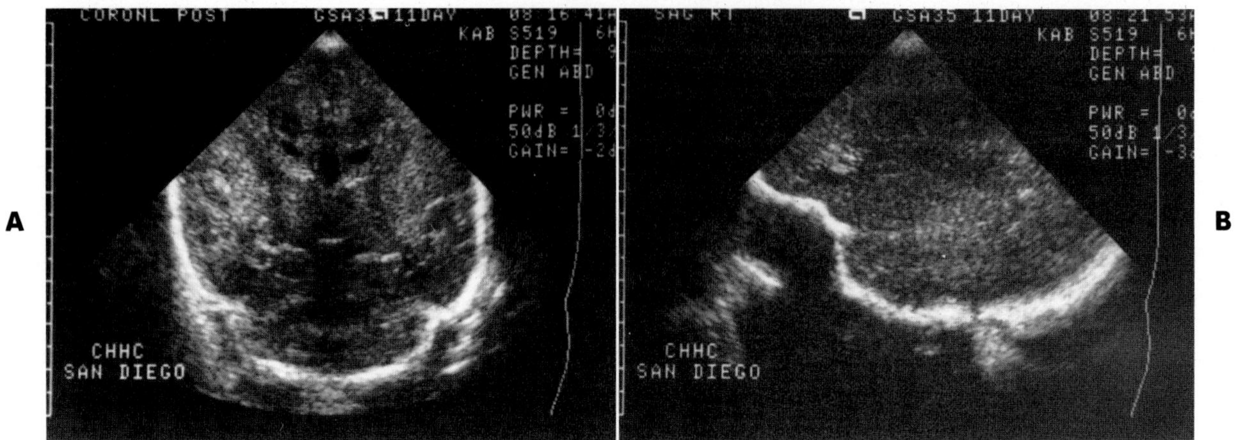

FIG. 16-51 A and B, Follow-up study of the patient in Fig. 16-50 shows a septal vein in the cavum septum pellicidum and increased ventricular size.

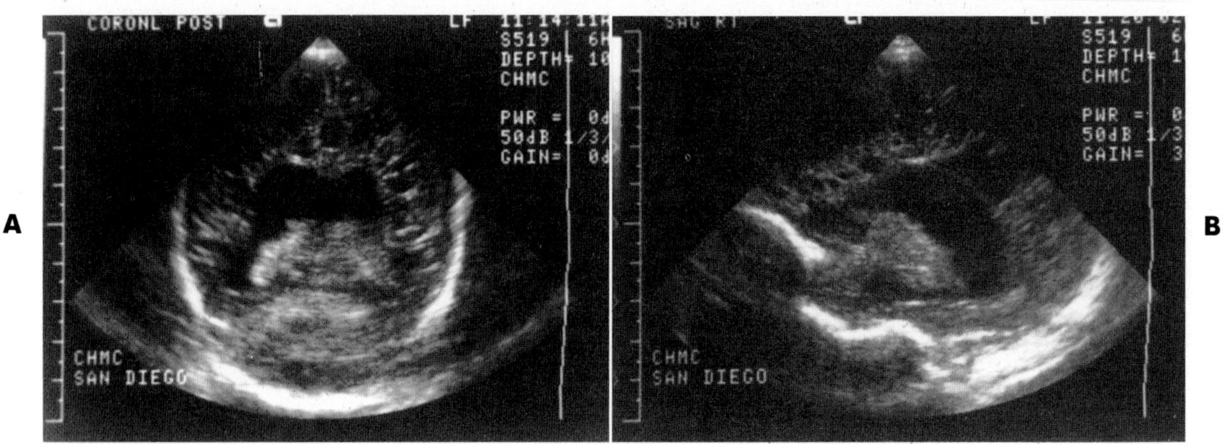

FIG. 16-52 A and B, Follow-up study 3 months later of the patient in Fig. 16-50 and 16-51 shows huge, dilated cystic changes throughout the brain parenchyma secondary to PVL.

infectious diseases, thromboembolism secondary to disseminated intravascular coagulation, and polycythemia have been implicated as etiologic factors in this condition.[39,45] These insults may occur prenatally or early in postnatal life, leading subsequently to the dissolution of the cerebral tissues and formation of cavitary lesions. The term *porencephaly* is used to describe a single cavity, multicystic encephalomalacia for multiple cavities, and hydranencephaly for a large single cavity with entire disappearance of the cerebral hemispheres.[39,45]

The images observed with ECHO in these injuries are very echogenic localized lesions within the distribution of the major vessel. The echo-dense lesions are considered to correspond to cerebral infarctions. After several days echolucencies appear within the echogenic areas. Subsequently the infarcted regions are replaced by cavities that may or may not communicate with the ventricle.

BRAIN INFECTIONS

Ventriculitis

Ventriculitis is a common complication of purulent meningitis in newborn infants. Ventriculitis probably is caused by hematogenous spread of the infection to the choroid plexus. The presence of a foreign body in the ventricular cavity, such as a catheter from a ventriculoperitoneal shunt, may provide a nidus for persistent infection of the ventricular cavities.

Ventriculitis leads to compartmentalization of the ventricular cavities by inflammatory adhesions extending from wall to wall. The first stage of ventriculitis is seen in ECHO as very thin septations extending from the walls of the lateral ventricles (Fig. 16-54). The septa become thicker and lead to multilocular hydrocephalus and extensive disorganization of the brain anatomy. Sequential studies in patients with meningitis or with ventriculoperitoneal shunts can provide early diagnosis of this severe complication.

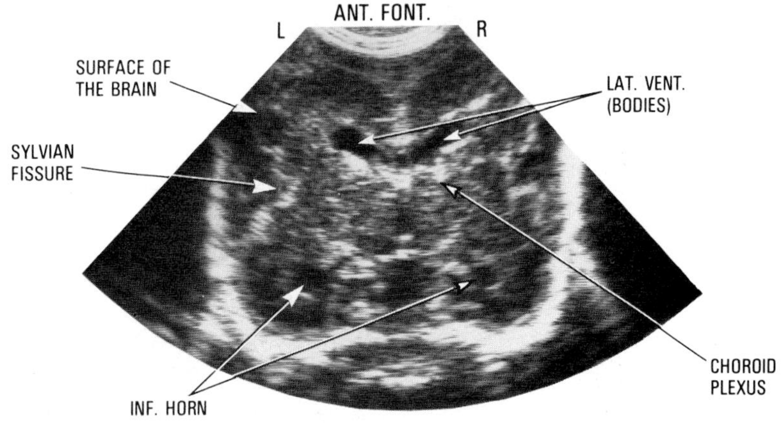

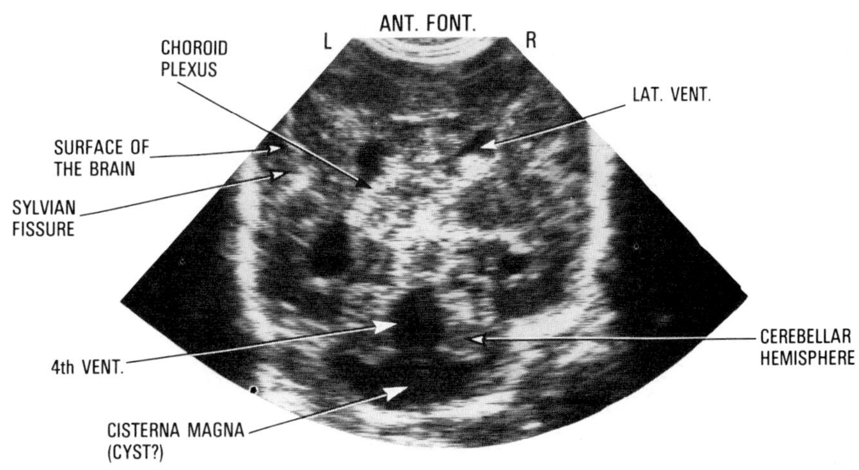

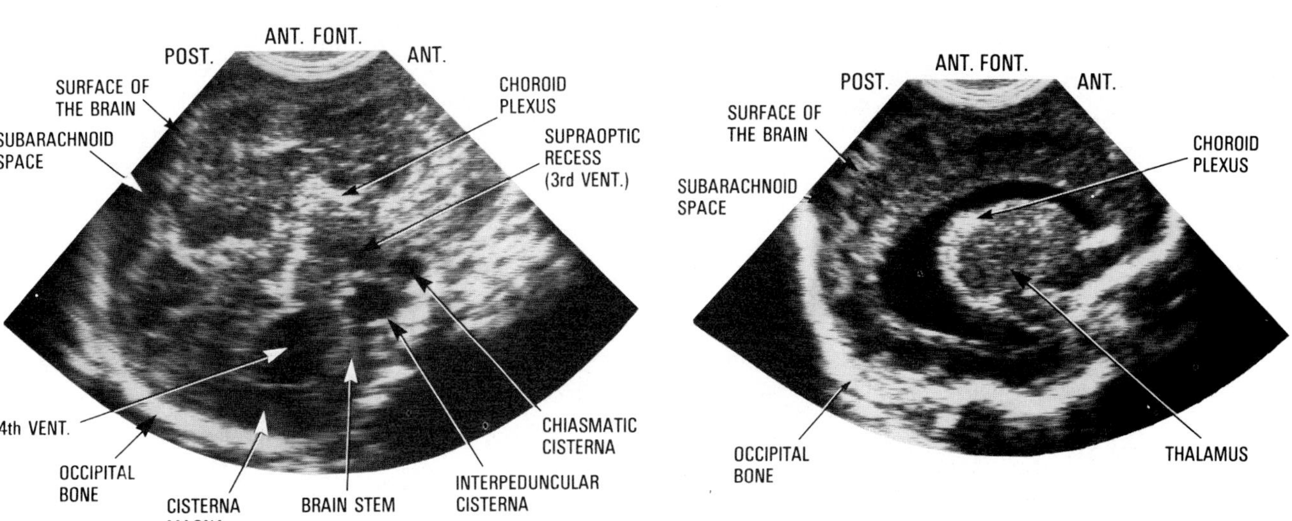

FIG. 16-53 Brain atrophy. Note the enlargement of the subarachnoid space, the widening of the Sylvian fissure, and the cisterns associated with moderate dilatation of the lateral ventricles. This patient had cerebellar infarctions imitating a Dandy-Walker malformation. *Continued.*

PARASAGITTAL PLANE (EXTERIOR)

POST.
ANT. FONT.
ANT.
SUBARACHNOID SPACE
SURFACE OF THE BRAIN
OCCIPITAL BONE

FIG. 16-53, cont'd. Brain atrophy.

CORONAL STUDIES

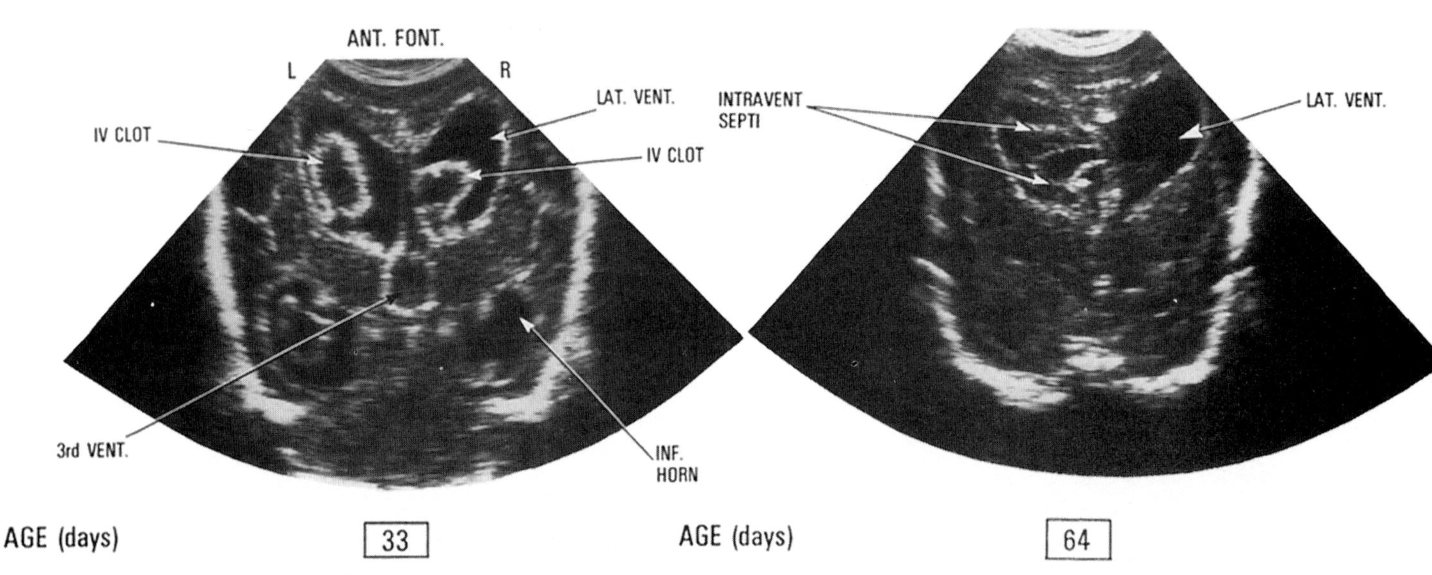

FIG. 16-54 Echoencephalograms in preterm infant with placement of a ventriculoperitoneal shunt. Note the septa extending from one wall to the other and eventual thickening of the septa with the formation of multiocular hydrocephalus and total disruption of the brain anatomy. *Continued.*

CORONAL STUDIES—cont'd

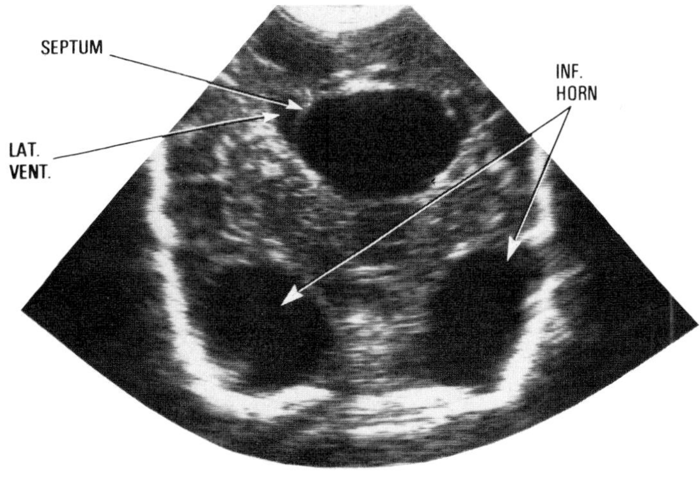

AGE (days) 96

PARASAGITTAL STUDIES

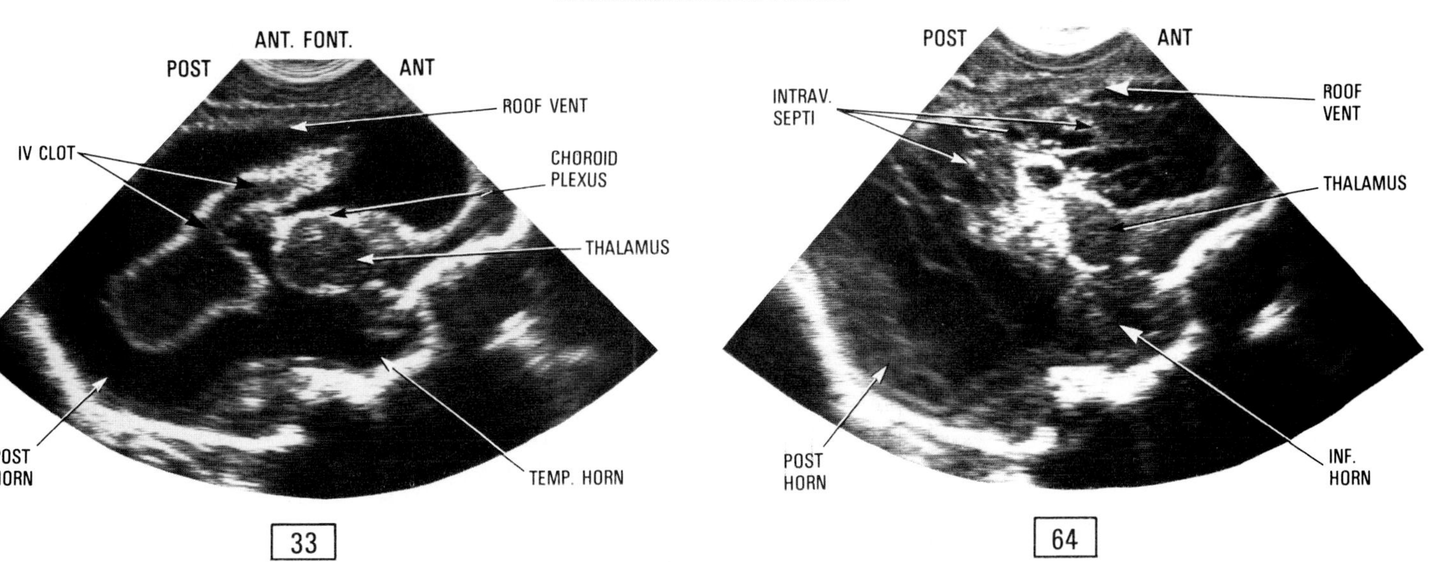

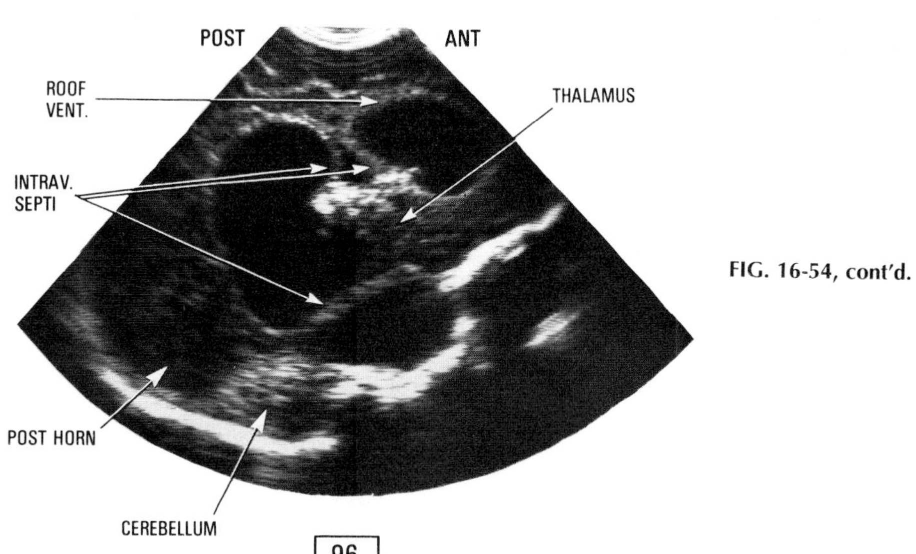

FIG. 16-54, cont'd.

Continued.

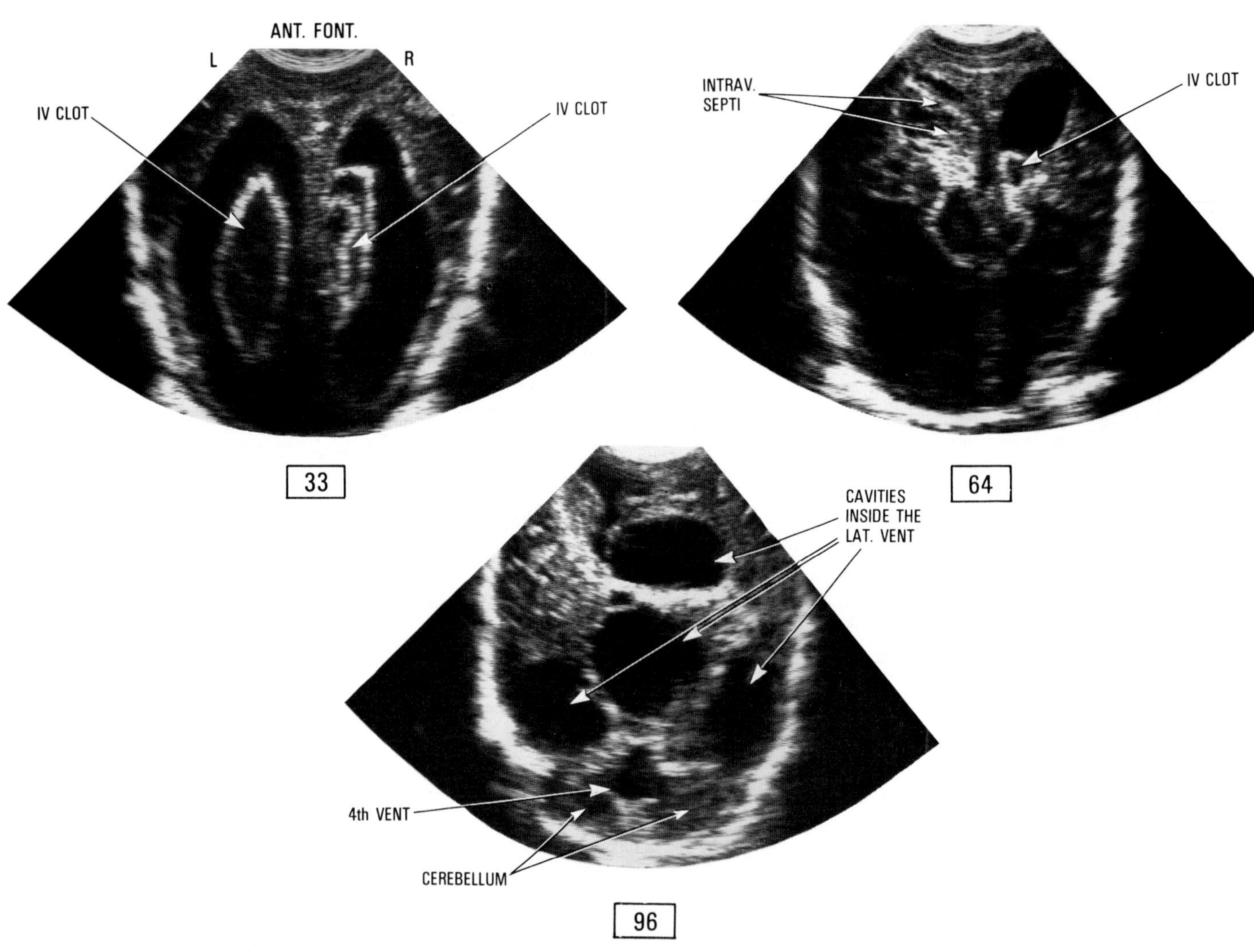

FIG. 16-54, cont'd. For legend see p. 16-46.

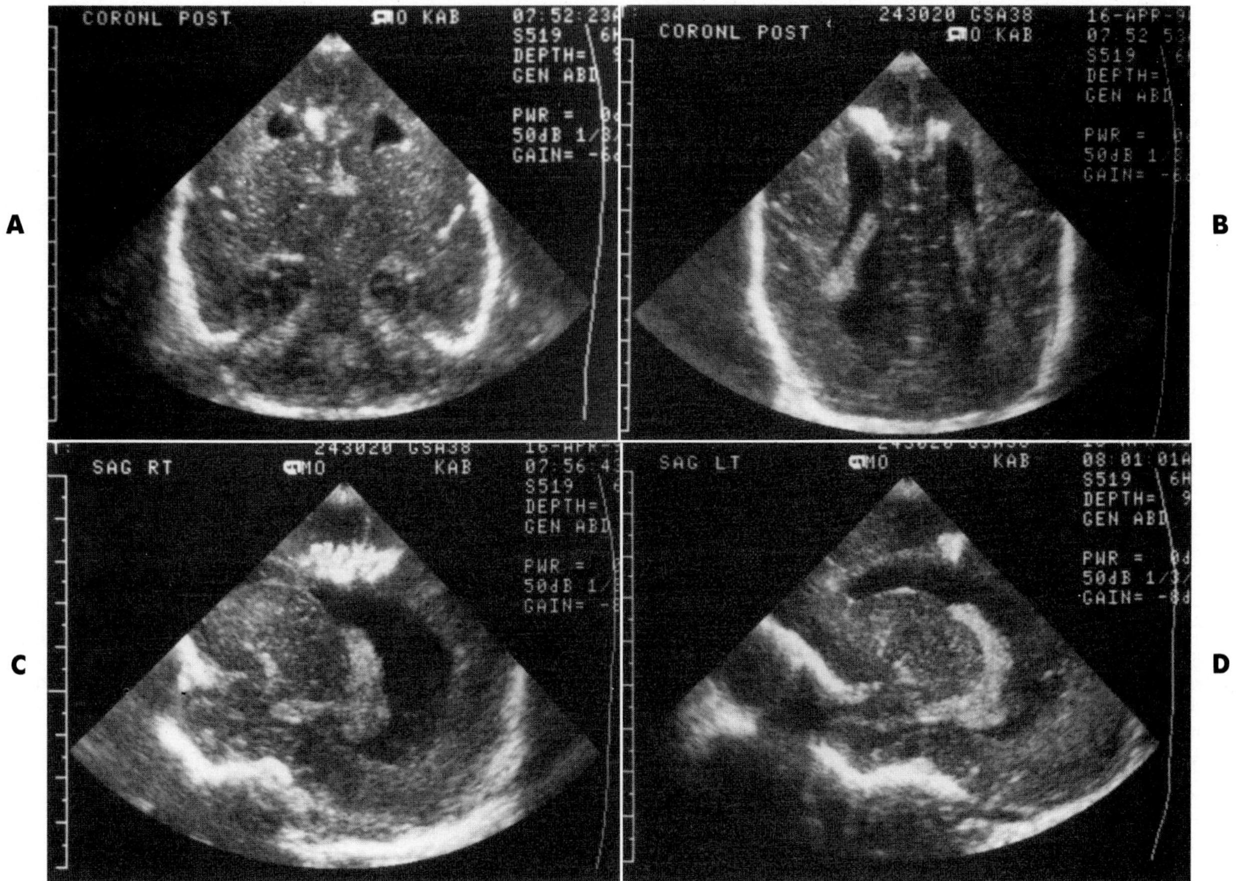

FIG. 16-55 A to **D,** A 1-month-old infant with bright calcifications bilaterally secondary to cytomegalovirus.

REVIEW QUESTIONS

1. What soft-tissue structure is seen within the third ventricle when it is dilated?
2. The lateral ventricles drain via what structure?
3. What connects the third and fourth ventricles?
4. What anatomic landmark within the brain is used to find the middle cerebral arteries?
5. Name the four segments of the lateral ventricles.
6. What transducer frequency is commonly used for neonatal brain echo studies?
7. Name the fontanelle through which the neonatal brain may be scanned.
8. Name four reasons why neonatal brains hemorrhage.
9. What is an Apgar score? Describe the scoring system.
10. A subependymal hemorrhage is found at what site?
11. List the grades of intracranial hemorrhage and define each.
12. Within what other structures does the choroid plexus lie?
13. Where is the most common site for a choroid plexus hemorrhage?
14. Define periventricular leukomalcia.
15. Name the etiologies for periventricular leukomalacia.
16. Define TORCH.
17. Define encephalitis.
18. What sonographic finding is seen in the neonatal brain with cytomegalovirus?
19. Agenesis of the corpus callosum may indicate what malformation?

REFERENCES

1. Armstrong D and Norman MG: Periventricular leukomalacia in neonates, Arch Childhood 49:367, 1974.
2. Armstrong E, Harwood-Nash D, Hoffman H, et al: Benign suprasellar cysts: the CT approach, AJNR 4:163, 1983.
3. Babcock D: Cranial ultrasonography of infants. Baltimore, Williams & Wilkins, 1981.
4. Babcock D and Han B: The accuracy of high resolution real time ultrasonography of the head in infancy, Radiology 139:664, 1981.
5. Barmada M, Moosy J, and Shuman R: Cerebral infarcts with arterial occlusion in neonates, Ann Neurol 6:495, 1979.
6. Barson A: Spina bifida: the significance of the level and extent of the defect to the morphogenesis, Dev Med Child Neurol 12:129, 1970.

7. Bejar R, Coen R, Merritt TA, et al: Focal necrosis of the white matter (periventricular leukomalacia): sonographic, pathologic, and electroencephalographic features, AJNR 7:1073, 1986.
8. Bejar R, Wozniak P, Allard M, et al: Antenatal origin of neurologic damage in newborn infants. Part I. Preterm infants, Am J Obstet Gynecol, 1987.
9. Bowerman RA, Donn SM, Silver TM, and Jaffe MH: Natural history of neonatal periventricular/intraventricular hemorrhage and its complications: sonographic observations, AJNR 5:527, 1985.
10. Bozynski MEA, Nelson MN, Matalon TAS, et al: Cavitary periventricular leukomalacia: incidence and short term outcome in infants weighing <1200 grams at birth, Dev Med Child Neurol 27:572, 1985.
11. Calame A, Fawer CL, Anderegg A, and Perenters E: Interaction between perinatal brain damage and processes of normal brain development, Dev Neruosci 7:1, 1985.
12. Calvert SA, Hoskins EM, Fong KW, and Forsyth SC: Periventricular leukomalacia: ultrasonic diagnosis and neurological outcome, Acta Paediatr Scan 75:489, 1986.
13. Chow PP, Horgan JG, and Taylor KJW: Neonatal periventricular leukomalacia: real-time sonographic diagnosis with CT correlation, Am J Roentgenol 145:155, 1985.
14. Donn S, Bowerman R, Dipietro M, and Gebarski S: Sonographic appearance of neonatal thalamic-striatal hemorrhage, J Ultrasound Med 3:231, 1984.
15. Dubowitz LMS, Bydder GM, and Mushin J: Developmental sequence of periventricular leukomalacia, Arch Dis Child 60:349, 1985.
16. Gilles FH, Levinton A, and Kerr C: Endotoxin leucoencephalopathy in the telencephalon of the newborn kitten, J Neurol Sci 27:183, 1976.
17. Gilles F, Price R, Kevy S, and Berenberg W: Fibrinolytic activity in the ganglionic eminence of the premature human brain, Biol Neonate 18:426, 1971.
18. Grant E, Schellinger D, and Richardson J: Real time ultrasonography of the posterior fossa, J Ultrasound Med 2:73, 1983.
19. Grant EG and Schellinger D: Sonography of neonatal periventricular leukomalacia: recent experience with a 7.5 MHz scanner, AJNR 6:781, 1985.
20. Hambleton G and Wigglesworth J: Origin of intraventricular hemorrhage in the preterm infant, Arch Dis Child 51:651, 1976.
21. Harwood-Nash D and Fitz C: Neuroradiology in infants and children. St. Louis, Mosby, 1976.
22. Hill A, Melson GL, Clark HB, and Volpe JJ: Hemorrhagic periventricular leukomalacia: diagnosis by real time ultrasound and correlation with autopsy findings, Pediatrics 169:282, 1982.
23. Icenogle D and Kaplan A: A review of congenital neurologic malformations, Clin Pediatr 20:565, 1981.
24. Jellinger K, Gross H, Kaltenback E, and Grisold W: Holoprosencephaly and agenesis of the corpus callosum: frequency of associated malformation, Acta Neuropathol 55:1, 1981.
25. Johnson ML, Dunne MG, Mack LA, et al: Evaluation of fetal intracranial anatomy by static and real-time ultrasound, J Clin Ultrasound 8:311, 1980.
26. Kreusser K, Schmidt R, Shackelford G, and Volpe J: Value of ultrasound for identification of acute hemorrhagic necrosis of thalamus and basal ganglia in an asphyxiated term infant, Ann Neurol 16:361, 1984.
27. Larroch J: Developmental pathology of the neonate. Amsterdam, Elsevier North Holland, 1977.
28. Levene M, Wigglesworth J, and Dubovitz V: Hemorrhagic periventricular leukomalacia in the neonate: a real time ultrasound study, Pediatrics 71:794, 1983.
29. Leviton A and Gilles FH: Acquired perinatal leukoencephalopathy, Ann Neurol 16:1, 1984.
30a. Matsumura G and England M: Embryology colouring book. England, 1992, Wolfe.
30b. McMenamin J, Shackelford G, and Volpe J: Outcome of neonatal intraventricular hemorrhage with periventricular echo-dense lesions, Ann Neurol 15:285, 1984.
30. Mealey J, Gimor R, and Bubb M: The prognosis of hydrocephalus at birth, J Neurosurg 39:348, 1973.
31. Moore KL: the developing human. Philadelphia, WB Saunders, 1992.
32. Naeye RL: Amniotic fluid infections, neonatal hyperbilirubinemia, and psychomotor impairment, Pediatrics 62:497, 1978.
33. Nelson KB and Ellenberg JH: Predictors of low and very low birth weight and the relation of these to cerebral palsy, JAMA 254:1473, 1985.
34. Rumack C and Johnson M: Role of computed tomography and ultrasound in neonatal brain imaging, J Comput Assist Tomogr 7:17, 1983.
35. Rumack C and Johnson M: Perinatal and infant brain imaging role of ultrasound and computed tomography. Chicago, Year Book, 1984.
36. Schellinger D, Grant EG, and Richardson JD: Cystic periventricular leukomalacia: sonographic and CT findings, AJNR 5:439, 1984.
37. Schelliner D, Grant EG, and Richardson JD: Neonatal leukoencephalopathy: a common form of cerebral ischemia, Radio Graphics 5:221, 1985.
38. Shemitt H: Multicystic encephalopathy, a polietiologic condition in early infancy: morphologic, pathogenic and clinical aspects, Brain Dev 1:1, 1984.
39. Schuman R and Selednik L: Periventricular leukomalacia: a one-year autopsy study, Arch Neurol 37:231, 1980.
40. Sims ME, Turkel SB, Halterman G, and Paul RH: Brain injury and intrauterine death, Am J Obstet Gynecol 151:721, 1985.
41. Sinha SK, Sims DG, Davies JM, and Chiswick ML: Relation between periventricular haemorrhage and ischaemic brain lesions diagnosed by ultrasound in very pre-term infants, Lancet 2:1154, 1985.
42. Trounce JQ, Fagan D, and Levene MI: Intraventricular haemorrhage and periventricular leukomalacia: ultrasound and autopsy correlation, Arch Dis Child 61:1203, 1986.
43. Volpe JJ: Normal and abnormal human brain development, Clin Perinatol 4:3, 1977.
44. Volpe JJ: Neurology of the newborn, Philadelphia, WB Saunders, 1987.
45. Weindling AM, Wilkinson AR, Cook J, and Calvert SA: Perinatal events which precede periventricular haemorrhage and leukomalacia in the newborn, Br J Obstet Gynaecol 92:1218, 1985.
47. Young RSK, Hernandez MJ, and Yagel SK: Selective reduction of blood flow to white matter during hypotension in newborn dogs: a possible mechanism of periventricular leukomalacia, Ann Neurol 12:445, 1985.

BIBLIOGRAPHY

Dimmick JE and Kolousek D: Central nervous system. Developmental pathology of the embryo and fetus. Philadelphia, JB Lippincott, 1992.

Evans DH: Doppler ultrasound and the neonatal cerebral circulation: methodology and pitfalls, Biol Neonate, 62:271, 1992.

Fenton AC, Papathoma E, Evans DH, and Levene MI: Neonatal cerebral venous flow velocity measurement using a color flow Doppler system, J Clin Ultrasound, 19:69, 1991.

Fenton AC, Shortland DB, Papathoma E, et al: Normal range for blood flow velocity in cerebral arteries of newly born term infants, Early Hum Dev 22:73, 1990.

van de Bor M, Walther FJ, and Sims ME: Acceleration time in cerebral arteries of preterm and term infants, J Clin Ultrasound 18:167, 1990.

Raju TN and Kim SY: Cerebral artery flow velocity acceleration and deceleration characteristics in newborn infants, Pediatr Res 26:588, 1989.

Horgan JG, Rumack CM, Hay T, et al: Absolute intracranial blood-flow velocities evaluated by duplex Doppler sonography in asymptomatic preterm and term neonates, Am J Roentgenol 152:1059, 1989.

Wong WS, Tsuruda JS, Liberman RL, et al: Color Doppler imaging of intracranial vessels in the neonate, Am J Roentgenol 152:1065, 1989.

CHAPTER 17

Pediatric Abdomen-Surgical Conditions

Suzanne M. Devine • Kate A. Feinstein • Arnold Shkolnik

In many institutions, sonography is now the initial imaging procedure used to evaluate infants and children with acute abdominal problems. This chapter focuses on sonographic examination techniques for detecting the more common surgical conditions that may be responsible for pain or vomiting and the ultrasound appearance of these entities. Hypertrophic pyloric stenosis, appendicitis, and intussusception are discussed.

Gaining the trust of the patient and the patient's family can do much to facilitate the examination. Therefore the sonographer should first allow sufficient time to explain the examination to the parents and to the child who is old enough to comprehend the proceedings. Sedation and immobilization techniques are generally not required. Toys, books, keys, mobiles, and a variety of other distracting devices can be very helpful in quieting the frightened young child. A pacifier or bottle feeding may likewise serve well when examining infants. Parents are encouraged to be present during the examination and can help reassure and quiet the patient.

Virtually no routine patient preparation is required. However, adequate distention of the urinary bladder is most desirable in some situations. This not only allows assessment of the bladder itself, but it facilitates identification of dilated distal ureters, free peritoneal fluid, the pelvic genitalia, and a pelvic mass. A urine-filled bladder may also help localize gastrointestinal abnormalities, such as appendicitis and intussusception.

HYPERTROPHIC PYLORIC STENOSIS

The pyloric canal is located between the stomach and duodenum. In some infants the pyloric muscle can become hypertrophied, resulting in significantly delayed gastric emptying. The pyloric canal itself is not intrinsically stenotic or narrowed, but it functions as if it were as a result of the abnormally thickened surrounding muscle.

Hypertrophic pyloric stenosis (HPS) presents most commonly in male infants between 3 and 6 weeks of age. Rarely, it becomes apparent at birth or as late as 5 months of age.[15] Bile-free emesis in an otherwise healthy infant is the most frequent clinical presentation.[6,25] As the pyloric muscle thickens and elongates, the stomach outlet obstruction increases and vomiting is more constant and projectile. Dehydration and weight loss may ensue. Peristaltic waves and reverse peristaltic waves crossing the upper abdomen may be observed during or after feeding as the stomach attempts to force its contents through the abnormal canal. In these infants, palpation of an olive-shaped mass in the right upper quadrant is diagnostic.[8,25] In infants with a suggestive history or an equivocal physical examination, diagnostic imaging is required (Fig. 17-1).[25,30]

In many pediatric radiology departments and in other radiology departments where there is appropriate expertise, sonography is the imaging method of choice to establish the diagnosis of HPS.* If HPS is not a primary diagnostic consideration or if the sonogram is not diagnostic, conventional contrast radiography of the upper gastrointestinal tract is necessary to assess for other potential causes of vomiting (e.g., gastrointestinal reflux, antral web, pylorospasm, hiatal hernia, and malrotation of the bowel) (Fig. 17-2).[8]

The neonate with projectile vomiting frequently is sent directly from the physician's office or the hospital emergency room. If the stomach is empty and HPS is not readily apparent, an oral feeding is given to facilitate comprehensive visualization of the pyloric area (Fig. 17-3).[9] Conversely, an overly distended stomach can displace the pyloric muscle posteriorly, making sonographic delineation virtually impossible (Fig. 17-4).[7] In this instance, aspiration of gastric contents via a nasogastric tube may be required.[3]

The infant is examined first in the supine and then in the right lateral decubitus position. A preliminary survey of the abdomen is performed to exclude abnormalities such as hydronephrosis or adrenal hemorrhage. Real time imaging is then performed using a 5-MHz or 7-MHz linear array transducer. Longitudinal images of the pyloric muscle are obtained by placing the transducer transversely across the right upper quadrant, just below the level of the xiphoid process. The transducer is then rotated obliquely until the pyloric muscle is visualized in its long axis (Fig. 17-5). Transverse short-axis images of the pyloric muscle are obtained from the right coronal plane. The gallbladder is initially identi-

*References 4, 5, 8, 9, 16, 27.

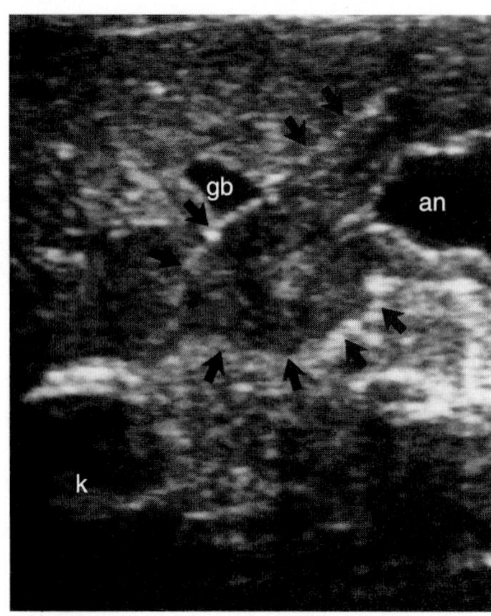

FIG. 17-1 Transverse image of the right upper quadrant using the liver as an acoustic window in a 5-week-old boy with hypertrophic pyloric stenosis shows a longitudinal view of an elongated thickened pyloric muscle *(arrows)*. The antrum, *an*, is filled with fluid. The gall bladder, *gb*, is anterior to the pyloric muscle, whereas the right kidney, *k*, is posterior and lateral.

fied, after which the transducer is angled medially until the bull's-eye appearance of the pyloric muscle and echogenic central canal is noted (Fig. 17-6).

If the diagnosis has not been established, the patient is then placed in a right lateral decubitus position and the transducer placed transversely in the right upper quadrant. This allows maximum visualization of the stomach and pyloric canal and is most advantageous for documenting the transit of gastric contents into the duodenum.

Pyloric muscle measurements can be made in both the short- and long-axis planes. Individual muscle wall thickness, total diameter, and length of the pyloric canal are measured. Thickness is measured from the periphery of the hypoechoic muscle to its junction with the echogenic central canal. Diameter is measured between the peripheral margins of the hypoechoic muscle layer. Length is measured from the proximal to the distal extremes of the echogenic central canal.

Sonographic diagnosis of HPS depends on the following findings: (1) visualization of a hypertrophied pyloric muscle with a canal measuring 17 mm or greater, (2) individual pyloric muscle wall thickness of 4 mm or greater, or (3) a pyloric diameter of 10 mm or greater.* An additional significant finding is the presence of active antegrade and reverse gastric peristalsis.[6]

APPENDICITIS

After gastroenteritis, appendicitis is the most common acute abdominal inflammatory process in children. Appendicitis occurs when the appendiceal lumen becomes obstructed and subsequently infected. In infants and young children the progression of acute appendicitis to perforation is more rapid than in older children and adults, sometimes occurring within 6 to 12 hours.[10] Classical physical and laboratory findings may be absent or confusing, making the diagnosis difficult.

Right lower quadrant pain and vomiting are a common clinical presentation. In addition to appendicitis, diagnostic considerations include enteritis, inflammatory bowel disease, and lymphoma. In girls the differential broadens to include gynecologic processes such as ovarian cysts and neoplasms as well as ovarian torsion.

Sonography has proven to be very accurate in confirming appendicitis.† As in virtually all conditions, a survey examination of the abdomen is first performed to assess the upper abdomen and the kidneys and bladder. In girls the adnexal areas should be examined. The right flank and right lower quadrant are reexamined using a 5-MHz or 7-MHz linear array transducer. The transducer is moved slowly over the abdomen using the graded compression technique described by Puylaert.[19] This technique enables the sonographer to visualize the appendix by displacing adjacent bowel loops. The appendix is usually seen anterior and medial to the psoas muscle and lateral to the iliac vessels.

Sivit et al. reported that of children with abdominal pain not resulting from appendicitis, 56% had a normal appendix.[23] Nonvisualization of the appendix may occur for multiple reasons and is not a definite indication of a normal appendix. Appendiceal nonvisualization may result from any of the following: (1) obscuration by overlying bowel, (2) retrocecal position of the appendix, (3) overdistention or nondistention of the urinary bladder, which alters the position of the appendix and overlying bowel, or (4) lack of sonographer experience.[22] Changing the patient's position and emptying or filling the urinary bladder may facilitate visualization of both the normal and abnormal appendix.[21]

The normal appendix appears as a blind-ending, long, tubular structure as seen in the longitudinal plane, and has a bull's-eye appearance in the transverse plane.[22,23] Peristalsis is not seen in the appendix, allowing differentiation of normal appendix and small bowel.[23] It may be tortuous and therefore difficult to visualize in its entirety. The walls are not thickened, and the normal appendix compresses easily.[21,23]

Sonographically the acutely inflamed appendix is noncompressible (Fig. 17-7). The appendix is measured in the transverse plane, across the short axis, using the maximum diameter. An outer diameter greater than 6 mm with compression is consistent with appendicitis both in children and adults.* Localized pain produced by overlying transducer pressure is an additional finding consistent with appendicitis. Other findings in appendicitis may include free perito-

*References 5, 9, 16, 17, 27

†References 10, 12, 21, 24, 32

*References 10, 13, 22, 23, 24

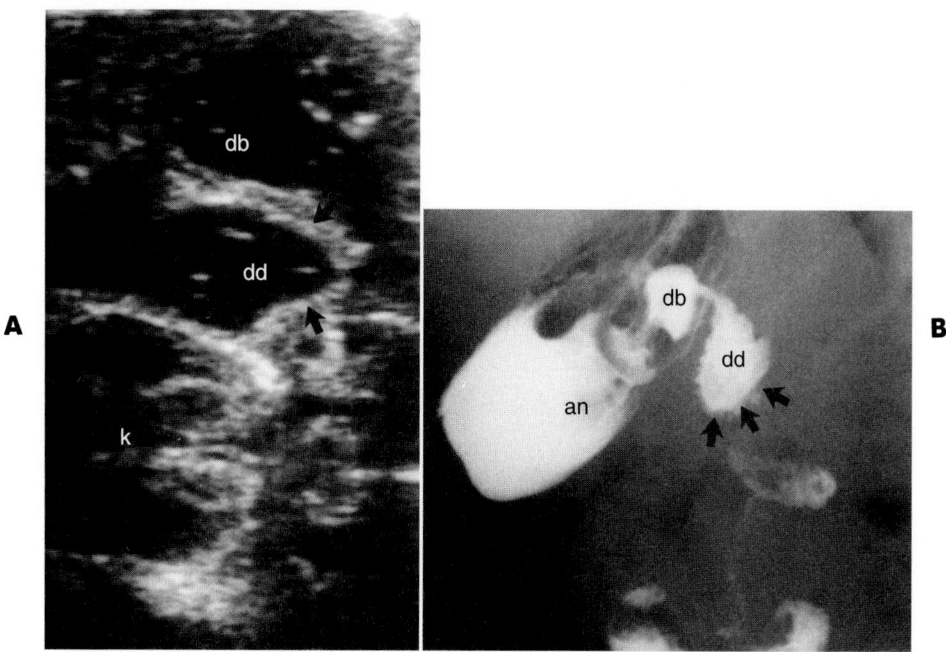

FIG. 17-2 A, Transverse image of the right upper quadrant using the liver as an acoustic window in a 4-week-old boy with projectile vomiting. There was to-and-fro peristalsis in the fluid-filled duodenal bulb, *db,* and descending duodenum, *dd*. The descending duodenum tapered abruptly *(arrows)* and could not be traced distally. The right kidney, *k,* is posterior to the descending duodenum. A hypertrophied pyloric muscle was not identified. **B,** Right lateral view from a barium examination in the same patient shows the stomach, antrum, *an,* duodenal bulb, *db,* and descending duodenum, *dd*. The descending duodenum tapers abruptly *(arrows)* and then spirals inferiorly. The barium examination delineates the surgically emergent malrotation, which could not be identified on the sonogram.

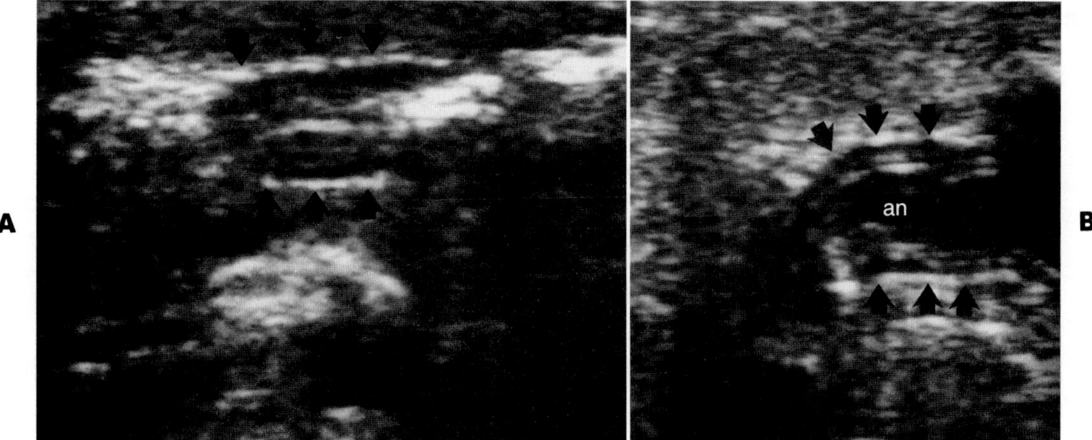

FIG. 17-3 A, Transverse view of the right upper quadrant in a 5-week-old boy. The antrum *(arrows)* is collapsed and contains a linear echogenic centrum representing the interface between the lumen and mucosa. **B,** Transverse view of the right upper quadrant shows the antrum *(arrows)* in the same patient after administration of glucose water by bottle. The antrum, *an,* is now filled with fluid and is easy to differentiate from a hypertrophied pyloric muscle.

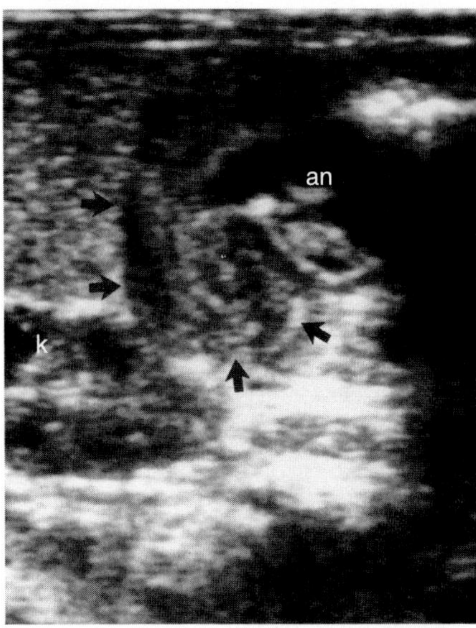

FIG. 17-4 Transverse view of the right upper quadrant in a 5-week-old boy with hypertrophic pyloric stenosis. The fluid-distended antrum, *an,* has pushed the elongated pyloric muscle *(arrows)* posteriorly, precluding accurate measurement of the length of the pyloric canal. The kidney, *k,* is lateral and slightly posterior to the pyloric muscle.

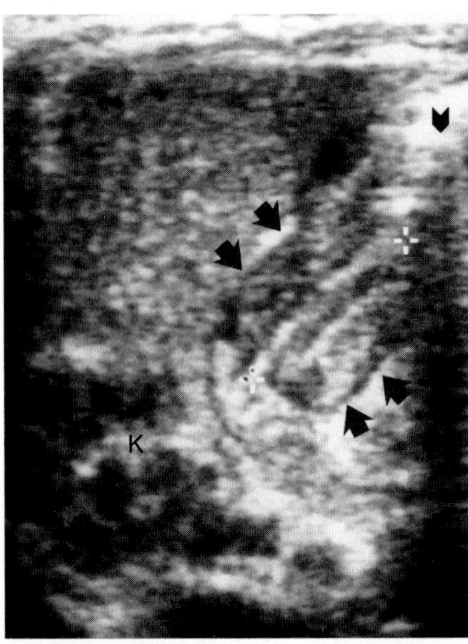

FIG. 17-5 Transverse view of the right upper quadrant shows the longitudinal extent of the hypertrophied pyloric muscle *(arrows).* The calipers measure the length of the pyloric muscle, which is 20 mm. The kidney, *k,* is posterior and lateral to the pyloric muscle. Gas *(arrowhead)* in the antrum is causing reverberation artifact.

neal fluid or a loculated fluid collection in the lower abdomen.[20,32] Confirmation of an appendicolith in a symptomatic patient is virtually diagnostic (Fig. 17-8). An appendicolith is densely echogenic, produces a classic acoustic shadow, may be single or multiple, and may be intraluminal or surrounded by a periappendiceal phlegmon or ab-

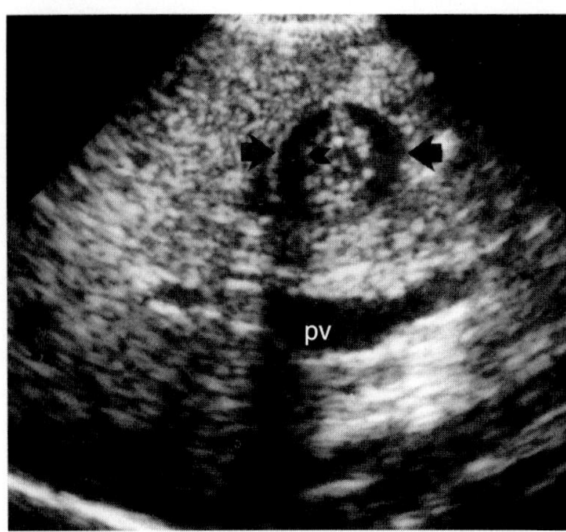

FIG. 17-6 Coronal view of the right upper quadrant shows the hypertrophied pyloric muscle in transverse section. The diameter of the muscle *(arrows)* is measured from the outer borders. The muscle thickness *(left arrow to arrowhead)* is measured from the outer border to the mucosal-muscle interface. The portal vein, *pv,* is posterior to the pyloric muscle in this plane.

scess.[23] The right kidney may at times be hydronephrotic because of ureteral inflammation.

The perforated appendix may or may not be visualized. If decompressed an abnormally thick bowel wall may be apparent.[10,20] A localized, well-defined right lower quadrant phlegmon or abscess with or without an appendicolith may be present (Fig. 17-9). Free peritoneal fluid may be the lone abnormal sonographic finding.[20] An abscess far removed from the right lower quadrant is another potential intraabdominal complication of an appendiceal perforation.

INTUSSUSCEPTION

Intussusception is the most common acute abdominal disorder in early childhood. This condition occurs when bowel prolapses into more distal bowel and is propelled in an antegrade fashion. Telescoping of bowel in this manner causes obstruction. The ileum may invaginate into more distal ileum, causing an ileoileal intussusception. If there is further progression through the ileocecal valve, an ileoileocecal intussusception results. Prolapse of the ileum into the cecum or beyond produces an ileocolic intussusception. Intussusception is usually seen in children between the ages of 6 months and 2 years. Bissett reported a higher incidence in males (2:1) and a seasonal prevalence.[2] Frequently, there is a history of an antecedent upper respiratory tract infection. Associated inflammation of lymphoid tissue in the ileocolic region may act as a lead point for the telescoping phenomenon.

Children may present with colicky abdominal pain, vomiting, and bloody (currant jelly) stools. An abdominal mass may also be palpable. In patients with this classic clinical presentation, in whom there are no peritoneal symptoms or fever, preliminary abdominal radiographs followed by a

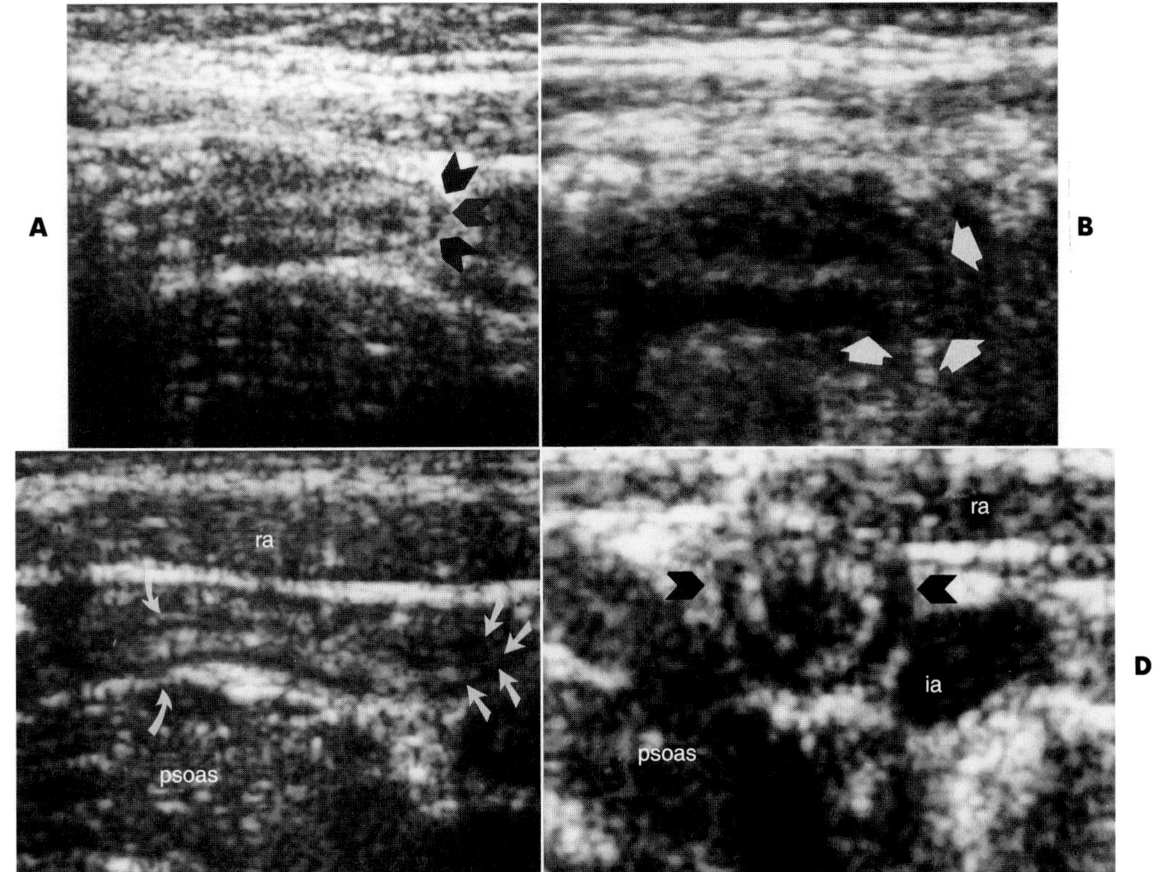

FIG. 17-7 A, Longitudinal view of an inflamed appendix using the graded compression technique. The bulbous tip *(arrowheads)* is clearly defined. **B,** Longitudinal view of a fluid-filled inflamed appendix in a different child. The bulbous tip *(arrows)* is less easily seen. **C,** Longitudinal image of the right lower quadrant in a boy with appendicitis. The rectus abdominis muscle, *ra,* of the anterior abdominal wall is being compressed with the transducer to delineate the longitudinal extent of the appendix to its blind ending tip *(arrows)*. The curved arrows demonstrate the alternating hyperechoic and hypoechoic bowel wall layers. The central echogenic band *(top curved arrow)* represents the interface between the lumen and mucosa. The most peripheral echogenic band *(bottom curved arrow)* represents the interface between the peripheral bowel wall muscle layer and the bowel wall covering. **D,** Transverse image of the right lower quadrant in the same patient demonstrates the inflamed appendix *(arrowheads)* in the transverse plane. The iliac artery, *ia,* and vein course parallel to the appendix. They can be differentiated from bowel by using Doppler imaging or tracing their course in the longitudinal plane.

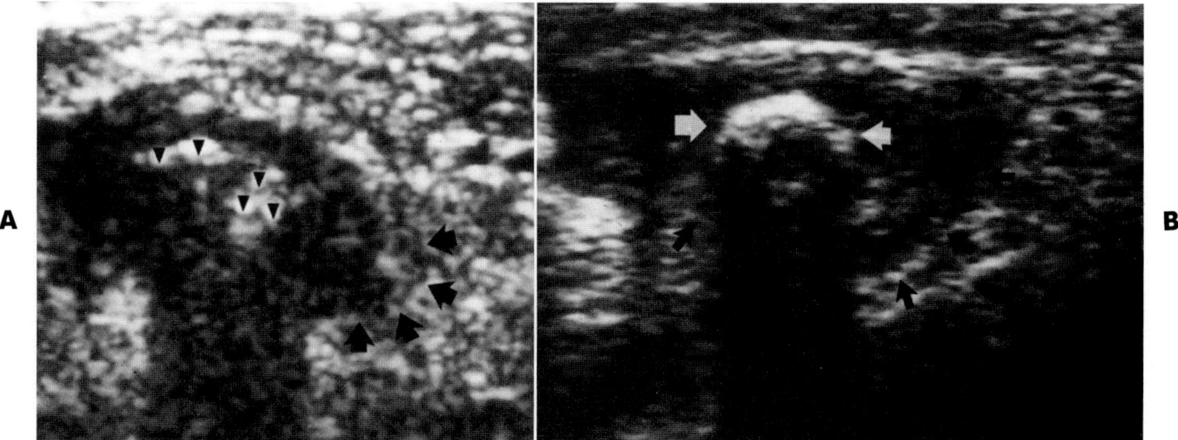

FIG. 17-8 A, Longitudinal image of an inflamed appendix containing multiple echogenic foci *(arrowheads)* consistent with appendicoliths, which cast acoustical shadows. The blind ending tip *(arrows)* confirms that the echogenic foci are within the appendix and are not gas moving through small bowel. **B,** Transverse image of an inflamed appendix in a different patient. There is a solitary appendicolith *(white arrows)* located centrally within the lumen. The hypoechoic periphery *(black arrows)* results from edema.

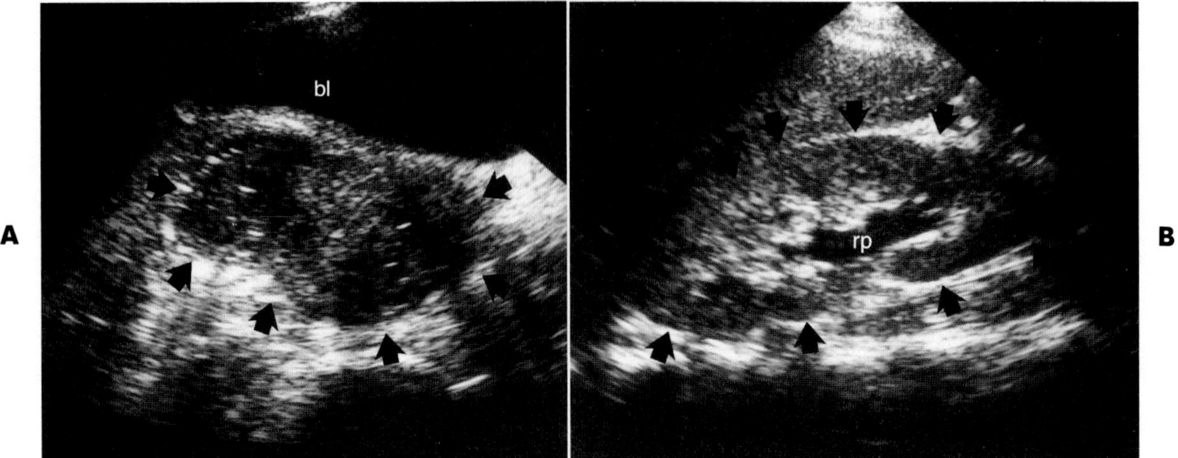

FIG. 17-9 A, Midline sagittal image in a boy with an appendiceal abscess *(arrows)* posterior to the urinary bladder, *bl*. The appendiceal abscess appears heterogeneous in echogenicity and is well demarcated from the surrounding bowel, which was actively peristaltic on real time examination. **B,** Coronal image of the right kidney *(arrows)* in the same patient shows moderate hydronephrosis because of distal ureteral inflammation from the abscess. A fluid-filled right renal pelvis, *rp,* may be a secondary sign of a right lower quadrant or pelvic process.

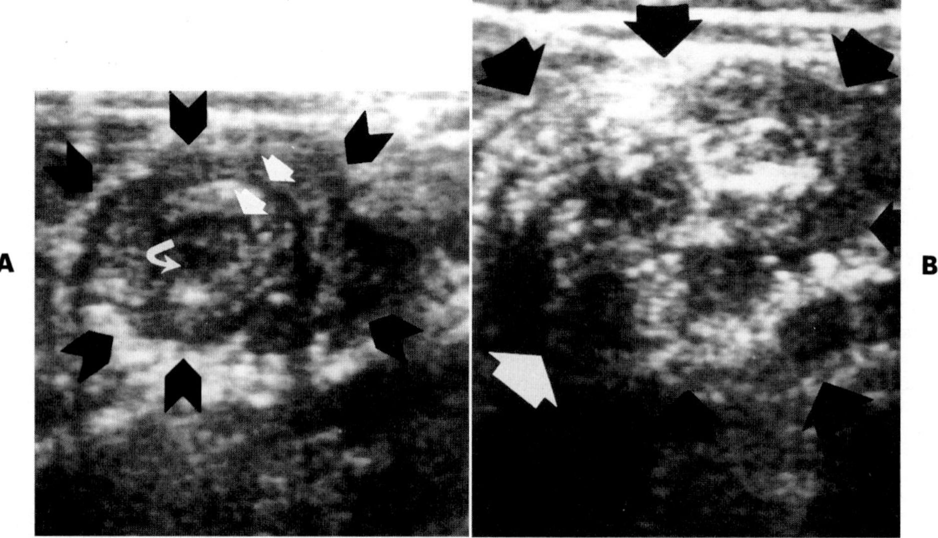

FIG. 17-10 A, Transverse image of an intussusception *(arrowheads)* showing a target sign. There are several circumferential layers of increased and decreased echogenicity *(arrows)* because of the telescoping bowel. The lumen *(curved arrow)* contains fluid. **B,** In an image at a more superior level in the same patient, intussusception *(arrows)* is identified. The target sign is present, but instead of being round, it is more C shaped because the bowel loop is coiled on itself.

barium or air enema are rapidly undertaken for both diagnostic confirmation and to attempt therapeutic reduction. Failure to thus reduce an intussusception mandates immediate surgical intervention. Likewise, in patients with a classical clinical presentation of intussusception who have developed fever and peritoneal signs, surgical intervention is indicated. In patients with a more vague clinical presentation, in whom intussusception remains suspect, an ultrasound examination is a helpful diagnostic undertaking.*

*References 1, 14, 24, 29, 31, 33

The patient is examined in the supine position. A survey of the entire abdomen is performed, followed by an examination focusing on the bowel using a 5-MHz or 7-MHz linear or curved array transducer.

The sonographic appearance of intussusception is of alternating hypoechoic and hyperechoic rings surrounding an echogenic center as seen in a short-axis view of the involved area. This is known as the *doughnut* or *target sign* (Fig. 17-10).[18] In the long axis, hypoechoic layers on each side of the echogenic center result in a pseudokidney or sandwich appearance (Fig. 17-11).[2,14,29] Free peritoneal fluid

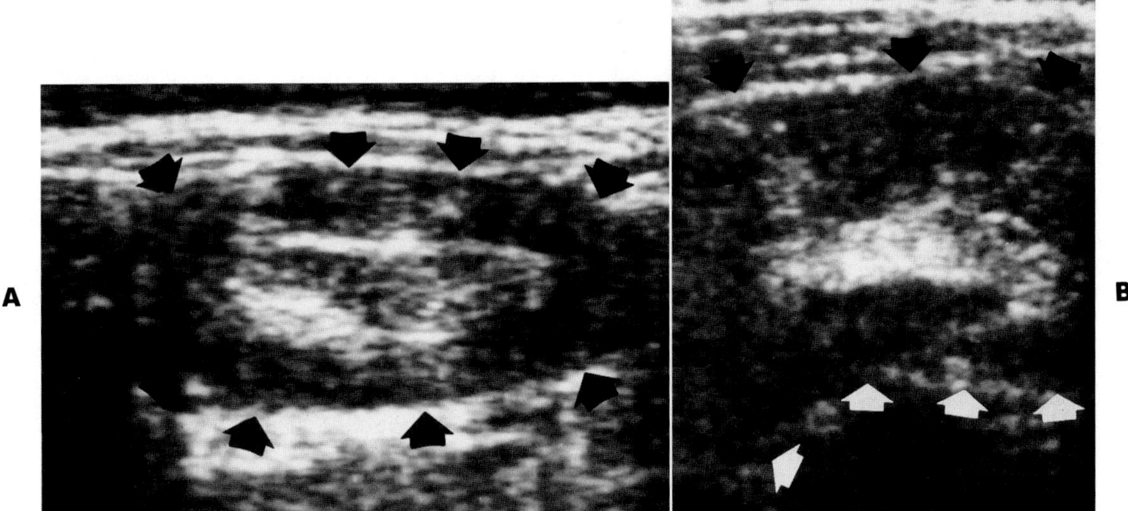

FIG. 17-11 A, Longitudinal image of the right lower quadrant demonstrates a pseudokidney appearance of an intussusception *(arrows)*. A normal kidney is present in each renal fossa, so this is not a pelvic kidney. **B,** Transverse image of the right lower quadrant in a different patient with intussusception *(arrows)*. The intussusception has a sandwich appearance.

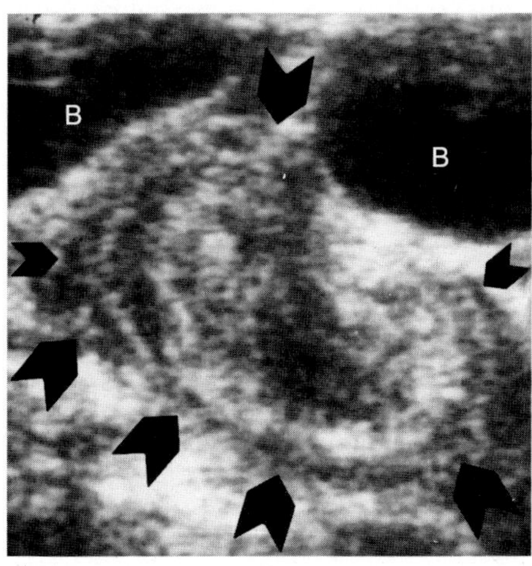

FIG. 17-12 There are multiple dilated fluid-filled bowel loops, *B*, located anterior to the intussusception *(arrowheads)*. The intussusception could not be reduced, a frequent occurrence when an ileoileocolic intussusception is encountered on contrast enema, mandating surgical intervention.

is not an uncommon finding with uncomplicated intussusception.[28,31]

When an intussusception is documented sonographically, an associated lead point, though relatively uncommon, should be sought. Itagaki reported a double target sign, diagnostic of an intussuscepted Meckel's diverticulum.[11] Other lead points, such as a small bowel tumor or duplication cyst, may likewise be identified.[26] Consideration of barium or air enema versus surgical intervention is as discussed previously (Fig. 17-12).

In addition to intussusception, conditions that can produce a targetlike sonographic appearance include primary bowel tumors such as lymphoma, and inflammatory bowel disease.[7,18]

REVIEW QUESTIONS

1. What are the most common age and gender for pyloric stenosis to occur?
2. Define the measurements used to evaluate a patient with pyloric stenosis.
3. What criteria are used to determine whether an infant has pyloric stenosis?
4. What method is used to identify the appendix?
5. What does the visualization of a normal appendix mean?
6. Define the measurement used to determine if appendicitis is present.
7. Describe intussusception in the infant and its occurrence.
8. What is the pseudokidney or sandwich sign?

REFERENCES

1. Bhisitkul DM, Listernick R, Shkolnik A, et al: Clinical application of ultrasonography in the diagnosis of intussusception, J Pediatr 121:182, 1992.
2. Bisset GS III and Kirks DR: Intussusception in infants and children: diagnosis and therapy, Radiology 168:141, 1988.
3. Blumhagen JD: The role of ultrasonography in the evaluation of vomiting in infants, Pediatr Radiol 16:267, 1986.
4. Blumhagen JD and Coombs JB: Ultrasound in the diagnosis of hypertrophic pyloric stenosis, J Clin Ultrasound 9:289, 1981.

5. Blumhagen JD and Noble HGS: Muscle thickness in hypertrophic pyloric stenosis: sonographic determination, Am J Roentgenol 140:221, 1983.
6. Bowen AD: The vomiting infant: recent advances and unsettled issues in imaging, Radiol Clin North Am 26:377, 1988.
7. Bowerman RA, Silver TM, and Jaffe MH: Real-time ultrasound diagnosis of intussusception in children, Radiology 143:527, 1982.
8. Breaux CW Jr, Georgeson KE, Royal SA, and Curnow AJ: Changing patterns in the diagnosis of hypertrophic pyloric stenosis, Pediatrics 81:213, 1988.
9. Haller JO and Cohen HL: Hypertrophic pyloric stenosis: diagnosis using US, Radiology 161:335, 1986.
10. Hayden CK Jr, Kuchelmeister J, and Lipscomb TS: Sonography of acute appendicitis in childhood: perforation versus nonperforation, J Ultrasound Med 11:209, 1992.
11. Itagaki A, Uchida M, Ueki K, and Kajii T: Double targets sign in ultrasonic diagnosis of intussuscepted Meckel diverticulum, Pediatr Radiol 21:148, 1991.
12. Jeffrey RB Jr, Laing FC, and Lewis FR: Acute appendicitis: high resolution real-time US findings, Radiology 163:11, 1987.
13. Jeffrey RB Jr, Laing FC, and Townsend RR: Acute appendicitis: sonographic criteria based on 250 cases, Radiology 167:327, 1988.
14. Lee HC, Yeh HJ, and Leu YJ: Intussusception: the sonographic diagnosis and its clinical value, J Pediatr Gastroenterol Nutr 8:343, 1989.
15. Lynn HB: The mechanism of pyloric stenosis and its relationship to preoperative preparation, Arch Surg 81:453, 1942.
16. Mollitt DL, Golladay ES, Williamson S, et al: Ultrasonography in the diagnosis of pyloric stenosis, South Med J 80:47, 1987.
17. O'Keeffe FN, Stansberry SD, Swischuk LE, and Hayden CK Jr: Antropyloric muscle thickness at US in infants: what is normal? Radiology 178:827, 1991.
18. Pracros JP, Tran-Minh VA, Morin De Finfe CH, et al: Acute intestinal intussusception in children. Contribution of ultrasonography (145 cases), Ann Radiol 30:525, 1987.
19. Puylaert JB: Acute appendicitis: US evaluation using graded compression, Radiology 158:355, 1986.
20. Quillin SP, Siegel MJ, and Coffin CM: Acute appendicitis in children: value of sonography in detecting perforation, Am J Roentgenol 159:1265, 1992.
21. Rioux M: Sonographic detection of the normal and abnormal appendix, Am J Roentgenol 158:773, 1992.
22. Siegel MJ: Acute appendicitis in childhood: the role of US, Radiology 185:341, 1992.
23. Sivit CJ: Diagnosis of acute appendicitis in children: spectrum of sonographic findings, Am J Roentgenol 161:147, 1993.
24. Sivit CJ, Newman KD, Boenning DA, et al: Appendicitis: usefulness of US in diagnosis in a pediatric population, Radiology 185:549, 1992.
25. Stevenson RJ: Non-neonatal intestinal obstruction in children, Surg Clin North Am 65:1217, 1985.
26. Stringer MD, Capps SNJ, and Pablot SM: Sonographic detection of the lead point in intussusception, Arch Dis Child 67:529, 1992.
27. Stunden RJ, LeQuesne GW, and Little KET: The improved ultrasound diagnosis of hypertrophic pyloric stenosis, Pedatr Radiol 16:200, 1986.
28. Swischuk LE and Stansberry SD: Ultrasonographic detection of free peritoneal fluid in uncomplicated intussusception, Pediatr Radiol 21:350, 1991.
29. Swischuk LE, Hayden CK, and Boulden T: Intussusception: indications for ultrasonography and an explanation of the doughnut and pseudokidney signs, Pediatr Radiol 15:388, 1985.
30. Teele RL and Smith EH: Ultrasound in the diagnosis of idiopathic hypertrophic pyloric stenosis, N Engl J Med 296:1149, 1977.
31. Verschelden P, Filiatrault D, Garel L, et al: Intussusception in children: reliability of US in diagnosis—a prospective study, Radiology 184:741, 1992.
32. Vignault F, Filiatrault D, Brandt ML, et al: Acute appendicitis in children: evaluation with US, Radiology 176:501, 1990.
33. Weinberger E and Winters WD: Intussusception in children: the role of sonography, Radiology 184:601, 1992.

CHAPTER

18

Neonatal Kidneys and Adrenal Glands

Suzanne M. Devine • Kate A. Feinstein • Arnold Shkolnik

Sonography is the initial diagnostic imaging method of choice when a renal or adrenal abnormality is suspected in the neonate. There are numerous indications for renal imaging in the newborn. One major indication is a renal abnormality detected during prenatal sonography. Some of the conditions or findings in the newborn associated with renal abnormalities are: flank masses, abdominal distention, anuria, oliguria, hematuria, sepsis or urinary tract infection, meningomyelocele, VATER (vertebral, anal, tracheoesophageal fistula, renal) anomalies, abnormal external genitalia, and prune belly syndrome.

EXAMINATION TECHNIQUES

General aspects of the ultrasound examination of the neonate are described in Chapter 17. Maintaining body temperature in the neonate is very important, since small infants can lose a potentially dangerous amount of body heat quickly. Whenever possible scanning through the portholes of an isolette provides an optimal environment for the premature or otherwise fragile neonate. When the examination is performed outside of the isolette, body heat loss can be minimized by the use of heat lamps and by exposing only the area of the trunk being interrogated.

Imaging of the urinary bladder, which includes assessment for distal ureteral dilation, is considered an important part of the renal sonographic examination (Fig. 18-1). Because of the infant's tendency to urinate spontaneously, scanning is gently initiated over the suprapubic region. If the urinary bladder is not distended at this time, or if voiding occurs before adequate detail can be obtained, this area can be examined after imaging of the kidneys and perirenal areas. Refilling of the urinary bladder is usually relatively rapid if the infant is fed and also when parenteral fluids are being administered.

Long- and short-axis views of the kidneys and of the perirenal areas are initially obtained by scanning via the flanks to obtain coronal and axial images, via the anterior abdomen for longitudinal and transverse images, or both. When necessary, additional transverse and longitudinal views can be obtained with the infant in a prone position. Renal scanning before and after the infant voids may provide useful information. For example, development of or increase in hydronephrosis after voiding would be very suggestive of high grade vesicoureteral reflux.

NORMAL KIDNEY AND ADRENAL GLAND

The normal kidney in the neonate is characterized by a distinct demarcation of the cortex and medullary pyramids. The medullary pyramids are large and hypoechoic, not to be mistaken for dilated calyces or cysts. The surrounding cortex is quite thin, with echogenicity essentially similar to or slightly greater than that of normal liver parenchyma (Fig. 18-2). Because of a paucity of fat in the renal sinus of the neonate, this area is generally hypoechoic and therefore indistinct. The arcuate arteries, which lie at the bases of the medullary pyramids, appear as punctate intensely echogenic structures. Renal cortical echogenicity normally decreases to less than that of liver parenchyma usually by 4 to 6 months of age.*

The normal adrenal glands are relatively larger and therefore more easily identified in the neonate than in the older infant or young child. Each gland lies immediately superior to the upper pole of the kidney. The left adrenal gland extends slightly medial. Sonographically, the gland has an inverted V or Y shape in the longitudinal plane (Fig. 18-3, *A*). In the transverse plane the portion of the gland delineated has a linear or curvilinear outline (Fig. 18-3, *B*). The adrenal medulla in the neonate is relatively thin, appearing as a distinctly echogenic stripe, surrounded by the more prominent and less echogenic adrenal cortex. When the kidney is absent or ectopic, the ipsilateral adrenal gland remains in the renal fossa but as a result may have an altered configuration (Fig. 18-4).[10,18,23]

The most common causes of renal and adrenal enlargement that can present as a palpable mass in the neonate are discussed next.

Hydronephrosis

Obstructive uropathy accounts for the vast majority of palpable abdominal masses in the neonate.[11]

*References 10, 17, 18, 19, 23

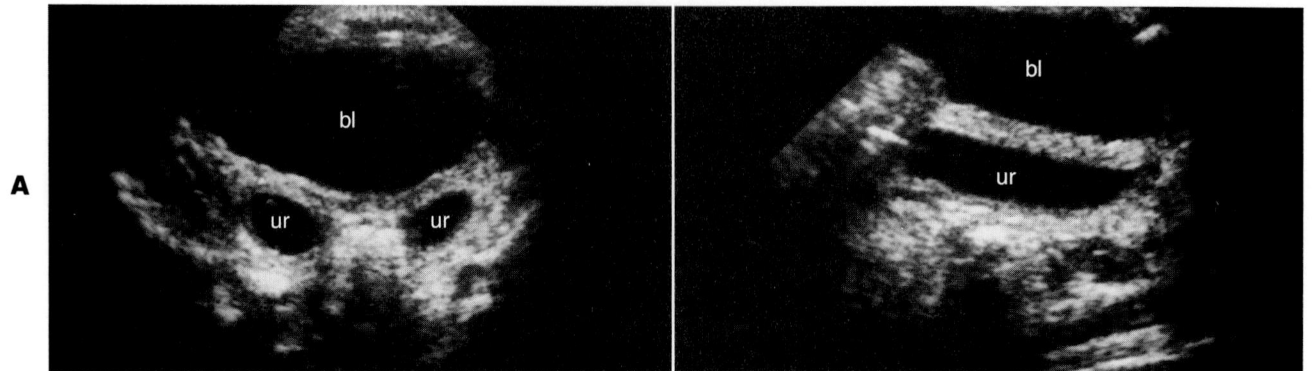

FIG. 18-1 **A**,Transverse image of the pelvis in a 2-day-old infant with bilateral primary megaureter (nonobstructive dilation of the distal ureter). The urinary bladder, *bl*, is well distended. Bilateral dilation of the distal ureter, *ur*, is seen posterior to the bladder. **B**, Longitudinal view of the same patient shows the distal ureter, *ur*, entering the urinary bladder, *bl*.

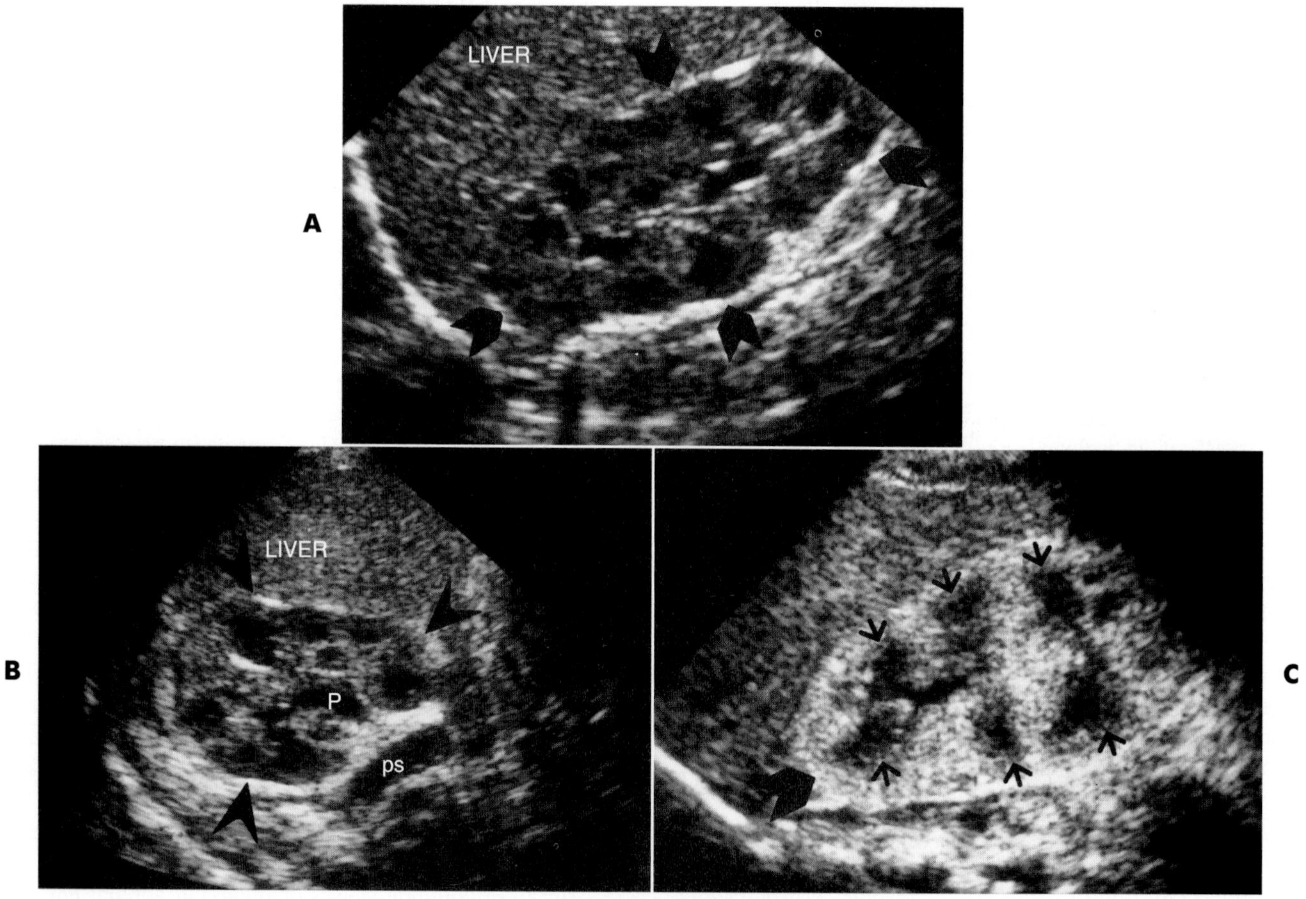

FIG. 18-2 **A**, Coronal view of a normal right kidney (*arrowheads*) in a 3-day-old male with a left multicystic dysplastic kidney. The medullary pyramids appear as triangular hypoechoic areas. The cortex has the same echogenicity as the liver. **B**, Transverse view of the same kidney (*arrowheads*). The hypoechoic psoas muscle, *ps*, is located posteromedial to the kidney. The nondilated renal pelvis, *p*, contains anechoic fluid. **C,** Normal kidney (*arrowheads*) in 13-day-old female. The increased echogenicity of the renal cortex compared to the normal liver parenchyma can be normal. The medullary pyramids appear large and hypoechoic (*arrows*).

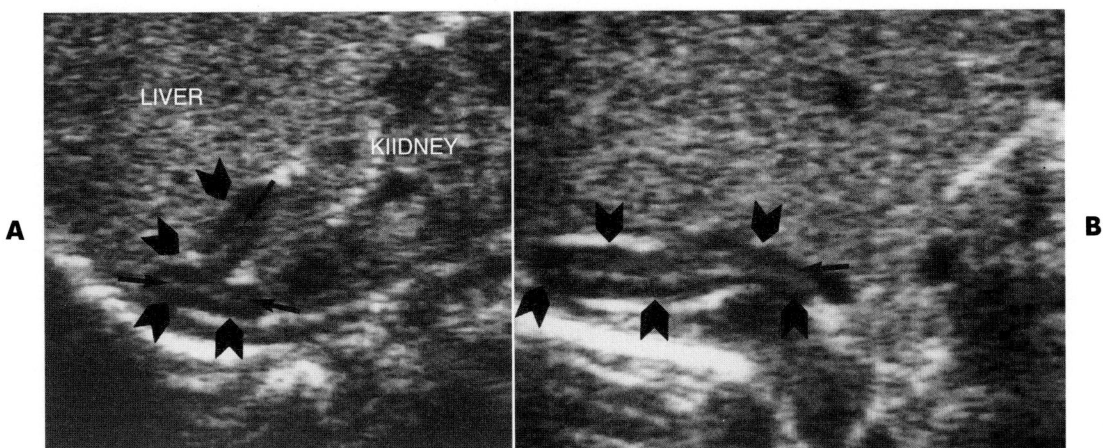

FIG. 18-3 **A**, Coronal view of a normal adrenal gland (*arrowheads*) in a 1-day-old infant with ambiguous genitalia. The adrenal medulla (*arrows*) appears as a central echogenic stripe, surrounded by the less echogenic cortex. The adrenal gland has an inverted Y configuration. **B**, Transverse view through a portion of adrenal gland (*arrowheads*) demonstrating the curvilinear shape in this plane.

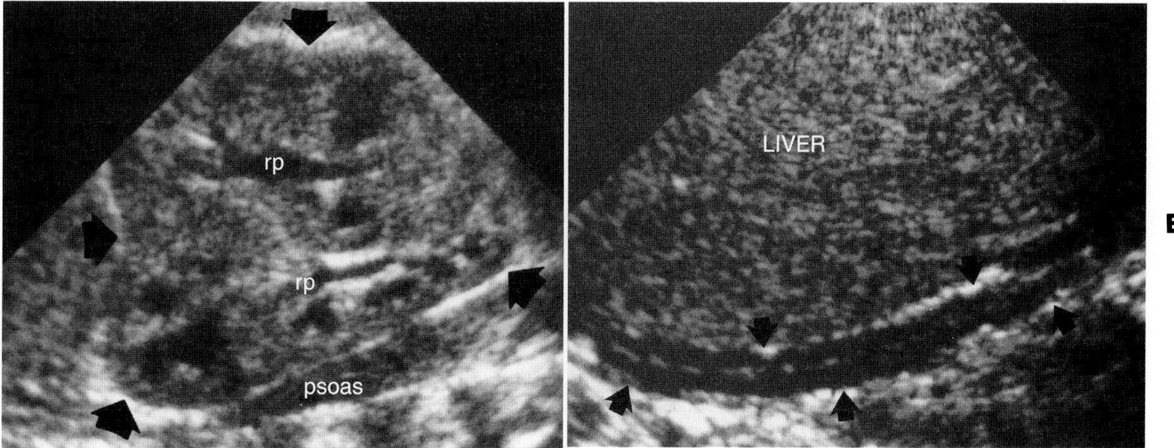

FIG. 18-4 **A**, Crossed-fused renal ectopia (*arrows*) in a 1-day-old male with imperforate anus. Sonogram through the right flank demonstrates the renal pelvis, *rp*, of each kidney. **B**, Coronal image through the right flank demonstrates an elongated adrenal gland (*arrows*) resulting from the absence of a kidney in this renal fossa.

Ureteropelvic Junction Obstruction

Ureteropelvic junction obstruction (UPJ) is the most common type of obstruction of the upper urinary tract; it most often results from intrinsic narrowing or extrinsic vascular compression.[2,6,9] Bilateral involvement may occur, as well as a contralateral multicystic dysplastic kidney or vesicoureteral reflux.[2,4-6] Sonographically, there is pelvocalyceal dilation without ureteral dilation (Fig. 18-5, *A*).[10,23] When the obstruction is pronounced, the dilated renal pelvis extends inferiorly and medially (Fig. 18-5, *B*). If vesicoureteral reflux or primary megaureter is present, the ureter may be dilated.[18,19]

Posterior Urethral Valves

Posterior urethral valves are the most common cause of bladder outlet obstruction in the male neonate.[9] The wall of the urinary bladder appears thickened and trabeculated (Fig. 18-6, *A*). Midline sagittal imaging with caudal angulation through the bladder may allow visualization of the distended posterior urethra.[18] Alternatively, the posterior urethra can be imaged directly from a perineal approach.[10] The resultant hydronephrosis and hydroureter may be asymmetric. Urinary ascites or a perirenal urinoma can result from high-pressure vesicoureteral reflux rupturing a calyceal fornix or tearing the renal parenchyma

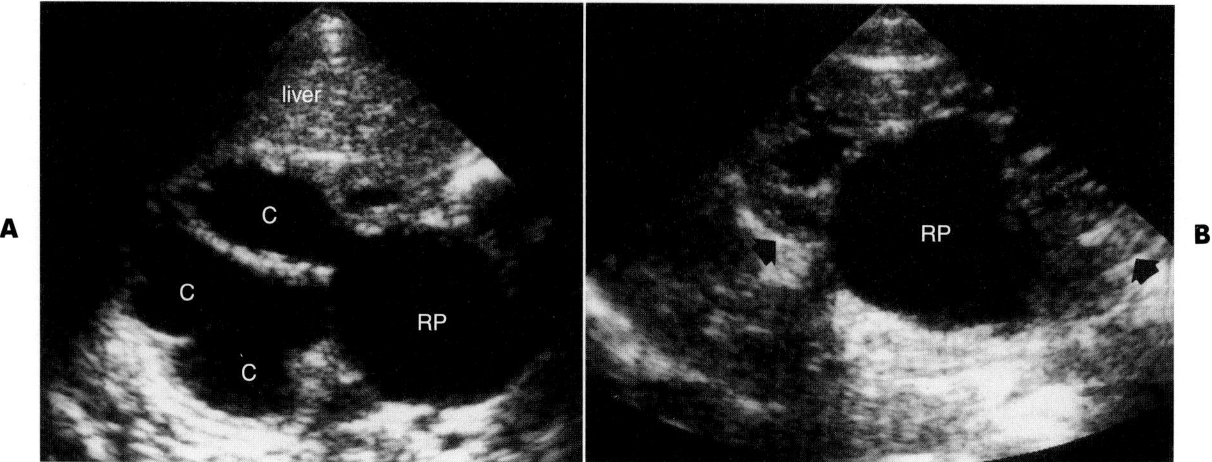

FIG. 18-5 **A**, Ureteropelvic junction obstruction in a 2-week-old female infant with an abnormal prenatal ultrasound. Marked dilation of the renal pelvis, *rp*, and calyces, *c*, is present. Parenchymal loss is also noted. The distal ureter was not identified. Radionuclide imaging confirmed the diagnosis. **B**, UPJ obstruction in a 1-day-old infant. Coronal image of the kidney (*arrows*) identifies marked dilation of the renal pelvis, *rp*.

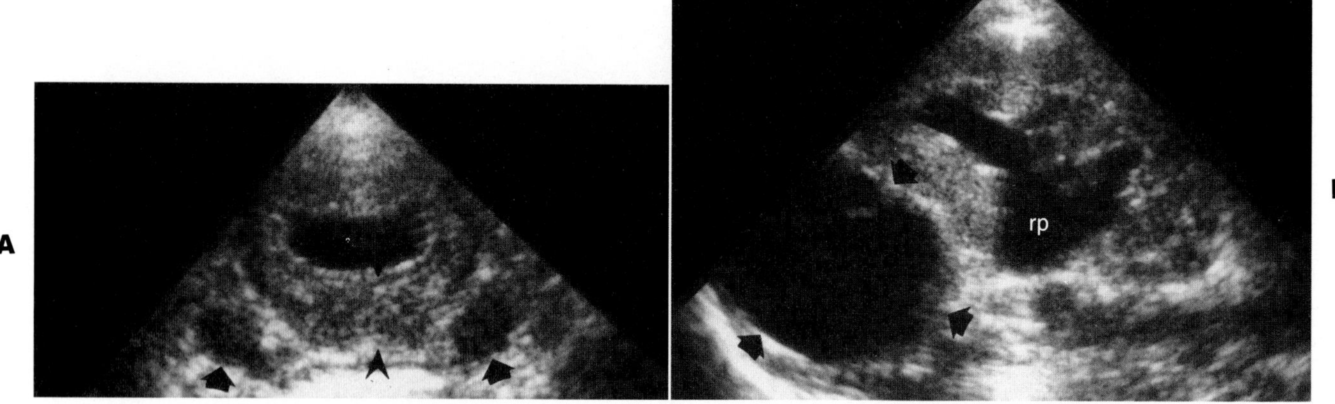

FIG. 18-6 **A**, Posterior urethral valves in a male infant. Transverse view of the urinary bladder shows the thickened bladder wall (*arrowheads*). Dilated distal ureters (*arrows*) are identified posterior to the bladder. **B**, Coronal view of the left kidney shows moderate pelviectasis, *rp*. A urinoma (*arrows*) is seen superior to the kidney.

(Fig. 18-6, *B*). The perirenal urinoma is usually anechoic, however, septations may be noted.[7,23] Other potential causes of perirenal urine extravasation include ureteropelvic junction obstruction, ureterovesical junction obstruction, and pelvic masses that obstruct the bladder or ureter (Fig. 18-7).[7,17]

Ectopic Ureterocele

Ectopic ureterocele occurs more commonly in females and more often on the left side. It results from an ectopic insertion and cystic dilation of the distal ureter of the upper moiety of a completely duplicated renal collecting system. The ectopic ureterocele, seen as a fluid mass within the urinary bladder, is located inferomedially to the ureteral insertion of the lower pole ureter (Fig. 18-8, *A* and *B*). The sonographic delineation of an upper pole fluid mass, in continuity with a dilated ureter, and the aforementioned ureterocele is diagnostic of this entity (Fig. 18-8, *C*).[10,17,18,23] Distention and effacement or contraction of the ureterocele may be evident during the real time study.[19,23]

Multicystic Dysplastic Kidney

Multicystic dysplastic kidney (MCDK) is the most common cause of renal cystic disease presenting in the neonate, and when hydronephrosis is excluded, it is the most common cause of an abdominal mass in the newborn.

Sonographically, the classic appearance of MCDK is of a unilateral mass resembling a bunch of grapes, which represents a cluster of discrete noncommunicating cysts, the largest of which are peripheral.[21] There is no identifiable

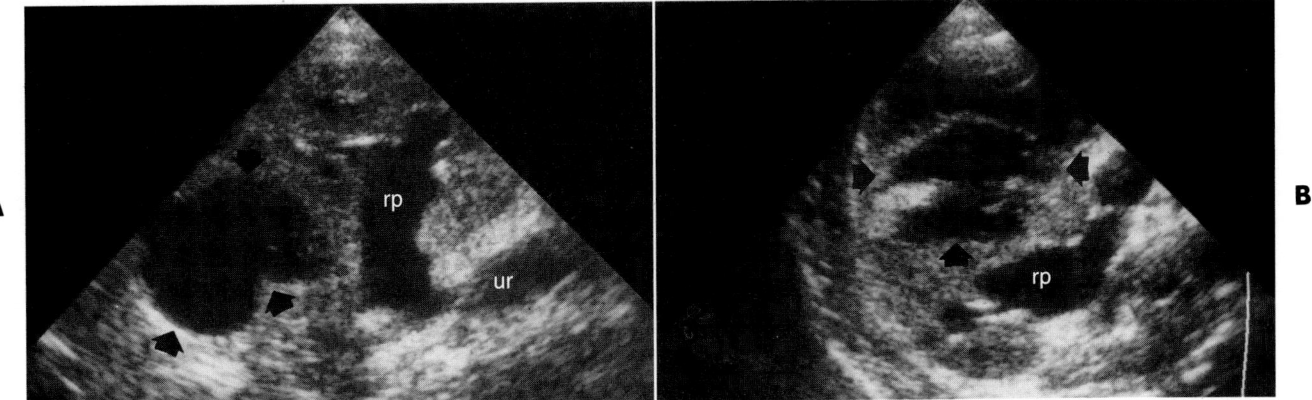

FIG. 18-7 A, Sonogram of urinoma (*arrows*) in a 5-week-old with bilateral ureterovesical obstruction. Moderate pelviectasis, *rp*, and dilation of the ureter, *ur*, is seen. **B**, Transverse image in the same patient identifies septations within the urinoma (*arrows*).

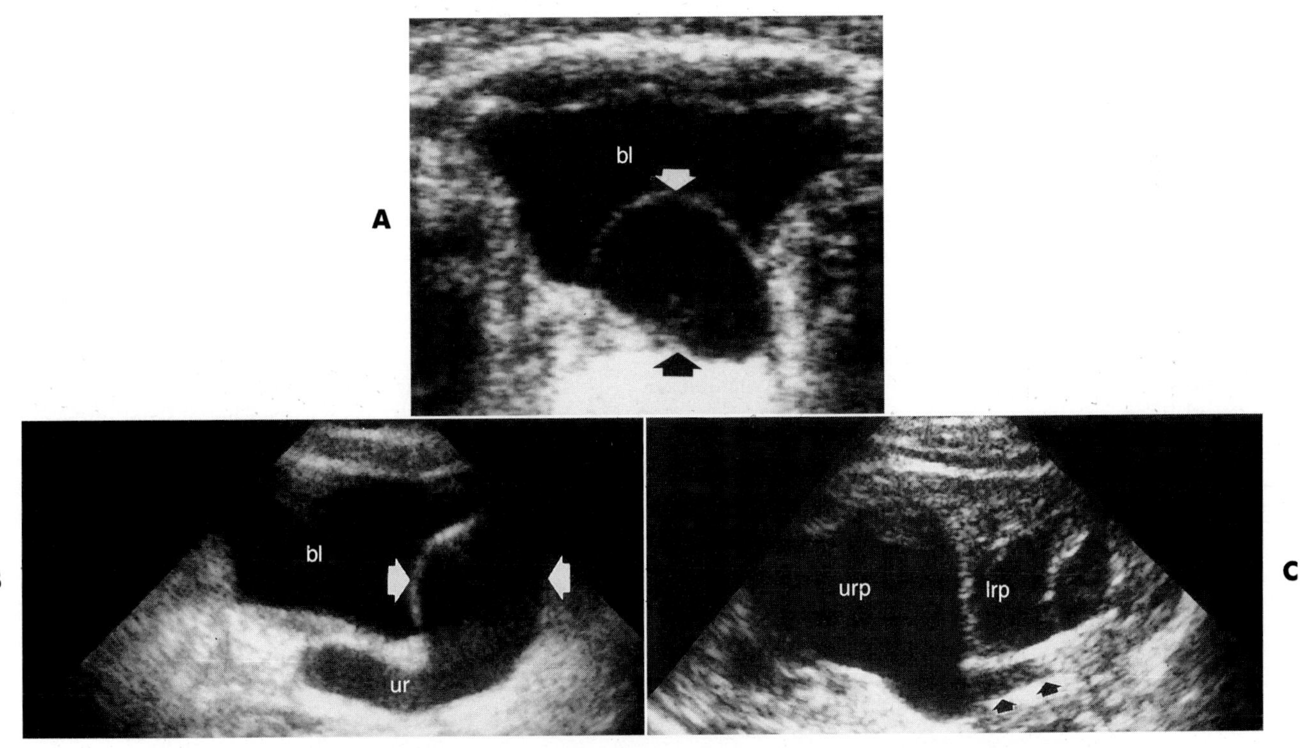

FIG. 18-8 A, Transverse image of the urinary bladder, *bl*, in a 2-month-old female with pyelonephritis. A large thin-walled ureterocele (*arrows*) is seen in the posterior aspect of the bladder. **B**, Longitudinal view of the bladder in the same patient shows the dilated ureter, *ur*, and ureterocele (*arrows*). Low-level echoes seen in the ureter and ureterocele represent debris. **C**, Coronal view of the kidney in the same patient demonstrates a duplicated kidney with marked pelvocaliectasis of the upper pole segment, *urp*, and moderate pelvocaliectasis of the lower pole segment, *lrp*. The ureter from the upper pole segment (*arrows*) is located medial to the lower pole renal pelvis.

renal pelvis (Fig. 18-9).[17,18] A less common hydronephrotic form of MCDK has been described in which a renal pelvis has been identified.[9,11,25] The association with contralateral UPJ has been noted. Bilateral occurrence of MCDK is fatal.[3,8,9,12]

At times, sonographic differentiation of MCDK from severe UPJ obstruction may be difficult. In such instances, radionuclide documentation of renal function usually indicates severe hydronephrosis. With the advent of sonography, there has been a growing trend toward conservative management of MCDK.[8,20] These abnormal kidneys most often involute and disappear completely or result in a small dysplastic kidney.[1,8,23] If there is evidence of growth, resection is usually undertaken.[19]

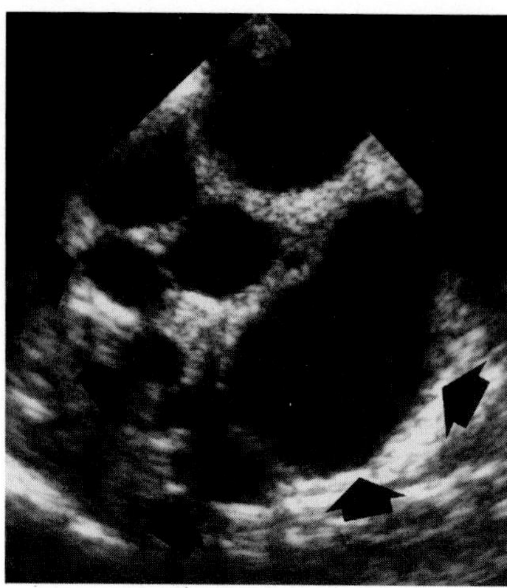

FIG. 18-9 Multicystic dysplastic kidney (*arrows*) in a 3-week-old male. Axial view of the left flank demonstrates multiple, noncommunicating cysts of varying sizes. There was no apparent renal pelvis. Radionuclide imaging confirmed the diagnosis.

Polycystic Kidney Disease

Polycystic kidney disease identified in the neonatal period is most often of the autosomal-recessive type (ARPKD). The typical presentation is that of poorly functioning, enlarged kidneys.[24] Pulmonary hypoplasia with respiratory distress and Potter's facies may be associated findings. The macroscopic cystlike appearance throughout both kidneys actually reflects dilated renal tubules that are generally less than 2 mm in diameter.[6,9,11,24] The innumerable acoustical interfaces that present because of this morphologic abnormality result in marked echogenicity obscuring corticomedullary demarcation. A thin peripheral hypoechoic renal rim may be demonstrated, representing either compressed renal cortex or elongated thin-walled cystic spaces (Fig. 18-10).[10,15] Associated mild hepatic fibrosis and ductal hyperplasia can produce a heterogeneous increase in echogenicity of liver parenchyma.[15]

In the juvenile form of ARPKD, symptoms can occur later in childhood.[6,13,26] The renal tubular ectasia and the resultant renal symptomatology are overshadowed by hepatic fibrosis leading to portal hypertension and gastrointestinal bleeding. In this condition the dilated renal collecting tubules produce an accentuated medullary echogenicity, and the renal cortex has an essentially normal appearance. Increased liver echogenicity reflects hepatic fibrosis.[10,14,15]

The autosomal-dominant form of polycystic kidney disease (ADPKD), the so-called adult type, has on rare occasions been reported in the young infant.[24,26] More typically it becomes manifest during adulthood, with hypertension and enlarged kidneys. On sonography, well-defined cysts can be identified in the kidneys. Cysts can also form in the liver, spleen, and pancreas.[9,10] Cerebral berry aneurysms are also known to occur in 10% to 15% of patients with ADPKD. Sonography of parents and siblings of patients with ADPKD has proven helpful in identifying this abnormality in afflicted persons who are asymptomatic.[22]

Renal Vein Thrombosis

Renal vein thrombosis is most likely to occur in the dehydrated or septic infant and is more prevalent in infants of diabetic mothers. One or both kidneys may be involved. There is renal enlargement, hematuria, proteinuria, and a low platelet count. Thrombosis occurs initially in the small intrarenal venous branches, and at this stage the enlarged kidney has a nonspecific disordered heterogeneous internal echogenicity corresponding to the extent and severity of the

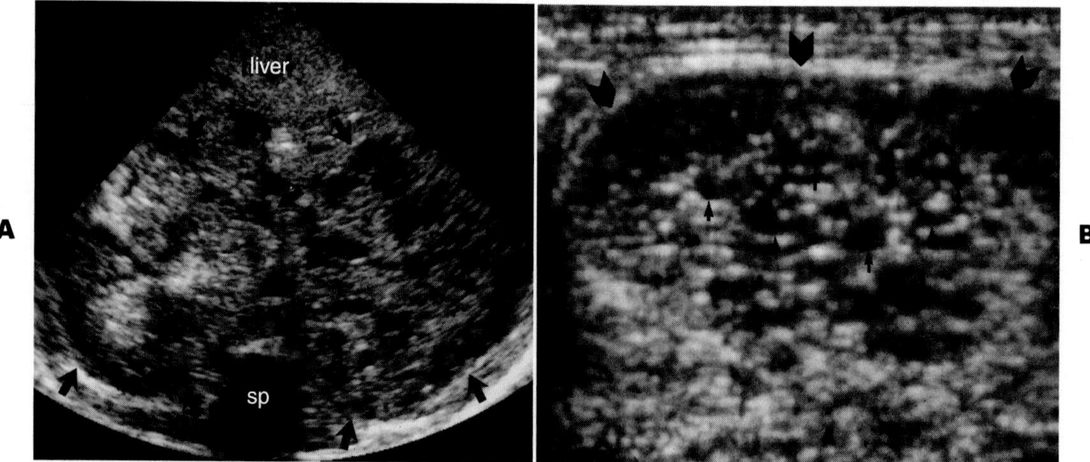

FIG. 18-10 A, Autosomal recessive polycystic kidney disease (ARPKD) in a 1-day-old male with abdominal distention. Transverse image of the upper abdomen using the liver as an acoustic window shows that the kidneys are enlarged and echogenic with a hypoechoic peripheral rim (*arrows*), spine *sp*. This appearance is typical for ARPKD **B,** A 7-MHz linear image of the kidney (*arrowheads*) in the same patient reveals multiple small cysts (*arrows*). The high frequency allows resolution of the cysts.

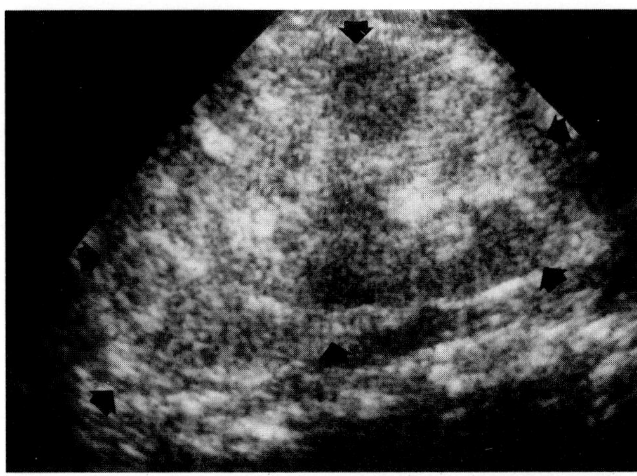

FIG. 18-11 Renal vein thrombosis in a 5-day-old term newborn with hematuria. Coronal sonogram of the left flank demonstrates an enlarged kidney (*arrows*) with patchy areas of increased echogenicity.

process (Fig. 18-11). If the thrombus reaches the renal vein or inferior vena cava, it may be directly visualized within these vascular structures.[11,16] There may be coexistent adrenal hemorrhage, particularly on the left side where the adrenal vein drains directly into the renal vein.[16] Calcification within the involved veins may eventually result.

Renal Tumors

Congenital mesoblastic nephroma is the most common renal tumor of the neonate and young infant. This tumor is benign but is indistinguishable from a Wilms' tumor by any method of imaging. Since the tumor may invade adjacent structures, nephrectomy is indicated. Sonographically, as with Wilms' tumor, this lesion may be hyperechoic, hypoechoic, or of mixed echogenicity (Fig. 18-12).[11,18] It is seen in children less than 1 year of age, whereas Wilms' tumor commonly occurs in children more than 1 year of age.[10,19]

Nephroblastomatosis is an abnormal persistence of fetal

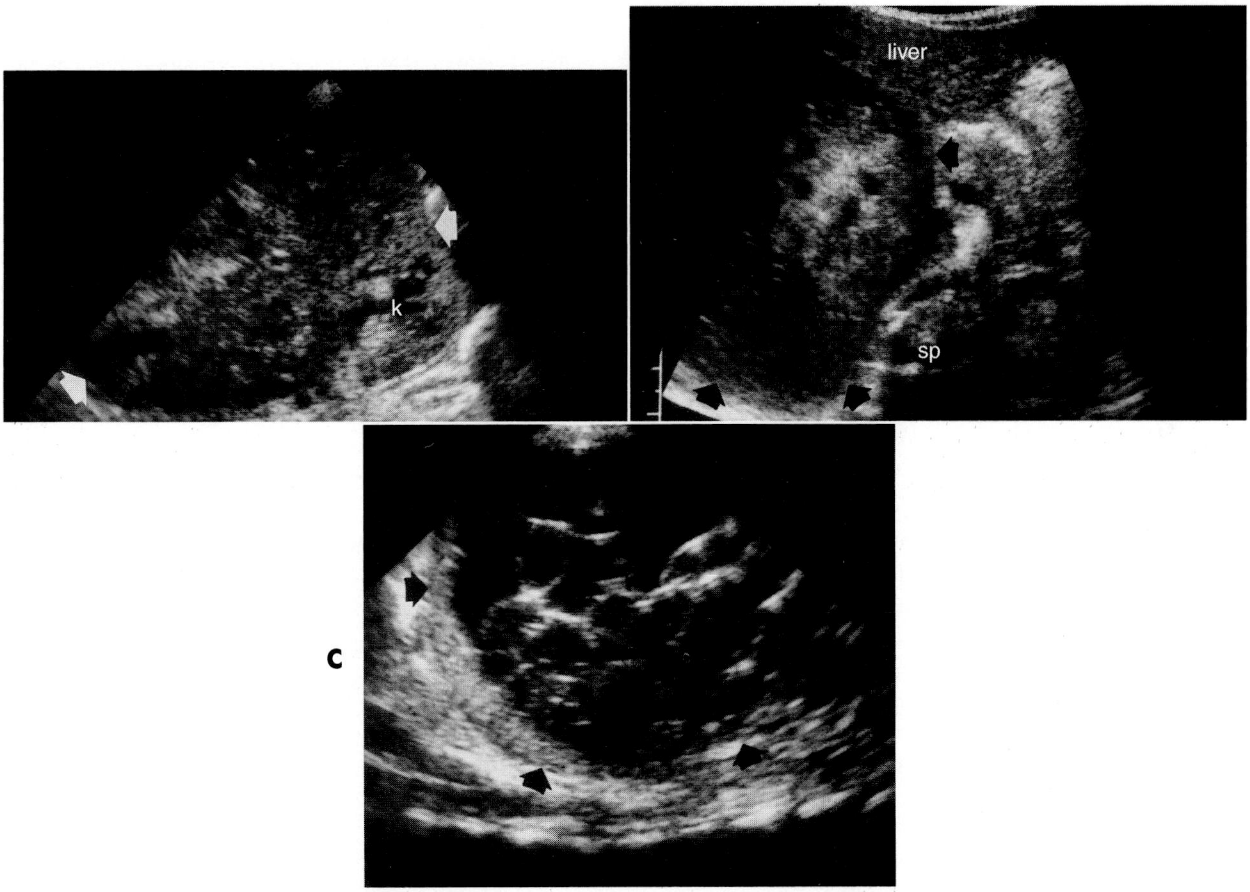

FIG. 18-12 A, Mesoblastic nephroma in an 11-week-old infant with a renal mass (*arrows*). Coronal image of the right flank identifies that the mass is predominantly solid, with some cystic areas, and arises from the right kidney, *k*. **B**, Transverse view shows the mass (*arrows*) posterior to the liver and anterior and lateral to the spine, *sp*. Nephrectomy and pathologic evaluation confirmed the diagnosis of mesoblastic nephroma. **C**, Wilms' tumor in a 7-month-old with an abdominal mass. Sonogram reveals a large mass with multiple cystic areas occupying the renal fossa. This represents an unusual presentation of a Wilms' tumor; more frequently a large solid component is present in these masses.

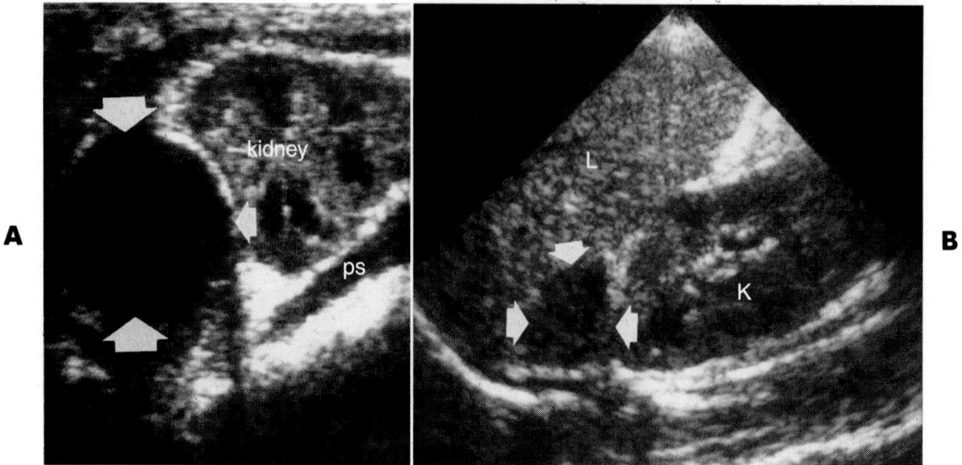

FIG. 18-13 A, Adrenal hemorrhage in a 2-week-old male with a history of neonatal infections, increased bilirubin, and an abdominal mass. Coronal sonogram demonstrates a cystic mass *(arrows)* superior to the kidney. A normal adrenal gland was not identified. The psoas muscle, *ps*, is located posteriorly. **B**, Adrenal hemorrhage in a jaundiced 3-week-old female. Coronal view of the right upper quadrant reveals an echogenic mass (*arrows*) superior to the kidney, *k*, and posterior to the liver, *l*.

renal blastema, which has the potential to develop into Wilms' tumor. A rare cause of bilateral renal enlargement in the neonate is diffuse nephroblastomatosis. It can occur in up to one third of kidneys with Wilms' tumor. An increased incidence of this abnormality is present in patients with Beckwith-Wiedemann and hemihypertrophy syndromes, as well as in patients with some major chromosomal abnormalities. In addition to renal enlargement, the involved areas may be hypoechoic, hyperechoic, or isoechoic compared with normal renal parenchyma. Although this abnormality may be evident sonographically, CT or MR imaging has been shown to be more accurate.[10,19]

Sonography is used for periodic renal monitoring in those at risk of developing Wilms' tumor, including patients with a previous Wilms' tumor or a family history of Wilms' tumor and patients who have sporadic aniridia.[6] Periodic sonographic monitoring is also performed in patients with either proven or potential nephroblastomatosis described previously.

Sonography is valuable in detecting Wilms' tumor extension into the renal vein, inferior vena cava, and right atrium.[10,19] Documentation of tumor extension can have a significant bearing on the surgical approach to the patient. When the tumor extends into the right atrium, cardiopulmonary bypass may be necessary to resect the tumor completely.

Adrenal Hemorrhage

Difficult delivery, large size, and neonatal hypoxia predispose to adrenal hemorrhage. However, the newborn with adrenal hemorrhage may have none of these associated factors but nonetheless present with an abdominal mass, jaundice, and anemia. Sonographically, adrenal hemorrhage results in ovoid enlargement of the gland or a portion of the gland. The appearance of the hemorrhagic gland can range from anechoic to hyperechoic, or a mixture of echogenicities, depending on the extent, age, and severity of the process (Fig. 18-13). When enlargement is significant, a characteristic blunting of the superior pole of the underlying kidney is produced, along with inferior displacement of the kidney. The initial appearance of adrenal hemorrhage may render it indistinguishable from an adrenal neuroblastoma. Follow-up sonography can differentiate these two entities. Unlike a neoplasm, a hemorrhagic adrenal gland does not enlarge but rather decreases in size. Generally within 4 to 6 weeks the lesion becomes appreciably smaller and subsequent calcification may be identified on the sonogram or radiographically.[10,13,23]

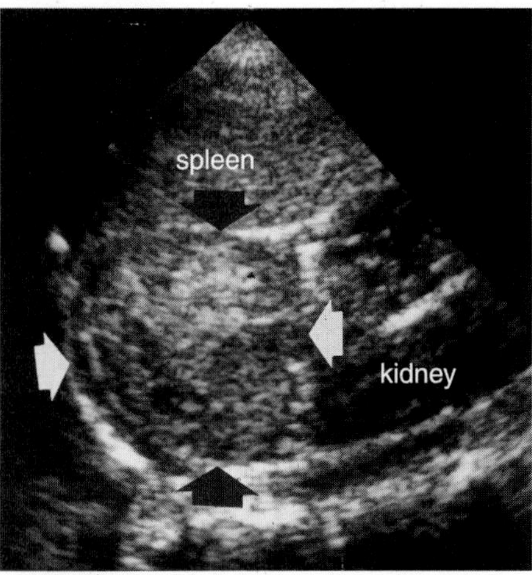

FIG. 18-14 Adrenal neuroblastoma in a 1-week-old female with history of a left kidney mass on a fetal sonogram. Coronal image through the left flank reveals a large heterogeneous mass (*arrows*) displacing the left kidney inferiorly.

Neuroblastoma

Neuroblastoma, a malignant tumor that arises in sympathetic chain ganglia and adrenal medulla, may be detected on antenatal sonography or at birth. The peak age of incidence is 2 years. Two thirds of cases arising in the abdomen originate in the adrenal gland. This neoplasm is usually highly echogenic. Intrinsic calcification may be identified (Fig. 18-14).[10,18] However, a cystic form of neuroblastoma has also been described. The adjacent kidney is displaced inferiorly and at times laterally.[10,23]

The disease is often disseminated at the time of presentation. Careful sonographic evaluation of the liver should be made for evidence of metastatic disease.[18] Since intraspinal extension is reported to occur in as many as 15% of patients and because ultrasonography can successfully define the spinal canal in young infants, such examination should be considered in the initial assessment of the infant with suspect neuroblastoma.

REVIEW QUESTIONS

1. Describe the procedure and protocol used to image the bladder and kidneys in the infant.
2. What is the appearance of a normal neonatal kidney and adrenal gland?
3. Name the abnormality responsible for the vast majority of palpable abdominal masses in the neonate.
4. What is the most common type of obstruction of the upper urinary tract in the infant?
5. What is the most common cause of bladder outlet obstruction in the male neonate?
6. What are the sonographic findings for a baby with posterior urethral valves?
7. Discuss the abnormality ectopic ureterocele and its sonographic appearance.
8. What is the sonographic appearance of multicystic dysplastic kidney in the neonate?
9. Name the two types of polycystic kidney disease and their appearance in the neonate.
10. What lesion is more likely to occur in dehydrated or septic infants, or in infants of diabetic mothers? Describe the sonographic appearance.
11. Discuss the findings of congenital mesoblastic nephroma in the infant.
12. What is a Wilms' tumor? Where is it found and what should the protocol be in evaluating a patient with a Wilms' tumor?
13. Discuss the sonographic features of an adrenal hemorrhage in the neonate.
14. What is the sonographic appearance of a neuroblastoma? What is the difference in sonographic texture over time between an adrenal hemorrhage and a neuroblastoma?

REFERENCES

1. Avni EF, Thoua Y, Lalmand B, et al: Multicystic dysplastic kidney: natural history from in utero diagnosis and postnatal followup, J Urol 138:1420, 1987.
2. Bernstein GT, Mandell J, Lebowitz RL, et al: Ureteropelvic junction obstruction in the neonate, J Urol 140:1216, 1988.
3. Blane CE, Ritchey ML, Di Pietro MA, et al: Single system ectopic ureters and ureteroceles associated with dysplastic kidney, Pediatr Radiol 22:217, 1992.
4. Brown T, Mandell J, and Lebowitz RL: Neonatal hydronephrosis in the era of sonography, Am J Roentgenol 148:959, 1987.
5. Clarke NW, Gough DCS, and Cohen SJ: Neonatal urological ultrasound: diagnostic inaccuracies and pitfalls, Arch Dis Child 64:578, 1989.
6. Donaldson JS and Shkolnik A: Pediatric renal masses, Semin Roentgenol 23:194, 1988.
7. Feinstein KA and Fernbach SK: Septated urinomas in the neonate, Am J Roentgenol 149:997, 1987.
8. Gordon AC, Thomas DFM, Arthur RJ, and Irving HC: Multicystic dysplastic kidney: is nephrectomy still appropriate? J Urol 140:1231, 1988.
9. Gray DL and Crane JP: Practical pediatric nephrology: prenatal diagnosis of urinary tract malformation, Pediatr Nephrol 2:326, 1988.
10. Hayden CK Jr and Swischuk LE: Pediatric ultrasonography, ed. 2. Baltimore, 1992, Williams & Wilkins.
11. Kirks DR, Rosenberg ER, Johnson DG, and King LR: Integrated imaging of neonatal renal masses, Pediatr Radiol 15:147, 1985.
12. Kleiner B, Filly RA, Mack L, and Callen PW: Multicystic dysplastic kidney: observations of contralateral disease in the fetal population, Radiology 161:27, 1986.
13. Lee W, Comstock CH, and Jurcak-Zaleski S: Prenatal diagnosis of adrenal hemorrhage by ultrasonography, J Ultrasound Med 11:369, 1992.
14. Margraf LR, Hawkins EP, Oshman DG, and Gilbert-Barness E: Diagnosis and discussion: autosomal recessive polycystic kidney disease, Am J Dis Child 147:77, 1993.
15. McAlister WH and Siegel MJ: Case 2: congenital hepatic fibrosis with saccular dilatation of the intrahepatic bile ducts and infantile polycystic kidneys, Am J Roentgenol 152:1329, 1989.
16. Orazi C, Fariello G, Malena S, et al: Renal vein thrombosis and adrenal hemorrhage in the newborn: ultrasound evaluation of 4 cases, J Clin Ultrasound 21:163, 1993.
17. Seeds JW, Mittelstaedt CA, and Mandell J: Pre- and postnatal ultrasonographic diagnosis of congenital obstructive uropathies, Urol Clin of North Am 13:131, 1986.
18. Shkolnik A: Applications of ultrasound in the neonatal abdomen, Rad Clin North Am 23:141, 1985.
19. Shkolnik A: Ultrasonography of the urogenital system. In Kelalis PP, King LR, and Belman AB, editors: Clinical pediatric urology,vol I, ed 3. Philadelphia, 1992, WB Saunders.
20. Strife JL, Souza AS, Kirks DR, et al: Multicystic dysplastic kidney in children: US follow-up, Radiology 186:785, 1993.
21. Stuck KJ, Koff SA, and Silver TM: Ultrasonic features of multicystic dysplastic kidney: expanded diagnostic criteria, Radiology 143:217, 1982.
22. Taitz LS, Brown CB, Blank CE, and Steiner GM: Screening for polycystic kidney disease: importance of clinical presentation in the newborn, Arch Dis Child 62:45, 1987.

23. Teele RL and Share JC: Evaluating an abdominal mass, In Teele RL and Share JC, editors: Ultrasonography of infants and children. Philadelphia, 1991, WB Saunders.
24. Wernecke K, Heckemann R, Bachmann H, and Peters PE: Sonography of infantile polycystic kidney disease, Urol Radiol 7:138, 1985.
25. Wood BP, Goske M, and Rabinowitz R: Multicystic renal dysplasia masquerading as ureteropelvic junction obstruction, J Urol 132:972, 1984.
26. Worthington JL, Shackelford GD, Cole BR, et al: Sonographically detectable cysts in polycystic kidney disease in newborn and young infants, Pediatr Radiol 18:287, 1988.

BIBLIOGRAPHY

Stark JE and Weinberger E: Ultrasonography of the neonatal genitourinary tract, Appl Radiol 22:50, 1993.

• PART FOUR •

Cerebrovascular and Peripheral Vascular Non-Invasive Evaluations

CHAPTER 19

Vascular Sonography and Plethysmography

Principles and Instrumentation

Richard E. Rae II

Throughout medical history the circulatory system has been a source of great mystery and puzzlement. Many diseases and conditions in the human body have led investigators to discover a vascular etiology where a completely different diagnosis was expected. Unfortunately the source often has not been found in time to save a diseased organ or limb or has been discovered only after the patient's death.

The introduction of radiographic imaging of the arterial system in 1923 made possible accurate vascular diagnosis and greatly enhanced the potential for surgical repair of vascular lesions. The first carotid arteriogram was performed in 1927,[8] and the first translumbar aortogram in 1929.[4] Many years were required to perfect angiographic equipment and techniques, but angiography has become the standard method for assessing vascular anatomy.

Angiography also has numerous drawbacks. There are risks resulting from reactions to the iodine-based contrast media. Furthermore, the examination is performed with the patient in an immobile position; needle punctures or cutdowns and rapid injections of contrast are required, all of which contribute to patient anxiety and occasionally result in patients refusing the examination.

The introduction of digital subtraction angiography (DSA) was originally hailed as a breakthrough in diagnosis; it was intravenous as opposed to intraarterial and could be performed on an outpatient basis. Various studies undertaken since its introduction, however, have shown as little as a 65% overall accuracy when compared with ultrasonic noninvasive findings and the true gold standard, the findings at surgery.[7] Intravenous Digital Subtraction Angiography has been supplanted by arterial injections in most institutions now, thus bringing the procedure full circle, back to the same risks found with conventional arteriography.

Many of the pitfalls of arteriography, venography, and DSA stem from the fact that these procedures are capable only of showing those structures that can be actively filled by the radiographic contrast material; thus, only filling defects can be interpreted as suspect (Fig. 19-1). The images are in two dimensions only and lack the ability to show the vessel from more angles without reinjection and running another film series. The contrast agents can often mask underlying anatomy, or "sneak by" low-density soft plaques that do not obstruct flow.

In addition to invasive procedures, many other noninvasive and nonangiographic methods are available, including ultrasonic techniques. In addition, techniques such as plethysmography correlate well and are often used within the specialty of vascular technology. Some of these techniques are discussed in detail in applicable sections of this and the next three chapters. The ideal noninvasive vascular diagnostic method is truly noninvasive, has a high overall accuracy, is atraumatic and comfortable to the patient, can be performed quickly, and does not require bulky equipment or long setup procedures.

Doppler and high-resolution duplex ultrasonic techniques fulfill these requirements. Doppler and duplex techniques have come a long way since their inception; Doppler techniques were first used for vascular purposes during the late 1960s and early 1970s, and commercial duplex scanners were developed and made available in the late 1970s. Initial physician wariness gave way to widespread acceptance as numerous papers and presentations began to document the accuracy and usefulness of these techniques. Among the pioneers in the vascular field are Eugene Strandness, Robert Barnes, and David Sumner, whose techniques and diagnostic criteria are still in use today. Hundreds of clinical and laboratory studies have been performed comparing noninvasive techniques to angiography and surgical findings, and high degrees of sensitivity, specificity, and overall accuracy have been reported over the years. The chapters in this part of the textbook describe Doppler, duplex sonography, color-flow imaging, and other noninvasive techniques for arterial and venous evaluation, including evaluation of the extremity vessels and the cerebrovascular system. Each vascular system is considered independently, including pertinent anatomy, pathology, and equipment needs, and commonly used examination procedures based

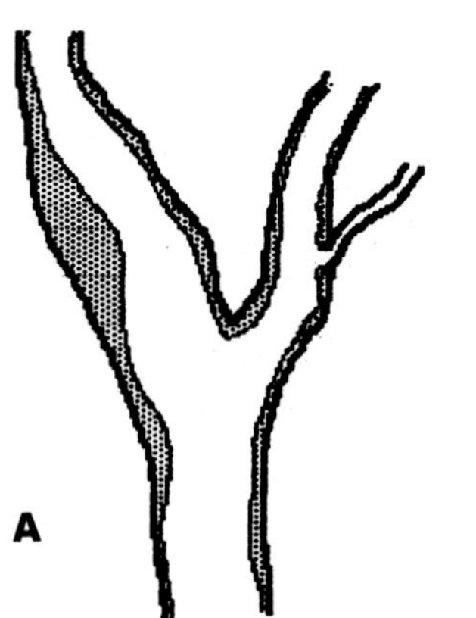

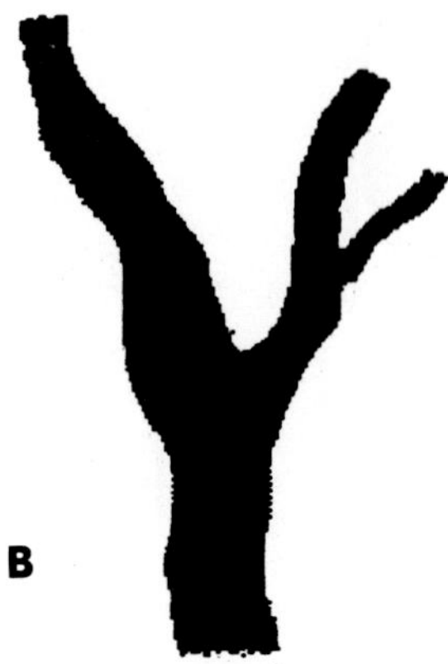

FIG. 19-1 The 50% smooth stenosis in **A** may not be adequately demonstrated by arteriography and be interpreted as normal, **B.**

on techniques described by Barnes, Strandness, Talbot, and others are explained. Data on examination variations, normal results, and interpretation of abnormal findings with examples of published diagnostic criteria are presented along with illustrative cases.

It is essential to understand the principles of a diagnostic procedure before becoming involved with it. This chapter considers the Doppler effect and how it applies to the vascular examination, along with the equipment and its use. The physiologic and mechanical principles of plethysmography will also be explained.

HISTORIC NOTE

The Doppler ultrasound apparatus makes use of the Doppler effect, which was described by the mathematician Christian Andreas Doppler in 1842. He observed that the frequency of sound waves varied depending on the speed of the sound transmitter relative to the listener.

About 2 years after Doppler's equation was developed to express the phenomenon, a scientific colleague of Doppler, Christoph Buys-Ballot, devised an experiment to test the equation's validity. He assembled a small group of musicians with perfect pitch and one horn player beside a railroad track. He then had a train pull a flatcar with another horn player past these musical observers. Each horn player played the same note, and the musical observers noted and recorded the differences in perceived pitch between the tone of the notes played by the musician going by on the flatcar at various speeds and the identical notes played by the musician in the stationary group. The resulting differences proved Doppler's theory.[6]

CONTINUOUS-WAVE DOPPLER

In the continuous-wave Doppler bloodflow device (Fig. 19-2) the sound source is a small probe housing one transmitting and one receiving crystal. Red blood cells reflect

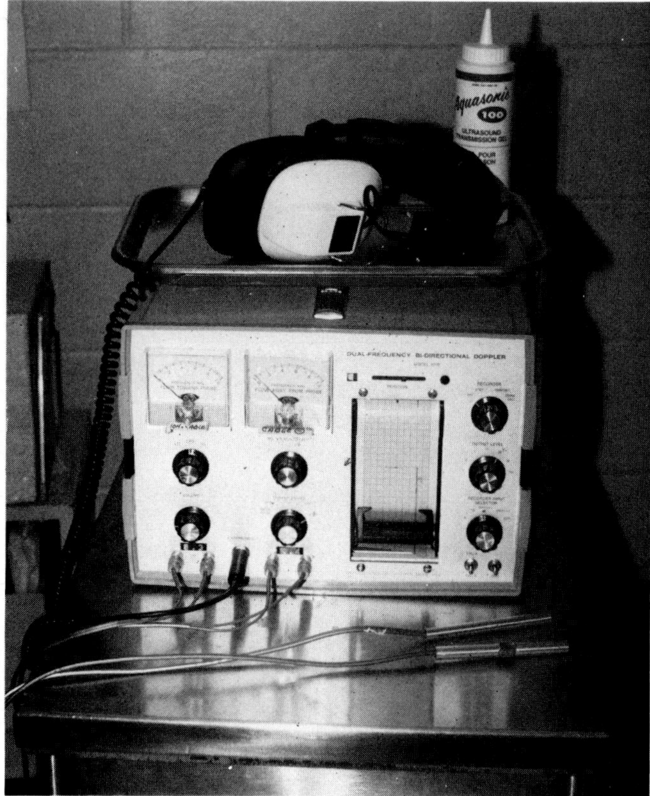

FIG. 19-2 Directional Doppler device.

ultrasound impulses, and the frequency of the reflected sound wave is shifted to either a higher or lower pitch depending on the flow velocity, as described by the Doppler equation:

$$F_d = 2F_cV\ (\cos \Theta)/C$$

where
F_d = Doppler-shifted frequency
F_c = stationary source center frequency
V = velocity
cos Θ = cosine of the beam angle
c = the propagation velocity of sound

Increasing the sound frequency, velocity of the source, or angulation changes the amount of Doppler shift, and increasing the propagation velocity of the sound decreases the Doppler shift.[12]

In all devices a change of shift in frequency is detected only if the flow velocity is greater than 4 to 6 cm/s, therefore an absent signal at a vascular site may imply anything from totally absent flow to flow moving at a velocity slower than 4 cm/s.[2]

In the directional Doppler device the probe is usually held so that the sound beam intersects the vessel at an angle of approximately 45 degrees to the plane of flow, which is the optimal angle for accurate measurement. Signals that do not intercept the flow at an angle other than perpendicular will not be Doppler-shifted, angles other than 30 to 50 degrees may result in false or erroneous readings. When the probe is oriented so that the flow is toward the probe face, this is usually interpreted as antegrade flow, and flow away from the probe face is usually considered retrograde flow (in certain circumstances and examination positions flow directions may be inverted, so sometimes the interpretation is reversed). A directional Doppler therefore is capable of showing the direction and the relative velocity of flow. Most equipment features two gauges, one for flow toward and one for flow away from the probe, and these gauges are calibrated to show relative velocity of the blood flow in the direction specified. It is important that the transducer be correctly directed relative to the direction of flow in the vessel being examined so that false diagnoses of flows seeming to go in the wrong direction are avoided.

In practice the probe is placed against the skin and is coupled by means of a water-soluble acoustic gel, which serves to eliminate air pockets and ensure optimal acoustic transmission and reception. The transmitted sound waves strike the red corpuscles and bounce back. The reflected signals are shifted in pitch, either higher or lower, depending on the relative velocity. The direction of flow also affects the reflected sound. As the reflected waveforms strike the receiving crystal, they are converted into electric signals via the piezoelectric principle. The circuitry of the Doppler device then separate the signals of increased frequency from those of decreased frequency and distinguishes between signals reflected by flow toward or away from the probe face. The signals are then fed to outputs that convert them to audible sound (heard by speakers or headphones) and also are fed to quadrature outputs for spectrum analyzers and zero-crossing strip chart devices.

Probes are available in frequencies manufactured in ranges from 2.25 to 10 MHz. The lower frequencies are usually found in fetal monitoring devices or Doppler stethoscopes intended for intraabdominal vessels, wherein sound penetration and large beam widths are desirable. The higher frequencies, from 5 to 10 MHz, are the ones most frequently used in extremity and cerebrovascular Doppler examination. The probes also vary in size and shape, from flat transducers with a fixed beam angle used often in surgery for brachial pulse monitoring to large pocket-sized devices that incorporate the transducer and signal processors into one unit.

The most versatile probe, and the one that is referred to exclusively in the discussion to follow, is the pencil-style probe. This probe is also available in many configurations, depending on the manufacturer. It can vary from a simple aluminum tube with the crystals epoxied into the end to a completely enclosed plastic probe with complex circuitry incorporated into the probe housing. The simpler the probe, however, the better, when maintenance and cost are prime concerns. The simple probes are light, practical, and easier to repair than complex probes. Their lower cost usually means that several can be placed in reserve for the same price as one more sophisticated probe. Usually the complex probes require attached modules to allow frequency-circuit matching. The simple probes are calibrated to one set frequency and are matched to calibrated input and output jacks. The latter system has advantages in that faulty frequency-matching modules may ruin both probe and Doppler devices whereas calibrated jacks and transducers require no modules between probe and Doppler system. Although the complex probe-module systems allow easier interchanging of different frequency probes, the devices using simpler probes are optionally equipped with two sets of calibrated outlets and a selection knob so higher and lower frequencies can be used alternatively.

The audible Doppler flow information requires a method of permanent recording if later interpretation and diagnosis are required. The most commonly used system is the strip-chart recorder. This device has a zero-crossing circuit, which discriminates between antegrade and retrograde flow, much as the directional gauges in the main device do. In the standard recording format, antegrade flow is placed on the positive (upward) side of a zero baseline and retrograde flow on the negative (downward) side. The examiner is thus able to determine the flow direction and flow patterns visually. Advances in computer technology have enabled serial interfaces to be used, which can take the positive-channel and negative-channel zero-crossing information and output it to portable computer systems with appropriate software. The versatility of these systems is considerable; one can watch the waveforms scroll by on the computer screen, freeze the display when an adequate range of waveforms has been obtained, scroll back to pick the specific group desired, and store them in the program for later printout. Some programs and devices can also save plethysmographic waveforms and store pressure readings from automatic cuff inflators connected to the interface. Once an examination is completed the sonographer or vascular technologist can simply enter a print command and the entire study, including patient data, history, pressure information, and graphically labeled and displayed waveforms, can be printed as a professional-appearing report. The savings in chart paper and sonographer time spent mounting the study can easily justify the extra expense for this enhancement.

Although a zero-crossing circuit and strip-chart recorder are more than adequate in general applications, the biggest disadvantage is created when two signals in opposite directions are of equal strength. The zero-crossing circuit averages the two outputs, and the net flow signal may average out to zero, creating an erroneous chart tracing. Unlike a zero-crossing circuit, a quadrature interface electronically isolates antegrade and retrograde signals and resolves this problem by displaying both sets of signals simultaneously in their respective directions and respective strengths (Fig. 19-3). Quadrature circuits are almost always used with spectrum analyzers, especially where critical flow information is important to diagnosis (see Spectral Analysis of Doppler Signals).

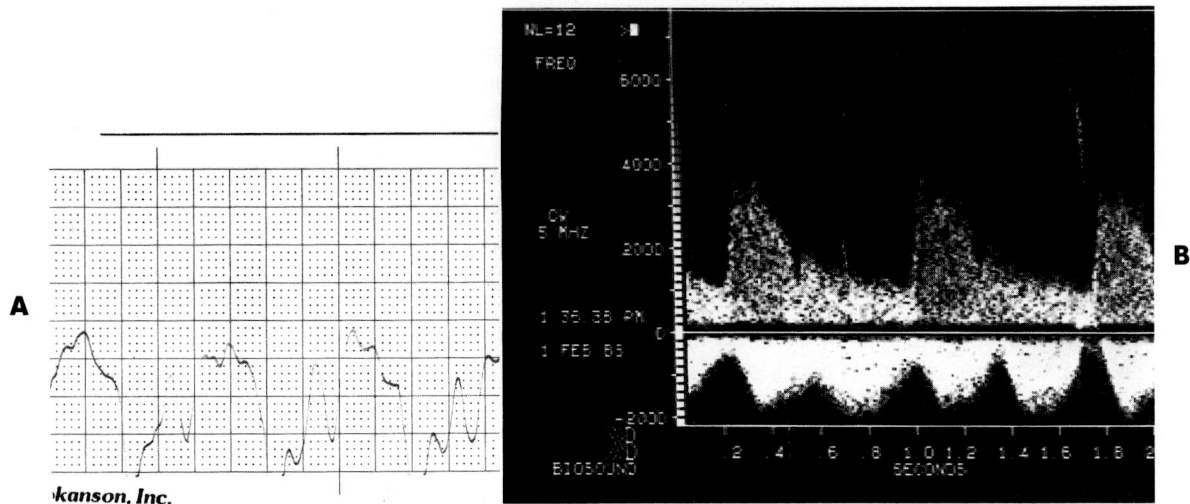

FIG. 19-3 Zero-crossing versus quadrature. Arterial and venous flow within the same beam path and in two directions is averaged together by the zero-crossing circuit, and discrimination is impossible, **A.** The same signals are easily discriminated on a spectrum analyzer and quadrature circuit, **B.**

Some Dopplers are equipped with a signal-select switch, which can be set to show retrograde flow on the positive side of the graph when depressed. In some devices this switch can completely shut off either the right or left channel to help facilitate determination of the amount of flow reversal, or help isolate information from one particular direction of flow. Other devices have a separate knob that allows only positive, only negative, inverted net flow, or normal net flow to be recorded.

Strip charts are usually single graph, but some recorders have provisions for two readouts simultaneously. One readout is usually set for net flow and the other for antegrade flow, retrograde flow, ECG, or any other tracing that may be useful while the Doppler examination is being recorded. For most purposes one graph is sufficient, and all strip-chart examples are shown with net flow on a single-graph chart.

PULSED DOPPLER

Continuous-wave devices are useful in many applications but have a few pitfalls in resolution because everything in the path of the beam is detected. This explains why arterial and venous signals are often detected simultaneously. Another problem with this is that signals from the multiple arteries in the beam path cannot be differentiated, so occasional errors are made. This is especially important when an occluded artery underlies a patent, unrelated vessel in the beam path. Pulsed Doppler devices enable discrimination to be made.

Pulsed Doppler devices are usually (but not exclusively) incorporated into real time imaging devices and work on principles more akin to B-scan imaging than Doppler. Whereas continuous-wave Doppler is, as the name states, continuous (one transducer always sending, the other always receiving), pulsed Doppler is pulsed (i.e., a signal is sent out in a pulse and then the transducer pauses to receive the signal). The advantage here is one of depth localization, using range gating. This means that while Doppler information from all levels is being received, the range gate can be set to detect only the information at a specific level. The sample volume, which does this, can be located anywhere along the beam path, and is shown on the A-mode as a gate or on an imager as a box on a line that shows the beam angle on those devices with a steerable Doppler. The sample volume can also be increased or decreased in size, meaning that flow can be sampled in a vessel within as small an area as 0.5 mm or enlarged to 2 cm or more to measure flow across an entire region. The sample volume is usually elliptic in shape. Beam angle is critical because it is in continuous-wave measurement; angles perpendicular to the flow do not give any useful flow-shifted information. In addition, many of the diagnostic criteria published for interpreting examinations assume that the insonation angle has been corrected to between 45 and 60 degrees. One drawback is that the pulse repetition frequency (PRF) may often be too high to detect slow-moving flow or too low to detect very high-velocity flow, resulting in inaccurate measurement at times. If a severe stenosis results in a severe flow velocity increase and frequency shift that exceeds half the PRF (The Nyquist limit), then the excessive frequencies may be "cut off" or transposed as spurious frequency readings. This is known as aliasing (see the Spectral Analysis of Doppler Signals and Color-Flow imaging sections). Pulsed Doppler is not always as convenient to use as a continuous-wave device and is generally not indicated for the routine examination of small peripheral vessels (unless imaging is required), since both hands are usually needed to adjust all the depth and volume factors.

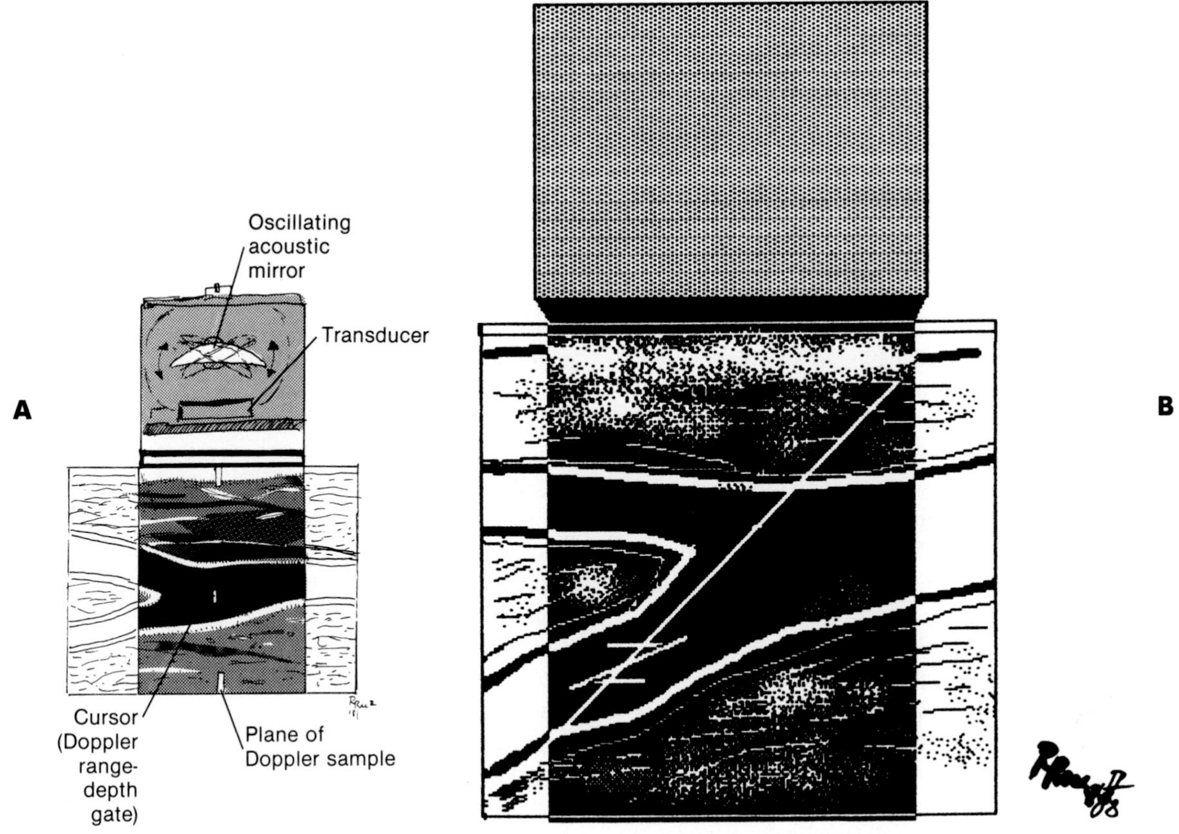

FIG. 19-4 Types of high-resolution scanner transducers. **A,** Oscillating acoustic mirror; **B,** Phased array with electronically steered Doppler.

The best results are often obtained with a combination of pulsed and continuous-wave Doppler techniques, since the two technologies are complementary and compensate for each modality's respective weaknesses.

HIGH-RESOLUTION DUPLEX REAL TIME ULTRASOUND EQUIPMENT

The introduction of high-resolution small-parts scanners has proved to be a definite breakthrough in the noninvasive examination of small or difficult-to-evaluate structures in the body. In the vascular field, these imaging devices are coupled with an integral pulsed Doppler device, a continuous-wave Doppler device, or both. Units that incorporate both imaging and Doppler are referred to as *duplex machines*. Units that can also perform color-flow imaging are occasionally called *triplex machines,* although this term has not found widespread acceptance. The most obvious benefit of a duplex scanner is the ability to image a vessel, then steer the Doppler sample volume to any area on the screen and obtain a flow sample. This allows the examiner to visualize a stenosis, then obtain flow samples proximal and distal to it to determine the hemodynamic effect of the stenosis. More recent devices are able to show the flow in color superimposed over the gray-scale image (see section on Doppler color flow).

Among the many uses of duplex scanners are the following:

- Carotid artery evaluation.
- Peripheral artery evaluation.
- Peripheral venous evaluation.
- Abdominal vessel evaluation.

Most of these applications are covered in depth later in this chapter.

Several companies manufacture small-parts scanners, and operator-oriented design and resolution improve constantly. Scanners used for vascular evaluation generally are either mechanical or electronically phased, and of two image-format types—sector and linear. Almost all modern ultrasound systems now use phased-array technology, but some systems that use mechanical sectoring still can be found. Most systems available use one of the methods described next to obtain a real time image of the area being examined and to obtain Doppler information (Fig. 19-4).

An older but still available system uses a fixed transducer with an oscillating acoustic mirror to sweep the beam through a fluid path.

Doppler in this system is obtained through the same transducer as is used for imaging. Activating the Doppler stops the mirror at the midline position and cuts in a simultaneous extended A-mode for reference when the Doppler sample depth is being range gated. The examiner can thus see changes in position and move the transducer to compensate. The "steerability" of the Doppler sample is limited in this system, since the mirror only traverses a 30-degree sector. The sample line can be angled 15 degrees in either direction from the centerline, however, and although angle vectoring is unavailable (see section on Spectral Analysis of Doppler Signals), the system is still flexible for peak frequency assessment. In addition, when the Doppler sample plane is centered, it is in the exact center of the image, and the entire probe can be angled in transverse or longitudinal positions and treated like a rather large handheld Doppler probe. The A-mode display can help with placement when the probe is used in this fashion, giving some degree of simultaneity but still not allowing a simultaneous image and Doppler display.

Another more commonly seen system uses a single-crystal mechanical transducer that rocks back and forth and provides a sector image. Doppler signals are obtained with the same crystal used for imaging or an integral separate crystal in the same place as the imaging crystal. The image can be set to update periodically as in other devices, and also lacks simultaneity of Doppler and image.

The most commonly available contemporary systems use a phased-array probe for imaging, but when a duplex mode is selected, certain crystals in the array can be set to provide only Doppler information, and the Doppler angle, depth, and sample volume can be electronically steered and adjusted (although one company uses a fluid-filled standoff wedge attached to the scanhead at an 18-degree angle for Doppler and color-flow acquisition), allowing the transducer to appear deceptively simple and to have no mechanical parts. In addition, these systems provide true simultaneous Doppler and imaging with little or no interference. Phased-array transducers can be in sector, linear, or curved linear formats. Among the advantages of these systems is the ability to evaluate abdominal vasculature, such as renal arteries, which can move in and out of the Doppler sample plane with each inspiration and which are almost impossible to evaluate for flow without this capability.

Most of these scanners have axial and lateral resolution capabilities of no less than 0.3 mm and can allow the image to be enlarged for evaluating the detail of the vessel walls or other area being examined. Their sizes vary from large to fairly compact; a few are portable enough for use in bedside examinations. Some companies have introduced miniature versions, enabling the device to be more easily transported and providing an equivalent or better image at roughly half the cost of the larger units.

As can be seen, the differing characteristics of the various machines available demand differing examination techniques. Discussion of the examination methods and idiosyncrasies present with each type is not practicable here. A general explanation and interpretation of typical applications for these systems is given in the body of the text, along with fairly flexible examination techniques that can be used with most of the systems currently available.

SPECTRAL ANALYSIS OF DOPPLER SIGNALS

The most common method of making a permanent record of Doppler flow signals has been through the strip-chart recorder. An organized set of flow tracings by this device also allows delayed interpretation and diagnosis of vascular flow abnormalities. The strip-chart tracing, however, shows only a mean flow velocity analog and does not reveal the complete range of frequencies present in the audible Doppler signal. Therefore the clinician interpreting the examination from tracings alone is unable to take into account the various sounds and frequency changes in the Doppler signal that may indicate flow obstructions and stenoses. This may lead to an incorrect diagnosis, especially in the cerebrovascular system, in which normal flow is of high velocity and always above the zero baseline. Unless a lesion occludes a vessel, the high-velocity and high-frequency jet effect distal to the obstruction may often have the parameters of a normal internal carotid signal. A well-trained examiner should be able to hear these changes; unfortunately, many times the examiner and the interpreting clinician are not the same person. The examiner may note, for the benefit of the interpreting clinician, where signals that are suggestive of disease occur; but any inexperience or uncertainty can confuse the diagnosis and cause erroneous interpretation.

Sound spectral analysis of Doppler signals is a technique that allows the information lost in strip-chart recording to be permanently recorded in a visual format. This method involves analyzing the frequencies present in a Doppler-shifted signal by fast Fourier transformation (FFT), with subsequent sorting of the frequencies by a series of filters.[2,12]

The relative strengths of the sorted frequencies are assigned respective brightness levels, or color codes on certain analyzers. They can also be displayed as a histogram of power levels at a given moment in the waveforms as a function of time. Note that the gradients of gray or color levels do not signify the relative velocity; this is shown as a deflection above (and below, on bidirectional devices) a zero baseline as in the strip-chart recorder, except that antegrade and retrograde flow can be shown simultaneously. Velocity or frequency or both are shown on the vertical axis of the display; time is displayed along the horizontal axis (Fig. 19-5).

Instrumentation

The spectrum analyzer has been available in many forms for a number of years. Early devices required recording several seconds of the signal intended for analysis on a built-in tape. The waveform was traced on a paper covered rotating drum as the tape played over and over, and the process usually took a minute or longer before the sonogram (or sonagram, as it was then called) was complete. This method is outdated now and had many disadvantages. The signals were not analyzed as they were being obtained (real time), and the process was not practical in a heavy case load since it meant tape recording the examination for later analysis

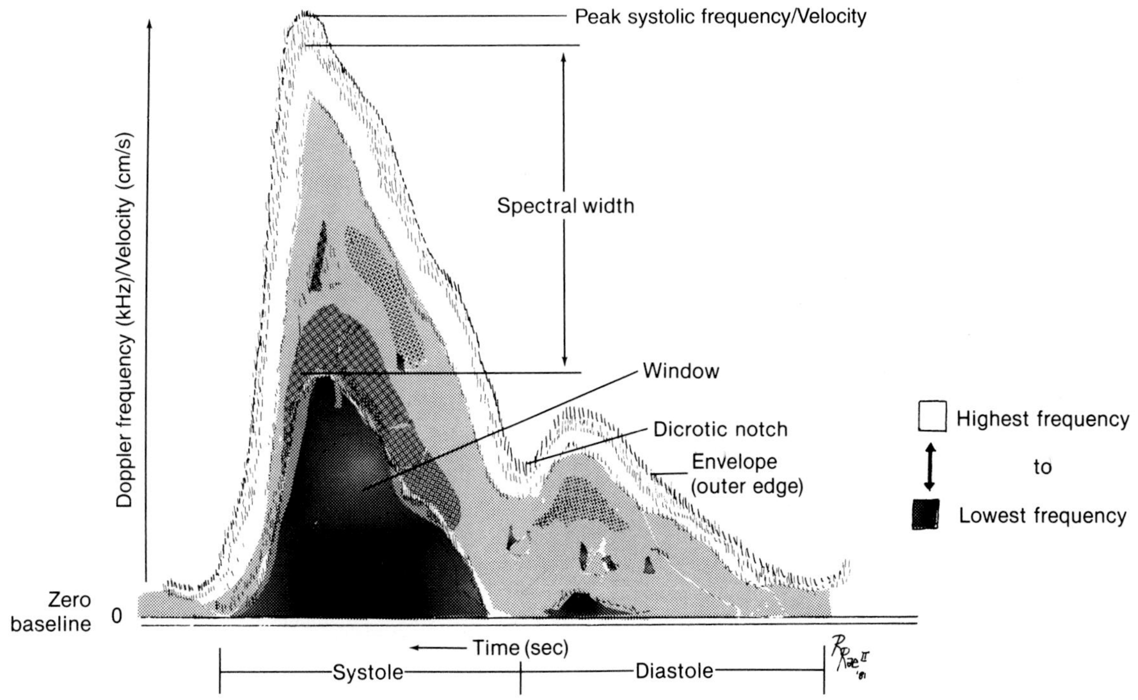

FIG. 19-5 Diagram of spectrally analyzed Doppler waveform, showing diagnostic characteristics.

processing. Another disadvantage was that many of the higher and lower frequencies were lost in the transfer from tape to tape. In addition, the frequency display on these older devices was extremely difficult to interpret, and is as far removed from today's spectral analysis displays as B-mode scanning with storage oscilloscopes is from today's digital gray-scale B-scanners.

Modern devices intended for Doppler flow analysis present the data in real time and allow high-quality calculations of flow velocities and frequency distribution. These devices are either incorporated into high-resolution B-scanners or are available as stand-alone units that can be attached to quadrature outputs or audio outlets defined for spectrum-analyzer use. They can display several seconds of signal data (some displays store up to a minute of data and allow scrolling backward) and can freeze the display for hard-copy recording. Some devices have gray-scale energy displays, some color-coded displays, and some both. Different displays can show peak frequency calculations, peak velocity calculations, spectral broadening levels, peak ratio comparisons, and a range of pulsatility indices, depending on the equipment used.

The majority of spectrum analyzers on the market are bidirectional, although unidirectional analyzes may be seen rarely. The unidirectional devices process both directions of flow together and show them superimposed on each other, making their use limited when analyzing extremity flow and of no use at all when making direction-critical assessments such as in a vertebral or carotid steal (Fig. 19-6).

The spectral display is basically the same regardless of whether incorporated into a duplex scanner or used with hand-held Doppler units. Velocity or frequency is displayed on the vertical axis. The display can be expanded to show a maximum shift of 22,000 Hz (22 kHz) or frequency reduced by steps to show frequencies as low as 2,000 Hz (2 kHz). Positive and negative flow velocity scales in m/s or cm/s will automatically vary as the angle vector is adjusted. The display scale can thus be adjusted as the examiner sees fit, ideally at the lowest setting that allows the peak of the systolic waveform to be completely seen on the screen. The zero baseline can be adjusted on many analyzers to allow retrograde flow shifts of an increased nature to be displayed. The display can be inverted to allow the proper directional orientation to be displayed, since probe and transducer angles must often be varied (especially in carotid examination) for easier access to the vessel in question, and flow toward the transducer may be considered retrograde, depending on the application. As mentioned when a pulsed Doppler is used and a severe stenosis results in a severe flow velocity increase or frequency shift that exceeds half the pulse repetition frequency (the Nyquist limit), then the excessive frequencies may be "cut off" or transposed as spurious frequency readings, and the true peak may be lost. This phenomenon is known as aliasing. Aliasing will not occur with a continuous-wave Doppler, so if high peak velocities or frequencies are detected, switching to a continuous-wave probe will allow display of the entire waveform (Fig. 19-7).

Most analyzers allow some degree of postprocessing.

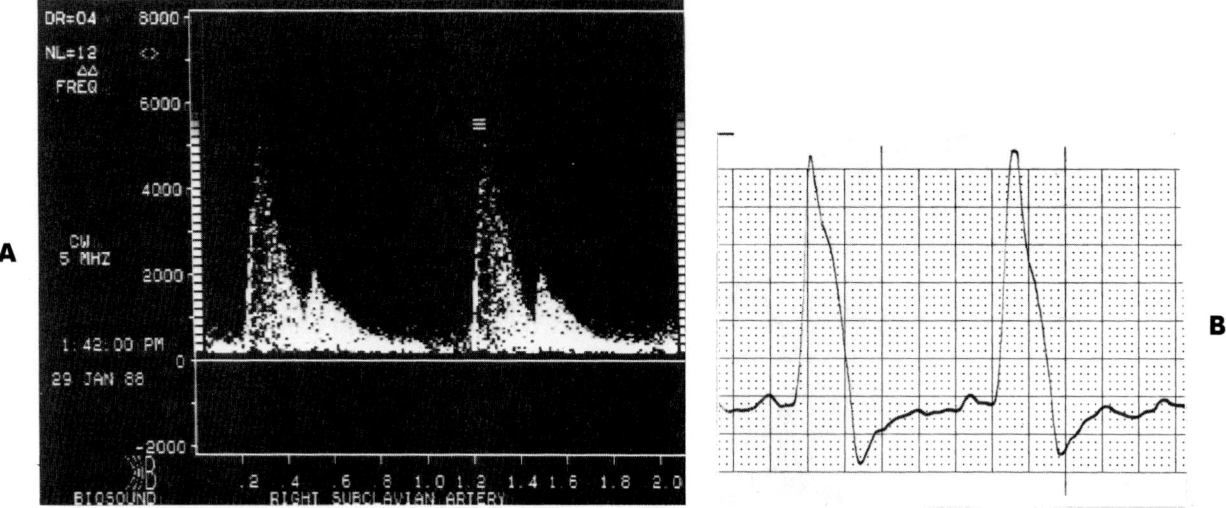

FIG. 19-6 Unidirectional spectrum analyzer. The spectrum analyzer waveform, **A,** does not accurately represent the triphasic analog waveform, **B;** the reversed second component is shown positively between the first and third components on the spectral display.

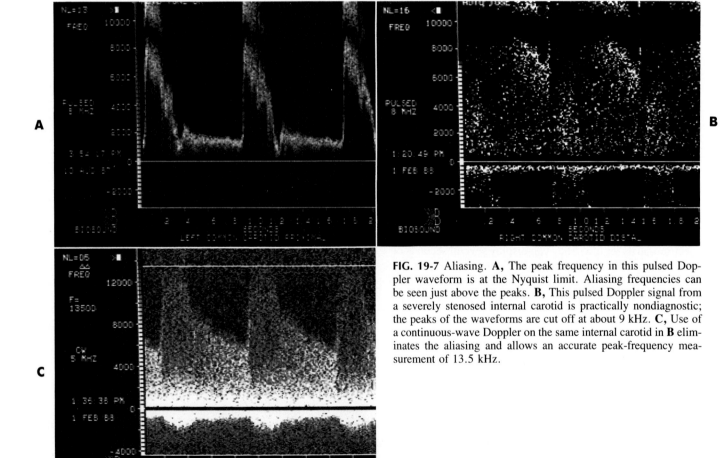

FIG. 19-7 Aliasing. **A,** The peak frequency in this pulsed Doppler waveform is at the Nyquist limit. Aliasing frequencies can be seen just above the peaks. **B,** This pulsed Doppler signal from a severely stenosed internal carotid is practically nondiagnostic; the peaks of the waveforms are cut off at about 9 kHz. **C,** Use of a continuous-wave Doppler on the same internal carotid in **B** eliminates the aliasing and allows an accurate peak-frequency measurement of 13.5 kHz.

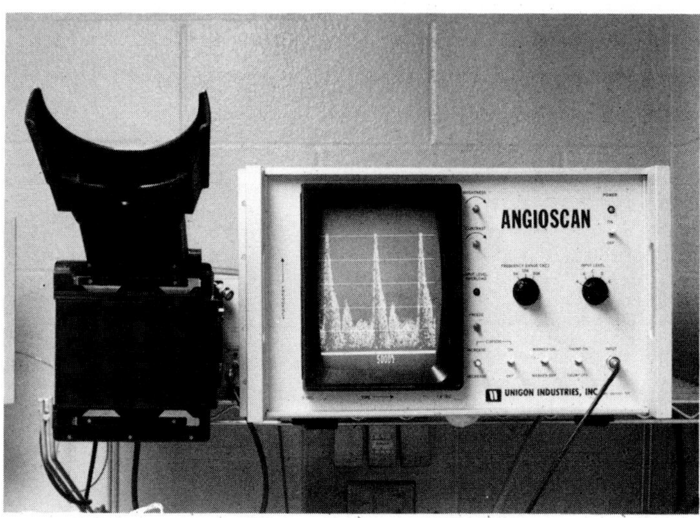

FIG. 19-8 Typical spectral analyzer (unidirectional, gray scale).

One or more cursors can be moved to anywhere along the vertical axis to allow velocity and frequency measurements, heart-rate calculation, spectral broadening indices, and pulsatility indices. These are very sensitive measurements and can help quantify the degree of flow disturbance or approximate percentage of stenosis, as we will discuss later. In addition, the display gain and background noise levels can be adjusted to allow the clearest waveform to be displayed or to enhance the waveform for critical analysis.

Peak frequency and peak velocity are two critical flow measurements that analyzers can be set to display. Which to use depends on the Doppler application or interpreter's preference. Peak velocity measurements are usually measured in meters per second (m/s) or centimeters per second (cm/s) and are accurate only when the precise angle of beam to flow direction is known and calculated from the Doppler equation. Analyzers in duplex scanners allow this to be calculated automatically using a flow vector line, which appears on the sample volume indicator and can be adjusted by the examiner on-screen. The examiner simply aligns the flow vector line parallel with the plane of flow in the vessel being sampled. The precise flow angle is displayed on-screen and can be adjusted through moving the Doppler angle line and adjusting the vector line. As the vector is altered the analyzer scale automatically updates. The most accurate velocity readings appear at a displayed vector angle of between 45 and 60 degrees, and almost all diagnostic criteria published take this range into account. Peak frequency is the mode of choice, however, when the beam-vessel angle cannot be precisely calculated as in a continuous-wave Doppler hand-held probe examination or with fixed-angle duplex and tortuous arteries. An example of a spectrum analyzer is shown in Fig. 19-8.

Interpretation of the Spectral Display

Several characteristics of the spectral waveform are analyzed when interpreting them[10] (see Fig. 19-5):

Initially the peak systolic frequency or peak systolic velocity is examined. This increases proportionally with the flow velocity, and higher readings correspond with luminal reduction; consider placing your finger over the end of a water hose. As you narrow the opening, the water velocity increases through the opening although volume does not. This high-velocity flow increase is called the *jet effect*. Peak end diastolic frequency and velocity are also significant, since increased diastolic flow readings can help narrow the range of suspected stenosis.

Next is the appearance of the waveform. The normal direction of systolic flow is conventionally displayed on the top half of the baseline and retrograde flow on the bottom half (note that if the probe is angled with the flow the display would then be inverted). Systole and diastole are displayed as concentrations of shades of gray or color levels ranging from dark gray to white, depending on the signal strength of the received velocity waveform. This display is a graphic representation of how the blood cells are moving through the vessel at a given moment in time. Normal laminar (smooth) flow has a bright concentration displayed near the outer edge of the waveform or envelope, indicating that most of the blood cells are moving at maximum velocity. There is a dark area in the center of the waveform, signifying a lack of low-velocity motion of blood cells during that phase of systole. This dark area is conventionally referred to as the window.

The shape of the waveform envelope is also a factor. A well-defined envelope is seen in cases of normal laminar flow. As flow is disturbed and turbulence increases, the envelope becomes ragged and less distinct.

During peak systole, the distance between the outer border at the peak of the waveform and the upper border of the window is considered the spectral width. This spectral width can be fairly narrow with a prominent window in a normal waveform, or it can be spread out and widened with filling-in or absence of the window when flow is turbulent

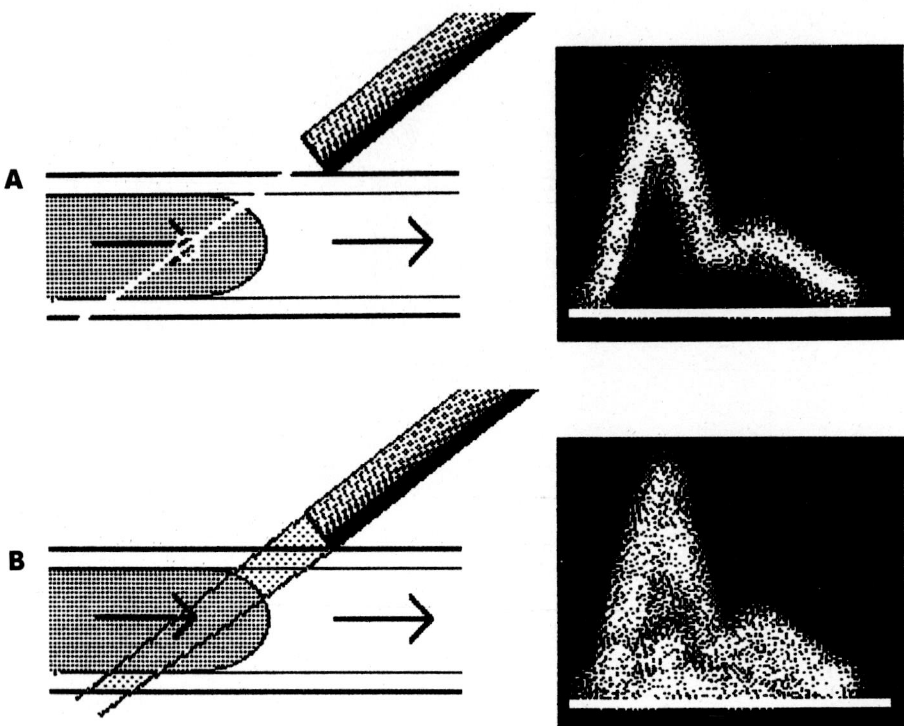

FIG. 19-9 Pulsed versus continuous-wave Doppler. The pulsed Doppler, **A,** allows discrete sampling of a particular flow stream from the center or edges of the vessel. The continuous-wave Doppler, **B,** samples the entire range of flow across the vessel and shows all the velocities present in the beam path at once.

or disturbed. This change in the spectral width increases with flow disturbance and is known as spectral broadening. As flow turbulence increases, eddying and severe flow disturbance may show a very bright concentration of flow at the baseline at peak systole and a poorly defined envelope with increased systolic velocity during the postsystolic/diastolic phase. This concentration corresponds with an audible bruit (see below).

Continuous-wave Doppler and pulsed Doppler waveforms are different on the spectral display and require modifying interpretive technique because of these differences. Continuous-wave spectrals almost always appear to have spectral broadening because flow across the entire vessel, as well as any other vessels in the beam path, is displayed, and the slower velocity flow along the vessel walls fills in the window. With a pulsed Doppler the sample is almost always taken from the center stream; thus the slower velocities along the walls are avoided. Pulsed Doppler spectra are inevitably cleaner and are more accurate indicators of turbulence and spectral broadening; however, continuous-wave Doppler spectra are better indicators of peak velocity and frequencies and for showing turbulence in the vessel, since pulsed Doppler sample placement may miss flow jets directed at areas other than where the sample is taken unless a color-flow imaging system is used, which allows the streamline to be seen (Fig. 19-9).

Note that there is always some spectral broadening near a flow divider (such as the carotid bifurcation). True flow samples should be taken at least 1 cm downstream for accurate readings (except when sampling at a site of focal stenotic velocity increase near the flow divider).

In situations of arterial stenosis the following diagnostic characteristics may be seen:

1. Proximal to the stenosis a normal or slightly blunted waveform may be seen. The peak frequency should be normal, and there may or may not be a rounding of the peak. The separation between the first and second components (dicrotic notch) may disappear because of vascular elastic changes along the stenosed area. The window may show some flow scattering throughout.
2. Across the stenosis an increased-frequency (higher-velocity) waveform will usually be seen. The same characteristics as in the proximal waveform may be noted, and the envelope may begin to break up. The velocity usually increases directly with the degree of stenosis. The window may also begin to disappear as spectral broadening increases. A corresponding increase in pitch is heard with the Doppler. It may help to remember that arterial flow remains nearly constant until a hemodynamically significant stenosis (at 60% to 70% luminal reduction) occurs.[2]
3. Immediately distal to the stenotic area, disturbed or turbulent flow may be found ranging from a strained burbling to a high-pitched hissing Doppler signal. Peak sys-

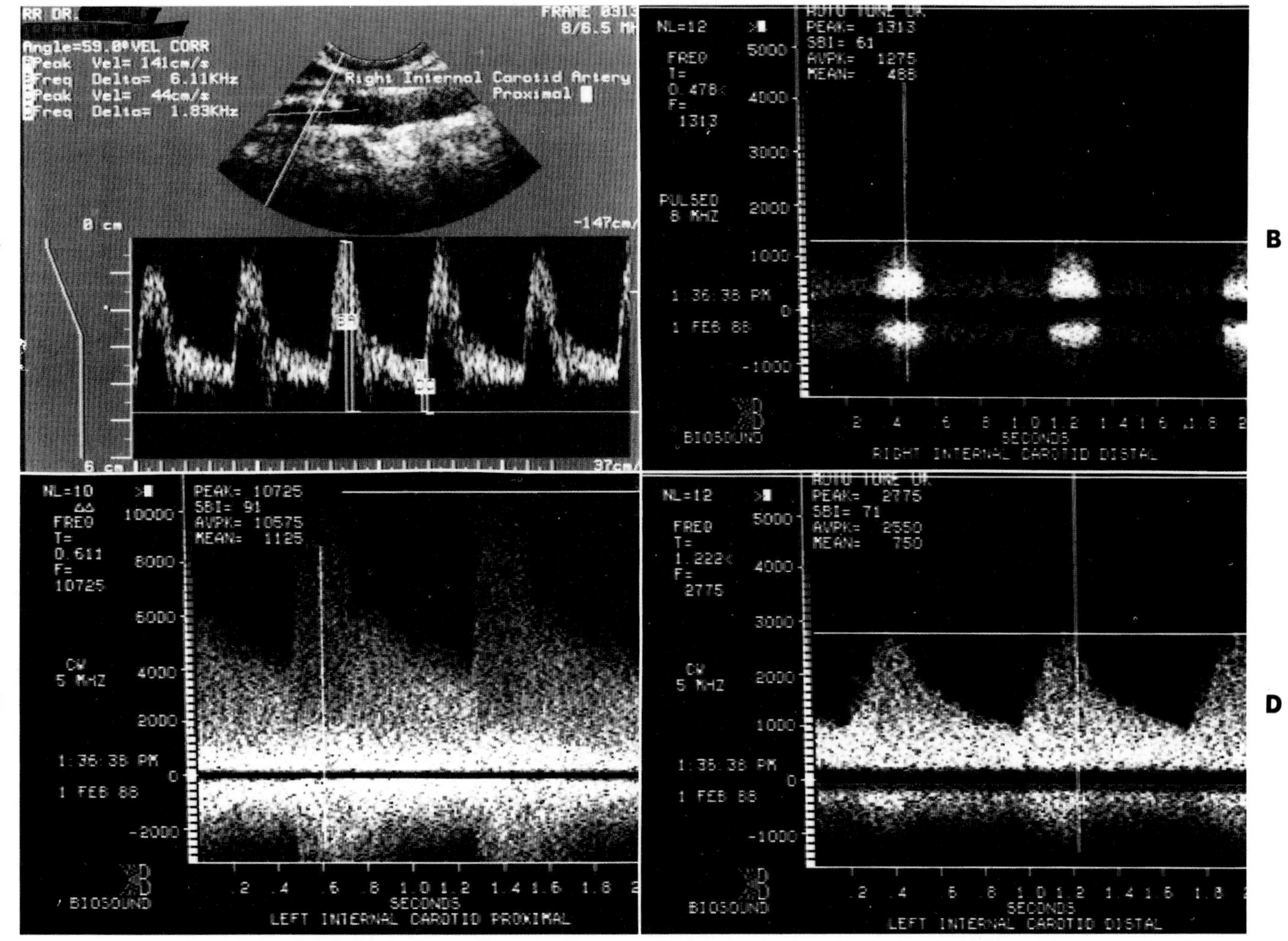

FIG. 19-10 Typical stenotic flow responses in an internal carotid artery on a spectrum analyzer. **A,** Moderate turbulence with velocity increase in a moderate stenosis. **B,** A severely turbulent and diminished pattern consistent with flow distal to a near-occlusion. **C,** Severely turbulent signal and velocity increase typical of a jet-effect response across a severe stenosis. **D,** Typical post-stenotic signal 2 cm distal to the signal in **C.**

tolic velocity and frequency increase as the flow stream increases by the jet effect, originating at the stenosis. An area of flow stagnation that occurs immediately distal to the plaque or lesion near the artery wall may cause turbulence during systole (Fig. 19-10). The spectral waveform will have a ragged-appearing indistinct envelope, with widely distributed frequencies, and a completely absent window. The severity of the stenosis may be judged from the level of envelope disruption and frequency distribution. Turbulence and eddy formation cause an increase in the higher-energy intensities at the baseline[10] and in severe cases may cause a completely disrupted waveform with apparent velocity reductions at systole in bidirectional analyzers. Pulsatility may be absent, and the pitch may either increase or decrease with the sound becoming rough and harsh.

4. A signal obtained more distally from the stenosis, away from the turbulent region, may assume the appearance of a reduced waveform with even intensity and broadening throughout, disturbed envelope edges, and no visible flow components. The peak frequency or velocity may be markedly diminished compared with the peak of the waveform seen directly at the level of stenosis. The peak frequency may be markedly rounded. Severely diminished flow may become almost flat in appearance.
5. In total occlusion a sharp thudding or thumping sound may be heard in the patent portion of the vessel immediately proximal to the block. Flow may actually drop to or below the baseline, and a very irregular-appearing spectral waveform with no distinguishing characteristics may be seen. This is caused from flow eddies within the stump.[1] No flow should be heard in the area of occlusion, although "blips" may sometimes be seen in visibly occluded arteries; these are artifactual and can be caused by vertical motion of the vessel detected by the Doppler or by nearby pulsatile vessels if the sample vol-

ume is set too wide or placed in an atrophied vessel. Diastolic flow proximal to a totally occluded vessel almost always drops to or even below the baseline. This finding of high-resistance flow is also suggestive of a distal obstruction especially when seen in a patent segment of a normally low-resistance vessel, such as the internal carotid artery.

The characteristics of flow increase across a stenosis apply to extremity arteries as well. Distal to the stenosis a rounded blunt waveform will be noted, with disappearance of the window and evidence of low flow velocities. As flow decreases, a flattened signal close to the baseline will usually be found. Remember that in the extremity arteries, loss of the second retrograde component signifies stenosis or occlusion proximally, and the flow envelope may remain well defined, regardless of the level of flow reduction.

COLOR-FLOW IMAGING

One of the disadvantages of any duplex ultrasound system is that although image data are displayed in high-resolution gray scale, the only way to determine the effect of any stenosis on the vessel's hemodynamics is to activate the pulsed Doppler and sample flow at different locations across the vessel, above and below the stenosis. It used to be assumed that flow patterns are parabolic and laminar throughout the vessel, and early pulsed Doppler sampling techniques often suggested placing the sample volume directly into the center of the visualized vessel, and angle correction instructions suggested that angle vector lines should be adjusted parallel to the sampled vessel's walls. Although this can work for unobstructed vessels with no stenotic processes, it does not work when stenoses are present. Hemodynamic studies performed on in vitro models of carotid artery bifurcations and other vessels show that discrete streamlines form, which can travel in numerous directions and at offset locations, depending on the architecture of both the vessel and any stenotic material within it. Without proper knowledge of the streamline location, the angle vector may not be set properly and subsequent velocity calculations may not be accurate (Fig. 19-11; see color images).

In the early 1980s a major advance was made in Doppler technology when systems were created that obtain Doppler shift information from returning echoes and then display that motion and direction information in color, superimposed over the image of the lumen. The earliest applications of color-flow imaging were performed in the cardiac field, but the technology was applied to analysis of other peripheral vascular structures soon afterward.

Color Flow and Hemodynamics

Before discussing color flow, it is important to discuss several hemodynamic factors that were unknown or poorly understood before the development of color-flow Doppler systems. Some new terms applicable to color flow also need defining.

In a straight tubular structure without abrupt curves or branches, flow tends to be laminar and parabolic in shape, slowing along the walls and becoming faster in the center stream. This concentration of faster velocities within a vessel is termed the *streamline*. When a streamline hits a flow divider or disruption, such as the Internal Carotid Artery/External Carotid Artery bifurcation, the flow streamline changes direction, sometimes moving to the inside of the vessel or at an angle. An area of slower velocities occurs away from the streamline, and an area of flow reversal and slow swirling may occur in an outer, dilated portion of a vessel (like the carotid bulb) or in a zone on the distal side of an obstruction. This type of flow reversal occurring simultaneously with antegrade systolic flow is termed *flow separation* (Fig. 19-12; see color image).

Most machines have the capability to display different color maps. Flow in one direction is usually displayed as a shade of red and in the other direction as a shade of blue. These shades become lighter as intensities increase. Positive velocities usually go from dark red toward near-white, or from dark red to bright yellow. Negative velocities go from dark blue toward white or from dark blue to light cyan. Conventionally, arterial flow is assigned the red value and venous flow the blue value; since this assignment can be reversed, however, it is possible to display blue arterial flow and red venous flow. In addition, since this is a function of direction, tortuous vessels may display both colors, depending on how the flow approaches or recedes from the transducer face.

Color-Flow Imaging Systems

Color-flow imaging devices use phased-array transducer technologies, and nearly all contemporary equipment has the capability to display color-flow information and gray-scale imaging data. However, manufacturers use different technology to obtain it.

There are currently two completely different methods of obtaining and displaying color-flow information; these methods are color Doppler flow imaging and time-domain flow imaging. There are advantages and disadvantages to both, and these are covered next.

Color Doppler Flow Imaging

The following Doppler equation should be familiar to all:

$$F_d = 2F_cV (\cos \Theta)/C$$

where
F_d = Doppler shifted frequency
F_c = stationary source center frequency
V = velocity
$\cos \Theta$ = cosine of the "look" angle
C = the propagation velocity of sound

Increasing the sound frequency, velocity of the source, or angulation changes the amount of Doppler shift, and increasing the propagation velocity of the sound decreases the Doppler shift.[12]

Color Doppler flow imaging systems analyze returning

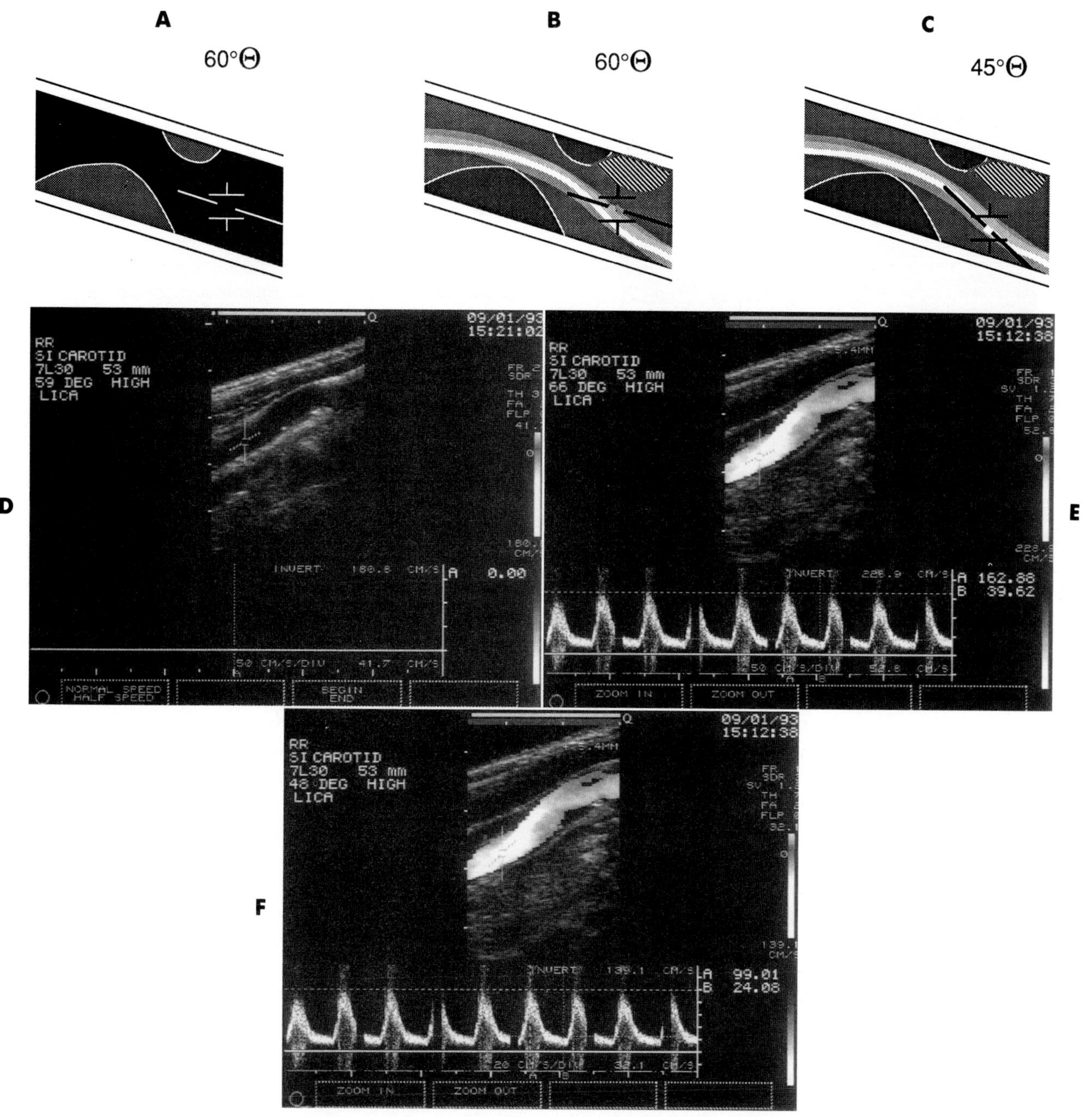

FIG. 19-11 A, In a conventional gray-scale duplex image, the sample volume is arbitrarily placed where a velocity increase is expected, and angle is corrected to place the vector line parallel with the walls. **B,** This sample placement and angle correction may not be accurate, as the streamlines defined with color-flow imaging show. **C,** With the streamline visible the sample can be accurately placed and the vector oriented with the angle of the flow streamline. **D,** To illustrate this principle and its effect on accuracy, a carotid artery image appears to have the sample and vector aligned correctly. **E,** With color flow on, the streamline is visible, the vector line does not align with it, and the velocity readings are artifactually elevated and could be interpreted as abnormal. **F,** Correcting the angle to parallel the streamline brings the velocities into a correct and more normal range.

echoes from both tissue and the moving red blood cells within the lumen. Usually on real time gray scale imaging the blood cells move too rapidly for their echoes to be discretely detected and displayed (unless the flow velocity is very low, as in veins). Color Doppler devices actually function additionally as multigated pulsed Doppler units, in that Doppler-shifted echoes at all depths can be displayed. As echoes return after the transmitted pulse, each displayed pixel location is analyzed for amplitude (stationary echoes, or what will appear as gray scale), frequency shift (move-

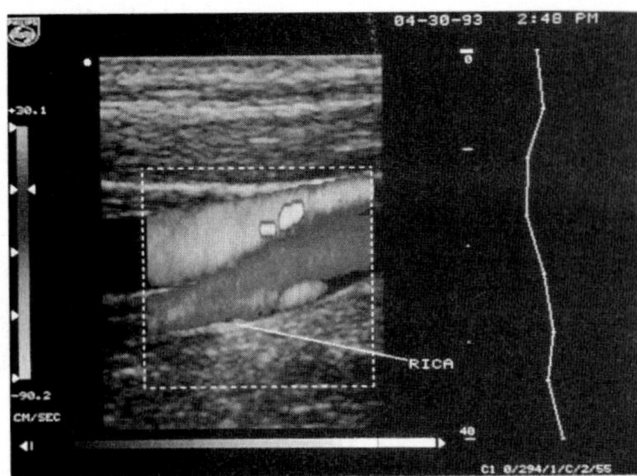

FIG. 19-12 An area of normal flow reversal appears as the blue area within the otherwise red internal carotid artery; this represents an area of flow separation.

ment and velocity), and phase (direction). Thus echoes that have no Doppler shift remain as different intensities of gray-scale pixels; echoes with Doppler-shifted information are assigned a color based on the detected direction (toward or away from the transducer face) and a value or intensity based on the return frequency shift proportional to the mean velocity at which the echo is traveling. Since every element of the transducer can thus function as a pulsed Doppler transducer, the effect is that of simultaneous blood flow in color displayed over the real time gray-scale image.

It is important to point out that pulsed Doppler used for spectrum analysis (referred to as *spectral Doppler* from here on) and color Doppler are different—a color display does not imitate exactly the same information seen when a single-point spectrum analysis is being performed (although there are often close relationships).[14]

Spectral Doppler calculates 128 to 256 points via FFT each time an ultrasound pulse is sent out and received (this is called a *look*). Very detailed high-quality flow information is obtained. There is a trade-off, however, in that the more FFT points that are calculated, the longer it takes to obtain the actual information (an increase in temporal resolution), so there is actually a delay from when the flow was sampled versus its actual dynamic state. This delay, however, is imperceptible to the observer because it occurs at a microsecond level. Spectral Doppler remains an ultrasonic standard for flow velocity because its accuracy has been documented.

Both spectral and color Doppler are affected by the frequency of the transducer and the bandwidth, since wide bandwidths are needed for better detection of tissue changes and the center frequency of a transducer is attenuated proportional to the depth of insonation. Wide bandwidths make calculation of the actual center frequency (F_c in the formula presented previously) very difficult, so many Doppler calculations assume a true frequency of 5 MHz.

Color Doppler averages between 10 and 32 looks to give a graphic estimation—an average—of the frequency shift that is not as accurate as pulsed spectral Doppler, since it does not display the strongest or peak velocity. It should be noted that for color Doppler to achieve the same accuracy as spectral Doppler, the device would have to perform the same 128 to 256 calculations on each displayed pixel, which would require unacceptably long processing times to display one complete frame of color and could not be done in real time.

A compromise must be reached between the frame rate (which determines the resolved detail of actual hemodynamic information) and the accuracy of velocities. High frame rates make the real time image appear more smooth and continuous but seriously affect color-flow information, which subsequently may appear jagged and lack streamline detail. High frame rates equal fewer looks per line of displayed information (usually about 50), and fewer looks decrease the accuracy of the detected velocities. Lowering the frame rate increases the accuracy of detected velocities and adds detail to the color-flow image display (because more looks can be obtained) but can slow the image down dramatically.

As stated, aliasing of both color Doppler and spectral Doppler occurs when the shifted frequencies reach half the PRF; the maximum velocities that can be displayed are determined by the displayed depth of the scan. Shorter scan depths increase the color and spectral velocities that can be displayed as the PRF increases. For more on color aliasing, see the section on Artifacts.

Color Doppler devices often must sacrifice gray-scale imaging quality for color-flow quality, and vice versa. This is because the axial resolution is determined by the transmitted pulse length. The longer the look, the better the Doppler shift information; the shorter the look, the better the axial resolution. So, a device with excellent axial resolution (and excellent gray-scale detail) often has decreased velocity accuracy (and poorer color-flow imaging); conversely, devices with excellent color-flow imaging may have poor gray-scale quality. Increased power levels increase the length of the pulse and can improve the color Doppler display since more looks are generated, but this can push the power level over the 100 mW/cm^2 safety standard. Gray-scale imaging and color Doppler are thus actually at opposite poles. Technologic advances and computer processing have permitted more balance between the two extremes, but some systems still do a much better job of it than others. A potential purchaser should evaluate all color-flow equipment carefully and, as with any other consumer product, not necessarily buy a product based on advertising or brand name alone.

There are two mechanisms for acquiring color Doppler information from the image. Since flow must intercept the ultrasound beam at an angle to detect a Doppler shift, there must be some provision for angulation of the ultrasound beam. A method used by one manufacturer is to actually angle the entire transducer face. This is done with a fluid-filled standoff wedge, which maintains the probe face at a constant 18-degree angle in relation to the skin during the

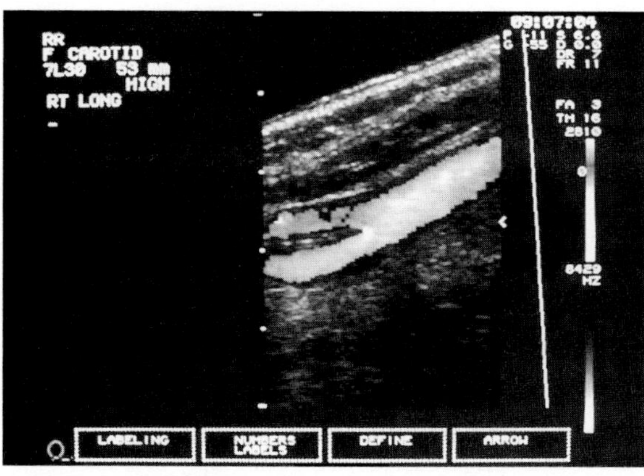

FIG. 19-13 An example image from a system that uses a standoff wedge to acquire color-flow Doppler imaging.

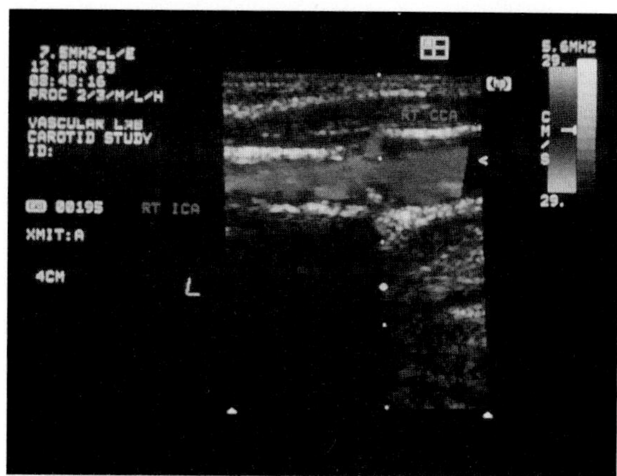

FIG. 19-14 An example image from a system that uses beam-steering to acquire color-flow Doppler imaging.

scanning procedure. The equipment is calibrated to expect the presence of this wedge, and Doppler flow and angulation information are displayed accordingly. This device can be used without the wedge if necessary. The operator simply selects a control to indicate that the wedge is not installed, and the software compensates to maintain the appropriate angulation and flow parameters. Surprisingly, the wedge does not interfere with the resolution of the displayed gray-scale image since it has been engineered into the design of the machine (Fig. 19-13; see color image).

The other method most commonly used is beam steering. Certain alternating elements of the phased-array transducer are electronically steered to reach the angle necessary to obtain the Doppler shift. This eliminates the need for a standoff wedge; but there is often a trade-off in speed and resolution, since some elements of the transducer are in effect reassigned to another purpose (Fig. 19-14; see color image).

All color Doppler devices have some limitations; display of the color-flow information is very processor-intensive. Color flow displayed across the entire image can dramatically slow the performance of the device to the point where the frame rates drop so low that the image no longer appears to be in real time. Reducing the depth of the image also often increases the frame rate. Many color Doppler devices try to compensate for this further by showing color flow only in a color box or flow window (Fig. 19-15; see color image). This box can be centered or steered to the left or right (the angle of the box is shown on screen) and sized so that the color-flow display is confined to the area of the box. Smaller boxes free up both the transducer elements that are obtaining Doppler shift information and the image processor that is converting the display to show color-flow information, so frame rates increase accordingly. The flow window can also help exclude unwanted flow patterns from nearby vessels or collaterals and can help minimize the flash artifact (see section on Color Artifacts).

Time-Domain Color-Flow Imaging[5,14]

The majority of color-flow devices available use color Doppler. One manufacturer, however, has adopted time-domain color-flow imaging, a technique that does not use Doppler at all to obtain color-flow information.

The equation used here is:

$$D = 2\,VT\cos\Theta/C$$

Where
D = distance
V = velocity
T = time
cos Θ = cosine of the "look" angle
C = the propagation velocity of sound.

Whereas each returning echo and pixel location in a color Doppler system is analyzed for amplitude, frequency, and phase, time-domain systems analyze each returning echo for amplitude and velocity.

The principle is that instead of using a defined Doppler sample, a packet, or group of red blood cells, is detected by the transmitted pulse and its repetition frequency (RF) signal stored. On additional looks, the technology can identify the same packet's RF signature and determine the distance the packet has traveled since the last look and how long it took to get there. Angulation is required to measure the directional shift and time-distance calculation, so angle dependence in the equation is identical to that in the Doppler equation. The relative distance, time, and direction traveled by the packet are converted to velocity, and colors corresponding to intensity and direction are assigned as with color Doppler devices. The resolution of the flow display corresponds to the size of the detected packet, which is adjusted in a fashion that corresponds to adjusting the size of a Doppler sample volume. There is less likelihood of color flash artifact (see section on Artifacts), since these artifacts are usually a function of Doppler-shifted echoes (Fig. 19-16).

Time-domain processing does not rely on the transducer

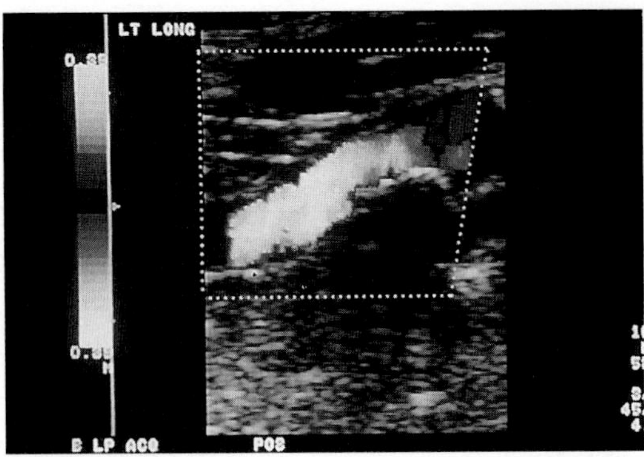

FIG. 19-15 An example image from a beam-steered system that makes use of a color box or flow window to display color-flow Doppler imaging information.

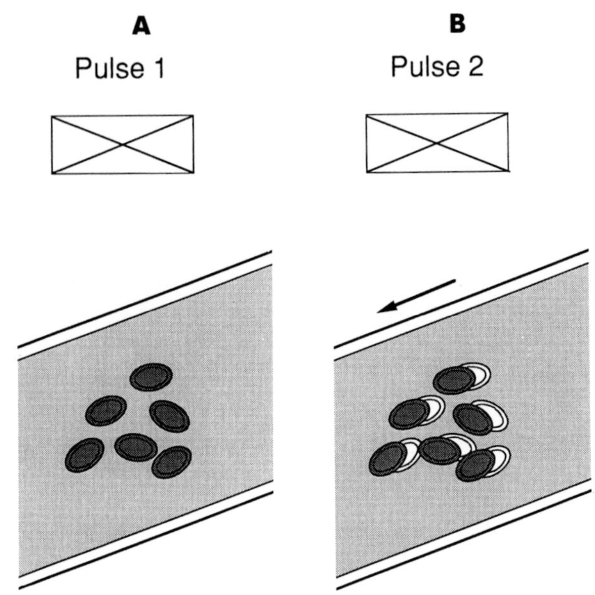

FIG. 19-16 A, In time domain color-flow imaging the first ultrasound pulse isolates a packet (group) of red blood cells and stores its pattern. B, The second pulse, which occurs microseconds later, identifies the same packet, determines how far it has moved and in what direction, and then calculates the velocity as a function of time and distance.

frequency or bandwidth, and requires fewer looks per line of information. The color pixel size and resolution of the color-flow image with time-domain processing usually depends on the packet size alone; thus, there is no sacrifice of gray-scale resolution or velocity accuracy. Transmit pulses are short, since no Doppler shift is being calculated, resulting in better axial resolution and velocity accuracy. Spatial resolution increases, allowing better streamlines to be defined at slower velocities. Since flow packet changes are being displayed over time, no FFT analysis is necessary and only 10 computations per look are performed rather than 256.

Since the peak velocities rather than average velocities are displayed in color with this method, correlation with spectral Doppler is almost exact.[14] These systems still incorporate a pulsed Doppler and FFT spectral analysis packet for conventional quantification and comparison, and are standardized with accepted diagnostic criteria.

Specific Features of Color-Flow Systems

Color Maps

Various color maps are provided by manufacturers and can be selected by the user to display the color-flow information in a visually interpretable format. Maps can be oriented toward several different arrangements.

- Hue maps assign each increased velocity level a completely different color.
- Saturation maps add white to the base color as velocities increase (slower velocities are darker, faster velocities are whiter). Some systems provide saturation maps that add yellow instead of white so the ranges appear as red-to-yellow or blue-to-cyan rather than red to pink-white and blue to blue-white. Saturation maps are among the easiest to visually interpret because of the visually logical gradient changes, and these are the most commonly used.
- Luminance maps simply increase the brightness of the basic color as velocities increase.
- Variance maps take scattered blood-flow reflectors into account and add shades of yellow or green to a current velocity level to indicate the variance of shifted frequencies around the mean;[9] these maps can help detect turbulence on the color-flow display but often can be difficult to interpret.

In all cases the brightest or whitest color in either direction occurs at the Nyquist limit and aliasing occurs above that point (see section on Artifacts). The color bar can be inverted to correctly reflect the direction of flow in angled or tortuous vessels or with reorientation of the transducer.

Flow Persistence

Color-flow displays are usually perceived as a smooth, pulsating uniform pattern in real time; when several seconds of recent imaging are displayed frame by frame (as in a cine-loop), it becomes obvious that certain areas of the vessel may or may not be uniformly filled or may fill only at a specific point of the cardiac cycle. Since it is sometimes difficult to determine if a specific area of a vessel does indeed fill with color or is patent, it is possible on most color-flow systems to adjust a factor known as *flow persistence*. This capability holds a displayed color on the screen for a length of time proportional to higher persistence settings, causing it to fade away slowly. This function can smooth out the color-flow display, making the color-flow image appear more uniform and diagnostic. Persistence can be set too high, however, causing the color pattern to appear blurry and unclear as systolic color patterns bleed into

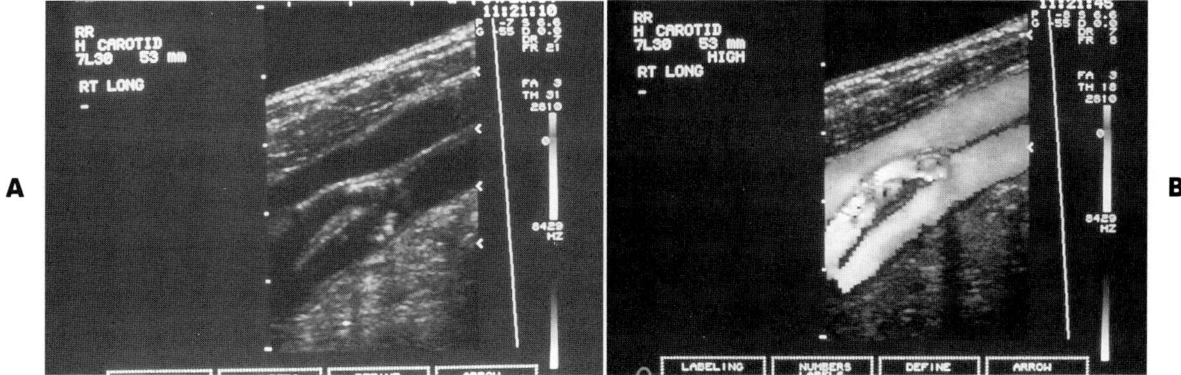

FIG. 19-17 Extensive plaque seen in gray scale within this carotid bifurcation (**A**) is obscured when color flow is turned on (**B**). This illustrates the need to evaluate a vessel both with and without color flow, unless write-prioritizing is available.

or over subsequent diastolic color patterns. Persistence should, therefore, be set as low as possible; in some cases, it is not necessary to use it at all.

Write Priority

When color-flow patterns are displayed over the gray-scale image, plaque imaged at an angle away from the perpendicular is occasionally obscured by the color display. Therefore plaque surfaces jutting into the lumen from a lateral or medial wall may not be detected or properly imaged. Imaging an area first with the color off and then with color on can rectify this situation (Fig. 19-17; see color image). In some color-flow ultrasound devices, however, specific thresholds can be set where gray-scale information displays take precedence over color pixels whenever a conflict between displaying the color flow and underlying image data occurs. This capability is termed *write priority-image* because color data is prioritized based on when it is to be "written" to the screen. It is important not to favor gray scale too much, however, since irregular plaques with many projecting surfaces could appear to be actually within the flow stream when in reality they are being picked up off of a lateral wall and do not obstruct the streamline.

Velocity Tagging

It is possible to tag or isolate a range of the velocities displayed in the color-flow image by using velocity tagging (also called *green tagging*). When tagging is selected, all velocities above or below a certain user-set breakpoint turn green instead of the color intensity corresponding to their velocity, which allows these velocities to be identified immediately within the red-and-blue color-flow image. A single velocity range can also be selected, so only velocities of that level are colored green. Diagnostically, tagging is useful for identifying the peak velocity points in a stenotic area or for detecting a specific level of abnormality. For example, the breakpoint for green tagging can be set at 130cm/sec, a common category boundary between a less-than-59% and greater-than-60% carotid stenosis. When set this way, only velocities in the greater-than-60% range will appear green. The tag can also be adjusted to locate the exact area where a high peak velocity is occurring to more accurately place Doppler sample volume or to define a streamline more clearly (Fig. 19-18; see color image).

Color Threshold and Gain

Color Doppler or time-domain intensities are often adjusted separately from image gain. Adjusting the threshold or gain control permits better detection of weak or low-intensity flow shifts, avoiding the need to increase power. The threshold level can be set too high, however; if color appears to be bleeding over the edges of the visible vessel walls or if stray color pixels begin appearing in non-flow-producing areas of the image, it is likely that threshold, color gain, or power is set too high. The best way to determine if the color gain or threshold is set correctly is to obtain a clear color-flow image, then increase the gain or threshold to a point of obvious bleed-through and oversaturation. Once this has been seen, back the control down gradually until color is seen within the walls of the vessel without it exceeding the limit of the intimal lining. Threshold and gain boosts are useful in cases where image penetration is adequate but color fill is poor, such as in deeply diving vessels or high bifurcations.

Color Velocity Range[9]

Another way to clarify color within a vessel is by raising or lowering the velocity range (which also changes the Nyquist limit). This feature is also referred to as *slow flow* on some devices. Slow flow reassigns the color intensities so that there is more balance in the color display, depending on the speed of the blood flow; for example, a low range setting may clearly show slow-moving venous and arterial flow without oversaturation and with a uniform color gra-

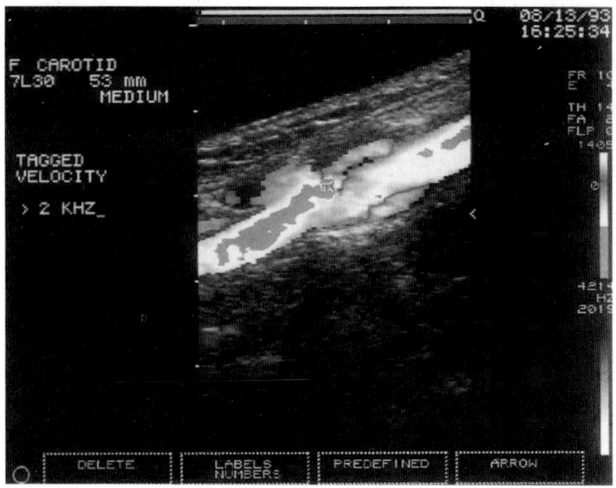

FIG. 19-18 All frequencies above 2019 Hz are tagged using a green color to distinguish them from slower velocities within the vessel in this image.

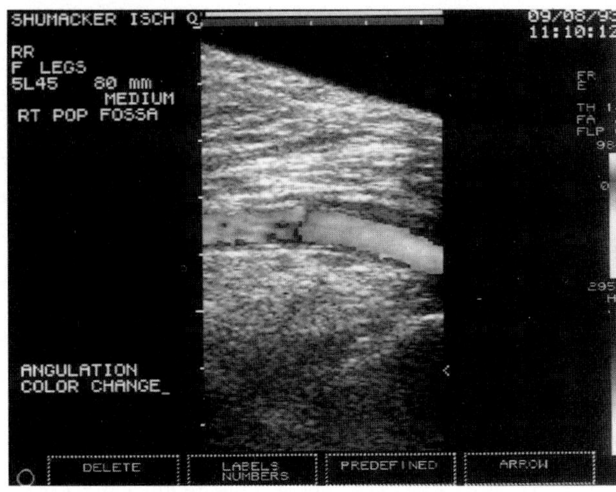

FIG. 19-19 If tortuous vasculature is present or if curvatures cause flow to move toward the transducer elements in one segment and away from the elements in another, both red and blue flow patterns may appear within the same vascular structure.

dient, but higher flow, such as occurs in a major artery, appears nearly white and may be aliasing (see section on Artifacts). Setting the range to a higher level balances the color-flow patterns and eliminates aliasing and stray color pixels. Conversely, velocity ranges set too high may exclude slower flow velocities and falsely imply that flow is not present in a patent structure. If the examiner is in doubt, he or she should obtain the best possible image and then evaluate color-flow patterns at the lowest velocity range, increasing the range scale to a point where there is no color aliasing, no extraneous artifactual pixels, and where streamlines are clear and defined. Pulsed Doppler sampling can also help determine whether peak or mean velocities are well within the displayed velocity range.

Baseline Shifting

As explained, the color-flow display and visible flow patterns correspond closely to the parameters of a spectral waveform, with forward intensities, a zero baseline, and reverse intensities. The baseline point between red and blue corresponds to the zero baseline on a spectral display and can be manually shifted or relocated to increase the displayed range of positive or negative color shift and eliminate color aliasing. It is especially important to note that in some color-flow ultrasound systems, shifting the baseline for color flow automatically moves the Doppler spectral baseline up or down, and vice versa; this is not undesirable, since it eliminates aliasing and shows the maximum range of displayed velocities in both displays. Some systems, however, allow the color baseline to be relocated independently of the Doppler spectral baseline. Shifting the baseline also has an effect on the color patterns seen on the display; as the baseline moves down, blue shades disappear until the color-flow image is full of red intensities. Moving the baseline up causes blue shades to dominate. The examiner must be certain that moving the baseline does not eliminate any blue or red shades that may be important diagnostic indicators of turbulence, flow separation, or reversed flow.

Color-Flow Artifacts

Color-flow imaging has its own set of artifacts that can cause problems and mislead interpreters if not corrected or noted.

Directional Artifacts.[9] As previously stated, the ultrasound beam must be steered to intersect blood flow at an appropriate angle for a doppler shift or time-domain shift to occur. Positive flow (normal arterial flow) is usually coded red, and negative flow (normal venous flow) is coded blue. Depending on the application and orientation of the transducer, flow moving away from the transducer surface is one color and flow moving toward the transducer surface is the other. If a vessel curves or branches in an unusual direction, positive flow may appear blue rather than red and vice versa. It is not uncommon to see flow in a tortuous vessel moving toward the transducer in a proximal segment and away from the transducer in a distal segment in the same image. In addition, if the beam is perpendicular to the blood flow, no color may be detected because there is no angulation and no Doppler shift or packet tracking (Fig. 19-19; see color image).

It is important to reinforce the fact that color flow is a dynamic modality. Since color-flow changes correspond to waveform changes, it is not a color artifact to see alternating red-blue-red patterns in normal extremity arteries because this reflects the normal triphasic flow pattern (see Chapter 20). A red pattern is seen for the first systolic component, a brief blue pattern is seen for the second diastolic reversal component, and a lesser-intensity red pattern is seen for the third diastolic antegrade component.

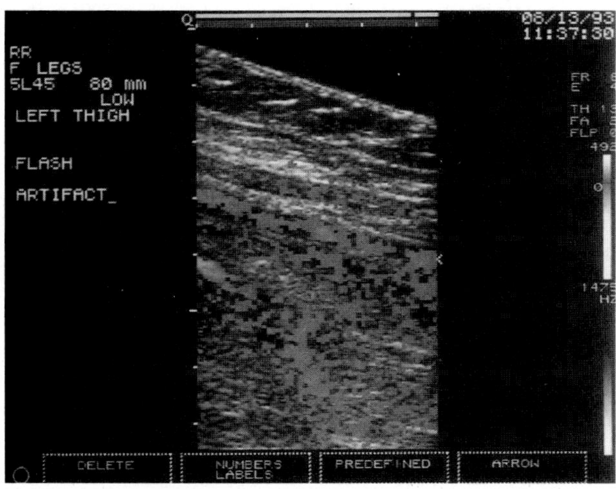

FIG. 19-20 Flash artifact (see text).

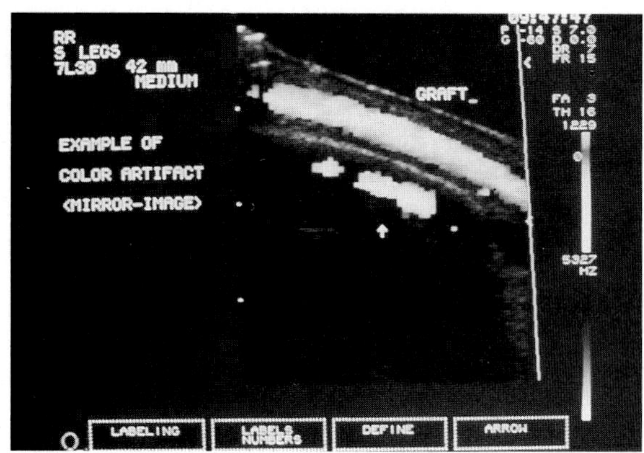

FIG. 19-21 Mirror-image color-flow artifact (see text).

It is also not a color artifact to see an area of blue or reversed flow separation in a normal carotid bulb alongside normal antegrade (red) flow. This is a normal finding resulting from the shape of the origin of the internal carotid (see Chapter 22). Carotid arteries after endarterectomy also have prominent swirling patterns (especially when a patch is used). The color-flow imager's ability to detect these areas of flow reversal and flow separation is important to the diagnosis of ulcerations, luminal irregularities, flow eddies along the vessel wall, and separations on the distal side of severe stenoses.

The examiner must be certain to know the proper direction of flow in the vessel to be examined, and make certain the color assignments reflect this. If in doubt, spectral pulsed Doppler can be used to check the vessel and confirm flow orientation. If videotaping, it is helpful to note any atypical flow patterns that occur.

Flash Artifact

When color-flow analysis is being performed over a sizable image area, the motion of the transducer and of patients (e.g., swallowing, talking, and coughing) may periodically cause extraneous color patterns to appear over the image in areas other than the vessel being interrogated. This color flash is referred to as a *flash artifact*. It occurs because any moving reflector within the ultrasound beam that generates a Doppler shift has a color pixel assigned to it, just as moving blood cells do. Flash artifacts can be minimized by avoiding abrupt and quick movements of the transducer and setting the color velocity threshold to a higher level (Fig. 19-20; see color image).

Mirror Image Artifact

The mirror image artifact produces a false, duplicated color-flow image (containing information from the true vessel on the near or superficial side) on the far or deep side of a strong reflecting surface such as bone or diaphragm (Fig. 19-21; see color image). An examiner can place a Doppler sample volume into this mirror image and even get a spectral waveform. The artifact can be minimized or eliminated by angling away from a direct perpendicular with the reflecting interface and by cutting back the power.

Aliasing

Color aliasing occurs when the Nyquist limit (half the pulse repetition frequency) has been reached and the waveform velocity exceeds it. As with spectral aliasing, the waveform goes "over the top" and wraps around to the bottom of the scale. In arterial flow situations, this appears as blue intensities occurring at peak streamline points in the middle of red intensities and vice versa in venous flow cases (Fig. 19-22; see color image). Aliasing can be compensated for by doing one or more of the following:

1. Adjusting the baseline to keep the flow peaks within the scale
2. Decreasing (or shortening) the image depth
3. Increasing the velocity threshold or pulse repetition frequency
4. Switching to a lower-frequency transducer

Bruits and Thrills

Bruits and thrills are not, by definition, artifacts, but they appear in an image and may be erroneously thought to be flash artifacts, directional artifacts, or complications of aliasing.

As discussed in the arterial and cerebrovascular chapters (see Chapters 20 and 22), a bruit (pronounced "BROO-ee," from the French word for "noise") is a harsh, turbulent, blowing sound akin to a cardiac murmur that can be auscultated with a stethoscope. They are caused by severe stenoses of the vessel (usually between 60% and 95% stenosis) that create strong turbulence and vibrations into the surrounding tissues. These vibrations create color-flow scatters in the image (similar to a flash artifact), which are centered around the stenotic source of the bruit. These

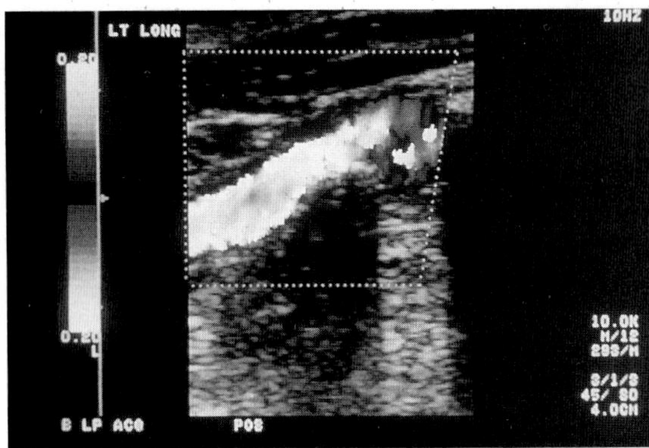

FIG. 19-22 Color aliasing. Normal flow away from the transducer should be coded as shades of red in this vessel; the velocity threshold is too low and higher forward velocities "wrap around" to the reverse, or blue, side of the color bar, as evidenced by the shades of blue in the center streamline area.

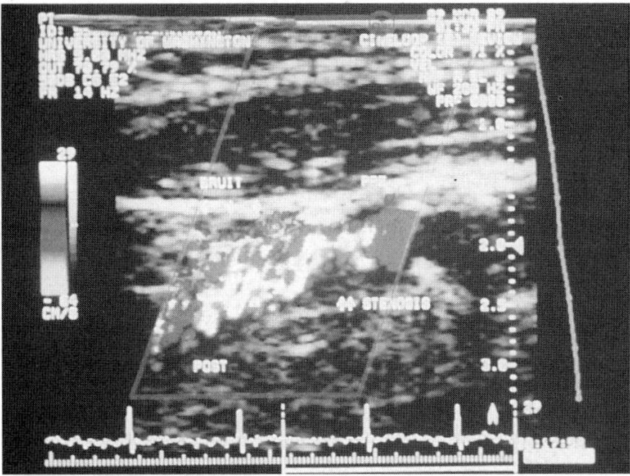

FIG. 19-23 A bruit from a stenosis may generate color disturbances around the vessel that are centered at the area of turbulence. (Courtesy Advanced Technology Laboratories.)

color-flow-displayed bruits can be extremely valuable from a diagnostic perspective because they help the examiner locate the stenotic area and determine which vessel is the source (important when distinguishing external carotid from internal carotid artery stenosis). They can be enhanced at lower velocity threshold settings or decreased at higher settings (Fig. 19-23; see color image).

Thrills differ from bruits in that the vibrations are so severe that one can actually palpate or even see the vibrations on the skin surface. Thrills typically occur in cases of violently turbulent conditions, such as irregular stenoses or, more commonly, arteriovenous fistulas (see Chapter 20). Although a bruit will accompany a thrill, it tends to sound more "musical" with harmonics occurring throughout. Whereas the color pattern in a bruit occurs with peak systole and goes away in diastole, thrill patterns tend to be rainbow-like mixed red and blue patterns that decrease but continue through diastole. This pattern often appears to be an artifact but once identified it is a definite indicator that an arteriovenous fistula may be present and should be sought (Fig. 19-24; see color image).

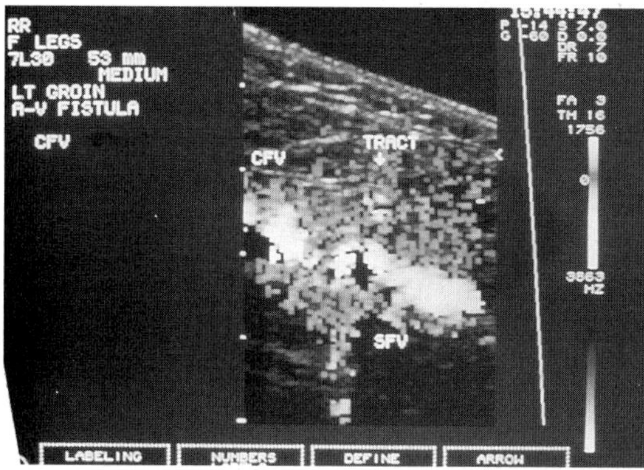

FIG. 19-24 An arteriovenous fistula or extremely turbulent vessel that causes a palpable thrill generates this type of mixed color pattern in its vicinity.

Color-Flow Summary

Color-flow imaging is a truly diagnostic enhancement that, when properly used, can provide the examiner with important dynamic information to help perform a more accurate and complete examination.

- It enables quicker identification of hemodynamic changes, anatomic stenoses, and occlusions.
- It increases operator accuracy by helping the examiner locate precisely where to place the sample volume for spectral Doppler waveform sampling.
- It enables rapid identification of arteries and veins, and can in some cases eliminate extravascular compression techniques or other methods to determine the presence of thrombosis or recanalization.

Color-flow imaging is not a shortcut to easy diagnosis. Familiarity with Doppler and vascular hemodynamics is much more important when using color flow, and these principles must be thoroughly understood to optimize color-flow parameters and maximize the use of the information obtained.

Illustrations of the clinical use of color-flow imaging can be found in the next three chapters.

BASIC PLETHYSMOGRAPHIC PRINCIPLES AND INSTRUMENTATION

Although plethysmography is not an ultrasound modality, it is used quite frequently in vascular laboratories around the world. Although it is seldom necessary to perform both Doppler and plethysmography on the same person, laboratories often use one modality or the other to obtain portions of their vascular evaluations. To this end, the equipment and basic principles of plethysmography are briefly covered here, and examples of waveforms and studies appear in subsequent chapters.

Plethysmographic techniques deal with recording volume changes in a limb or digit (from the Greek *plethysmos,* or "increase," and *graphein,* or "write"). There are currently five plethysmography techniques (four in general use), almost all of them interchangeable. Water systems, the earliest form, record changes in fluid-volume displacement by the expansion of a limb contained within a rigid water-filled container. This is considered the most direct technique for evaluating volume changes but is prone to possible errors caused by uneven water temperatures and hydrostatic pressure. Air systems indirectly measure volume changes by air displacement and the use of pressure transducers in a closed system. The most common method today is to use a pressure cuff wrapped around the limb that is inflated to about 40 to 65 mm Hg to keep the cuff in contact with the skin. These techniques are easy to perform and the equipment is simple to operate, but it is important to use the same amplitude settings and inflation pressures for each segment to ensure accuracy and consistency. Strain-gauge systems use a small silastic rubber tube filled with mercury that contacts electrodes at either end. These strain gauges are available in many lengths and are wrapped and slightly stretched around the limb or digit being evaluated. The length of the gauge is varied proportionally as the limb volume increases or decreases. The electrical changes in resistance and voltage reflect the limb circumference changes. Impedance systems indirectly measure volume changes by corresponding changes in electrical resistance from electrodes attached to the limb. Two electrodes transmit an electrical current through the part being examined and two more record voltage changes. Impedance devices are most commonly used in venous applications, since they can easily measure venous outflow versus venous capacitance. Photophlethysmography does not measure volume change and thus is not technically a plethysmographic technique. It measures the reflectance of light emitted by a light-emitting diode (LED) from the skin by means of a photosensor. Blood is more opaque than surrounding tissues to infrared light, and the relative changes in perfusion of red blood cells in the skin cause corresponding changes in reflectivity. These changes can be displayed by a waveform or graph.[13]

Plethysmography devices are usually oriented around either air plethysmography (often called volume pulse recording [VPR]), or strain-gauge plethysmography as their primary function, but almost all devices also provide photoplethysmography. The volume change data is displayed as a waveform and can be recorded on a strip-chart recorder much as Doppler signals are.

Two typical strain-gauge and photoplethysmographic devices are shown in Fig. 19-25.

The output of plethysmography units can be run through amplifiers to enhance the detection capability and improve the waveform recordings. There are two amplification modes available—alternating current (AC) and direct current (DC) modes. AC amplification is used to detect rapid changes in pressure or blood flow states, such as in arterial evaluation. DC amplification is used with slower volume changes or flow states, such as in venous evaluation. DC amplification also can be used in cases of diminished arterial perfusion where pulsatility cannot be readily detected, such as in extremely ischemic digits.

In general, all base plethysmography devices have connection ports for the input sources, AC- and DC-mode amplifiers for both arterial and venous applications, and a strip-chart recorder, computer interface, or external recorder output. The strip-chart or computer program should ideally have selectable recording speeds of 1 mm/sec, 5 mm/sec, and 25 mm/sec.

Air plethysmographs use two or more connecting air hoses and cuffs of various sizes and lengths as input sources. The plethysmograph is connected to a manual sphygmomanometer inflation bulb or to an automatic cuff inflator with adjustable inflation controls and pressure meters. This enables cuffs to be inflated, inflation pressures to be monitored, and the pressure held while the waveform tracings are made. Once a base level has been calibrated, a consistent standard cuff inflation pressure should be maintained and the size or position of the trace pen should not change.

Photoplethysmographs use one or more photocells for input. Some devices include a sensitivity switch to boost faint AC-mode waveform amplification. An examiner should note that photocells are extremely light-sensitive. A baseline strip should be run before any permanent recordings are made to properly set the size and location of the chart pen or zero line so that the entire waveform will fit on the strip. Once the baseline has been stabilized and calibrated, the examiner needs to avoid changing the room light levels or passing a hand or body shadow over the probe accidentally to avoid skewing the waveform printouts. Photoplethysmograph examinations are often best performed in a dimly lit room or with the photocell covered so external light is blocked.

Strain-gauge plethysmographs use two or more strain gauges of various lengths and sizes as input. The examiner must avoid choosing strain-gauges that are too short when placing them on a limb or digit, since they can be overstretched and broken; likewise, the gauge must not fit too loosely because some stretch is necessary for uniform contact. Because they are so sensitive to volume changes, however, in practice they can be slightly difficult to calibrate or use compared with air plethysmographs.[13]

The applications of plethysmographic methods and examples of their use can be found within the next two chapters.

MAGNETIC RESONANCE ANGIOGRAPHY

In addition to ultrasonic and plethysmographic methods, a relatively new development in noninvasive vascular assessment has recently become available to the diagnostician. Magnetic resonance angiography (MRA), is an out-

A

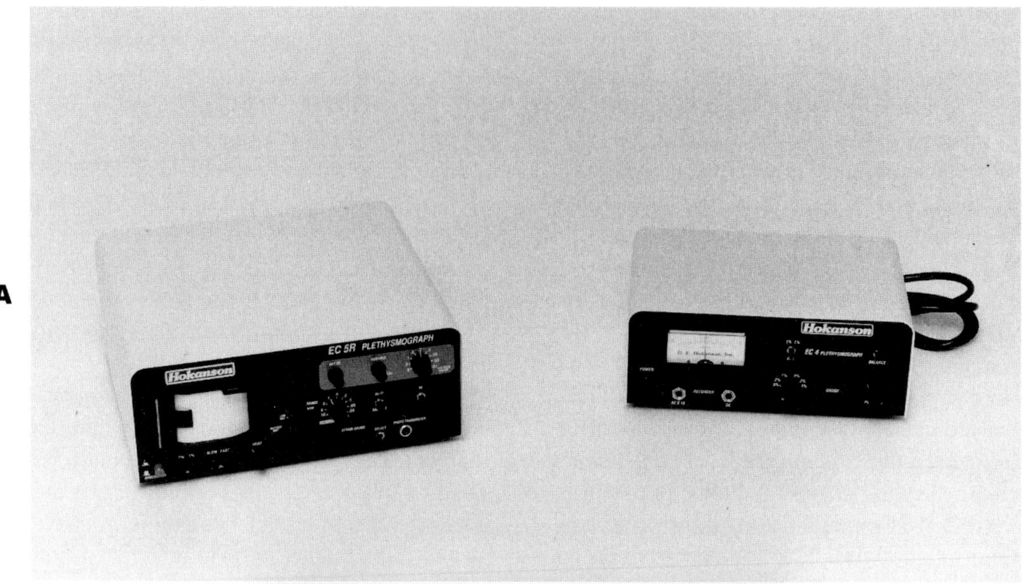

B

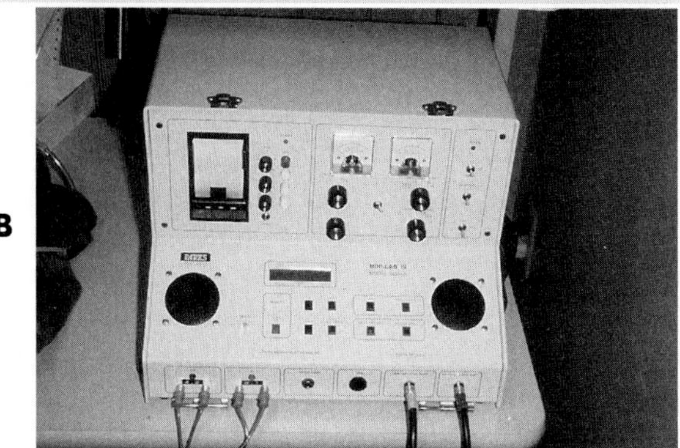

FIG. 19-25 Plethysmograph devices. **A,** Two examples of dedicated plethysmography units. The unit on the left has an integral chart recorder and can perform strain-gauge plethysmography and photoplethysmography. The unit on the right performs strain-gauge plethysmography only and can be connected to an external recorder or a larger integrated system. **B,** An example of a device that combines continuous-wave Doppler, air plethysmography (volume pulse recording), photoplethysmography, and an integral automatic cuff inflator into one unit. (**A** courtesy D. E. Hokanson.)

growth of magnetic resonance imaging that uses two-dimensional time-of-flight pulse sequencing to selectively enhance moving spins (flow) while suppressing stationary spins (tissue) to create both transverse and reconstructed longitudinal images of arteries and veins. Because of the flexible technology and software, the subsequent maps of vascular trees can be converted to three-dimensional maps and rotated for specific identification of vessels and separation of overlying branches, which is difficult or impossible with conventional uniplanar or biplanar angiography. Because the tissue echoes are suppressed but not fully eliminated, the anatomic relationships of the vessels can be evaluated, especially in transverse cuts. This is especially important in evaluating distal runoff in the lower leg and foot.[11]

Although detailed discussion of MRA is not practical here, investigators are claiming results that rival those of contrast angiograms.[11] The procedure does, however, have the following drawbacks:

1. The acquisition time for an MRA slice can be upwards of 7 minutes, with a reconstruction time of 1 minute. If the patient moves during this time span, jumps in the flow course can mimic occlusions or stenoses on the reconstructed images. To do complete evaluations of both legs may take upwards of 2 hours of acquisition time. Claustrophobic patients cannot generally be examined with MRA.
2. If pulse sequence timing does not match the periodicity of blood flow, ghost vessels at regular intervals may surround the native vessel. This is corrected with cardiac gating with seeded reconstruction algorithms.[3]
3. Bands or stripes may appear in the vessel that may mimic stenosis because of reversal of flow spins (e.g., triphasic flow patterns). The saturation band must be moved to rectify this.[3]
4. Metallic clips and prostheses from previous surgery may cause areas of signal void or dropout that can mimic an occlusion.[3]

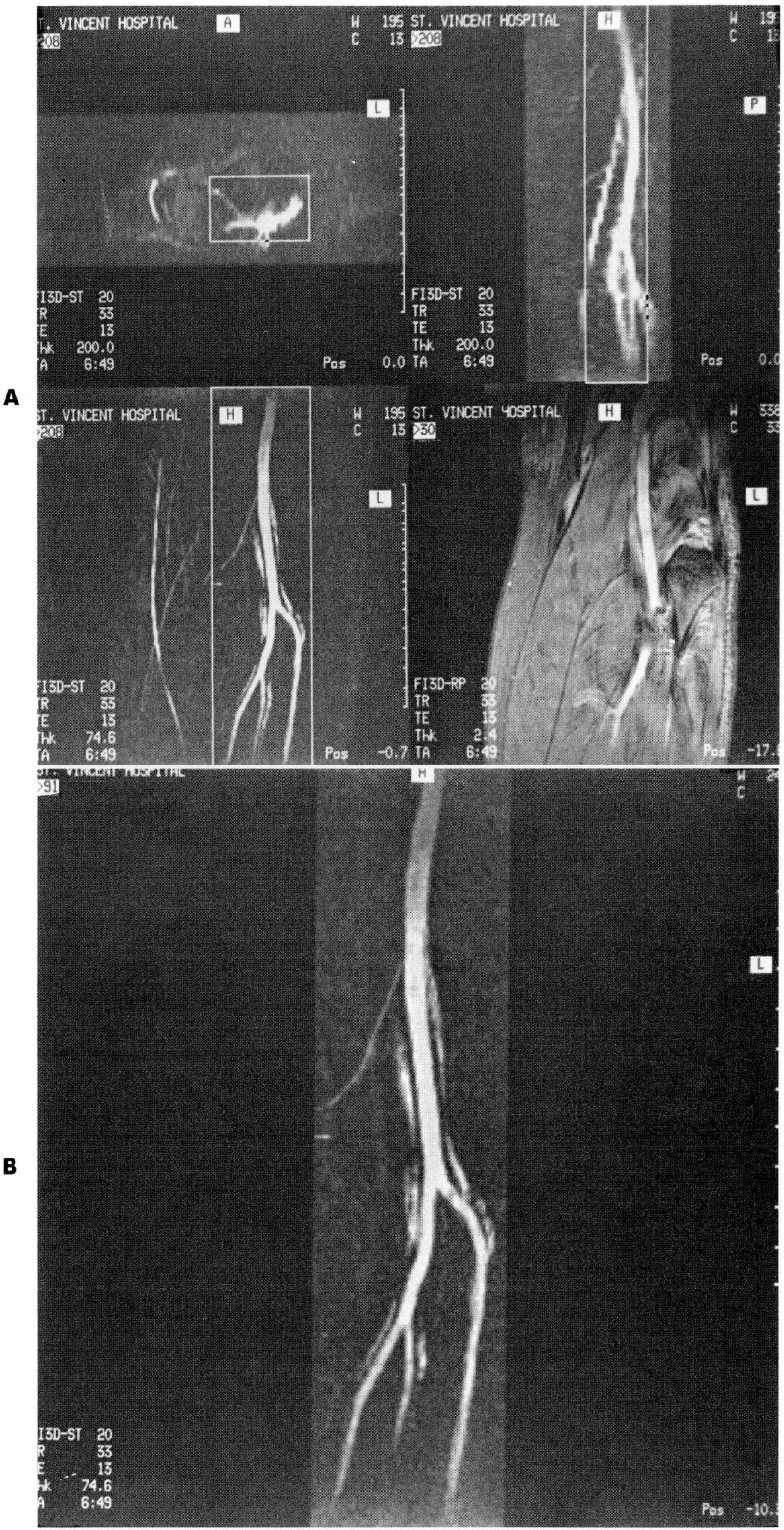

FIG. 19-26 Lower-extremity magnetic resonance angiograms. Flow information from sections of transverse cuts is isolated **(A),** and the data are reconstructed to create an AP view of the trifurcation arteries below the knee **(B).**

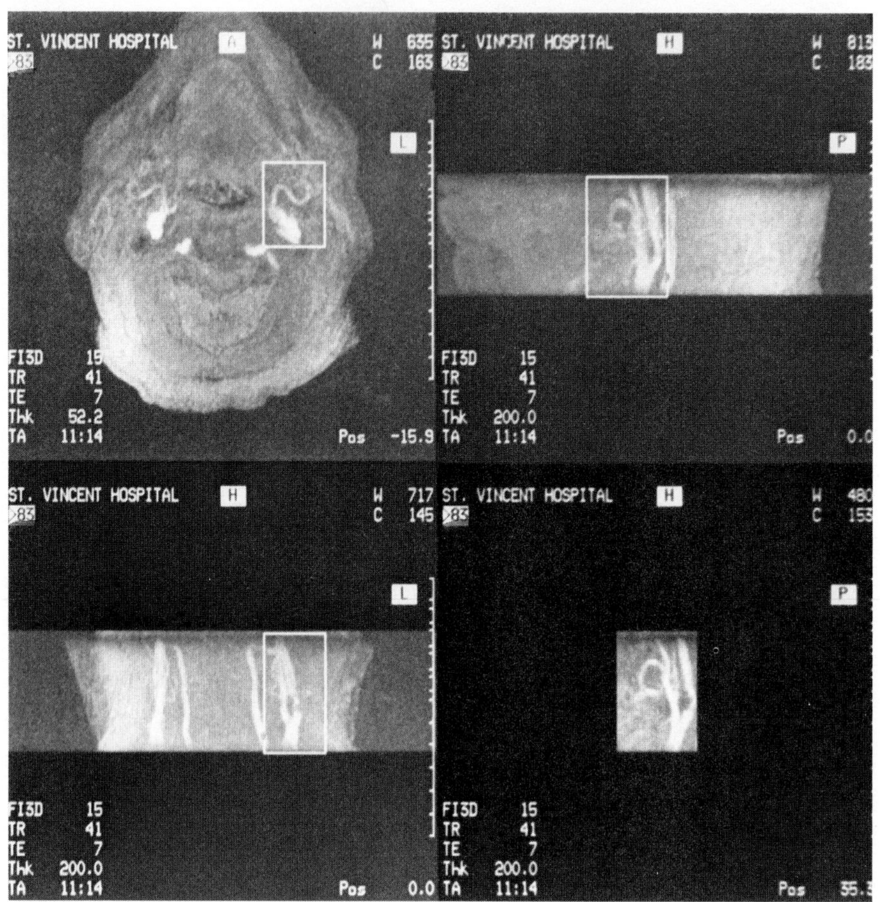

FIG. 19-27 Carotid magnetic resonance angiograms. Flow information from segmental transverse cuts is isolated and compiled to create a reconstructed image of the carotid bifurcation (see also Fig. 19-28).

5. The MRA procedure can cost about $1000 per hour, whereas complete arterial Doppler and/or duplex can be performed for about $150 to $200 for 30 minutes to 1 hour of examination.

Technology seldom stands still, and it is likely that resolution and acquisition times will improve and that costs will decrease with time and advancements in the technique. At present, MRA is still considered cumbersome and is not fully accepted as a replacement for contrast angiography. Examples of MRA images are shown in Figs. 19-26 to 19-28 (see color images of Fig. 19-28).

CONCLUSION AND GENERAL COMMENTS

Doppler techniques are accurate, sensitive, and completely noninvasive methods for evaluation of the peripheral arterial and venous systems, the cerebrovascular systems, and major portions of the abdominal vascular system. The techniques are indeed somewhat involved and are often confusing to the beginner, especially sonographers who have suddenly been told that they will "learn Doppler" and are thrown into a new environment. Many die-hard vascular technologists are in the same boat when they are pressed by current trends or physicians to learn their way around the abdomen to perform visceral vascular duplex examination. The techniques are often learned best by on-the-job training or attendance of any number of excellent courses that are available, often by the companies that make the equipment.

Probably the most important fact about Doppler techniques that can be stressed here is that the sonographer or vascular technologist must know the basics thoroughly. Since the physician who interprets the examination often reads it at a later time, the sonographer is the direct link to the quality and accuracy of the examination. If the sonographer is unable to produce an accurate and diagnostic evaluation, then the quality of care the patient receives suffers. I personally have seen many false diagnoses result from poor technique and lack of attention to the quality of the signals recorded. There is no excuse for performing a poor-quality examination, since there are educational courses, numerous books available, and competent vascular technologists who can give helpful advice. Membership in professional organizations that deal primarily with noninvasive

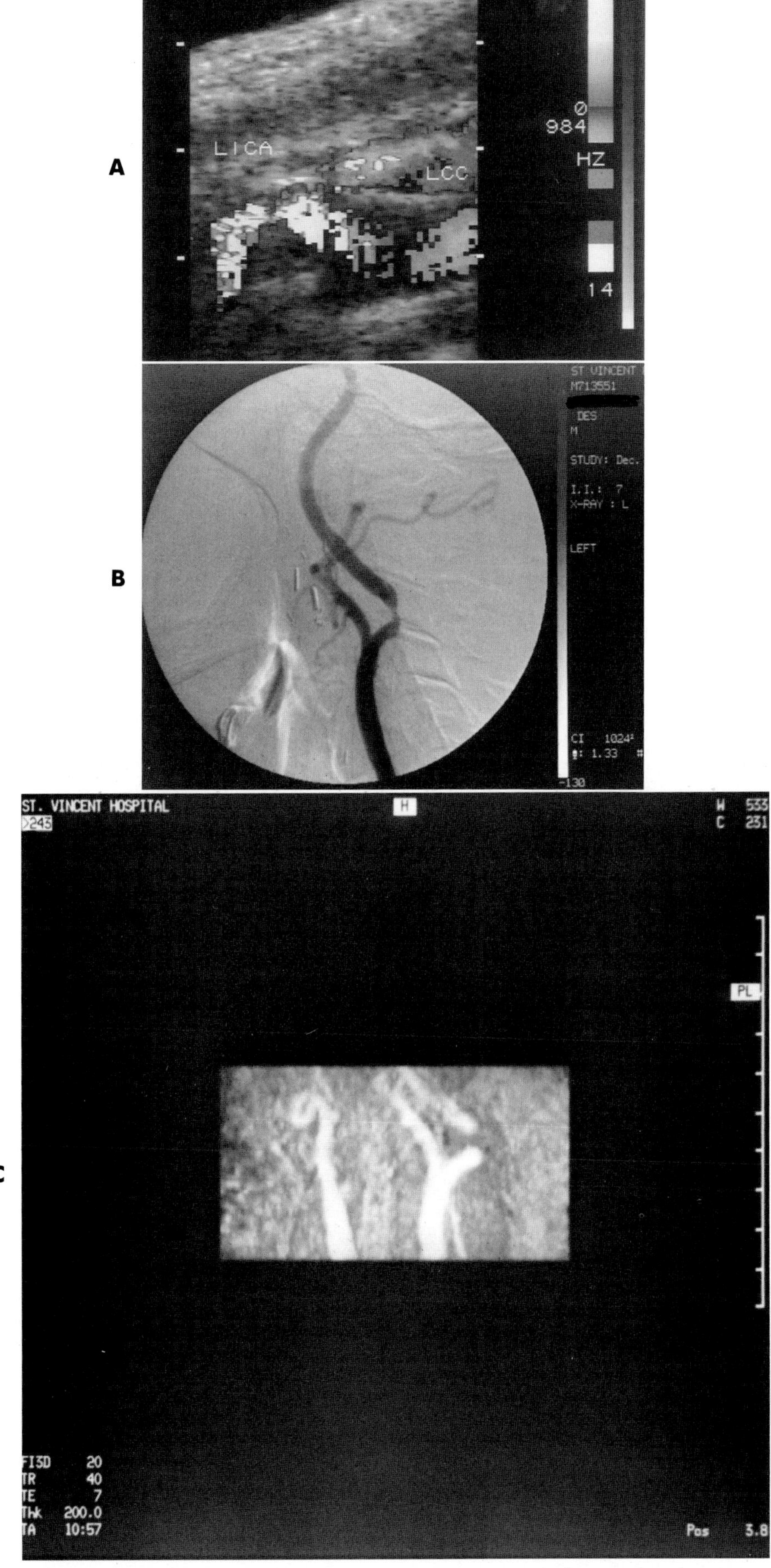

FIG. 19-28 Comparison between digital subtraction arteriography, color-flow duplex sonography, and magnetic resonance angiography on the same patient. A severe internal carotid stenosis is identified by duplex **(A)** and is clearly shown in the digital subtraction arteriogram **(B)**. **C,** The image data acquired from a magnetic resonance angiogram shows the same stenotic area.

vascular testing can provide a wealth of knowledge and information. A typical organization is the Society of Vascular Technology, which publishes a quarterly journal for its members and has courses and seminars across the country that can help train the sonographer in nearly every form of invasive testing available.

A sonographer should thoroughly know the following before performing an examination:

1. *Vascular anatomy.* This is an absolute must. If a sonographer does not know where a specific artery or vein lies and where branches are given off, then doing a Doppler study is a hopeless endeavor and is also going to be nondiagnostic or even detrimental to the patient. Study the vascular anatomy thoroughly and imagine the course of the artery or vein in question superimposed on the skin. Follow it with a Doppler to see if you envision it correctly. This simple technique can speed up the learning process immeasurably.
2. *"Knobology."* If the sonographer does not know what the controls do or how the Doppler or duplex device works, then the results will show it. Take the time to read the manuals and practice whenever possible—there are simple controls on every Doppler that can do tremendous things for the quality of the examination, provided they are used. Study the examinations of others and feel free to contact an applications technologist from the com pany that manufactures your machine for information and help regarding image quality and equipment use.
3. *Hemodynamics.* Know the flow direction in the vessel being examined. Be aware of what changes will occur if disease processes or collaterals are present. Learn the ranges of normal and abnormal flow velocities and frequencies. Learn the normal sound patterns and spectral appearances of arteries and veins. Learn to expect the type of flow signal that can occur if a significant-appearing stenosis is seen.
4. *Disease conditions.* Learn about the types of vascular disease and their appearance and effect on the circulation. Be aware of these while doing an examination so that the condition is thoroughly documented and all appropriate arteries or veins involved are adequately assessed.

Almost all of the points above are thoroughly covered in the following chapters. Although this does not purport to be a definitive text regarding peripheral vascular Doppler and duplex vascular scanning, no text can truly be that since there are numerous ways and approaches of evaluating the vascular system and new advances are being made every day. Although some techniques may become obsolete within a very short period, some remain the "state of the art," and it is likely that many of the techniques discussed here will remain in the latter category. A sonographer can only be made a better diagnostician by knowing and practicing the material presented here.

Whether these techniques are used by a vascular technologist or sonographer, a vascular surgeon or radiologist, remember that the ultimate beneficiary of the techniques and technology of noninvasive vascular diagnosis is the patient.

REVIEW QUESTIONS

1. What are some of the problems that can occur with angiographic techniques? What does angiography actually show compared with ultrasound?
2. List three noninvasive techniques that are not ultrasound-based but that are used in vascular technology.
3. How was Doppler's theory first tested, and by whom?
4. What are some of the differences between continuous-wave Doppler and pulsed Doppler?
5. Would continuous-wave or pulsed Doppler be better for sampling flow in an artery that has a large vein just below it? Why?
6. What is the Nyquist limit? What is aliasing?
7. What is the main difference between a zero-crossing display and a spectrum analyzer display? Which would be better for displaying turbulent, disturbed blood flow?
8. What is the proper angle range for accurate Doppler measurement with both continuous-wave and pulsed Doppler equipment?
9. What is a sample volume? What is a flow vector line?
10. How does the examiner indicate the proper Doppler angle-to-flow relationship for automatic flow velocity calculation when using a duplex scanner?
11. When are velocity scales accurate, and when should frequency scales be used?
12. What do color-flow imaging devices do that strictly gray-scale duplex devices do not?
13. Name the two different principles of obtaining color-flow information used by current manufacturers.
14. What are some differences between color Doppler imaging and spectral pulsed Doppler?
15. Name the two transducer mechanisms used to obtain color Doppler shifts.
16. How does time-domain flow processing differ from Doppler?
17. What are the two factors that make gray-scale imaging and color Doppler combinations difficult to reconcile?
18. Name three color-flow imaging artifacts.
19. Name the three forms of plethysmography most commonly used in the vascular laboratory setting.
20. Would AC or DC amplification be used for arterial volume-pulse wave recording? How about for venous outflow studies?
21. What is MRA? What are some of its advantages? What are some of its disadvantages?

REFERENCES

1. Barnes RW, Wilson MR: Doppler ultrasonic spectrum analysis of carotid velocity signals; a programmed audiovisual instruction. Richmond, Va: Medical College of Virginia, 1980.
2. Barnes RW, Wilson MR: Doppler ultrasonic evaluation of peripheral arterial disease; a programmed audiovisual instruction. Iowa City, Iowa, 1975, University of Iowa Press.
3. Baum RA, Holland GA, Carpenter JP, et al: MR angiography of peripheral vascular disease, Radiology 185(proceedings), 1992.
4. Bergan JJ and Yao JST: Gangrene and severe ischemia of the lower extremities. New York, 1978, Grune and Stratton.
5. Bonnefous O and Pesqué P: Time domain formulation of pulse-Doppler ultrasound and blood velocity estimation by cross correlation, Ultrason Imaging 8:73, 1986.
6. Eden A: Christian Doppler; thinker and benefactor. Salzburg, Austria, 1988, Christian Doppler Institute for Medical Science and Technology.
7. Johnson J: Angiography and ultrasound in diagnosis of carotid artery disease; a comparison, Contemp Surg 20, 1982.
8. Juergens JL, Pittell JA, and Fairbairn JF: Peripheral vascular diseases. Philadelphia, 1980, WB Saunders.
9. Kremkau FW: Principles of color flow imaging, J Vasc Technol 15(3):104, 1991.
10. Myers L, Avecilla LS, et al: Correlative studies of color-coded real-time spectral analysis of flow in model arterial systems and selected cerebrovascular pathology. Scientific poster. Bowman Gray School of Medicine (personal communication).
11. Owen RS, Carpenter JP, Baum RA, et al: Magnetic resonance imaging of angiographically occult runoff vessels in peripheral arterial occlusive disease, N Engl J Med 326(24):1624-6, 1992.
12. Powis RL and Powis WJ: A thinker's guide to ultrasonic imaging. Baltimore, 1984, Urban and Schwarzenberg.
13. Sumner DS: Volume plethysmography in vascular disease: an overview. In Bernstein EF, editor: Noninvasive diagnostic techniques in vascular disease, ed 3. St. Louis, 1985, Mosby.
14. Tegelin CW, Kremkau FW, and Hitchings LP: Color velocity imaging: introduction to a new ultrasound technology, J Neuroimag 1:85, 1991.

CHAPTER 20

Arterial Sonography, Doppler, and Plethysmography Examinations

Richard E. Rae II

The Doppler examinations pertaining to the arterial system are probably the simplest to learn and interpret. The techniques still require a high degree of examiner familiarity and a thorough knowledge of the arterial anatomy to enable confident and accurate diagnoses to be made. This section discusses basic arterial occlusive syndromes and disease processes, Doppler signal characteristics, flow physiology, anatomy, examination of the lower and upper extremities, and related studies.

TYPES OF ARTERIAL OCCLUSIVE CONDITIONS

Occlusive diseases and other pathologic conditions are common to arteries anywhere in the body and present clinically in various manners. Extensive coverage of these is beyond the scope of this work, but several of the more common diseases and pathoses that the examiner is likely to encounter are discussed.

Atherosclerosis accounts for the greatest percentage of occlusive diseases in which the arteries are constricted or narrowed, preventing adequate flow to the distal portion of the arterial tributaries. Atherosclerosis is distinguished from arteriosclerosis by the fact that the former is usually a focal accumulation of lipids, calcium, fibrous tissue, and blood products in the intima of an artery, whereas the latter is a generalized aging process in the entire system, shown by intimal thickening, calcification, and loss of vascular wall elasticity.

Focal atherosclerotic areas are also known as *plaques*. Plaques are usually elevated lesions of the intima that can be fatty or fibrous and that project into the lumen of an artery, narrowing the flow path and reducing flow. They have amorphous or atheromatous cores and may calcify or become ulcerated and thromboembolic. Cast-off emboli from plaques may occlude distal capillaries and tributaries, causing ischemia (deficiency of blood) to the areas they supply. These thrombi are composed of platelet material, and it is thought that platelet secretions may interact with vessel walls and actually initiate atherosclerosis. The causes of arterial thrombosis are often related to plaque formations, but it may also be due to embolization from cardiac diseases, such as occurs in subacute bacterial endocarditis with vegetation formation or myocardial infarctions with an accompanying thrombus. Atherosclerosis may also be referred to in severe cases as *atherosclerosis obliterans*.[4,14]

Congenital arterial anomalies, such as congenital arteriovenous fistulas that cause abnormal communication between arteries and veins, can occur. Coarctation, or kinking, of an artery is also possible. Some other anomalies include variations in the anatomic course of an artery, absence of a normal vessel, and separate branches appearing in different locations or at unusual origins. The use of real time sonography may help in questionable cases.[5]

Raynaud's phenomenon is related to cold and abrupt temperature changes that cause vascular spasm in the digits and resulting obstruction. Fingers and toes are often purplish in this disorder. Vasospasm occurring by itself is termed *Raynaud's disease,* whereas vasospasm resulting from another condition is called *Raynaud's phenomenon*. The latter is often seen in lupus erythematosus, arthritis, and other diseases.[14]

Buerger's disease is a form of presenile spontaneous gangrene that affects the distal arteries in the digits and toes. It is caused by heavy cigarette smoking and can be distinguished from atherosclerotic disease on an arteriogram by a smooth, well-defined artery proximal to a distant occlusion point. The fingers and toes are usually involved simultaneously, and Raynaud's phenomenon may also occur with this syndrome. The onset is much more acute than that of atherosclerotic occlusion and usually presents a sudden total arterial occlusion. Intense rest pain may occur independently in Buerger's disease, rather than as a progressive process after claudication. (See Symptoms of Arterial Disease.) This disease is also termed *thromboangiitis obliterans*. It is treated by selective amputation and/or sympathectomy in extreme cases.[14]

Frostbite involves the actual freezing of tissue. The cause of arterial occlusion has been attributed to permanent vasoconstriction in response to the cold with or without freezing of blood or fluids. The exact cause of tissue injury is not fully understood. The emergency treatment of warming the affected part is an attempt to restore circulation by relaxing the vasospasm. If flow is not restored in time to save viable tissue, necrosis of the ischemic parts occurs and amputation may be necessary.[14]

Arteritis is usually caused by collagen-related diseases. In cases such as Takayasu's syndrome the media of the artery becomes thickened and swollen, occluding the arterial lumen without changing the external configuration of the vessel itself. This process is usually detected by a diminishing pulse noted over time. Takayasu's Syndrome does not localize but usually occurs in the entire arterial system from the aortic root outward. Other types may occur in isolated vessels.[5,14]

Mechanical compression of an artery involves obstruction by compression of the vessel between or against another part of the body. Examples are thoracic outlet syndrome, in which the arteries, veins, and nerve plexuses are compressed against the first rib or muscle groups by arm flexion and abduction, and malignant tumors (such as chemodectomas and specifically carotid body tumors) and loculated infections that produce purulent lesions or masses, both syndromes that can compromise nearby vasculature and compress the vessels against other areas of the body.

Entrapment syndromes cause problems in a similar manner to mechanical compression syndromes but are often related to congenital anomalies or trauma and usually involve muscle fascia or ligament obstructions in areas such as the popliteal artery or the anterior compartment of the lower leg.

SYMPTOMS OF ARTERIAL DISEASE[4-6,14]

Claudication. The term *claudication* comes from the Latin verb "to limp" and was first coined, and the condition described, by Jean-Marie Charcot in his treatise on limping as a symptom of arterial obstruction in horses and in humans.[8b] Patients with claudication notice tiring and pain in the limb distal to the occlusion with exertion. A walking patient may feel pain in the calf first, often within a measurable distance. The pain and tiring progress to muscle cramping if the patient persists (e.g., for a city block). If the patient rests, the cramping and pain resolve completely. The symptoms resume with the onset of activity. In the arms a patient may feel pain, tiring, and cramping after extensive lifting or elevation of the affected arm. In either legs or arms the affected limb may give way if too much demand is placed on it.

Dependent Rubor and Elevation Pallor. Erythema is often seen in patients with advancing arterial disease, along with drying and flaking of skin and thickening of the nails. If the extremity is hung dependent, it usually presents puffy and red digits and even the entire forefoot or hand in advanced disease. If the limb is elevated, the redness disappears and the limb becomes increasingly pale.

Ischemic Rest Pain. Ischemic rest pain is a symptom of very severe arterial insufficiency and is usually found in cases of lower-than-normal resting blood flow. The pain is localized in specific areas of inadequate perfusion (e.g., toes, heel, or calf). It manifests as a constant, severe pain present regardless of activity and is not relieved by normal means. It is often described as a burning pain that keeps the patient awake at night. The skin is red and thin and is often shiny. This symptom is a definite sign that arterial reconstruction or some other means must be undertaken to prevent loss of the limb.

Coldness of the Limb. Coolness of the limb results from inadequate arterial flow and is readily noticed by the examiner.

Gangrene. When the disease advances to near cessation of flow, circulation to the distal portion of the digits (with the most easily occluded vessels) is often blocked completely. The tissue necroses and gangrene sets in, appearing as a black shriveling spot or region that progresses and from which fluids exude. Amputation is often the only course, although recent advances in hyperbaric pressure chamber medicine have enabled many largely necrosed limbs to be saved in whole or in part.

Regardless of the symptoms and signs, arterial disease is a dangerous entity. It depletes the blood flow to vital organs, impairs normal activity, and often acts as a precursor to more serious conditions.

FLOW DYNAMICS IN THE PERIPHERAL ARTERIAL SYSTEM

The normal arterial Doppler flow signal is evaluated by the chart tracing and audio signals. Both positive and negative chart deflections exist in the arterial signal, again with antegrade flow being positive and retrograde flow being negative. Probe position is critical in the arterial examination. If the sound beam is perpendicular to the direction of flow, no Doppler shift occurs and a flat tracing results. The examiner should use the flow direction gauges and the signal strength as heard through the speakers to determine the precise angle for optimal blood flow sampling.

The normal arterial Doppler flow signal in the extremities consists of three components: a large positive deflection with systole, a period of net flow reversal to the negative side of the zero line, and a lesser diastolic positive deflection (Fig. 20-1). The period of reversal results from the high resistance of the vascular bed in the extremities. In vasodilated conditions the flow is seen primarily on the positive side, but the three deflections are still present. The normal arterial flow signal, because of the three components, is said to be *triphasic*.[5]

In cases of arterial obstruction the flow signal begins to lose one or more components, becoming biphasic or monophasic. The flow pattern tends to remain triphasic proximal to the obstruction but begins to show diminished systolic components and lose the diastolic component distally, secondary to narrowing across the occlusion site and in some cases to ischemia-induced vasodilation in the distal vascular bed (Fig. 20-2). Spectral arterial waveforms

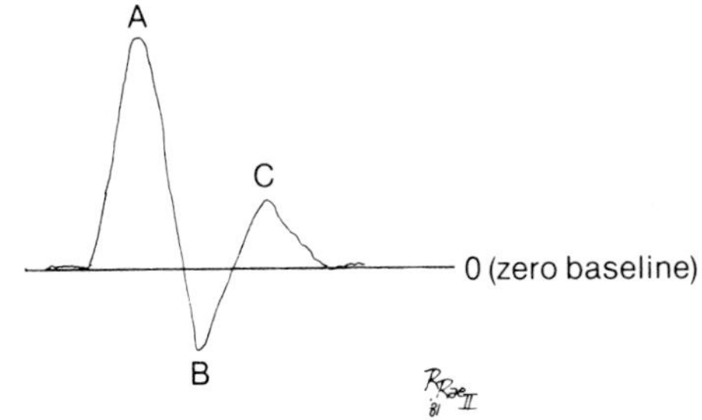

FIG. 20-1 Normal arterial waveform in the extremities. *A* is the first diastolic component, *B* the brief period of reversal, and *C* the diastolic component.

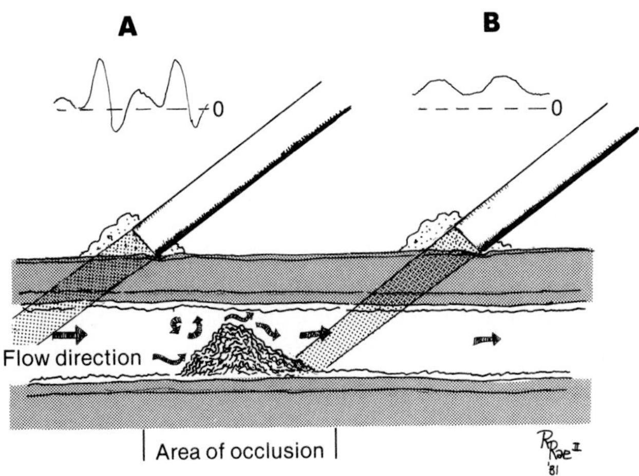

FIG. 20-2 Diagram of flow patterns proximal and distal to an occlusion. **A** shows the waveform obtained proximally, with all normal components present. **B** shows the characteristic loss of components and flow diminishing found in the segment distal to the block.

show an increase in spectral broadening, with increased peak velocity at the stenosis and a disruption of the envelope distal to the stenosis.

PHYSIOLOGY OF FLOW PRESSURES[5]

Segmental blood pressure measurement in the limb is the basis of the Doppler examination in the extremities. To understand what happens, the examiner must understand some basic physiology of blood flow dynamics.

Poiseuille's law pertains to pressure gradients of fluids through arterial segments in the body. Two factors determine the flow: (1) the pressure difference across the segment and (2) the resistance of the segment. Poiseuille's law is stated as the following equation:

$$\Delta P = Q8Lv/\pi r^4$$

where the flow, Q, as determined by the length of the segment, L, viscosity of the blood, v, and radius of the segment, r, varies directly with the pressure gradient, ΔP, across the segment and indirectly with the resistance (interaction of L, v, and r) across it. ($8/\pi$ is a mathematic constant.) This can best be applied physiologically to arteries in which the pressure gradient across the segment can be increased by increasing the flow through the segment or decreasing the radius of the lumen.

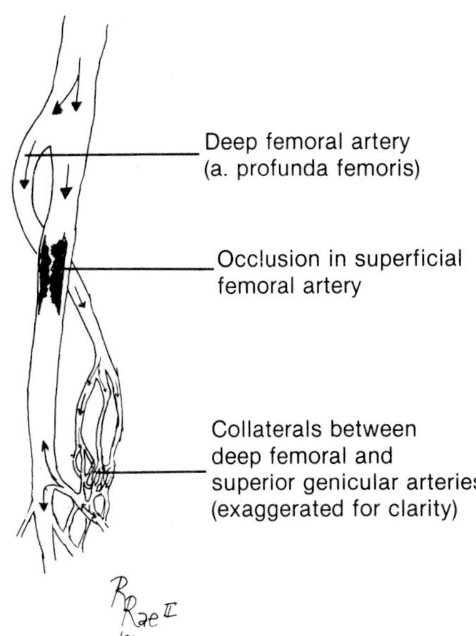

FIG. 20-3 Diagram of recovery in a segment distal to a superficial femoral occlusion resulting from collateralization from the profunda femoris.

When obstructions are present, blood is forced through collateral channels, where the resistance is higher than the normal vessel (Fig. 20-3). Thus, as flow is forced around the obstruction and into collaterals, the pressure drop along that segment is increased. This information is important for the arterial Doppler examination, since the examiner must be aware of pressure drops that can occur and must understand the mechanism of the pressure drop distal to an occlusive site.

DOPPLER LOWER EXTREMITY ARTERIAL EXAMINATION

Arterial Anatomy of the Lower Extremities[11]

To understand the Doppler lower extremity examination, thorough knowledge of the vascular anatomy as it pertains to the Doppler examination is necessary. Only the arteries that are directly accessible and that figure into the examination are discussed.

Flow to the extremities comes from the abdominal aorta. The aorta bifurcates about the level of the umbilicus to form the common iliac arteries. The common iliac vessels then bifurcate into the internal and external iliac arteries. The internal iliac (hypogastric) supplies the buttock and genital area. The external iliac supplies the leg and becomes the common femoral artery at approximately the level of the inguinal ligament. Several branches are given off, of which the profunda femoris is the most important. It comes off about 2 to 5 cm below the inguinal ligament and supplies the bone and muscles of the thigh.

At this point the common femoral becomes the superficial femoral artery. It runs along the medial surface of the thigh and curves posteriorly behind the knee to become the popliteal artery.

The popliteal artery continues behind the knee joint and gives off the anterior tibial artery 3 to 6 cm below the popliteal fossa. The popliteal then terminates as the posterior tibial and peroneal arteries (Fig. 20-4).

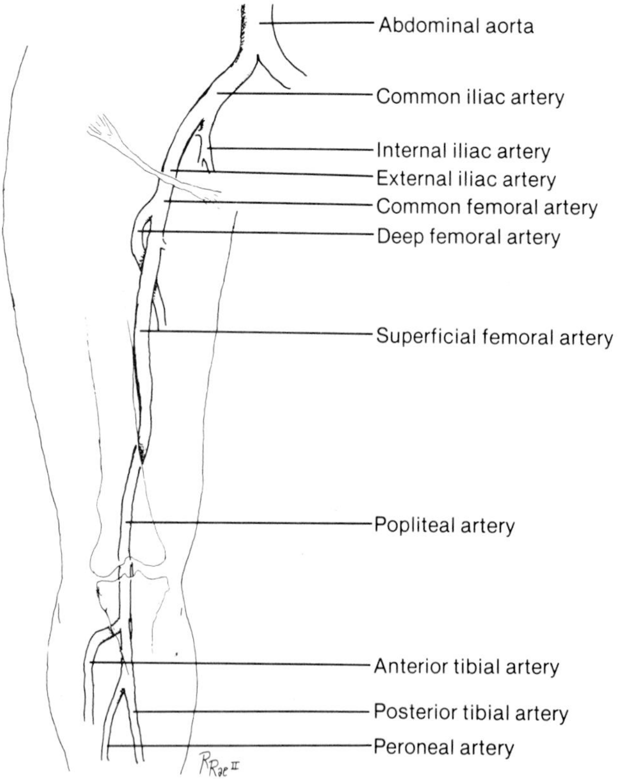

FIG. 20-4 Arterial blood supply to the lower extremity.

The anterior tibial descends through muscles along the tibia and becomes the dorsalis pedis at the level of the ankle. The dorsalis pedis then runs superficially and dorsally on the medial side of the foot to terminate in the deep plantar arch between the first and second metatarsals.

The posterior tibial artery descends along the posterior surface of the tibia to run posterior to the medial malleolus.

The peroneal artery descends deeply on the fibular side of the leg and becomes accessible anterior to the lateral malleolus (Fig. 20-5).

LOWER-EXTREMITY ARTERIAL EXAMINATION TECHNIQUES

Before beginning any examination of the lower extremities, the first step is to obtain as complete a history as possible from the patient, the patient's chart, or both. The emphasis should be placed on the following information:

1. If the patient is claudicating, note whether one or both legs are affected, where the pain is felt (e.g., calf, thigh, hip), and if it is a tiring or a cramp in the muscle. The distance the patient can ambulate before stopping because of the pain should be noted and whether the symptoms are relieved by rest.
2. Palpate the pulses at the femoral, popliteal, posterior tibial, and dorsalis pedis arteries. Weak or absent pulses should be noted.
3. Check for *night cramping* or *ischemic rest pain*. Remember that simple aching or pain at rest may not constitute the specific diagnosis of rest pain unless the other criteria of critical ischemia are met (e.g., skin changes, absent pulses, limited mobility).
4. Note the *skin color and condition*. Check for dry skin,

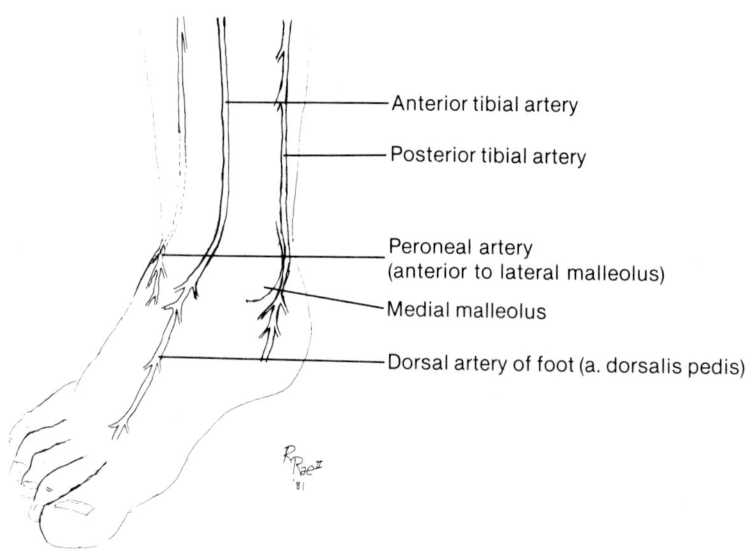

FIG. 20-5 Arteries of the ankle that are accessible to the Doppler probe.

erythema of the toes, thickened nails, gangrenous spots, and unhealed ulcers.

5. Check for *known vascular diseases, past bypass surgeries, diabetes, cardiac disease, smoking, hypertension,* and any *family history* of these atherosclerotic risk factors. Also, when a patient states that he or she has had a "bypass," inquire further as to whether this means a *peripheral arterial bypass* in the extremity or a *coronary bypass*. This is important, since scars from the harvesting of saphenous veins for coronary artery bypass grafting often appear identical to those encountered in peripheral arterial bypassing (see Doppler Examination of the Postoperative Patient).

Several different component methods can make up an evaluation of the lower-extremity arterial system. Usually one or more of these is used in combination with segmental pressure measurement. The four techniques described here are considered the primary diagnostic methods by the Essentials and Standards of the Intersocietal Commission for the Accreditation of Vascular Laboratories.[10]

DOPPLER VELOCITY WAVEFORM ANALYSIS

Continuous-wave Doppler waveforms can be taken in any order and at any time or can be integrated with the segmental pressure technique. The procedure below follows one logical progression.

The patient should lie supine and be made comfortable. The femoral arteries are first accessed by palpating the superior border of the inguinal ligament and placing the probe in position just above the ligament to determine the proper site for monitoring of the femoral artery (Fig. 20-6). The external iliac is actually being monitored at this level rather than the common femoral, but it is better to obtain the signal here than to listen below the ligament, where the bifurcation of the profunda femoris can cause confusion. The common femoral arteries are then monitored and recorded bilaterally. Some pressure on the probe may be needed to obtain a clear signal. The signals are found lateral to the common femoral venous signals (heard as a "windstorm" sound). An arterial signal found medial to the vein is probably the hypogastric artery and must not be mistaken for the femoral. If in doubt, move the probe laterally and medially to locate the vein and determine the vessel's relationship. The hypogastric artery also may appear as a retrograde signal when the probe is angled cephalad.

The popliteal arteries are next to be examined and are found at their sites behind the knees. There are two methods of examining the popliteal arteries: supine and prone.

In the supine position the knees are bent to about a 75-degree angle and are relaxed laterally ("frog-leg" position) and the probe is placed in the popliteal fossa and angled cephalad (Fig. 20-7). An ample quantity of gel is required to ensure good probe-skin contact. Firm pressure may be needed to displace fat and tissue. Be careful not to occlude the artery. The probe should be angled to obtain the clearest signal with distinct waveform patterns. This segment of the study requires an accurate tracing, since the popliteal signal may be the determining factor in deciding whether an occlusion exists above the knee or in the trifurcation vessels below the knee. The best signal is obtained with the probe more toward the calf than toward the knee, to avoid catching the flow at an angle that could suggest occluded flow or even retrograde flow in the artery (Fig. 20-8).

In the prone position the patient's legs are elevated 30 to 45 degrees and are supported with a bolster or pillow (Fig. 20-9). The same basic examination technique is used as in the supine position, and the probe is angled cephalad. The advantage of this position is the ability actually to see the relationship of the popliteal fossa and the probe. It is a good position to use for the examiner-in-training.

Both positions give excellent results. A major advantage

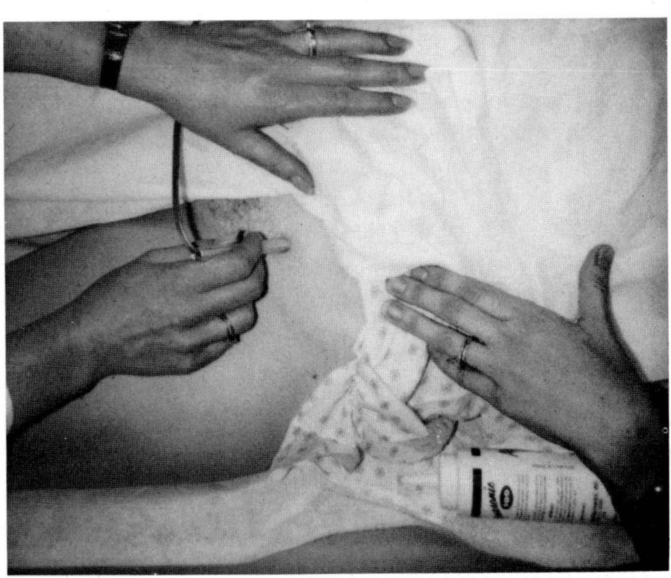

FIG. 20-6 Examining the common femoral artery.

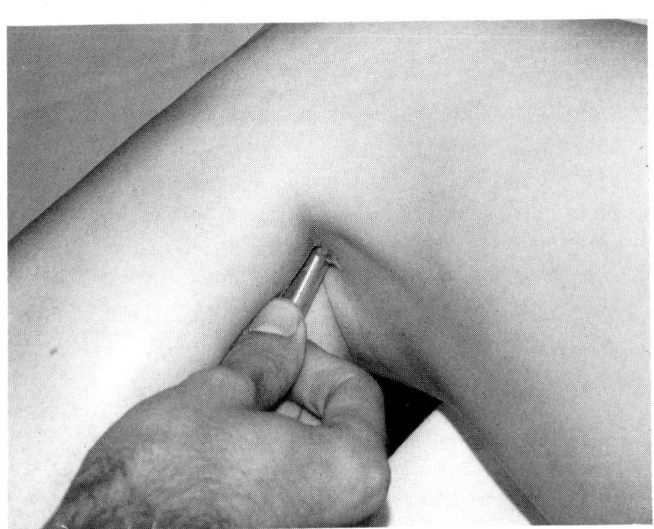

FIG. 20-7 Supine examination of the popliteal artery.

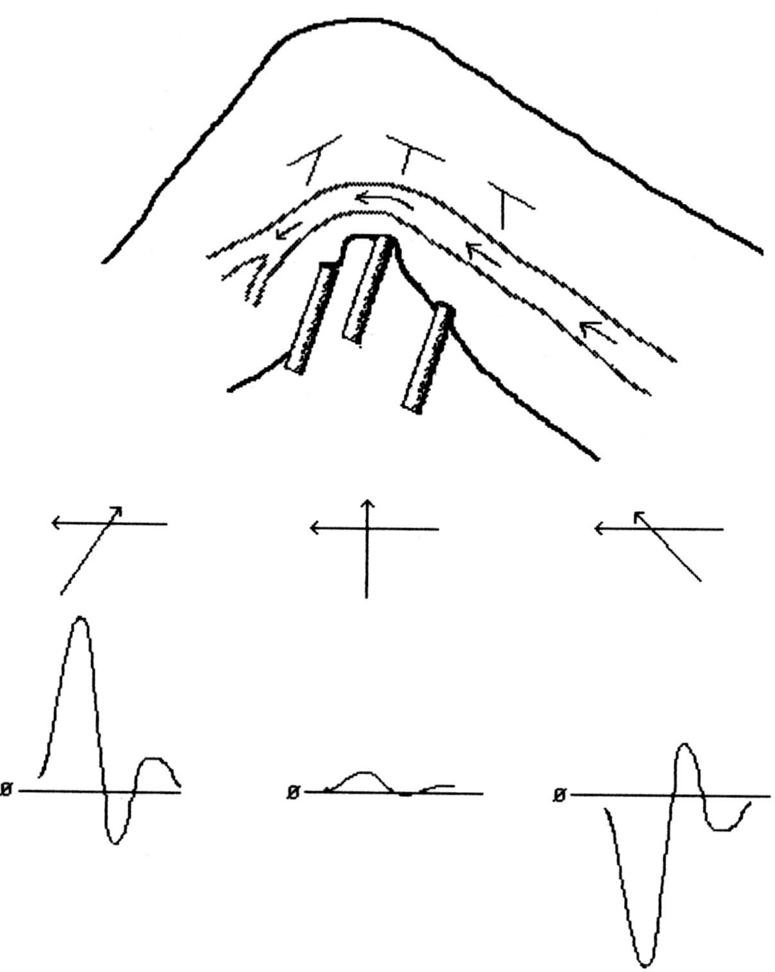

FIG. 20-8 How improper probe placement can cause a false reading of retrograde or diminished flow if the beam is not angled against the flow of the vessel.

of the supine position is that the patient does not need to move after the initial portion of the examination has been completed. This is especially beneficial to the postoperative or invalid patient who cannot turn over. The choice of examination positions is best left to the examiner's preference.

If there is a discrepancy in the signal quality between the femoral and popliteal sites, the superficial femoral artery can be examined by palpating the femur on the anterior aspect of the leg and placing the probe medial to it in the muscle groove, angling cephalad. The superficial femoral artery can be examined anywhere along the region shown in Fig. 20-10. This can help localize the level of stenosis more accurately.

To summarize the technique:

1. Obtain Doppler waveforms from the femoral artery above the inguinal ligament.
2. Obtain waveforms from the popliteal artery behind the knee, either with the patient in a supine position with knee bent (preferred) or with the patient prone, knee flexed, and with the lower leg supported by a bolster or pillow.
3. Obtain waveforms from the posterior tibial artery at its site medial and posterior to the medial malleolus.
4. Obtain waveforms from the dorsalis pedis artery along the midpoint of the volar surface of the foot, in line with the space between the first two toes and the ankle.
5. If necessary, obtain a waveform from the peroneal artery anterior to the lateral malleolus at the ankle.
6. Optionally, a waveform can be obtained from the superficial femoral artery in the midthigh medially along the sartorius groove.

The waveforms can be obtained in any order, and each of the steps should be performed bilaterally when possible.

Interpretation of Doppler Waveforms

A normal arterial signal is triphasic. Diminution or loss of any of the components implies obstruction proximal to the probe site. If flow is triphasic at the ankle, it must be triphasic at all sites above the ankle. The absence of a

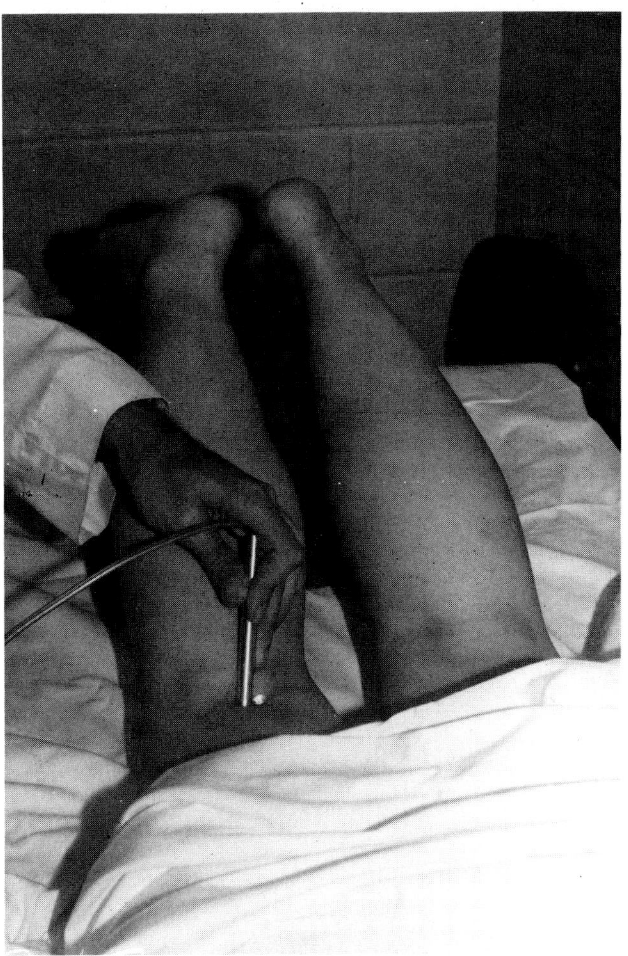

FIG. 20-9 Prone examination of the popliteal artery.

triphasic pattern in the popliteal artery in the presence of a normal triphasic pattern in the femoral and ankle areas implies technical error, and the artery should be re-checked.

Following is a guide to interpretation of the waveforms in cases of disease:

1. If the waveforms are triphasic in the femoral, popliteal, dorsalis pedis, and posterior tibial arteries, the flow in the leg is within normal limits.
2. If the waveforms are triphasic in the femoral and popliteal but biphasic or monophasic in either of the ankle vessels where the other is triphasic, the abnormal artery is probably the only one diseased.
3. If flow is triphasic in the femoral and popliteal but biphasic or monophasic in both ankle arteries, there is probably disease within the distal popliteal or below the popliteal involving the trifurcation vessels.
4. If flow is triphasic in the femoral but biphasic or monophasic at the popliteal and ankle vessels, this implies superficial femoral artery or popliteal artery stenoses or occlusions. Examination of the proximal and distal superficial femoral artery can help locate the level of obstruction.
5. Biphasic or monophasic flow at the femoral and all sites below implies an iliac artery or distal aortic stenosis or occlusion.
6. Finally, absence of a signal in any artery with no detectable distal flow implies a complete occlusion or thrombosis of the artery. This diagnosis can be made most reliably in the trifurcation vessels; but see below.

The additional use of segmental pressures compared with the waveform readout and audible information is quite accurate in helping to determine the relative flow status of the extremity. However, errors in interpretation can occur and are often the result of poor examination technique. The next section discusses these problems.

False-Positive Conditions and Their Rectification[5]

Absent signal. The Doppler signal may be absent in cases of extreme atherosclerosis obliterans. The examiner must be aware, however, that absence of flow should not be observed in patients with strong pulses. The probe site should be re-checked and a careful search made for the artery by slowly moving the probe laterally and medially. Care must also be taken that an even but not extreme amount of pressure is being applied; otherwise the vessel may be occluded by the force on the probe. Careful examination is often required to register flow when there is not enough pressure in the segment to create a palpable pulse. One suggestion is to apply a generous amount of acoustic couplant to the skin at the various probe sites along the arterial segment and place the probe within the mound of gel without actually touching the skin. The gel acts as an acoustic path, allowing minimal flow information to be obtained without inadvertent pressure on the artery being examined, which might occlude it (Fig. 20-11).

False diagnosis of biphasic or monophasic flow at the popliteal site. False diagnosis of biphasic or monophasic flow at the popliteal site is most often a result of poor technique and is usually noticed because the femoral and ankle arteries exhibit normal triphasic flow. Precise positioning of the probe, careful pressure judgment, moving the probe more toward the calf than toward the thigh, and angling cephalad with respect to the course of the artery should resolve this problem. If in doubt, another attempt should be made.

False diagnosis of biphasic or monophasic flow at the femoral site. False diagnosis of biphasic or monophasic flow at the femoral site occurs when triphasic signals are found in the distal vessels in the postsurgical or obese patient. It is a result of fatty tissue or scarring in the groin. The probe should be moved lateral to the vein and placed on either side of the scar, or with the fat held back out of the way. Angling medially or laterally into the desired area should give good results. Remember also that the beam should be 45 degrees to the flow, not to the skin surface. If it is impossible to obtain an accurate signal above the ligament, the report form should be noted to that effect and

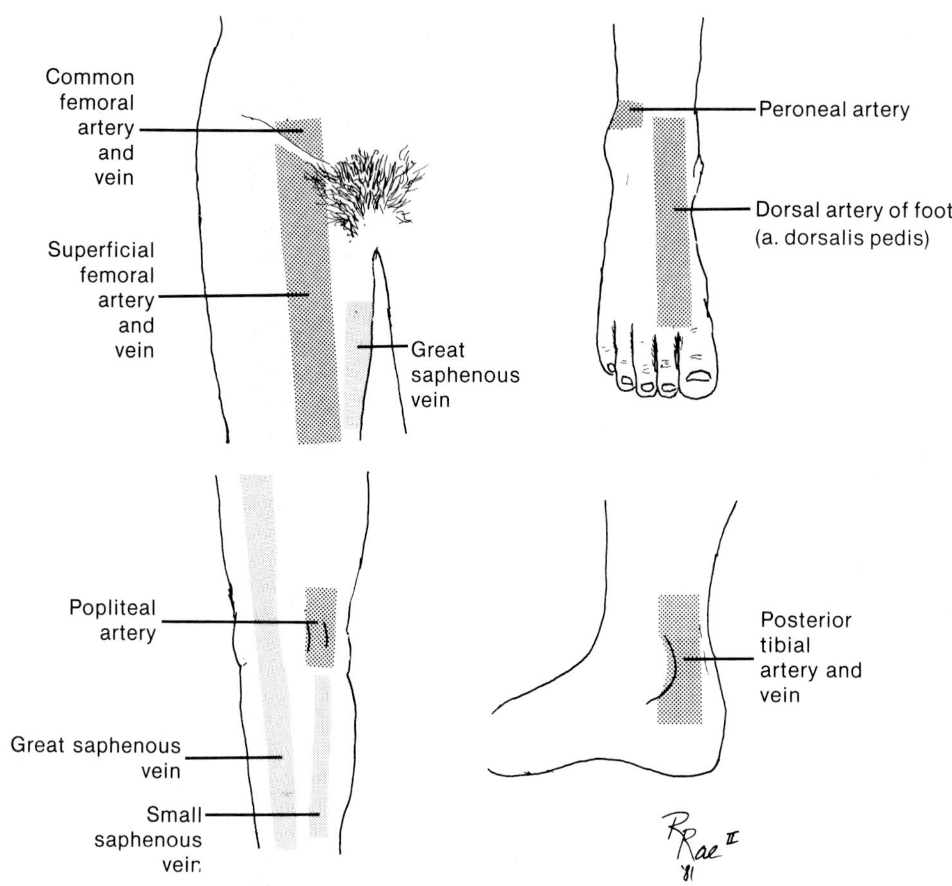

FIG. 20-10 Sites where both arterial and venous signals can be obtained in the lower extremity.

the proximal segment of the superficial femoral artery away from the profunda bifurcation should be obtained.

False diagnosis of retrograde flow in a major limb artery. False diagnosis of retrograde flow in a major limb artery occurs when the beam is angled through a segment at a point where flow is perceived as receding from the probe. In the femoral region the hypogastric artery can be wrongly monitored medial to the common femoral vein. The probe should be moved lateral to the vein for the correct signal. This can also occur if the probe is angled incorrectly. In the popliteal area the probe should be moved toward the calf to allow the beam to intersect flow at the correct angle.

False reversal in the posterior tibial artery and the dorsalis pedis occurs most often when flow below the knee is so reduced that pulsatility nearly vanishes and the accompanying vein sounds are mistaken for those from the artery. Careful listening is necessary to detect any trace of a pulse. The vein can be ruled out by squeezing the fleshy part of the foot and listening for a rush of flow, which does not occur in the artery.

SEGMENTAL PRESSURES

Measuring pressure gradients at four or more different levels in the legs is considered by many to be an important part of the evaluation of arterial flow; whereas Doppler velocity waveform analysis is a qualitative examination of blood flow and hemodynamics of a stenosis, segmental pressure gradients are quantitative in that they can show and document the physiologic effect of a stenosis or occlusion on the perfusion pressure in the distal extremity. These gradients and regional perfusion states cannot be assessed by Doppler or duplex alone.

Segmental pressures are usually (but not always) assessed in conjunction with Doppler velocity waveform analysis, arterial duplex scanning, or volume pulse recording. In all cases, some method must be used to insonate the ankle vessels to audibly monitor the waveforms and obtain pressure measurements. The technique described below uses a continuous-wave Doppler probe, but a duplex scanner can also be used (although this method can be cumbersome).

The patient lies in a supine position and blood pressure cuffs are applied to the legs for measuring the pressure gradients (except in certain postoperative cases; see Doppler Examination of the Postoperative Patient.) The cuffs are placed in four locations on each leg: one on the ankle, one just below the knee on the calf, one just above the knee on the lower thigh, and one just below the groin on the upper thigh (Fig. 20-12).

The main requirement is that the cuffs be long enough to wrap around the patient's legs. Narrow cuffs should be

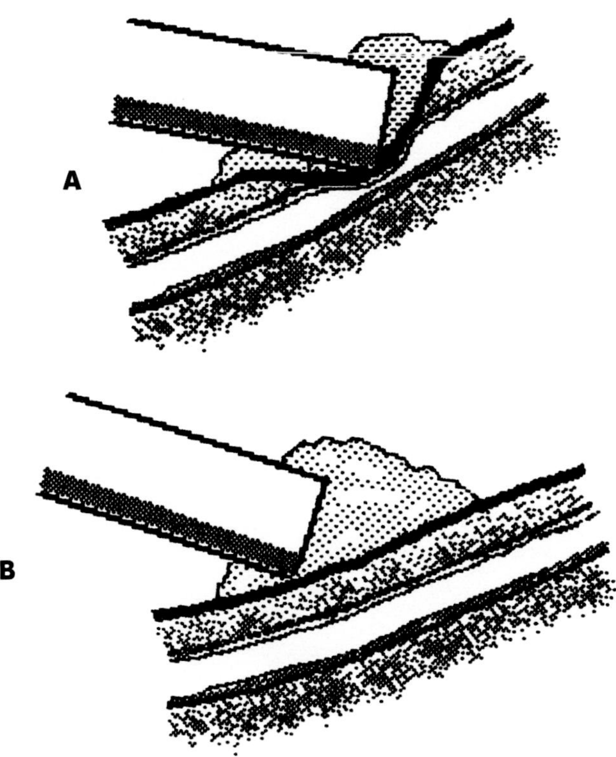

FIG. 20-11 Probe compression. **A,** Too much pressure with the probe can occlude a superficial artery, falsely implying an absent signal. **B,** Light contact with ample gel as a coupling window allows a signal to be obtained.

used for the thigh pressures despite the higher-than-normal pressure readings that can be expected there. An aneroid sphygmomanometer can then be attached to each cuff, or one manometer or automatic cuff inflator can be easily transferred from cuff to cuff using a Luer-Lok or friction type of connector.

When the four cuffs have been placed on the legs, another one is placed on the arm to take a brachial blood pressure.

The brachial artery is examined at its site on the medial side of the antecubital fossa, and the probe is angled cephalad until the most satisfactory signal is obtained. A tracing is made of the Doppler signal. With the probe still in place, the cuff is inflated above the point at which the signal disappears. It is then deflated about 2 to 4 mm/sec until the systolic pulse is heard. This breakthrough point is the systolic pressure. Deflation continues until the fourth returning sound corresponding to the diastolic antegrade component on the waveform is heard and the flow resumes its normal pattern. The point where the "slurred" sound of the third and fourth component is heard marks the diastolic pressure. Recording the pulse tracing is not necessary but can help the examiner locate the point where the flow resumes its normal pattern until proficiency or "ear training" is attained. For purposes of the Doppler examination, recording the diastolic pressure is not necessary since the systolic pressure is the only component needed for calculation of the ankle-brachial index.

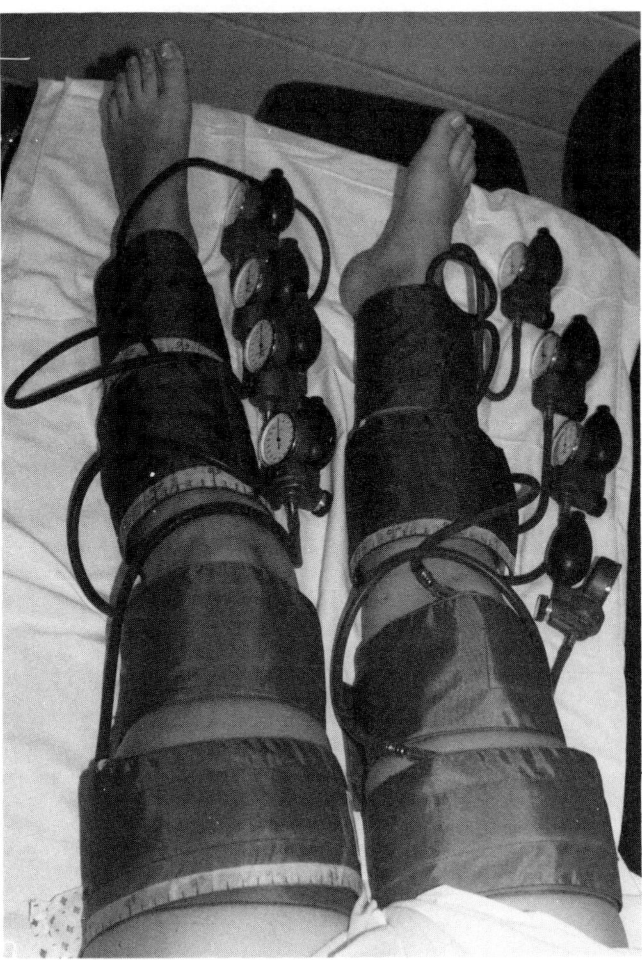

FIG. 20-12 Pressure cuffs in place on the legs for the lower-extremity arterial study.

The foregoing steps are repeated for the other arm. The examiner then moves to the patient's feet to commence examination of the ankle arteries and pressures.

The posterior tibial artery is monitored at its site posterior to the medial malleolus. The probe is angled until the strongest signal is obtained. It is then kept in place, and the ankle cuff is inflated past the point where the signal disappears. Deflation begins until the systolic signal is heard, and the pressure at that point is recorded (Fig. 20-13).

The examiner then moves the probe to examine the dorsalis pedis at its sites on the dorsum of the foot. Once again, the best signal is obtained and an ankle pressure is recorded in the same manner as for the posterior tibial artery (Fig. 20-14).

Before continuing, the examiner should compare waveforms and pressures of the two arteries. The artery with the higher pressure should be used to take the remaining pressures in the leg.

If flow in either the dorsalis pedis or the posterior tibial artery is unsatisfactory or absent, the peroneal artery should

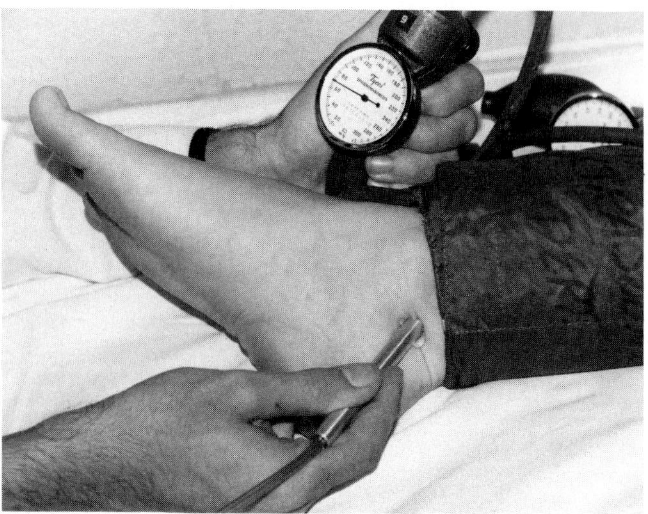

FIG. 20-13 Examining the posterior tibial artery.

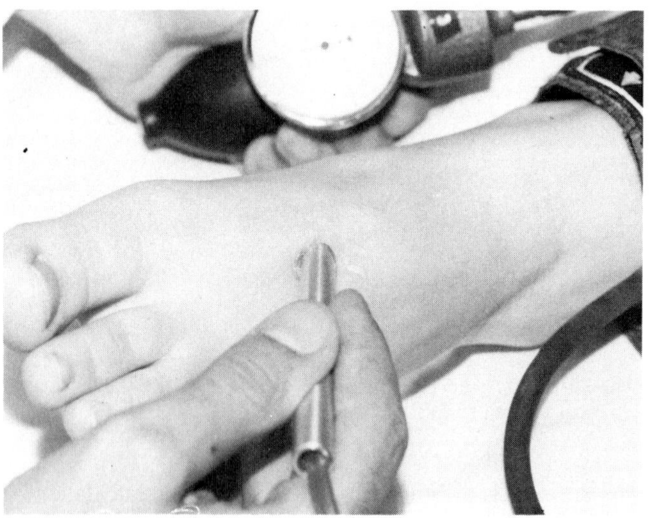

FIG. 20-14 Examining the dorsalis pedis artery.

be examined at its site anterior to the lateral malleolus. It is examined in the same manner as the other ankle vessels (Fig. 20-15).

The artery that is selected is then monitored. Each cuff from calf to upper thigh is inflated and deflated in turn, and the systolic blood pressure is taken at each level. It is a must to keep the probe stationary and motionless to prevent the systolic signal from being lost as the cuff is deflated.

When the tracings and pressures from one extremity have been taken, the procedure is repeated for the other.

After pressures have been taken at all cuff sites in both legs, the cuffs are removed. If further information about the foot and digit perfusion is required, additional cuffs can be used. A transmetatarsal cuff can be applied across the instep of the foot, as well as a digit cuff around the base of the big toe. Flow is monitored with a Doppler probe in the

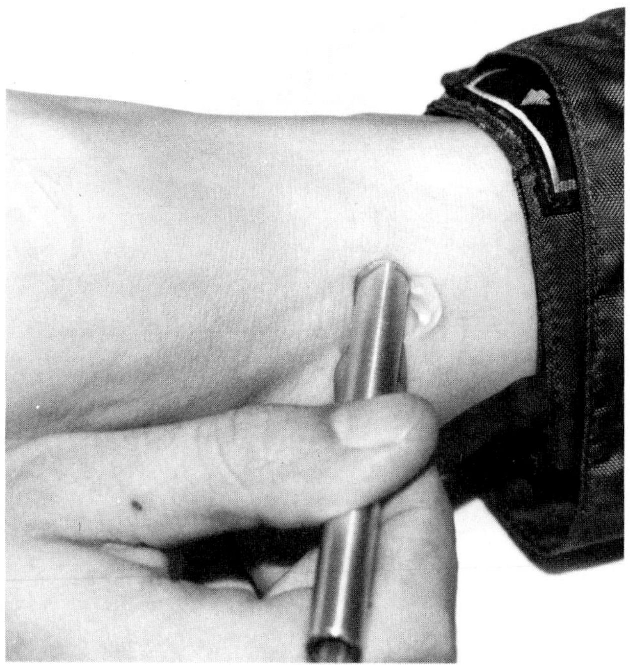

FIG. 20-15 Examination of the peroneal artery.

dorsalis pedis artery below the cuff, and pressures are acquired as with the other cuffs. Flow in the toe is monitored either with a Doppler probe or with a photoplethysmography photo cell. If using a Doppler, listen for a faint pulse in the center of the plantar surface of the toe distal to the digit cuff and slowly inflate the cuff, preferably by hand to avoid cuff bladder damage. This method may not work if there is digital ischemia or calcified vessels. An easier and somewhat better method is to obtain the toe pressure using either a photoplethysmography (PPG) photo cell or strain gauge (SPG) that does not rely on audible flow. The photo cell should be attached to the plantar surface of the toe distal to the cuff using double-sided cellophane tape. If a strain gauge is used, it should be looped around the end of the toe. If a multifunction system is used instead of a standalone photoplethysmograph, it should be switched to the PPG or SPG mode, depending on the method used. The amplifier mode switch should be set to AC and the chart sizes and sensitivity adjusted until a uniform and readable waveform is obtained. The digit cuff is inflated until the waveform disappears and a flat line trace is seen. The cuff is then slowly bled until a peak is seen on the tracing indicating the return of systolic flow. At that precise moment of waveform return, the pressure reading from the manometer should be recorded.

Interpretation of Segmental Pressure Measurements

To determine the flow status of the extremities, one must calculate ratios of the ankle systolic pressures divided by the brachial systolic pressures. The ankle-brachial index is thus obtained. The higher systolic pressure of the two arteries examined at the ankle is divided by the higher systolic pressure of the two arms. This is done for each leg. The higher brachial pressure should be used for both legs to ensure uniformity.

In normal individuals the ankle-brachial index should be greater than 1. Patients who are asymptomatic or with slight symptoms have indices from 0.90 to 1. Patients with claudication show indices of 0.4 to 0.85. Anything less than 0.4 implies rest pain or severe ischemia.[5]

Using this criteria, the ankle-brachial ratio also can be used in categorizing the severity of flow impairment to the distal extremity.

- Indices running between 0.85 and 1 imply mild impairment.
- Indices running between 0.4 and 0.85 imply moderate impairment.
- Indices running between 0.1 and 0.4 imply severe impairment.

Readings falling on the borderline between categories are often interpreted as "mild to moderate," "moderate to severe," and so on.

Experience with follow-up studies has shown that in normal individuals the ankle-brachial index can vary from 0.85 to as much as 1.1. This factor seems to depend on the relative blood pressure that a patient may have on the day of examination and whether it may change between the time the arm is checked and when the ankle pressures are taken. Therefore the examiner and interpreting physician should not expect the same index in a normal patient to be completely reproducible from examination to examination and should be aware that a lower index may not imply disease if a strong triphasic signal is found.

It should also be noted that patients with calcific arteries often have abnormally or unusually high ankle-brachial indices, such as 1.2 to 3. In these individuals the quality of the waveform is the best indicator of occlusion since the vessels are incompressible. Patients with extremely obese legs or diabetes also may have abnormally high indices.[4,5]

Further information about the circulation may be obtained by comparison of the segmental pressures. In a normal patient, there is usually no greater than 40 mm Hg of difference between any two cuffs. The pressure reading increases as the circumference of the extremity increases. An accurate pressure at the thigh could be obtained only with an extremely wide cuff, but it is unnecessary for Doppler readings because the difference between cuffs is used as an indicator of a pressure drop. The upper thigh pressure should not exceed 50 mm Hg above the brachial pressure.

As mentioned, extremely high pressures (as in noncompressible arteries or other situations with pressures greater than 300 mm Hg) in the ankle or calf imply a calcified segment. This should be noted on the report form so there will be no confusion during interpretation.

If an upper thigh pressure is significantly less than the brachial pressure, this implies iliac artery stenosis.

If there is a significant pressure drop between the lower and upper thigh cuffs, this implies a superficial femoral artery obstruction.

If there is a significant pressure drop between the lower thigh and calf cuffs, a popliteal artery stenosis is implied.

If there is a significant pressure drop between the ankle and calf cuffs, this implies stenosis of the anterior tibial, posterior tibial, or peroneal arteries. Marked pressure drops between metatarsal-toe pressure and ankle pressure may indicate small-vessel disease in the forefoot or digits. This finding is not uncommon in cases of diabetes or Buerger's disease.

It is important to correlate segmental pressure findings with the results of duplex, Doppler velocity waveform analysis, or volume pulse recording, if available, to obtain a more complete picture of hemodynamic and perfusion conditions in the leg.

VOLUME PULSE RECORDINGS (AIR PLETHYSMOGRAPHY)

Volume pulse recording provides an alternate qualitative method of obtaining waveform from arteries in the lower extremity. It can easily be performed on patients who have already had segmental pressures, since both the cuffs used and their placement sites are exactly the same.

To obtain volume pulse waveforms, the patient should lie supine, and the examiner should place cuffs at the upper thigh, lower thigh, below-knee calf, ankle, and metatarsal positions bilaterally. Again, cuffs should be no more than 12 cm wide and should be long enough to wrap around the leg (Fig. 20-16).

An air supply hose is connected from the plethysmograph to the cuff at the location being examined. Some devices can connect four or five cuffs simultaneously (although only one or two at a time are inflated). Once the hoses are connected, the examiner can begin the study. The examiner needs to be certain the system is set to evaluate volume pulse recording and that a manual aneroid sphygmomanometer, regulated air compressor, or automatic cuff inflator is

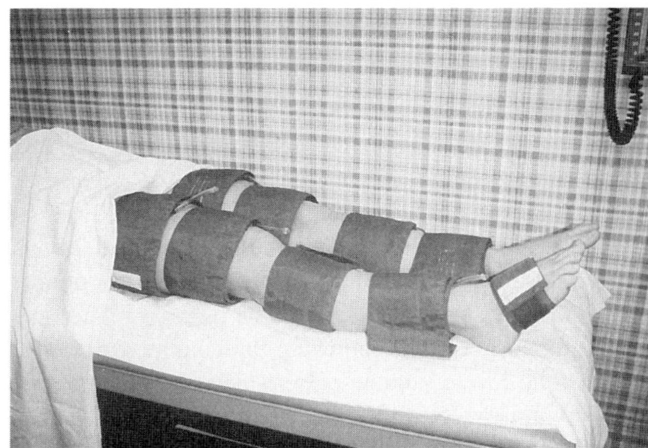

FIG. 20-16 Positioning of cuffs for volume pulse recording (air plethysmography).

attached to the air input port (some devices have automatic cuff inflators built in). The examiner must then perform a calibration run before actually recording waveforms. This is done by inflating a cuff to a pressure of 60 mm Hg, observing the displayed waveform, and adjusting the pen position and tracing size on the chart recorder or computer display to ensure that the waveform is displayed fully and accurately. It is best to start at the upper thigh and work distally since the thigh waveform is almost always the largest or strongest volume wave obtained. Once the size and position have been established, the examiner must not change these settings and must use this standard pressure in all cuffs (although some suggest differing ranges of pressure, a 60 mm Hg is presented here and in the example cases).

Once the system and chart recorder are calibrated, the high-thigh cuff is inflated to 60 mm Hg and the pressure is held. Once a stable waveform is seen on the tracing or computer display, roughly five to six stable waveforms should be recorded. This procedure is repeated until waveforms have been bilaterally recorded from:

1. The high-thigh cuffs
2. The low-thigh cuffs
3. The calf (below-knee) cuffs
4. The ankle cuffs
5. The metatarsal cuffs

If digit waveforms are desired, a PPG photocell or strain gauge can be used (preferably after all volume pulse recording tracings are complete to avoid recalibration). The photocell should be attached to the plantar surface of the toe distal to the cuff using double-sided cellophane tape. If a strain gauge is used, it should be looped around the end of the toe with a slight stretch to ensure contact. The amplifier mode switch should be set to AC, the device switched to photoplethysmography or strain gauge recording, and the chart sizes and sensitivity adjusted until a uniform and readable waveform is obtained. Roughly five or six waves should be obtained. PPG waves sometimes rise and fall along the course of the tracing, and it sometimes helps if the patient avoids deep breathing or holds their breath during recording.

Interpretation of Volume Pulse Recordings

It is important to remember that all forms of plethysmography, in principle, measure changes in volume. The displayed wave does not indicate blood flow but rather indicates changes in limb diameter as a result of increase and decrease of blood in the segment being examined. In systole, blood flows in via the arteries faster than it is drained by the veins, causing a rapid volume increase. After systole the opposite occurs, allowing the volume to return to the diastolic level. Volume pulse waves can be compared readily with Doppler velocity waveforms. The peak systolic upslope of the normal volume pulse recording wave corresponds to the first systolic component of a triphasic Doppler waveform. As the volume falls, there is a retrograde wave, which is seen on a normal volume pulse recording waveform as the dicrotic notch and as the second or reverse component in a Doppler waveform. The volume pulse recording downslope in diastole then corresponds to the third component of the Doppler waveform (Fig. 20-17).

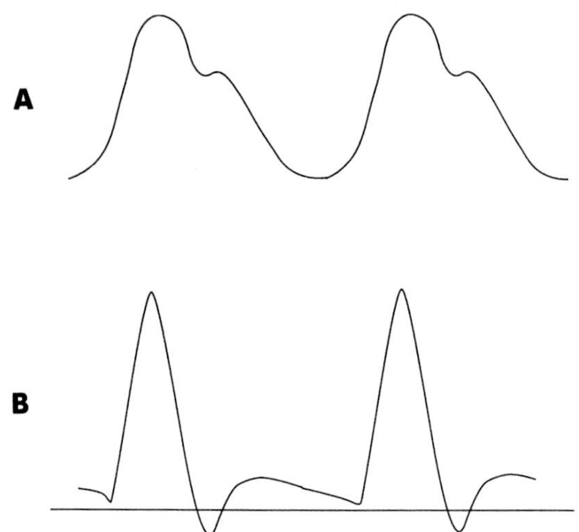

FIG. 20-17 Comparison of normal extremity plethysmographic arterial volume pulse waveforms, **A,** with normal extremity arterial Doppler waveforms, **B.** Note that there is no zero baseline in the plethysmographic waveform and that the plethysmographic waveform shows volume changes during a cardiac cycle, whereas the Doppler waveform corresponds to direct blood flow velocities and flow direction in the artery.

Volume pulse waveforms decrease in amplitude as perfusion is decreased. Although this can be quantified by trying to class the wave chart deflection into one of five categories,[19] this is seldom done. Volume pulse recordings and strain-gauge waveforms are generally diagnosed as normal, abnormal, or flat.

Please note that although photoplethysmography waveforms are functionally different (because they measure reflected light from the skin microvasculature), the waveforms are interpreted by the same criteria and appear very similar:

- A normal volume pulse recording waveform has a quick inflow upstroke with an initial downslope, a dicrotic notch, then a slower outflow downstroke.
- An abnormal volume pulse recording waveform has less amplitude and a less-rapid upslope in the peak upstroke with loss of the dicrotic notch, depending on the severity of disease, corresponding to loss of the second component in a stenotic Doppler waveform. Amplitude may decrease as inflow decreases (Fig. 20-18).
- A flat volume pulse recording waveform indicates poor filling and perfusion, with possibly absent flow.

The level of obstruction can be discerned by comparing the waveform contours at each cuff level.

- Iliac stenosis is indicated by abnormal waveforms at and below the high-thigh level.
- Superficial femoral stenosis is suggested by normal waveforms at the high-thigh level with abnormal waveforms distally.

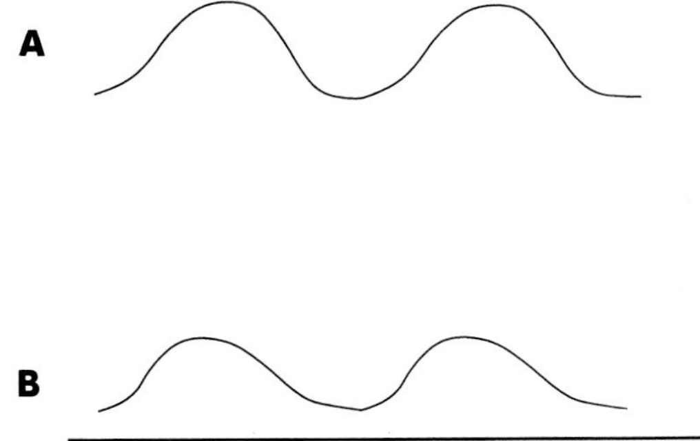

FIG. 20-18 Comparison of abnormal extremity plethysmographic arterial volume pulse waveforms, **A**, with abnormal extremity arterial Doppler waveforms, **B**. Note that there is a similarity in the contour, but the upslope (filling volume) is of a slower rise in the stenotic plethysmographic wave in **A** compared with the more direct Doppler measurement of arterial flow in **B**.

- Popliteal stenosis is suggested by normal waveforms at the high-thigh and low-thigh levels with abnormal waveforms distally.
- Tibial vessel stenosis is suggested by normal waveforms at the high-thigh, low-thigh, and calf levels with abnormal waveforms distally.
- Small-vessel disease in the foot is suggested by normal waveforms proximal to the metatarsal cuff, digit PPG, or both. Normal flow except in the digit implies regional ischemia.

The following examples of arterial lower-extremity cases use combinations of these technologies. Doppler velocity waveform analysis and segmental pressures appear in all examples; the last two cases additionally feature volume pulse recordings; the reader may wish to compare them with the accompanying Doppler waveform patterns to aid in understanding the interpretation criteria.

Arterial Lower-Extremity Doppler/Segmental/VPR Cases

Case 1 (Fig. 20-19): Normal. This is an example of a normal Doppler examination of the lower extremities. Note that the waveforms are triphasic at all sites and that there are no significant segmental pressure drops between cuff sites. High-thigh pressures are well above the brachial artery pressures. The ankle-brachial indices are 1.05 bilaterally, well within the normal range.

Case 2 (Fig. 20-20): Normal with tibial artery stenosis. In this case the examination is essentially normal, as with case 1, except that there is evidence of bilateral anterior tibial artery stenoses. Note that the ankle pressures at the posterior tibial artery are slightly elevated with a slightly elevated ankle-brachial index. This patient also received a postocclusive hyperemic study (see Case 2, Fig. 20-64).

Case 3 (Fig. 20-21): Right—severe superficial femoral artery stenosis; left—mild iliofemoral artery stenosis. In the right leg, there is a relatively normal femoral signal. There is a severely turbulent signal in the right superficial femoral artery with a dramatic reduction in flow (monophasic signal) at the popliteal and anterior tibial/dorsal pedal artery. There is no signal at the right posterior tibial artery, implying possible occlusion of this vessel. The segmental pressures are consistent with the waveform analysis, because there is a significant drop in pressure between the high-thigh and low-thigh readings and distally. The right ankle-brachial index of 0.22 indicates severe impairment of flow.

In the left leg, biphasic waveforms can be seen at the femoral, popliteal, posterior tibial, and dorsal pedal sites. Pressures suggest a mild drop between the low-thigh and calf cuff readings. The left ankle-brachial index of 0.93 is in the range of mild flow impairment.

Case 4 (Fig. 20-22): Right leg, normal. Left leg, moderate subpopliteal stenosis or tibial artery stenosis. This claudicating patient shows normal right leg waveforms, with a normal ankle-brachial index of 1.02.

The left leg, however, was symptomatic below the knee. Although normal femoral and popliteal waveforms are seen, no signal was detectable in the left posterior tibial artery and there was a monophasic waveform present in the left dorsalis pedis artery. The waveform analysis coupled with the ankle-brachial index of 0.58 strongly implies a stenosis in the distal popliteal or tibial arteries with a possible posterior tibial occlusion.

Case 5 (Fig. 20-23): Distal aorta and/or bilateral iliac stenosis, moderate. Monophasic waveforms can be seen at all the artery sites here, and although there are no significant pressure drops within the leg, the high-thigh pressures are markedly below the systolic pressures in the brachial arteries, which is a significant finding for iliac femoral disease. Note that the ankle-brachial indices bilaterally are 0.57, in the range of low-moderate flow impairment.

Case 6 (Fig. 20-24): Distal aorta and/or bilateral iliac stenosis, severe. Again, monophasic waveforms can be seen at all the artery sites here, but the amplitude is extremely low and diastole is almost flat. There are no significant pressure drops within the leg in this case either, and the high-thigh pressures are severely lower than the systolic pressures in the brachial arteries. There is additionally either bilateral anterior tibial stenosis or flow velocities in them are too slow to be detected. The ankle-brachial indices bilaterally are 0.22, in the range of severe (almost dire) impairment.

Case 7 (Fig. 20-25): Arterial examination with Doppler velocity waveforms, segmental pressures, and volume pulse recordings, normal. This 52-year-old patient was evaluated 1 month after a right femoral artery thrombectomy. The patient was asymptomatic and this study was done as a postoperative follow-up. All volume pulse recording waveforms are of normal contour and amplitude, although the dicrotic notch is not prominent.

Case 8 (Fig. 20-26): Arterial examination with Doppler velocity waveforms, segmental pressures, and volume pulse recordings, bilateral iliac stenosis or occlusion. This 54-year-old patient complained of bilateral claudication occurring at approximately half a block, with progressive calf pain and numbness. The abnormal monophasic Doppler

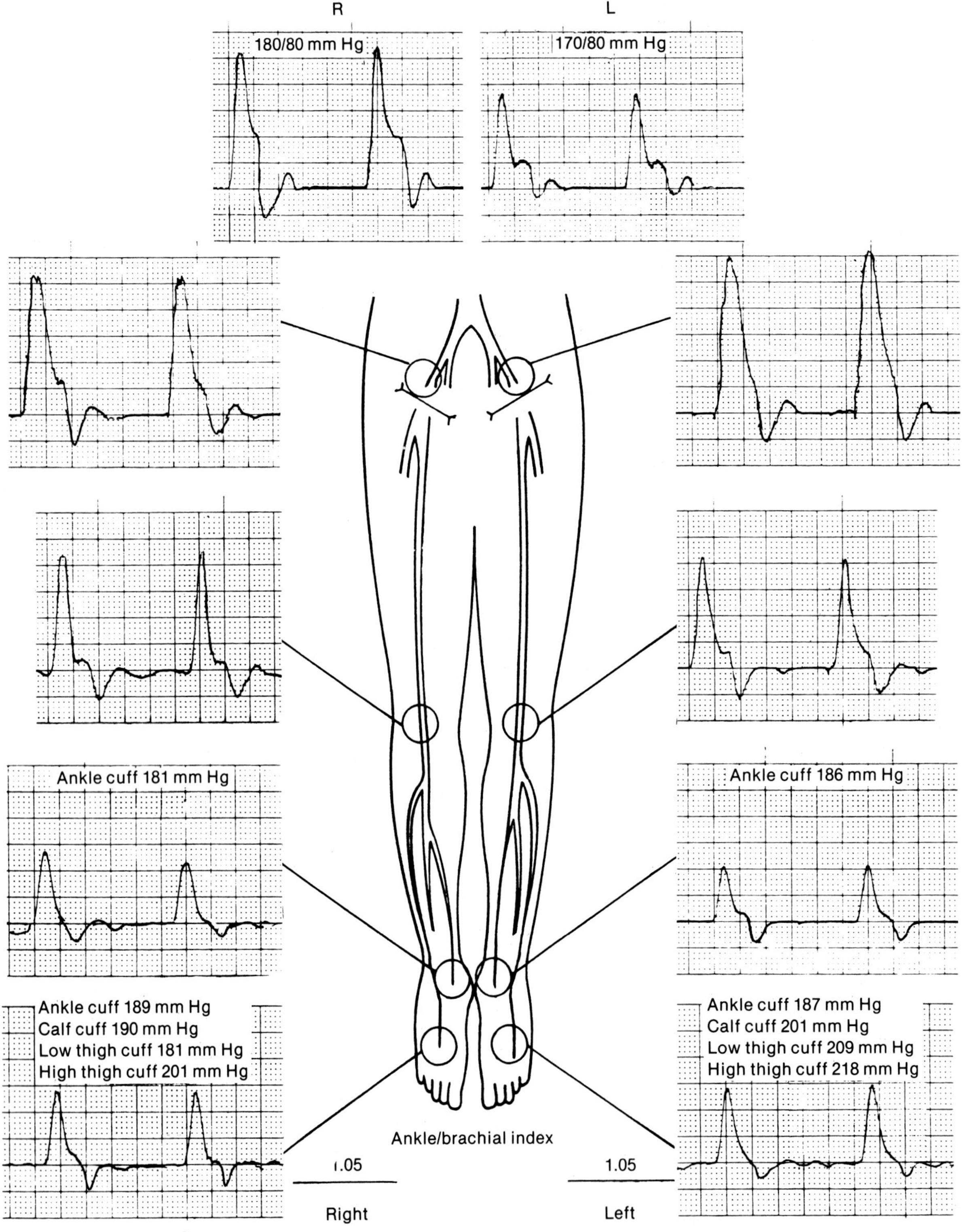

FIG. 20-19 Normal Doppler examination of lower extremities.

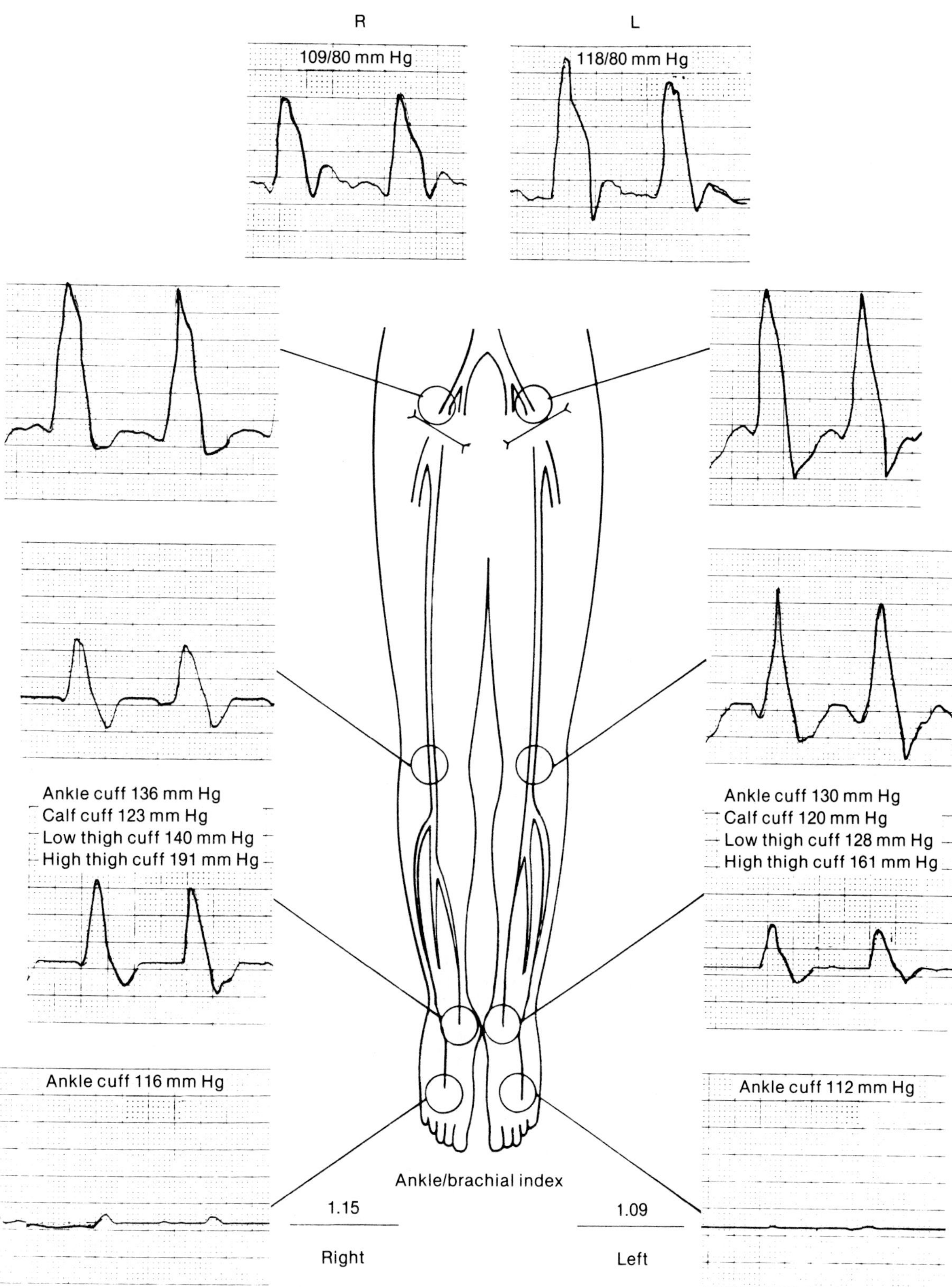

FIG. 20-20 Normal examination except for tibial artery stenosis.

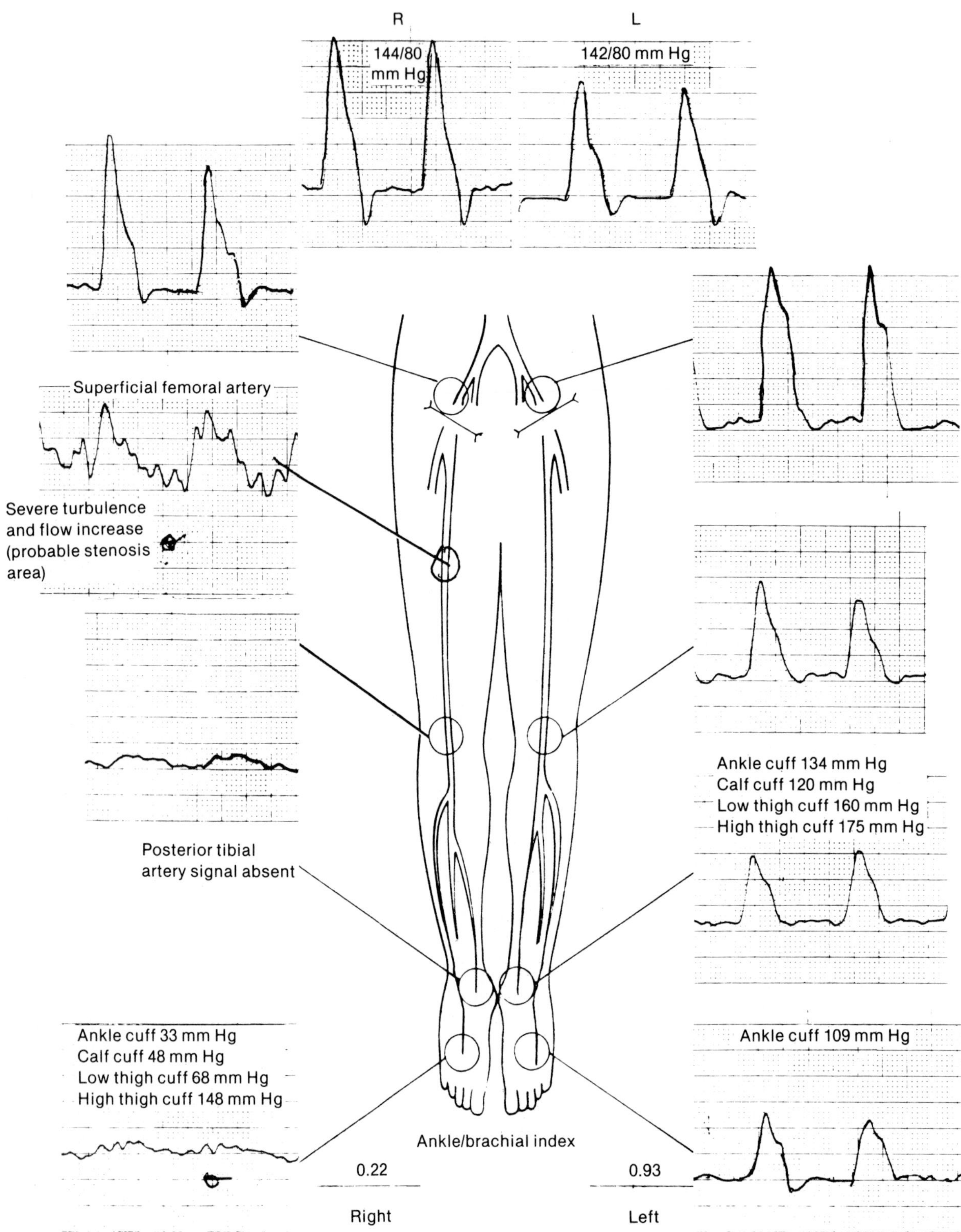

FIG. 20-21 *Right,* severe superficial femoral artery stenosis. *Left,* mild iliofemoral artery stenosis.

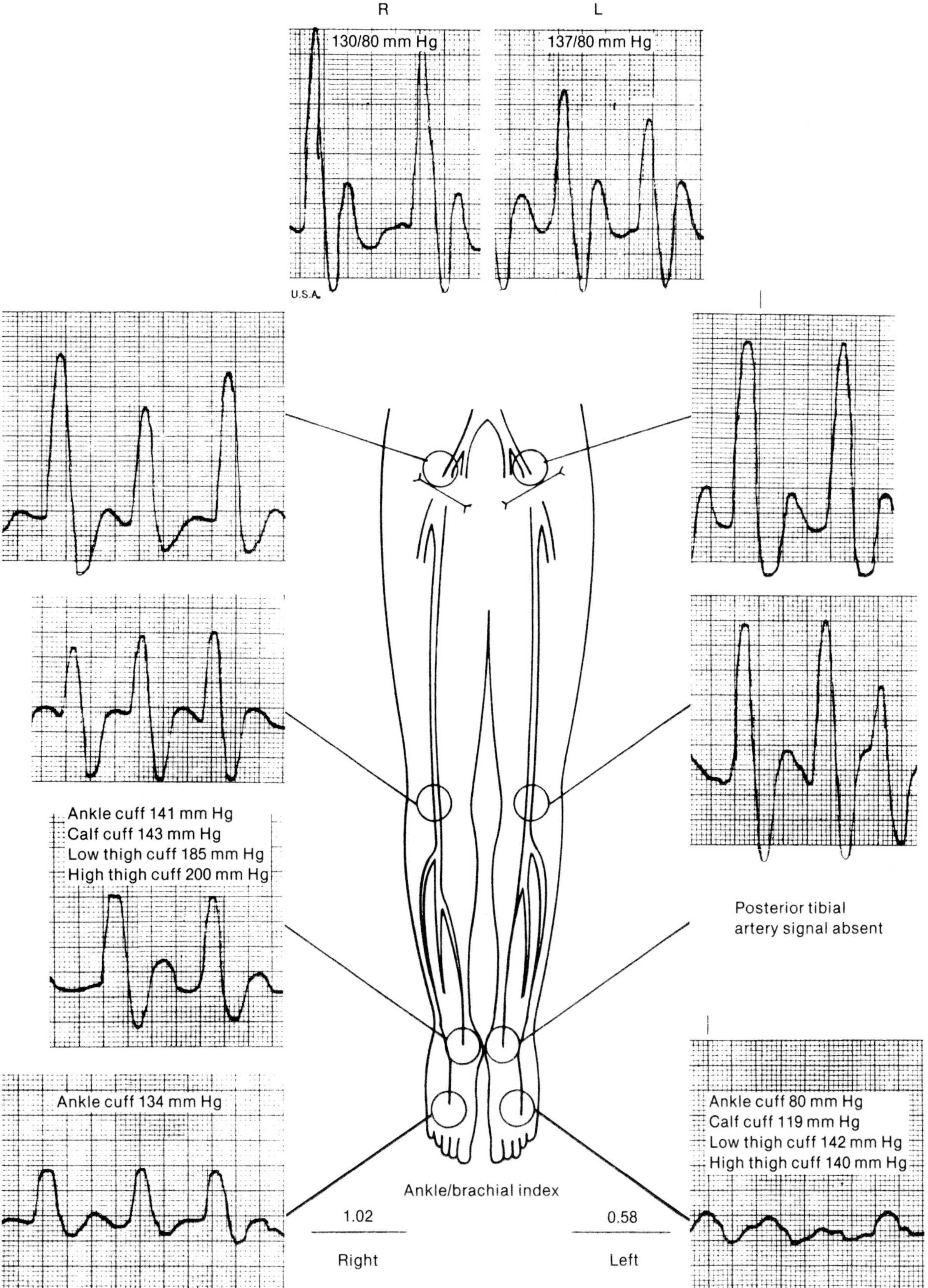

FIG. 20-22 Right leg normal. Left leg exhibits moderate subpopliteal stenosis or tibial artery stenosis.

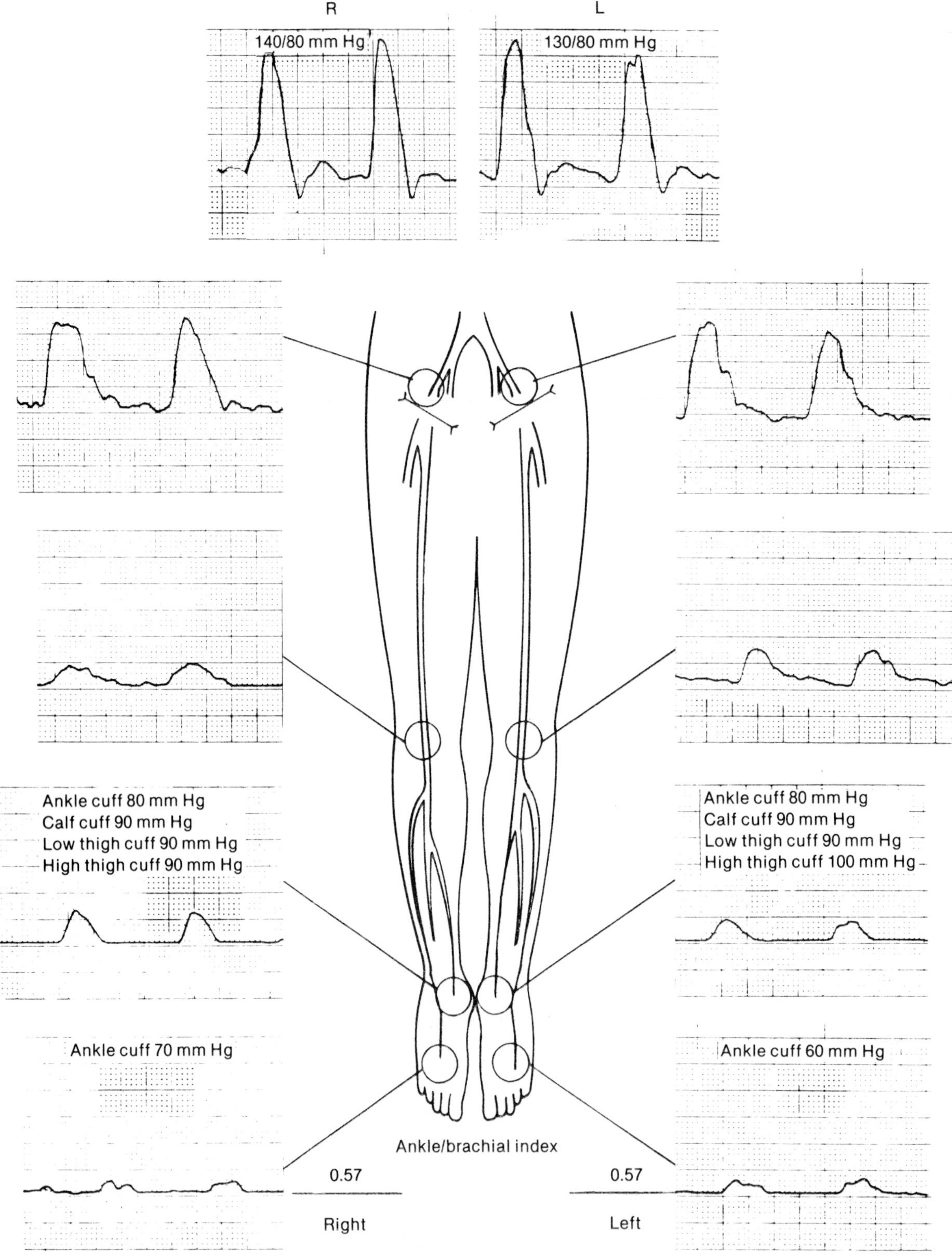

FIG. 20-23 Distal aorta or bilateral iliac stenosis, moderate.

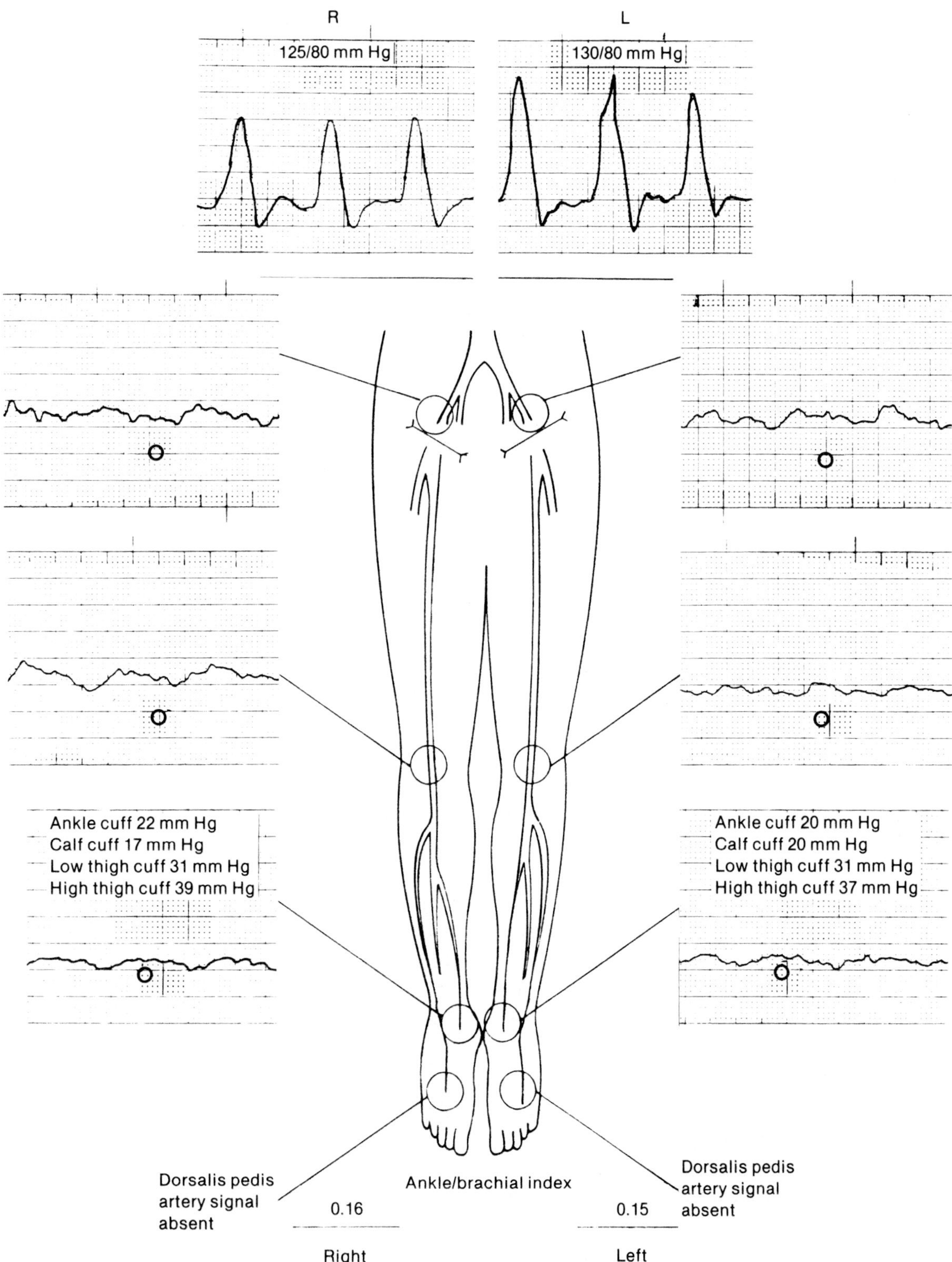

FIG. 20-24 Distal aorta or bilateral iliac stenosis, severe.

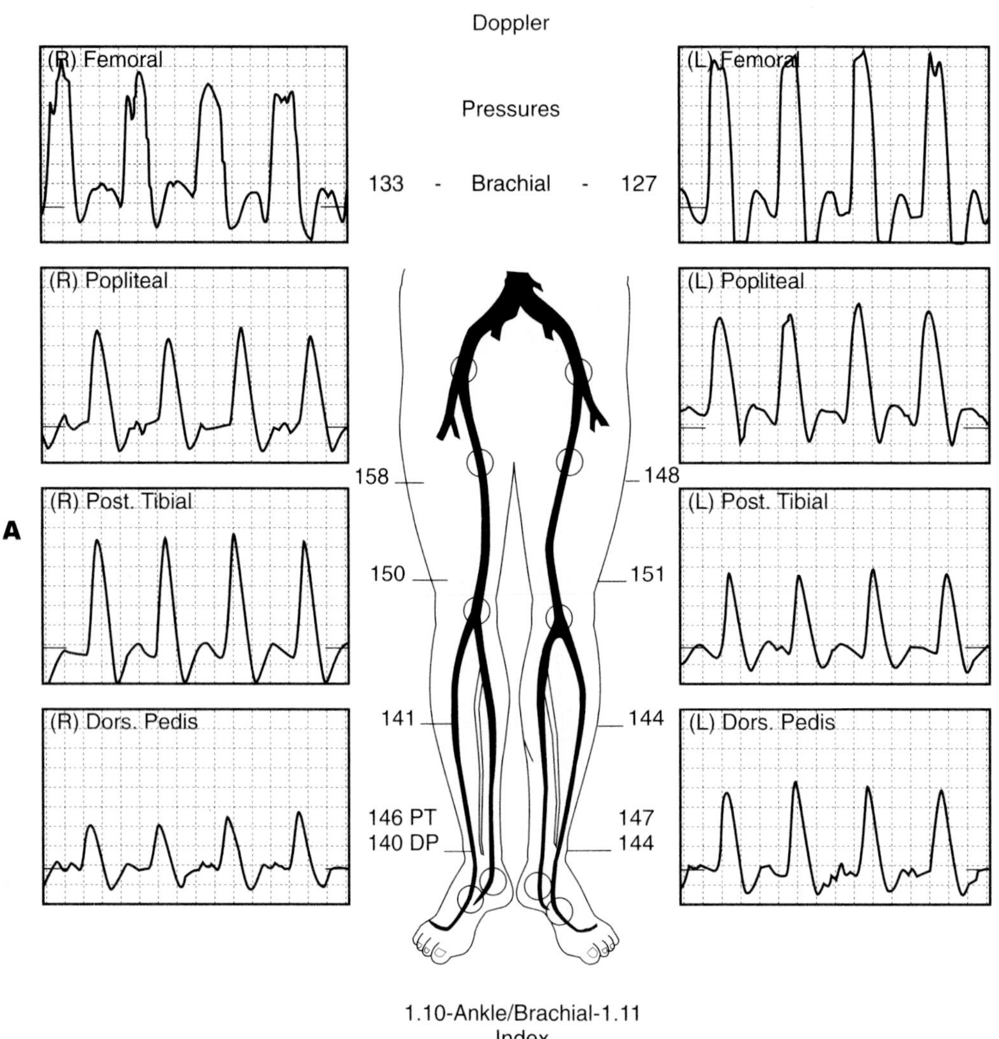

FIG. 20-25 A, Normal Doppler waveforms (compare with the volume pulse recording in **B**).
Continued.

waveforms and ankle-brachial indices of 0.57 on the right and 0.55 on the left, as well as the low high-thigh pressures, confirm the presence of a bilateral iliac or distal aortic obstruction. The volume pulse recording waveforms appear abnormal at all levels with loss of the dicrotic notch and a decreased upslope; note that they do not provide as much information about the arterial stenotic state as the Doppler waveforms, however.

See also Case 7 under Examination of the Postoperative Patient, which features side-by-side Doppler waveform and volume pulse recording comparison of a normal leg and one with a severe superficial femoral artery (SFA) stenosis (see Fig. 20-58).

ARTERIAL DUPLEX SONOGRAPHY

Arterial duplex sonography involves direct imaging of the arterial structures in the leg, with an emphasis on visualizing stenoses or occlusions and detecting their location. The hemodynamic effect of any stenoses can additionally be measured by color-flow imaging, spectral Doppler, or both. Aneurysmal vessels, arteriovenous fistulas, and iatrogenic arterial injuries (e.g., pseudoaneurysms) can be evaluated. Assessing patency and flow in arterial reconstructions and bypass grafts is also an important application of duplex (see Examination of the Postoperative Patient).

The duplex examination of the lower extremities, whether of arteries or veins, demands a great deal from the examiner. He or she must have a very thorough knowledge of the normal arterial anatomy and hemodynamics and be familiar with what would constitute an abnormal finding. It is also important to know how the vessels are oriented in the calf to avoid misinterpreting the image. The reader may wish to review the segment on arterial anatomy of the lower extremities on p. 475 before studying this section.

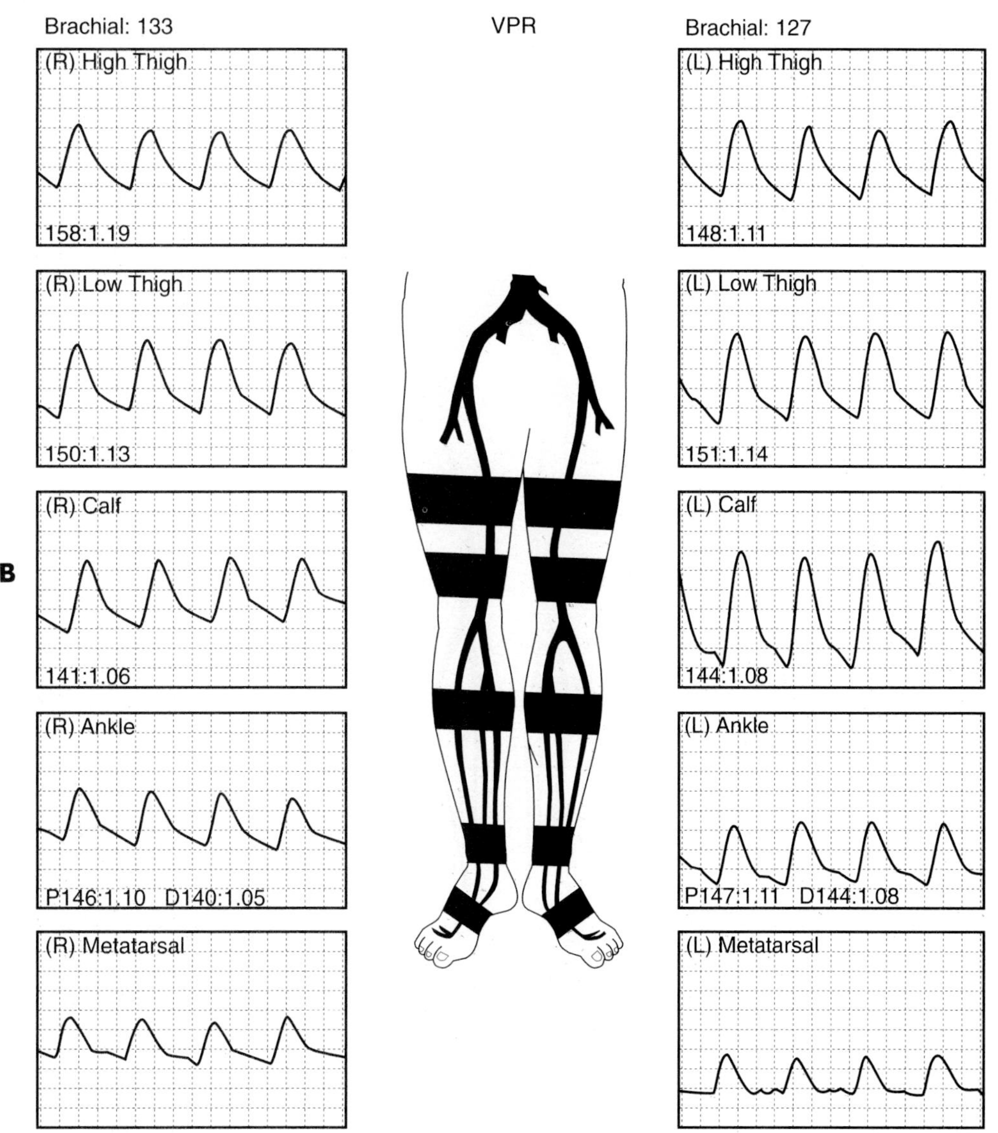

FIG. 20-25 cont'd. B, Normal volume pulse recording waveforms on the same patient (compare with Doppler in **A**).

Duplex and Color-Flow Vascular Image Characteristics

Specific sonographic and color-flow appearances of arteries and veins should be kept in mind when evaluating the extremity. A normal peripheral artery appears sonographically as a vessel with bright, even walls and a pulsatile red-blue-red color-flow pattern on color-flow imaging. In a transverse image, the artery has a definite circular appearance. The artery does not change its diameter if compression is applied on it by the transducer.

The normal vein may appear as a vascular structure with definite walls but a somewhat unevenly bordered appearance; if color-flow imaging is used, the blue flow pattern does not pulsate with the cardiac cycle but rises and falls in intensity with respiration. In transverse the outline is oblong and the vein dilates if probe pressure is lightened or flattens out (compresses) if firmer pressure is applied.

These characteristics and differences are applicable when using duplex to evaluate arteries and veins in all peripheral locations. There are some subtle differences in arterial flow in the cerebrovascular system, which are discussed in Chapter 22. The venous hemodynamics are detailed further in Chapter 21.

Basic Lower-Extremity Arterial Duplex Technique

Examination of the lower-extremity arteries should begin with the patient in a supine position. It is often easier to start proximally and work down the leg to the ankle. A 5-MHz-frequency transducer is recommended because it allows excellent penetration and visualization in most patients.

The examiner first should locate the external iliac artery

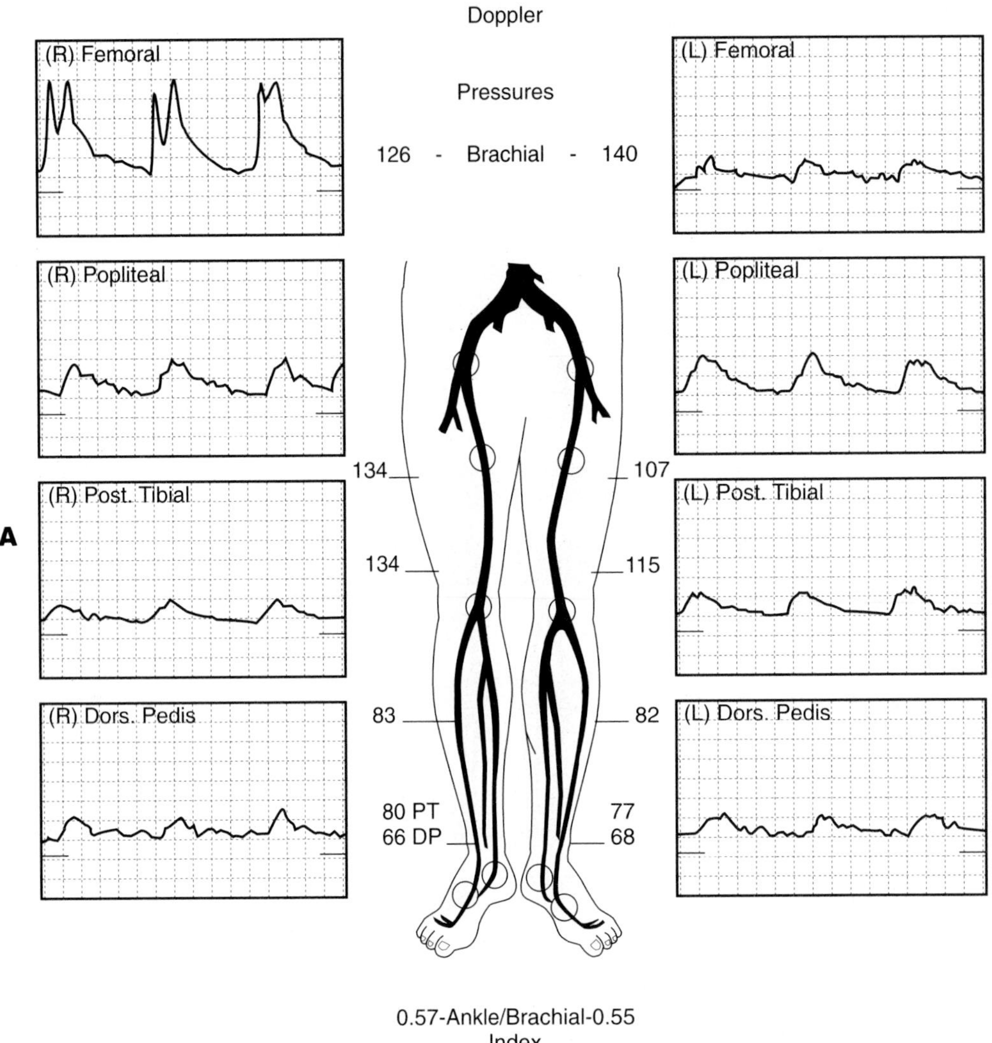

FIG. 20-26 A, Bilateral iliac or aortic stenosis or occlusion, Doppler waveforms. Note turbulence in right femoral signal and diminished left femoral signal. *Continued.*

in the groin above the inguinal ligament. Gray-scale image factors, such as time gain compensation (TGC), overall image gain, and focal transmit zones, should be adjusted at this time. If color-flow imaging is used, the color thresholds and power levels should be adjusted so that color fills the lumen but does not extend beyond the intimal lining or outside the walls.

Once these image factors are set, the external iliac artery is evaluated in a longitudinal plane beginning above the inguinal ligament (Fig. 20-27; see color image). The examiner should make certain that the artery being examined is lateral to the external iliac vein by moving the transducer back and forth, laterally and medially, and checking with color flow if available. Turning the probe transversely also helps identify the vessels.

The external iliac becomes the common femoral at about the level of the inguinal ligament. It should be followed and imaged in a caudal direction across the pubic crest and inguinal ligament until the bifurcation of the profunda femoris artery and superficial femoral artery is seen (Fig. 20-28; see color image). Spectral Doppler waveforms should be obtained within the femoral, profunda, and proximal superficial femoral arteries and across any areas of stenosis identified.

The superficial femoral artery is examined and followed distally along the sartorius groove in the medial thigh to just above the knee, continuing distally and medially from the position shown in Fig. 20-28. At this level, the artery appears to dive deeply and may be difficult to visualize as it enters the adductor hiatus. The use of color-flow imaging and increased depth can help the examiner image the vessel in this area. The superficial femoral vein appears below the artery. Spectral Doppler waveforms should be obtained to document flow (Fig. 20-29; see color image). The vessel should be imaged in both longitudinal and transverse planes.

The examiner should now have the patient flex the knee slightly and rotate the leg laterally into a "frog-leg" posi-

B

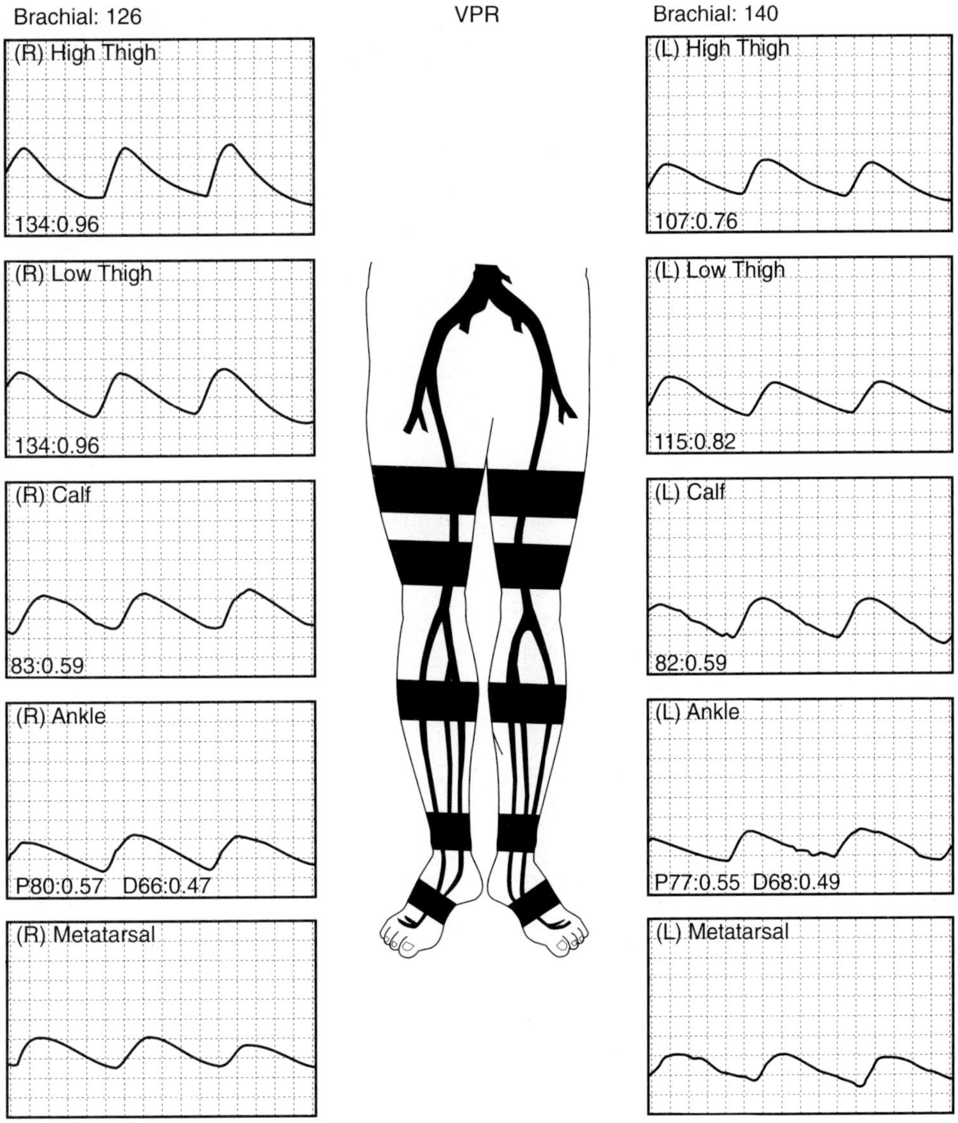

Brachial: 126
VPR
Brachial: 140
(R) High Thigh
134:0.96
(L) High Thigh
107:0.76
(R) Low Thigh
134:0.96
(L) Low Thigh
115:0.82
(R) Calf
83:0.59
(L) Calf
82:0.59
(R) Ankle
P80:0.57 D66:0.47
(L) Ankle
P77:0.55 D68:0.49
(R) Metatarsal
(L) Metatarsal

FIG. 20-26 cont'd. B, Abnormal volume pulse waveforms on the same patient as in **A.** Note the roughly equal perfusion levels and loss of dicrotic notch.

A

04-30-93 2:20 PM
R CFA
PEAK 169.3
SD
RI
AS
PI
PEAK: 169.3 CM/S

B

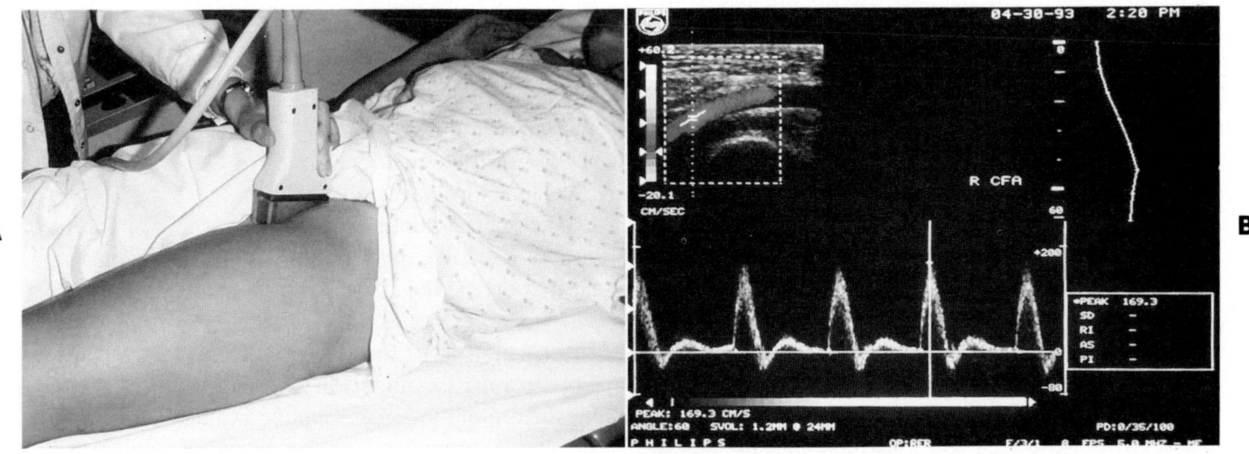

FIG. 20-27 A, Transducer position for long-axis imaging of the external iliac and common femoral artery. **B,** Color-flow image of distal external iliac-common femoral artery with normal duplex spectral Doppler waveform.

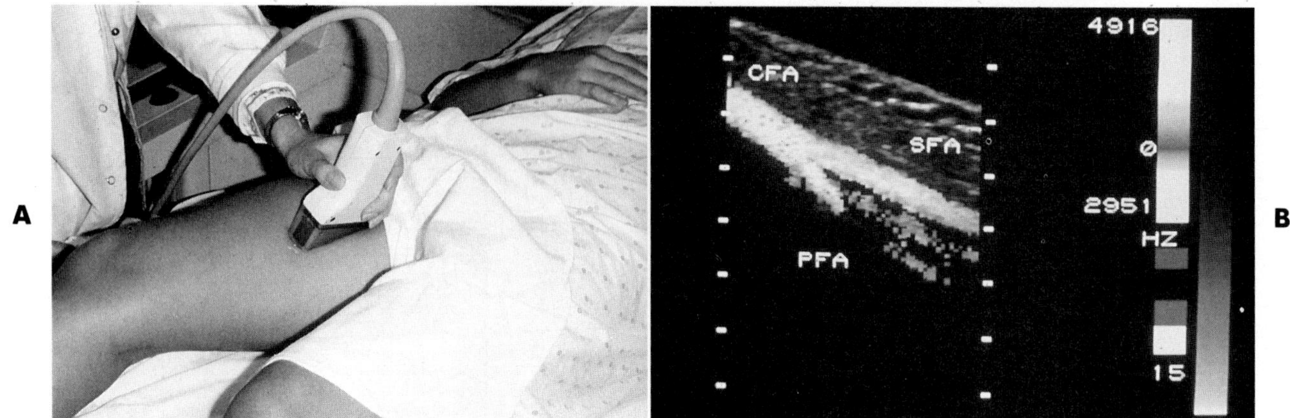

FIG. 20-28 **A,** Transducer position for long-axis imaging of the common femoral–profunda femoris bifurcation and the superficial femoral artery. **B,** Color-flow image of the superficial femoral artery common–profunda femoris artery bifurcation off the common femoral artery.

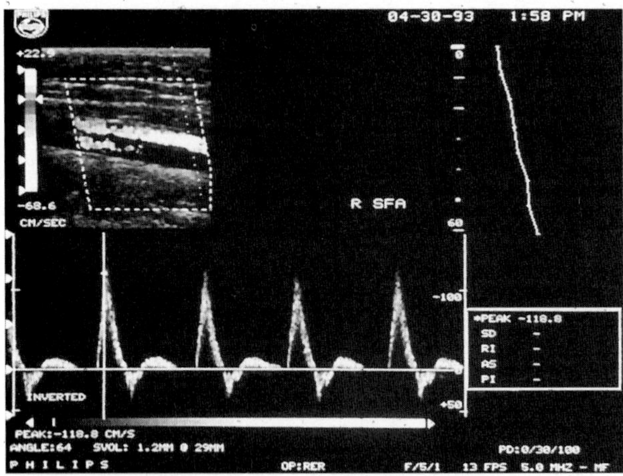

FIG. 20-29 Color-flow image of superficial femoral artery with normal duplex spectral Doppler waveform.

tion. The popliteal artery can now be examined from the posterior side of the leg. Remember that the orientation of the image now changes, with the posterior skin surface now at the top of the display; the popliteal vein appears to be above the popliteal artery instead of beneath it as was seen in the thigh (Fig. 20-30; see color image). The popliteal artery should be examined from the posterior distal thigh, across the popliteal fossa, and into the proximal posterior calf. Spectral Doppler waveforms should be recorded from this area also. Longitudinal and transverse images should be obtained.

Just distal to the popliteal fossa, the examiner may notice an artery branch coming off the popliteal artery that appears to dive deep; this is the origin of the anterior tibial artery. A spectral Doppler waveform may be taken at this site if desired. Longitudinal and transverse images should be obtained.

The examiner now moves the transducer to the medial calf, insonating in the groove between the tibia and gastrocnemius muscle. The distal popliteal artery and peroneal-tibial bifurcation can be identified in this area (Fig. 20-31).

The posterior tibial artery can be followed and examined along the medial calf to the medial malleolus, coming straight in and angling to bring it into view (Fig. 20-32; see color image). The peroneal artery can also be seen running deep to the posterior tibial artery depending on the angle of the transducer, or can be isolated by scanning posteriorly along the fibular area. Longitudinal and transverse images should be obtained.

The anterior tibial artery is followed on the lateral anterior side of the tibia by aiming the transducer straight back and moving laterally away from the bone until the artery is seen. It is best to start just below and lateral to the patella then move distally. The peroneal artery also can be seen in this view, deep to the anterior tibial artery (Fig. 20-33; see color images). The scan can be continued down into the foot to follow the dorsalis pedis artery if the transducer can resolve very superficial structures, has a standoff wedge, or if there is a standoff gel pad available. Longitudinal and transverse images should be obtained.

If the peroneal artery cannot be seen deep to the anterior tibial artery or to the posterior tibial artery, it can be seen by scanning the posterior calf medial to the fibula and aiming toward the anterior surface of the lower leg (Fig. 20-34; see color image).

The arterial duplex exam can be recorded on videotape, or representative images and spectral waveforms can be recorded on a printer or multiformat camera.

Interpretation of the Lower-Extremity Arterial Duplex Sonography Examination

The arterial images should be evaluated for the presence of plaque formations and the degree of luminal reduction, if any. (For more information on plaque morphology and surface characteristics, see Chapter 22). Stenoses can occur at almost any location and it is possible that several tan-

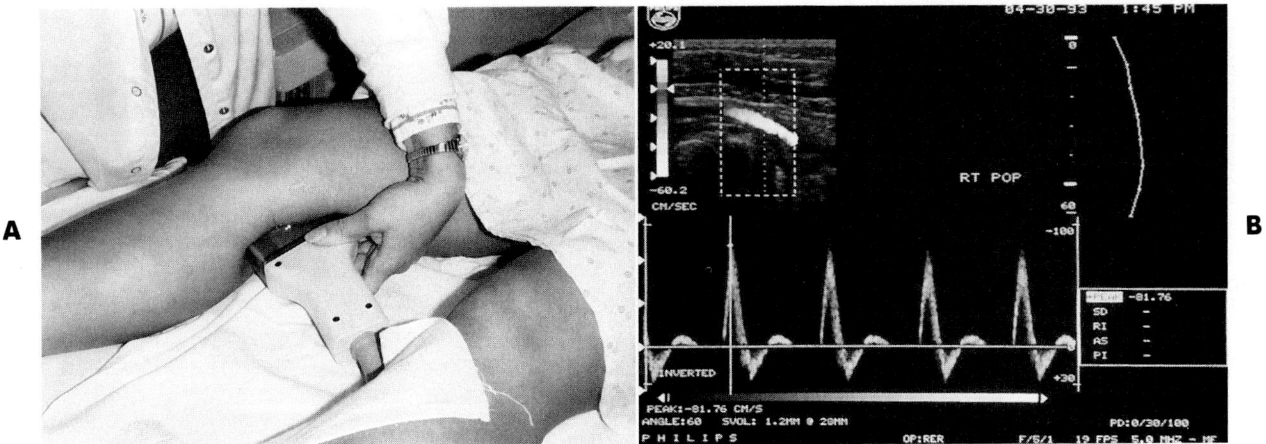

FIG. 20-30 **A,** Transducer position for long-axis imaging of the popliteal artery. **B,** Color-flow image of the popliteal artery with normal duplex spectral Doppler waveform.

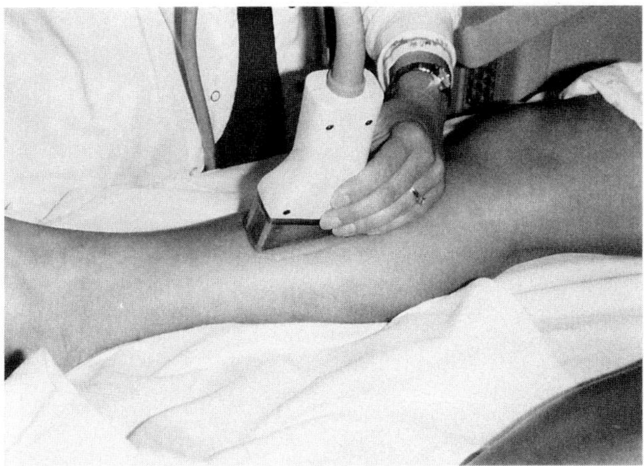

FIG. 20-31 Transducer position for long-axis imaging of the peroneal-tibial trunk and posterior tibial artery.

dem stenoses can cause a severe reduction of flow to the lower leg. The best way to determine the significance of a stenosis is to look for filling defects in the color-flow pattern and evaluate the color-flow streamlines to see if areas of increased turbulence and velocity increase are occurring (Fig. 20-35; see color image). Once an area of increased velocity is isolated, a Doppler spectrum should be obtained at that site. The sample volume should be sized accordingly and then placed within the streamline slightly distal to the most reduced portion of the lumen. Please note that gray-scale or color-flow imaging alone is insufficient to diagnose hemodynamically significant stenoses and pulsed Doppler spectrum analysis must be used in conjunction. Areas of suspected stenosis must be evaluated in transverse as well as longitudinal planes to check for asymmetry and irregularities that may not be seen directly in the longitudinal plane.

Luminal-reduction caliper measurements can be obtained but are generally not pertinent because of difficulty correlating these measurements with angiography.

Diagnostic Velocity Criteria

Diagnosis of the degree of stenosis is based on velocity increases at the stenotic site with turbulence and disturbed flow downstream, much as has been discussed in the earlier portions of this chapter. Many published diagnostic criteria[7,13] base estimates of stenotic significance on spectrally demonstrated hemodynamic changes, with a luminal reduction of greater than 50% corresponding to an increase in the peak systolic velocity double that of the segment proximal to the stenosis. In addition, the spectral changes described earlier occur: increased spectral broadening, disruption of the envelope, and progressive loss of waveform components distal to the stenosis as severity increases (Fig. 20-36).

Total occlusion of a segment manifests as homogeneous or heterogeneous echogenic material filling the entire lumen (Fig. 20-37; see color image); color-flow imaging shows flow abruptly stopping with some retrograde flow turbulence at the point where the flow stream hits "a dead end." An occluded segment may not cause proximal loss of diastolic flow if collateralization has occurred. Color-flow imaging often enables the actual collateral branches and pathways to be traced around the blockage and then followed distally to a patent, reconstituted segment (Fig. 20-38; see color image) as was described in Fig. 20-3.

Occluded segments with no collaterals show an abrupt flash of systolic color on color-flow imaging with no color in diastole; this is seen mostly in tibial vessels or in bypass grafts (see Examination of the Postoperative Patient). Spectral Doppler waveforms show a high-resistance "whipcrack" waveform in patent segments proximal to the occlusion in these cases.

Summary of Diagnostic Criteria

1. Stenoses appear as homogeneous or heterogeneous echogenic areas projecting into the lumen; a stenosis may not have a significant effect on the hemodynamics

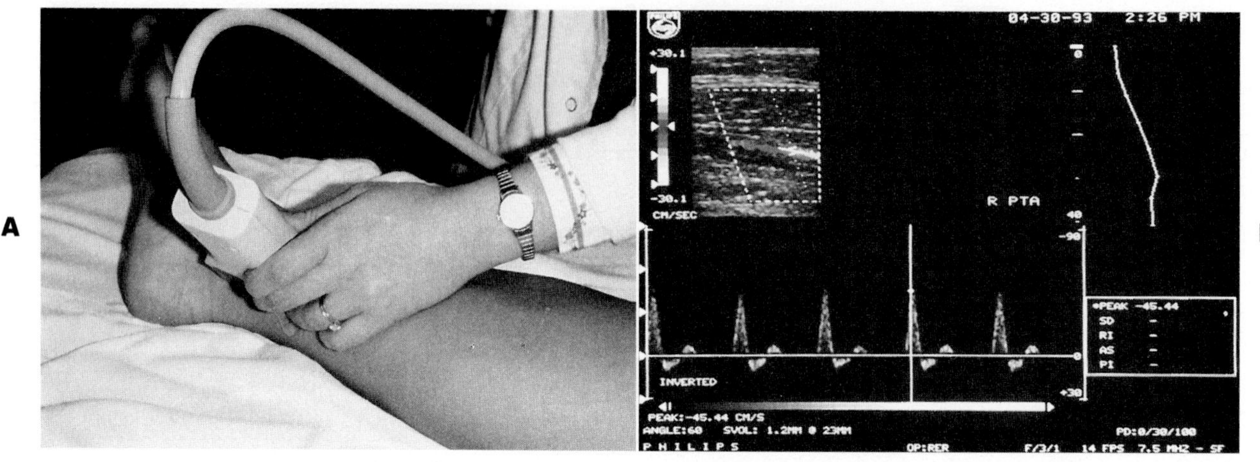

FIG. 20-32 A, Transducer position for long-axis imaging of the distal posterior tibial artery. **B,** Color-flow image of the posterior tibial artery with normal duplex spectral Doppler waveform.

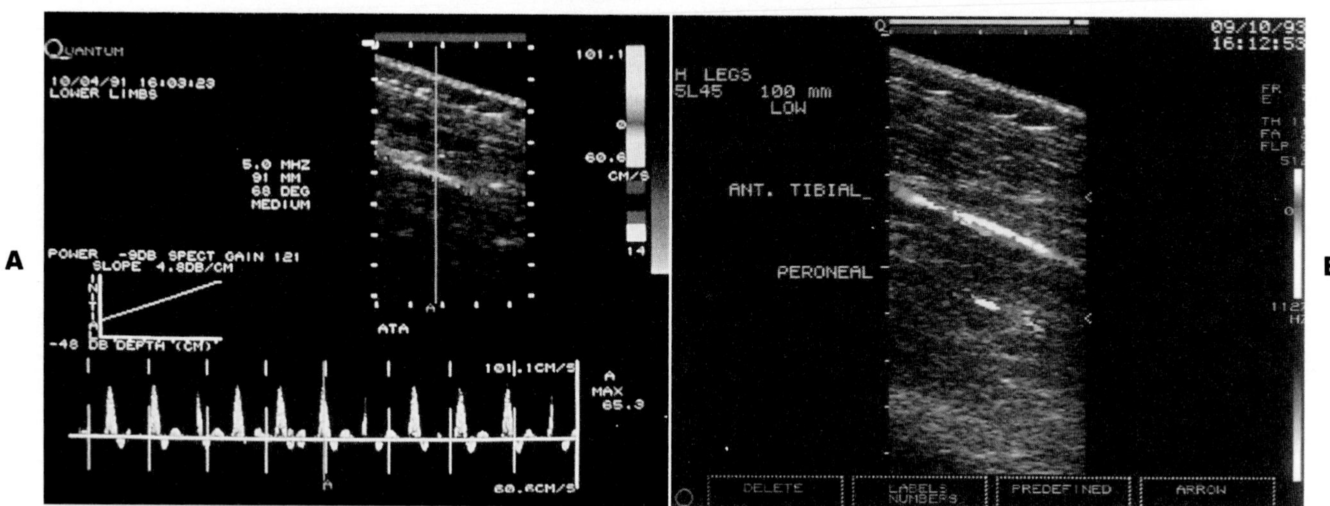

FIG. 20-33 A, Color-flow image of anterior tibial artery with normal duplex spectral Doppler waveform. **B,** Color-flow image of anterior tibial artery showing the peroneal artery deep to it in the anterior scanning position.

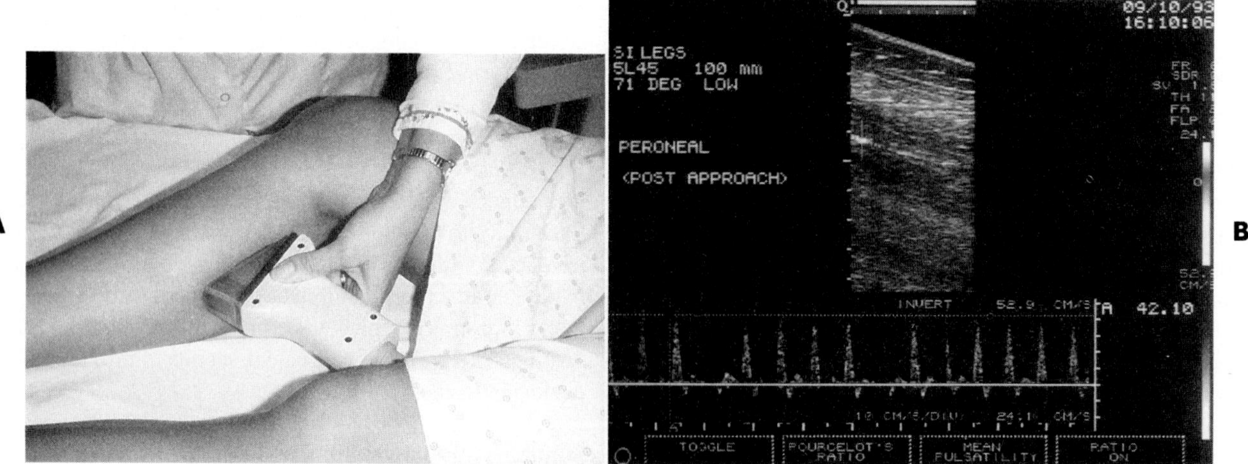

FIG. 20-34 A, Transducer position for long-axis imaging of the peroneal artery from a posterior approach. **B,** Color-flow image of the peroneal artery with normal duplex spectral Doppler waveform.

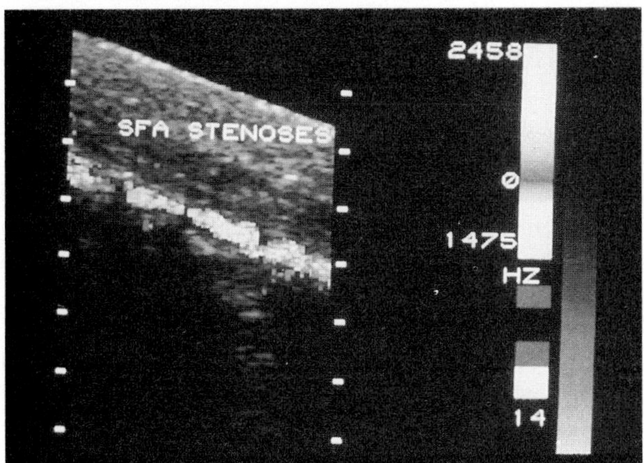

FIG. 20-35 A longitudinal color-flow image of a superficial femoral artery showing multiple irregular stenoses within the segment. Note the acceleration of the color-flow streamlines and the presence of flow disturbances.

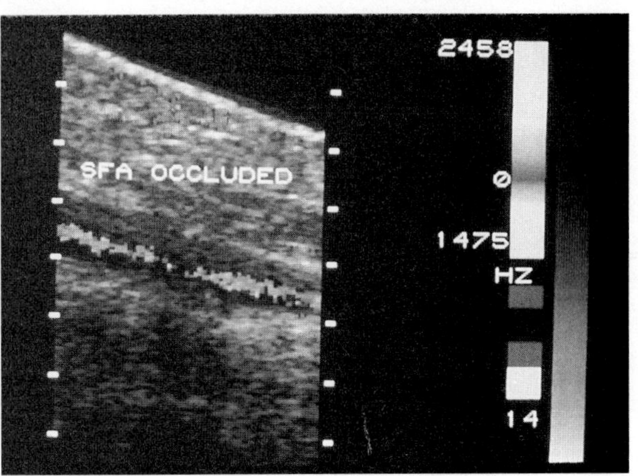

FIG. 20-37 Occluded superficial femoral artery (note patent superficial femoral vein deep to the artery with normal blue venous color flow).

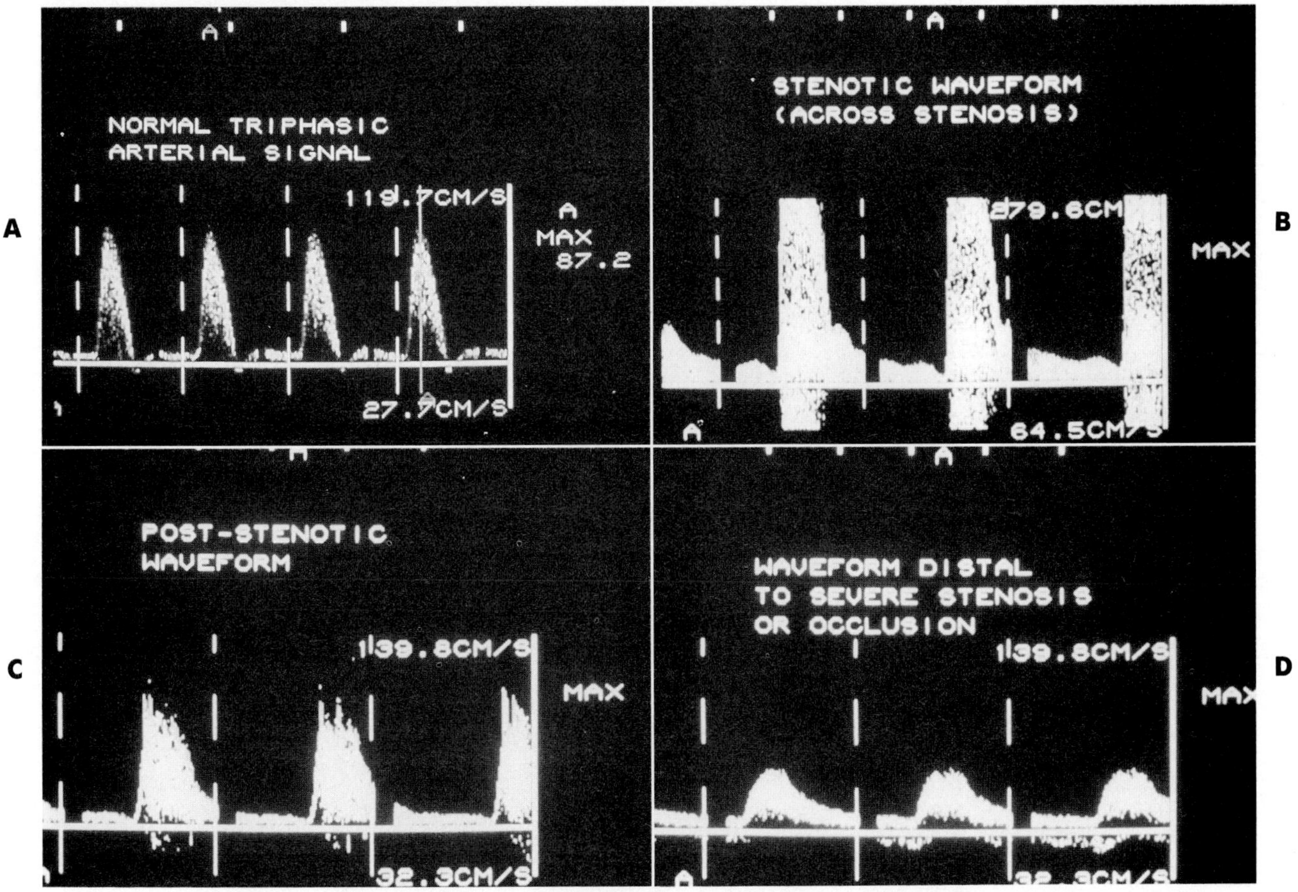

FIG. 20-36 **A,** Normal triphasic duplex Doppler spectral waveform. **B,** Stenotic Doppler spectral waveform at the area of peak stenosis (note velocity is aliasing off the scale, over 279 cm/sec). **C,** Poststenotic Doppler spectral waveform just distal to the area of stenosis in **B. D,** Monophasic and blunted Doppler spectral waveform in a patent segment several centimeters distal to the stenosis in **B.**

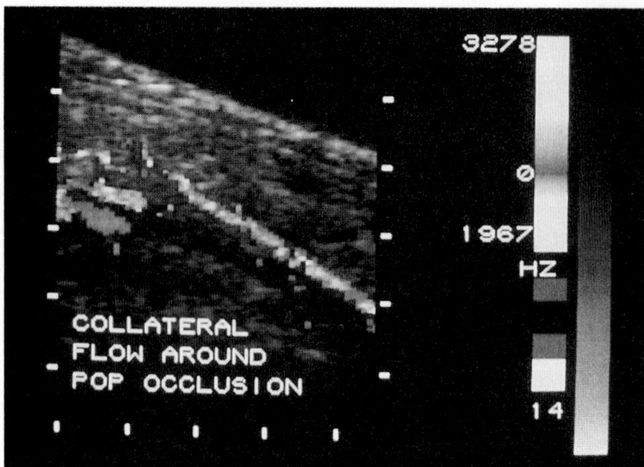

FIG. 20-38 Color-flow imaging example showing collaterals directing flow from a patent proximal popliteal artery around an occluded distal segment.

of the artery until a 50% to 60% luminal reduction occurs.[3,5] The presence of a stenosis can be identified more easily at times with color-flow imaging, as can the presence of hemodynamic streamline effects and turbulence caused by the stenosis. Color-flow imaging and gray-scale imaging alone are not sufficient to grade the significance of a stenosis.

2. Hemodynamic changes can be determined by pulsed Doppler and spectral analysis. Stenoses of greater than 50% have a doubling of the peak segment proximal to the stenosis.[7] Flow distal to the stenosis shows a decrease in peak velocity with rounding and blunting of the peak and progressive loss of the second and third components as the severity increases.

Arterial Aneurysm Evaluation

Aneurysms and ectasia of arterial segments can occur without significant stenosis. Although the basic techniques

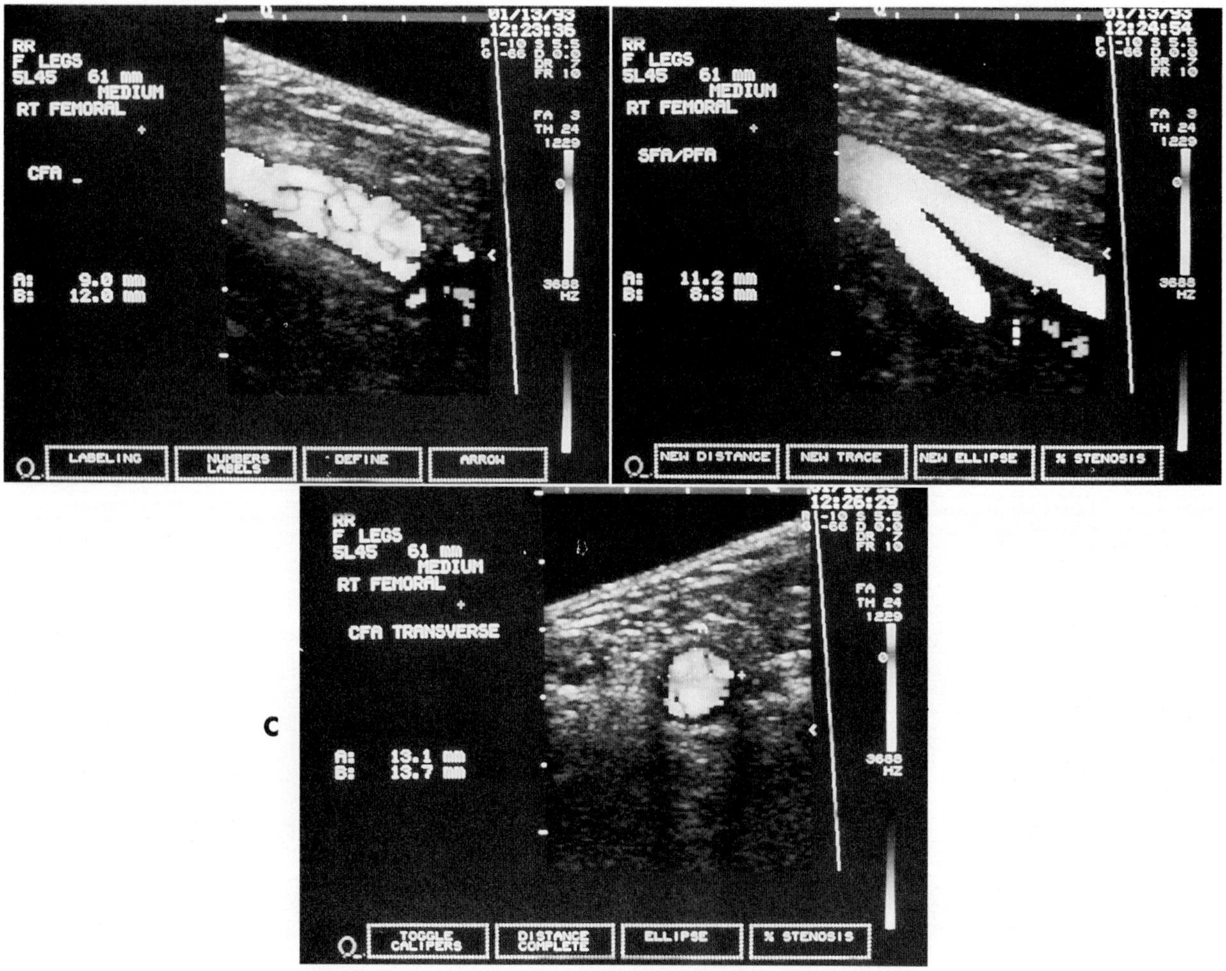

FIG. 20-39 Common femoral ectasia. This common femoral artery measures 9 mm proximal to an area of dilation, **A,** with an increase to 12 mm across the ligament. This tapers to 11.2 mm just above the superficial femoral–profunda femoris bifurcation. The superficial femoral artery distal to the bifurcation measures 8.3 mm, *B*. Transverse measurement of the ectatic area is 13.1 by 13.7 mm, **C.**

of imaging, color flow, and Doppler acquisition apply, it is important to evaluate the arterial segment in longitudinal and transverse planes and take respective images of segments at the proximal, central, and distal portions of the area in question. Electronic calipers should be used to record the anteroposterior and lateral diameters for comparison.

In general, peripheral arteries are normally smaller than 1 cm in diameter, although this varies; a segment with a slight measurable dilation compared with a proximal or distal segment may be classed as ectatic (Fig. 20-39; see color images), and a focal enlargement approximately double the size of a normal proximal or distal segment may be considered a true aneurysm (Fig. 20-40; see color images). Aneurysms can be additionally classed as saccular (where they appear as a focal bulging central to proximal and distal segments of normal caliber) or fusiform (where the aneurysm appears to be a gradual tapered expansion of the vessel over several centimeters). Examiners should be aware that arterial segments that have had balloon angioplasty have focally dilated segments because of the expansion of the balloon and compression of the plaque (Fig. 20-41; see color image). These do not represent aneurysms. This underscores the importance of obtaining a complete surgical and procedural history before examination, being aware of percutaneous transluminal angioplasty (PTA) sites can avoid interpretation errors of this type.

Arterial Duplex Sonography—Important Considerations and Applications

Arterial duplex sonography is a very time-consuming and involved examination. Although the format for a complete examination has been described, it is not always practical to examine everyone who presents with arterial complaints with arterial duplex sonography (although this point can be argued both ways[7,8a]). A lower-extremity arterial examination using Doppler velocity waveform analysis and segmental pressures, for example, can be accomplished in less than 30 minutes by a practiced hand. Complete duplex arterial studies can take more than an hour. Patients with negative results do not benefit from duplex sonographic evaluation, and no physiologic data can be derived from duplex alone. Duplex sonography is also difficult to correlate with arteriography because only a small segment of the arterial tree is examined at a time, and sonographic landmarks are not readily available that can help identify levels when com-

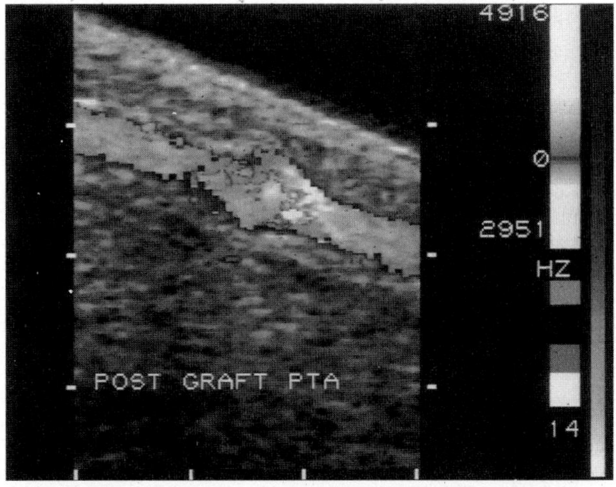

FIG. 20-41 This arterial in situ graft segment received a percutaneous transluminal balloon angioplasty for a focal stenosis, causing normal postangioplasty dilation of the artery. Note that this does *not* represent an aneurysm.

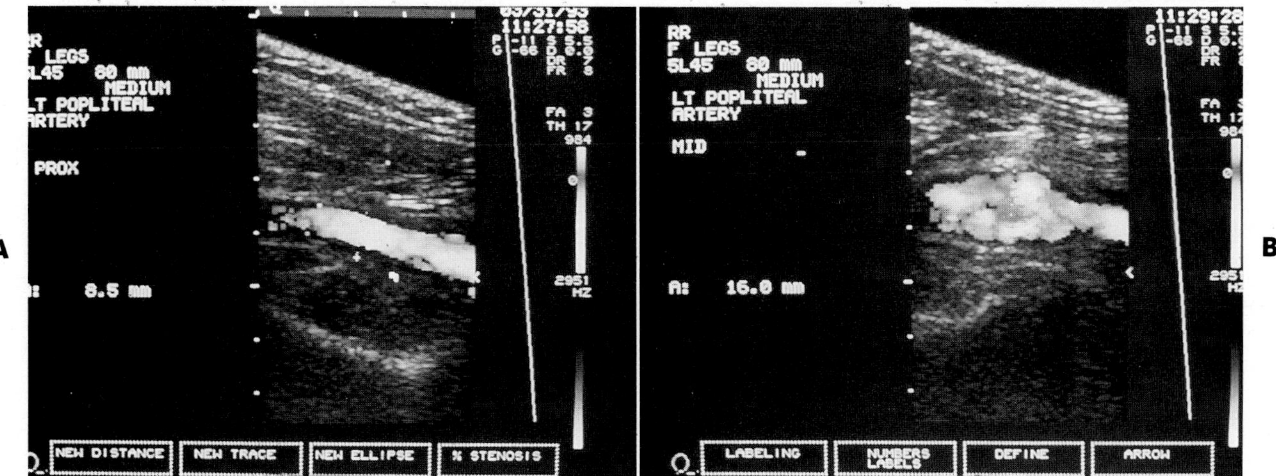

FIG. 20-40 Popliteal aneurysm. This popliteal artery measures 8.5 mm in a straight segment proximal to the popliteal fossa, **A.** Just distal to this, the artery has an aneurysmal segment that measures 16 mm in anteroposterior diameter, **B.** Note that the vessel assumes a normal diameter distal to the aneurysm (right side of **B**).

paring arteriography with duplex images. Surgeons in general often still order an arteriogram before performing any form of bypass surgery, and duplex sonography of the arteries in these cases is sometimes redundant. Routine follow-up of patients with regular complete duplex sonography studies also is not cost- or time-effective and is difficult in the immediate postoperative period because of the presence of surgical clips, dressings, and incisions.

With all of these points in mind, the best routine application of arterial duplex sonography may be as a secondary adjunct to performance of arterial waveforms (Doppler or volume pulse recording) and segmental pressures. If an area of suggested stenosis is implied by the indirect tests' waveform and pressure gradient findings, then limited duplex evaluation using the described methods should be done to locate and evaluate the areas of stenosis. In addition, arterial duplex sonography should be the primary method of choice when evaluating for aneurysms, pseudoaneurysms (see Evaluation of Iatrogenic Arterial Injuries), and patency of bypass grafts (see Examination of the Postoperative Patient).

ARTERIAL DUPLEX SONOGRAPHY CASES

Case 1 (Fig. 20-42: Superficial femoral artery stenosis. This 63-year-old patient presented with left-calf claudication. The duplex examination showed tandem irregular stenoses within the left superficial femoral artery (see Fig. 20-35) with a high-velocity stenotic jet of over 270 cm/sec at a point of maximal stenosis and color aliasing *(A)*. Just distal to the stenosis, a disturbed flow pattern was seen *(B)*. The popliteal artery runoff was monophasic and of a lower velocity (42 cm/sec) *(C)*; this monophasic flow continued into the distal vessels *(D)*.

This case is a good example of how tandem stenoses can cause diminished distal flow; the patient subsequently received an angioplasty of the superficial femoral artery stenoses with a good result.

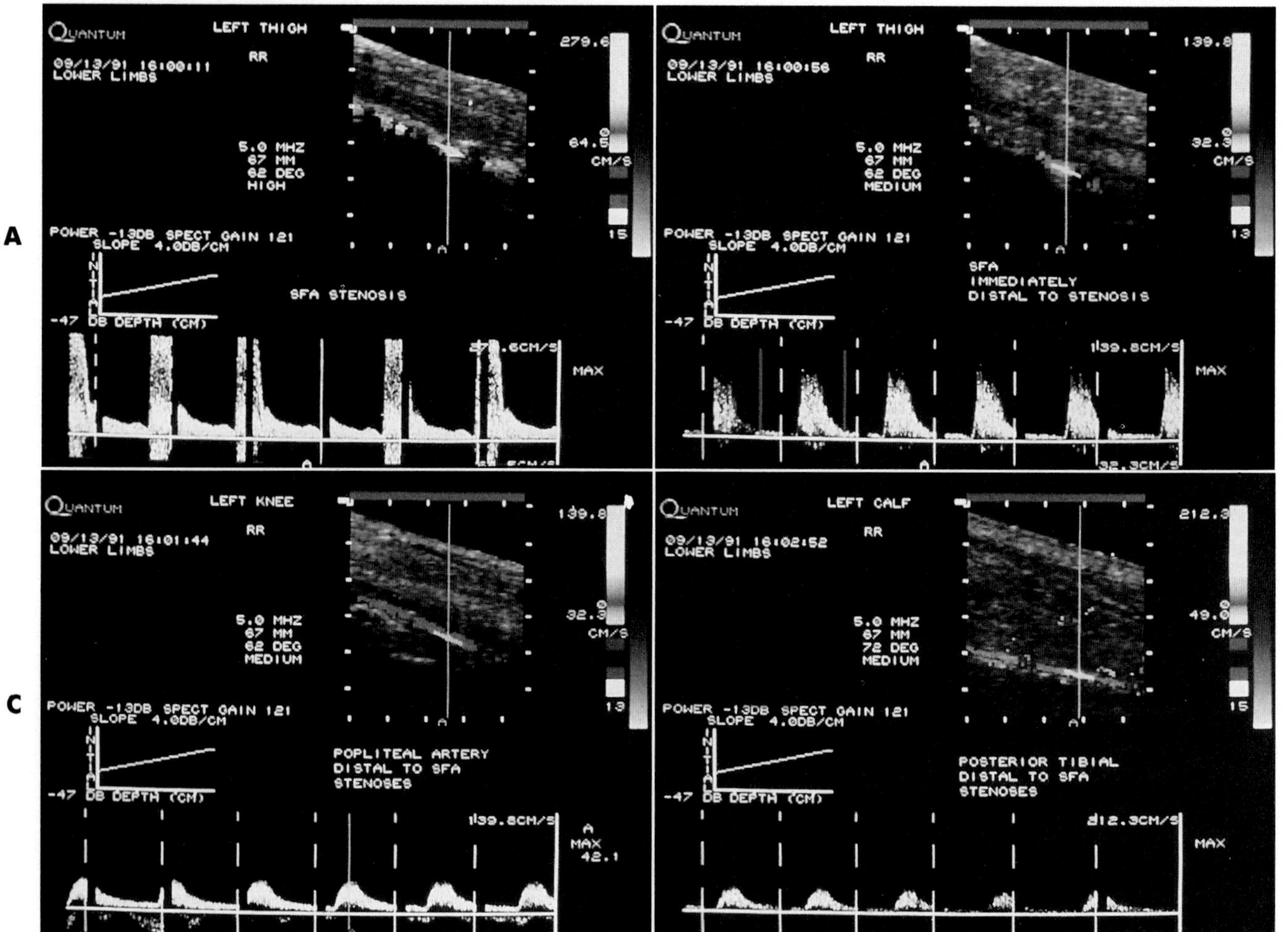

FIG. 20-42 A, Superficial femoral artery stenosis, Doppler spectral pattern at stenosed segment (see text). **B,** Superficial femoral artery stenosis, Doppler spectral pattern just distal to stenosed segment (see text). **C,** Superficial femoral artery stenosis, Doppler spectral pattern at popliteal artery (see text). **D,** Superficial femoral artery stenosis, Doppler spectral pattern at posterior tibial artery (see text).

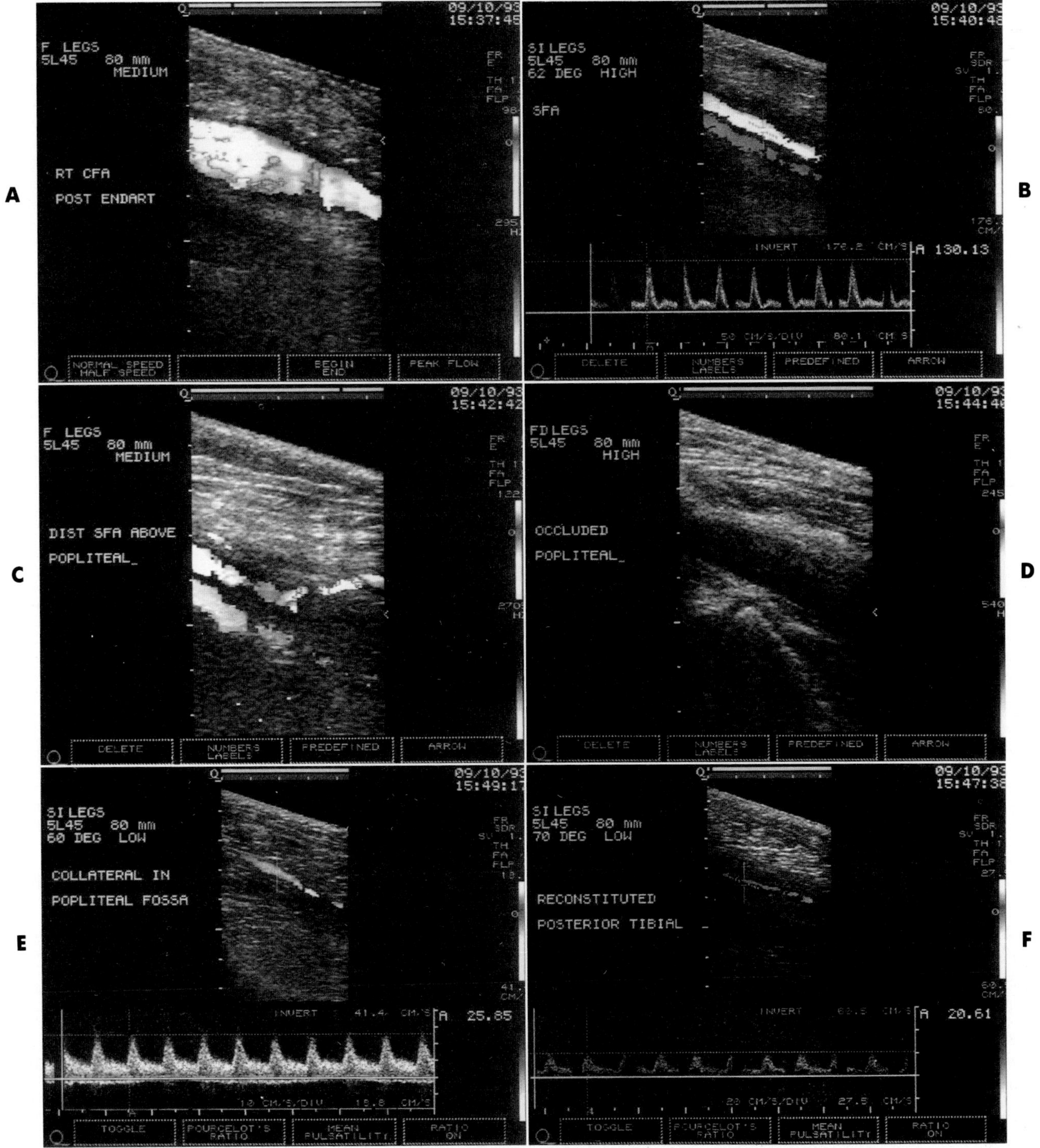

FIG. 20-43 A, CFA endarterectomy and popliteal occlusion—common femoral artery (see text). **B,** CFA endarterectomy and popliteal occlusion, superficial femoral artery and corresponding Doppler spectral waveform (see text). **C,** CFA endarterectomy and popliteal occlusion, distal superficial femoral artery (see text). **D,** CFA endarterectomy and popliteal occlusion, occluded popliteal artery (see text). **E,** CFA endarterectomy and popliteal occlusion, popliteal collateral and corresponding Doppler spectral waveform (see text). **F,** CFA endarterectomy and popliteal occlusion, posterior tibial artery and corresponding Doppler spectral waveform (see text). **G,** Doppler waveform analysis and segmental pressures (see text). *Continued.*

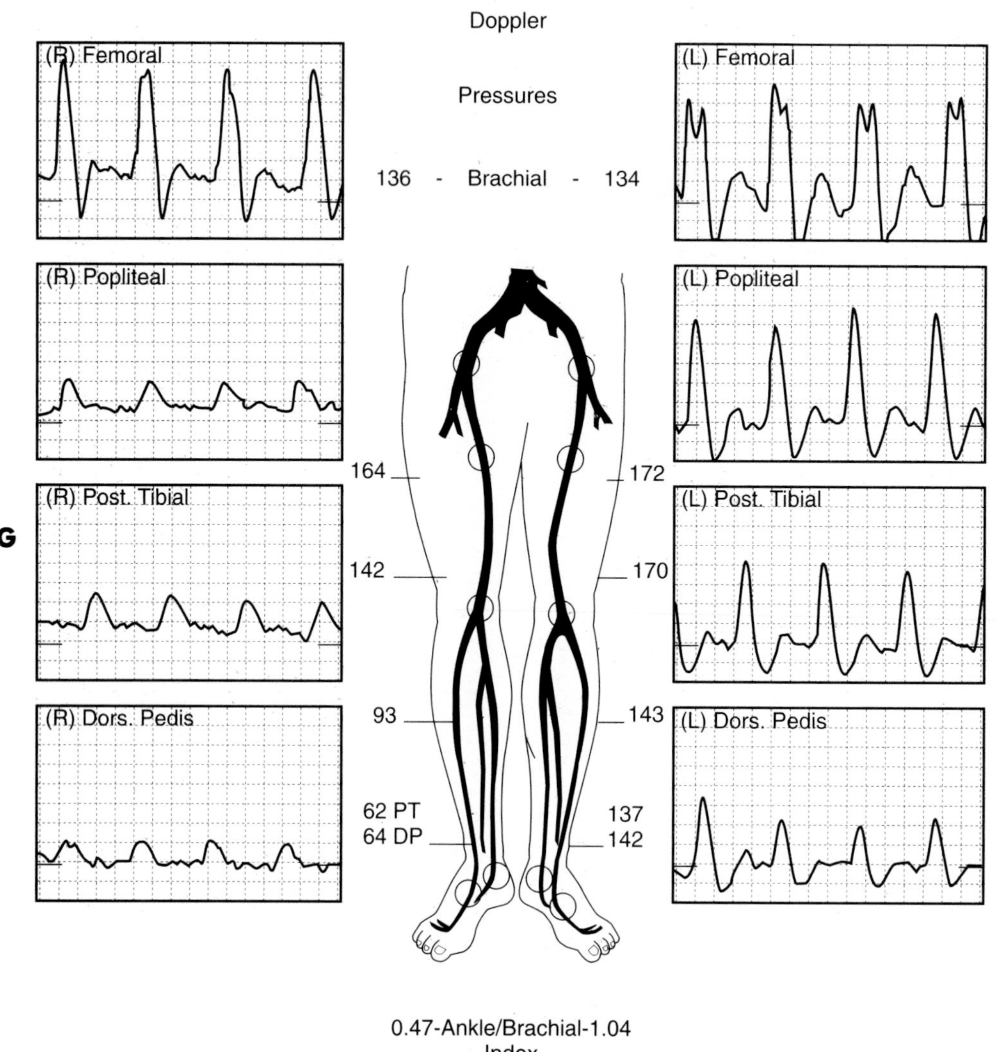

FIG. 20-43 cont'd.

Case 2 (Fig. 20-43; see color images): common femoral artery (CFA) endarterectomy, popliteal artery occlusion. This 43-year-old patient had had an acute right arterial lower-extremity embolus that necessitated a femoral embolectomy, a femoral endarterectomy that was extended to the iliac, and a popliteal embolectomy all during the same procedure on the right leg. He recovered but noticed a resumption of right claudication at one block within the first month after surgery; he ignored it until he was evaluated at 3 months for follow-up.

Duplex imaging of his right femoral area showed a typical postendarterectomy dilated appearance with normal color flow, *A*, and normal but slightly hyperemic flow in the superficial femoral artery, *B*. At the distal superficial femoral near the adductor hiatus, the artery became irregular and was occluded at the popliteal, with a large collateral branch coming off posteriorly, *C*. The popliteal artery was seen to be occluded throughout the popliteal fossa and to the peroneal-tibial area, *D*, but a large patent collateral with monophasic flow was noted running posteriorly, *E*. It reconstituted the posterior tibial and anterior tibial artery through runoff branches, *F*, both with monophasic and diminished flow.

The Doppler analog waveform analysis and segmental pressure study that was done before duplex imaging *(G)* correlates with the duplex examination, showing similar waveforms and an ankle-brachial index of 0.47 in the right leg. The left leg is normal at all levels.

It is important to note that the right popliteal analog waveform actually reflects the collateral and not the occluded popliteal artery. It is possible that by analog waveform analysis alone the popliteal might have been interpreted as patent but with stenotic flow, thus pointing out one of the benefits of duplex imaging.

THE BASIC ARTERIAL EXAMINATION

The best arterial lower-extremity evaluation incorporates two or more of the components described in detail above. Here is a basic suggested protocol for evaluating a patient.

1. Obtain as complete a history as possible from the patient or from accompanying records, emphasizing the

patient's symptoms, past surgical procedures, and vascular risk factors.

2. Obtain Doppler waveforms from the femoral, popliteal, posterior tibial, and dorsalis pedis arteries. Optionally, obtain waveforms from the superficial femoral arteries, big toe, or both.

   OR

   Obtain VPR waveforms from the high-thigh, low-thigh, calf, ankle, and metatarsal areas using appropriate cuffs. Optionally, obtain a PPG or strain-gauge waveform from the big toe.
3. a. Perform segmental pressures by applying blood-pressure cuffs to the arms, high thighs, lower thighs, calves, and ankles.
   b. Obtain bilateral systolic brachial blood pressures.
   c. Obtain pressures from the ankle using the dorsalis pedis and posterior tibial arteries, or if necessary, the peroneal artery. Compare the ankle systolic pressures at these sites to each other and then use the artery with the highest pressure to sequentially obtain pressures at the other three sites. Repeat for both legs.
   d. If desired, obtain a pressure from the big toes bilaterally using a digit cuff and a plethysmographic or Doppler method.
   e. Document the pressures at each location, and calculate the ankle and brachial indices.
4. Briefly compare waveforms with each other, looking for abnormal waveforms, and look for interval pressure drops between the segmental blood-pressure cuffs.
5. Use arterial duplex sonography, color-flow imaging, or both to investigate any arterial segments where a potential stenosis is implied by the indirect methods. Obtain images and spectral Doppler velocities from any areas of stenosis.

Fig. 20-10 illustrates some sites where arteries and veins can be evaluated using continuous-wave Doppler waveforms and duplex imaging.

Miscellaneous Factors

Several mechanical and technical factors should be constantly checked to ensure accuracy in performing these evaluations. Doppler probes and photocells should be monitored periodically for wire and electric damage, epoxy decay, or crystal damage. Manometers and cuffs should be calibrated and checked for leakage every 2 or 3 weeks. Regularly scheduled preventative maintenance should be performed on duplex, Doppler, and plethysmographic equipment to ensure safety and accuracy.

The examiner's skills need to be fine-tuned as well. In Doppler and segmental pressure examinations, concentration is required, as well as practice at keeping the probe in place with one hand while inflating and releasing the cuff with the other. Cultivation of ambidextrous independence is useful to provide flexibility. Maintaining constant probe position also should be practiced to avoid losing the signal during cuff inflation and release. Careful calibration and adjustment of patient and pressure factors are important when performing plethysmographic techniques. Mastery of the use of color-flow imaging and spectral Doppler is vital to maximize the information that can be obtained with these techniques. In short, although the tool may be at fault occasionally, any tool is only as good as the user. Experience and practice are the best ways to develop the examination technique.

EVALUATION OF THE POSTOPERATIVE PATIENT

This section deals with the variations in the examination needed to provide adequate results in the patient who has recently undergone vascular surgery. The basic formats of the routine Doppler waveform and segmental pressure examinations are adhered to by the sonographer. The brachial arteries are examined as in the routine examination unless an arterial monitor line or IV prevents it. One of the two arms is required for the ankle-brachial index determination, especially since the success or failure of the surgery often depends on the results obtained by the examiner. Again, either the higher of the two arm pressures or the single arm pressure is used. Note, however, that if the only available brachial artery signal appears stenosed or occluded, the index will be inaccurate (see Upper Extremity Arterial Examination).

The history is taken, and the type of surgery and graft material (either the patient's own vein or a synthetic) is noted. If possible, a drawing of the surgical connections should be made for future reference if included in the patient's chart, showing the vessels that were resected or ligated, the levels where the graft is attached to the artery, and the course of the graft in the extremity. It is often beneficial to review the surgeon's operative notes, since these tell when the procedure was performed and exactly what was done. These also can help the examiner determine where the proximal and distal anastomoses actually are located and what type of graft materials were used.

There are many different methods of bypass grafting and types of graft materials;[20,21] materials used for grafts are either of organic or synthetic origin. Organic grafts include human allografts, human prepared umbilical vein, and a patient's own autogenous superficial veins. Synthetic grafts are made of materials such as Dacron, Gore-Tex, or PTFE (Teflon).

Their purpose is to shunt the main blood flow around the obstructed area to the patent sections of the artery at a lower level. Fig. 20-44 illustrates several of the most common bypasses in the lower limb.

Types of grafts and the surgical conditions for which they are used include the following:

1. *Aortoiliac*. Commonly a synthetic bifurcated graft, employed in cases of abdominal aortic aneurysm at the bifurcation of the common iliac arteries.
2. *Aortofemoral*. Also synthetic, either unilateral or bilateral, used to bypass iliac obstructions or aneurysms extending past the common iliac regions.

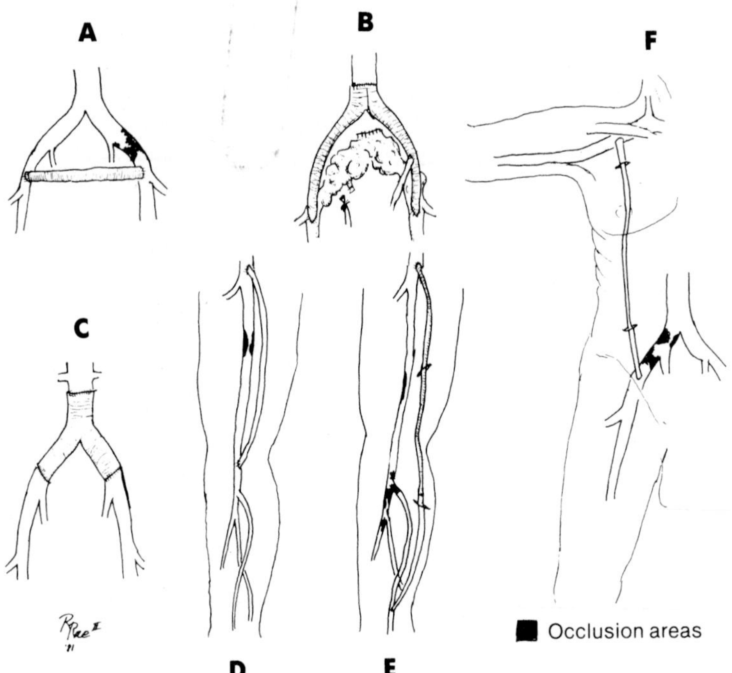

FIG. 20-44 Various types of bypass graft operations. **A,** Femorofemoral. **B,** Aortofemoral. **C,** Aortoiliac. **D,** Femoropopliteal. **E,** Femorotibial. **F,** Axillofemoral.

3. *Femorofemoral.* Synthetic, placed subcutaneously across the lower abdomen to shunt flow from a patent femoral to a point distal to the obstruction in the opposite femoral artery.
4. *Femoropopliteal.* Synthetic graft, or (preferred) autogenous saphenous vein. In the latter case the patient's own greater or lesser saphenous veins are used. The great saphenous, for example, can be used in the following ways:
   a. The great saphenous is physically removed, the small branches are ligated, and the vein is turned backward and then anastomosed to the native artery above and below the obstruction. It is often placed deep in an anatomic tunnel or routed through the tissues to protect it (reversed saphenous vein).
   b. The great saphenous is physically removed and has the small branches ligated, a valvulotome (valve cutter) is passed through, then the vein is anastomosed to the native artery above and below the obstruction without being reversed. It is sometimes relocated deep in the leg (nonreversed-nonreversed translocated saphenous vein).
   c. Sections of greater or lesser saphenous vein from either leg, or basilic or cephalic vein from the arm, may be attached to each other end to end to form a longer bypass (composite vein).
   d. The great saphenous vein is left in situ; in this method the vein is not removed from the thigh, but the proximal and distal ends needed for anastomosis are exposed, a valvulotome is passed through (sometimes under angioscopic guidance), and feeding branches are ligated (Fig. 20-45). The proximal and distal ends are then reanastomosed to the native artery above and below the obstruction (in situ vein).
5. *Femorotibial.* The same materials are used as in the femoropopliteal graft, but insertion is in either the anterior or the posterior tibial arteries; it is often passed subcutaneously on the medial (infrequently the lateral) surface of the leg and may be palpated easily at the

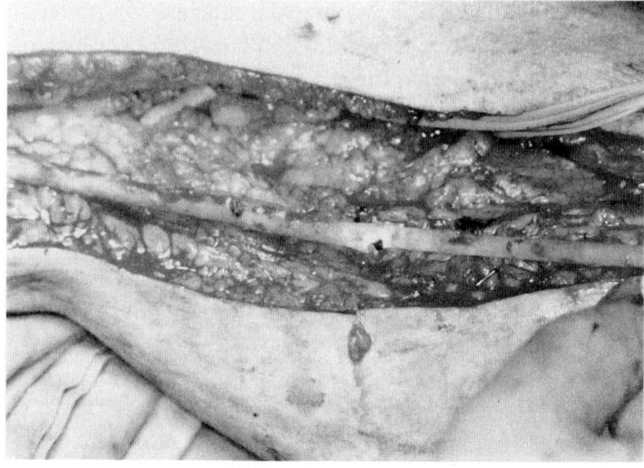

FIG. 20-45 In situ bypass graft. In this figure the great saphenous vein has been exposed and the small branches ligated. The light in the center of the graft is from an angioscope; the valves are being cut under angioscopic guidance.

knee area; used to bypass obstructions extending through the popliteal artery or involving the trifurcation vessels.

6. *Femoroperoneal.* Used in the same circumstances as the femorotibial graft but may be passed through the popliteal fossa rather than the medial side of the knee.
7. *Axillofemoral.* Usually synthetic, passed from the axillary artery subcutaneously across the chest and lower abdomen to the ipsilateral femoral artery; can also be palpated along its length.

There are many variations on these methods.[6] To avoid confusion, the examiner should be aware of the extent and exact type of surgery performed.

There is a definite rule to follow in postoperative examination, and although this suggestion is not often followed in many institutions, it is sound nevertheless. Never put a pressure cuff over a graft whether new or old, because you might occlude the graft. It is far safer to use just the ankle and calf cuffs or just the ankle cuff if the graft extends that far down (as in femorotibial bypasses). If ankle cuffs should not be used (as in cases of femorotibial bypasses that anastomose in the foot area or to the dorsalis pedis), then velocity waveforms should be obtained as described below (see Duplex Evaluation of Vein Bypass Grafts). One factor that is not often considered is the patient's potential reaction to postoperative pressure cuffs. A patient tends to be somewhat protective of the graft, especially considering that he or she has already undergone a traumatic procedure and may have noted a marked improvement. If the graft fails or complications with it develop, it is not uncommon for the patient to believe (albeit probably incorrectly) that the use of a pressure cuff occluded the graft; this can lead to a number of uncomfortable situations for the examiner and laboratory alike. Using velocity measurements and duplex sonography can obviate this reaction and still obtain more diagnostic information about the graft.

In addition, many synthetic graft materials, such as PTFE or Gore-tex, can be obtained with rigid rings spaced evenly along the length of the graft to prevent inadvertent compression or kinking of the graft and to preserve the lumen shape. These grafts are usually used in stress or flexion points, such as at knee joints, or when added protection is required (such as an axillofemoral segments along the superficial abdominal wall). These grafts often resist compression and do not yield accurate results in any case.

Only the ankle pressure is required for the ankle-brachial index. The use of segmental cuffs is not actually necessary in the immediate post-operative period since in most patients a prior examination or arteriogram has confirmed the occlusion preoperatively. If the patient has undergone an endarterectomy or embolectomy rather than a bypass, the same guidelines should be observed.

Duplex Evaluation of Vein Bypass Grafts

Graft surveillance is a common application of duplex sonography, and one that has been very successful. Vein

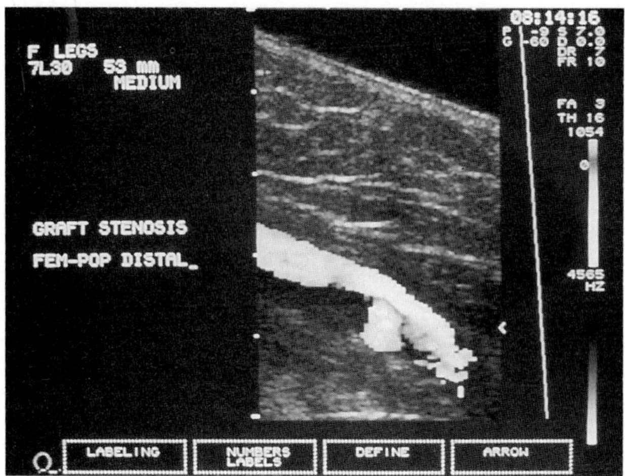

FIG. 20-46 This stenotic area in a vein bypass graft is occurring at a valve sinus, with thrombotic material lodged in a residual valve cusp. Note the hemodynamic flow streamline, and the area of flow separation on the distal side of the stenosis.

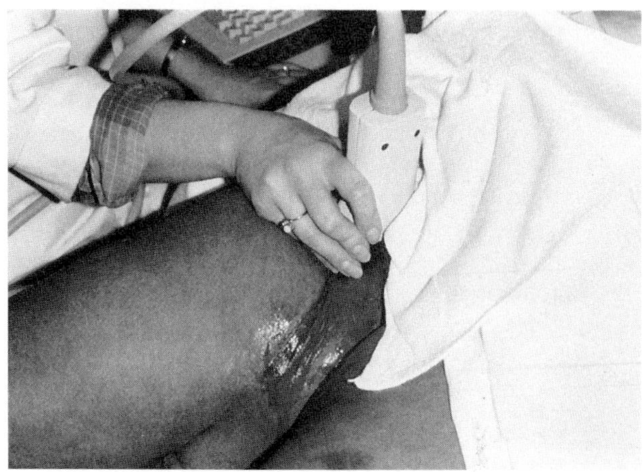

FIG. 20-47 Scanning the area of the proximal anastomosis of an in situ bypass graft.

grafts have their own set of idiosyncrasies, any of which can cause failure or perfusion problems.

1. Arteriovenous fistulas can occur in in situ grafts when one or more feeder branches of the saphenous vein have not been ligated (See Case 5, below). These fistulas can cause local varicosities and discomfort and sometimes "steal" flow from the graft causing a decrease in distal perfusion and runoff.
2. Valve cusps that have been insufficiently cut can act as sites for thrombus formation and can cause focal stenotic changes (Fig. 20-46; see color image).

To evaluate the graft, the examiner first should adjust the technical factors as described earlier (see Arterial Duplex Sonography). The examiner then locates the native artery proximal to the graft (above the incision) longitudinally and progresses distally until the proximal anastomosis is visualized (Fig. 20-47). The anastomosis should be evaluated for the presence of stenosis, then the graft itself should be steadily followed, moving distally (Fig. 20-48) until the distal anastomosis is reached. When examining the graft, the transducer should be moved from side to side to look for tell tale signs of arteriovenous fistulas or intact valve cusps; color-flow imaging is extremely beneficial in these cases. Once the distal anastomosis has been evaluated (Fig. 20-49), the distal native vessel should also be briefly examined to check for extension of plaque. Spectral Doppler velocity measurements should be taken in the native vessels above and below the graft anastomoses, and (at minimum) proximally and distally within the graft. If areas of suspected stenosis or intact cusps are detected, velocity measurements must be recorded at the stenotic area and downstream from it. Transverse images should also be obtained if necessary.

If an arteriovenous fistula in the graft is detected, the patent branch should be followed in both longitudinal and transverse planes into the leg, and spectral Doppler velocities should be obtained in the graft above the fistula, below the fistula, and within the fistula branch itself. Sometimes it is even possible to track a branch to its insertion in a major vein (see example, Case 5, Postoperative Cases). Fistulas planned for focal surgical ligation can be marked by this using a waterproof surgical dye once the origin has been identified.

Since graft imaging is usually performed along with Doppler waveforms and an ankle-brachial ratio, the examination can sometimes be abbreviated to just a proximal and distal graft waveform coupled with an ankle-brachial ratio if ankle flow appears to be within normal limits.

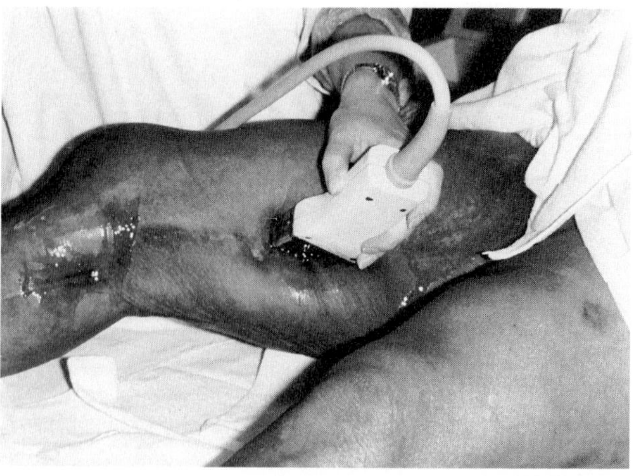

FIG. 20-48 Scanning the central section of an in situ bypass graft.

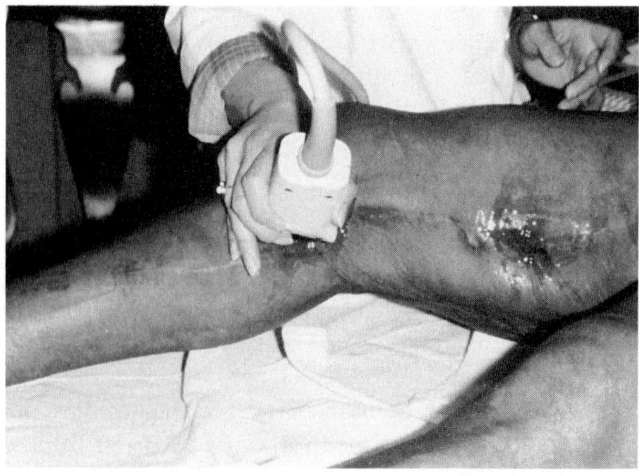

FIG. 20-49 Scanning the area of the distal anastomosis of an in situ bypass graft.

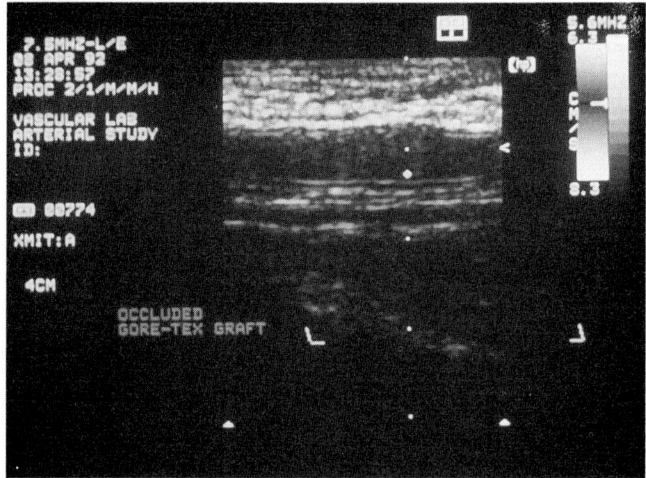

FIG. 20-50 Appearance of an occluded Gore-Tex bypass graft. Note absence of color flow within and the bright walls of the synthetic material.

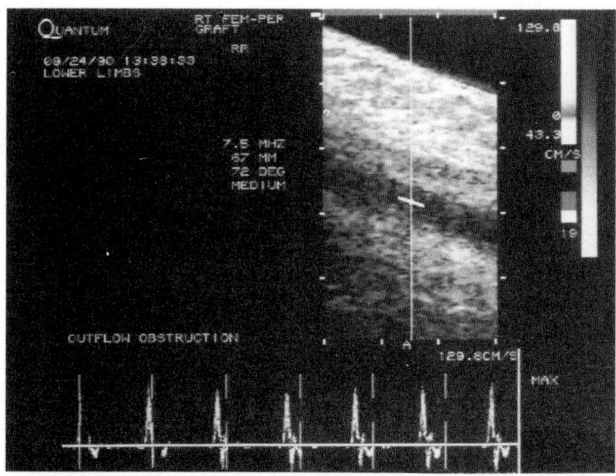

FIG. 20-51 Doppler signal in outflow obstruction or distal occlusion. The graft here is patent, but flow is abrupt and resistant. Note the narrow systolic peak and the absence of any diastolic component; on color-flow imaging, the graft had no color present during diastole.

Graft Stenosis and Velocity Criteria

The duplex criteria for evaluating in situ grafts is the same as that for the rest of the arterial system,[7] as described in Arterial Duplex Sonography previously. One difference, however, is that a graft velocity of less than 45 cm/sec in the smallest-diameter graft segment has been suggested to predict potential graft failure if it is obtained after a 2-month postoperative period.[2,3,9] (Normal graft velocities of less than 45 cm/sec can occur, however, if grafts are large in diameter.) Occluded grafts show a graft lumen filled with echogenic thrombotic material (Fig. 20-50; see color image), and a high-resistance waveform with a complete absence of diastolic flow may be present in a segment either proximal to an occlusion or in cases of outflow obstruction distal to a graft (Fig. 20-51).

PROCEDURE SUMMARY

The following procedure for the postsurgical patient can be used:

1. Obtain the patient's history, concentrating on the operative notes (if available) and incisional locations to determine the levels and extents of any bypass grafts.
2. Obtain Doppler velocity waveforms from all sites as in a routine study (see Doppler Velocity Waveform Analysis). Take waveforms from specific axillofemoral segments, femorofemoral segments, and peripheral grafts. Note: if evaluating a below-knee femoropopliteal or femorotibial graft, do not try to obtain a popliteal waveform at the conventional site behind the knee unless the graft has been routed through the popliteal fossa. Waveforms obtained otherwise do not reflect the true hemodynamic state of the lower leg, since it is possible for a

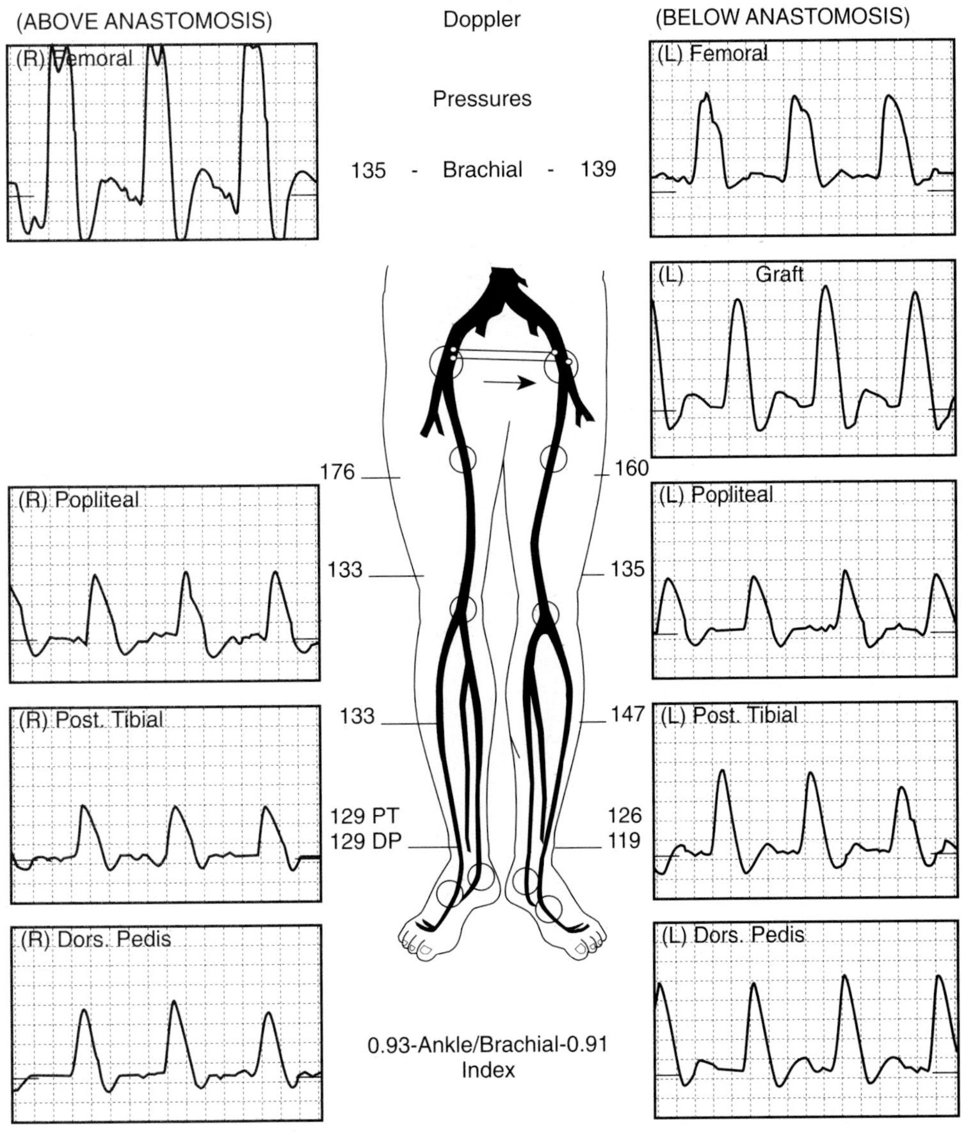

FIG. 20-52 Femorofemoral bypass, Doppler analog waveforms and segmental pressures (see text).

patent native popliteal artery to be monophasic from collaterals although triphasic flow reaches the rest of the leg through the graft.

3. Apply pressure cuffs to the arms and the ankles (when possible). Obtain ankle pressures and brachial pressures and calculate the ankle-brachial indices.
4. If a vein graft is in place, perform duplex and/or color-flow imaging of the graft and obtain spectral Doppler waveforms and velocities from the proximal and distal sections, anastomoses, stenotic areas, and native vessels.

If dressings, skin closures, surgical clips, or other interfering items are present, the examination may have to be abbreviated. Some waveforms or images may not be taken in these cases, and the presence of these limiting factors should be noted on the report forms.

Postoperative Cases

Case 1 (Fig. 20-52): Femorofemoral bypass graft. This 69-year-old patient had a right-to-left femorofemoral bypass with a right iliac percutaneous transluminal angioplasty (PTA) and a redo right-to-left femorofemoral bypass 2 years later and has been asymptomatic since.

The Doppler analog waveform analysis and segmental pressure study shown here shows triphasic flow through the graft and bilaterally at all levels in the legs. There are relatively normal ankle-brachial indices of 0.93 and 0.91 in the right and left legs, respectively. Note that there is some slight decrease in the ankle-brachial indices, which is consistent with the hemodynamic changes that occur distal to the graft anastomoses.

Case 2 (Fig. 20-53): Axillobifemoral bypass graft. This 67-year-old patient had an axillobifemoral graft with a sub-

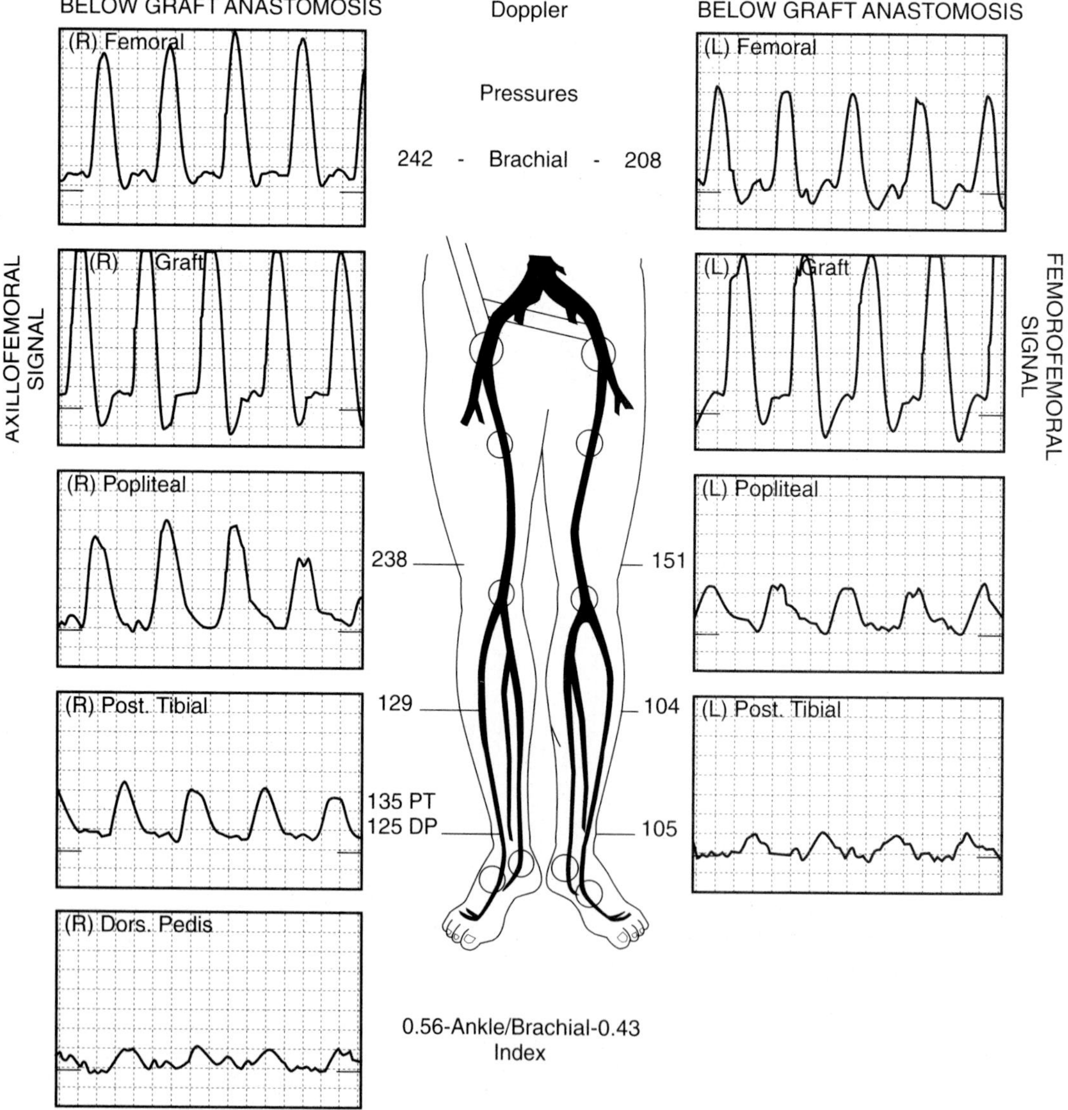

FIG. 20-53 Axillobifemoral bypass—Doppler analog waveforms and segmental pressures (see text).

sequent redo 4 years later after graft infection. Postoperatively, he had no complaints for his level of activity.

The Doppler analog waveform analysis and segmental pressure study shown here shows triphasic flow through the axillofemoral and femorofemoral segments to both legs, with slightly decreased triphasic flow in the superficial femoral segments below the distal graft anastomoses. Waveforms distal to this level in the popliteal and ankle arteries are monophasic, reflecting known chronic bilateral superficial femoral artery occlusions, also evidenced by the significant pressure drops between the high-thigh and low-thigh cuffs. The ankle-brachial indices are 0.56 and 0.43 in the right and left legs, respectively.

Case 3 (Fig. 20-54; see color images): Normal femoropopliteal in situ graft. These images are from a 70-year-old patient and represent normal proximal and distal Doppler waveforms and velocities in a patent in situ femoropopliteal bypass graft.

Case 4 (Fig. 20-55; see color images): Multiple stenoses in composite femorotibial in situ graft. This 65-year-old patient had a composite in situ–reversed saphenous vein graft running from the femoral artery to the peroneal artery near the foot. During a 2-year period, the patient developed at least four stenoses at various points in the long graft. *A* shows the proximal stenosis with the occluded superficial femoral artery (SFA) visible below it; *B* shows a stenosis just above the knee; *C* shows a stenosis just below the knee; *D* shows a stenosis at the midcalf level at a residual valve sinus; *E* shows a stenosis at the distal graft just above the anastomosis with an associated bruit and turbulence; *F* shows the Doppler spectral waveform in this stenotic segment with velocities exceeding 280 cm/sec (the native vessel can be seen just to the right).

All the stenoses were either atherectomized or angioplastied with very good results; see Fig. 20-41, which shows the postangioplasty result of *C* above.

Case 5 (Fig. 20-56; see color images): Arteriovenous fistula in in situ graft. This 72-year-old patient had received a femoroperoneal in situ bypass graft and was noted to have a palpable thrill in the leg near the graft during examination. Duplex examination of the graft was performed, and a residual vein branch forming an arteriovenous fistula off the graft was detected in the area of the thrill. The graft was imaged and Doppler spectral waveforms were taken above, *A* and below the fistula takeoff, *B*. Velocities were 80 cm/sec and 85 cm/sec respectively with little change to the normal postsurgical hyperemic waveform; this indicated that the fistula was not causing a significant reduction in flow to the distal graft. Velocities in the graft at the ankle level were 80 cm/sec as well.

Flow within the fistula branch itself was turbulent and of high velocity, well over 257 cm/sec *(C, D)*. The fistula was marked and subsequently ligated.

Case 6 (Fig. 20-57; see color images): Occluded superficial femoropopliteal reversed saphenous vein graft. This 42-year-old patient had had bilateral femoropopliteal bypass with occlusive disease of the right tibial vessels. His right femoropopliteal bypass was revised to a superficial femoral artery-popliteal bypass and urokinase infusions were done for thrombolysis of the anterior and posterior tibial arteries. The patient did well until about 5 months after the last procedure when he presented with an ischemic right foot and an early foot toe ulceration. Duplex scanning of the native superficial femoral artery above the graft, *A,* showed a patent superficial femoral artery with some visible luminal irregularity. The proximal anastomosis, *B,* showed a patent proximal anastomosis with a swirling "dead-end" flow pattern proximal to an occlusion. The graft was examined in the central portion across the knee (*C*—note the collateral below) and to the distal anastomosis *(D)*. The graft was totally occluded as was the popliteal artery above and below the distal anastomosis. No color-

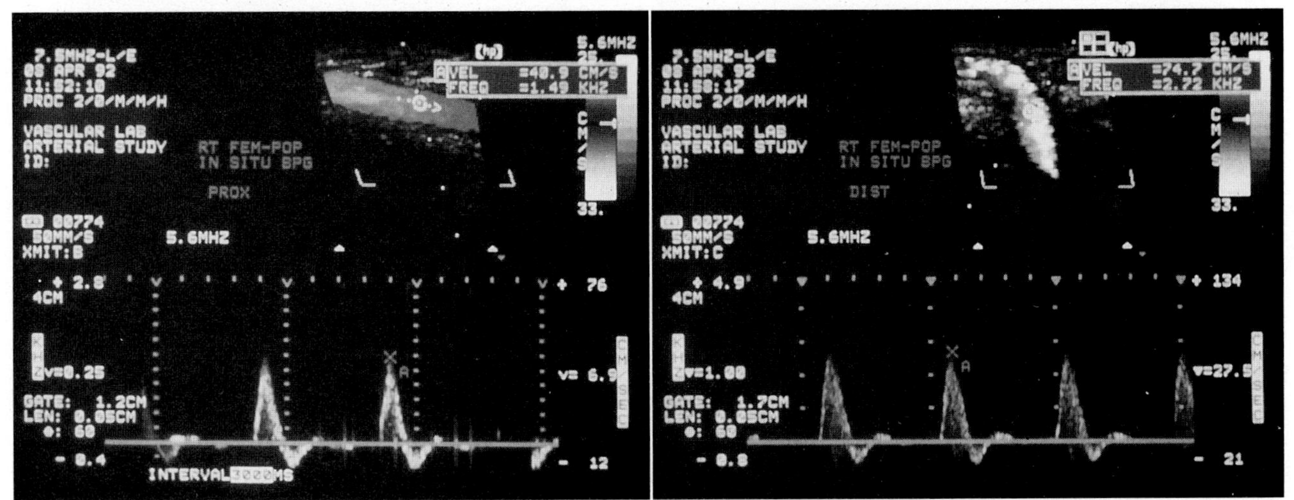

FIG. 20-54 A, Normal femoropopliteal graft, proximal segment (see text). **B,** Normal femoropopliteal graft, distal segment (see text).

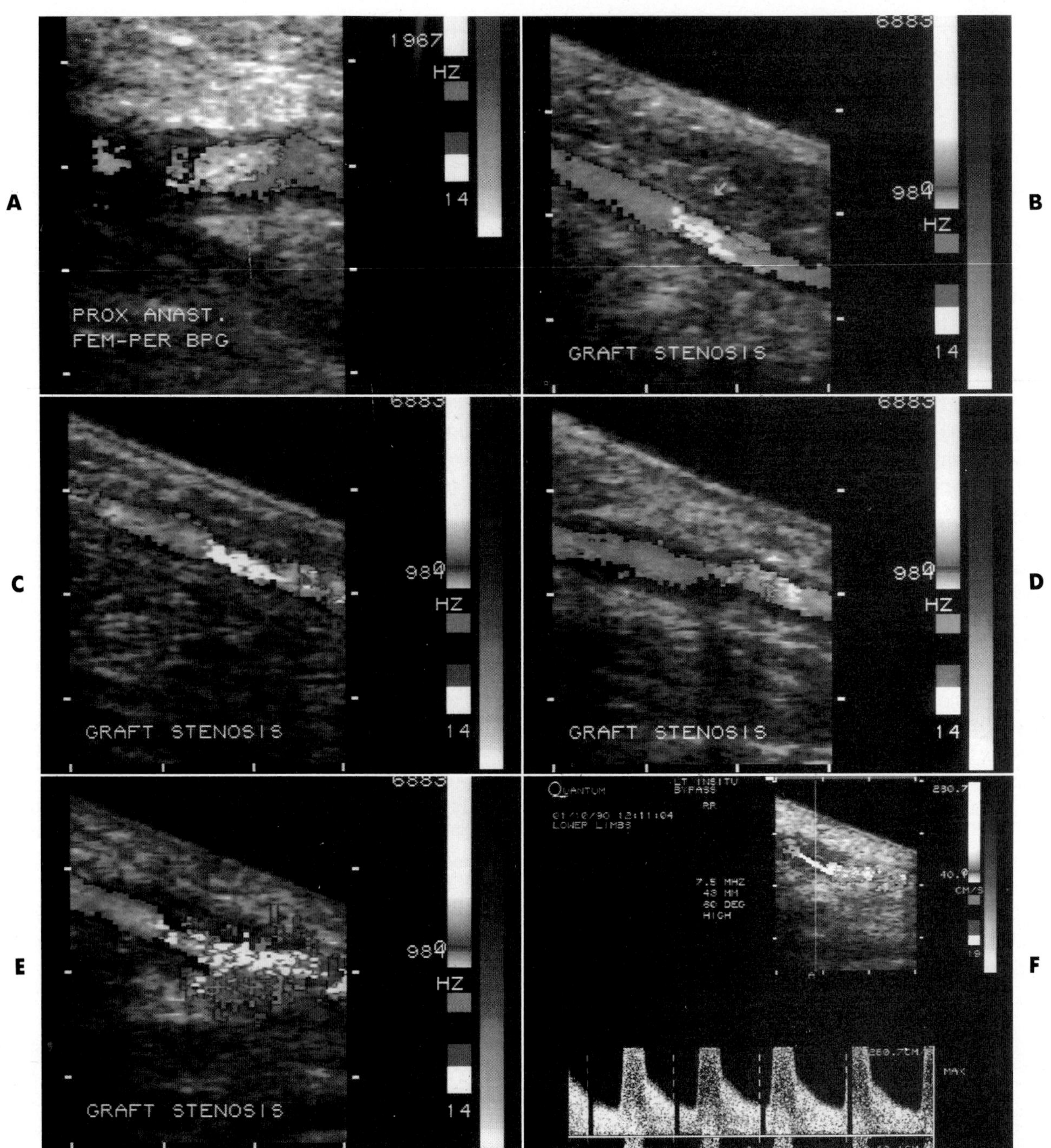

FIG. 20-55 A, Multiple graft stenoses, proximal graft anastomosis (see text). **B,** Multiple graft stenoses, above-knee graft stenosis (see text). **C,** Multiple graft stenoses, below-knee graft stenosis (see text). **D,** Multiple graft stenoses; midcalf level graft stenosis (see text). **E,** Multiple graft stenoses, graft stenosis above distal anastomosis (see text). **F,** Multiple graft stenoses, Doppler spectral waveforms at distal stenosis shown in **E** (see text).

flow or Doppler signals could be detected in these areas. An ankle-brachial index on the same leg 1 month later showed blunted monophasic distal waveforms and an index of 0.58, indicating some collateral reconstitution to the foot.

Case 7 (Fig. 20-58): Aortoiliac graft with left limb and superficial femoral artery occlusion. This 59-year-old patient was examined 3 years after an aortoiliac bypass and presented with a recent onset of left claudication at less than 1 block distance. The right limb of the aortoiliac graft is patent with normal Doppler waveforms and segmental pressures on the right and an ankle-brachial index of 0.96. The left femoral signal, however, shows a slightly resistant waveform with blunted and diminished second and third

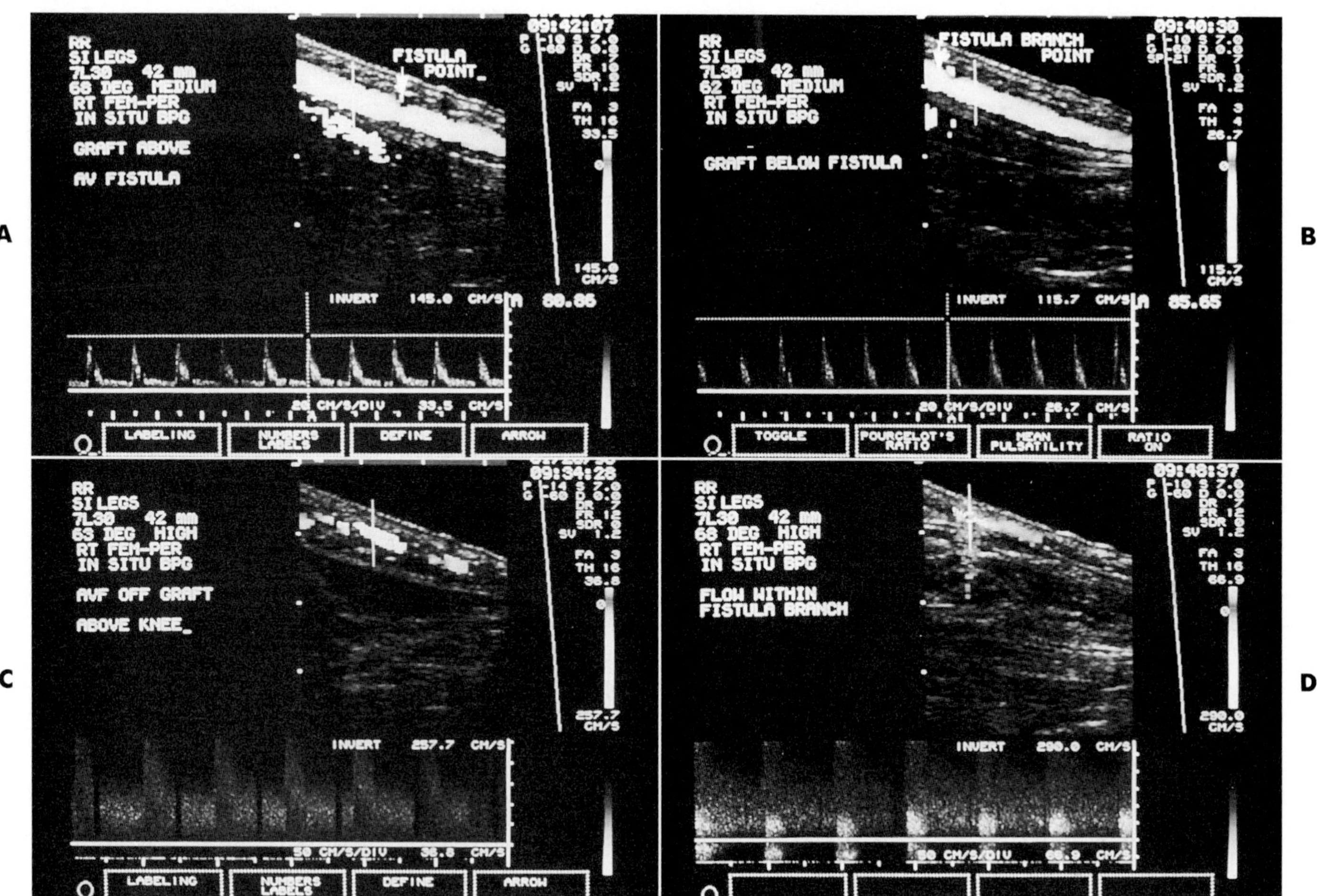

FIG. 20-56 A, In situ graft with waveforms and velocity proximal to arteriovenous fistula takeoff (see text). **B,** In situ graft with waveforms and velocity distal to arteriovenous fistula takeoff (see text). **C,** Waveform in the proximal segment of the arteriovenous fistula (see text). Note the elevated velocity scale. **D,** Waveform in a distal segment of the arteriovenous fistula (see text).

components. Flow below this site is severely decreased with monophasic waveforms at all distal levels and an ankle-brachial index of 0.48 VPR. Waveforms are normal at all levels on the right with visible dicrotic notches; waveforms on the left show a mild decrease (nearly normal waveform) at the high-thigh level. Below this, there is a decrease of the upslope, deterioration of the downslope, and loss of the dicrotic notch that progresses distally at all levels to the left ankle. Note the nearly flat waveform at the left metatarsal position.

EXAMINATION OF THE PATIENT AFTER PERCUTANEOUS BALLOON ANGIOPLASTY, BALLOON THROMBECTOMY, ATHERECTOMY, OR ENDARTERECTOMY

Many obstructive cases have been found to be of a nature that does not necessarily indicate bypass surgery as the only method of relief. There are many cases where a thrombus or clot forms within an artery, most often occurring in an acute situation and causing a sudden onset of symptoms or occasionally a complete and dire loss of flow to the extremity. When the artery is obstructed by a thrombus as opposed to atherosclerotic plaque, the typical procedure is a thrombectomy. Thrombectomies typically are done by performing an arteriotomy superior to the clot and by inserting a short balloon catheter into the lumen and forcing it through the jellylike clot material. Once the catheter is on the distal side of the clot, the balloon is inflated and the catheter is withdrawn, extracting the clot with it (Fig. 20-59). When the plaque is soft and atheromatous, a technique known as *percutaneous transluminal angioplasty* may be used. This involves methods similar to those used for arteriography; special catheters, fluoroscopic guidance, and contrast injections are needed. A catheter designed by Gruntzig that has a balloon in its tip with the boundaries marked radiopaquely is used. This balloon catheter is threaded through the artery along a guide wire to the point of obstruction or stenosis. It is then threaded through the obstructed section until the balloon lies along the area marked for dilation. The balloon is inflated to a pressure of 5 to 10 atm. This compresses and disperses the plaque against the arterial walls, stretching the artery to some extent as well (Fig. 20-60). The method does not work well with calcific, severe, or multiple obstructions. In some cases of focal obstruction (and often during a bypass surgery above or below the point of implantation) an endarterectomy may be performed. In this technique the artery is opened across the area of stenosis. An intimal elevator is used to dissect the intimal layer and area of plaque away from the walls, and this area is cut away. The loose ends of the residual intima are tacked down with sutures, remaining bits of plaque in the area are removed, and the vessel is closed.

Although a direct endarterectomy is often a fairly aggressive approach short of bypassing, in certain situations an atherectomy may be performed. Atherectomy catheters are of two types, directional and rotational. The atherectomy catheter is thin and is somewhat similar in design to the angioplasty catheter, except that there is an opening on one side of the catheter and a balloon opposite. The atherectomy catheter is threaded through the negotiable lumen and is placed across the plaque section. The balloon is inflated and the opening in the catheter is forced over a portion of the plaque. Once this is done and checked under fluoroscopic guidance, an integral blade slices off the section of plaque encompassed by the catheter. The catheter is then withdrawn, the section of atheromatous material extracted, and repeated passes are made until the lumen is enlarged to the guiding physician's satisfaction (Fig. 20-61).

Rotational atherectomy catheters have an abrasive cone-like tip (Rotoblator) or spiraling cutter; although FDA approved, these methods are not considered acceptable by many interventional radiologists. Neither rotational method can remove atheroma plugs larger than the tip of the catheter itself. The Rotoblator is promoted as having the ability to grind the atheroma down to particles as small as blood cells, thus eliminating emboli, but in practice this is considered too risky. This method does not have the practical applications that the directional method does and is deemed by many to be no more useful than the vascular laser (which is no longer in active use in many institutions).

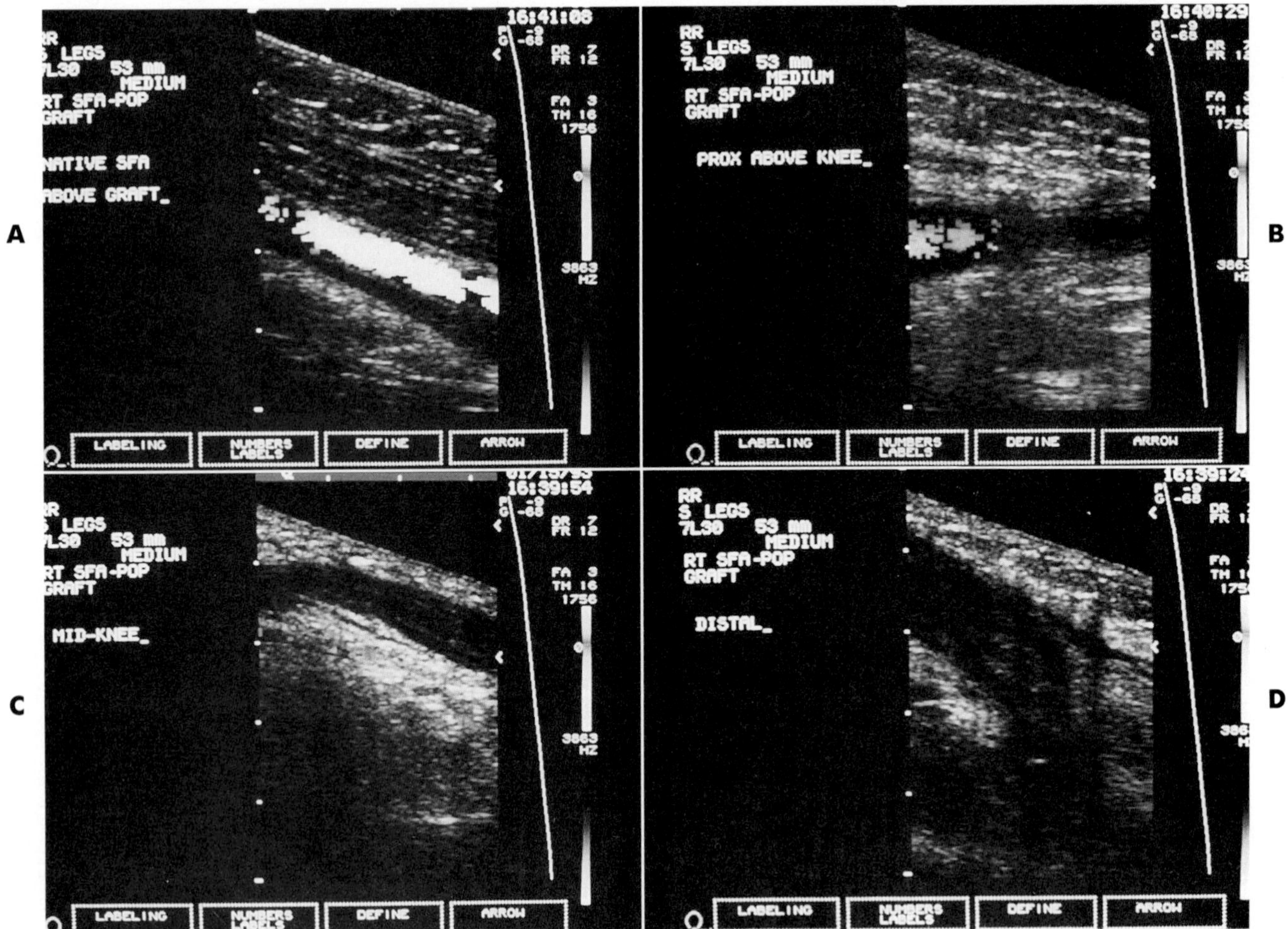

FIG. 20-57 A, Occluded superficial femoropopliteal graft, Native SFA (see text). **B,** Occluded superficial femoro popliteal graft, proximal anastomosis (see text). **C,** Occluded superficial femoro popliteal graft, center graft (see text). **D,** Occluded superficial femoro popliteal graft, distal anastomosis (see text).

Of course, many lesions or multiple areas of stenosis or occlusion are not amenable to any of the above techniques, and bypassing is indicated in these cases.

The Doppler examination after endarterectomy, angioplasty, thrombectomy, or atherectomy does not differ from the normal examination, except that thigh cuffs and tracings in the region of the catheterization site may be omitted if the patient is feeling tenderness in that area or if a cutdown wound would interfere with cuff or transducer placement.

EXAMINATION OF THE PATIENT WITH A FALSE-NEGATIVE RESULT

Occasionally the examiner encounters a patient who presents with the typical symptoms of lower-extremity claudication (often severe) but has normal tracings and indices. This type of symptomatic patient is difficult to evaluate, because the pain and claudication present only with exercise. The symptoms often result from a neuropathic rather than a vascular disorder.

In these patients, either an exercise stress test or hyperemic test frequently determines whether obstruction is present. The main aim is to increase demand for blood flow in the extremity either by exercising the patient on a treadmill or by inducing hyperemia through transient application of a tourniquet (inflated blood pressure cuff). The intention in both cases is to recreate or simulate the conditions that bring on the claudication and then measure the amount of time required for normal flow patterns to resume.

Although there are many different attitudes concerning the treadmill versus the hyperemic test, [1,12] the final decision is based on individual opinion, and further reading is encouraged on these subjects.[1,12]

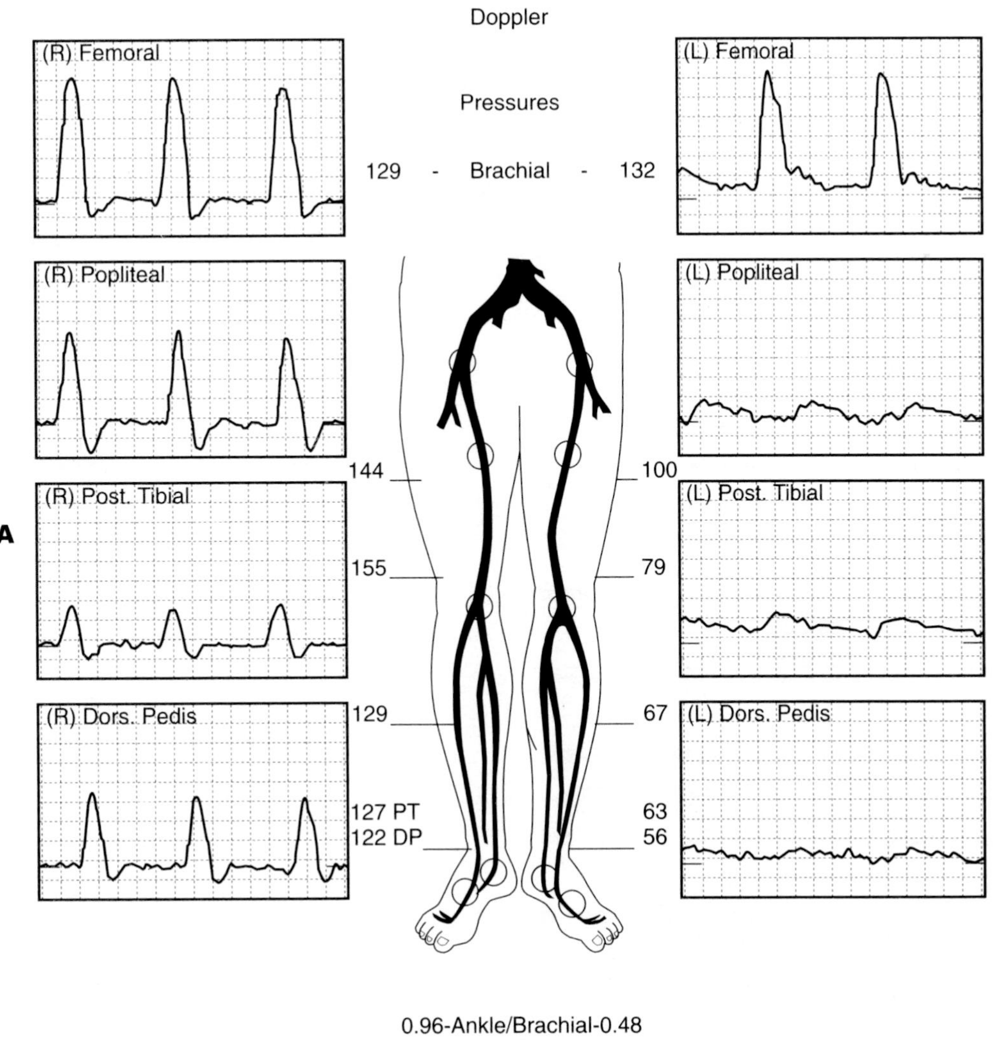

FIG. 20-58 A, Stenosis of left limb of aortoiliac graft with left SFA stenosis or occlusion. Doppler waveforms and segmental pressures (see text).

Continued.

Brachial: 129 VPR Brachial: 132

B

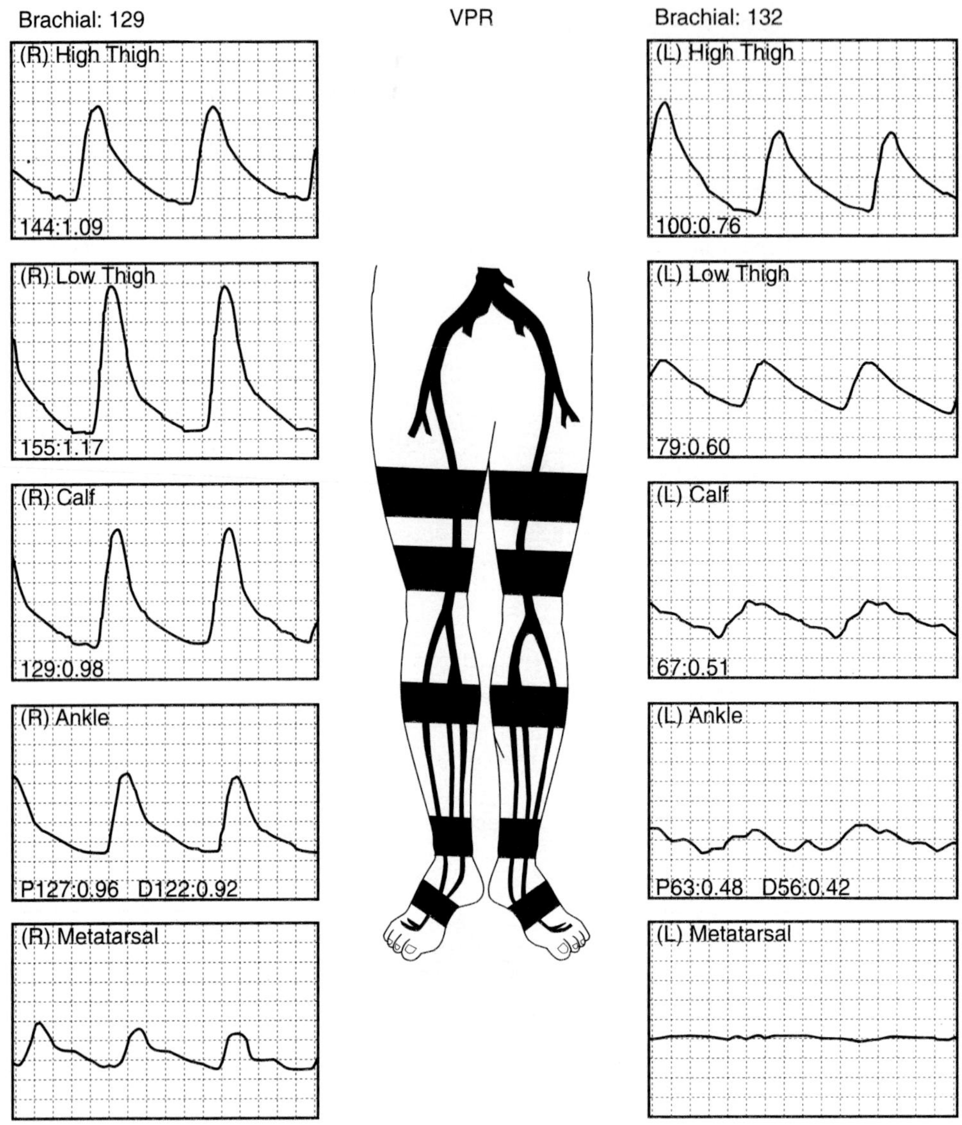

(R) High Thigh 144:1.09 | (L) High Thigh 100:0.76

(R) Low Thigh 155:1.17 | (L) Low Thigh 79:0.60

(R) Calf 129:0.98 | (L) Calf 67:0.51

(R) Ankle P127:0.96 D122:0.92 | (L) Ankle P63:0.48 D56:0.42

(R) Metatarsal | (L) Metatarsal

FIG. 20-58 cont'd. B, Stenosis of left limb of aortoiliac graft with left SFA stenosis or occlusion. Volume pulse recording waveforms (see text).

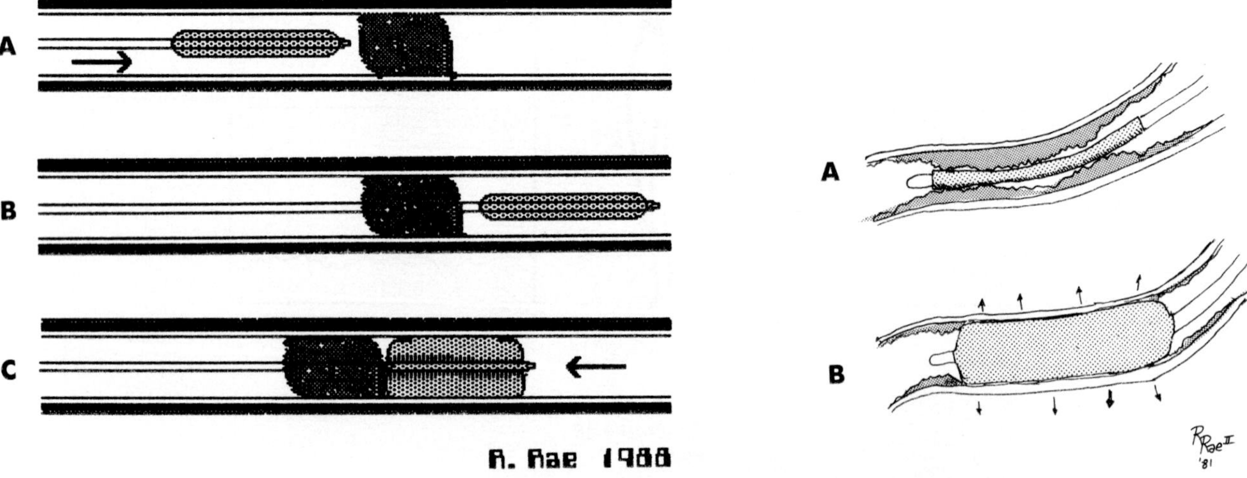

FIG. 20-59 Embolectomy. **A,** The catheter is pushed through the embolus, and the balloon is inflated distal to it, **B.** The catheter is withdrawn, pulling the embolus with it, **C.**

FIG. 20-60 Percutaneous transluminal angioplasty. **A,** Positioning the balloon along the diseased segment. **B,** Inflation of the balloon, compression of the atheroma, and dilation of the artery.

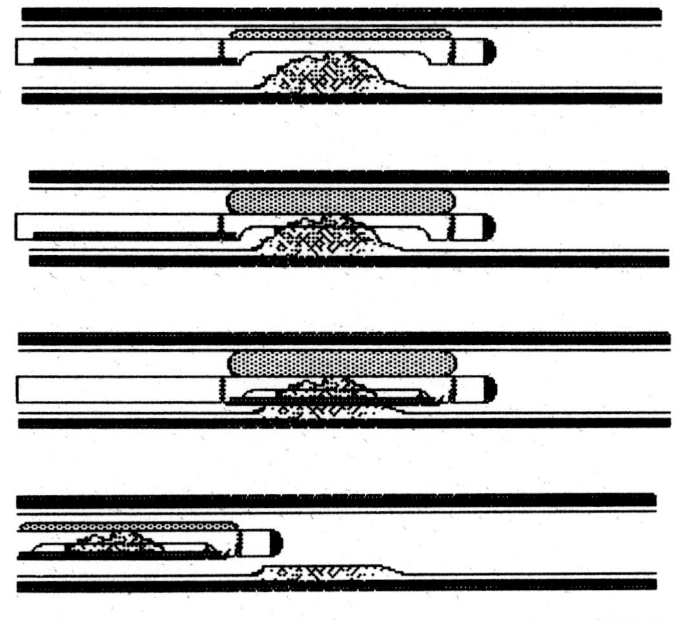

FIG. 20-61 Atherectomy. **A,** The catheter inserted to a point where the opening approximates the plaque. **B,** The balloon forces the opening in the catheter over the plaque. **C,** The blade cuts off the section of the plaque within the catheter. **D,** The catheter with the plaque specimen is then withdrawn.

Physiologic Responses to Exercise[5,14]

The normal response to exercise in the leg is a demand for increased blood flow in the muscular vascular bed, causing decreased vascular resistance. Flow is increased in the main arteries of the leg, and an adequate oxygen supply is thus provided. The normal muscular metabolism is maintained, as is the flow pattern.

In cases of obstruction, however, exercise results in the same demand for blood in the vascular bed and decreased resistance but the obstructed vessels and collaterals cannot supply enough blood to meet the demand. The pressure in the major arteries (including the ankle arteries) drops, and the waveform diminishes. Metabolic waste products accumulate, causing the pain, cramping, and muscle tiring of claudication.

Doppler Treadmill Examination

The criteria and examination techniques quoted here are based on information given by Barnes et al.[1,5]

The Doppler treadmill examination requires a stopwatch, three pressure cuffs, and a treadmill set for a constant load of 2 mph at a 12% grade.

Brachial and ankle systolic pressures are taken as in the routine examination, and recorded. The patient keeps the ankle cuffs in place and walks on the treadmill for 5 minutes or until claudication forces him or her to stop. The patient should tell the examiner where and when pain is noticed and then walk until he or she would normally stop because of the pain.

At the end of 5 minutes, or when the patient reaches his or her tolerance limit, the treadmill is stopped and the patient resumes the supine position. The arm with the higher pressure and both ankle pressures are taken and recorded at 1, 2, 4, 6, 10, 15, and 20 minutes after the exercise. Ankle pressures are usually taken until either the preexercise pressure or the time limit is reached (Fig. 20-62).

It should be noted that experience with patients with neuropathic etiologies has shown a return to normal pressures and waveforms within the first minute after exercise, making the first time measurement on the scale of Barnes et al.[5,18] almost unusable, especially since the patient must be asked to quickly resume a supine position on the examining table. This obviously can take longer than 1 minute, depending on the patient's condition. The severely obstructed or neuropathic patient may take longer than 2 minutes to recover, but the preexercise level is reached usually in less time. Shorter intervals may be required for determining the recovery rate within the first minute after exercise.

If an ECG treadmill examination is also performed, it is often advantageous to do the Doppler treadmill simultaneously; but cardiac and respiratory factors may not allow the patient to lie quickly supine, especially if the heart rate is being evaluated.[5]

Doppler Hyperemic Postocclusion Examination

This method requires the thigh and ankle cuffs and is often performed after the routine Doppler resting examination.

Instead of ambulation, the patient rests supine and the femoral artery is occluded at the upper thigh to simulate exercise and induce metabolic changes. This examination is advantageous when the patient is unable to walk.

Pressure cuffs are placed bilaterally on the ankles and high thighs, and the brachial pressure is taken and recorded. The higher of the two systolic arm pressures is again used for the ankle-brachial indices. One leg is examined at a time.

Before the thigh cuff is inflated, a preocclusive resting waveform and ankle pressure should be taken in the ankle vessels and recorded. The artery with the higher pressure is used for the examination. The probe is held in place, and the thigh cuff is inflated well above the point at which the signal disappears. The pump is then locked off, and the stopwatch is started. It is important to monitor the artery and maintain the occlusive pressure for 3 minutes. After that time, the thigh pressure is released all at once and an immediate waveform and ankle pressure are taken and recorded. Waveforms and pressures are continually taken every 15 seconds until the artery reaches its preocclusion pressure and waveform pattern. The technique is repeated for the other extremity.

Most patients resume normal pressures and waveforms within 30 to 60 seconds. The individual pressures at each interval are divided by the brachial pressure to give sequen-

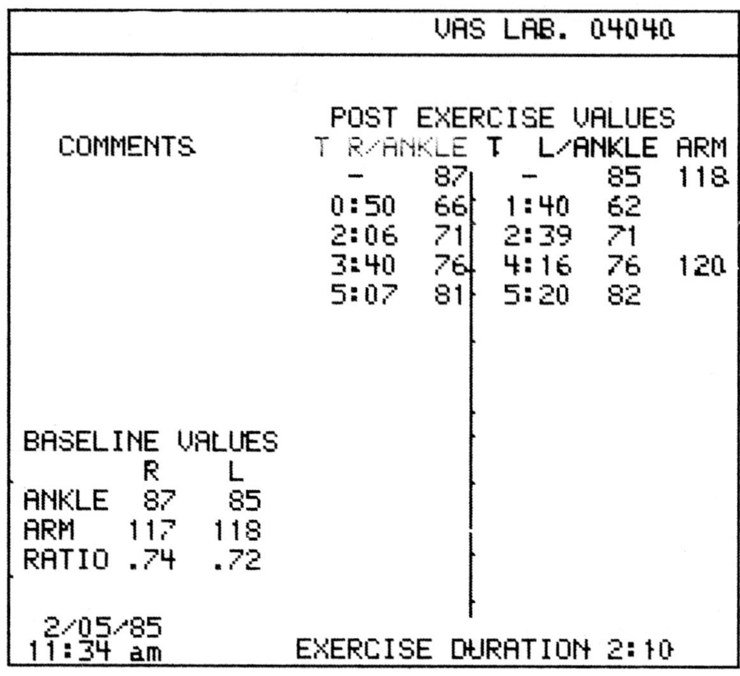

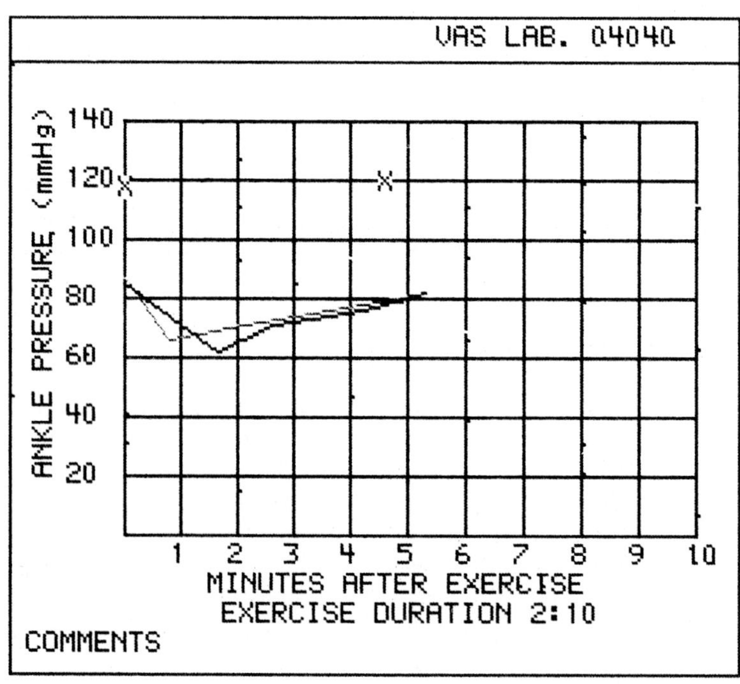

FIG. 20-62 Typical postexercise values and graphic representation.

tial ankle-brachial indices up to the preocclusion level. Normal ratios taken immediately after occlusion should be above 0.8. Lower indices or recovery times in excess of 1 minute imply neurologic or obstructive disease.

The disadvantages to this method include possible probe slippage during the occlusive period, intolerance of high-thigh cuff pressure by some individuals, and varying results depending on the examiner's ability to take tracings and cuff pressures one after the other every 15 seconds.

This examination also fails to work on patients with obese thighs, noncompressible or calcified arteries, or patients with femoropopliteal bypass grafts.

It is not really diagnostic to exercise or perform a hyperemic test on any patient who has an abnormal resting study, especially if moderate to severe occlusive disease is obviously present by waveforms and ankle-brachial index. Doing stress procedures in these cases can cause further discomfort to the patient, and a majority of patients almost always cannot tolerate or complete the exam.

There are other methods of hyperemic and treadmill test-

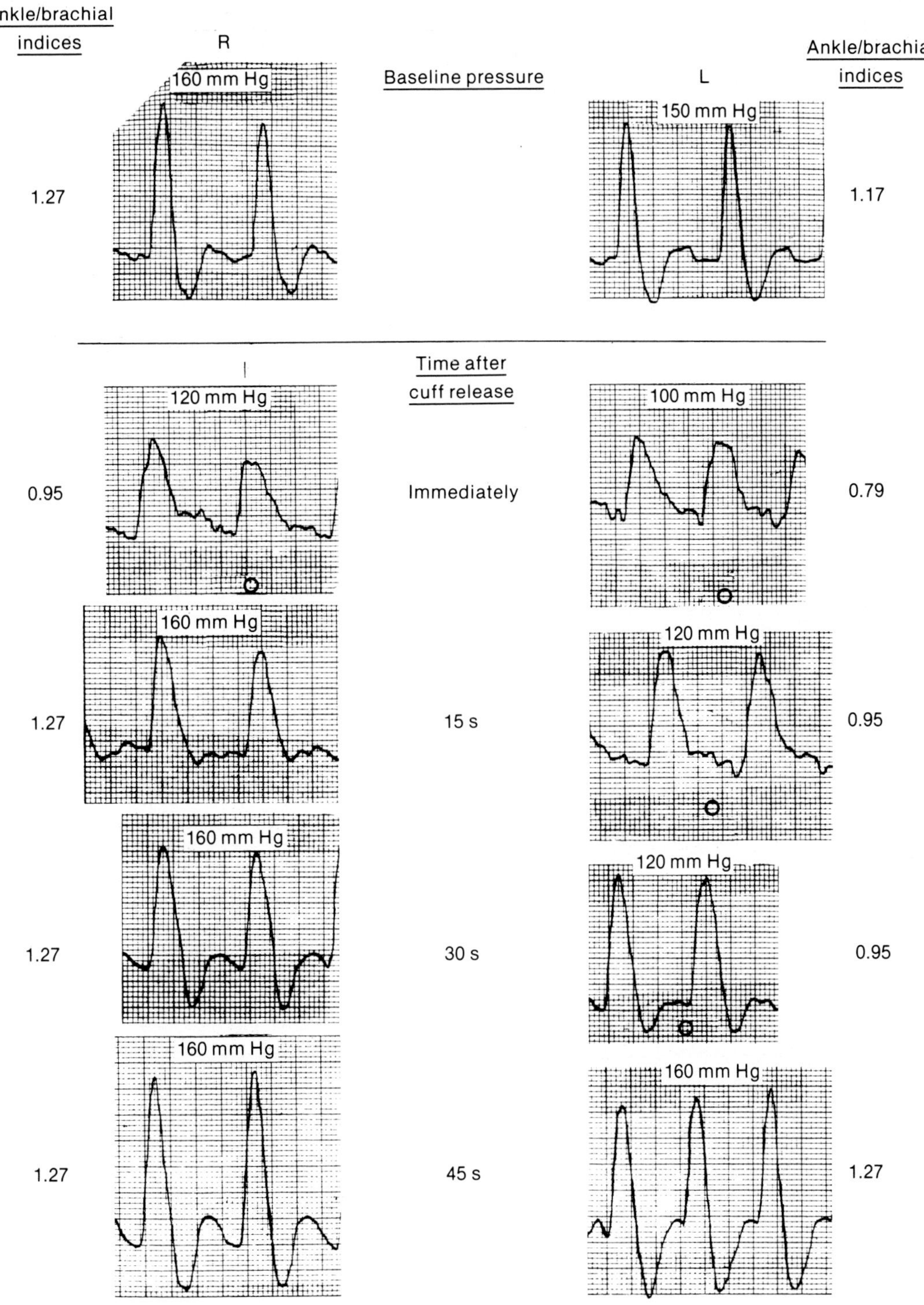

FIG. 20-63 Normal postocclusive hyperemia study.

ing as well as studies that have used treadles pumped by the patient in a supine position. However, the results are similar to those reported.[1,14]

Hyperemia Cases. Both patients in the following examples had normal waveforms and indices at rest but claudication complaints.

Case 1 (Fig. 20-63): Normal. As can be seen at the top of Fig. 20-63, the resting posterior tibial artery signals are triphasic and normal, with baseline indices of 1.27 on the right and 1.17 on the left. After thigh occlusion and release, waveform progression and baseline pressure values are reached well within 1 minute (45 seconds bilaterally). Immediate indices are within normal limits of 0.95 and 0.79, respectively.

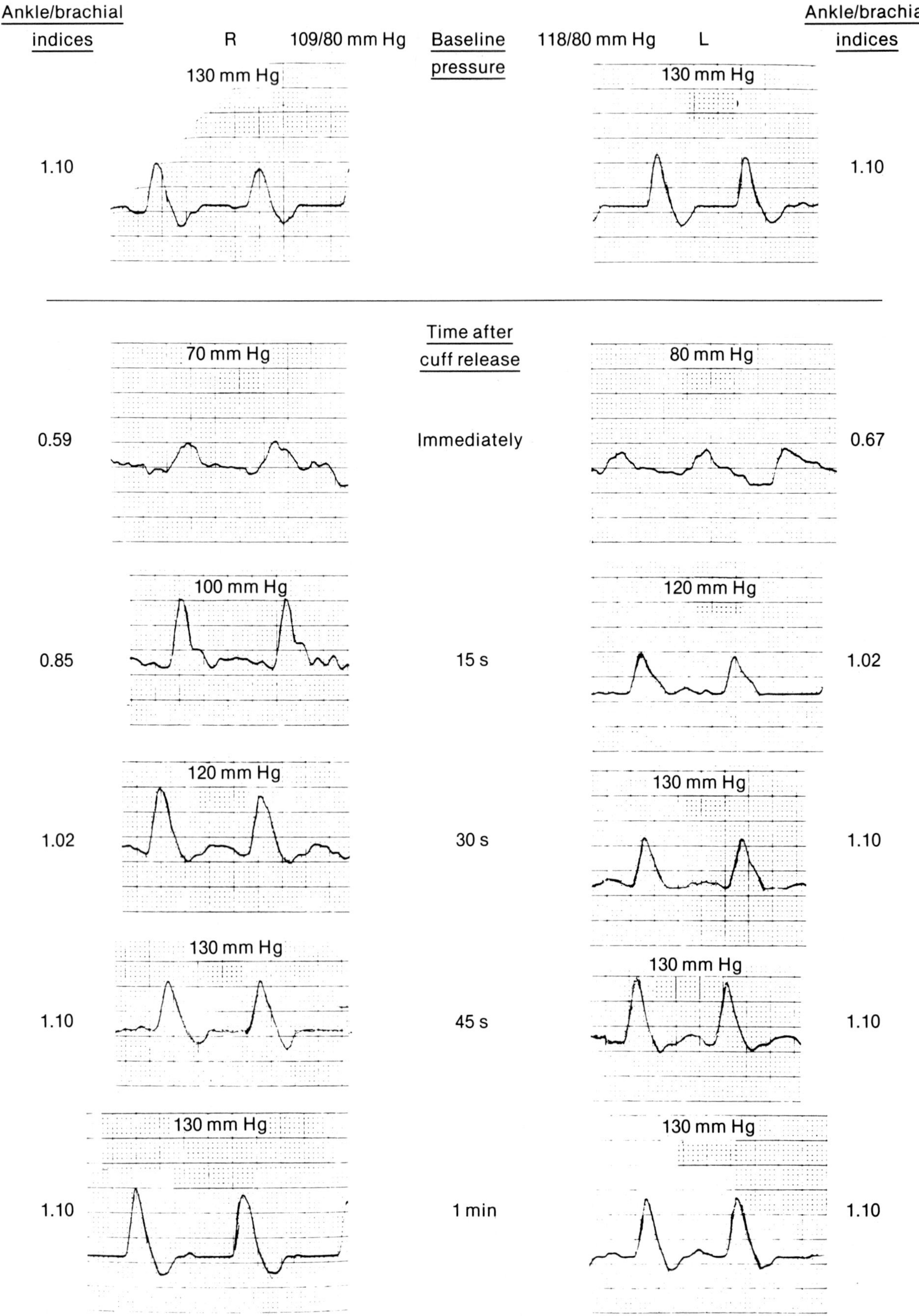

FIG. 20-64 Abnormal postocclusive hyperemia study (see indices on the right).

Case 2 (Fig. 20-64): Abnormal. Again, the resting signals are triphasic and baseline indices are within normal limits (1.1).

After thigh occlusion and release, the waveform progressions and baseline pressures are again achieved within 1 minute. The left posterior tibial signal in this case recovers after hyperemia much more quickly (30 seconds), whereas the left does not achieve the baseline index until 45 seconds. Indices immediately after cuff release are, however, abnormal: 0.59 on the right, 0.67 on the left. Immediate waveforms also indicate a slower response than those in the normal case.

DOPPLER PENILE BLOOD FLOW TEST

Recently studies have been undertaken to show that impotence is not always psychologic but is often physical in nature. Tests have shown that many patients with arteriosclerotic vascular disease present with reduced or nonexistent sexual function. Doppler has been a great aid in the noninvasive diagnosis of physical impotence resulting from impaired blood flow.

Blood to the penis comes from the right and left cavernosal (profunda) arteries, the right and left dorsal arteries, and the right and left spongiosal arteries. These branches of the internal pudendal arteries arise from their respective internal iliac arteries [11,15] (Fig. 20-65).

The dorsal arteries have no part in the erectile function and lie superficially on the dorsum of the penis.[15] The cavernosal arteries run through the center of their respective corpora cavernosa. During sexual arousal, if either or both arteries are occluded, a reduced amount of blood pools in the corpus and erection of the occluded sides does not occur. Lopsided erections result.

The penile Doppler examination begins with a history obtained as in the lower-extremity examination, with attention paid to claudication and arterial insufficiency symptoms. Buttock cramping is often a sign of internal iliac occlusion.

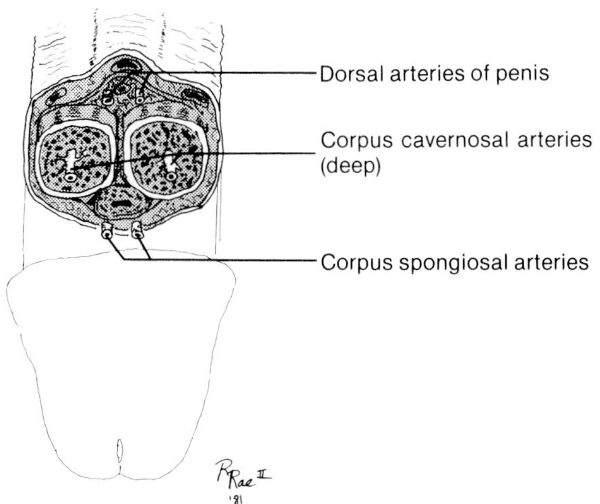

FIG. 20-65 Arterial blood supply to the penis.

Next, a specific set of questions is asked pertaining to the patient's impotence.[15]

1. Is he able to obtain and maintain erections, and are they full or partial?
2. Do positional changes or activity cause a loss of function?
3. How long has the dysfunction been occurring, especially if it coincides with the onset of claudication?
4. Does erection occur on waking up, and does it disappear with urination?
5. Does he have spontaneous nocturnal erections?
6. How is his libido?
7. Is he able to ejaculate?
8. Is there a history of diabetes? What about alcohol intake? What medications is he presently taking?
9. Has he had any testosterone therapy, and if so, how long and what effect did it have?
10. Has he ever had any kind of back injury or possible neurologic damage?
11. Has he ever had a vasectomy or a trans urethral resection (TUR) of the prostate?

The patient first should receive a routine arterial lower-extremity Doppler examination to determine the state of his limb circulation, especially concentrating on the iliofemoral region, since the internal iliacs may also be affected if this area is diseased.

When the lower-extremity examination is completed, a small digit cuff is placed around the base of the penis. It should be strong enough to withstand pressures greater than 250 mm Hg and have extra-strong Velcro fastenings to prevent its coming undone. A regular manometer is used with the cuff.

For purposes of hygiene the examiner should wear rubber gloves during the examination. Gel is applied to the probe sites, and the vessels are monitored.

The cavernosal vessels are examined close to the glans of the penis bilaterally (Fig. 20-66). When an adequate tracing is obtained, the cuff is slowly inflated to the point at which the signal is obliterated. (Be careful not to inflate the cuff too far beyond this point to avoid unnecessary discomfort to the patient and avoid overstressing the cuff.) The examiner should slowly deflate the cuff and note the point where the systolic component returns. This is done three times, and the pressure is obtained by averaging the three readings.

The dorsal arteries may next be examined by checking their sites carefully on the dorsum of the penis. Pressures are taken as with the cavernosal arteries. It should be reiterated that the dorsal arteries are not involved in the erection mechanism and are not diagnostic in determining vasculogenic impotence.[11,15] Flow decrease in these arteries should not be considered significant if the cavernosal arteries are patent and show good pressure indices.

In addition to the Doppler procedure described, color-

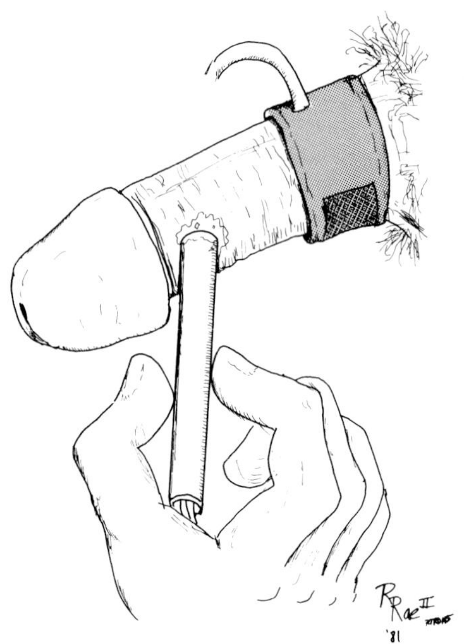

FIG. 20-66 Doppler examination of the cavernosal arteries.

flow imaging and duplex sonography have been used increasingly in some institutions since they provide an effective means of visually evaluating flow in the cavernosal arteries; the procedure involves tourniquet placement around the base of the penis and injections of papaverine directly into the cavernosa to create a pseudoerection. Flow and patency of the cavernosa arteries can thus be directly visualized and sampled with spectral pulsed Doppler, and areas of insufficiency or decreased flow can be appropriately evaluated.

Interpretation of the Penile Examination

A penile-brachial index is obtained by dividing the systolic brachial pressure into the averaged pressure for each artery. On the basis of studies performed by various vascular laboratories, an index of less than 0.86 implies vascular impotence, with indices of less than 0.60 diagnostic or adrenal obstruction.[15] Current studies also show that a variety of normal waveforms exist in the penile arteries and that monophasic and biphasic waveforms should not be automatically interpreted as diseased. However, there is usually a noticeably diminished signal strength on a stenosed side and a significant pressure drop. Both factors can help confirm a suspected vascular problem in the cavernosal arteries.

Penile Cases

Case 1 (Fig. 20-67): Unilateral pudendal or cavernosal artery stenosis, severe. This 39-year-old man complained of lopsided erections, with the left side of the penis remaining flaccid but normal erectile qualities on the right. No equality had been obtained at any time for 1 year. He had no claudication symptoms.

The ankle-brachial index was 1.08 bilaterally; the penile-brachial indices were 1.28 on the right and 0.61 on the left. Normal brachial artery signals were obtained, with a pressure of 130/80 on the right and 120/80 on the left. Normal femoral, popliteal, and posterior tibial signals were also obtained. There may or may not have been anterior tibial disease, for the dorsalis pedis signals were not well heard. In light of the other tracings the dorsal pedal signals were not considered abnormal. Normal pressure gradients were obtained bilaterally.

The penile study showed normal antegrade flow in the right cavernosal artery, with a pressure of 180. The left cavernosal, however, showed some diminishing of the second component and a pressure of only 80. This implied a left internal iliac or pudendal artery stenosis.

It is not known whether any surgical correction was performed.

Case 2 (Fig. 20-68): Bilateral internal iliac and/or cavernosal artery stenosis. This patient presented with a long history of impotency and had documented internal iliac stenoses by arteriography. Percutaneous transluminal angioplasty of the lesions had been performed, but the patient's impotence had not resolved.

The normal lower-extremity examination on this patient is case 1 under the arterial lower extremity cases. His penile flow test shows monophasic waveforms with cavernosal indices of 0.55 bilaterally, well below the normal value of 0.86.

EVALUATION OF IATROGENIC ARTERIAL INJURIES

A very common complication that can occur after any vascular radiologic procedure involving catheterization is the formation of pseudoaneurysms (false aneurysms) or acquired arteriovenous fistulas. These occur because of an incomplete seal of the arteriotomy or venotomy. Inadequate duration of pressure sometimes prevents a seal, or occasionally the arteriotomy reopens. Sometimes both the arterial and venous lines have been pulled simultaneously during cardiac catheterization, enabling a tract to form between the adjacent artery and vein. Pseudoaneurysms also can occur at anastomotic sites of bypass grafts where part of the graft anastomosis becomes detached from the native artery.

Pseudoaneurysms appear sonographically as small or large pulsatile areas anterior to the native artery (commonly the femoral or superficial femoral artery in catheterization cases). Usually a visible tract can be identified linking the mass to the artery. The outer margins of pseudoaneurysms may have thrombus surrounding a false lumen that contains pulsatile, swirling flow; color-flow imaging shows the hemodynamics of these structures in amazing detail. Note that in many cases hematomas may be found that are not pseudoaneurysms; these can be identified as such because of the absence of a visible tract and of pulsatile flow within them. The characteristics and examples of arteriovenous fistulas resulting from this type of injury are described next (see Arteriovenous Fistulas, p. 527).

Examination Techniques. The techniques for examin-

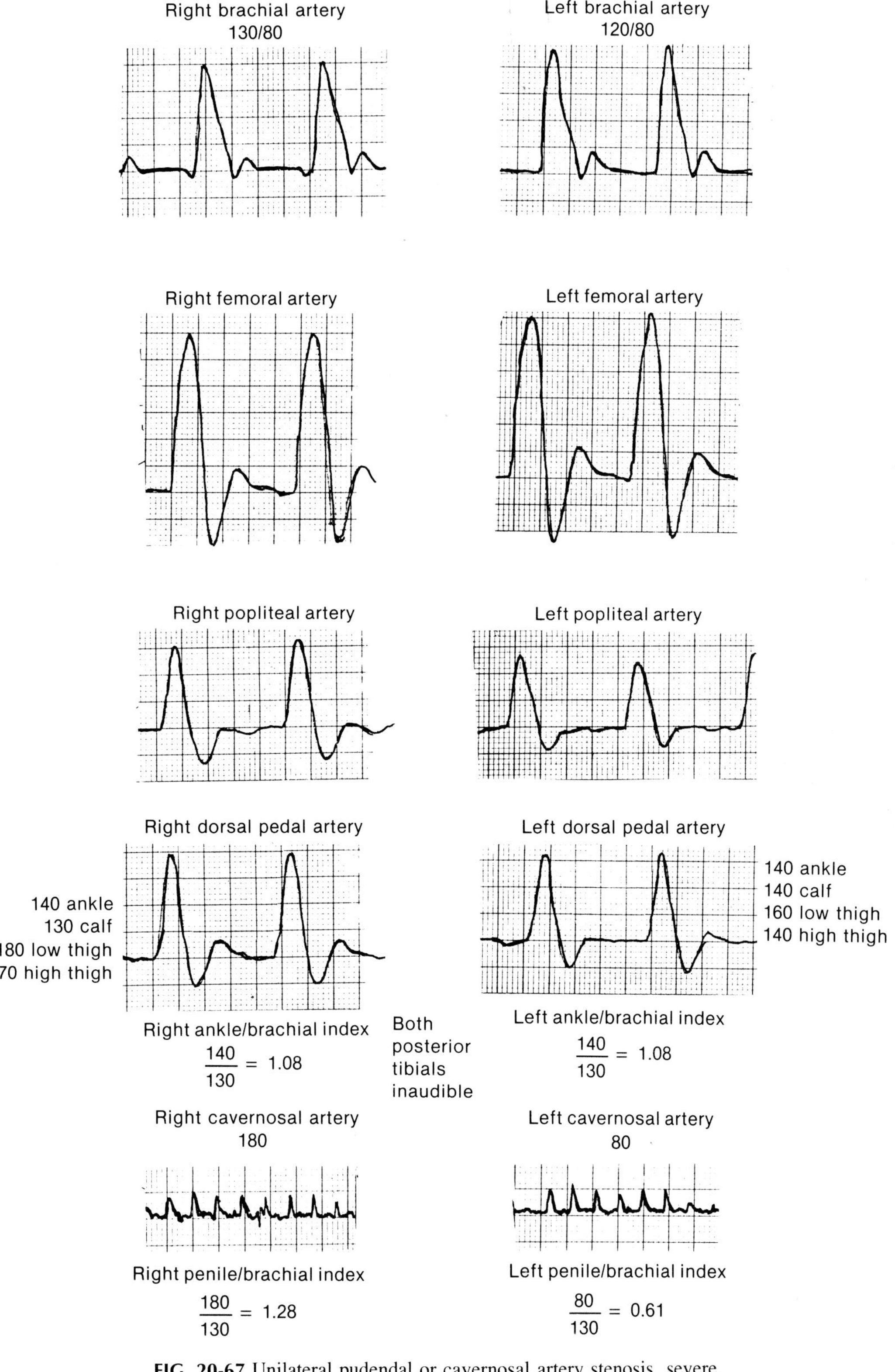

FIG. 20-67 Unilateral pudendal or cavernosal artery stenosis, severe.

ing areas of suspected pseudoaneurysm or fistula formation are basically the same as those described in Arterial Duplex Sonography on p. 492.

Before scanning, the examiner should palpate the pulsatile mass and determine where it lies in relation to the inguinal ligament. Any areas of excessive ecchymosis into the leg tissues should be noted. Any palpable thrills should be identified and bruits should be localized using a stethoscope. The date of any catheterization procedures, the length of time the patient has had the noticeable discom-

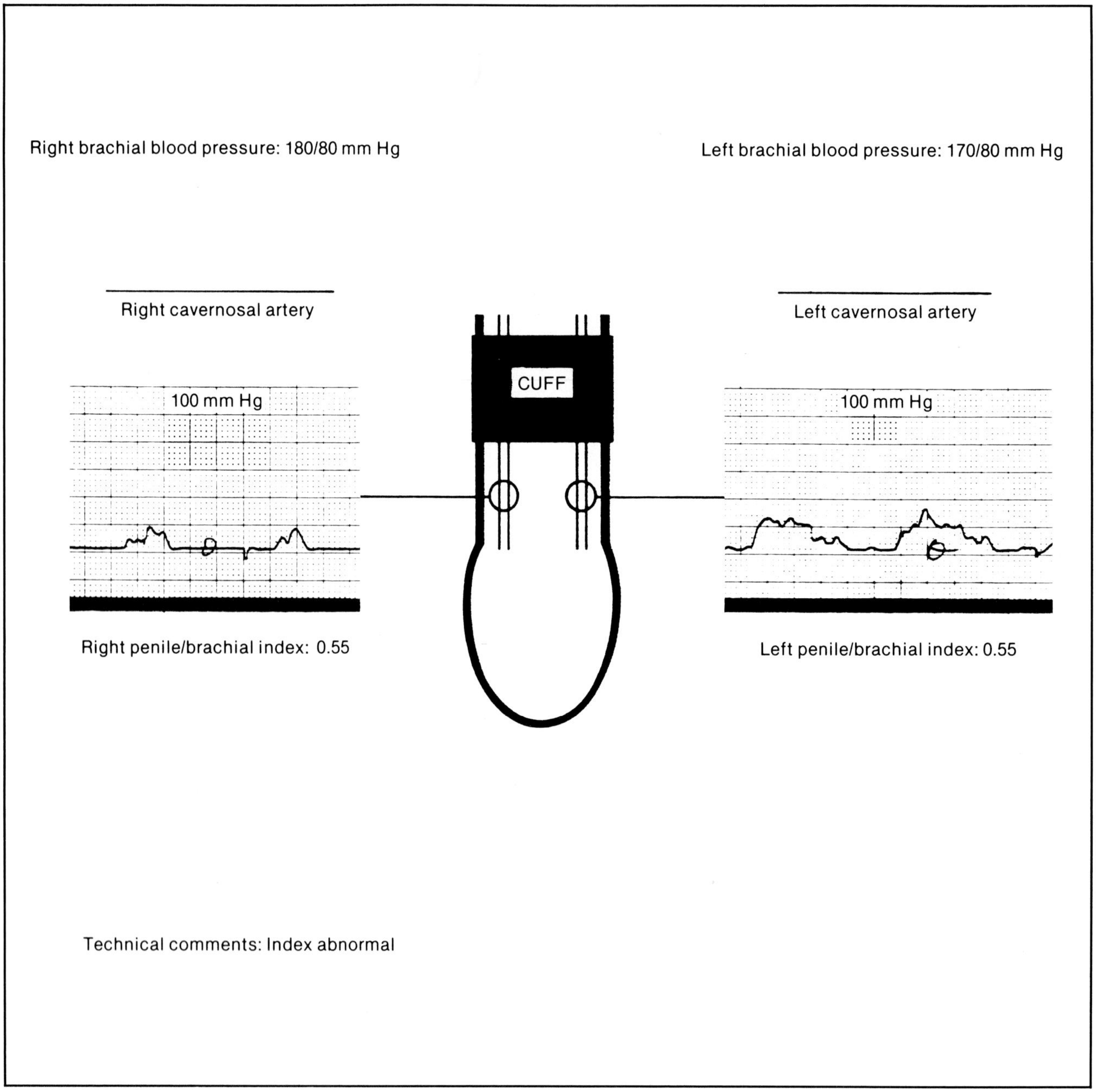

Right brachial blood pressure: 180/80 mm Hg

Left brachial blood pressure: 170/80 mm Hg

Right cavernosal artery

Left cavernosal artery

CUFF

100 mm Hg

100 mm Hg

Right penile/brachial index: 0.55

Left penile/brachial index: 0.55

Technical comments: Index abnormal

FIG. 20-68 Bilateral internal iliac or cavernosal artery stenosis.

fort, and whether it is perceived to have enlarged over time should be recorded.

The external iliac and common femoral areas should be evaluated with duplex sonography and color-flow imaging as described earlier, with an emphasis on locating any pulsatile areas, their relationship to neighboring vessels, and their extent. The presence of a communicating tract should also be shown. Spectral Doppler waveforms should be obtained in the native artery above and below the tract location and additionally within the pseudoaneurysm tract. The areas should be evaluated in both longitudinal and transverse planes, and caliper measurement should be performed on the mass itself.

Flow Characteristics and Diagnostic Criteria

Pseudoaneurysms have swirling, multicolored flow patterns seen within on color-flow imaging, with flow intensities increasing near the inflow site (Fig. 20-69; see color image). On gray-scale imaging, blood flow within the pseudoaneurysm may be swirling so slowly that blood particle motion may be seen. A high-velocity streamline is usually seen within the tract on color-flow imaging, although tracts can be easily identified on gray-scale imaging as well (Fig. 20-70; see color images).

Doppler spectral patterns in pseudoaneurysm tracts are very distinctive, high-velocity, to-and-fro pulsatile jets (Fig. 20-71; see color image). A sample volume size of be-

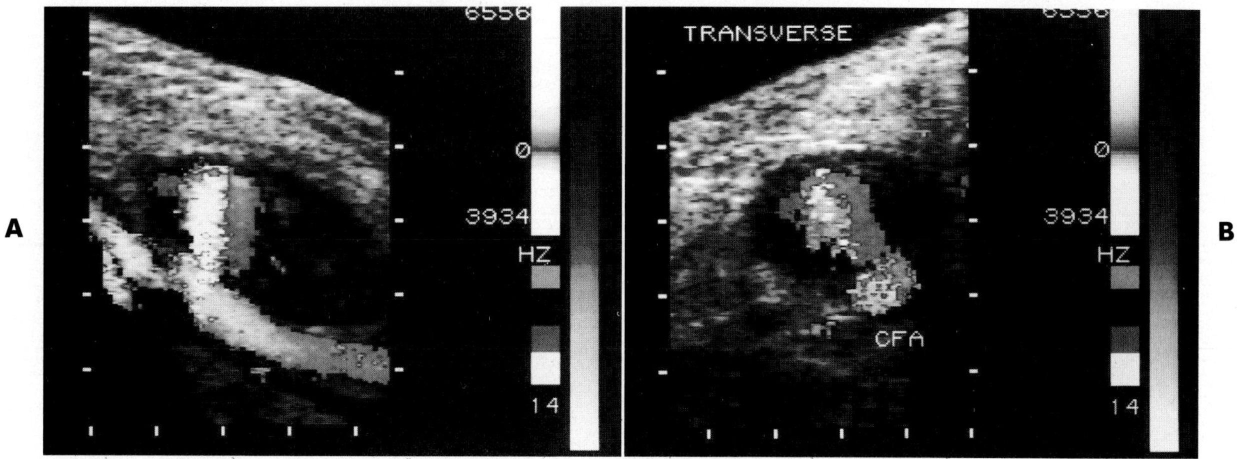

FIG. 20-69 "Swirling" color-flow patterns in a pseudoaneurysm. **A,** In this common femoral artery pseudoaneurysm, an axial jet from the tract is directed toward the transducer (which appears as blue color flow). This subsequently causes multidirectional "swirling" flow in the false lumen, seen more clearly in the transverse view of the same pseudoaneurysm, **B.**

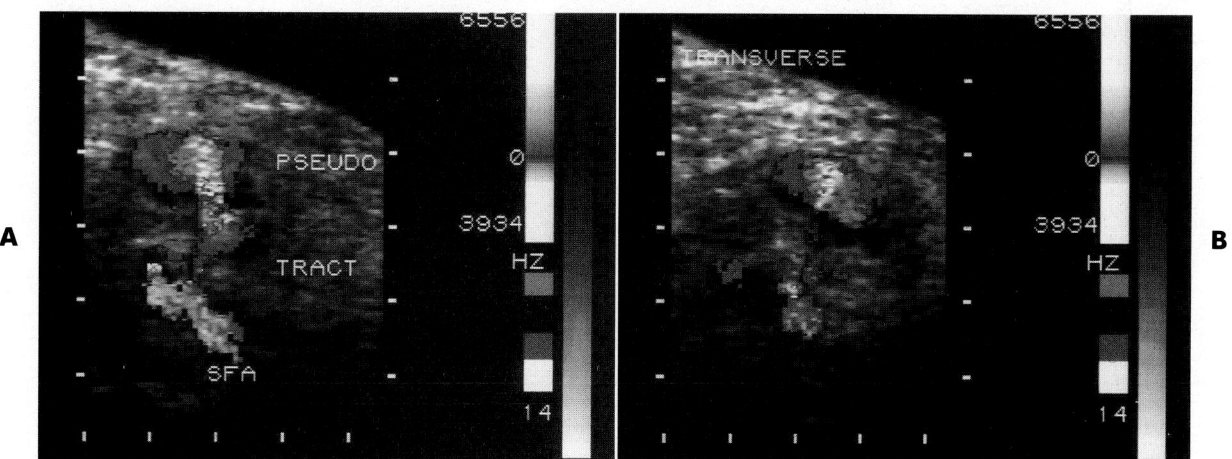

FIG. 20-70 Color-flow appearance of the pseudoaneurysm tract. This superficial femoral artery pseudoaneurysm has a clearly defined tract that can be identified in both the **A,** longitudinal and **B,** transverse planes.

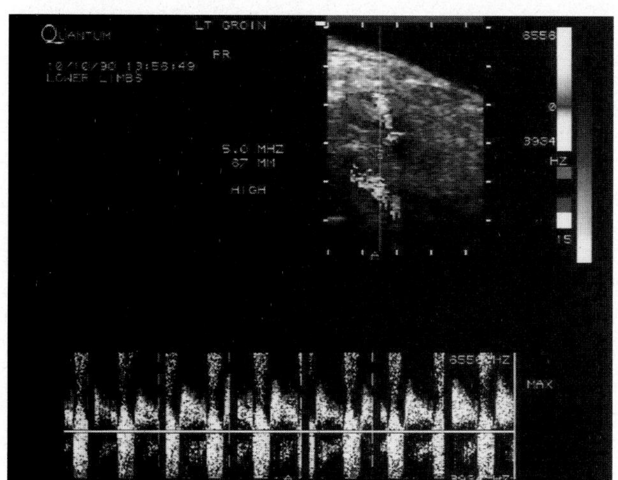

FIG. 20-71 Characteristic bidirectional to-and-fro flow pattern in the tract of the pseudoaneurysm shown in Fig. 20-70.

tween 1 and 2 mm should be adequate for measurement of most tracts. Suspected tracts that lack a back-and-forth pattern and appear as unidirectional arterial patterns are probably small arterial branches and not fistula tracts, which can always be traced to the pseudoaneurysm.

Pseudoaneurysm Case

Case 1 (Fig. 20-72; see color images). Bilateral anastomotic pseudoaneurysm. This 65-year-old patient had a aortobifemoral bypass and a previous occurrence of bilateral anastomotic pseudoaneurysms, which were repaired 7 years later. He presented 8 years later with pulsatile masses in both groins, with the left much larger and more prominent; he had no recent catheterization procedures.

Duplex imaging of the right groin showed a 2.6-cm pseudoaneurysm of the distal anastomosis of the right aortofem-

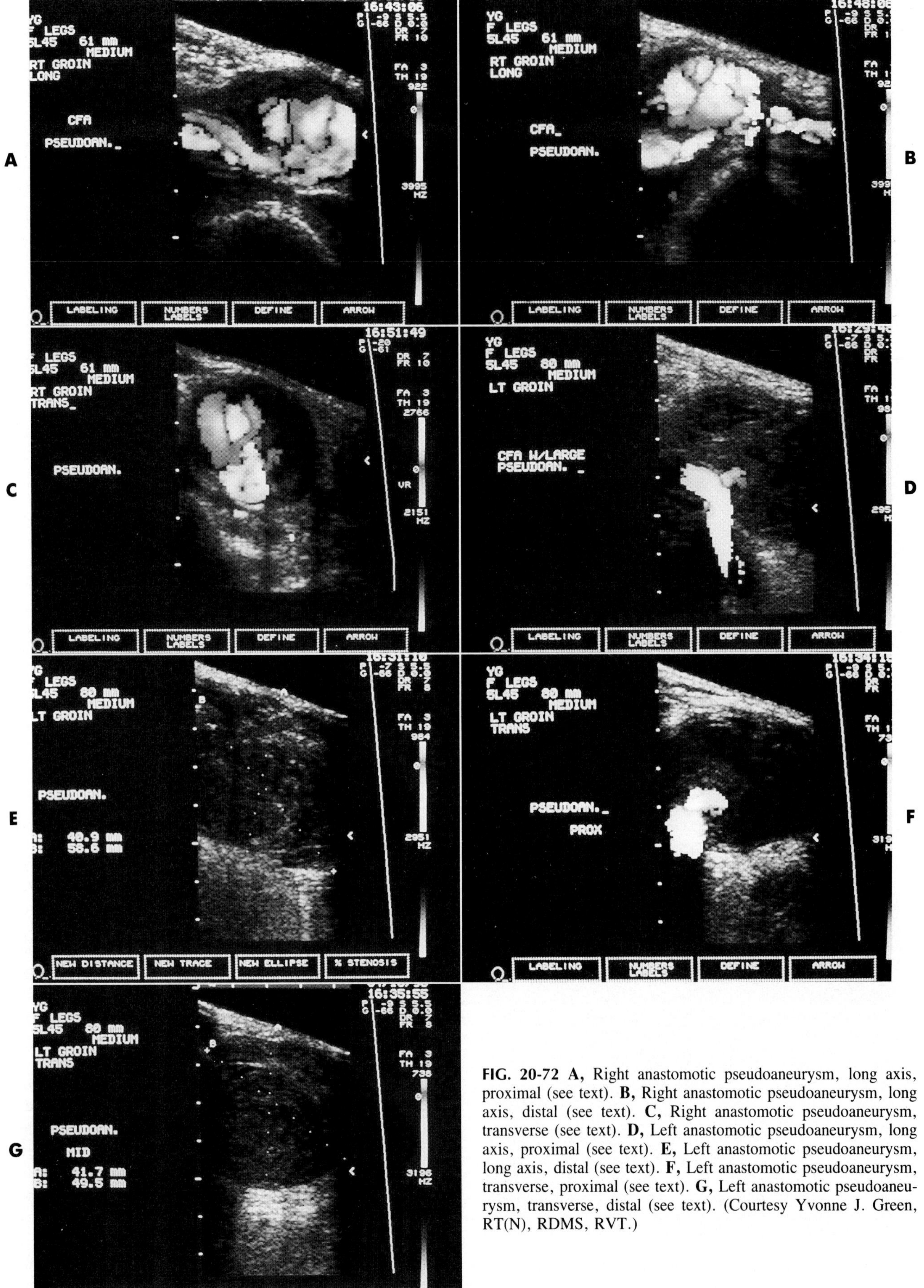

FIG. 20-72 A, Right anastomotic pseudoaneurysm, long axis, proximal (see text). **B,** Right anastomotic pseudoaneurysm, long axis, distal (see text). **C,** Right anastomotic pseudoaneurysm, transverse (see text). **D,** Left anastomotic pseudoaneurysm, long axis, proximal (see text). **E,** Left anastomotic pseudoaneurysm, long axis, distal (see text). **F,** Left anastomotic pseudoaneurysm, transverse, proximal (see text). **G,** Left anastomotic pseudoaneurysm, transverse, distal (see text). (Courtesy Yvonne J. Green, RT(N), RDMS, RVT.)

oral limb and the native common femoral artery (CFA) (*A,to B*). In image *A* the proximal limb of the graft with hematoma can be seen to the left; in *B* the native CFA is seen to the right. In this transverse image *(C)* the laminated thrombus and false lumen are shown.

Duplex imaging of the left groin showed a huge 4.2 × 5.0 × >6.0–cm thrombosed pseudoaneurysm of the distal anastomosis of the left aortofemoral limb and the native CFA. In image *D,* the patent proximal limb of the graft and native CFA are seen, with a small tract marking the point of graft detachment. The size of the pseudoaneurysm precluded it being shown all in one view; following even more distally, *E,* the extended thrombosed lumen continues into the upper thigh. In the transverse plane, *F,* the extent of thrombus and its relationship to the inflow point false lumen are shown proximally. The transverse diameter of the distal segment is shown in *G*.

The patient subsequently had bilateral surgical repair of the pseudoaneurysms and evacuation of the left thrombus collection.

Compression Repair of Pseudoaneurysms

The appearance of a pseudoaneurysm traditionally meant a trip to the operating room for a surgical ligation; this is becoming less frequent nowadays because of the development of ultrasound-guided compression techniques.

Many pseudoaneurysms spontaneously thrombose on their own; others may simply get larger. If a pseudoaneurysm has not thrombosed after a 2-week period, or is symptomatic, compression repair may be attempted as the first stage before surgery.

This procedure involves imaging the pseudoaneurysm, with color flow on. Once the pseudoaneurysm is located, however, the examiner increases pressure with the transducer until the pseudoaneurysm and tract are obliterated without completely occluding the native artery. Pressure is held at this level and the artery monitored in real time for 10 to 15 minutes, then compression is released to see if thrombosis is occurring. If there is still a patent pseudolumen, tract, or both, the compression procedure is repeated at 10- to 15-minute intervals until four to six compression periods have occurred or the pseudoaneurysm or tract has thrombosed and no further flow is identified within. Images should be taken after each compression cycle to document progress.

Special clamps along the lines of C-clamps used in radiology angiographic suites are available that lock around the transducer with a base beneath the patient. Once the pseudoaneurysm has been compressed and the ideal on-screen result achieved, the examiner can tighten several locks, which keeps the transducer in this position and can stop manual compression. This saves the technologist's arms and avoids some of the physical problems described below.

This procedure has met with great success in many institutions, but it has the following drawbacks:

1. It can be very uncomfortable to the patient (unless a mild sedative has been prescribed).
2. It is hard on the arms, wrists, and back of the person performing the compressions, and the transducer can slip off accordingly.
3. The procedure ties up an imaging system and technologist for anywhere from 15 minutes to 2 hours, because constant monitoring is necessary. Evidence of progress may not be attained until after the first two compression cycles.
4. Patients on heparin, warfarin, or other blood-thinning agents may not achieve any measurable level of thrombosis.
5. A flat linear-array transducer must be used; transducers with rounded contact surfaces do not work as well.

Large pseudoaneurysms cannot often be successfully compressed, and those with a narrow visible length of tract often thrombose much more successfully than pseudoaneurysms that arise directly off an opening in the artery wall.

ARTERIOVENOUS FISTULAS

An arteriovenous fistula is an abnormal direct communication between an artery and an adjacent vein. AV fistulas can be either congenital or acquired.[5,20] Congenital arteriovenous fistulas involve multiple communications with arteries and veins in a specific area of the body and are present at birth. Acquired arteriovenous fistulas are localized communications that may have been caused by trauma, aneurysmal erosion, or infection.[5,20]

Arteriovenous fistulas are also classified by size. Microfistulas are too small to be seen with the naked eye. Macrofistulas are readily seen.[5]

Congenital AV Fistulas. The flow dynamics of congenital arteriovenous fistulas are extremely complicated, involving turbulence and cross-channeling of oxygenated and nonoxygenated blood between the two systems (Fig. 20-73). Physical symptoms in the extremities usually consist of swelling, purplish discoloration, prominent varicosities, focal tangled-appearing varicose areas, pallor, palpable thrills and bruits, and pain. The limb may or may not become incapacitated and may develop ischemia, depending on the extent of the fistula.

By using Doppler, duplex sonography, and color-flow imaging, an examiner can map out the major arterial and venous pathways to show areas of increased turbulence and changes in flow dynamics. A characteristic Doppler examination may show signs of turbulence, monophasic and biphasic flow in arteries, retrograde flow in arteries resulting from collaterals and venous connections, absence of flow in a major vessel, pulsatile flow in a vein, and so on. These may occur individually or in combination.

Surgical intervention is almost always required, with amputation often being necessary in severely affected limbs.[20] Because of the extensive network found in patients with congenital arteriovenous fistulas, individual ligation of the site is usually impractical and nearly impossible. Microfistulas pose the biggest problem in this regard. A recent technique that has had varying success is therapeutic emboliza-

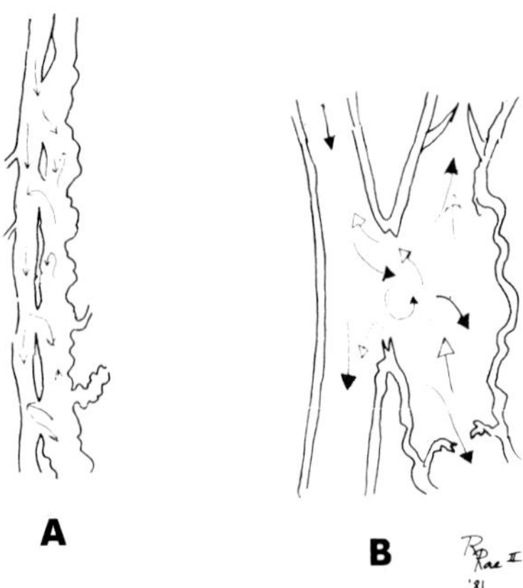

FIG. 20-73 Arteriovenous fistulas. **A,** Multiple connections in a congenital malformation. **B,** Flow dynamics occurring in an AV fistula. Arterial flow *(black arrows)* progresses partly through the arterial segment and partly through the fistula to move either antegrade or retrograde in the vein. The pressure can destroy the valves in the distal venous segment and create insufficiency in the veins. Venous flow *(white arrows)* can also enter the arterial segment and disrupt the flow of oxygenated blood to the distal arterial branches.

tion, which involves injecting a saline solution of tiny sponge balls (Ivalon or other materials) or using microcoils into the main connecting arteries. The suspension travels to the various fistula points and occludes them, sealing many of the more threatening connections and allowing easier ligation or revascularization. The microcoils induce a thrombosis that occludes larger communicating pathways.

Acquired Arteriovenous Fistulas. Arteriovenous fistulas that are acquired occur from trauma or disease processes, as mentioned earlier. Common causes of acquired arteriovenous fistulas include postcatheterization fistula formation, inadvertent puncture of an artery and vein after phlebotomy, and remaining venous branches in an arterialized saphenous vein bypass segment.

One of the first clinical signs of an arteriovenous fistula presence is the bruit or thrill that a physician may notice. Once a patient has been referred for evaluation, it is important that the examiner try to determine a possible cause—recent cardiac catheterization, percutaneous transluminal angioplasty (PTA) or percutaneous transluminal angioplasty (PTCA), arteriogram, in situ bypass surgery, or a similar factor. Duplex sonography and color-flow imaging should be the primary techniques to evaluate these types of fistulas. Imaging methods were described previously (see Arterial Duplex Sonography, p. 492).

With color-flow imaging, an examiner first notices a scattered area of mixed red and blue in the tissues near the bruit site, centering on the actual arteriovenous fistula itself. An area of increased velocity and very turbulent flow marks the tract location, and flow changes are seen in the native artery and vein at the outflow and inflow points along the vessel walls. Arteriovenous fistulas are seldom uniform in appearance and may communicate at lateral or medial walls, as well as anterior and posterior locations. It may be necessary to increase the color and Doppler velocity thresholds to exclude as much of the bruit or thrill scatter as possible. Spectral Doppler waveforms should be obtained in the native artery, the fistula tract, and the native vein. Abnormal arterial flow in the vein may cause local flow disturbances that can be detected and displayed.

Acquired arteriovenous fistulas generally need focal surgical ligation to be repaired. In some cases where the tract is long, ultrasound-guided compression repair procedures can be performed as described previously (see Compression Repair of Pseudoaneurysms, p. 527).

Arteriovenous fistulas are often surgically created in patients for renal dialysis. Unfortunately, these shunts often experience problems, and Doppler and imaging assessment can help localize obstructions, stenoses, defects, hematomas, or other abnormalities. In these shunts, the characteristic turbulence and "hissing" or "burbling" sounds may occur in normal patients; care must be exercised. A beginning vascular technologist can often gain a great deal of experience in learning typical arteriovenous fistula sound and flow patterns by examining a shunt patient.

The general technique for Doppler examination of a patient with suspected or known arteriovenous fistulas varies with the individual. When examining a suspected arteriovenous fistula patient, follow the normal paths of the arteries and veins and look for specific areas of focal turbulence and abnormally high flow velocities. Bear the following criteria in mind:

1. Collateral channels may exist that shunt flow around a fistula and cause retrograde flow in a given segment immediately distal to the fistula.
2. Venous valves become incompetent. Thus flow will be reversed in the venous segment *distal* to the fistula and may mimic arterial flow, whereas it will be continuous in the *proximal* venous segment.
3. Manual occlusion of the fistula causes flow in the distal arterial segment to resume normal characteristics.
4. If the standard Doppler extremity examination is performed, there will be a pressure drop distal to the fistula.

Knowledge of these characteristics facilitates discrimination among arteriovenous fistulas.

Arteriovenous Fistula Cases. The reader may wish to refer to the Upper Extremity Arterial Examination Techniques section below before analyzing the next four cases.

Case 1 (Fig. 20-74): Congenital multiple arteriovenous fistulas in the right arm (normal left arm). This 40-year-old woman had a history of congenital arteriovenous fistulas of the right subclavian, brachial, and radial artery-vein systems. She had also had congestive heart failure because of the flow problems. A macrofistular area was repaired at the elbow level.

At the time of this examination, she had had intermittent pain and swelling in the right hand for 2 weeks. The right arm itself was swollen, with dilated and tortuous superfi-

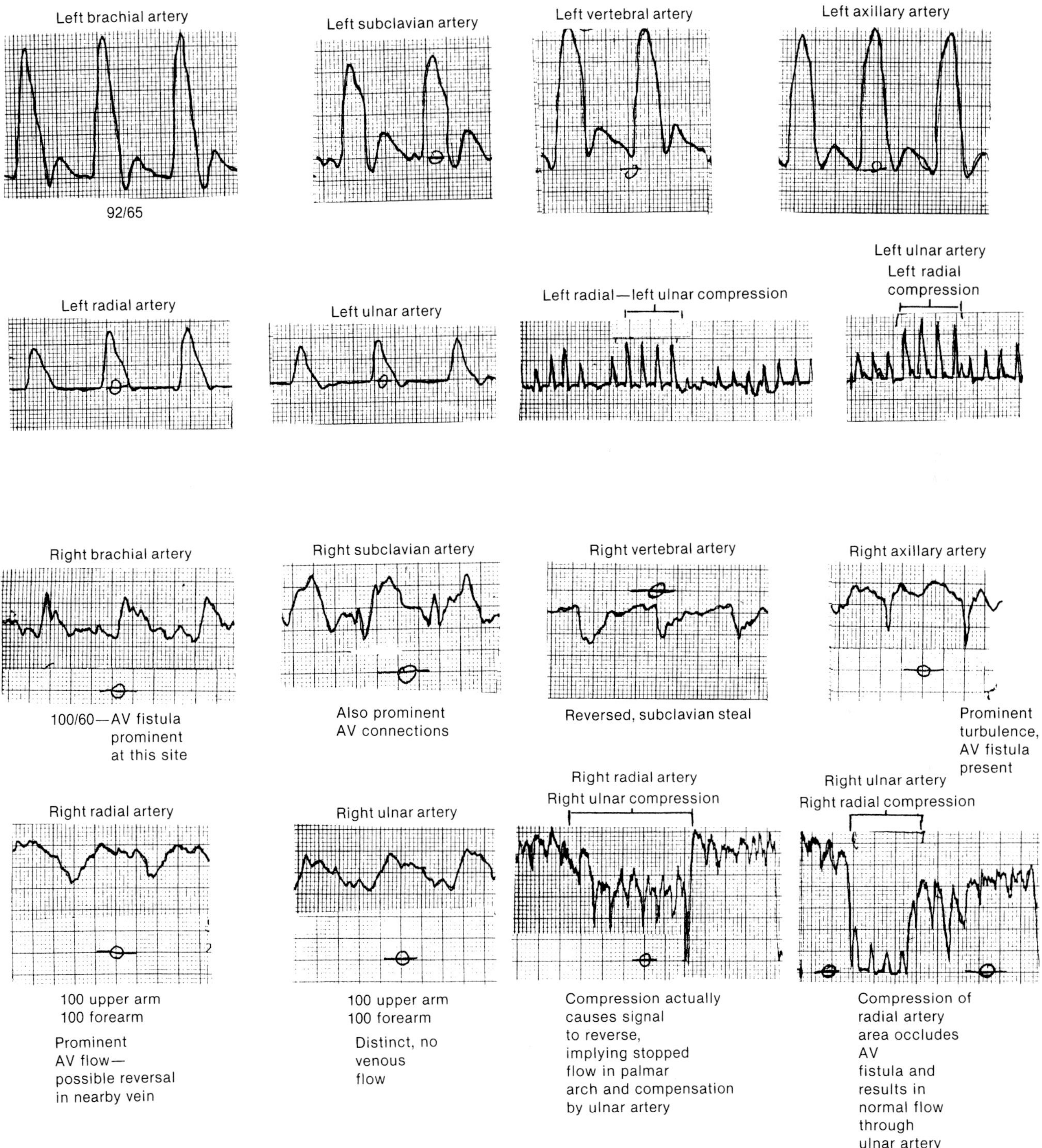

FIG. 20-74 Normal left arm. Abnormal right arm with multiple congenital arteriovenous fistulas.

cial varices, and large purplish-green blotches on the right chest, shoulder, and arm. The hand at the base of the thumb was greatly swollen, and the patient could move her fingers only weakly. Amputation had been declined.

The right forearm-brachial index was 1.00, the left 0.92.

On the left side characteristic normal tracings can be seen at the brachial, subclavian, vertebral, axillary, radial, and ulnar arteries. The compression responses show normal flow through the left palmar arch.

On the right side the brachial shows a prominent signal indicative of obstruction and turbulence. The subclavian signal also shows proximal venous connections reducing the flow. The vertebral shows a subclavian steal present, regardless of the normal blood pressure in the arm. The ax-

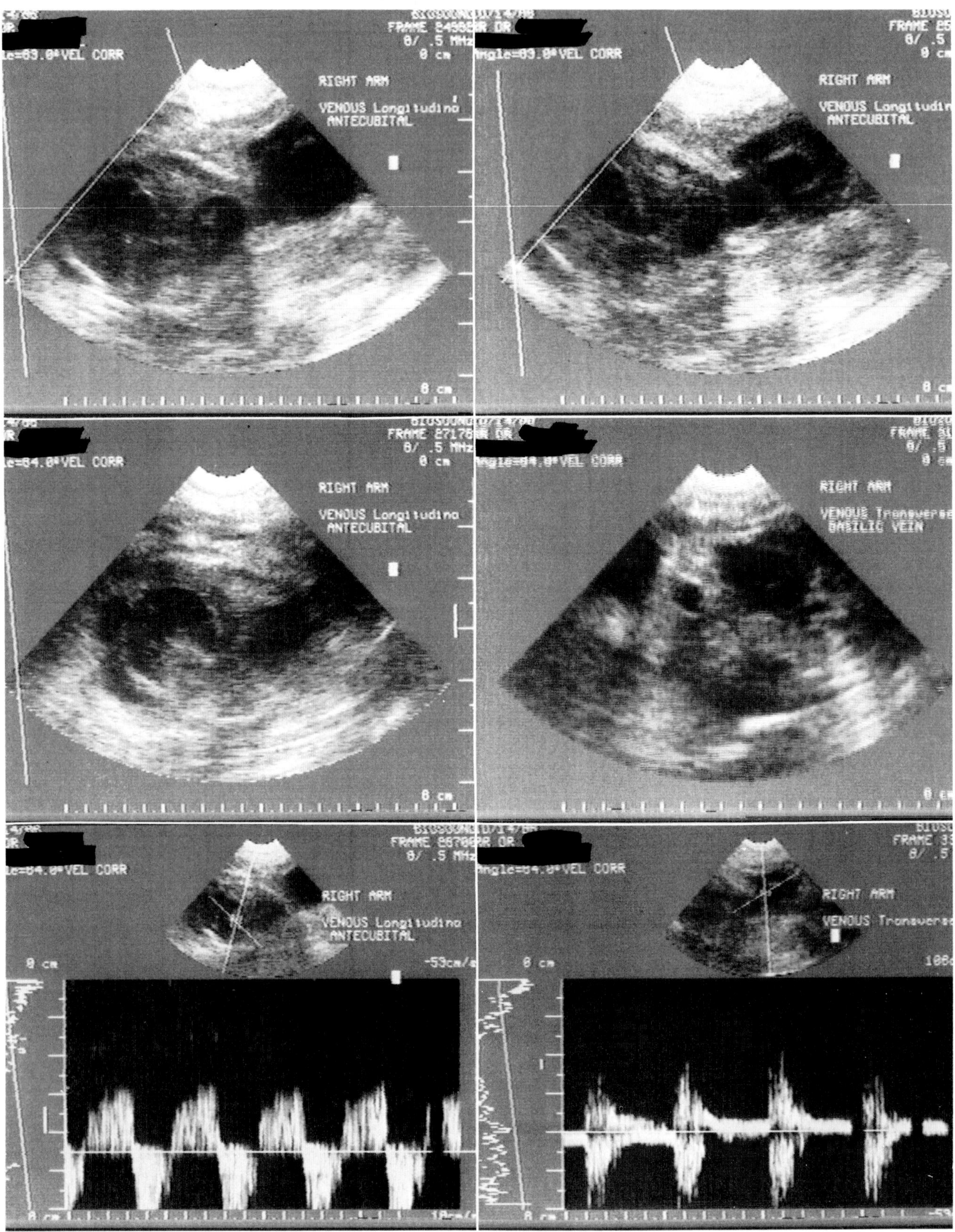

FIG. 20-75 Acquired arteriovenous fistula and pseudoaneurysm.

Continued.

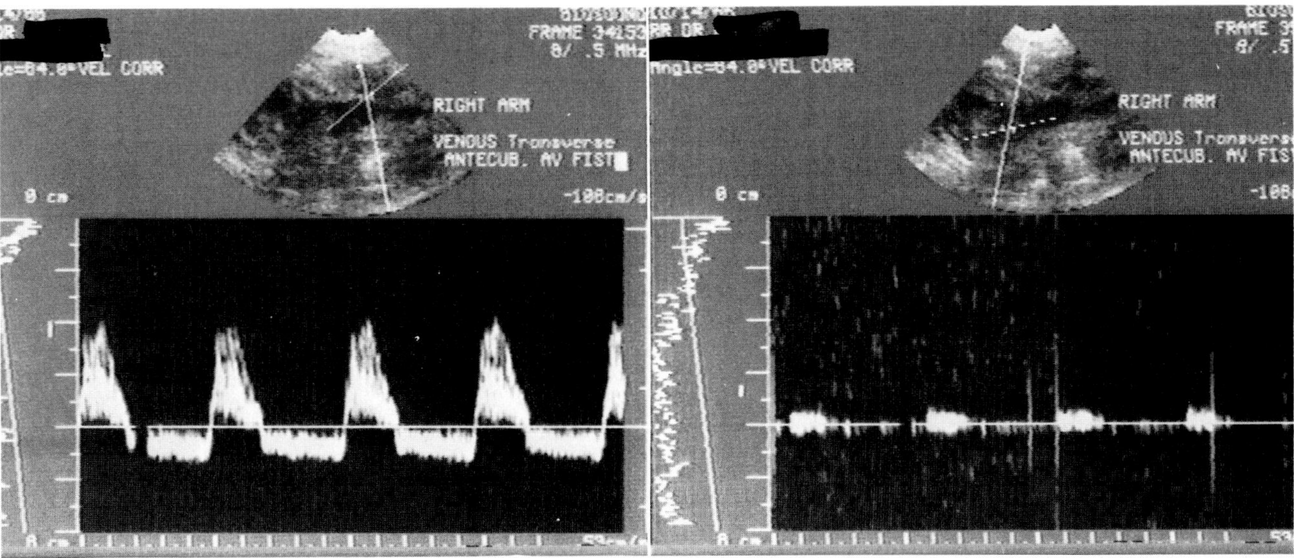

FIG. 20-75 cont'd.

illary artery also has a turbulent signal, showing flow problems. The radial arterial signal was turbulent and difficult to interpret, for reversed flow in the accompanying vein possibly prevented normal flow to the hand. Compression of the ulnar artery resulted in retrograde flow in the artery, implying a prominent arteriovenous connection. The ulnar signal also indicated flow discrepancies, with high-pitched turbulence present. Compression of the radial artery occluded the arteriovenous fistula and resulted in resumption of normal flow through the ulnar artery segment.

At surgery the radial artery was ligated and the arteriovenous fistula and palmar arch injected and blocked with Ivalon sponge solution. The patient's symptoms subsided, and she was released.

Case 2 (Fig. 20-75): Acquired arteriovenous fistula in brachial artery and/or vein. This patient had blood drawn from his right arm 2 days before being examined. He presented with a severely painful right arm, which had a hard, slightly swollen area in the antecubital fossa. Examination with a real time scanner showed a massive acquired arteriovenous malformation with encapsulated hematomas apparently connecting the arterial and venous systems in the antecubital region (*A* to *C*). Flow patterns within the visualized masses showed equally bidirectional flow in the venous components (*E* and *G*) and turbulent flow in the arterial components (*F* and *H*). Because of the complexity of the malformation it was difficult to establish which vessels were actually involved, although a definite uninvolved vein was traceable between the masses *(D)*. An arteriogram confirmed that the brachial and basilic veins were involved and that the formation had been apparently caused by the phlebotomy needle penetrating both the artery and vein in that area.

Case 3 (Fig. 20-76; see color images): Congenital upper extremity arteriovenous malformation. This 15-year-old patient presented with a progressively enlarging pulsatile mass in the left supraclavicular area bordering on the anterior shoulder. A bruit was noted over this area and a faint thrill could be palpated. Color-flow duplex imaging of this area revealed a large aneurysmal arteriovenous fistula with feeding arterial branches from the subclavian artery and venous branches that could be traced back to the subclavian artery and venous branches that could be traced back to the subclavian vein. *A* shows the aneurysmal region with a collateral branch in a sagittal plane, and *B* shows the same area from a transverse angle. The fistula branches can be identified near the aneurysm and the typical turbulent bruit or thrill color-flow pattern can be seen surrounding the involved vessels. Swirling, disturbed flow is seen within the vascular structures.

A subclavian arteriogram indicated that the fistula involved branches of the ascending cervical artery and collaterals from the internal mammary artery, which formed a fistula communication with venous branches of the subclavian vein. The arterial feeding branches were embolized with Hilal mini- and microcoils of varying sizes; the venous branches could not be embolized because a valve in the subclavian vein prevented passage of the catheter. Nevertheless, a good thrombosis result was obtained with the exception of the venous collaterals, *C, D*. Compare the postembolization image in *C* with the preembolization view in *A*, and the postembolization image in *D* with the preembolization view in *B*.

Case 4 (Fig. 20-77; see color images): Acquired lower-extremity arteriovenous fistula. This 54-year-old patient was referred approximately 1 month after having had a cor-

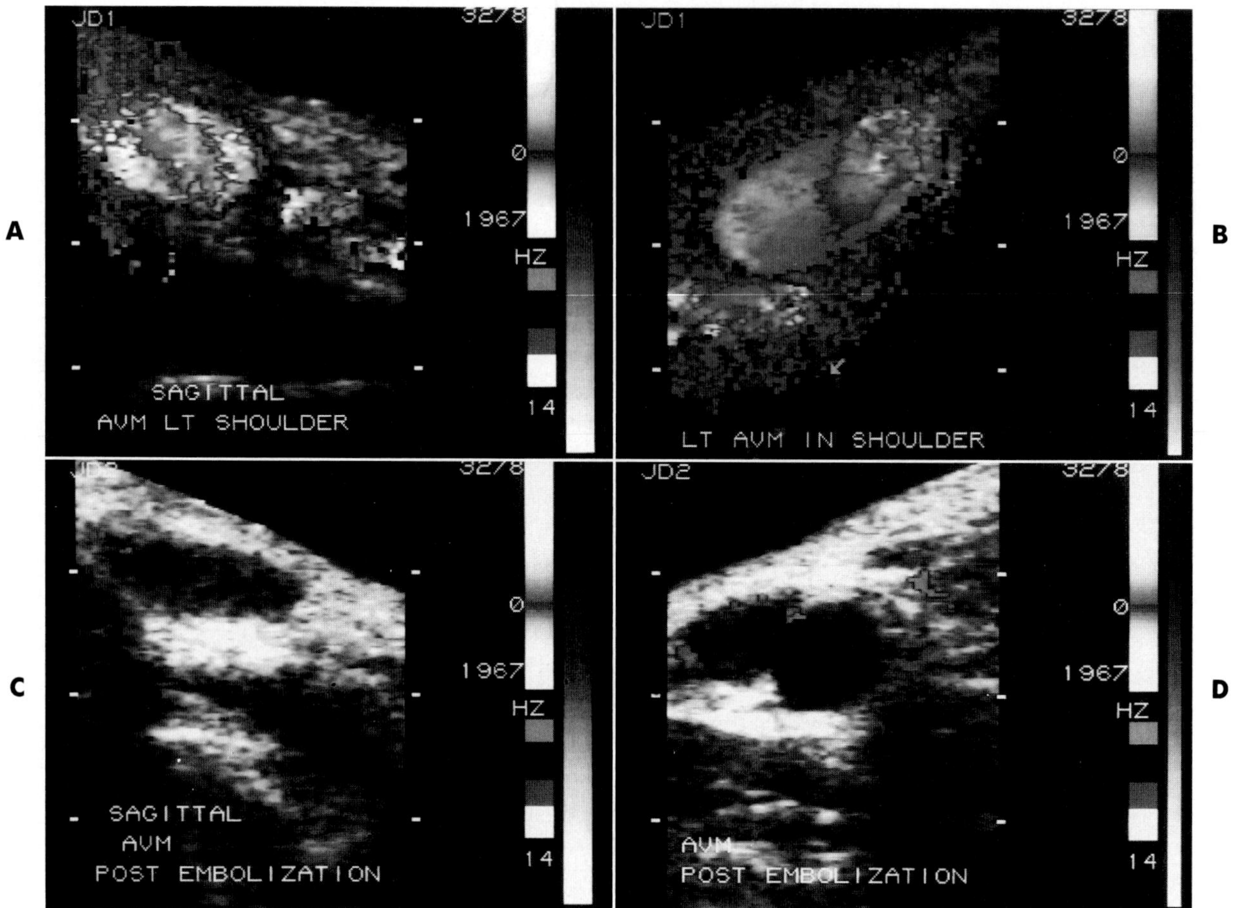

FIG. 20-76 A, Upper-extremity arteriovenous fistula, aneurysmal fistula and branches, sagittal plane (see text). **B,** Upper-extremity arteriovenous fistula, aneurysmal fistula and branches, transverse plane (see text). **C,** Upper-extremity arteriovenous fistula, aneurysmal fistula and branches, sagittal plane, postembolization (see text). **D,** Upper-extremity arteriovenous fistula, aneurysmal fistula and branches, transverse plane, postembolization (see text).

onary angioplasty procedure. Although he was asymptomatic, his cardiologist had noted a pitched, harmonic bruit in the right groin. Duplex examination revealed an arteriovenous fistula near the catheterization site. Longitudinal imaging of the origin of the superficial femoral artery bifurcation *(A)* showed mildly disturbed flow in the proximal segment; a Doppler signal taken in the superficial femoral artery (SFA) distal to the fistula origin *(B)* showed triphasic flow with evidence of a color-flow thrill scatter in the tissues nearby. Medial motion of the transducer in the long axis *(C)* revealed the tract communicating between the SFA and the common femoral vein (CFV). Doppler spectral flow patterns within the tract were typically disturbed and of high velocity at the insertion into the CFV *(D)*. High-velocity arterialized disturbed flow was also present in the CFV proximal to the fistula insertion *(E)*.

Transverse imaging shows the tortuous fistula with its associated bruit pattern and its relationship to the SFA and CFV *(F)*. Doppler signals are easier to obtain in these fistulas in transverse imaging *(G)*, and again a high-velocity turbulent signal was obtained.

The fistula was subsequently surgically ligated.

UPPER-EXTREMITY ARTERIAL EXAMINATION TECHNIQUES

Evaluation of the upper-extremity arteries differs little from the examination in the lower extremities; the same Doppler, segmental pressure, plethysmographic, and duplex sonography techniques can be used with similar diagnostic criteria. The specifics of upper-extremity evaluation are covered in some detail here. Upper-extremity examinations are performed less often in general vascular laboratories than are lower-extremity studies, but there are subtleties in technique and diagnoses of conditions unique to the arms and hands that all vascular technologists and sonographers should know. Some of the techniques and conditions described here also have a bearing on the cerebrovas-

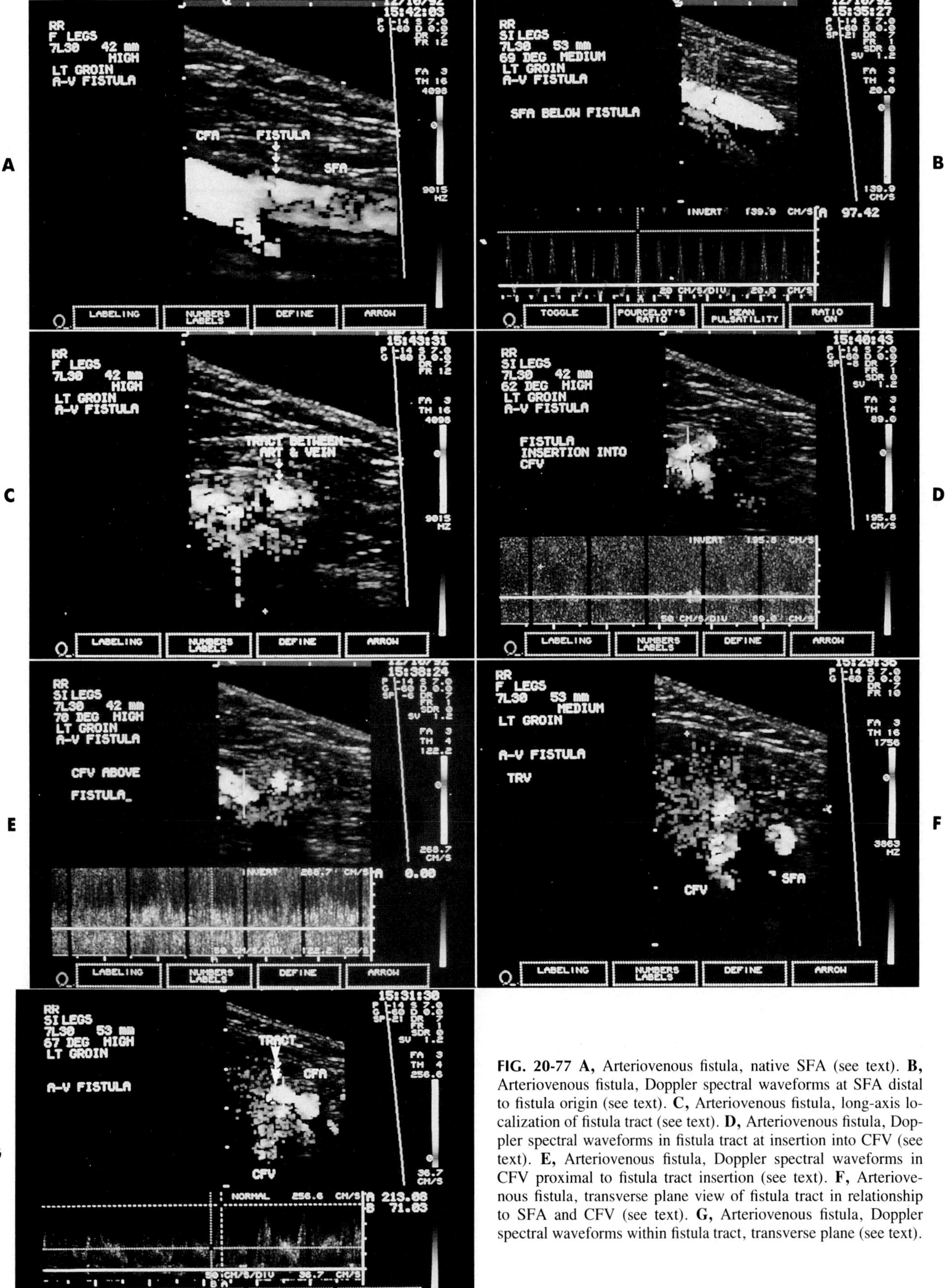

FIG. 20-77 **A,** Arteriovenous fistula, native SFA (see text). **B,** Arteriovenous fistula, Doppler spectral waveforms at SFA distal to fistula origin (see text). **C,** Arteriovenous fistula, long-axis localization of fistula tract (see text). **D,** Arteriovenous fistula, Doppler spectral waveforms in fistula tract at insertion into CFV (see text). **E,** Arteriovenous fistula, Doppler spectral waveforms in CFV proximal to fistula tract insertion (see text). **F,** Arteriovenous fistula, transverse plane view of fistula tract in relationship to SFA and CFV (see text). **G,** Arteriovenous fistula, Doppler spectral waveforms within fistula tract, transverse plane (see text).

cular evaluation, and the examiner should be aware of those appropriate relationships.

Arterial Anatomy of the Upper Extremities[11]

This section covers Doppler-related anatomy in the upper extremity and upper thorax.

The subclavian artery is the first major artery to arise from the aortic arch. It has a different origin on each side. On the right it arises from the brachiocephalic (innominate) artery, and on the left directly from the aortic arch.

The first branch of the subclavian artery is the vertebral artery. Its anatomy is discussed in more detail in the cerebrovascular anatomy section.

Many other arteries are given off between the arch and the shoulder. At the level of the first rib, the subclavian becomes the axillary artery. The axillary artery tends to run superficially through the axilla and then slightly more deeply at the tendon of the teres major. Here it becomes the brachial artery (Fig. 20-78).

The brachial artery runs medially along the arm to the elbow. Approximately 1 cm distal to the elbow, it bifurcates into the radial and ulnar arteries.

These continue on to the wrist on the anterior surface of the arm, the radial on the radial side and the ulnar on the ulnar side. The ulnar artery gives off a medial interosseus branch, which may occasionally be heard between the radial and ulnar. Each artery passes into the hand and terminates at respective radial and ulnar palmar arches, which are connected by collaterals (Fig. 20-79).

BASIC UPPER-EXTREMITY EXAMINATION TECHNIQUES

The same basic primary techniques and instrumentation used for lower-extremity evaluation are applied to the upper extremities.

The first step is again to take a detailed history from the patient and from the chart, with emphasis on upper-extremity occlusive disease. The classic symptoms consist of claudication of the arm that occurs with lifting objects or holding the arms raised over the head for short periods. The afflicted arm also feels colder to the touch than the unobstructed arm, and occasionally numbness and discoloration of the fingers occur. Systolic blood pressures usually show a discrepancy between the two sides. Microembolic activity, digital artery or palmar arch stenosis, or vasospastic phenomena can be suspected in cases of digital discoloration when the rest of the arm is normal. Note should be made also of whether the patient notices discoloration with exposure to cold or temperature changes.[6,14]

A patient with dizziness accompanying the extremity problems can be suspected of having a subclavian steal syndrome. This is always a possibility when there is a pressure difference of greater than 20 to 40 mm Hg between the two arms.[17,21]

After the history is taken, the patient should lie supine on the examination table prior to the examination.

DOPPLER VELOCITY WAVEFORM ANALYSIS

Doppler waveform characteristics in the arms are no different than those in the legs. A triphasic waveform is obtained in a normal individual, and the waveform loses amplitude and the second and third components and deteriorates progressively distal to a stenosis.

As in the lower extremities, the waveforms can be obtained and recorded in any order. An examiner should listen to and record signals from the following vessels, the Doppler and duplex access sites of which are illustrated in Fig. 20-80:

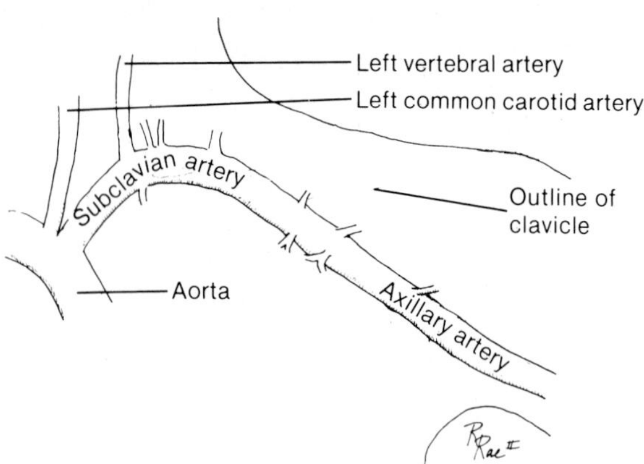

FIG. 20-78 Arteries of the upper extremity from the aorta to the axilla.

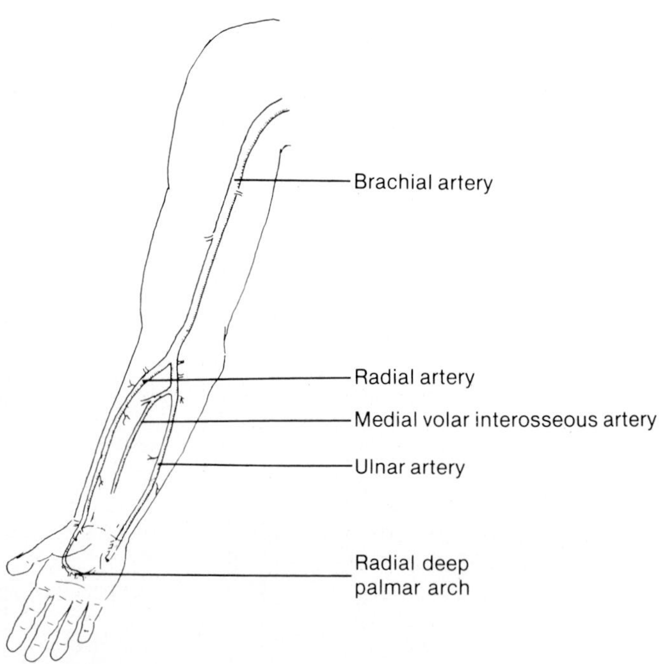

FIG. 20-79 Arteries of the upper extremity from the axilla to the hand.

1. *Both subclavian arteries*. The subclavian artery can be heard by one of two methods. The probe can be placed in the supraclavicular fossa angling medially, slightly anteriorly, and downward (Fig. 20-81, *A*). The probe can also be placed just beneath the clavicle but medial to the shoulder and angled deep, medially, and slightly superiorly toward the clavicle (Fig. 20-81, *B*). A strong triphasic signal should be heard, but slight angle adjustments may have to be made to eliminate venous interference.

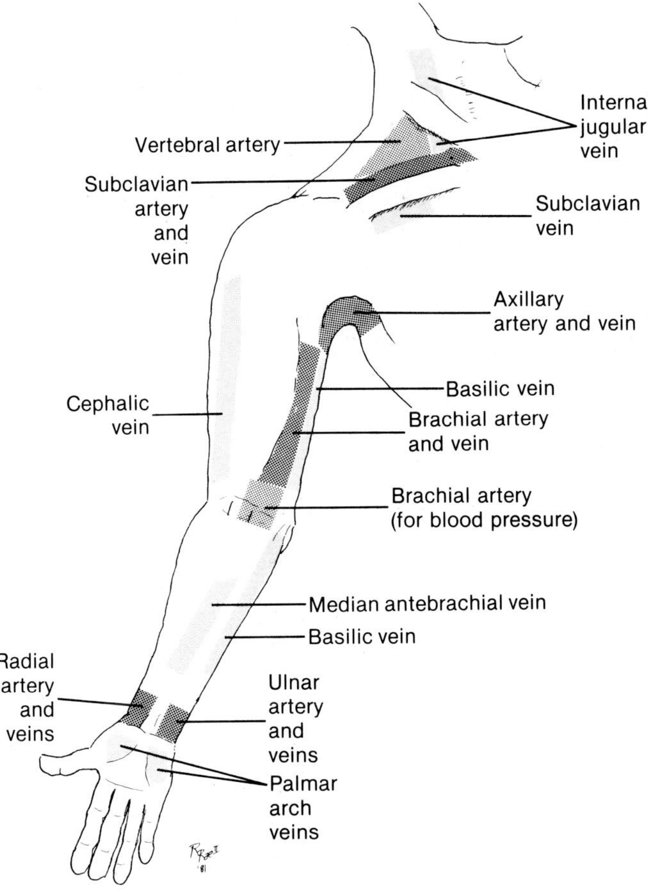

FIG. 20-80 Sites for both arterial and venous examinations of the upper extremity.

2. *Both axillary arteries*. The axillary artery can be best heard by having the patient raise the upper arm and then placing the probe into the axilla, angling medially and cephalad with the probe against the axillary surface of the upper arm (Fig. 20-82). The axillary artery can also be accessed by listening at the fleshy part of the shoulder below the clavicle and shoulder joint, angling the probe medially.
3. *Both brachial arteries*. The brachial artery is heard best in the antecubital fossa, usually on the medial side of the fossa, angling the probe cephalad (Fig. 20-83). Some side-to-side searching may have to be done since the artery location can vary slightly in some individuals.
4. *Both radial arteries*. The radial artery is found on the lateral, or radial, side of the wrist (with the palm turned out in the anatomic position) (Fig. 20-84).
5. *Both ulnar arteries*. The ulnar artery is accessed on the medial, or ulnar, side of the wrist (Fig. 20-85).
6. *The vertebral arteries* should be included in the evaluation when there is an ipsilateral significant blood pressure difference between the two arms (of more than 20 mm Hg), an abnormal (monophasic or biphasic) signal in the subclavian artery on one side, or both. This is important to rule out subclavian steal syndrome and also to determine whether the stenosis is proximal or distal to the vertebral origin. The vertebral arteries can be evaluated with a continuous-wave probe but are most easily examined with a duplex scanner and spectral Doppler (see below). Color-flow imaging is very beneficial because the direction of flow in the vertebral artery and its degree of patency are immediately apparent.

If using a continuous-wave Doppler, place the probe on the proximal neck just above the supraclavicular fossa but just posterior to the sternocleidomastoid muscle (Fig. 20-86). Angling medially and caudally, listen for a distinct low-

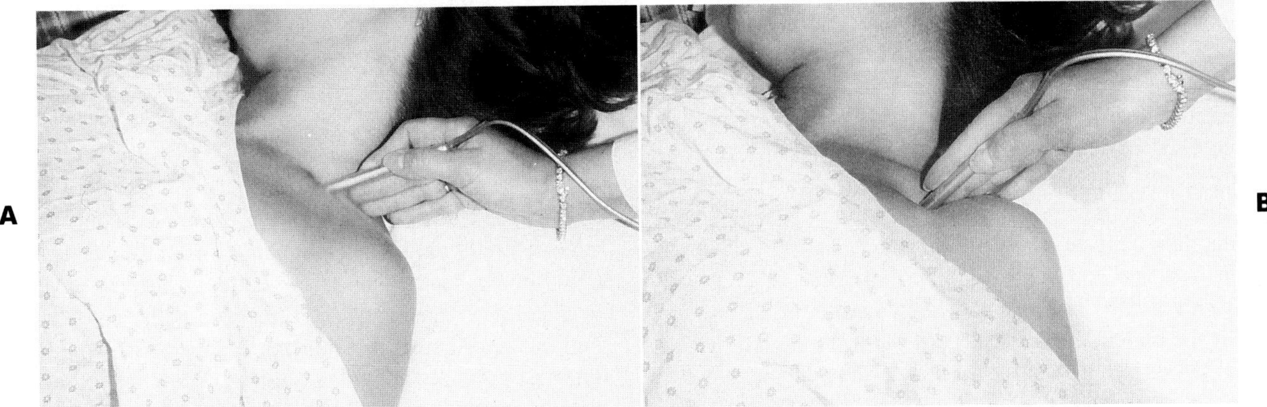

FIG. 20-81 Probe placement for continuous-wave Doppler evaluation of the subclavian artery. **A,** Supraclavicular approach. **B,** Infraclavicular approach.

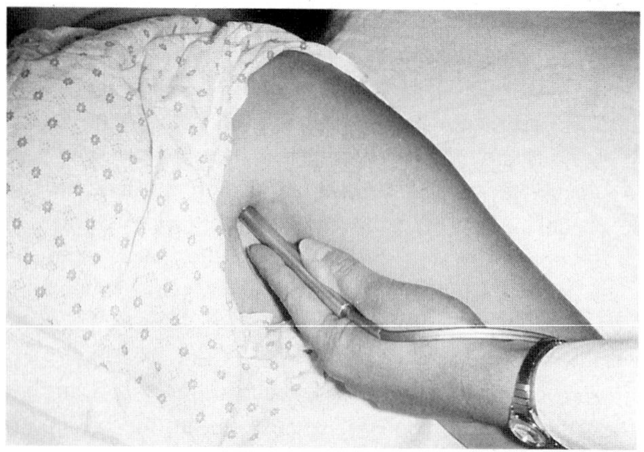

FIG. 20-82 Probe placement for continuous-wave Doppler evaluation of the axillary artery.

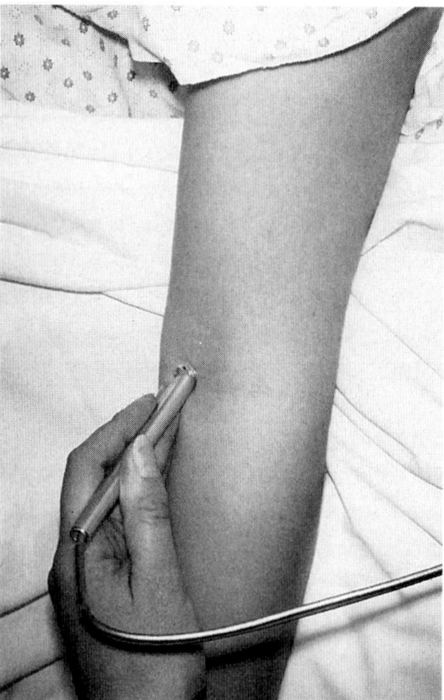

FIG. 20-83 Probe placement for continuous-wave Doppler evaluation of the brachial artery.

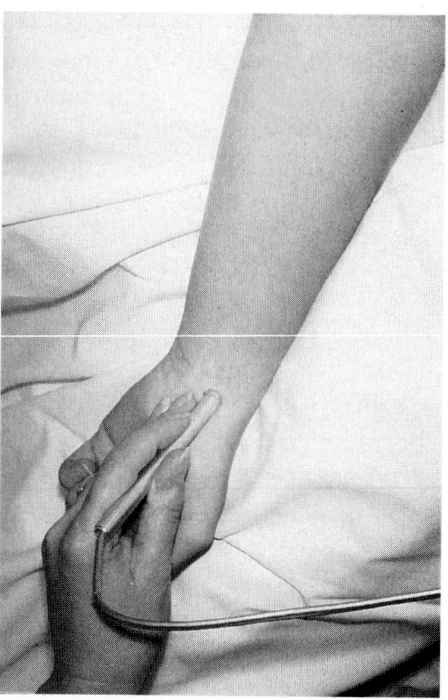

FIG. 20-84 Probe placement for continuous-wave Doppler evaluation of the radial artery.

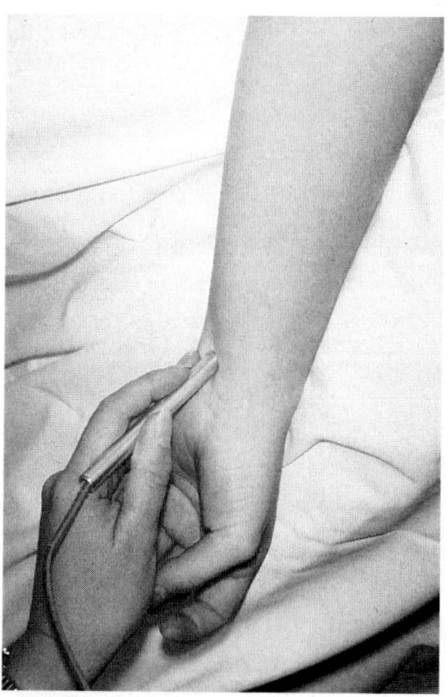

FIG. 20-85 Probe placement for continuous-wave Doppler evaluation of the ulnar artery.

resistance waveform that is similar to a carotid waveform but *is not in the same area as the common carotid*. It is possible to be insonating on top of a vertebra, so it is important to move up and down to try to get a signal proximal to C-6 or between the vertebral interspaces. A triphasic signal more than likely represents the subclavian artery and not the vertebral. Biphasic signals or high-resistance signals may indicate distal vertebral stenosis or occlusion.

The best way to obtain the vertebral signals is by using a duplex scanner. The examiner should seat himself or herself at the patient's head, and turn the head slightly away from the side being examined. Imaging should be done with the head of the patient oriented toward the left side of the image per general ultrasound convention. The examiner needs to locate the common carotid artery first by scanning in a longitudinal and anterior plane (Fig. 20-87) (for more details, see Chapter 22), then the examiner should slowly angle laterally until the bright echoes from the cervical vertebral bodies (seen deep to the common carotid) give way to a series of interrupted bony echoes with vessels identified between them (the transverse processes). Color-flow imaging normally shows pulsatile red flow from the vertebral artery and phasic blue flow from the vertebral vein (Fig. 20-88; see color image). Spectral pulsed Doppler waveforms should be obtained from the vertebral artery to indicate the direction and velocity of flow. Retrograde or

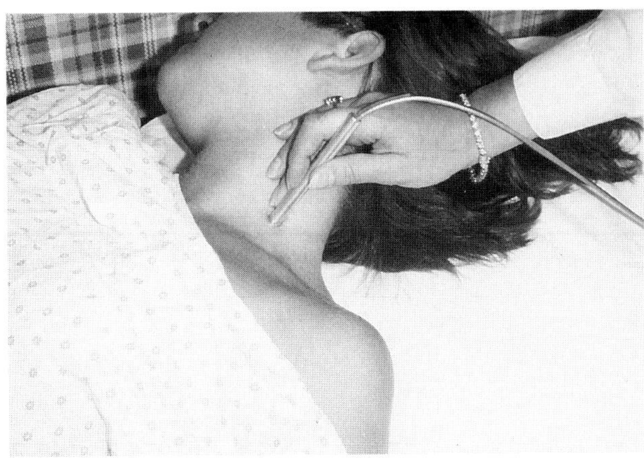

FIG. 20-86 Probe placement for continuous-wave Doppler evaluation of the vertebral artery.

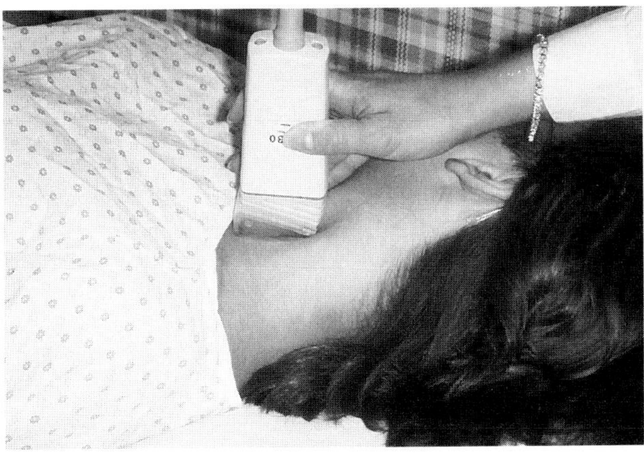

FIG. 20-87 Transducer placement for duplex scan and Doppler spectral evaluation of the vertebral artery.

reversed flow in one vertebral artery is suggestive of subclavian steal.

Evaluation of the hand and digits is covered separately below.

Interpretation of Upper-Extremity Doppler Velocity Waveforms

Waveform interpretation in stenosis follows the same guidelines as in the lower extremities (see the lower-extremity Doppler waveform criteria earlier in the chapter).

1. Normal flow at all sites will be triphasic; if spectral pulsed Doppler is used, there will be little or no spectral broadening.
2. Triphasic patterns in the subclavian, axillary, and brachial arteries with abnormal waveforms in the radial and/or ulnar arteries indicate focal stenosis or occlusion of the respective radial or ulnar vessels.
3. Normal waveforms in the subclavian and axillary arteries with abnormal brachial, radial, and ulnar artery waveforms suggest a brachial artery stenosis or occlusion.

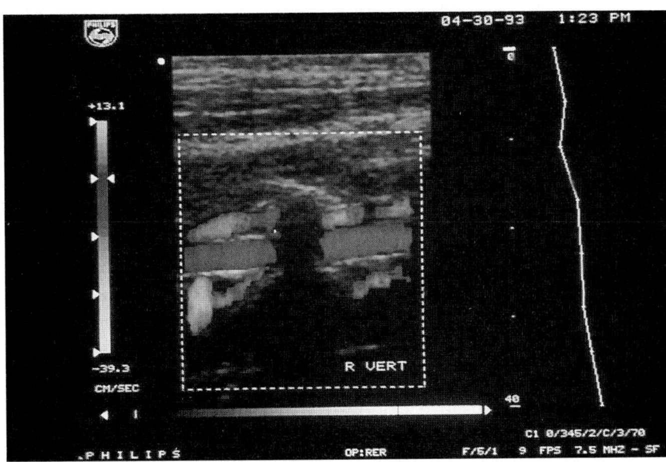

FIG. 20-88 Normal color-flow appearance of the antegrade vertebral artery (red) and vertebral veins (blue). Note the shadow from the transverse vertebral process.

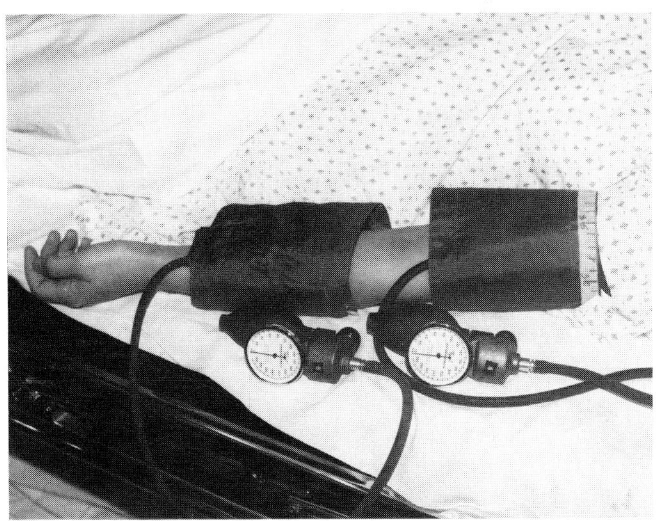

FIG. 20-89 Pressure cuffs in place for the upper-extremity arterial study.

4. A normal subclavian waveform with abnormal waveforms at the axillary artery and distal to it implies a stenosis or occlusion of the distal subclavian and/or axillary artery.
5. Abnormal waveforms from the subclavian distally indicate a probable subclavian artery stenosis or occlusion; if the vertebral artery is antegrade with normal flow, the obstruction is probably distal to the vertebral origin. If the vertebral is partially or totally retrograde, a proximal subclavian stenosis or occlusion can be suspected.

SEGMENTAL PRESSURES

The same techniques for cuff placement and obtaining pressures in the lower extremities are applicable in the arms.

1. Pressure cuffs are applied to the upper arm and forearm (Fig. 20-89).

2. Doppler signals are monitored in the brachial artery and a systolic pressure is obtained and recorded bilaterally.
3. Signals are located in the radial artery at the wrist, and a systolic pressure is obtained and recorded using the forearm cuff first, then a systolic pressure is obtained and recorded from the brachial cuff bilaterally.
4. Signals are located in the ulnar artery, and a systolic pressure is obtained and recorded again using the forearm cuff first, then a systolic pressure is obtained and recorded from the brachial cuff bilaterally.
5. The highest of the two brachial artery systolic pressures is divided into the systolic pressures at each wrist artery to obtain forearm-brachial indices for each forearm artery:

Forearm/brachial index = radial pressure/highest brachial pressure

or

ulnar pressure/highest brachial pressure

Do not use the brachial cuff segmental pressures that were taken using the radial or ulnar artery; use the ones obtained from the brachial cuff with the probe at the brachial artery in the antecubital fossa (2 above).

Evaluation of the hand and digits is covered separately below.

Interpretation of Upper-Extremity Segmental Pressures

The same criteria for comparing pressure differences in the legs applies to the study in the arms. A pressure drop of more than 30 mm Hg implies the presence of a significant focal stenosis in the arteries between the two cuffs; a difference between sides implies a stenosis or occlusion on the side with the lower brachial pressure.

It is possible for both arms to have equal or comparable pressures with normal forearm-brachial indices but be abnormal. This can occur when there is an aortic arch problem or bilateral subclavian or axillary stenoses or occlusions: The waveforms must be relied on in this case, so segmental pressures should not be performed without using some method of obtaining waveform patterns for segment comparison.

VOLUME-PULSE RECORDINGS (AIR PLETHYSMOGRAPHY)

Volume-pulse recording can also be performed on arteries in the upper extremity. It can again easily be performed on the patient after segmental pressures have been obtained.

To obtain volume-pulse waveforms, the examiner should place cuffs on the upper arm and high forearm bilaterally; an additional cuff should be placed on the lower forearm near the wrist (Fig. 20-90). Placement of forearm cuffs is easier if 10-cm-wide cuffs are used in this test. As before, an air supply hose is connected from the plethysmograph to the cuff at the location being examined. The examiner needs to set the equipment up by ensuring that AC amplification is selected, that the system is set to evaluate volume pulse recording, and that a manual aneroid sphygmomanometer, regulated air compressor, or automatic cuff inflator is attached to the air-input port. As in the lower-extremity arterial exam, the examiner must perform a calibration run and adjust the recorder output before actually recording waveforms. (See the procedure in the lower-extremity section).

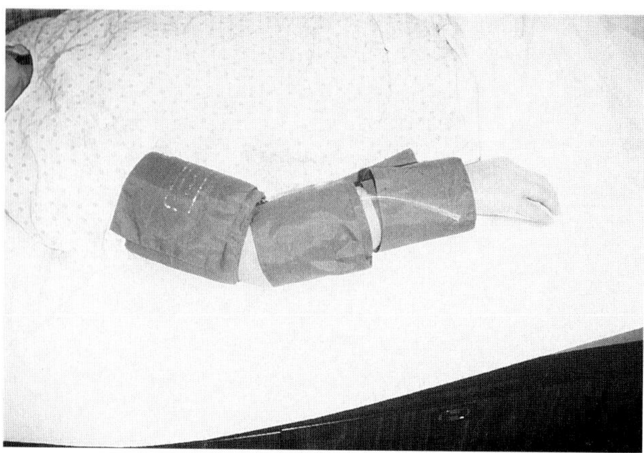

FIG. 20-90 Cuff placement for volume pulse recording of the upper extremity.

After calibration, each cuff is inflated to 60 mm Hg and the pressure is held. Once a stable waveform is seen on the tracing or computer display, roughly five to six stable waveforms should be recorded. This procedure is repeated until waveforms have been recorded from:

1. The upper arm cuffs bilaterally
2. The forearm cuffs bilaterally
3. The wrist cuffs bilaterally

Evaluation of the hand and digits is covered separately below.

Interpretation of Upper-Extremity Volume Pulse Recordings

Volume pulse waveforms decrease in amplitude as perfusion decreases. Volume pulse recording waveforms in the arm are generally diagnosed as normal, abnormal, or flat. To review, a normal volume pulse recording waveform has a quick inflow upstroke with an initial downslope, a dicrotic notch, then a slower outflow downstroke. The loss of the dicrotic notch in a volume pulse waveform corresponds to the loss of the second component in a Doppler waveform. Amplitude may decrease as inflow decreases. A flat volume pulse recording waveform indicates very poor filling and perfusion, with possibly absent flow.

The level of obstruction can be discerned by comparing the waveform contours at each cuff level.

1. A normal waveform at the upper arm and forearm lev-

els with abnormal waveforms at the wrist level indicates segmental forearm artery stenosis (or stenoses).
2. A normal waveform at the upper arm cuff with abnormal waveforms at the forearm and wrist levels indicates stenosis or occlusion of the distal brachial artery or arteries at the antecubital level.
3. Abnormal waveforms at all cuff sites imply proximal stenosis or occlusion of the subclavian or axillary artery or both.

Volume pulse waveforms are less diagnostic for isolating disease locations than Doppler waveforms are, since relative perfusion is being measured, but it is impossible to tell where a proximal stenosis is located or, in the forearm, whether the decrease results from one or both forearm arteries.

Arterial upper-extremity continuous-wave Doppler, segmental pressures, and volume pulse recording cases.

Case 1 (Fig. 20-91): Abnormal moderate segmental forearm stenosis. This patient presented with right forearm and hand numbness after exertion (the left arm had been amputated). Triphasic waveforms can be seen in the subclavian, axillary, and brachial arteries, and monophasic waveforms are present in the radial and ulnar arteries. The Allen's test shows normal augmentation with arterial compressions indicating a normal patent palmar arch system. There is a marked pressure drop between the arm cuff and the forearm cuff, confirming the presence of stenosis implied by the waveforms. In addition, the forearm-brachial indices are 0.67 in the radial and 0.53 in the ulnar, both within the range of moderate impairment.

Case 2 (Fig. 20-92): Doppler, segmental pressures, and volume pulse recording of arms—left normal, right subclavian stenosis. This 53-year-old patient had placement of a right subclavian interposition graft, with subsequent thrombectomy of the right subclavian, axillary, and brachial arteries 6 months later, and a right subclavian percutaneous transluminal angioplasty (PTA) 7 months later. During follow-up of the patient in the 5 years after PTA, she complained of steadily progressive claudication of the right arm.

The Doppler analog waveform analysis *(A)* showed monophasic flow at all sites in the right arm, with normal triphasic flow at all locations in the left arm. Volume pulse recordings *(B)* show markedly diminished abnormal waveforms at all cuff sites in the right arm, and normal waveforms with prominent dicrotic notches at all cuff sites in the left arm. Segmental pressures (shown on *B*) indicated a pressure difference between the right and the left arms of 41 mm Hg (right arm 87 mm Hg, left arm 128 mm Hg), with a forearm-brachial index of 0.66 on the right and 1.04 on the left.

Note that the decreased forearm-brachial index in the right arm reflects overall pressure differences from the stenosed subclavian artery. There is no significant segmental pressure difference between the two right arm cuffs to imply the presence of a brachial or forearm artery stenosis.

ARTERIAL DUPLEX SONOGRAPHY

Duplex sonography and color-flow imaging are less frequently used in the upper-extremity arteries than in the cerebrovascular system or lower-extremity arteries, except to evaluate renal dialysis access fistulas, pseudoaneurysm, or aneurysm.

All arteries in the upper extremity can be evaluated with color-flow imaging and gray-scale duplex sonography, but the main requirement in the arm is that the transducer's near-field focal zone be able to show structures within the top centimeter of the visual display. Higher-frequency transducers should be used. Transducers with wedges seldom have a problem, but other devices may require a standoff or gel pad to see such superficial structures. Arteries in the shoulder and infraclavicular areas may be best imaged with lower-frequency transducers.

As mentioned in the section on imaging the lower-extremity arteries, the best use of duplex and color-flow imaging may be as an adjunctive study to a Doppler waveform and segmental pressure evaluation. It is important, however, to know the sonographic appearance and patterns in normal arteries in the arm. If an examiner is uncertain as to the identity of a vessel, color-flow imaging can easily enable identification by color and flow pattern, as can the use of spectral pulsed Doppler.

1. The subclavian artery is accessed in the longitudinal plane by scanning beneath the clavicle (Fig. 20-93, *A*) and rotating and angling the transducer until the artery and vein are visualized (Fig. 20-93, *B*; see color image). The artery can be more readily identified and distinguished from the vein using color-flow imaging.
2. Following the subclavian artery laterally across the anterior shoulder into the arm (Fig. 20-94, *A*) brings the axillary artery into view (Fig. 20-94, *B*; see color image); this can be traced into the upper arm distally into the biceps groove (Fig. 20-95, *A*), where the brachial artery can be visualized (Fig. 20-95, *B*; see color image), and tracked to the antecubital fossa.
3. Just below the inner bend of the elbow, the radial and ulnar bifurcation off the brachial artery can be identified and examined.
4. The radial artery is found laterally in the forearm (Fig. 20-96; see color image) and can be followed to the wrist.
5. The ulnar artery can be traced medially (Fig. 20-97, *A*) and usually dives deep (Fig. 20-97, *B*; see color image) before moving superficially to the wrist. At about the upper third of the forearm, the bifurcation of the median volar interosseous branch off the ulnar is visual-

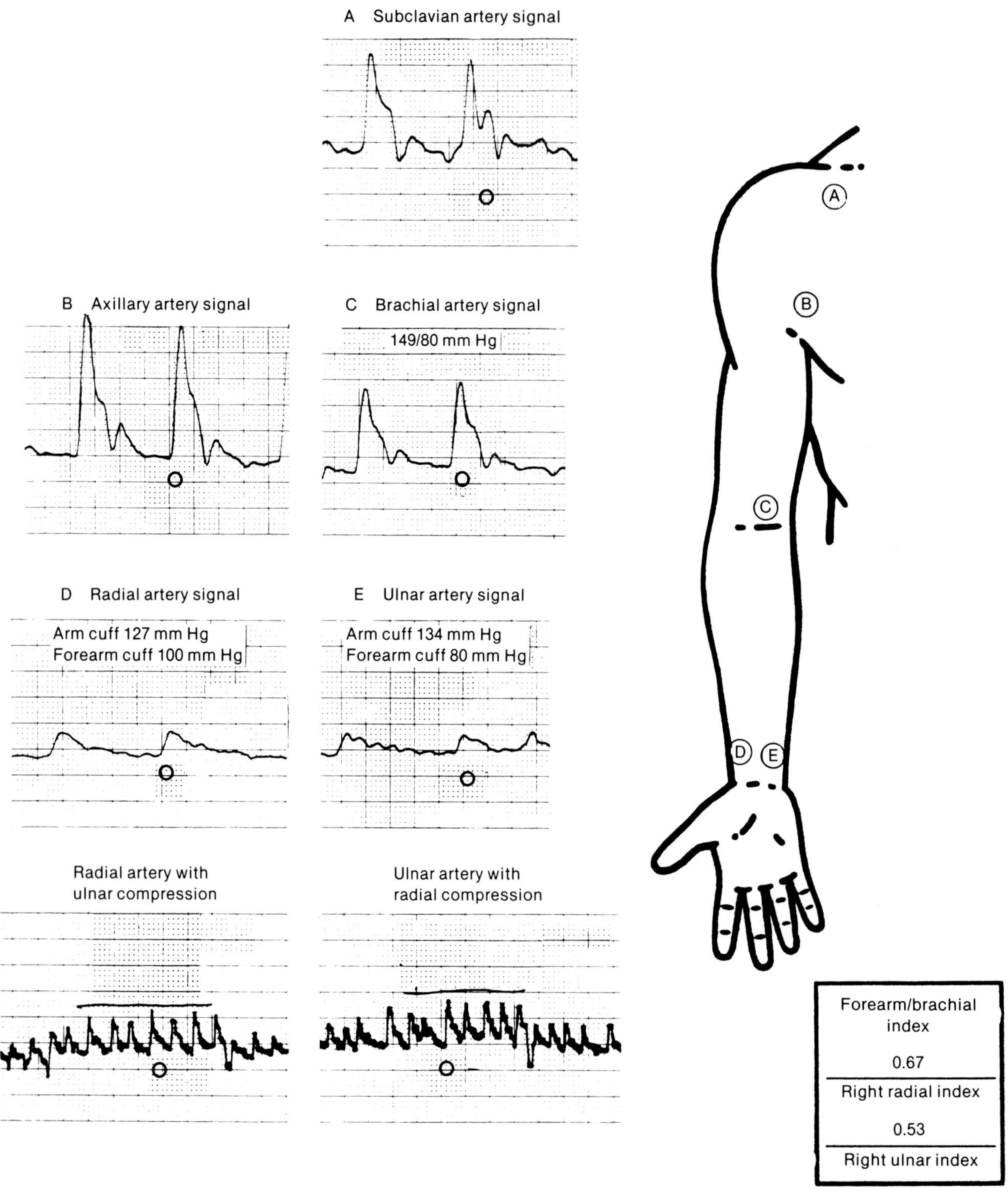

FIG. 20-91 Moderate segmental forearm stenosis.

ized and, if desired, the artery can be followed distally in the center of the forearm.

Images of each artery should be obtained in both longitudinal and transverse planes.

Spectral pulsed Doppler waveforms will be triphasic and should be obtained from each artery as necessary.

Any given segment can be measured using electronic calipers in longitudinal and transverse planes if attempting to rule out ectasia or aneurysm.

Hemodialysis grafts are generally looplike grafts easily visible under the skin of the forearm (a common placement site), connecting a superficial vein or the brachial vein with

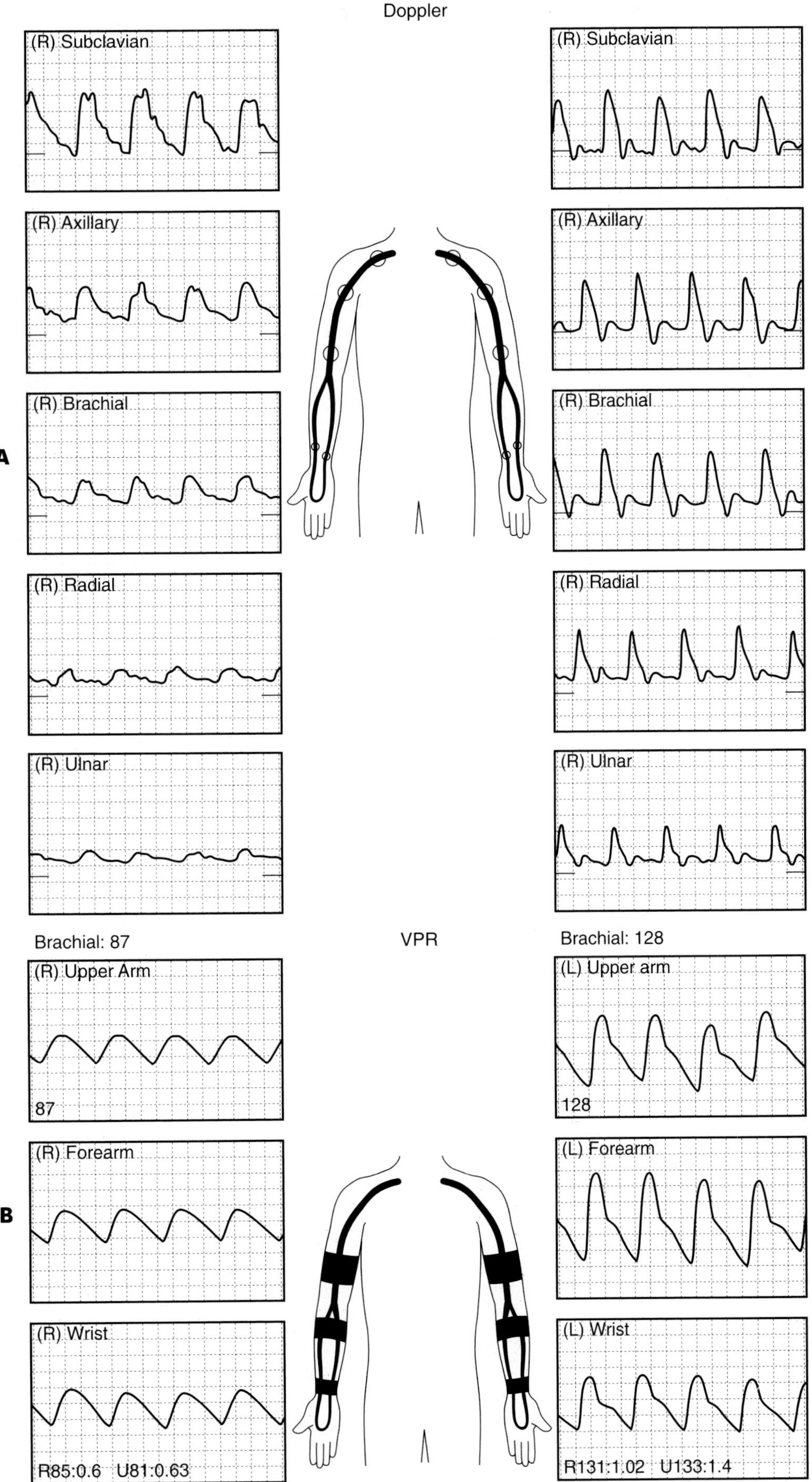

FIG. 20-92 A, Right subclavian stenosis, Doppler analog waveform analysis (see text). **B,** Right subclavian stenosis, volume pulse recordings and segmental pressures (see text).

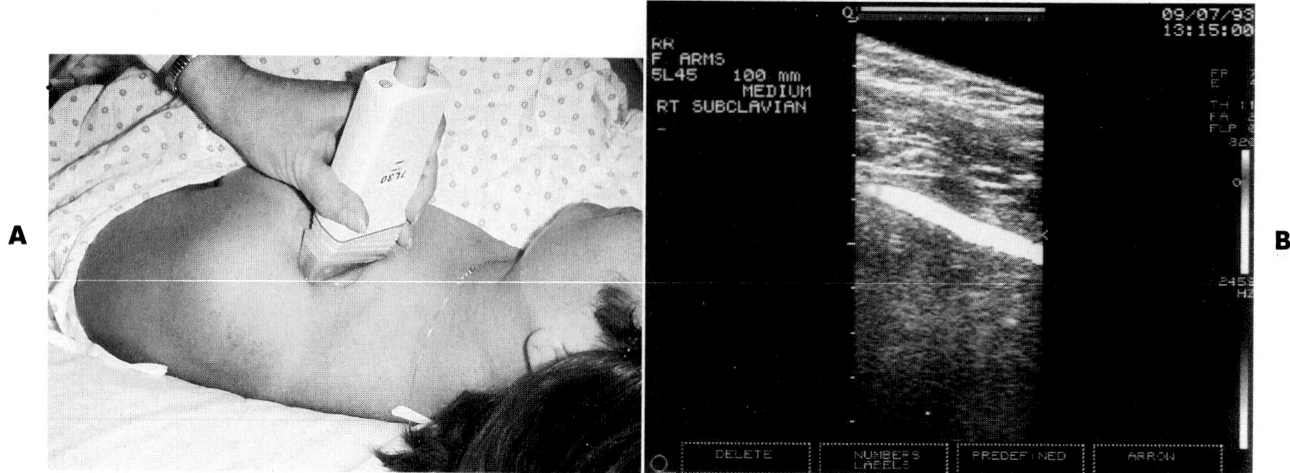

FIG. 20-93 A, Duplex scanning position for the subclavian artery. **B,** Color-flow duplex appearance of a normal subclavian artery.

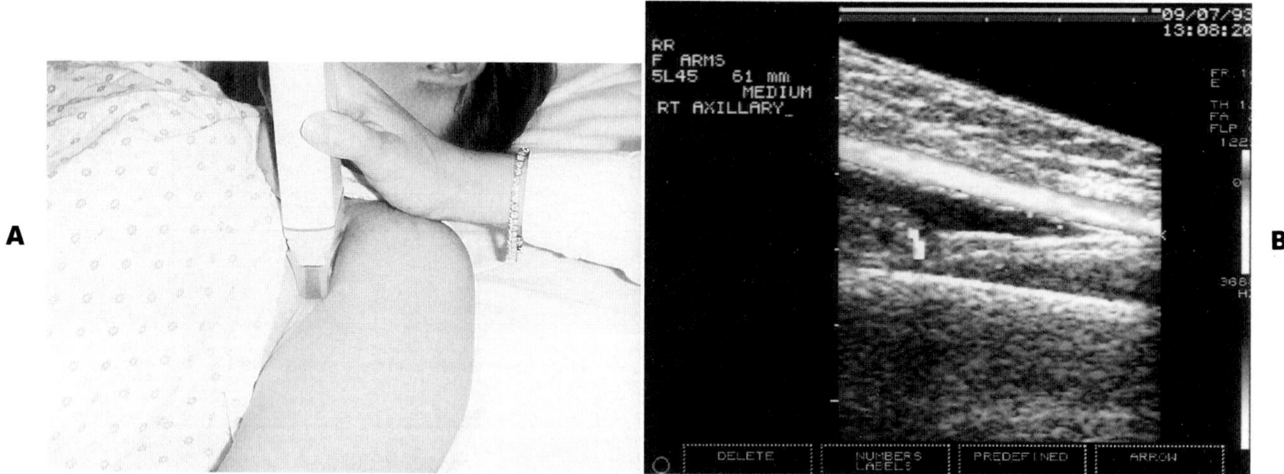

FIG. 20-94 A, Duplex scanning position for the axillary artery. **B,** Color-flow duplex appearance of a normal axillary artery.

the brachial artery. The basic techniques for evaluating them are the same as for evaluating any other artery, but there is a focus on identifying any stenoses or kinks by gray-scale imaging, color-flow imaging, and Doppler spectral analysis. The normal color-flow and Doppler patterns are pulsatile but have a characteristic high-velocity turbulent and disturbed quality similar to those found in other non-surgically created arteriovenous fistulas.

The graft should be followed in longitudinal and transverse planes from one anastomosis to the other, and areas of stenosis, occlusion, kinking, or flow decrease should be identified and documented.

Upper-Extremity Arterial Duplex Interpretation Criteria

The same interpretation criteria concerning plaque identification, stenosis determination, waveform appearances, and flow velocities in the lower extremities can be applied to the upper extremities (see p. 475). In review, echogenic material is present, color-flow velocities increase, and the peak velocity is double that of the prestenotic artery across a stenosis of more than 50%. Waveforms degrade with turbulence.

No velocity criteria can be applied to dialysis grafts because of the extreme turbulence and high velocities normally seen. Efforts to quantify and grade flow volume in milliliters per minute by calculations of velocity compared with cyclic wall diameter are, however, being done for future potential applications.

Aneurysmal dilation is diagnosed by comparing segment size, often with accepted norms. In general, if a maximal arterial diameter is 1.5 times that of a straight, uniform normal segment, it may be classed as ectatic or mildly aneurysmal; if greater than that, it may be aneurysmal.

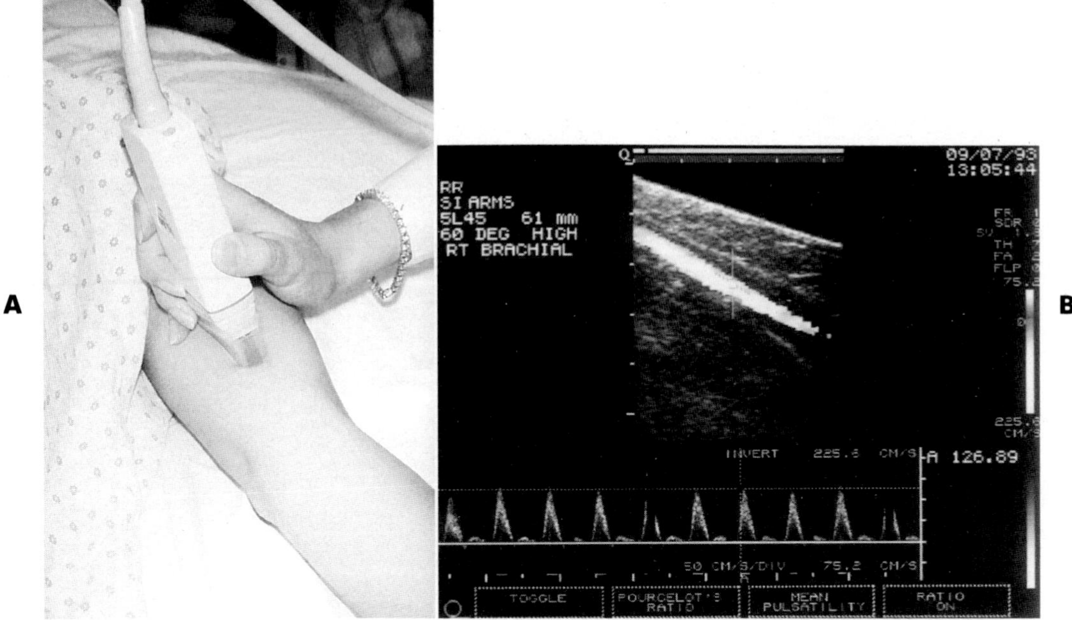

FIG. 20-95 A, Duplex scanning position for the brachial artery. **B,** Color-flow duplex appearance of a normal brachial artery with a normal Doppler spectral waveform.

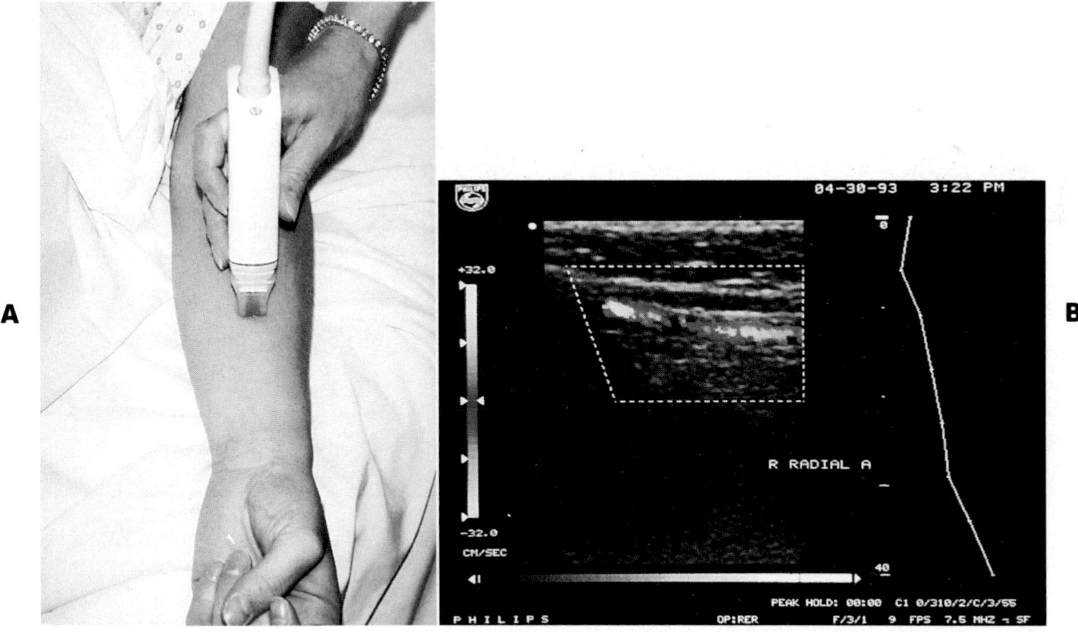

FIG. 20-96 A, Duplex scanning position for the radial artery. **B,** Color-flow duplex appearance of a normal radial artery.

Thoracic Outlet Syndrome Examination

Patients often show completely normal resting upper-extremity pressures even though they have difficulty only when their arms are raised or placed at an unusual angle. These patients usually complain of numbness, tingling, and discoloration if the arm is abducted, lain on, pulled back behind the shoulder, or held over the head. Changing the position of the arm to a more forward or neutral position resolves the symptoms completely.[14] In these patients a routine upper-extremity examination should be performed and then a more specialized examination of the thoracic outlet.

Photoplethysmography can be used as a waveform monitoring device in the thoracic outlet examination, as well as a Doppler probe; the photocell can be taped with double-sided cellophane tape to a digit or strapped on using a Vel-

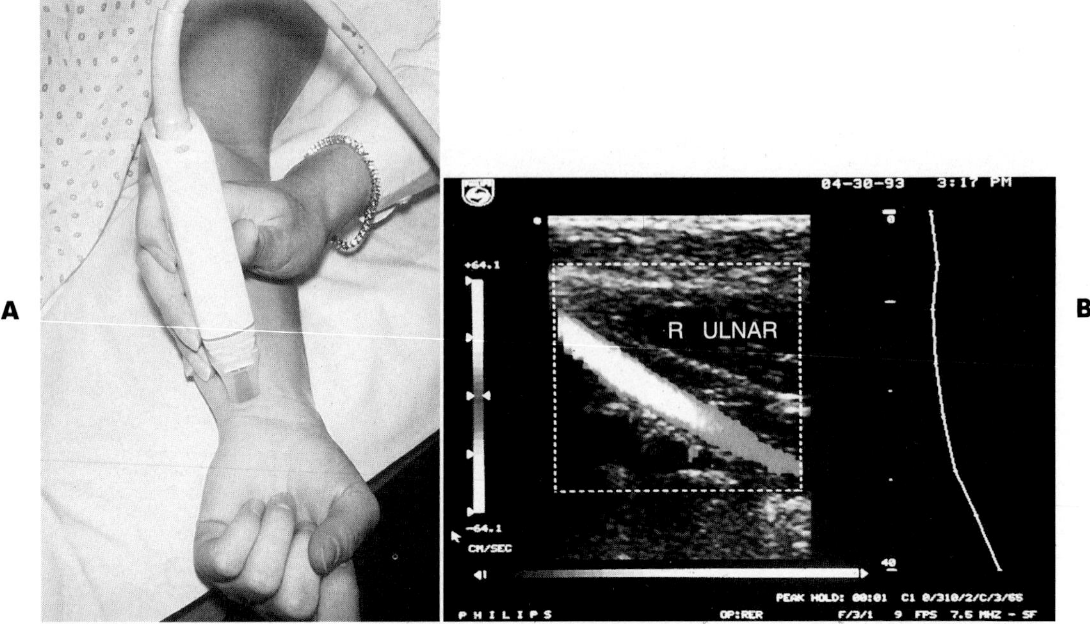

FIG. 20-97 **A,** Duplex scanning position for the ulnar artery. **B,** Color-flow duplex appearance of a normal ulnar artery.

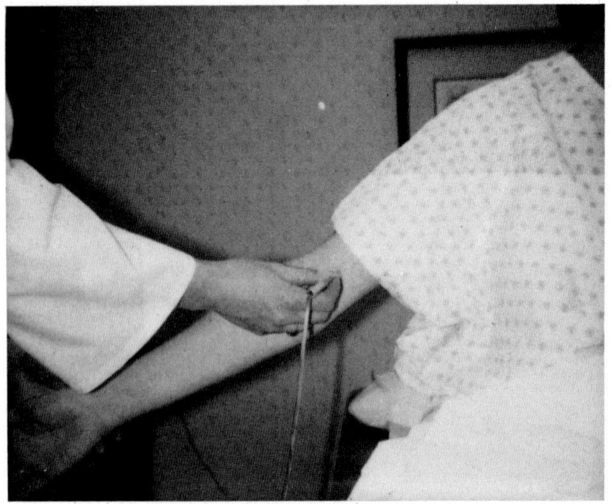

FIG. 20-98 Thoracic outlet examination. Examining the arm at 45-degree angle.

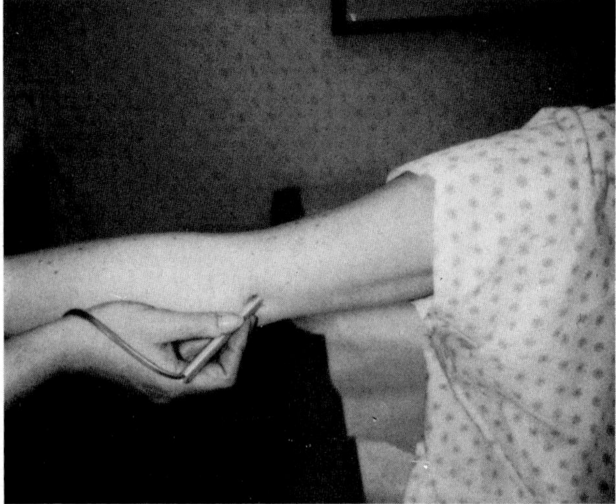

FIG. 20-99 Thoracic outlet examination. Examining the arm at 90-degree angle.

cro strip. The tracing should be calibrated before the testing maneuvers described below are performed. A benefit of using a photocell is that both of the examiner's hands are free to support the patient's arm during the examination. If a Doppler probe is used, it must be held against the brachial artery with one hand while the arm is supported with the other.

Thoracic outlet syndrome occurs when the arteries, veins, and/or nerves supplying the arm are obstructed by compression between the clavicle and first rib, a cervical rib and the scalene muscles, or the pectoralis minor with hyperabduction of the arm. The vessels usually involved are the subclavian artery and vein and the brachial nerve plexus where it leaves the chest and goes to the arm.[14]

In the thoracic outlet examination the patient should sit either in a chair or on the edge of the examination table with the arms completely relaxed. The examiner takes a tracing from the brachial artery with a Doppler probe (or from the digit if a PPG is used) with the arm in a neutral position. Then, the patient's arm is raised to a 45-degree angle (Fig. 20-98). The patient is instructed to let the arm go limp and offer no assistance at all; it should be supported by the examiner. A tracing is taken from the arm in this position and is marked accordingly. With the arm in this

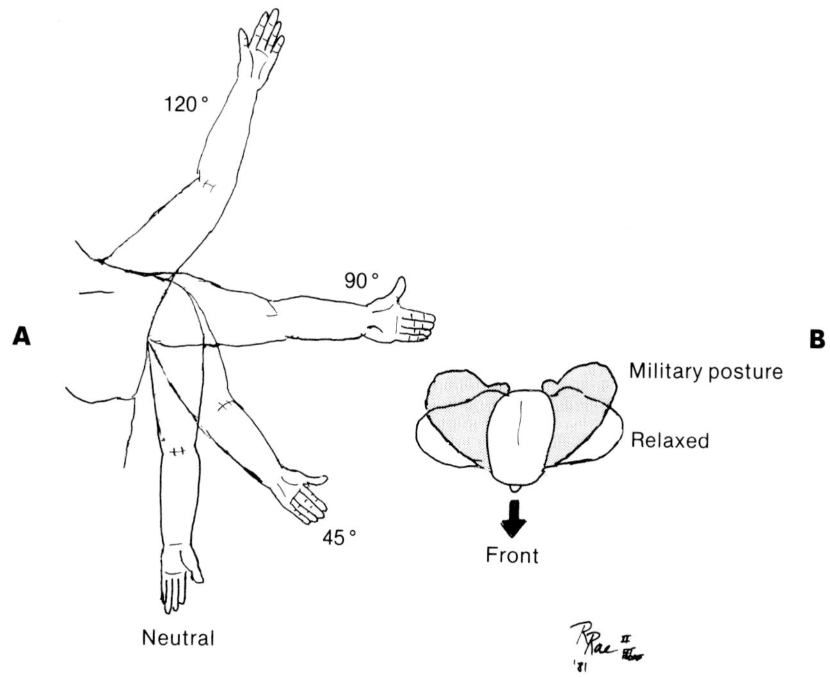

FIG. 20-100 Positions for examination of the patient with thoracic outlet syndrome. **A,** Arm and angles. **B,** Shoulders in relaxed and military postures.

position the patient then is instructed to pull the shoulders back into a military posture and perform a Valsalva maneuver. The examiner keeps the probe in place during the Valsalva and records any changes that occur.

The arm is raised to a 90-degree angle, and the procedure is repeated (Fig. 20-99). A tracing is made both neutrally and with the patient in military posture performing a Valsalva maneuver. The arm is then raised to a 120-degree position and the same steps are repeated. The arm can also be raised to a 180-degree angle if symptoms warrant.

Additional maneuvers can include hyperabduction, hyperadduction, and Adson's test. In Adson's test, the patient hyperabducts the arm over the head and turns the head toward the side being examined. This position can help reveal the presence of a cervical rib.[14]

Positive findings in thoracic outlet syndrome will be a reduction or cessation of flow at or above a specific degree of elevation or abduction, diminution or cessation with military posturing, and with the application of Adson's test. Any comments the patient makes concerning the onset of symptoms with the assumption of a particular position should be noted on the report form.

The positions for the thoracic outlet examination are shown in Fig. 20-100.

Thoracic Outlet Case. The case presented here uses a Doppler probe to obtain the brachial waveform.

Case 1 (Fig. 20-101): Normal right arm—abnormal left arm. This patient suffered pain and numbness in the left arm when it was raised above the shoulder level, after an industrial accident.

On the right side, normal triphasic brachial waveforms are seen that do not diminish or significantly alter as the arm is raised from hanging through 180 degrees. Application of military postures in each position also has no effect with the exception of some mild flow diminution without alteration of the flow pattern when military posturing is applied at 90 degrees.

On the symptomatic left side, there is a normal, triphasic pattern in the brachial artery in the hanging and 45-degree positions with complete compression and loss of signal occurring as the arm is brought to the 90-degree position and is elevated higher. Compression at this level was confirmed by lowering the arm slowly through 90 degrees while continually monitoring the brachial artery. The strip at the bottom shows the gradual return of flow to normal triphasicity during this latter step.

EXAMINING FOR SUBCLAVIAN STEAL SYNDROME

Subclavian steal syndrome occurs when there is an obstruction in the subclavian or innominate artery, which is proximal to the vertebral origins. If flow to the arm is compromised significantly enough, flow from the contralateral patent vertebral is "stolen" around the vertebrobasilar junction reversing down the ipsilateral vertebral artery into the subclavian artery to help supply the arm (Fig. 20-102). In complete steal a fully retrograde flow pattern is seen in the vertebral artery (a pulsatile blue-dominant pattern on color-flow duplex) with an antegrade pattern in the opposing vertebral in this condition (Fig. 20-103, *A, B*). In latent steal (where the subclavian stenosis may be moderate) flow reverses in systole but recovers antegrade in diastole (an al-

A Right arm UE-TOS

R

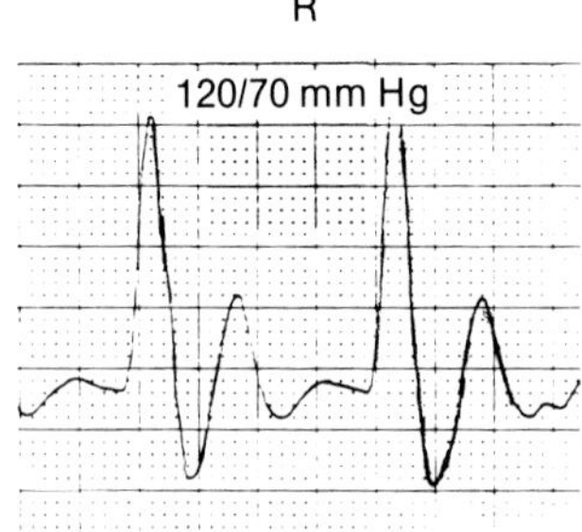

Arm hanging

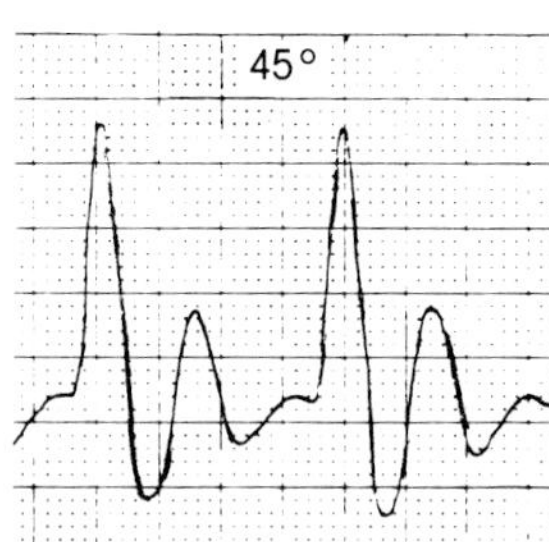

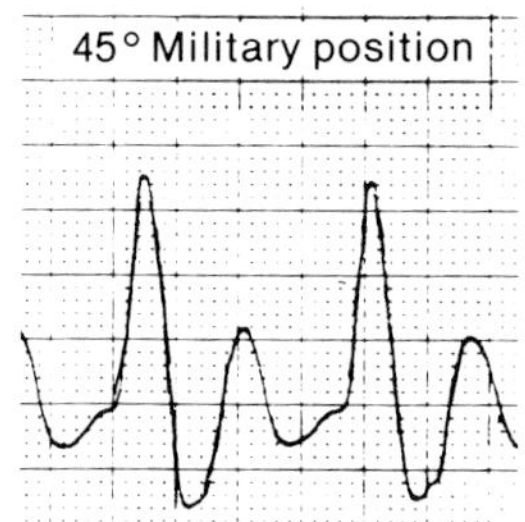

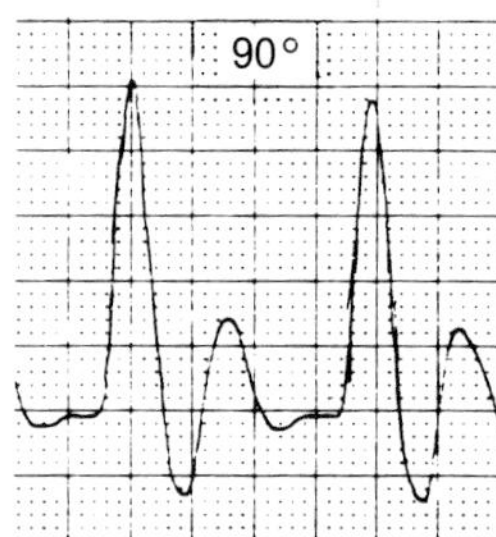

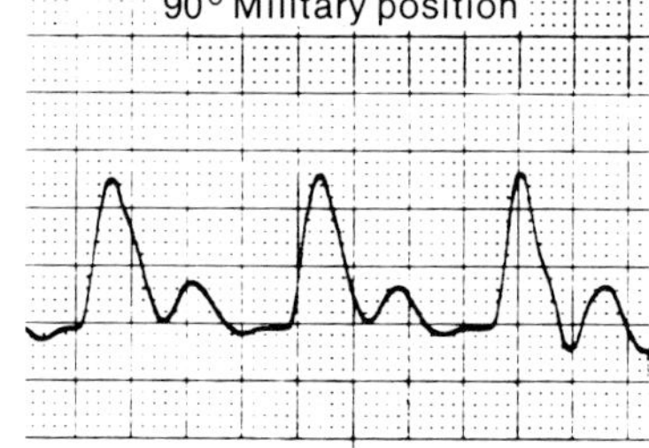

Mild compression with military position at 90°

No effect with Adson's maneuver

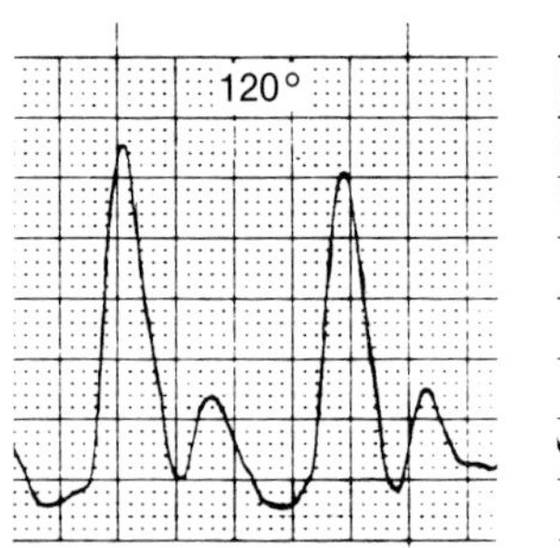

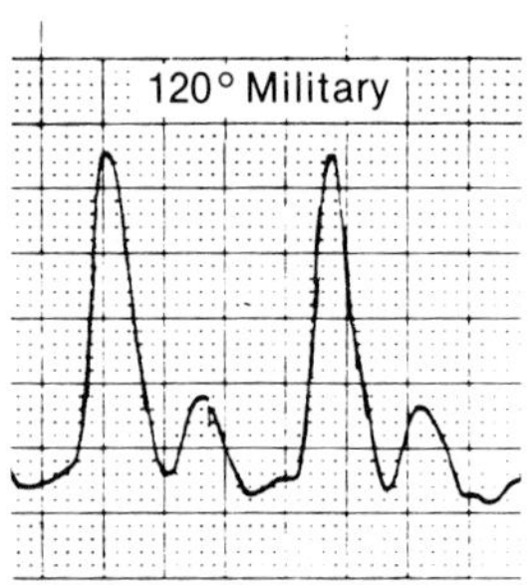

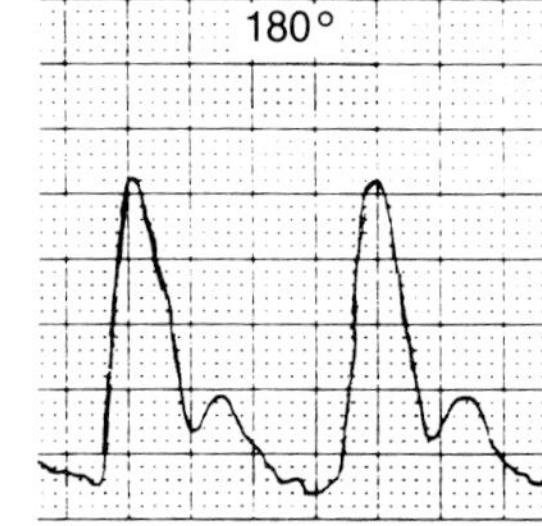

FIG. 20-101 A, Normal right arm. *Continued.*

ternating blue-red-blue-red pattern in color flow) (Fig. 20-103, *C, D*).

If the proximal innominate artery becomes severely stenosed or occluded, it is possible for a carotid steal to occur, where flow from the left vertebral is shunted via the circle of Willis to the right side of the body and travels retrograde in both the vertebral and carotid systems; this occurs rarely but knowledge of its characteristics helps the examiner if it is encountered. For more information on the hemodynamics of carotid steal and some examples of cases, please see Chapter 22. In a patient with vertebral steal, a well-defined reversed vertebral signal on the side with a

B Left arm UE-TOS

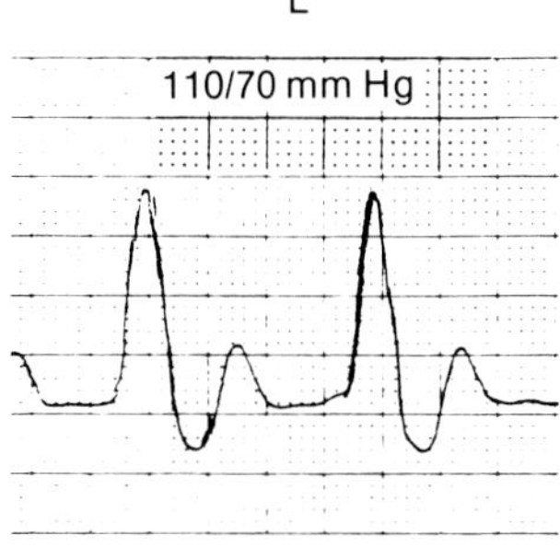

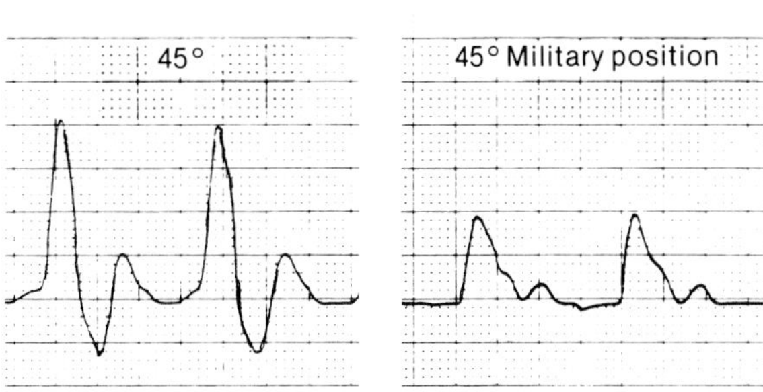

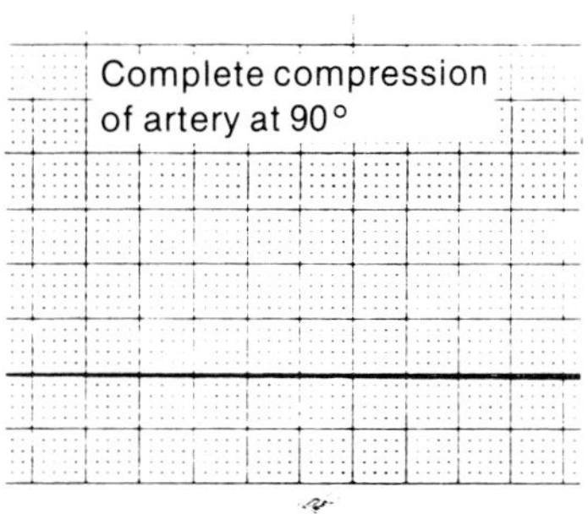

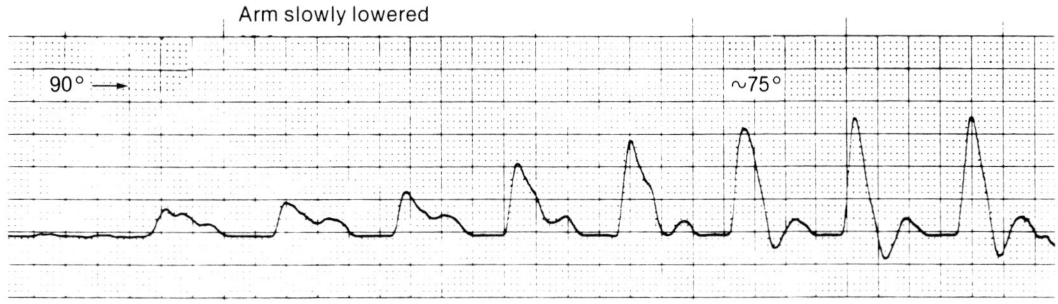

FIG. 20-101 cont'd. B, Abnormal left arm.

subclavian stenosis is often more than sufficient to imply a probable steal. In a patient presenting with questionably reversed or weak but antegrade vertebral flow, steal presence should be verified. To check for steal syndrome, the examiner has the patient lie supine and places a pressure cuff on the *arm with the occlusion*. The vertebral artery is monitored with either Doppler or a color-flow duplex scanner with the cuff inflated to at least 50 mm Hg above the systolic pressure to occlude flow to the arm and induce hyperemia. The monitoring continues with the cuff inflated for 3 minutes. At the end of that time, the cuff pressure is released. The chart recorder or spectrum analyzer display should be running before release of the cuff to show any changes that occur.

In a patient with vertebral steal a reversed signal augments for a short period. An antegrade signal momentarily

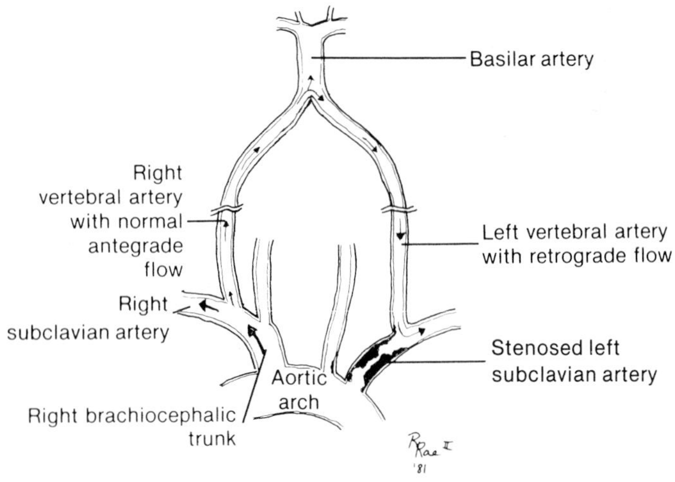

FIG. 20-102 Stenosed left subclavian artery and mechanism of subclavian steal syndrome.

reverses below the zero line for several beats within the first 5 to 15 seconds (Fig. 20-104; see color images); if monitored longer, the examiner sees the waveform return to its preocclusive state.

EVALUATION OF THE HAND AND DIGITAL ARTERIES

Doppler Examination of the Digital Arteries

Many patients present with focal ischemia of the fingers and hand resulting from trauma, frostbite, microvascular obstruction, and Raynaud's phenomenon. In these patients the problem may affect the entire hand, one or two fingers only, or just a fingertip. These problems also may be traced to obstruction of the palmar arch, especially if the arch is

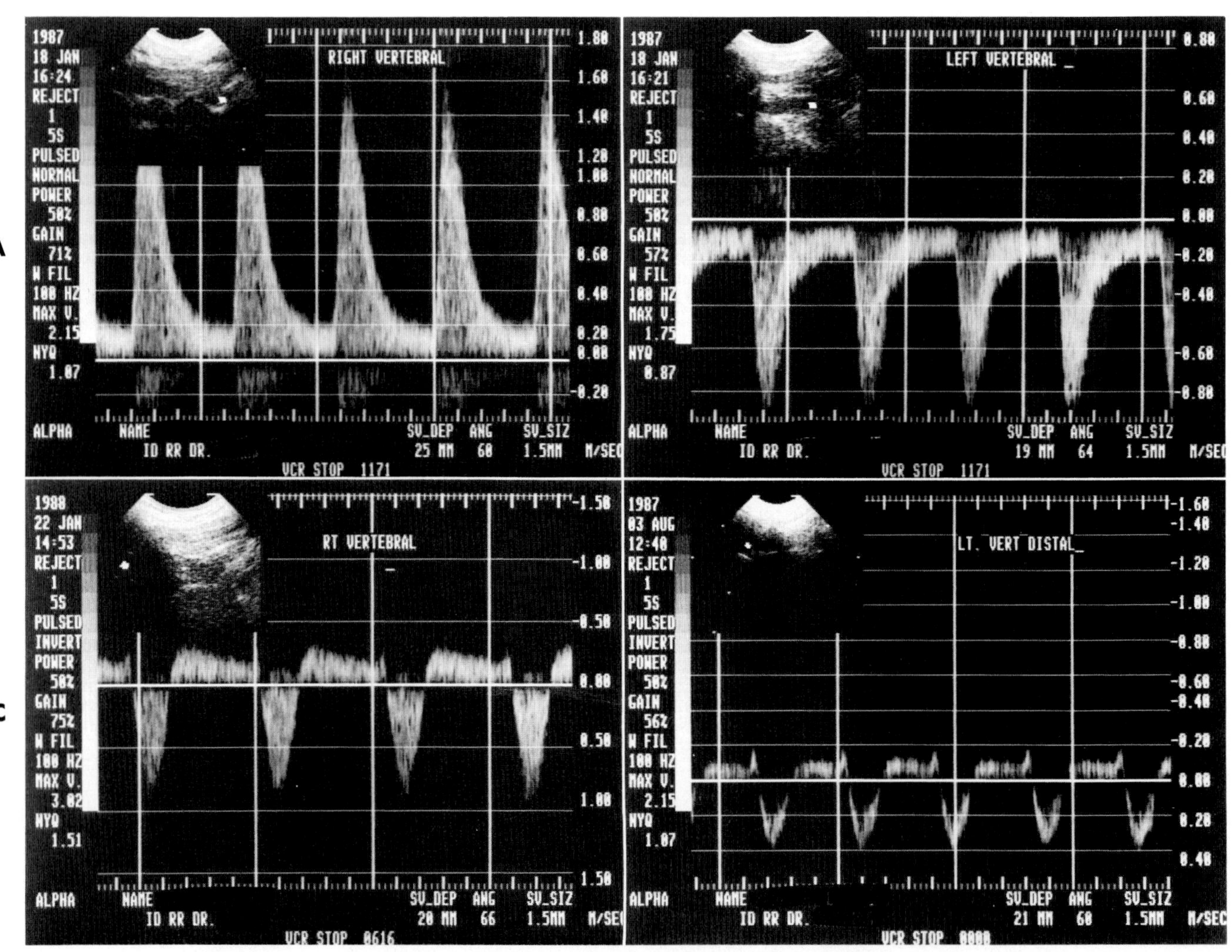

FIG. 20-103 Vertebral steal. **A,** Normal but elevated signal typical of compensatory response from unaffected side. **B,** Strongly reversed signal indicative of frank vertebral steal on affected side in same patient. **C,** Moderate latent vertebral steal (note bidirectional flow and recovery in diastole). **D,** Mild latent vertebral steal.

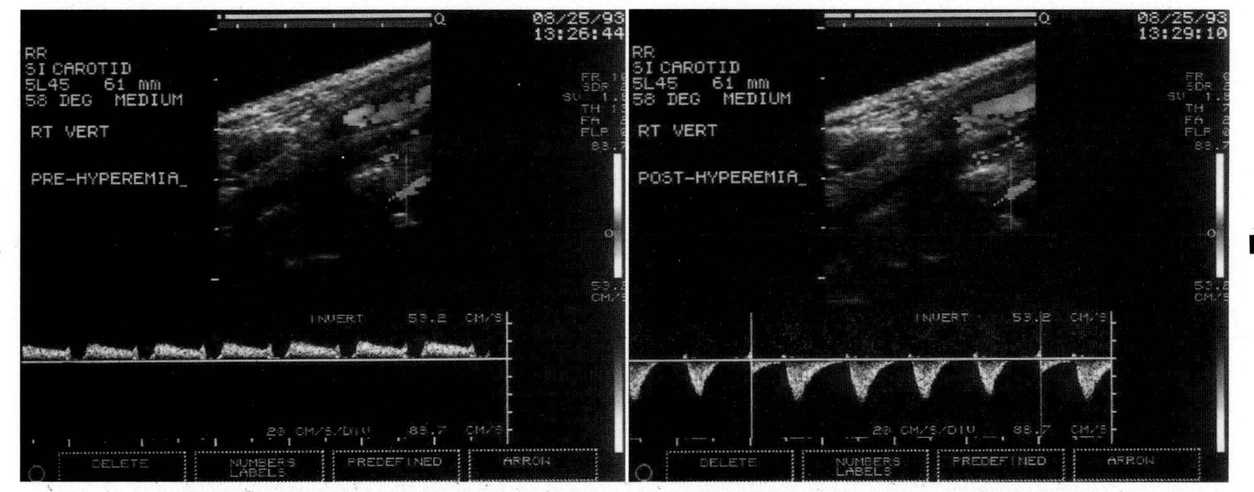

FIG. 20-104 Subclavian steal hyperemia test. The transient vertebral signal in **A** reverses in systole but does not go below the baseline. After 3 minutes of brachial occlusion with a pressure cuff and release, reactive hyperemia in the arm causes the signal to fully reverse below the baseline in systole and diastole, **B.**

incomplete. Vasospasm, whether focal or general, is often corrected microsurgically by digital nerve sympathectomy where the microconnections between the digital artery and nerve are severed, allowing flow to resume. Carpal tunnel syndrome can also cause a neurologic vasospasm, and a carpal tunnel release can often restore digital flow.

A standard Doppler upper-extremity arterial exam does not generally assess the hand, and although photoplethysmographic and temperature-sensing probes may be used to confirm an ischemic problem, these techniques do not pinpoint the level of stenosis or give pressure information.

Angiography is still the best way to show the digital tree and palmar arch, but again there is a noninvasive Doppler technique that, when used as a screening and follow-up tool, can spare the normal patient an angiogram.

Anatomy of the Arterial Circulation to the Hand

The radial and ulnar arteries terminate into the radial and ulnar palmar arches, as shown in Fig. 20-79. The common digital arteries arise from the palmar arches, which then terminate into the proper digital arteries, one on each side of the finger. Barring a developmental anomaly, the radial arch generally supplies the digital arteries on the radial (lateral) side of the digit and the ulnar arch the digital arteries on the medial (ulnar) side.

Hand and Digital Artery Examination Techniques

Evaluation of the palmar arch is important because the arch may be either incomplete (the radial and ulnar sides each supplying two or three fingers) or complete (communicating as a closed loop). To evaluate its patency and whether it is complete or incomplete, two methods can be used.

1. A modified Allen's test can be performed with a Doppler probe; the radial side of the arch is accessed by placing the tip of the probe into the fleshy part at the base of the thumb angled toward the radial artery at the wrist. The ulnar side of the arch is located by placing the probe into the fleshy area at the ulnar side of the hand angling toward the ulnar artery. A triphasic signal should be heard at both locations. While monitoring the radial portion, the examiner should manually occlude the ulnar artery by pressing down with the free hand or thumb. The normal response in a complete arch is augmentation of the radial signal. The same method is used to check patency from the ulnar side; in this case the radial artery is compressed, and again flow should augment in the ulnar artery. Lack of augmentation during compression from one side or the other implies an incomplete or occluded arch (Fig. 20-105).
2. Photoplethysmography can be used to evaluate the palmar arch segments as well. In this method, photocells are taped or strapped to the fingertips of the second and fourth digits. PPG waveforms from the second digit are monitored first. The radial and the ulnar arteries are individually compressed while watching the waveform for changes. The fourth digit is evaluated the same way.

Normally, when one artery is compressed, the other artery compensates and maintains flow in the digit being examined via the palmar arch. If the digit PPG waveform signal is obliterated (goes flat) when either the radial or ulnar artery is compressed, then the palmar arch is incomplete (either congenitally or from stenosis or occlusion). If one digit remains patent and the other occludes, this implies that the radial or ulnar palmar arch segments may not communicate and each may supply only specific digits of the hand.

Plethysmography of the Digits. To determine the general perfusion of flow to the fingers, photoplethysmography or strain-gauge plethysmography can be used effectively, since these tests are simple to perform. The photo-

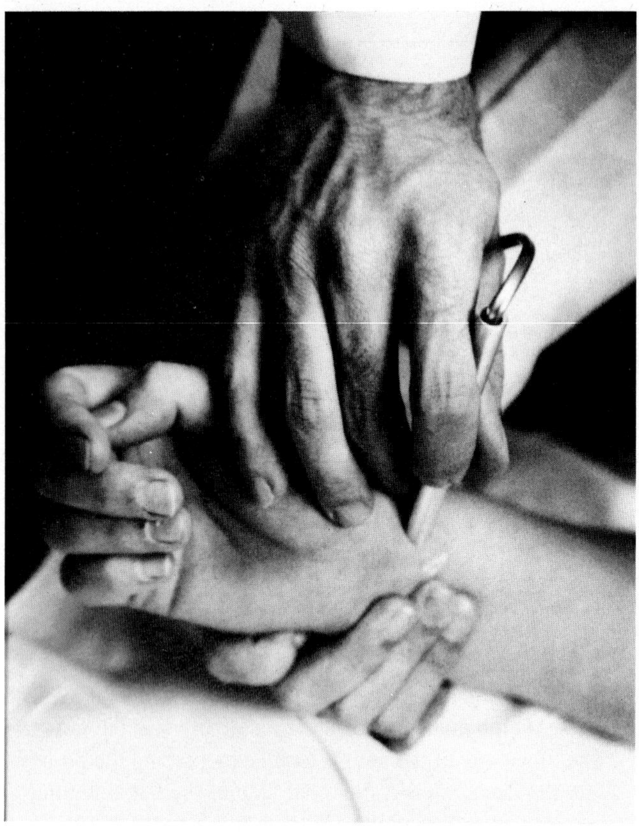

FIG. 20-105 Performing the Allen's test.

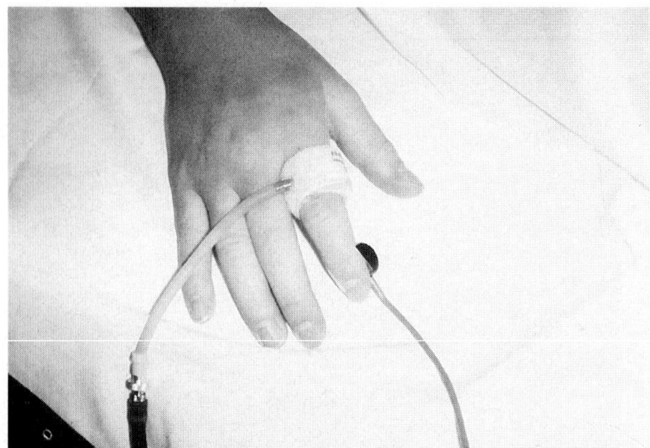

FIG. 20-106 Technique of obtaining digital pulse waveforms and pressures using photoplethysmography.

cell is taped or strapped to the fingertip of the digit being examined, or an appropriately sized strain gauge is looped around the fingertip; the plethysmography device is set to acquire PPG or SPG waveforms, the mode switch is set to AC, and the waveform display or chart recorder is calibrated as previously described.

Once a suitable stable waveform has been recorded, a digit pressure cuff can be placed on the proximal phalanx (Fig. 20-106), and the digit cuff is inflated with a manual sphygmomanometer until the waveform disappears and a flat line trace is seen. The cuff pressure is then slowly bled off until a peak is seen on the waveform display indicating the return of systolic flow. At that precise moment of waveform return, the pressure reading from the manometer should be recorded.

This procedure should be repeated for all digits of the hand being examined. Again, pattern recognition of normal and abnormal pulse contours should be used as explained. Interpretation of pressure criteria is discussed in the next subsection.

Doppler Examination of the Digits. The protocol below was developed by me based loosely on work done by Thulesius, Nielsen, and Lassen,[16] and the developmental study was presented at the Thirteenth Annual Meeting of the Society of Diagnostic Medical Sonographers (SDMS) in 1984.[18]

The patient first receives a limited upper-extremity arterial examination on the symptomatic side or sides, using segmental pressures and brachial radial ulnar waveforms as outlined previously (see Routine Upper Extremity Arterial Examination) but without axillary, subclavian, and vertebral waveforms being taken. An Allen's test for palmar arch patency is done as well. The examiner then should use an ample amount of gel and monitor the waveforms of the digital arteries on both the lateral and medial sides of the thumb and each finger in turn (Fig. 20-107). When doing this the examiner should angle the probe caudally and listen between the phalangeal joints of each digit, noting whether a signal is heard. The most distal extent to which a signal is detected in the finger is then mapped out on a report form, using the creases in the fingers as a landmark for the level of patency. If a flow signal is detected at the fingertip or distal phalanx but not in the proximal phalanx on the side being examined, there is probably a technical error. Once the arteries are mapped, the examiner should then place a digit pressure cuff around the proximal phalanx of the digit being examined and record the pressures and a waveform in each digital artery, repeating until the entire hand has been evaluated. Pressures will probably not be obtainable in digits with suspected distal occlusion. Forearm-brachial and digital-brachial ratios are calculated.

If the patient shows signs of ischemia only under exposure to cold, a vasospastic phenomenon such as Raynaud's must be suspected and ruled out, using a simple cold stress test.

Although sophisticated equipment exists for cold stress of digits, in reality little more is required than a glass of water, ice, and the Doppler to achieve similar results. A preimmersion signal is obtained in the symptomatic digits, and then the digit is immersed in the ice water for a maximum of 3 minutes or until severe pain occurs (Fig. 20-108). The digits are then removed and are immediately examined with the probe to see whether an audible signal is detected at preimmersion sites. Note: Do not perform cold stress evaluations on any digits with prominent evidence of spastic or occlusive disease (absent distal flow) regardless

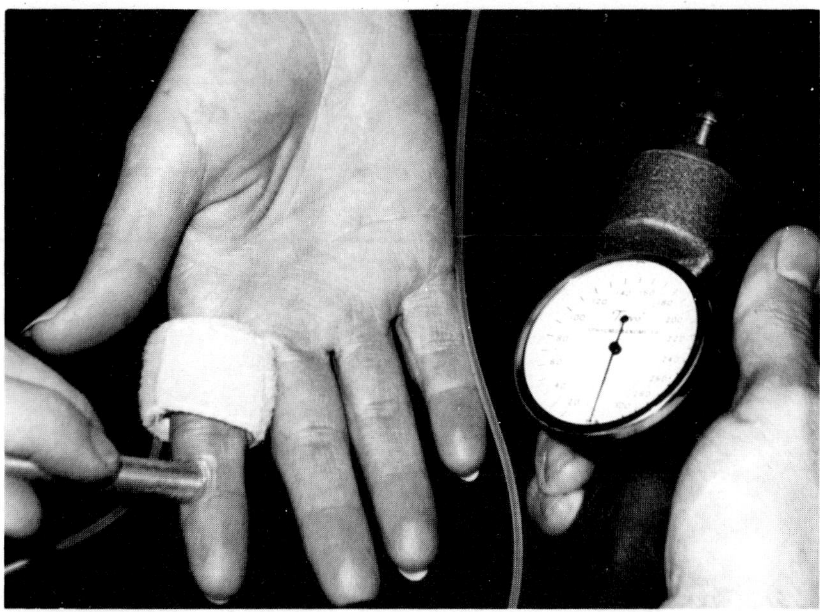

FIG. 20-107 Technique of obtaining individual digital artery waveforms and pressures using continuous-wave Doppler.

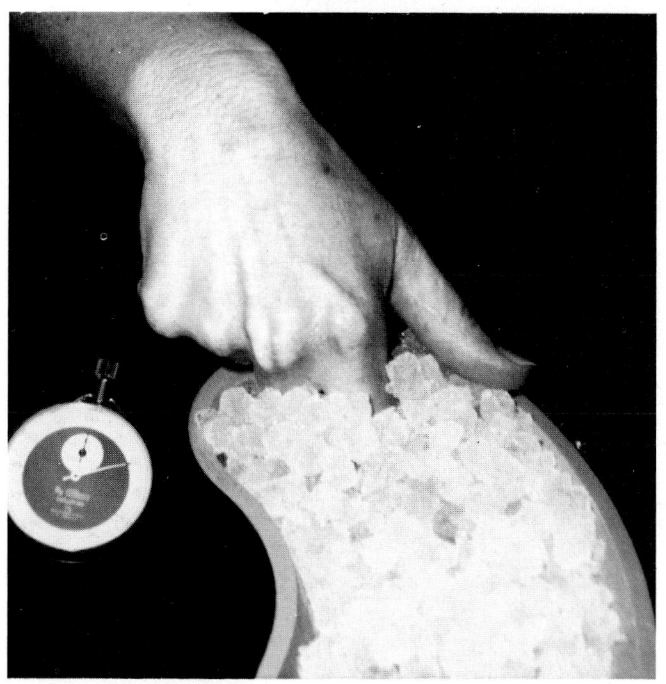

FIG. 20-108 Digital cold stress using ice water.

of symptoms; this may cause further damage to the already ischemic tissue.

Following is a summary of the steps required in digital artery evaluation:

1. Obtain a specific history, concentrating on any trauma to the digit or digits of interest, evidence of pain or numbness with exposure to cold, discoloration, ulceration, or ischemic changes.
2. Perform a limited upper-extremity examination, taking tracings and segmental pressures from the brachial, radial, and ulnar arteries.
3. Map flow from the base of finger to the fingertip, following the digital artery and noting any areas of absent flow on the mapping form. Use the creases of the fingers on the palmar side to help localize areas of obstruction or spasm; the obstruction usually occurs close to the joint.
4. Take pressures and waveforms from any detectable digital arteries on both sides of each finger using a digit cuff.
5. Calculate the forearm-brachial index and digital-brachial indices for each digital artery recorded.
6. If Raynaud's phenomenon is present, do a cold stress examination.

Interpretation of the Doppler Digital Examination

As with the routine upper-extremity exam, wave morphology and pressure change diagnoses are identical to those listed under Interpretation of the Upper Extremity Arterial Examination.

Flow patterns in the digits tend to be of a lower resistance pattern than those in the arm, and to have higher pressures. Digit-brachial indices from 1.0 to greater than 1.2 are considered normal.

Absence of flow at any distal segment of a digital artery is positive for focal digital artery occlusion at the mapped point.

Lack of augmentation of either the radial or ulnar artery with opposing compression during the Allen's test is consistent with palmar arch stenosis, occlusion, or congenital incompletion. The arch side affected often affects its respective digital arteries as well.

After cold stress, the absence of a signal where one was previously located is positive for cold-induced vasospasm. After warming the digit, the digit signal should be located again to confirm its presence and rule out technical error. The severity of vasospasm is often directly proportional to the amount of time needed for signal recovery.

Digital Examination Cases

Case 1 (Fig. 20-109): Normal. This is an example of a normal Doppler digital artery study. Brachial, radial, and ulnar waveforms are triphasic and the Allen's test is normal. Note that the digital flow is mapped as patent to the fingertips on both sides of each digit, and representative

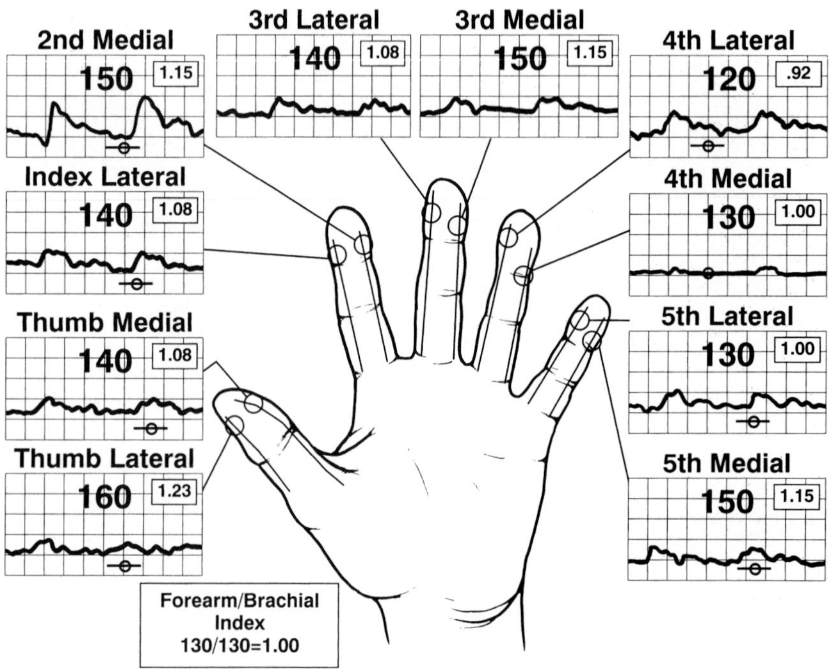

FIG. 20-109 Normal Doppler digital artery study.

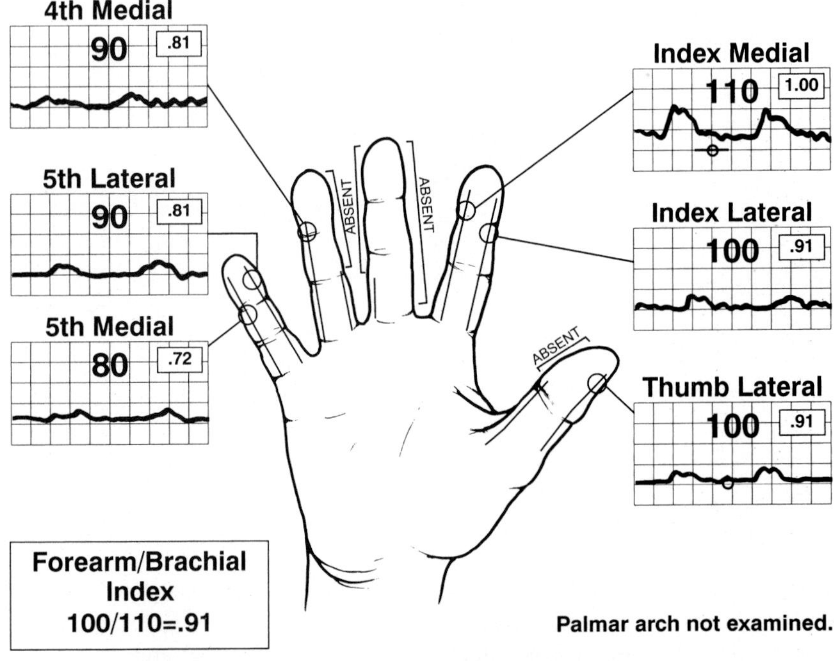

FIG. 20-110 Multiple areas of digital artery occlusion.

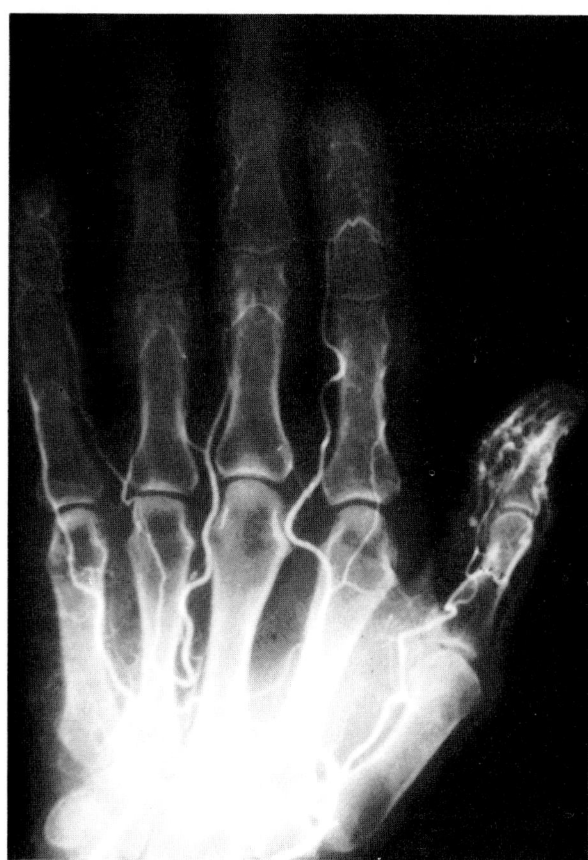

FIG. 20-111 Arteriogram confirming Doppler findings shown in Fig. 20-110 before digital sympathectomy.

waveforms are not diminished in appearance. The forearm-brachial indices are 1.00, and digital-brachial indices are not below 0.90.

Case 2 (Figs. 20-110 to 20-111): Multiple focal digital artery occlusions—predigital and postdigital sympathectomy. The first examination (Fig. 20-110) shows a patient with multiple areas of digital artery occlusion occurring in the medial thumb, lateral index finger, distal two thirds of the lateral third finger, and the distal third of the medial fourth and fifth fingers. Brachial, radial, and ulnar arteries are normal, and the Allen's test had no changes with compression. The forearm-brachial indices were normal. The Doppler findings were confirmed by an arteriogram (Fig. 20-111).

After digital sympathectomy to eliminate vasospastic responses and dilate the digital arteries, a dramatic improvement can be seen as flow is returned to all the digital arteries and normal digital-brachial indices are obtained (Fig. 20-112).

Case 3 (Fig. 20-113): Doppler—digital artery occlusion, fourth and fifth digits. This 61-year-old patient was referred with bluish discoloration, coldness, and pain of the fourth and fifth digits of the right hand.

An upper-extremity Doppler and segmental pressure examination showed normal flow patterns and pressures with no abnormality within the right arm *(A)*. The forearm-brachial indices were 1.06 (radial) and 1.10 (ulnar).

Doppler examination of the digital arteries *(B)* showed normal patent flow on both sides of the first three digits but only in the lateral proper digital arteries in the fourth and

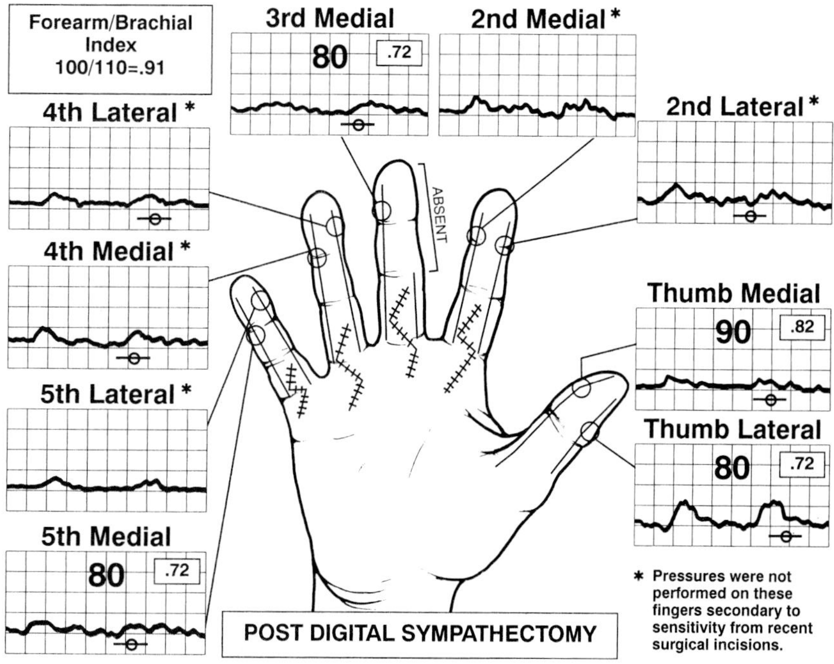

FIG. 20-112 Post-operative follow-up. Doppler digital artery study showing improvement of post-digital sympathectomy (compare with Fig. 20-110).

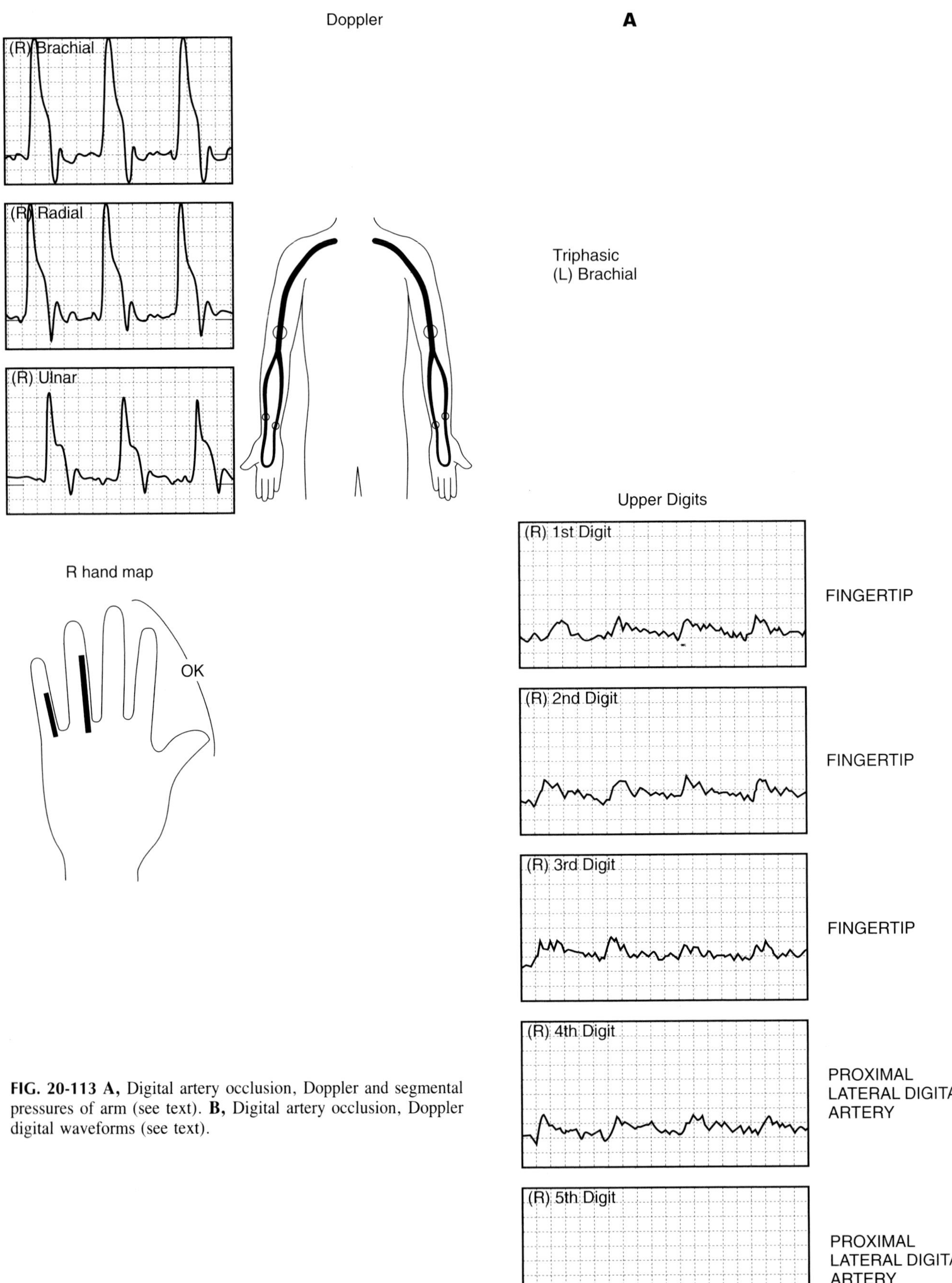

FIG. 20-113 A, Digital artery occlusion, Doppler and segmental pressures of arm (see text). **B,** Digital artery occlusion, Doppler digital waveforms (see text).

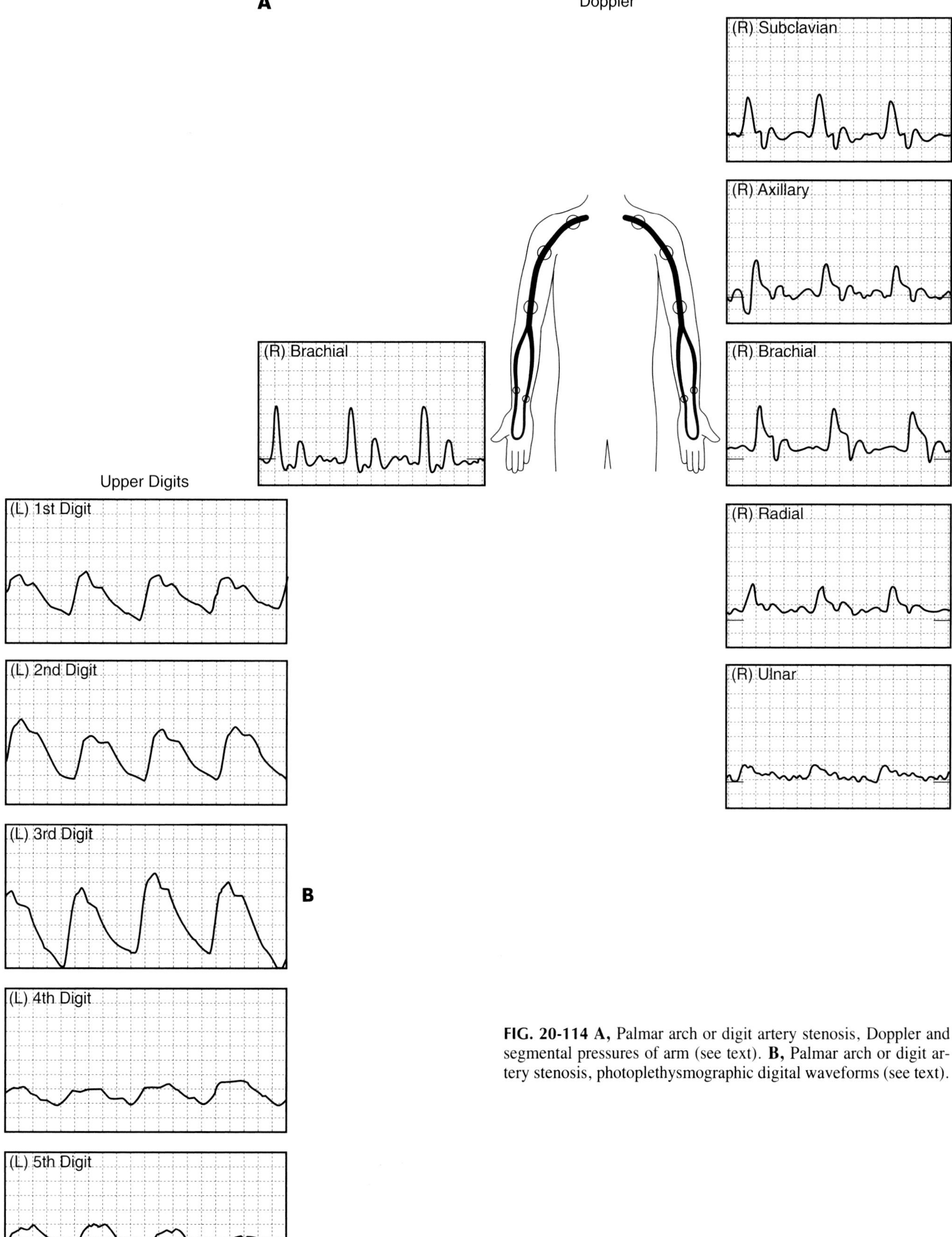

FIG. 20-114 A, Palmar arch or digit artery stenosis, Doppler and segmental pressures of arm (see text). **B,** Palmar arch or digit artery stenosis, photoplethysmographic digital waveforms (see text).

fifth fingers with the medial artery occluded and the distal arteries in the fourth and fifth fingertips occluded above the distal PIP joint. Pressure indices in the digits were normal in the first three fingers (1.05, 1.16, 1.13, respectively); pressure indices in the proximal patent lateral digital arteries were 0.88 (fourth digit) and 0.51 (fifth digit), implying proximal stenosis. The palmar arch was incomplete on Allen's testing.

Arteriography confirmed the digital artery occlusions and the patient was referred to a hand surgeon for digital sympathectomy.

Case 4 (Fig. 20-114): Photoplethysmography—digital artery or palmar arch embolic stenosis. This 57-year-old patient was referred with left arm aching and left hand pain with ischemic fourth and fifth digits; distal embolization to the fingers was suspected.

An upper-extremity Doppler and segmental pressure examination showed no abnormality within the left arm, although the radial and ulnar signals were slightly diminished *(A)*. The forearm-brachial indices were 1.06 (radial) and 0.96 (ulnar).

Photoplethysmographic examination of the digits *(B)* showed normal pulse waveforms in the first three digits with good dicrotic notches and upstroke. The waveforms in the fourth and fifth digits, however, were abnormal with decreased upstroke and blunted peaks; the fourth-digit waveform was markedly abnormal. Pressure indices in the digits were mildly abnormal in the first three fingers (0.81, 0.89, and 0.89, respectively); the pressure index in the fourth digit was severely diminished at 0.49. The fifth-digit pressure index was moderately abnormal at 0.73. The palmar arch was incomplete on Allen's testing, but was radial-dominant.

FINAL COMMENTS

No single modality provides the "best" arterial vascular examination; the "big picture" is only obtained through combinations of the techniques described in this chapter. It is up to the technologists or vascular laboratory physicians to set what they feel is a suitable protocol for effective diagnosis, but at the same time redundant tests should not be performed, nor should a large battery of noninvasive tests be used to prove something that could be diagnosed by one test alone. If the reader reviews the material in this chapter and becomes familiar with the modalities and techniques described herein, he or she will be well prepared for arterial evaluations in any vascular laboratory. Numerous other books and journal articles delve deeper into the techniques described here; I encourage the reader to investigate further.

REVIEW QUESTIONS

1. Name six conditions or processes that cause arterial occlusive disease.
2. What does claudication signify? List the symptoms or signs of arterial disease in order of progressive severity.
3. What does a normal Doppler waveform look like? What do each of the components signify?
4. What does Poiseuille's law, in principle, pertain to? Why is it important in the arterial system?
5. What factors should be evaluated in the preliminary history for patients with suspected arterial disease?
6. List the sites where Doppler waveforms are normally obtained in the lower extremities.
7. What findings should you expect to obtain in patients with:
   a. Distal aortic occlusion?
   b. Superficial femoral artery occlusion?
   c. Anterior tibial artery occlusion with a patent posterior tibial artery?
8. Where should segmental pressure cuffs be placed on the legs? How many are normally used?
9. Look at the pressure examples listed below. Specify where you think the stenosis or occlusion may be located in each case:
   a. Brachial 150, high thigh 120, low thigh 110, calf 100, DP 90, PT 90
   b. Brachial 120, high thigh 160, low thigh 150, calf 100, DP 90, PT 90
   c. Brachial 120, high thigh 160, low thigh 110, calf 90, DP 80, PT 80
   d. Brachial 140, high thigh 180, low thigh 180, calf 160, DP 160, PT 90
10. Calculate the ankle-brachial index for the following sets of numbers:
    a. Right arm 150, Left arm 130, Right PT 120, Right DP 120, Left PT 80, Left DP 112.
    b. Right arm 120, Left arm 160, Right PT 120, Right DP 130, Left PT 150, Left DP 140.
11. What are the differences between volume pulse recording and Doppler waveforms? What information is each method really showing?
12. How are stenoses identified with color-flow imaging? What color characteristics would you expect to see with a severe stenosis?
13. Describe the appearance of an occlusion in an artery. What might you see on Doppler spectral waveforms and on color-flow imaging?
14. What methods can be used to evaluate patients with normal resting Doppler and segmental findings who claudicate?
15. What range of penile-brachial index is significant for vasculogenic impotence?
16. Name some causes of arterial injury that can cause pseudoaneurysm formation. What characteristics do you expect to see sonographically and with color-flow imaging in a suspected pseudoaneurysm?
17. Name the two classifications of arteriovenous fistula. What can cause some acquired fistulas? What flow patterns should you expect to see?

18. What findings should you expect to obtain in patients with:
    a. Proximal subclavian artery stenosis?
    b. Distal subclavian artery stenosis?
    c. Brachial artery occlusion?
    d. Radial artery stenosis?
19. What causes thoracic outlet syndrome? What positions are used to evaluate it with Doppler or PPG?
20. What methods can be used to evaluate flow to the fingers?

REFERENCES

1. Baker JD: Post-stress Doppler ankle pressures; a comparison of treadmill exercise with two other methods of induced hyperemia, Arch Surg 113:1171, 1978.
2. Bandyk DF, Cato RF, and Towne JB: A low flow velocity predicts failure of femoropopliteal and femorotibial bypass, Surgery 98:799, 1985.
3. Bandyk DF, Seabrook GR, Moldenhauer P, et al: Hemodynamics of vein graft stenosis, J Vasc Surg 8:688, 1988.
4. Barnes RW: Axioms on acute arterial occlusion of an extremity, Hosp Med 14:34, 1978.
5. Barnes RW, Wilson MR: Doppler ultrasonic evaluation of peripheral arterial disease: a programmed audiovisual instruction. Iowa City, Iowa, 1976, University of Iowa Press.
6. Bergan JJ and Yao JST: Gangrene and severe ischemia of the lower extremities. New York, 1978, Grune & Stratton.
7. Burnham CB: Color Doppler duplex arterial scanning, J Vasc Tech 15:129, 1991.

8a. Burnham CB and Cummings C: Should arterial duplex imaging replace segmental pressures? J Vasc Tech 17:49, 1993.

8b. Charcot J-M: Sur la claudication intermittente observé dans un cas d'oblitration complète de l'une des artères iliaques primitives, Comptes Rendus de la Société de Bidogie, p.225, 1858.

9. Edwards J, Cato R, Bandyk DF, et al: Vascular laboratory surveillance of infrainguinal bypass: the role of early postoperative duplex scanning. J Vasc Tech 15:241, 1991.
10. Interscoietal Commision for the Accreditation of Vascular Laboratories: Essentials and standards for noninvasive vascular testing. Vascular Laboratory Operations, Part II (Peripheral Arterial Testing). Rockville, Md: 1993, The Commission.
11. Gray HC and Carter HV: Gray's anatomy. St. Louis, Mo, 1992, Mosby.
12. Hummel BW, Hummel BA, Mowbry A, et al: Reactive hyperemia versus treadmill testing in arterial disease, Arch Surg 113:95, 1978.
13. Jager KA, Ricketts JH, and Strandness DE: Duplex scanning for the evaluation of lower limb arterial disease. In Bernstein EF, editor: Noninvasive diagnostic techniques in vascular disease, ed 3. St. Louis, 1985, Mosby.
14. Jürgens JL, Spittell JA, and Fairbairn JF: Peripheral vascular diseases. Philadelphia, WB Saunders, 1980.
15. Nath RL, Menzoian JO, Kaplan KH, et al: The multidisciplinary approach to vasculogenic impotence, Surgery 89:124, 1978.
16. Nielsen SL and Lassen NA: Finger systolic pressures in upper-extremity testing for cold sensitivity (Raynaud's phenomenon). In Bernstein EF, editor: Noninvasive diagnostic techniques in vascular disease, ed 2. St. Louis, 1982, Mosby.
17. Platz M: Doppler ultrasound studies of subclavian steal hemodynamics in subclavian stenosis, J Thorac Cardiovasc Surg 27:404, 1979.
18. Rae R: Doppler examination of the digital arteries: a reliable method of evaluating focal ischemic phenomena in the hand. Proceedings of 13th Annual Convention of the Society of Diagnostic Medical Sonographers, J Ultrasound Med 3:186, 1984 (abstract).
19. Raines JK: The pulse volume recorder in peripheral arterial disease. In Bernstein EF, editor: Noninvasive diagnostic techniques in vascular disease, ed 3. St. Louis, 1985, Mosby.
20. Rutherford RB: Noninvasive testing in the diagnosis and assessment of arteriovenous fistula. In Bernstein EF, editor: Noninvasive diagnostic techniques in vascular disease, ed 3. St. Louis, 1985, Mosby.
21. von Reutern GM, Budingen HJ, Freund HJ, et al: Dopplersonographische diagnostik von Stenosen und Verschlussen der Vertebralarterien und des Subclavian-Steal-Syndroms, Arch Psychiatr Nervenkr 222(2-3):209, 1976.

BIBLIOGRAPHY

Stanley JC, Lindenauer SM, Graham LM, et al: Vascular grafts. In Moore WS, editor: Vascular surgery: a comprehensive review, ed 2. Orlando, Fla, 1986, Grune & Stratton.

CHAPTER

21

Venous Sonography, Doppler, and Plethysmography Examinations

Richard E. Rae II

The incidence of venous disease has been estimated to surpass that of cardiac disease and stroke.[2] Venous thrombosis, varicose veins, and pulmonary embolism are among the most common problems encountered in both outpatients and inpatients.

Pulmonary embolism is among the most dangerous venous diseases. It occurs as a result of venous thrombosis and can especially affect bedridden, paraplegic or quadriplegic, and comatose patients in whom clots develop because of a lack of muscular activity leading to venous stagnation.[10,15,20] An embolus can detach itself from the intimal wall in an area of thrombosis and can travel superiorly or inferiorly through the vena cava to the pulmonary arteries, where the thrombus can occlude any portion of the pulmonary vasculature and cause severe damage or death. Thrombi that cause pulmonary embolism very rarely travel from calf veins; the majority of these clots come from the femoral, iliac, or inferior vena cava.

Thrombophlebitis is the main reason for evaluating the venous system. A thrombus or clot can form almost anywhere within the venous system, and usually arises as the result of intimal damage to the vein wall with a subsequent platelet response resulting in a focal coagulation of blood. Inflammation of the vein can result. Stagnant venous flow from insufficient venous return also can compound the problem and enlarge the thrombus. A thrombosis can be of an acute or chronic nature; fresh or new (acute) thrombus tends to be less organized and may be easier to resolve with anticoagulant therapy or lysis. Clot that remains in a vein for a long period (chronic) becomes more organized and firm. Chronic thrombi also increase the flow pressure required to move blood toward the heart and often force collaterals to develop and shunt the blood around the obstruction. Thromboses also can form in the venous valve sinuses where flow slows or stagnates. Progression of these thrombi can freeze the venous valves in an open or partially open position, resulting in venous insufficiency and backflow as well as damage to the valve cusps themselves from the inflammation and flow pressure. A damaged valve usually becomes incompetent, and the distal portion of the vein may deform and dilate because of increased venous back pressure. When this occurs in a superficial vein, this can result in varicose veins (although heredity can also contribute to their formation).[3] After treatment of a venous thrombosis with anticoagulants, lytic agents, or both, these damaged valves may remain insufficient and cause pooling of blood in the dependent veins and thus swelling or edema. When this occurs after resolution of a prior case of thrombophlebitis, this condition may be termed *postphlebitic syndrome*. If severe valvular incompetence threatens the deep system, a surgical anastomosis of the superficial femoral vein with proximal great saphenous vein below the valve can restore some sufficiency.

The diagnosis of venous disease based on physical examination has proved to be one of the most difficult areas for the physician, exceeding a 50% error margin.[2,10] Fortunately many of the classic methods of diagnosis have now been supplemented with newer techniques designed to rule out venous thrombosis or insufficiency.

Contrast phlebography (venography) is the standard method of diagnosing venous thrombosis or embolism.[2,10] This is, again, an invasive technique, with many of the same risks found in arteriography (e.g., contrast media reactions, radiation risks). A further complication is that the patient must support his or her own weight and attempt to remain immobile while tourniquets are applied and irritating contrast medium is injected. The position may, understandably, be difficult to maintain. Venography can also be performed in the supine position, but this does not often result in satisfactory filling of calf or foot veins, since the leg or extremity is not dependent. The examination may also, in rare cases, cause a thrombus to form. Venography is considered by many to be the gold standard, since small thrombi can be readily detected throughout the entire superficial and deep venous systems even with no flow obstruction. It should be noted, however, that the efficacy and accuracy of venous duplex sonography and color-flow imaging have caused many to question whether venography remains the gold standard.

Nuclear medicine techniques are also used to diagnose sources of venous emboli (thrombi).[2,10] These involve injecting radionuclides, which are either followed through the deep venous system by a gamma camera or absorbed by the thrombus and shown on a static scan. The former method uses technetium-99^m pertechnetate and is more efficient for veins above the knee; discrimination of calf veins is impossible because of the diminished resolution. The latter method, using I-125 fibrinogen, allows discrimination of isolated calf thrombi but is not successful in veins above the knee because of the higher background activity from the radionuclide absorption. Both methods eliminate the irritation of the venographic contrast media and are accurate but are not feasible for routine screening of symptomatic patients. Other methods are indicated in these patients.

Plethysmographic techniques are also widely used as adjunctive procedures in the venous system. Some of these methods are discussed later in this chapter.

The venous system can be examined ultrasonically in two ways: the first and simplest method requires only the use of the Doppler device. Small, pocket-sized instruments can be carried for bedside examination to avoid patient transportation. Strip-chart recording is optional if a record of flow is desired. The use of a stethoscope or low-frequency sensitive headphones is imperative, because venous velocity signals tend to be very slow and low pitched and could be missed if external speakers alone are used. The second, and most thorough, method requires the use of a high-resolution real time duplex scanner, which is much more accurate than venous Doppler alone, since venous Doppler is inaccurate for assessing calf vein thrombosis and is more accurate above the knee. Venous duplex sonography combined with color-flow imaging and Doppler spectral flow analysis is proving to be more reliable than contrast venography alone and has resulted in much more accurate and specific diagnoses. Venous duplex sonography, unlike venography, shows the full extent of a clot and enables some age determination (acute versus chronic). In addition, long-term follow-up is more practical with venous duplex sonography than by radiographic means and also gives important information about the valves and perforator veins unobtainable with venography. Many clinical centers are beginning to hail venous duplex sonography as the new gold standard.[22,23]

The Intersocietal Commission for the Accreditation of Vascular Laboratories has identified venous duplex ultrasonography (or B-mode imaging supplemented by continuous-wave Doppler) as the primary noninvasive diagnostic method to be used in accredited noninvasive vascular laboratories to evaluate peripheral venous disease. Other noninvasive techniques (plethysmography and photoplethysmography methods, phleborheography, continuous-wave Doppler without imaging, and B-mode imaging without continuous or pulsed Doppler) are considered secondary techniques that may provide further information but should not be individually used to diagnose venous disease.[13]

Although a technologist will undoubtedly encounter laboratories that use one or more of the secondary techniques in addition to venous duplex sonography, the body of this chapter concentrates on the primary methods: venous duplex sonography techniques, color-flow imaging, B-mode imaging characteristics, and the continuous-wave Doppler venous examination. The other secondary modalities are briefly discussed but some techniques are not covered in depth; the reader may wish to refer to other detailed texts that cover these nonimaging methods.

CHARACTERISTICS OF THE NORMAL VENOUS VELOCITY SIGNAL[2]

Physiologically, flow dynamics of the venous and arterial systems differ because of the methods by which the blood is moved through them. In the arterial system, blood is pumped directly by the heart, and a pulsatile pattern of flow corresponding to the cardiac cycle is heard. In the venous system, however, there is no pump to force the blood back toward the heart so there should be no pulsatility.

Unlike the arteries, the veins possess valves along their courses that prevent blood from backing up into the more distal segments and ensure a steady flow of blood. The blood is moved through the veins by respiratory variations in intraabdominal and intrathoracic pressure. During inspiration the pressure is increased, the valves close, and flow stops. During expiration the pressure eases, the valves reopen, and blood flows forward once again (Fig. 21-1).

Familiarity with the normal arterial signal can help the examiner locate the venous signals at their various sites. The venous signal has been described as windlike; it is of a lower velocity than the arterial signal and rises and falls in pitch with expiration and inspiration, respectively. This quality of variation with respiration is called *phasicity*.

There are six normal qualities in the veins that are checked by an examiner at all examination sites.

The first quality is patency. This means that a vein allows blood to flow through it without obstruction of the lumen. Flow heard or seen by color-flow imaging through a venous segment implies patency of that portion of the vein. Complete absence of a flow signal at any given site implies occlusion of that segment.

The second quality is *spontaneity*. This means that a signal is heard or flow patterns visualized through the vein without manipulation of the limb to force flow through the

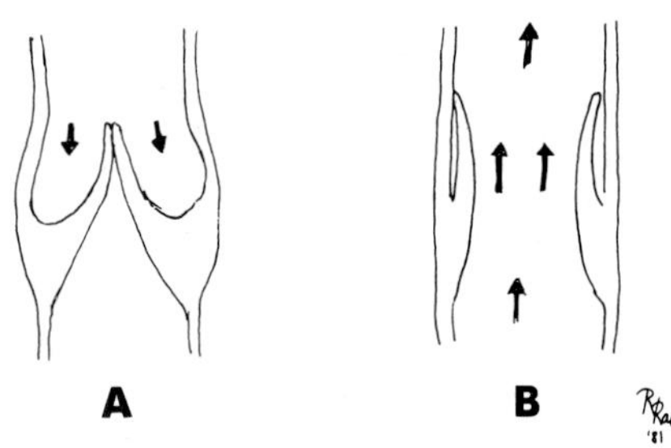

FIG. 21-1 Venous valves. **A,** Closed with inspiration. **B,** Open with expiration.

segment being examined. Spontaneity does not occur in vasoconstricted veins (e.g., those in a cold leg), nor in veins that are drained of blood, as in an elevated leg. Only the posterior tibial vein may not be normally spontaneous and may require compression of the foot to augment flow.

The third normal quality is *phasicity*. As mentioned earlier, this means that normal variations with respiration should occur in a normal vein. Loss of phasicity results in a steadily rushing, unchanging, continuous flow pattern. This always implies disease.

The fourth normal quality is called *augmentation*. This is the technique of compressing the venous pools in the distal portion of the limb to increase, or augment, the flow. Augmentation can also be created by compressing the segment of the vein proximal to the probe site, holding it for several seconds, and then releasing. This creates a backup of flow, shutting competent valves and stopping flow briefly, which then rushes forward on release of compression. Lack of augmentation implies occlusion or thrombus between the probe and the compression site.

The fifth quality concerns *competence* of the valves in the limb, or their normal ability to prevent retrograde flow in the venous system. If the valves are destroyed by thrombus or disease, leakage occurs and flow backs up into the distal segment of the vein. Incompetence is often found after treatment of deep-vein thrombosis and in varicose veins. Competency is checked by listening for reflux, which may occur with release of distal compression or the act of proximal compression. Any reflux implies lack of valvular competence between the probe and the compression site. The Valsalva maneuver is also a good test for the valves since it should also stop flow and shut the venous valves.

The sixth and final quality is *nonpulsatility*. It is usually abnormal for the venous system to vary with the cardiac cycle in the lower extremities. A patient with congestive or right heart failure may have pulsatility as a result of increased pressure within the venous system. A patient with an extremely irregular breathing pattern may also show a similar pattern to pulsatility. The veins in the upper extremity thoracic area do not show this quality, and pulsatility is a normal quality there because of reflected pulsatility from the heart through the superior vena cava.

In summary, the six qualities of the normal venous velocity signal are:

1. Patency. Flow can be heard through the venous segment spontaneously or with augmenting.
2. Spontaneity. Flow is heard without manipulation of the limb, except in the posterior tibial vein occasionally.
3. Phasicity. Flow varies with the respiratory cycle.
4. Augmentation. Flow increases normally with distal compression and also with release of proximal compression.
5. Competence. The valves prevent retrograde flow or reflux in the vein.
6. Nonpulsatility. The venous flow is not affected by the cardiac cycle, except in the upper extremities.

LOWER-EXTREMITY VENOUS EVALUATION TECHNIQUES

Venous Anatomy of the Lower Extremity[15]

There usually is a corresponding vein for every artery evaluated in the lower extremities; thus ultrasonic or Doppler access sites usually apply to venous evaluations as well. Although it is a conventional practice to refer to, for example, a posterior tibial vein, in reality the major deep veins are paired plexuses that parallel the arteries (often referred to as venae comitantes). The veins, unlike the arteries, are divided into superficial and deep systems. A third system, the perforating veins, connects the superficial and deep veins at several levels in the leg.

Deep Veins

In the deep system various plantar veins anastomose into larger tributaries that unite with the deep venous plantar arch. These veins come together to form the posterior tibial veins.[6]

The posterior tibial veins run along the medial surface of the leg superiorly and are superficially accessible directly posterior to the medial malleolus and along the calf to just below the knee, where they join the peroneal vein at the peroneal-tibial junction with the popliteal vein.

The anterior tibial veins follow the course of the anterior tibial artery, lateral to the tibia from the ankle to the knee. They are superficially accessible along the anterior surface of the leg just lateral to the tibia. Although they are evaluated by venous duplex sonography, they are seldom included in the continuous-wave Doppler examination.

The peroneal veins run posterior, deep in the calf muscles along the fibula, joining with the posterior tibial vein just below the knee to form the peroneal-tibial junction with the popliteal vein.

The popliteal vein runs alongside the popliteal artery behind the knee and continues upward into the thigh, where it becomes the superficial femoral vein. The superficial femoral vein continues cephalad and becomes the common femoral vein at the point of anastomosis of the deep femoral (profunda femoris) vein, which drains the muscles and bone.

The common femoral vein continues cephalad and becomes the external iliac vein, which anastomoses with the internal iliac vein to form the common iliac vein. The common iliacs from each side come together to join with the inferior vena cava (Fig. 21-2).

Superficial Veins

The superficial system, for Doppler and imaging purposes, consists mainly of the great and lesser saphenous veins.

The great saphenous vein arises from the dorsum of the foot and ascends anterior to the medial malleolus. It runs along the medial surface of the leg superficially, outside the knee to the thigh, and anastomoses with the common femoral vein at the *saphenofemoral* junction. Accessory saphe-

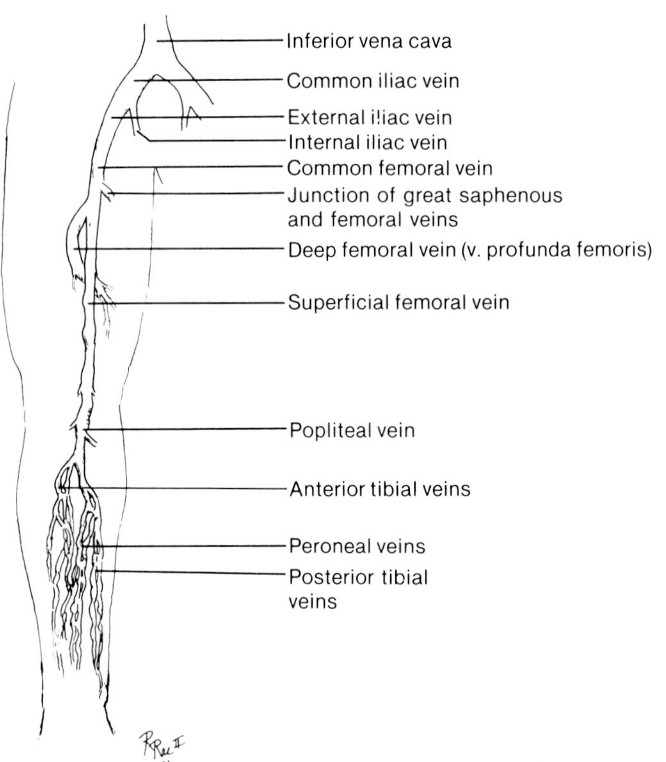

FIG. 21-2 Deep venous system of the lower extremity.

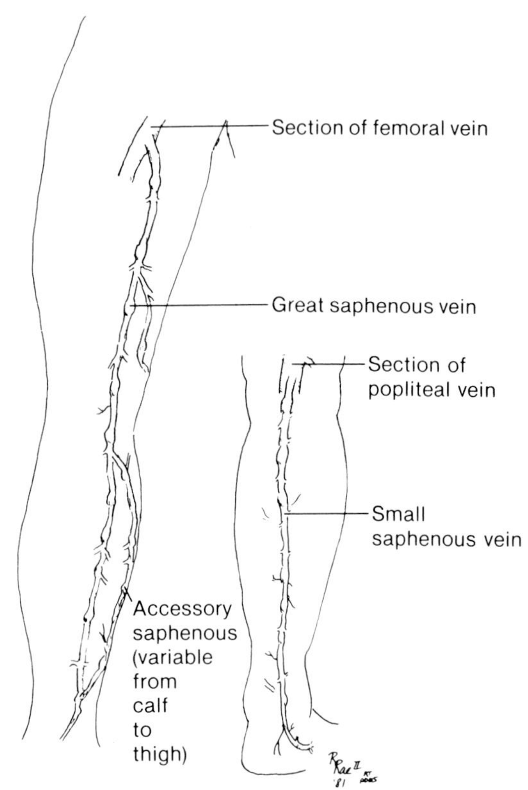

FIG. 21-3 Superficial venous system of the lower extremity.

nous veins can occur randomly along the thigh or calf and empty into the great saphenous vein.

The saphenous vein arises posterior to the lateral malleolus. It progresses superficially up the back of the calf to the knee, where it penetrates the deep fascia and empties into the popliteal vein (Fig. 21-3).

An important superficial vein that may be encountered and that can affect diagnosis is the Giacomeni vein, which has a distal anastomosis with the popliteal vein and leaves the popliteal vein above the saphenopopliteal junction and travels medially along the thigh to join the great saphenous;[3] in some cases the Giacomeni vein can arise from the saphenopopliteal junction (Fig. 21-4).

Perforating Veins

The perforating veins are important because they can cause superficial varicosities and venous stasis ulceration. They connect the superficial veins with the deep veins, and each perforating vein group has a different name depending on its location. In general, there are one to three main perforators in the medial lower calf near the ankle (Cockett perforators), two perforators just below the knee in the anteromedial calf (Boyd perforators), one or more perforators above the knee in the distal third of the thigh (Dodd perforators), and one or more perforators at the midthigh level (Hunterian perforators).[3] All these connect superficial branches of the great saphenous or of arch veins with the deep veins, and they all are usually best seen with color-flow duplex sonography (Fig. 21-5).

Anomalies

Examiners should be aware that duplication of major veins does occur, mostly in the legs; it is not uncommon to find two superficial femoral veins, two popliteal veins, or two great saphenous veins that originate and insert into normal single segments. It is important to remember this because one venous limb may be thrombosed, whereas the other is patent. This bears on mapping of the great saphenous vein as well. Either saphenous limb may be unsuitable for bypass use and surgeons need to be aware of multiple branches, especially when creating in situ bypasses.

At times, other anomalous communications may occur, for example, between the deep femoral vein and the superficial femoral vein or between the great saphenous vein and the Giacomeni vein, and others. An examiner should carefully image all suspect vessels in longitudinal and transverse planes to show their course and extent.

Before the Noninvasive Examination

Most patients presenting with venous disease require lower-limb examination. One of the best ways to determine the presence of venous disease is to check for arterial symptoms first and determine whether a pulse is felt.[10] Purplish discolorations, dark spots in the calf, and dark ulcerated ar-

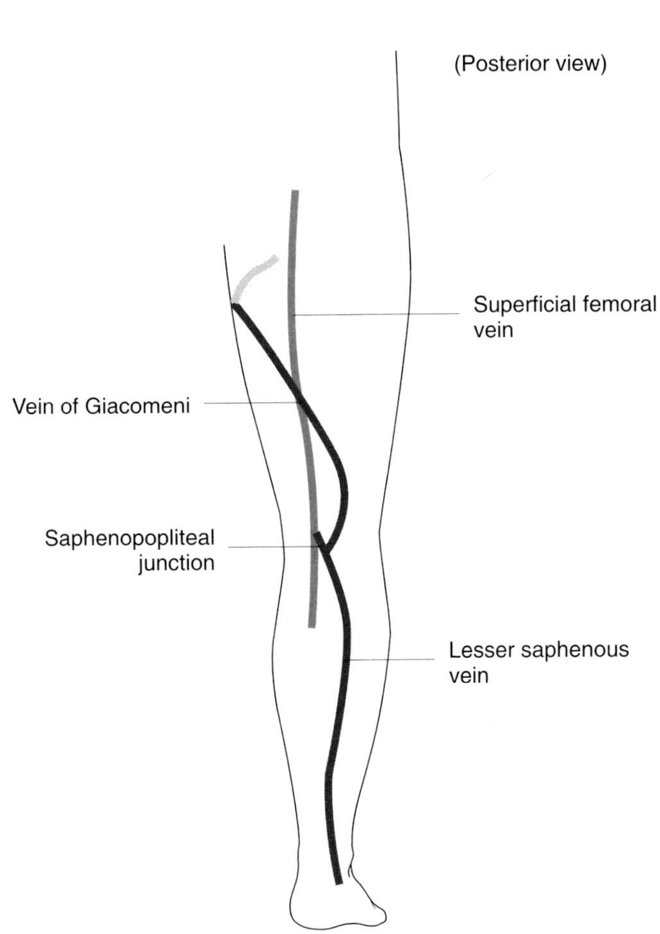

FIG. 21-4 Posterior view of the leg showing the superficial Giacomeni vein and its relationship to the lesser saphenous vein, the saphenopopliteal junction, and the deep veins.

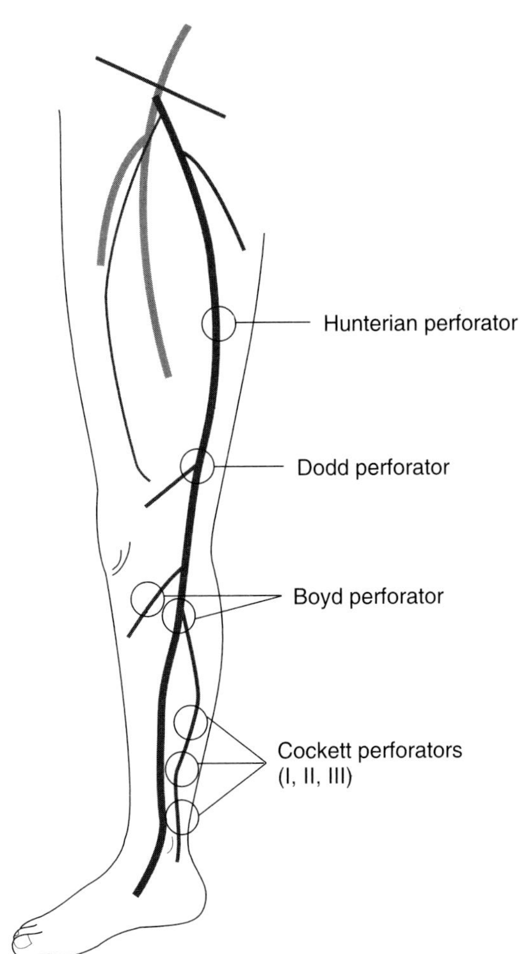

FIG. 21-5 Anterior view of the leg showing the great saphenous vein and the locations of the major perforating veins (see text).

eas near the medial malleolus all characterize venous disease, as do swelling and edema of the ankles and legs. The leg will be warm rather than cool as in arterial disease. Pain occurs with dependence of the limb, and relief is obtained by elevation. Swelling also diminishes with elevation of the extremity. Pain also appears regardless of whether the patient is walking or resting, and walking may actually alleviate the symptoms. Varicosities and red streaks on the limbs also characterize venous disease. Pulling the toes of the foot back toward the leg (dorsiflexion) may cause sharp pain in the calf if calf-vein thrombosis is present (Homan's sign),[10] but it should be noted that Homan's sign is positive in 65% of normal patients. These symptoms should help the examiner make a differential determination.

As in all examinations, the first step is to obtain a thorough history from the patient or the chart. Special attention must be paid to the location of the pain, whether it occurs with walking or rest, and whether elevation relieves the discomfort. Areas of swelling are checked. If unilateral disease is present, one leg appears larger than the other. Areas of dark almost greenish color are signs of venous insufficiency, as are purple patches and prominent varicose veins. Red streaks imply superficial disease. The patient should also be questioned about past surgeries, especially if arterial or coronary artery bypasses have been performed. In these cases the saphenous vein is removed in whole or in part and is used for the bypass. A high percentage of postcoronary bypass patients develop venous disease or marked swelling in the leg 6 months to 1 year after surgery because of the loss of this superficial vein. It is important to ask the patient if any superficial vein strippings, varicose vein ligations, or sclerotherapy injections have been performed, especially because this may affect the image findings on duplex examinations.

Finally, it is helpful to document any past history of phlebitis or deep vein thrombosis and determine whether the patient is currently taking anticoagulants, such as heparin or warfarin, or underwent treatment with lytic agents, such as streptokinase or urokinase.

The patient should remove all clothing from the lower extremities, including stockings and underwear, and lie supine with the head raised 20 to 30 degrees to ensure venous pooling in the legs.[2] The legs should not be elevated and should be relaxed and slightly flexed at the knees to allow good flow dynamics and prevent compression of the popliteal vein against the condyles of the knee joint. The room should be warm to prevent vasoconstriction. If venous studies other than duplex evaluation are being done, it sometimes helps to have the patient lie supine for 10 to 15 minutes to allow the veins to stabilize before beginning the other tests.

CONTINUOUS-WAVE DOPPLER LOWER-EXTREMITY VENOUS EVALUATION

To perform the continuous-wave Doppler examination, the examiner needs a bidirectional Doppler, preferably equipped with both a high-frequency and low-frequency probe and headphones (since the pitch of venous signals is often too low to be readily heard without them). Waveforms can be documented by chart recorder or by computer software, but many examiners simply record the audible findings in a matrix that lists the basic six venous flow characteristics and summarizes the information at a glance (Fig. 21-6).

Legs - Doppler

	CFV		SFV		PV		ATV		PTV		GSV	
	R	L	R	L	R	L	R	L	R	L	R	L
Spontaneous	+	+	+	0	+	0	+	+	+	+	+	+
Phasic	+	+	+	0	+	0	+	0	+	0	+	0
Augmented	+	-	+	0	+	-	+	-	+	-	+	+
Competent	+	+	+		+	+	+	-	+	+	+	0
Nonpulsatile	Y	Y	Y	Y	Y	Y	Y	Y	Y	Y	Y	Y

+ = Present - = Reduced 0 = Absent Y = Yes N = No

CFV = Common Femoral
PV = Popliteal
PTV = Posterior Tibial
SFV = Superficial Femoral
ATV = Anterior Tibial
GSV = Greater Saphenous

FIG. 21-6 Typical example matrix for indicating venous findings by continuous-wave Doppler.

The first vein to be examined is the posterior tibial vein at its site posterior to the medial malleolus. Gel is applied to the site, and the probe is angled caudally. The posterior tibial artery can be used as a landmark for locating the area. The patient is instructed to take in exaggerated breaths to accentuate the phasicity in the veins. A patient with cold feet may have vasoconstriction, and a spontaneous signal may not be heard.

When the site has been determined, the foot may be squeezed to augment flow if spontaneity is not present (Fig. 21-7). The examiner listens for phasicity and nonpulsatility. The amount of augmentation with distal (foot) compression is evaluated; then the leg is grasped at the calf proximally to the probe, compressed for several seconds, and released to elicit augmentation (Fig. 21-8). The flow signal should stop with proximal compression, then resume in a rush, and return to normal with release. Lack of response with either distal or proximal compression implies disease.

The popliteal vein is the next vein to be examined. As with the popliteal artery, there are two ways to position the patient—supine or prone. If the prone method is preferred, examination of the popliteal can be performed as the last step in the examination.

In the supine position the patient's knee should be flexed a bit more, and the probe is placed in the popliteal fossa and angled caudally. (See Fig. 21-9 for relative positioning.) The arterial signal is located, and the probe is angled medially and laterally until a distinct venous signal is heard.

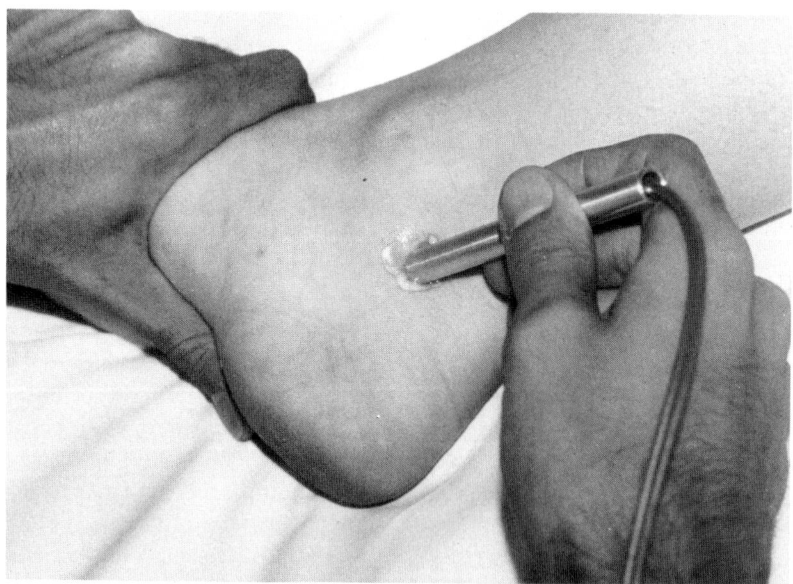

FIG. 21-7 Posterior tibial vein examination with distal (foot) compression. Note that the probe is angled against the flow.

The amount of pressure required can vary, because venous collaterals in the fossa should be stopped but the popliteal vein should not be occluded. Gentle pressure usually will not occlude the deep vein.

When the signal has been found, the examiner checks for patency, spontaneity, phasicity, and nonpulsatility. Augmentation is evaluated by distal compression of the foot and calf (Fig. 21-10) and by proximal compression of the thigh. A Valsalva maneuver may be performed at this point to demonstrate the competence of the proximal venous valves.

In the prone position the patient's feet are elevated approximately 30 degrees by pillows. With this exception, the examination is performed in the exact sequence as described above for the supine position (Fig. 21-11).

The common femoral vein is examined next. The best site to examine the vein is superior to the inguinal ligament. The common femoral artery is first located, and the probe is moved medially and angled caudally to obtain the venous signal. Pressure may be applied to the probe gently to occlude the superficial venous collaterals, since the femoral vein is not as easily compressed. Once again, the signal is evaluated for patency, spontaneity, phasicity, and nonpulsatility. Augmentation is elicited by distal compression (calf, thigh) and proximal compression of the vein superior to the probe site by Valsalva maneuver. Competence is assessed by listening for reflux with compression and by the response to the Valsalva.

If a discrepancy between the groin and knee is noted, the superficial femoral vein may be examined in the groove

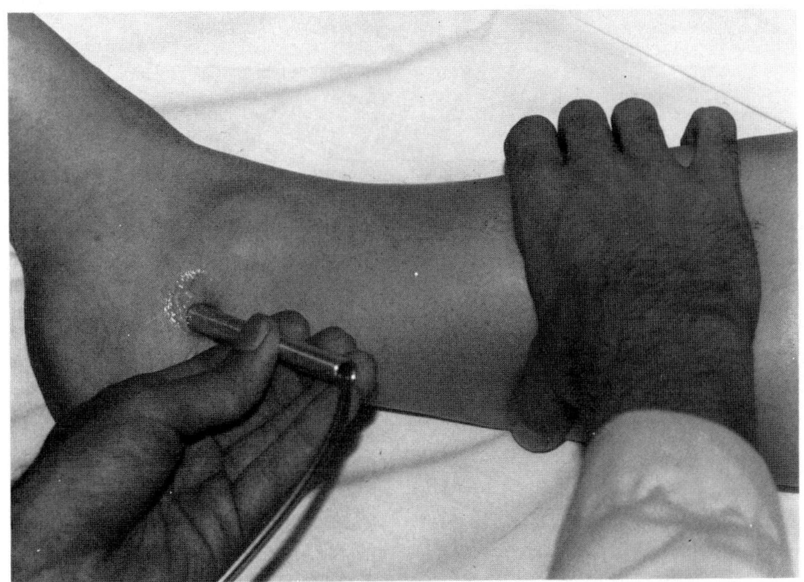

FIG. 21-8 Examination of the posterior tibial vein, with proximal calf compression.

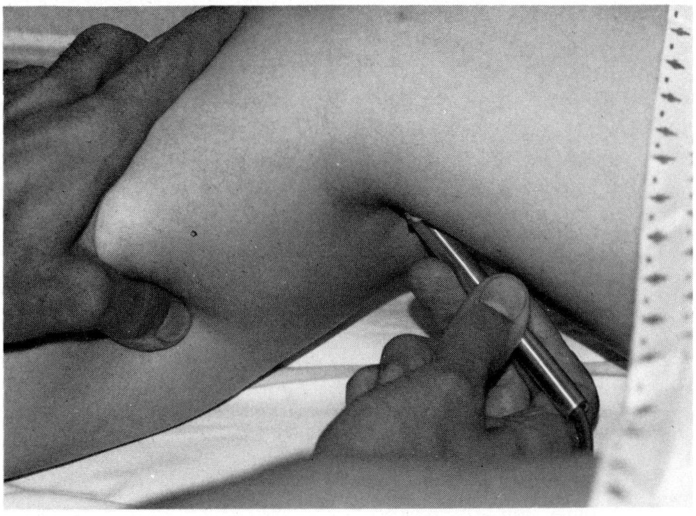

FIG. 21-9 Supine examination of the popliteal vein, with distal calf compression. Note that the transducer is angled against the flow.

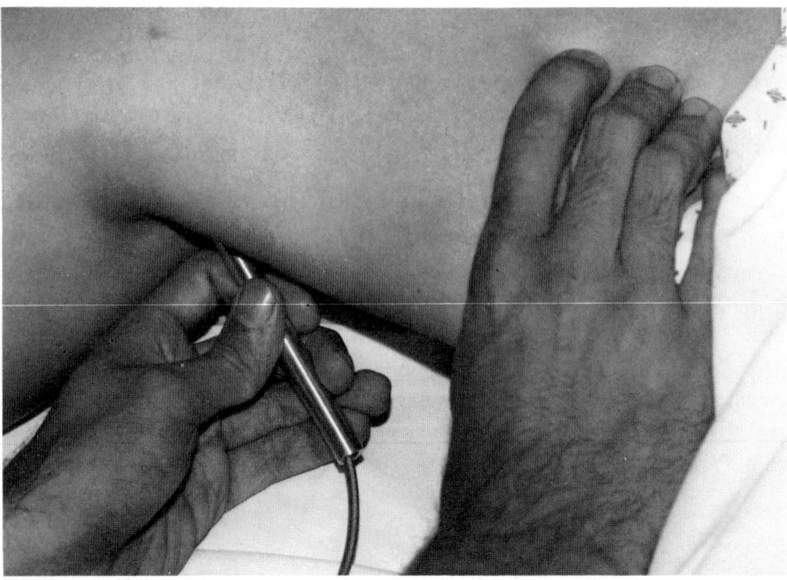

FIG. 21-10 Examination of the popliteal vein with thigh (proximal) compression.

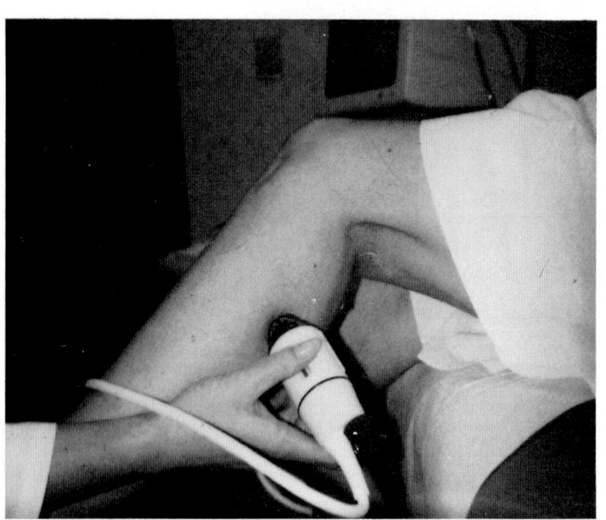

FIG. 21-11 Prone examination of the popliteal artery.

superior to the vastus medialis and the sartorius on the thigh. The examination should follow the same procedure of signal evaluation, distal and proximal compression, and the Valsalva as used at the other sites. This completes the examination of the deep veins.

The superficial system examination is less involved but requires a finer degree of awareness on the part of the examiner.

The great saphenous vein can be examined anywhere along its course from ankle to the saphenofemoral junction. A light probe pressure is required to avoid compression of the vessel. Flow may or may not be spontaneous or phasic through the saphenous systems. It is helpful to position the probe at the site on the inside medial thigh and percuss or milk the distal vein to augment its flow.

Whether the responses obtained by augmentation and the relative flow dynamics signify disease depends on whether a predisposing factor is suspected. Femoral thrombosis extending into the saphenofemoral junction, varicose veins, and evidence of superficial venous thrombotic symptoms are all predisposing factors that affect the flow, occlude the vein, or both. Following the saphenous along its length may help localize small thrombi.

The lesser saphenous follows the same criteria and can be examined along its course at the back of the calf from the lateral malleolus to the knee. Be careful when evaluating this vein in the popliteal area to avoid confusing it with the popliteal venous signal; conversely, a patent small saphenous vein in the presence of a thrombosed popliteal vein distal to the lesser saphenous insertion can also create a false-negative response regarding the popliteal vein's patency. Venous duplex sonography should be ideally used to avoid this occurrence (see below).

The above deep and superficial vein examination is repeated for the other leg.

In summary, the following are the steps in the routine lower-extremity venous examination:

1. Obtain a history, with emphasis on past phlebitis, graft surgery, pain location, swelling, and discoloration.
2. The patient lies supine with the knees flexed and the head elevated 30 degrees.
3. Examine the posterior tibial vein for flow pattern abnormalities, with distal compression of the foot and proximal compression of the calf to augment flow.
4. Examine the popliteal vein in the supine position. Check the signal for abnormalities and perform distal and proximal compression.
5. Examine the common femoral vein. Check the signal for abnormalities and perform distal compression. Proximal compression, Valsalva, or both can also be used for augmentation.

6. Examine the superficial femoral vein if there is evidence of thrombosis between the knee and groin.
7. Check the superficial veins to determine whether thrombosis exists either within or at the points where they anastomose with the deep veins.
8. Repeat steps 1 through 7 for the other leg.
9. If popliteal examination was not performed in the supine position, have the patient turn over, elevate the feet, and examine the vein in the prone position.

See Fig. 21-12 for examination sites in the lower-extremity venous study.

Interpretation of the Lower-Extremity Venous Examination. It may be helpful to reiterate the normal responses obtained in the examination at each site:

1. All deep veins should be patent and phasic, respond well to augmentation, be nonpulsatile, have competent valves, and, with the exception of the posterior tibial vein, be spontaneous.
2. If no spontaneous flow is heard, the vein should be augmented to determine whether flow is present and the vessel patent.
3. Normal distal augmentation results in an abrupt increase in flow that then returns to normal. Normal proximal augmentation results in stopping of flow with the act of compression, and a sharp increase in flow with a return to normal follows release of compression.
4. The normal superficial venous system may or may not be spontaneous and/or phasic but should augment well and allow patency to be determined.

In calf vein thrombosis the posterior tibial signal is less phasic or continuous if it is spontaneous. Distal compression will be normal unless the ankle veins are occluded. There will be decreased augmentation on release of calf compression.

The popliteal signal will usually be continuous or less phasic, depending on whether the thrombus extends into the distal popliteal. The signal may not be spontaneous, and there will be decreased augmentation with foot compression. Foot compression will not result in any augmentation of flow through the calf veins.

Both the superficial and the common femoral signals will be normal, with normal responses to augmentation except by calf compression. It may help to compare the affected leg with the unaffected leg if the disease is unilateral.

In femoropopliteal vein thrombosis the posterior tibial vein signal is continuous, with normal distal and decreased proximal augmentation.

The popliteal vein will have either no signal or markedly reduced flow. Usually high-pitched collaterals will be heard in the popliteal fossa. Distal and proximal augmentation maneuvers will result in either extremely reduced or absent augmentation.

The common femoral vein will be continuous or less phasic, again depending on whether the thrombus extends into the proximal femoral segment. The superficial femoral will be absent, or reduced and continuous. Abnormal augmentation responses can be anticipated. An increased flow signal at the femoral may be a result of saphenous shunting around the thrombus.

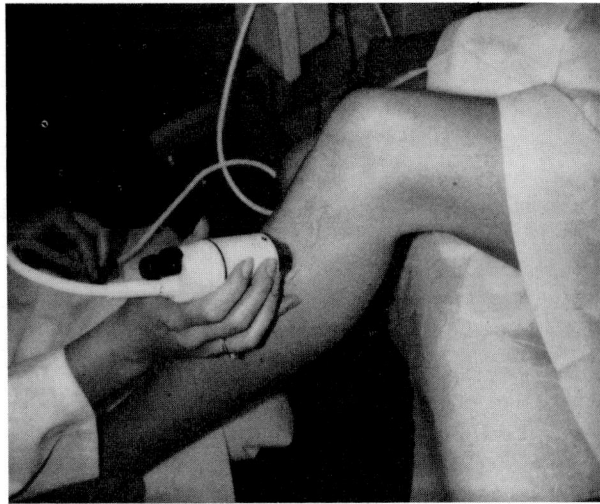

FIG. 21-12 Sites where both arterial and venous signals can be obtained in the lower extremity.

In iliofemoral thrombosis the posterior tibial, popliteal, and superficial femoral veins are continuous, with reduced augmentation at all sites. The common femoral will have absent or reduced continuous flow with poor or absent responses to augmentation maneuvers. Prominent collaterals may exist in the groin.

The diagnosis of superficial vein thrombosis by Doppler alone is often difficult, for spontaneous or phasic flow may or may not be present. The determination of disease should be based on the predisposing factors mentioned earlier and on reduced or absent augmentation.[2,10]

Occasionally patients present with diminished-sounding flow or flow that seems continuous where normal responses to compression are noted. The examiner should recheck results for the presence of collaterals, by applying gentle pressure to the probe at the site, and should check the patient's breathing pattern and have him or her inspire more deeply and exhale more forcibly to be certain that a phasic pattern does not exist in the veins.

Findings in Postphlebitic Patients and Examination Additions. Postphlebitic syndrome occurs in patients who have had deep-vein thrombosis at one time but have undergone anticoagulation treatments or other methods of thrombolysis. These patients may have a recurrence of symptoms because of insufficiency resulting from the destruction of the valves by the earlier thrombus. When assessing these patients, the examiner must check their history to help determine whether the insufficiency may result from a new thrombus or from the destruction of the old valves from the previous phlebitis.

The normal Doppler examination is done with attention given to reflux heard after proximal compression or the release of distal compression. The area of reflux enables one to pinpoint the site of the old thrombus. Valsalva maneuvers do not stop the flow if there are no competent valves proximal to the thrombus site.

In the superficial system, reflux through the great saphenous implies destruction of the valves at the saphenofemoral junction.

Perforating veins can be evaluated if located at their approximate sites with a continuous-wave Doppler probe, but evaluation of their incompetence is more accurate and easier with venous duplex, especially if color-flow imaging is used. Scanning over a stasis ulcer or site of induration often reveals an incompetent perforator beneath it. The leg can be squeezed above and below the imaged site to determine the presence and degree of reflux through the perforator.

Venous Lower-Extremity Doppler Cases

Case 1 (Fig. 21-13): normal responses and flow in right leg, abnormal responses in left leg

This 23-year-old woman was admitted to the hospital with left leg pain and swelling of 2 weeks' duration. She had recently had hepatitis. There was marked tenderness of the calf and thigh but no red streaking. Thrombophlebitis was suspected.

The right leg showed normal responses and qualities at the posterior tibial, popliteal, and femoral veins.

The left leg had phasic flow at the posterior tibial, with normal responses. At the popliteal, superficial femoral, and femoral sites, however, there was definite continuous flow with only a vague hint of phasicity. Valsalva maneuvers did not stop the flow as they did in the right leg. Iliofemoral thrombophlebitis and valvular incompetence were implied by these findings and confirmed by a subsequent venogram.

The patient was given anticoagulant therapy, which resolved the problem and dissolved the thrombus. Illustrated in Fig. 21-13 are typical normal and abnormal responses in the lower limb.

Venous Duplex Examination of the Lower Extremities

Duplex assessment of the lower extremity veins is a relatively recent development, but it is one that has shown remarkable diagnostic capabilities and has begun to challenge the ascending contrast venogram as the gold standard. Techniques for evaluating the venous system by imaging differ considerably from assessment with Doppler alone, but with practice and patience examinations of superb diagnostic quality can be performed. Color-flow imaging has been shown to be extremely beneficial in the venous duplex examination, especially of the calf veins. It can save time and speed identification of flow presence and vasculature, and it also enables identification of a patent lumen versus a thrombosed one without the need to always use extrinsic compression.

The earliest technique of venous duplex was described by Talbot in 1984 and remains one of the standard methods of gray-scale evaluation.[25] It is based on the use of transverse imaging and venous compression maneuvers. In 1986, Semrow[23] described an alternative technique that is well suited to the evaluation of calf veins; it is based on leg dependence and longitudinal imaging.[23]

The technique described here is a synthesis of the best features of these two techniques, enabling thorough evaluation of the entire deep, superficial, and perforator systems of the legs.

It should be noted that many institutions do not routinely evaluate calf veins. This is because the reported incidence of focal calf vein thrombosis is very low and not always considered worth aggressive treatment. Recent studies, however, show that nearly 20% of patients with initial, isolated calf vein thrombus had propagation into the popliteal vein on follow-up duplex scans performed within 24 hours of the initial study.[18b] Thus, while calf vein thrombus may initially seem nonthreatening for pulmonary embolus, the evolution and propagation of the thrombus may result in a potentially dangerous situation. This possibility in itself forms a strong case for inclusion and through evaluation of the calf veins.

Venous Landmarks. A brief review of the lower extremity venous anatomy may help you locate veins in relationship to nearby bone structures and arteries. Calf veins are usually, but not always, paired and run alongside their respective arteries. The posterior tibial vein is accessible on the medial side of the leg posterior to the medial malleolus and runs superiorly along the tibia to its insertion in the deep calf. The peroneal vein runs close to the fibula and lies in the posterior portion of the calf. The anterior vein follows the lateral side of the tibia. The popliteal vein can be found behind the knee in the popliteal fossa and can be traced posteriorly and on the medial side of the leg where it joins the superficial femoral vein. The superficial femoral vein runs medial to the femur and becomes the femoral vein around the pubic crest. Above the pubic crest, the external iliac vein is seen medial to the iliac artery.

Here is a summary of bone-vein relationships (Fig. 21-14):

- Iliofemoral: above the pubic crest in line with the medial border of the femur
- Superficial femoral: medial to the femur
- Popliteal: posterior to the condyles of the femur
- Posterior tibial: medial to the tibia
- Anterior tibial: lateral to the tibia
- Peroneal: posterior and medial to the fibula

Veins are usually deep to or flanking the corresponding artery.

For more information, see the venous anatomy section previously discussed.

Preparation. Preliminary procedures are as with the lower-extremity continuous-wave Doppler examination.

Equipment. A 7.5-MHz transducer should be used for superficial veins, and a 5-MHz transducer for deep calf and thigh veins; some "frequency-agile" transducers may enable

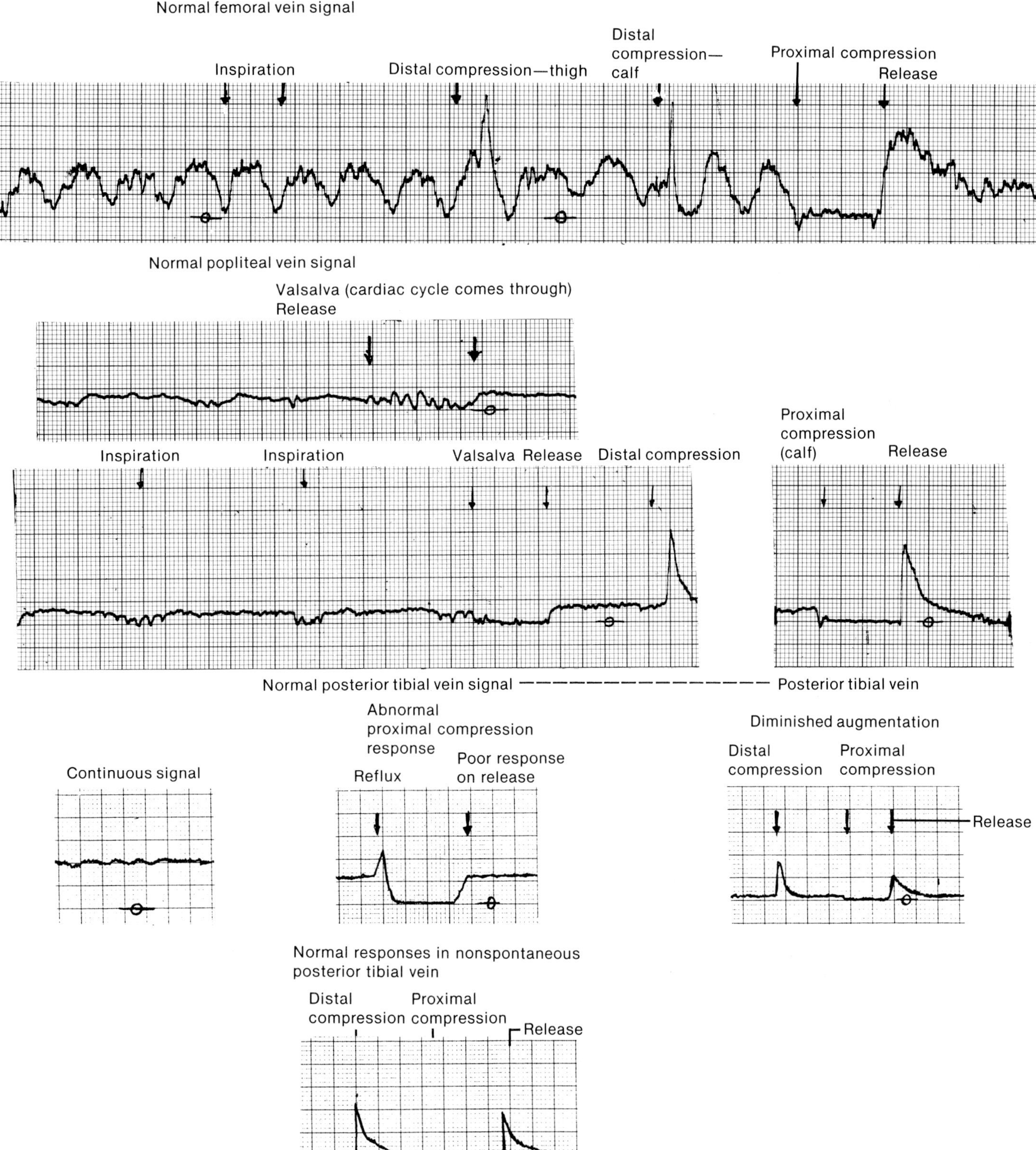

FIG. 21-13 Normal responses and flow in right leg, abnormal responses in left leg.

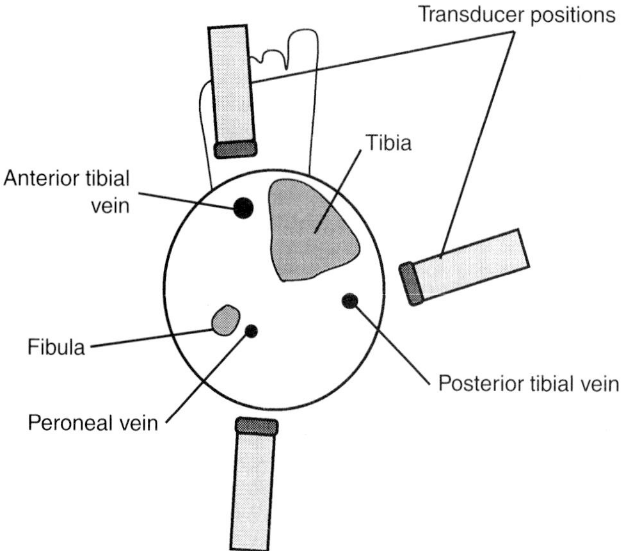

FIG. 21-14 Cross-sectional graphic of the lower leg looking caudally, showing the relationships between bones and calf veins and appropriate duplex imaging planes.

evaluation of all depths without switching probes. Color-flow imaging windows should be as large as practicable without a noticeable slowing of the image, and velocity thresholds should be set to low-flow levels. Linear or sector scanheads can be used, but there may be some lateral distortion of the vein caused by the probe shape or scan field with a sector scanhead, and compressions may be less even. Start at a field depth of 5 cm for superficial veins and 10 cm for calf and thigh veins; this depth may be increased or decreased as necessary.

Positioning. When examining the calf veins, the patient should be sitting on the end of an examination table with the back of the knee off the edge. The examiner should sit on a chair in front of the patient and rest the foot of the leg being examined on a towel placed on his or her knee. The leg may thus be easily rotated to various positions for access to the leg veins during the examination. The dependent position helps distend and fill the veins for better visualization and flow determination.

When examination of the calf veins is completed, the patient should move up on the examination table and lie su-

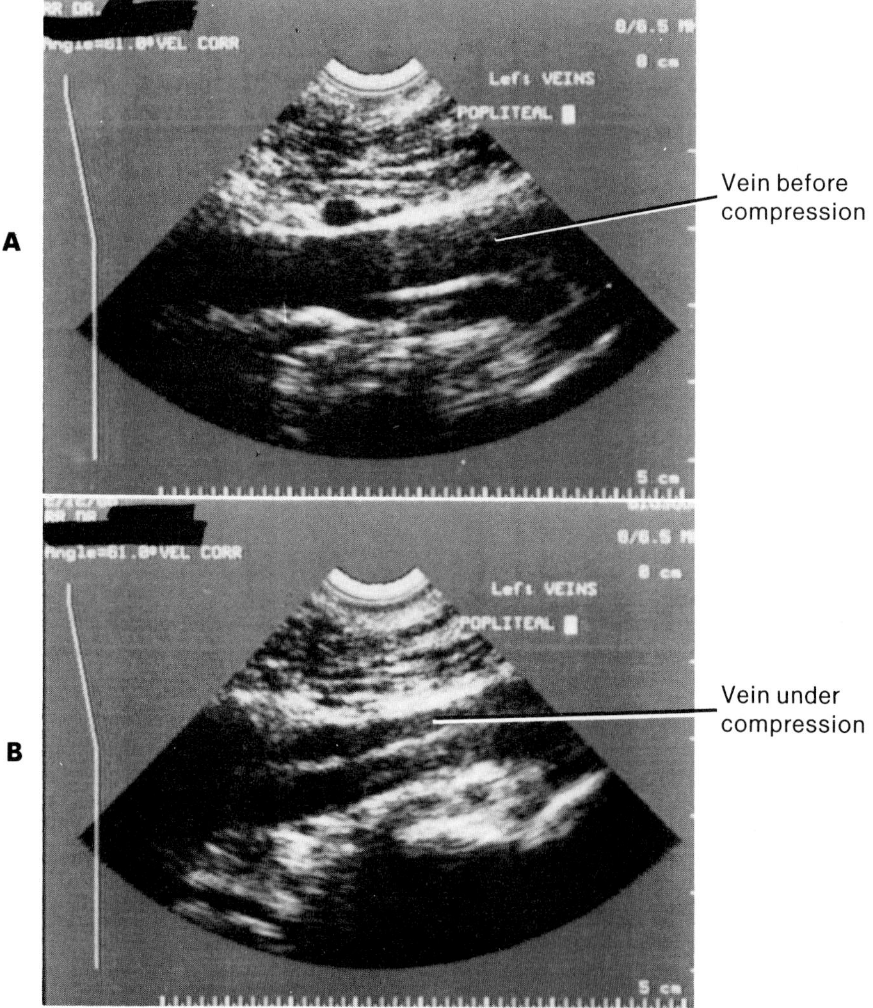

FIG. 21-15 Normal popliteal vein before, **A**, and during, **B**, compression. Note that the walls meet smoothly, implying an absence of lumen-occupying clot.

pine with the head and thorax elevated about 20 to 30 degrees. This enables easier evaluation of the veins of the thigh and pelvic area.

Scanning Procedure. For each vein being visualized, look for the following criteria:

1. Compressibility. The vein walls should meet when compressed with the probe (Fig. 21-15). Firm pressure may be required. This can best be seen by doing this in transverse, especially with a sector probe.
2. Valves should coapt (when seen) and should have thin leaflets.
3. Flow should be spontaneous and phasic (augmentation may still be necessary).
4. Perforator veins should not be enlarged, when seen.

Remember that veins may be paired in the calf and may also be doubled even in the popliteal and superficial femoral vein regions. Both sections should be evaluated in these cases to avoid missing a thrombosis that may be in one limb of the vein and not the other. Blood echoes can usually be seen moving through the vein, and phasicity can be assessed visually with color-flow imaging as well as audibly with Doppler spectral waveforms.

Before scanning, it is important to remember that the veins parallel the arteries; it is often helpful to use the arteries as landmarks to find the concomitant vein. With color flow, arteries can be easily distinguished from veins or venous branches. An artery also does not compress under probe pressure as easily as a normal vein; thus the examiner should apply only enough transducer pressure to maintain contact with the skin during the basic scan when not compressing for thrombus detection. It is recommended that the examiner record the examination on videotape, and document all normal and abnormal findings with hard copies of representative images and of Doppler spectral waveforms showing appropriate flow responses (especially in the evaluation of valvular reflux). When performing compressions of veins in transverse, it is often helpful to use the side-by-side or dual-image mode if the ultrasound system provides it. In this way the uncompressed vein can be shown on the left side of the image and the compressed vein on the right for easy interpreter comparison (see Fig. 21-25, *C*).

Start the examination by examining the calf veins; as described, have the patient sit on the edge of the examination table with the foot on the examiner's knee. Start by scanning the posterior tibial vein or veins on the medial side of the leg, starting at the ankle. Place the transducer posterior to the medial malleolus and aim laterally (Fig. 21-16); initially searching for the posterior tibial artery can help. Follow the veins (Fig. 21-17; see color image) from the ankle to the knee at their insertion at the peroneal-tibial junction at the popliteal vein, starting in the longitudinal plane and moving from the ankle to just below the knee. Evaluate the image and flow characteristics using Doppler spectral waveforms and color-flow imaging. Perform proximal and distal augmentation maneuvers periodically during the scan. After evaluating in the longitudinal plane, go back to the ankle, then turn the transducer to the transverse position and again progress from ankle to knee, compressing the vein area sequen-

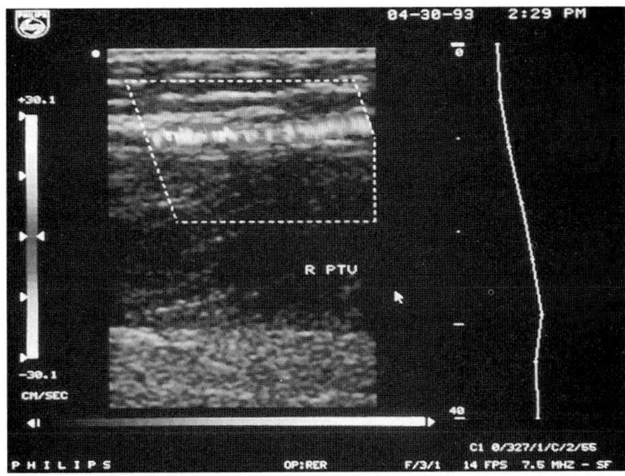

FIG. 21-17 Longitudinal color-flow duplex appearance of a normal posterior tibial vein.

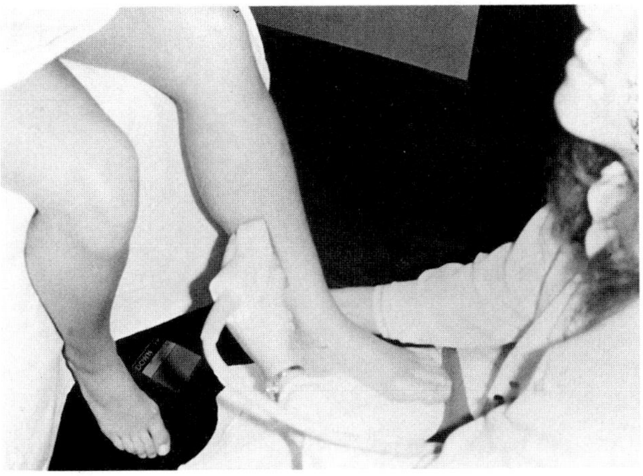

FIG. 21-16 Mediolateral longitudinal scanning position for the posterior tibial veins.

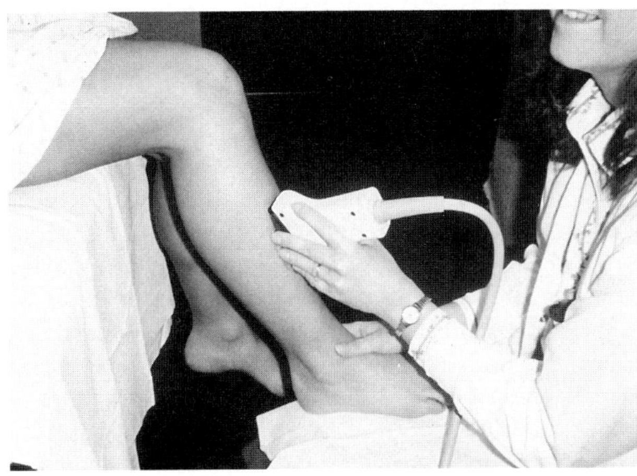

FIG. 21-18 Anteroposterior longitudinal scanning position for the anterior tibial veins.

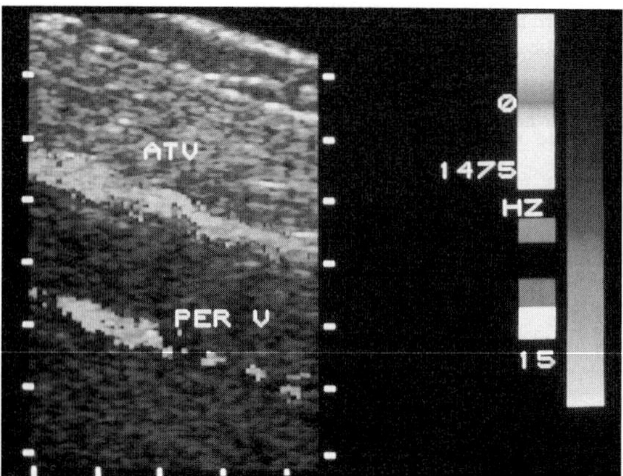

FIG. 21-19 Longitudinal color-flow duplex image of a normal proximal anterior tibial vein (note the relationship of the peroneal vein visualized deep to it in the anteroposterior scan plane).

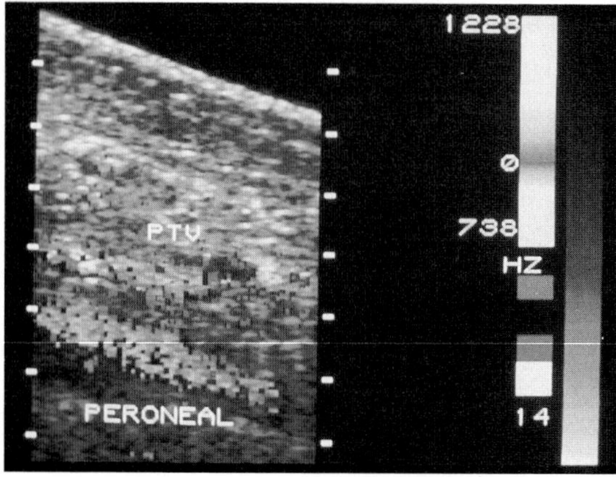

FIG. 21-20 Longitudinal color-flow duplex image showing relationship of the peroneal vein deep to the the posterior tibial vein in the mediolateral scan plane.

tially to rule out the presence of thrombus (the compression effect and the presence of thrombus on the walls are easier to assess in the transverse plane).

The anterior tibial vein or veins are evaluated by placing the transducer lateral to the tibia on the anterior surface of the lower leg, then aiming anteroposteriorly (Fig. 21-18). Start just below the patella and look for the anterior tibial artery as it arches anterior; a good way to begin is to move medially until the bone reflector is seen, then slowly move the transducer laterally until the tissues, the artery, and accompanying veins are identified (use of color flow and augmentation is extremely helpful here) (Fig. 21-19; see color image). Start in the longitudinal plane and move from the knee to the ankle, following the vein and evaluating image and flow characteristics using Doppler spectral waveforms and color-flow imaging patterns. Perform proximal and distal augmentation maneuvers periodically during the scan. After evaluating in the longitudinal plane, go back proximally and look transversely, again progressing from knee to ankle and compressing the vein area sequentially to rule out the presence of thrombus.

The peroneal vein is usually seen deep to the posterior tibial veins when examining the posterior tibial area, and deep to the anterior tibial vein when scanning in that plane (Figs. 21-19 and 21-20; see Fig. 21-20 color image). Considering the peroneal vein as the apex of a triangle (see Fig. 21-14), one can angle back and forth to identify and follow it in both positions without necessarily having to evaluate it separately. If it is necessary (because of a patient's habitus or if there are questionable findings), the peroneal vein can be examined by placing the transducer posterior to the fibula and angling anteriorly toward the lateral side of the tibia (Fig. 21-21). One can either follow the vein or veins from the peroneal-tibial junction to the ankle or scan from the ankle superiorly to the peroneal-tibial junction. After evaluating in the longitudinal plane, go back proximally, then turn the probe transversely, again scanning from knee

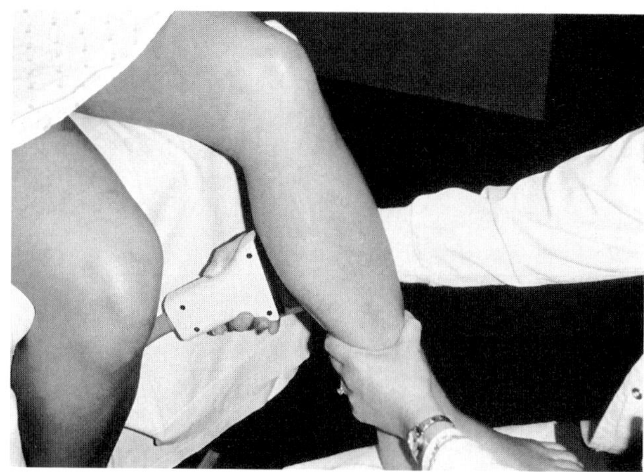

FIG. 21-21 Posteroanterior longitudinal scanning position for the peroneal veins.

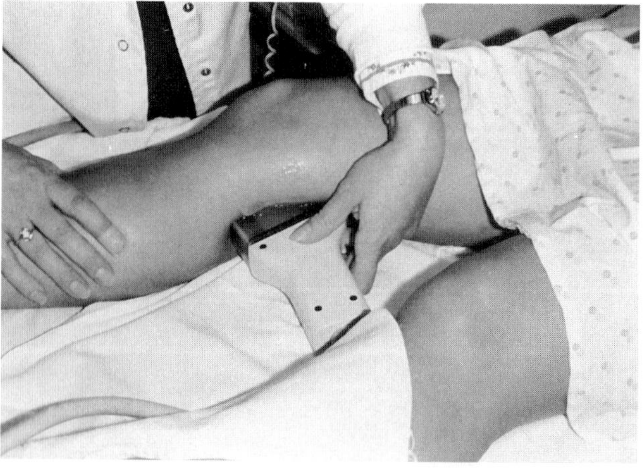

FIG. 21-22 Posterior longitudinal scanning position for the popliteal vein. Note the method of applying distal calf augmentation while scanning.

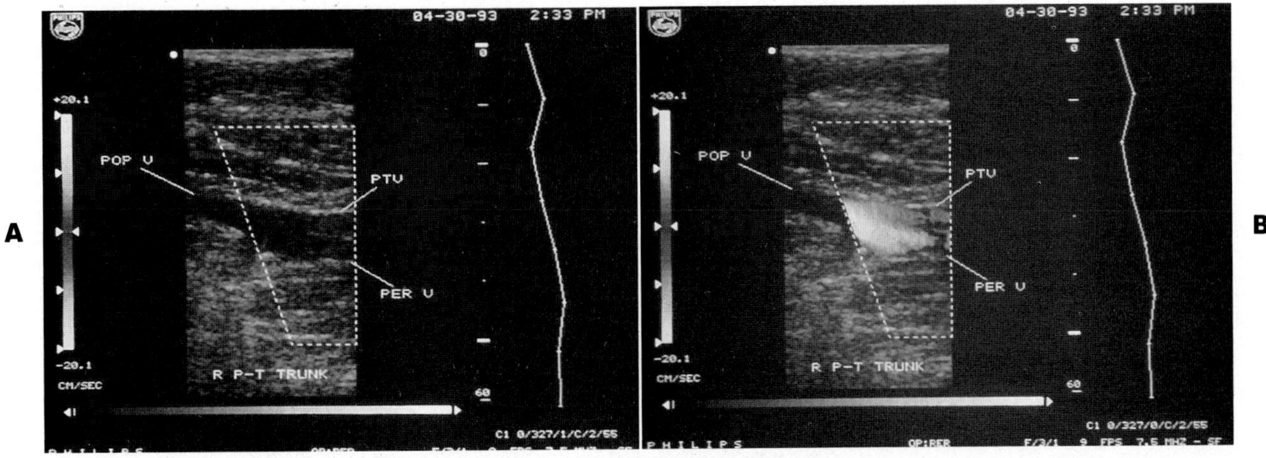

FIG. 21-23 Longitudinal duplex images showing the appearance of the normal peroneal-tibial junction with the distal popliteal vein **(A)** in gray scale **(B)** with color-flow imaging on.

to ankle and compressing the vein area sequentially to rule out the presence of thrombus.

After the calf veins have been imaged and recorded, the patient should move up on the examination table and lie supine with the head and thorax elevated about 20 to 30 degrees. Slightly flex the knee and have the patient rotate the leg being examined into a frog-leg position.

Scan the popliteal area from the proximal calf to the distal posterior thigh by placing the transducer in the popliteal fossa and aiming anteriorly (Fig. 21-22). Evaluate the distal popliteal vein in the proximal calf first, looking for the peroneal-tibial junction (Fig. 21-23; see color image) and the insertion of the anterior tibial vein (which appears to be posterior to the popliteal vein) (Fig. 21-24; see color image). Move proximally to the center of the fossa and then to the proximal thigh. The popliteal vein may lie directly above the artery or lateral to it in this examination plane (Fig. 21-25; see color images). Scan the entire vein area first in the longitudinal and then in the transverse plane, adjusting color-flow directions as needed and compressing the vein area in transverse to coapt the walls and rule out the presence of thrombus. If possible, evaluate the saphenopopliteal junction area (see later discussion of imaging the lesser saphenous vein on the superficial surface of the posterior calf). Use Doppler spectral waveforms and color-flow imaging patterns with proximal and distal augmentation maneuvers to evaluate the flow characteristics.

The superficial femoral vein is followed superiorly along the medial side of the leg from the adductor hiatus area to the superficial femoral-deep femoral junction with the common femoral vein. Place the transducer anteriorly on the thigh and then aim straight in or angle medial to the femur along the sartorius groove (Fig. 21-26). The superficial femoral artery appears to lie above or lateral to the superficial femoral vein in this scan plane (Fig. 21-27; see color image). Just below the area of the inguinal ligament, the junction of the profunda femoris (deep femoral) vein and

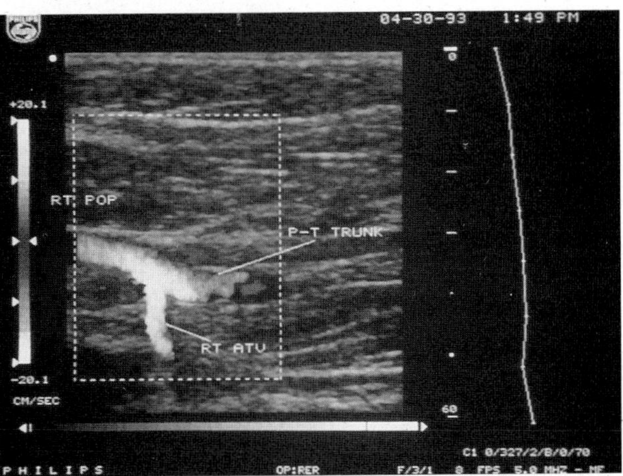

FIG. 21-24 Longitudinal color-flow duplex appearance of the normal distal popliteal vein, showing the insertion of the anterior tibial vein.

superficial femoral vein with the common femoral vein is seen (Fig. 21-28; see color image). Start in the longitudinal plane and move from the knee to the groin, following the vein and evaluating image and flow characteristics using Doppler spectral waveforms and color-flow imaging patterns. Perform proximal and distal augmentation maneuvers periodically during the scan. After evaluating in the longitudinal plane, go back distally, then look transversely, again progressing from knee to groin and compressing the vein areas sequentially to rule out the presence of thrombus.

After evaluating the area of junction of the superficial femoral, deep femoral, and common femoral for the presence of thrombus and normal or abnormal flow characteristics, the examiner should move the transducer up into the common femoral vein area (Fig. 21-29) and above the inguinal ligament and pelvic brim to evaluate as much of the distal external iliac vein as possible (Fig. 21-30; see color image). If iliac veins are imaged, it is best to do so with

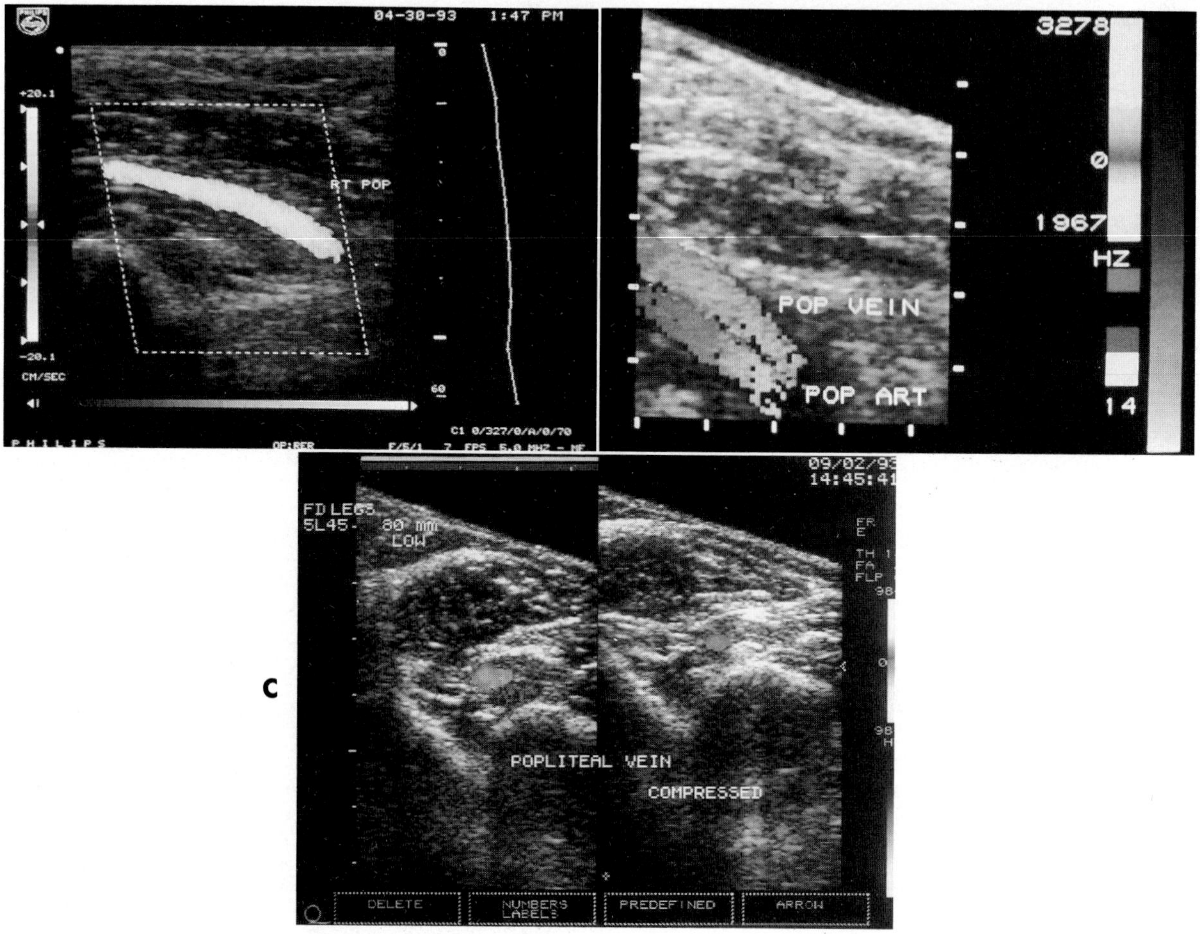

FIG. 21-25 A, Longitudinal color-flow duplex appearance of the normal popliteal vein across the central popliteal fossa. **B,** Longitudinal color-flow image of the popliteal vein showing its relationship with the popliteal artery in the posterior imaging plane. **C,** Transverse view of a normal popliteal vein in "side-by-side" mode, showing the uncompressed vein on the left image and the vein compressed by the transducer on the right image. Note that the walls coapt easily (compare with Fig. 21-71, *B*).

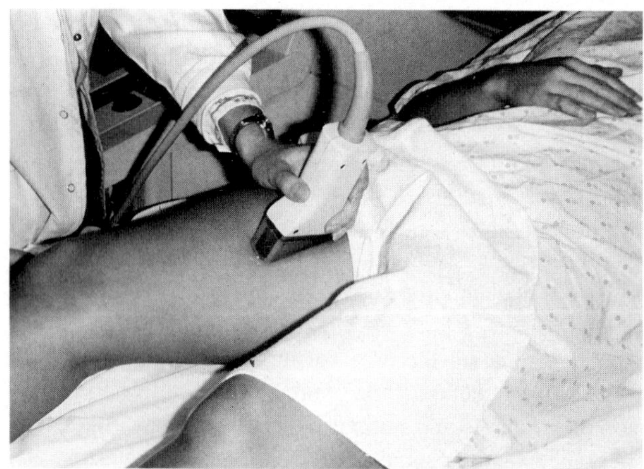

FIG. 21-26 Anterior longitudinal scanning position for the superficial femoral vein.

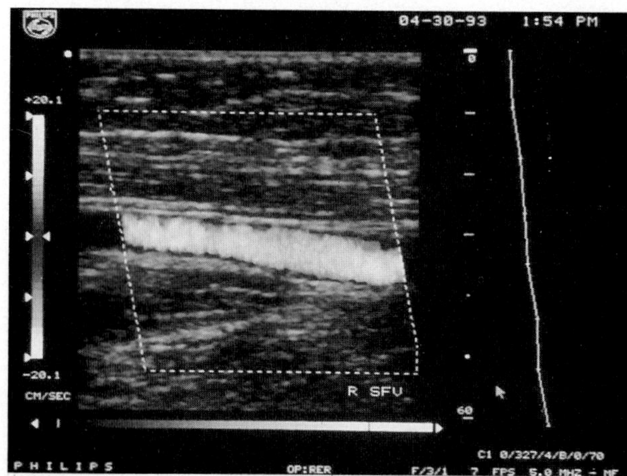

FIG. 21-27 Longitudinal color-flow duplex appearance of the normal superficial femoral vein.

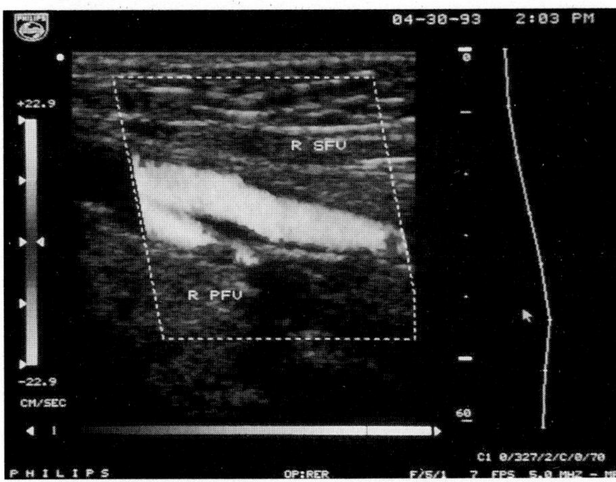

FIG. 21-28 Longitudinal color-flow duplex appearance of the superficial femoral–deep femoral junction with the common femoral vein.

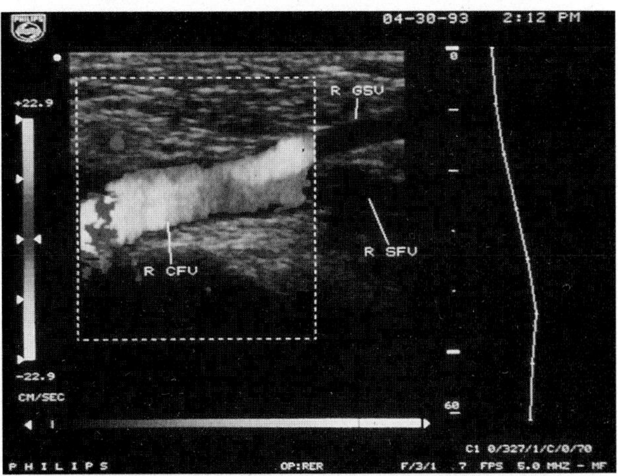

FIG. 21-30 Longitudinal color-flow duplex image of the normal common femoral vein (note the saphenofemoral junction to the right).

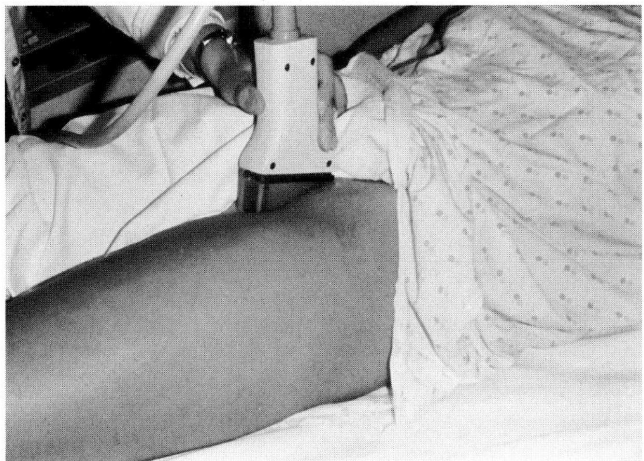

FIG. 21-29 Anterior longitudinal scanning position for the common femoral vein across the inguinal ligament.

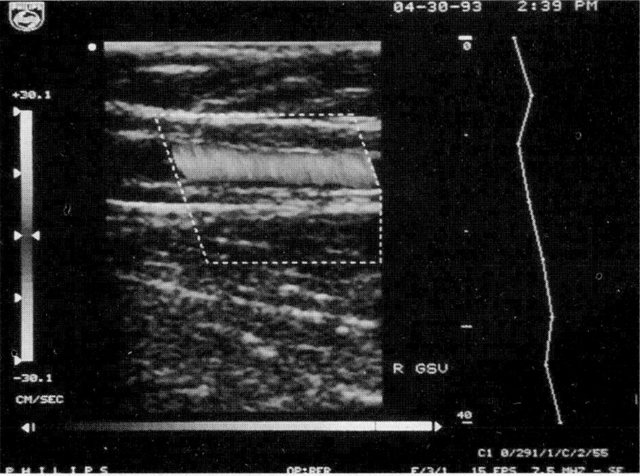

FIG. 21-31 Longitudinal color-flow duplex appearance of the great saphenous vein.

either a linear- or phased-array sector probe with adequate penetration. Using the ligament as the landmark, scan below and above it in both the longitudinal and transverse planes, again compressing the veins sequentially to rule out thrombus and using Doppler spectral waveforms and color-flow imaging patterns with proximal and distal augmentation.

The superficial veins can be either imaged separately at this point or included during the deep imaging of the femoral and popliteal veins. The greater saphenous vein is imaged on the medial side of the leg and normally lies within 2 cm of the skin surface. It can be followed from the saphenofemoral junction with the common femoral in the groin to the ankle level in most patients (Fig. 21-31; see color image). This vessel may split into one or more accessory branches and each branch should be followed. A very important valve at the saphenofemoral junction should particularly be checked. When the patient is supine the saphenofemoral junction is more easily seen. The lesser saphenous vein is imaged on the superficial surface of the posterior calf in line with the popliteal vein (Fig. 21-32; see color image). It should be followed from its easily seen insertion at the popliteal vein as far distal as possible.

Perforator veins should be evaluated at their approximate locations in the leg during the main examination (see Fig. 21-5 for locations). If they are identified and visualized by color-flow imaging, compress the leg above and below the perforator while observing it. Using Doppler sample volume or color flow to monitor the vein, flow should normally move from the superficial vein to the deep vein without reflux.

Interpretation of the Lower-Extremity Venous Duplex Examination

Normal veins

1. Easy compressibility, smoothly meeting walls under compression (Fig. 21-33).

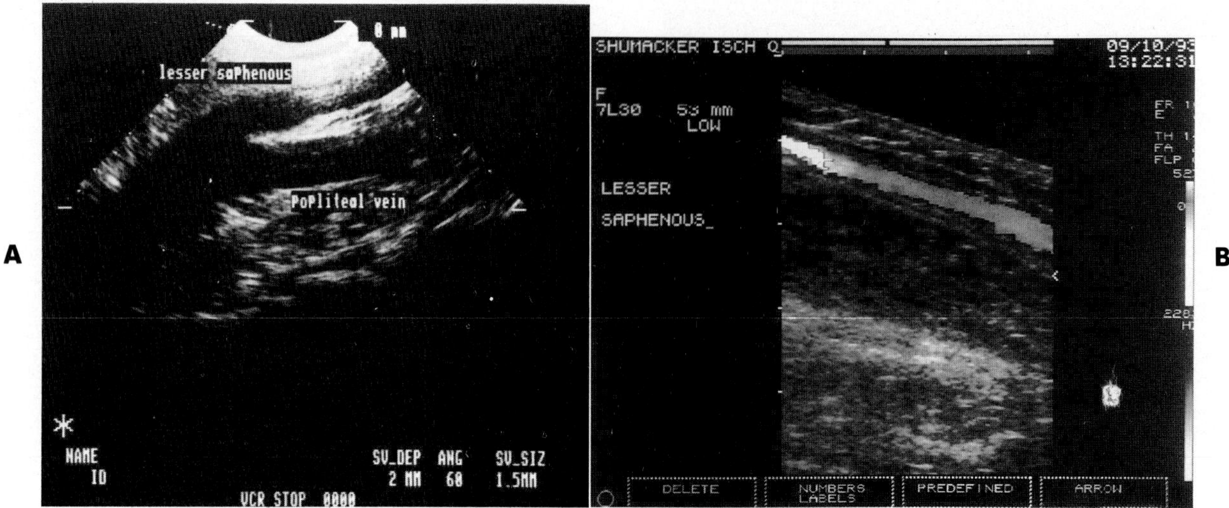

FIG. 21-32 **A,** Gray-scale duplex appearance of the saphenopopliteal junction. **B,** Color-flow duplex appearance of the lesser saphenous vein distal to the saphenopopliteal junction.

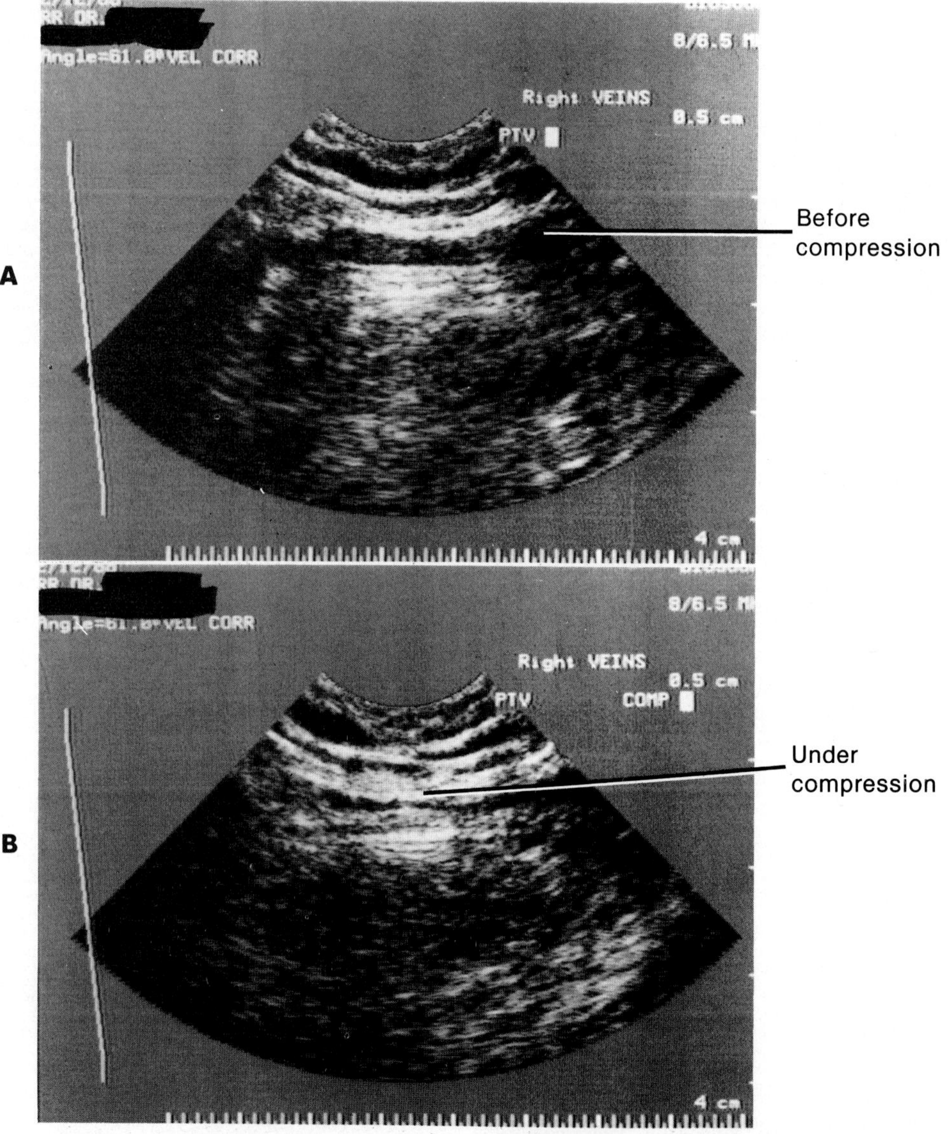

FIG. 21-33 Compression response of the normal posterior tibial vein. **A,** Before, and **B,** during.

2. Competent, coapting valves; thin leaflets (when valves are seen) (Fig. 21-34).
3. Phasic and spontaneous Doppler flow patterns. Color-flow imaging patterns should fill the visible lumen without defects in the color display.
4. Perforator veins should be competent with no reflux and not markedly dilated.

Abnormal findings

1. Veins that do not allow the walls to meet under transducer compression or that do not show normal color-flow filling from wall to wall may have thrombus present. Completely thrombosed segments have obvious echogenic material filling the lumen with no color flow within (Fig. 21-35; see color image); partially thrombosed segments show evidence of flow passing around the thrombus. The degree of echogenicity and compressibility can assist in aging the thrombus to determine whether it is acute or chronic (see below). Patent veins usually are dilated distal to the obstruction and Doppler flow patterns show decreased phasicity or continuous flow, depending on the degree of obstruction.
2. Thickened, stiff, or nonfunctioning valves may imply the presence of disease on gray scale; color flow often shows filling defects in the color patterns and abnormal hemodynamics (including reflux) around abnormal valves. Thrombus may also occur in and around the valves and valve sinuses that can "freeze" the valve open (Fig. 21-36; see color image). Doppler and color-flow patterns demonstrate evidence of reflux during standard proximal and distal augmentation maneuvers. Valves also may occasionally be seen to prolapse with proximal augmentation.
3. Reflux through a venous segment can imply proximal valvular insufficiency; this can easily be assessed using duplex Doppler and color-flow imaging. Significant reflux can be identified by a flow or color reversal lasting over 1 second after release of proximal or application of distal compression (Fig. 21-37; see color images). Reflux time and degree, however, are best assessed using a Doppler spectral display (Fig. 21-38). Reflux can be enhanced by having the patient stand with the leg dependent during the examination. Further information re-

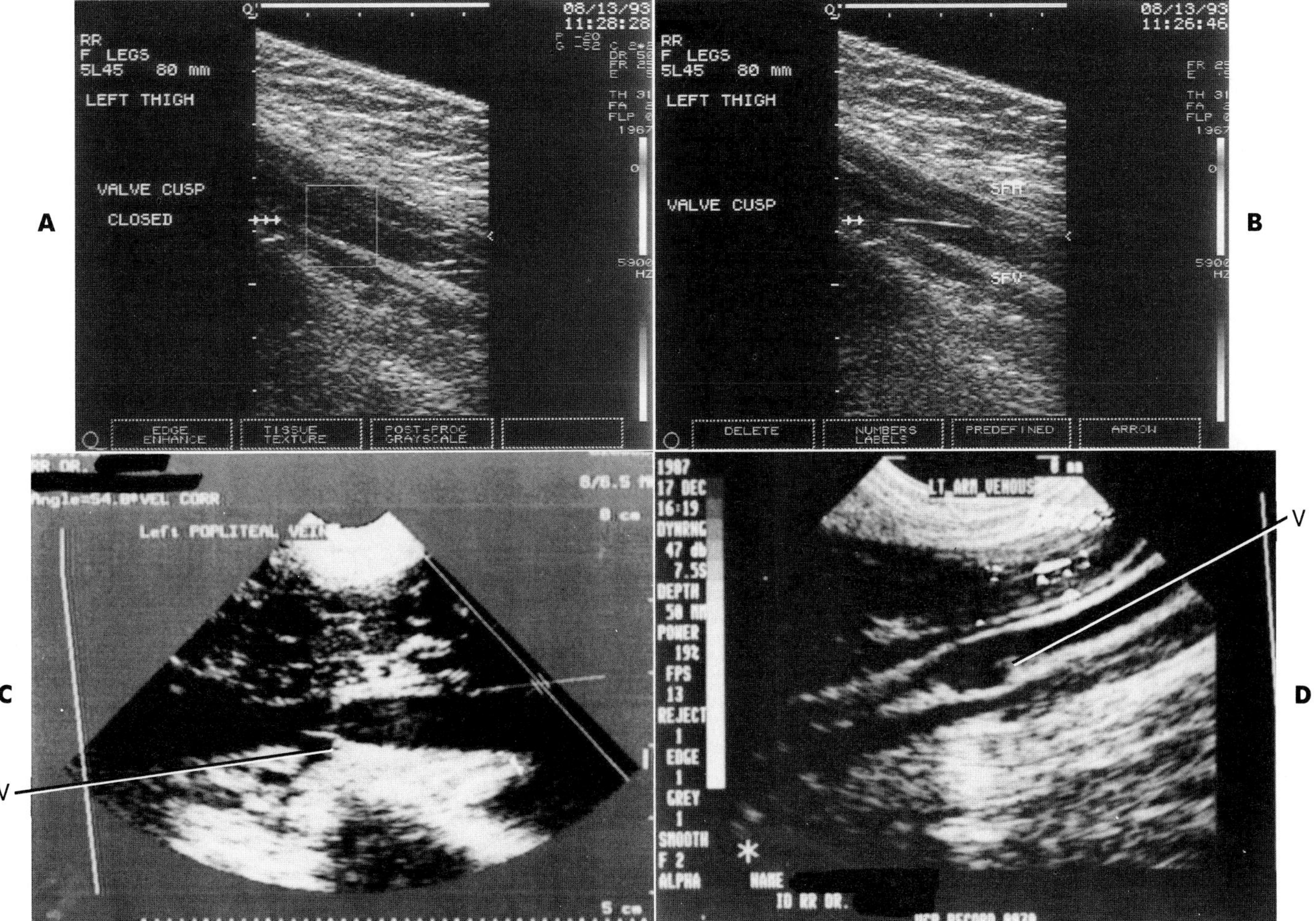

FIG. 21-34 Valves. Normal appearance of venous valve cusps in the **A,** open, and **B,** closed states in a superficial femoral vein. **C,** Appearance of a thickened valve cusp. **D,** An unusually well-defined valve and valve sinus in a brachial vein.

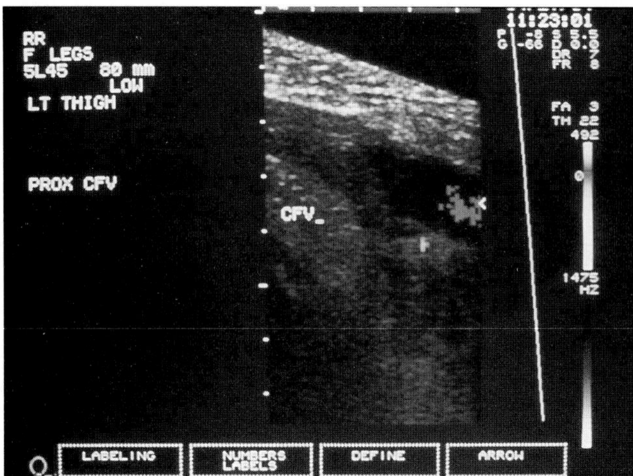

FIG. 21-35 Appearance of thrombosis. The proximal portion of this common femoral vein is filled with echogenic homogeneous thrombus; note the patent distal segment to the right, which has some evidence of low-velocity color flow (blue).

garding specific superficial incompetence can be gained by having the patient stand erect while scanning over the saphenofemoral or saphenopopliteal junctions. During the scan, a pressure cuff can be placed around the calf below the junction or segment being scanned and then inflated to a pressure of around 45 mm Hg. The cuff is rapidly deflated while monitoring the veins and the degree of reflux is recorded and documented by either color-flow imaging or (preferably) Doppler spectra.[3]

4. Reflux in perforator veins and superficial veins must be documented because it can be linked to complications from varicose veins or venous insufficiency (Fig. 21-39; see color images). Noting both the severity and the location of superficial and perforator incompetence may help a surgeon determine the appropriate course of therapy for the patient, which many times may not involve lysis or ligation.

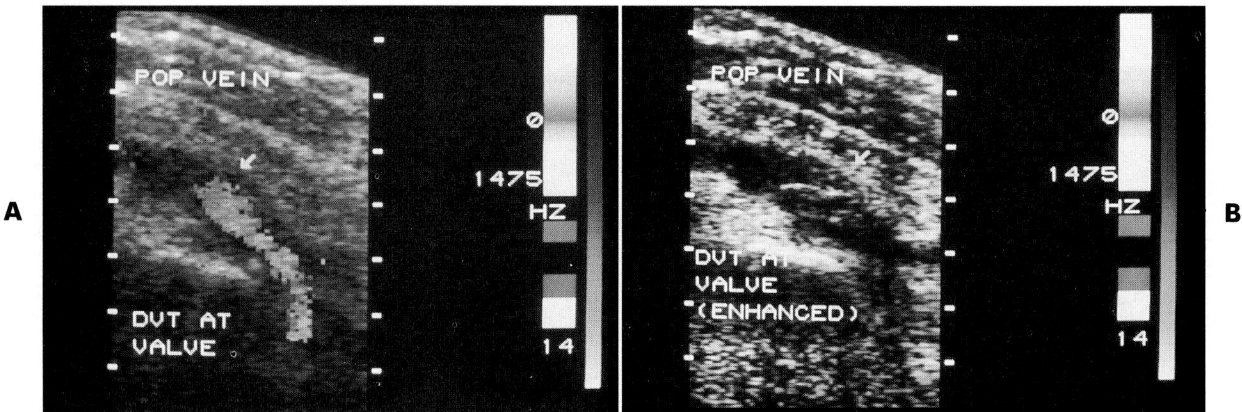

FIG. 21-36 Thrombus at a valve. **A,** A popliteal vein has thrombus concentrating near what appears to be a valve *(arrow)*. **B,** Under image enhancement and with color flow turned off, the valve can be seen with chronic thrombus in the sinus and acute thrombus propagating proximally to the left of the valve.

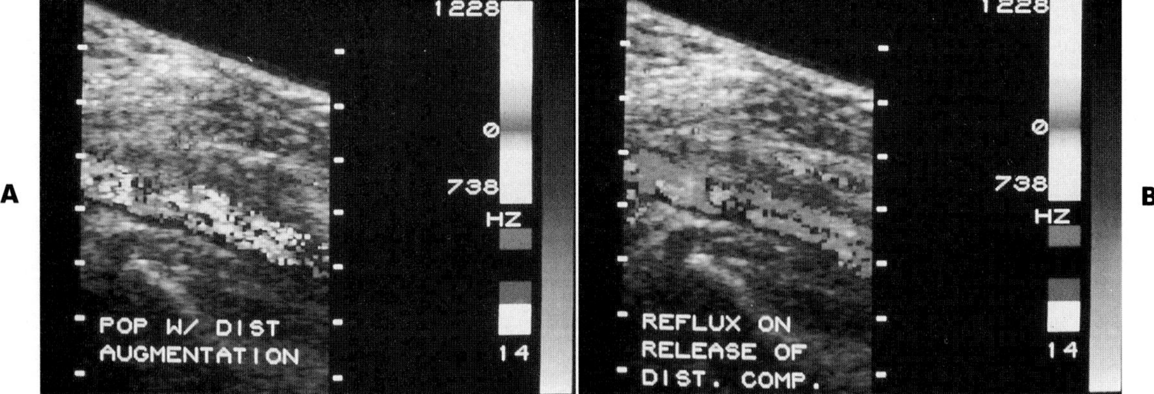

FIG. 21-37 A, Color-flow appearance of reflux. In this patient with severe postphlebitic syndrome, distal calf augmentation shows normal blue antegrade flow through this chronically recanalized popliteal vein. **B,** On release of calf compression, strong red retrograde flow is seen rushing back through the venous segment.

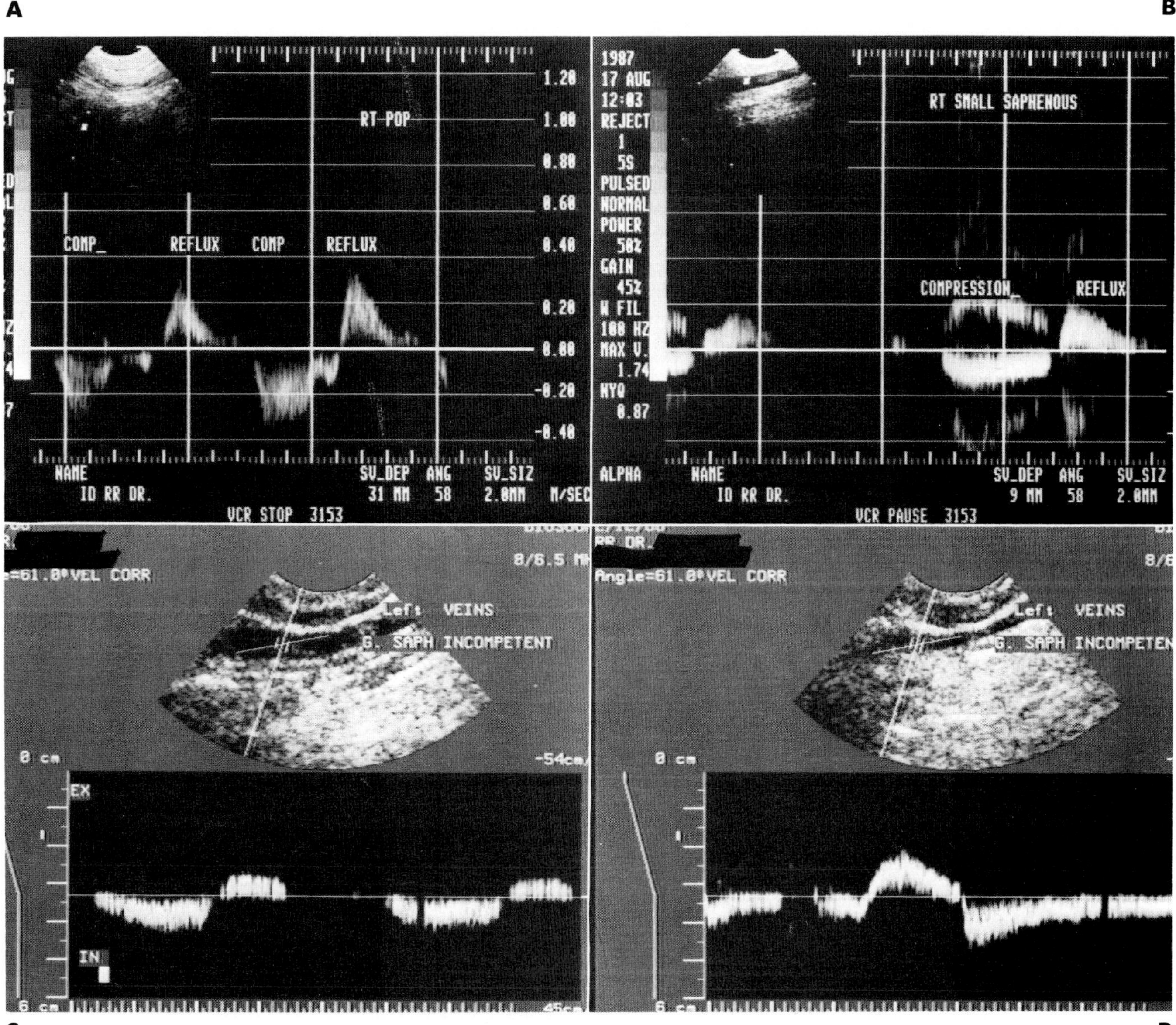

FIG. 21-38 Doppler reflux patterns in the popliteal, **A**, and lesser saphenous, **B**, veins showing venous insufficiency. The great saphenous venous signal in **C** shows severe incompetence with reflux occurring during simple respiration. With calf compression and release, the signal shows moderate to severe valvular incompetence, **D**.

Classification of thrombus. The morphology of a thrombus that is visualized may often be a diagnostic indication of whether the venous disease is of a recent or long-standing etiology. Whether the thrombus is acute or chronic also influences the type of therapy the patient receives.

The following criteria can be used to grade, or "age," a thrombus:

1. Acute
   a. Acute thrombus may be focal in nature, with patent segments above and below (Fig. 21-40; see color image). Thrombus may occupy the entire venous lumen, be partially occlusive and adherent to one wall, or be free-floating in the center of the lumen (Fig. 21-41; see color images). It may be slightly (but not completely) compressible under the transducer.
   b. The thrombus generally has a smooth surface.
   c. The thrombus has a "soft," homogeneous appearance (see Fig. 21-40).
   d. Patent vein segments are distended below the thrombus.
2. Chronic
   a. Chronic thrombus is firm, stationary, and incompressible under the transducer (Fig. 21-42; see color image).
   b. The thrombus has an irregular surface.
   c. The thrombus has a very echogenic heterogeneous appearance (see Fig. 21-42).

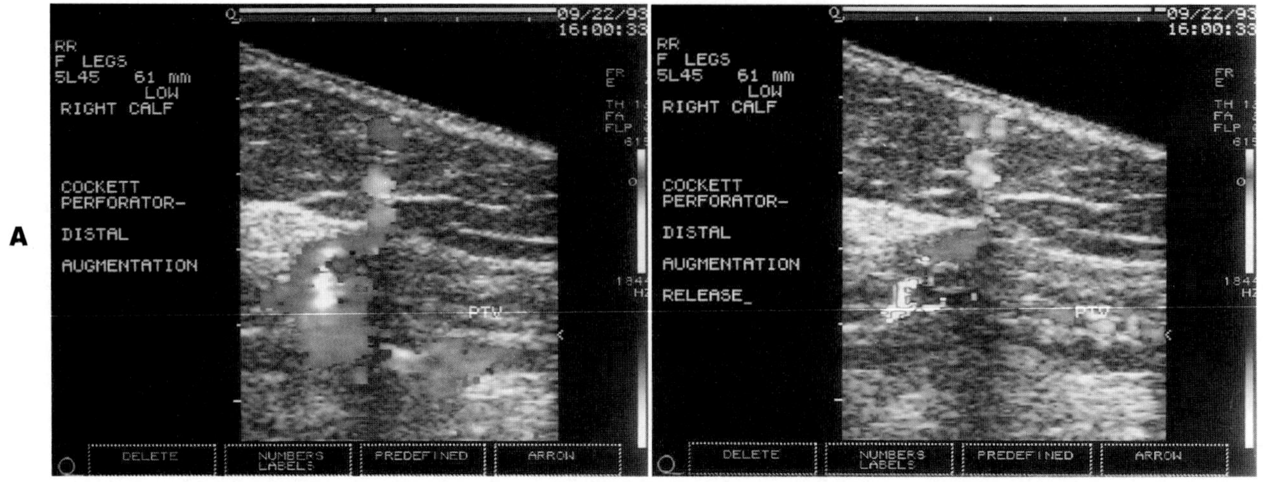

FIG. 21-39 Reflux in an incompetent perforating vein. The Cockett perforating vein shown in this series communicates between an incompetent great saphenous vein and the posterior tibial vein. **A,** With distal compression of the foot, flow travels normally through the perforator from the superficial vein to the deep vein (flow is away from the transducer, thus is coded red-see scale to the right). **B,** On release of distal compression, flow becomes retrograde in the perforator (flowing back toward the transducer and thus coded blue), flowing back into the superficial vein.

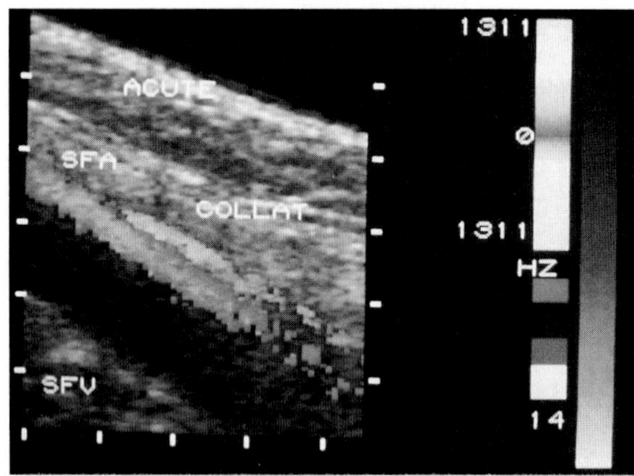

FIG. 21-40 Acute thrombus. Note the homogeneous appearance of the thrombus and the dilated vein.

d. Prominent collateral veins may be seen around the thrombosed segment and recanalization may occur through the thrombus (Fig. 21-43; see color images).

Technical Factors. Carefully adjust the time-gain compensation and slope, as well as the near and far gain and contrast controls, to give the best image possible, free of artifact and reverberation. This is important, since inadequate gain settings prevent the visualization of acute thrombus, and overcompensated gain creates artifacts that may be misinterpreted as thrombus, especially if a vein proves difficult to compress because of improper technique. The ideal setting allows the intimal linings to be distinctly seen, and there are some faint specular echoes of moving blood in the veins. If using color-flow imaging, make certain that the velocity thresholds are set low enough to ensure that flow is detected from wall to wall and that little or no aliasing occurs during augmentation maneuvers. Compression of the vein may not be necessary if flow is well visualized to the walls in both the longitudinal and transverse planes, but compression should always be used in situations where the absence of visualized color flow resulting from slow-flow states may be mistaken for the presence of thrombus. This method ensures confirmation of patency or obstruction.

Mapping Saphenous Veins for Conduit

One other application of venous duplex ultrasonography in the lower extremities is in evaluating superficial veins for use as conduit, such as for coronary artery bypass grafting, in situ saphenous vein bypass grafting, surgical patch angioplasty, or other bypass purposes. To do this, the examiner can follow the same procedures to visualize and trace the saphenous vein as far distal as possible. In addition, the examiner should have some sort of indelible marker dye or permanent marking pen to define the course of the vein on the skin surface. To summarize the technique and procedure:

1. Have the patient lie supine with the torso elevated. Locate the great saphenous vein in a longitudinal plane at the saphenofemoral junction with the common femoral vein near the groin. Mark the groin with a dot at the location of the junction, then mark a dot below the transducer where the length of the vein segment lies in line with the junction. Measure the vein's diameter with electronic calipers to determine its relative size (Fig. 21-44; see color image). Measure from either inner wall to inner wall or outer wall to outer wall, but be consistent.
2. Keeping the long-axis view of the saphenous vein, move

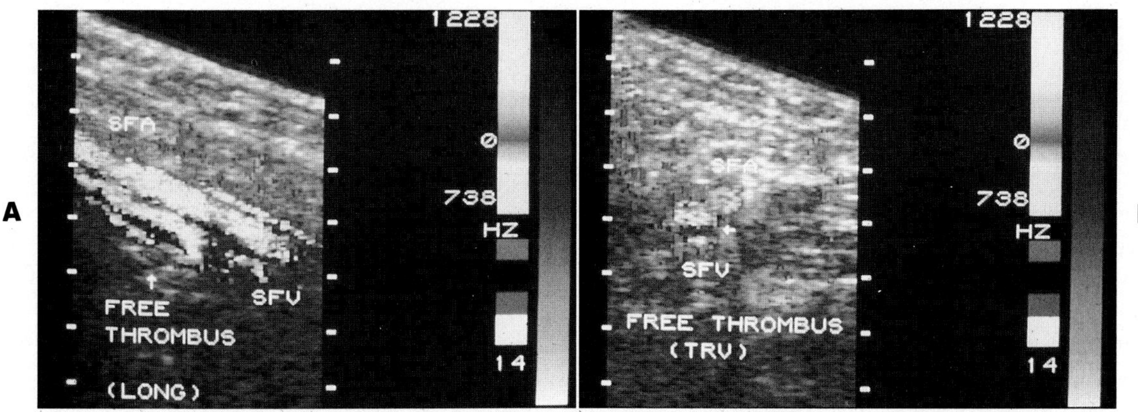

FIG. 21-41 Adherent or free thrombus. **A,** In longitudinal section, note the "tongue" of thrombus in the superficial femoral vein, which is adherent to the wall proximally but appears to "float" within the color-flow pattern, almost giving a double-lumen appearance. **B,** The true nature of the thrombus becomes more apparent in the transverse plane, where it is surrounded on three sides by color flow and adheres to the lateral wall (to the right).

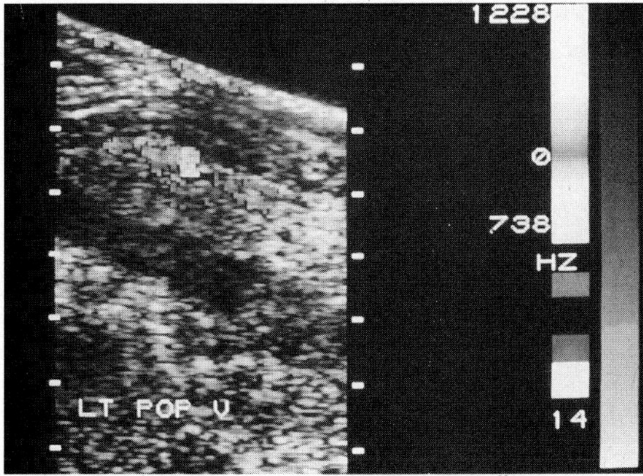

FIG. 21-42 Chronic thrombus. Note the heterogeneous appearance of the thrombus and the irregular, nondilated appearance of the vein. (Compare with Fig. 21-40.)

below the inferior dot above and localize the segment in long axis, again marking a dot below the transducer where the next length of vein lies in line with the previous dot. Measure the vein again.

3. Continue visualizing and measuring the vein and marking the leg, progressing distally, below the knee if possible, until the vein terminates or branches.
4. Once completed, connect the dots from proximal to distal with a single line of dye. The location of any duplicated vein segments or prominent branches should also be mapped out and marked on the leg.
5. If necessary, the lesser saphenous vein can be followed and marked in a similar fashion, starting at the saphenopopliteal junction and moving distally down the center of the calf. It may help to have the patient lie prone with the knees flexed slightly.

Most saphenous veins are considered suitable for coronary artery bypass if they are not varicose and measure between 2 and 3 mm in average diameter. Vascular surgeons generally prefer veins 3.5 to 4.5 mm (or slightly larger) for in situ use, although this is variable.

Examining the Venous Patient After Lysis, Ligation, Stripping, Bypass, or Sclerotherapy

Lytic Therapy

Acute deep venous thromboses or obstructions are typically treated by lysis with heparin or warfarin derivatives, often under hospitalization to head off the threat of potential pulmonary embolus. Some institutions lyse thrombi directly using catheter-delivered urokinase, streptokinase, or other lytic agents. Superficial thromboses are generally treated with low-level anticoagulants, heat, and elevation of the extremity.

Follow-up venous duplex examinations may be performed to determine the effect of lysis; sometimes the comparative findings can be quite dramatic (Fig. 21-45; see color images). The basic examination protocols can be used with no changes.

Ligation and Stripping

Patients with severe varicose veins or saphenous vein incompetence may require surgical ligation of the great saphenous vein or large varicosities to treat the symptoms; in certain other cases, stripping of the vein or veins may be the method of choice (although this procedure is less frequently performed today). In this technique, incisions are made at both ends of the varicose venous segment (which can include an entire saphenous vein), and a stripper is then passed through the vein from the distal end to the proximal end (or vice versa). The stripper catches the proximal end of the vein to be removed; the stripper is then pulled back subcutaneously through the leg to the entry point, pulling out the vein along with it.[5] Patients who have had strippings can usually be identified by a series of numerous short scars along the thigh and calf in the areas of their former varicosities.

Stab avulsion may be performed on small varicosities; in this technique a small incision is made over the varicosity and the vein is grasped by a hemostat. The vein is pulled out slightly and clamped on both sides, then cut in the center. One end of the segment is then grasped with the hemostat, and the veins are pulled out.[5] Another method uses an avulsion hook; it is inserted into the leg at the point of the varicosity, the vein is hooked and twisted around the shaft end (such as in winding spaghetti around a fork), and then the hook with the vein wound around it is pulled out of the leg.[5]

In these patients the duplex examination protocol is again the same as in routine evaluation. The examiner should look for any hematoma or focal thromboses in adjoining residual veins or alternate systems that might have gone undetected during ligation or other treatment (especially after avulsion or stripping), since some trauma to the vein branches and tissues can occur.

Venous Surgery. In many cases, patients with severe deep venous insufficiency or chronic proximal venous occlusion can have some semblance of normal venous hemodynamics returned by creative surgical techniques. Many techniques and procedures can be performed, as determined by the patient's situation. For example, patients without intact valves in the superficial femoral and distal veins in a leg can be helped by venous transposition surgery. In one approach the superficial femoral vein below the junction of the superficial femoral and profunda femoris is transected and anastomosed to either the distal profunda femoris vein or the proximal great saphenous vein below the saphenofemoral junction to provide a competent, functioning valve to the distal deep system.[17] Occasionally focal direct valve repair is performed as well.

In another example a femorofemoral venous bypass can be created in cases of chronic unilateral iliac occlusion to shunt flow from the patent distal veins in the ipsilateral obstructed leg to the contralateral patent side. This is done in one method by transecting the great saphenous vein in the contralateral patent leg low in the thigh and leaving the proximal portion (including the saphenofemoral junction) intact. This section of great saphenous vein is brought across the pubic area through an anatomic tunnel and anas-

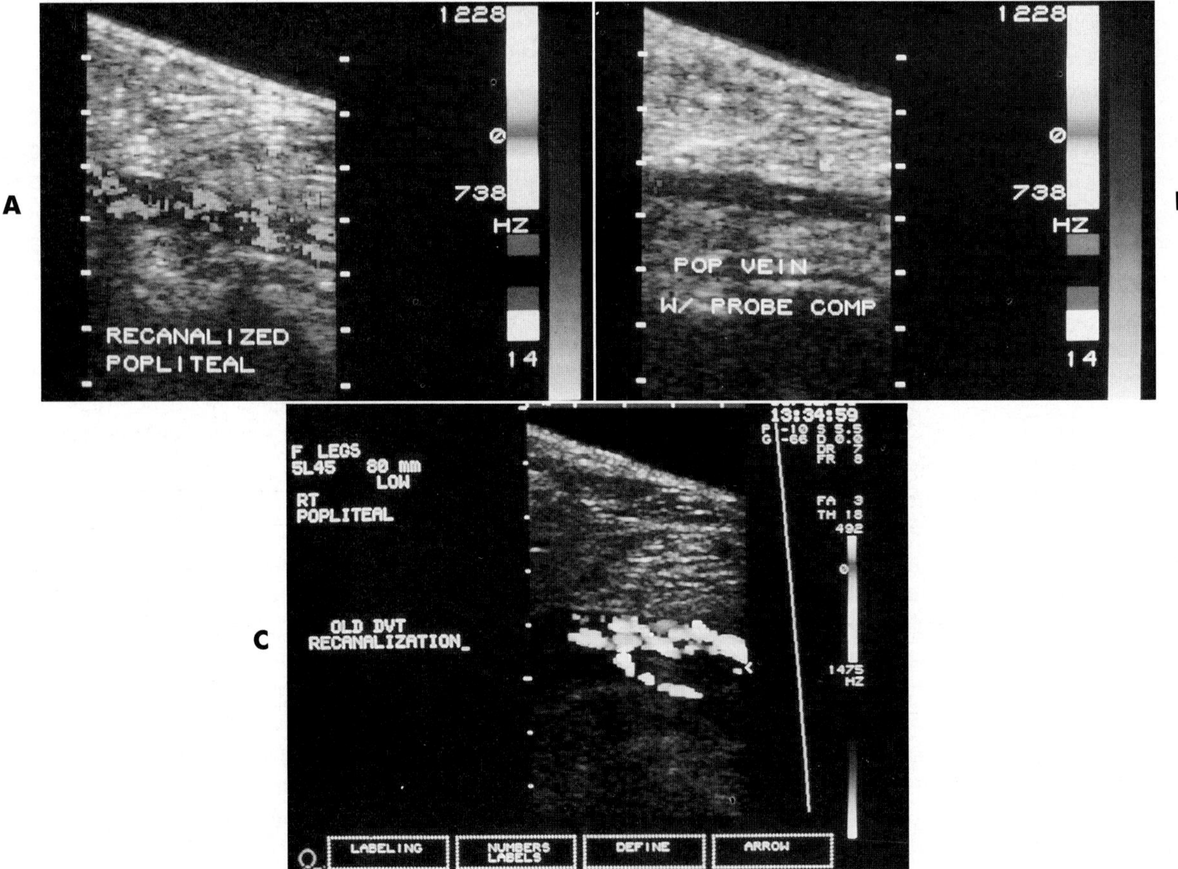

FIG. 21-43 Recanalized thrombus. **A,** The popliteal vein in this segment has old chronic thrombus through which numerous pathways have developed (seen with color-flow imaging). A continuous-wave Doppler examination might not detect any flow abnormality. **B,** Transducer compression of the vein in **A** closes the pathways but the walls do not meet because of the presence of the thrombus. **C,** This popliteal vein has recanalized almost completely from an old thrombosis; note the turbulent flow pattern, the irregular walls, and the presence of a patent collateral.

tomosed to the ipsilateral obstructed leg below the level of the obstruction (Fig. 21-46). Venous flow then can travel up the ipsilateral leg, across the bypass, and dump into the contralateral common femoral vein, which can restore venous drainage to the formerly occluded side[4] (see also Lower-Extremity Venous Duplex Case 2, Fig. 21-49).

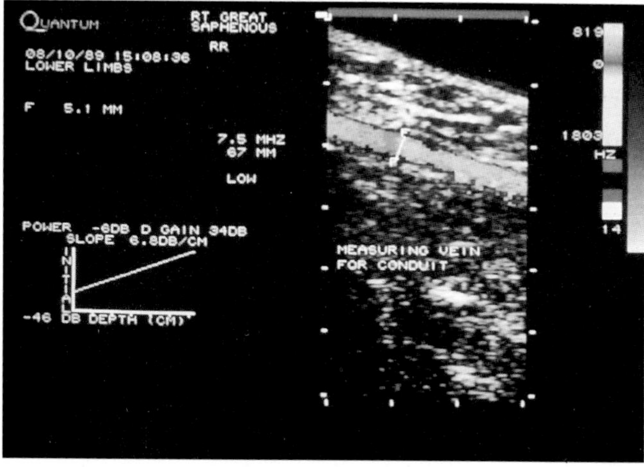

FIG. 21-44 Measuring the size of the great saphenous vein to determine suitability for bypass conduit.

The duplex examination protocol is the same as in routine evaluation, but the examiner needs to read the patient's operative note and surgical history to become familiar with the actual procedure that was done before scanning. He or she should take additional time to evaluate any bypasses and proximal or distal venous anastomoses, concentrating especially on the level of valvular competence and the flow characteristics.

Sclerotherapy

Sclerotherapy is identified by many as a cosmetic procedure performed on small and unsightly spider telangiectasias; it can, however, be used in some cases to sclerose and obliterate significant varicosities or even entire saphenous veins.[21] The procedure generally involves isolating the teleangiectasia or varicosity, then compressing the proximal and distal ends of the isolated vein segment with the fingers of one hand. As much blood as possible is evacuated from the segment (by digital compression or cannulation), then a sclerosing agent (such as saline or sodium tetradecyl sulfate) is injected directly into the isolated empty vein. The sclerosing agent actually irritates and inflames the vein walls, causing a focal phlebitis. After injection, the treated area of the leg is compressed by tightly wrapping it with an elastic bandage or by having the patient don a pre-

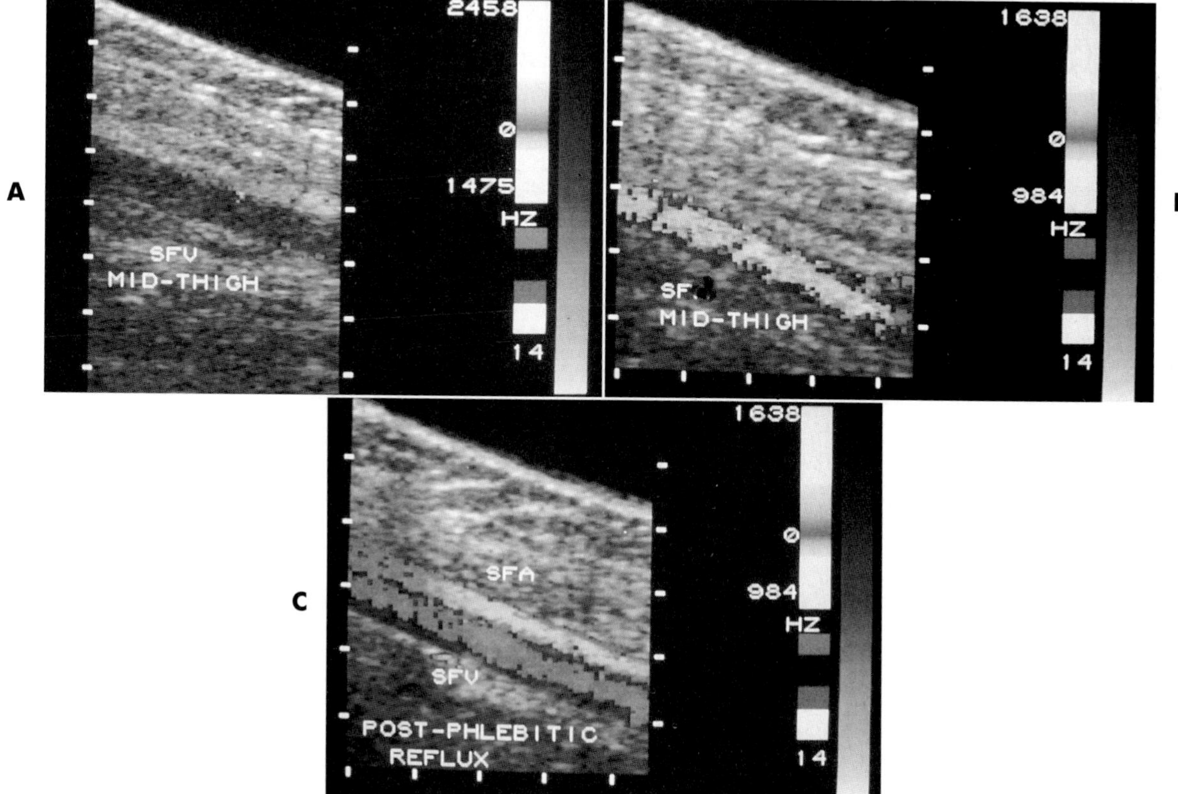

FIG. 21-45 Before and after lysis. The following images are taken from a patient with recurrent deep-vein thrombosis. **A,** The superficial femoral vein is completely thrombosed. **B,** In a follow-up examination 6 months after anticoagulation therapy the same segment is now patent with some residual irregularity, although postphlebitic reflux is present, **C.**

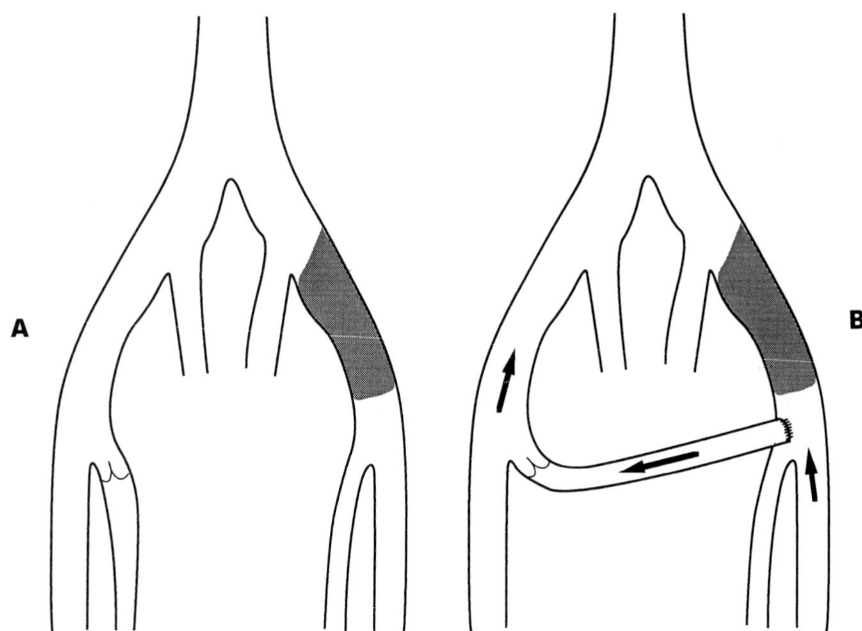

FIG. 21-46 Femorofemoral venous bypass. **A,** Before bypass. There is a complete occlusion of the left external iliac vein with normal patency on the right. **B,** After bypass. The right great saphenous vein has been divided distally, brought across the pubis, and anastomosed to the left femoral vein below the occlusion. Venous drainage is thus restored to the left leg as illustrated.

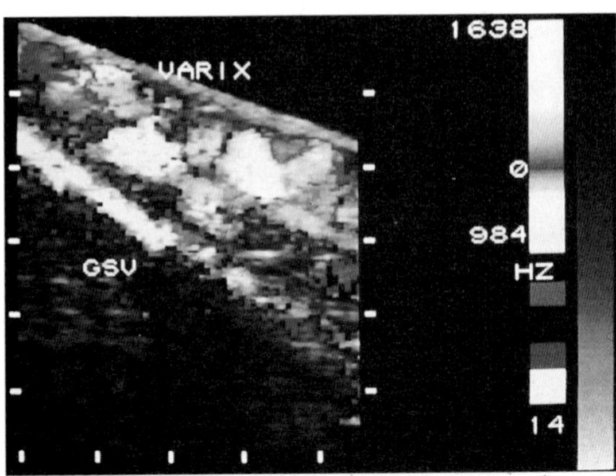

FIG. 21-47 This large dilated varicosity appeared on external physical examination to involve the great saphenous vein; duplex sonography shows the varix to be an entirely separate, and thus focally treatable, venous branch (note the normal saphenous vein deep to the varix).

scription venous compression stocking (20 to 30 or 30 to 40 mm Hg compression). The wrap or stocking is used to collapse and keep the the treated veins flattened so that the irritated walls stick together, thrombosing and ultimately destroying the vein.[9] The bandage or hose is kept on for 48 hours, then worn daily for up to 2 weeks to achieve the desired result. The treated veins ideally fibrose and are reabsorbed. Some investigators advocate sclerotherapy for large veins as an alternative to stripping or ligation.[21]

The duplex examination protocol again is unchanged from routine evaluation. Examinations before sclerotherapy may be required to help determine whether the varicosity being treated is a branch of a more significant venous tributary or instead is contiguous with an incompetent saphenous vein (Fig. 21-47; see color image); if so, surgical ligation might be considered instead of sclerotherapy. Duplex is also used to rule out the presence of existing deep vein thrombosis or superficial thrombosis that could cause complications and contraindicate sclerotherapy.[9] Duplex can also be used as a follow-up to check the result of treatment, especially of larger varicosities.

Lower-Extremity Venous Duplex Sonography Cases

In these cases the images are described and arranged in sequence from the groin to the ankle to make comparisons easier and for reader clarity; in practice the protocol of scanning from the ankle level to the groin that was described previously was followed during all of the cases presented here.

Case 1 (Fig. 21-48): normal deep-system, thrombosed lesser saphenous vein

This 46-year-old patient had recent sclerotherapy treatment of a large dilated lesser saphenous vein and was examined after he noticed an area of recurrent inflammation of the posterior calf.

The evaluation of the deep veins showed exceptionally well-defined veins with normal flow patterns and characteristics in the junction of the superficial femoral, profunda femoris, and common femoral veins (Fig. 21-48, *A*; see color image), superficial femoral vein (Fig. 21-48, *B*; see color image), junction of the popliteal and peroneal-tibial

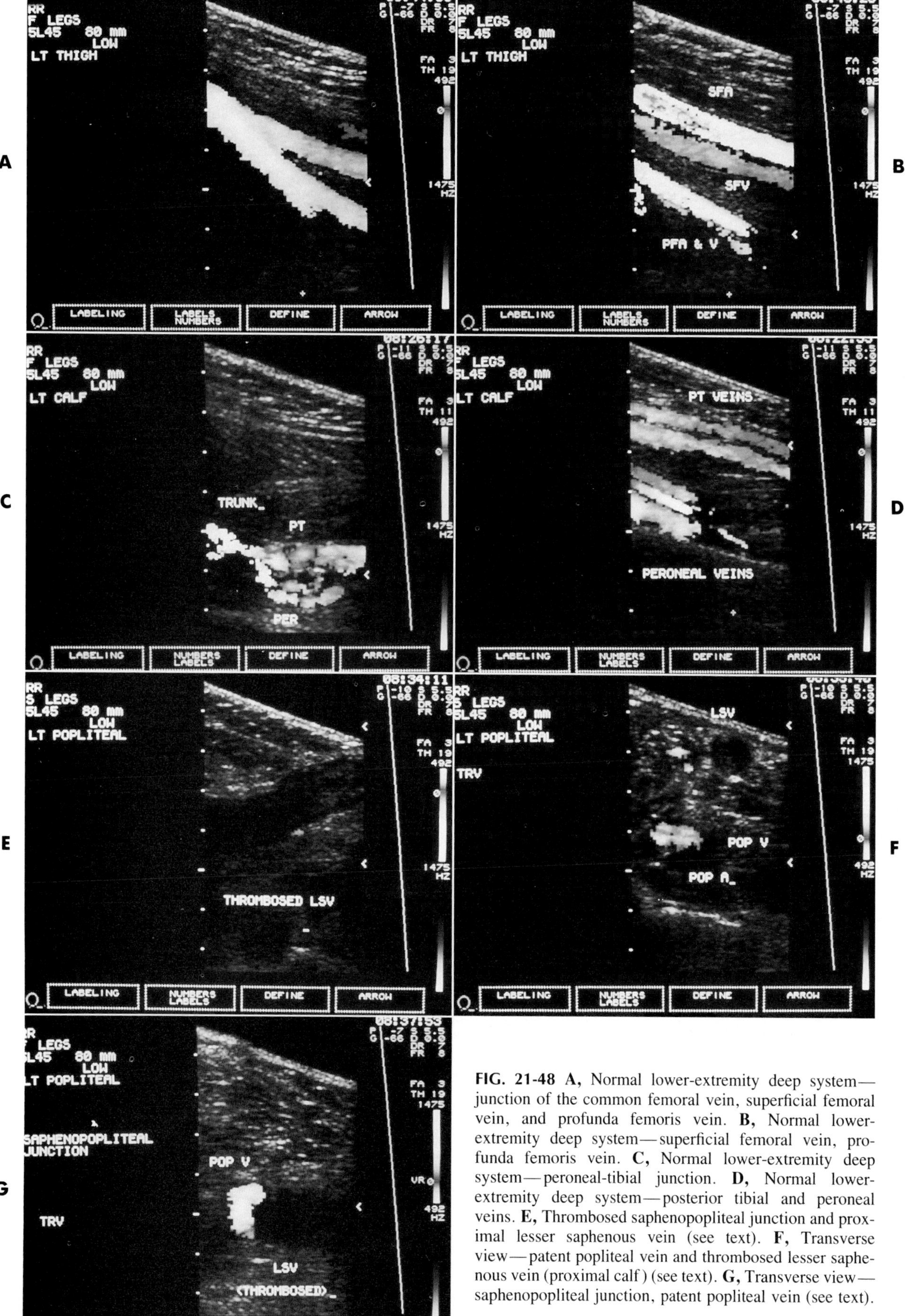

FIG. 21-48 **A,** Normal lower-extremity deep system—junction of the common femoral vein, superficial femoral vein, and profunda femoris vein. **B,** Normal lower-extremity deep system—superficial femoral vein, profunda femoris vein. **C,** Normal lower-extremity deep system—peroneal-tibial junction. **D,** Normal lower-extremity deep system—posterior tibial and peroneal veins. **E,** Thrombosed saphenopopliteal junction and proximal lesser saphenous vein (see text). **F,** Transverse view—patent popliteal vein and thrombosed lesser saphenous vein (proximal calf) (see text). **G,** Transverse view—saphenopopliteal junction, patent popliteal vein (see text).

veins (Fig. 21-48, *C*; see color image), and calf veins (Fig. 21-48, *D*; see color image). The lesser saphenous was full of very echogenic irregular thrombus after the sclerotherapy treatment (Fig. 21-48, *E*; see color image); in transverse the thrombosed saphenous lumen could be easily followed in the posterior calf (Fig. 21-48, *F*; see color image) and at the laterally placed saphenopopliteal junction (Fig. 21-48, *G*; see color image). Note that the border of the lesser saphenous thrombosis fortunately stops right at the junction and does not propagate into the popliteal vein.

The symptoms were felt by the surgeon to be sequelae to the extensive thrombosis in the lesser saphenous. In later clinical follow-up the patient had no further complaints with an excellent fibrous cord after sclerosis.

Case 2 (Fig. 21-49): femorofemoral venous bypass

This 33-year-old patient had a history of chronic left iliac vein occlusion with a markedly swollen left leg. Preoperative venous duplex sonography revealed a patent deep system below the iliac with poor collateral drainage. A femorofemoral cross-pubic bypass was performed as described above and illustrated in Fig. 21-46.

The left-side anastomosis of the distal great saphenous vein is shown in Fig. 21-49, *A* (see color image). Note the strong flow in the common femoral vein below the anastomosis and the flow that is visualized in the bypass, traveling superiorly and medially (coded blue).

The right side anastomosis (Fig. 21-49, *B*; see color image) shows the patent right common femoral vein with the visualized saphenofemoral junction. Note that the great saphenous vein has been reflected proximally to cross the pubic region, and that flow is traveling away from the transducer (coded red) into the junction from the left side, denoting a properly functioning venous bypass.

This patient has had a normal lifestyle with no recurrent problems over a 3-year follow-up period.

Case 3 (Fig. 21-50): chronic and acute distal common femoral vein, superficial femoral vein, popliteal vein, and calf vein thrombosis

After a long overseas airplane trip, this 75-year-old patient presented with a markedly swollen right leg of about 2 weeks duration with tenderness in the popliteal area and calf.

Longitudinal examination of the proximal common femoral vein was normal. Evaluation of the distal common femoral vein and the superficial femoral vein–profunda femoris vein–common femoral vein junction, however, revealed a combination homogeneous-heterogeneous thrombosis of the superficial femoral vein (Fig. 21-50, *A*; see color image), which propagated with asymmetric homogeneous thrombus into the common femoral vein, partially obstructing it; this was best appreciated in transverse (Fig. 21-50, *B*; see color image). The profunda femoris vein was patent (see *A*). The superficial femoral vein was completely thrombosed in the thigh (Fig. 21-50, *C*; see color image), as was the proximal popliteal vein (Fig. 21-50, *D*; see color image). The distal popliteal vein was also occupied by homogeneous thrombus but some flow could be seen around the periphery of the thrombus near the posterior wall and distally (Fig. 21-50, *E*). Although the peroneal-tibial junction was thrombosed, some recanalization or collateralization was taking place, mostly from peroneal branches through echogenic thrombus (Fig. 21-50, *F*); the posterior tibial vein was thrombosed to the ankle.

The patient was subsequently admitted to the hospital for anticoagulation therapy.

Case 4 (Fig. 21-51): acute distal superficial femoral vein, popliteal vein, and posterior tibial vein thrombosis

This 37-year-old patient presented with a markedly swollen right calf of about 5 days' duration, with tenderness in

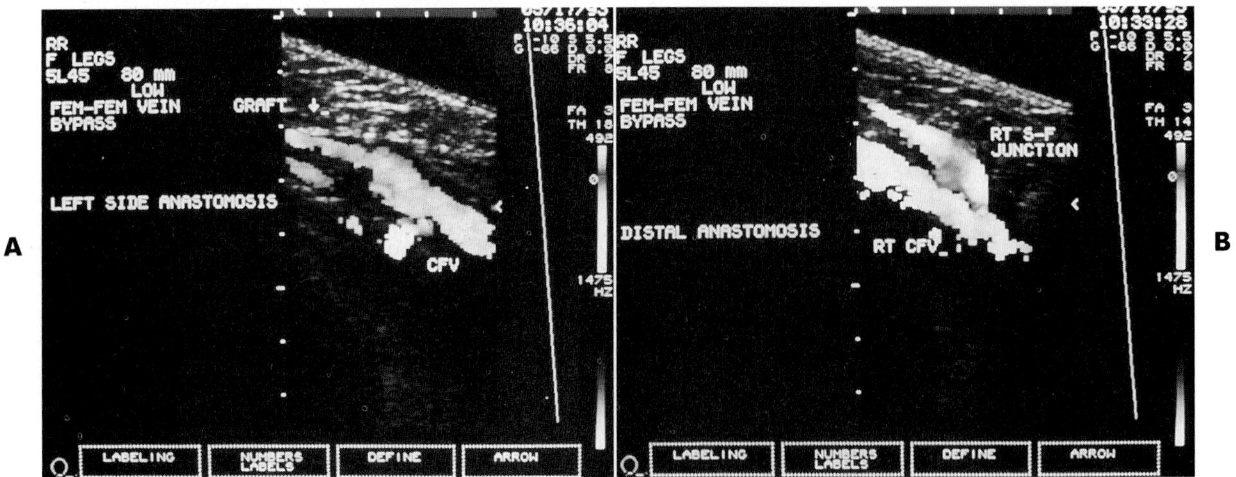

FIG. 21-49 A, Femorofemoral venous bypass—left anastomosis, left common femoral vein (see text). **B,** Femorofemoral venous bypass—right saphenofemoral junction, right common femoral vein (see text).

the popliteal area and calf. He had a history of prior deep-vein thrombosis of the left leg.

Evaluation of the common femoral vein (Fig. 21-51, *A*; see color image), profunda femoris vein, and proximal superficial femoral vein showed patent veins with fairly normal flow, although there was some flow diminution in the proximal superficial femoral vein (Fig. 21-51, *B*; see color image). Evaluation of the saphenofemoral junction (see Fig. 21-51, *A*) and great saphenous vein (Fig. 21-51, *C*; see color image), however, revealed the presence of high-velocity continuous flow from the calf level to the groin. This implied that the great saphenous vein was draining the majority of flow from the distal leg. Imaging of the midthigh portion of the superficial femoral vein (Fig. 21-51, *D*; see color image) showed an occluded distal superficial femoral vein with a single active collateral reconstituting the proximal superficial femoral vein. The superficial femoral vein was completely thrombosed distal to this (Fig. 21-51, *E*; see color image), as was the popliteal vein (Fig. 21-51, *F*; see color image) and the posterior tibial vein (Fig. 21-51, *G*; see color image).

The patient was admitted to the hospital for anticoagulation therapy.

Case 5 (Fig. 21-52): superficial thrombosis of great saphenous vein

This 72-year-old patient presented with a markedly swollen right leg and a tender, palpable cord along the medial calf; the referring physician stated that the patient had been undergoing radiation therapy to the pelvic area. He had had two previous examinations before this, 1 month apart, and had gone from a patent deep system with a superficial phlebitis to acute onset of the symptoms.

The patient was noted to have an acute superficial femoral vein thrombosis (Fig. 21-52, *A*), but of primary significance was the presence of a thrombosed segment of the great saphenous vein in the calf. Above the knee, the great saphenous had some chronic and acute thrombus

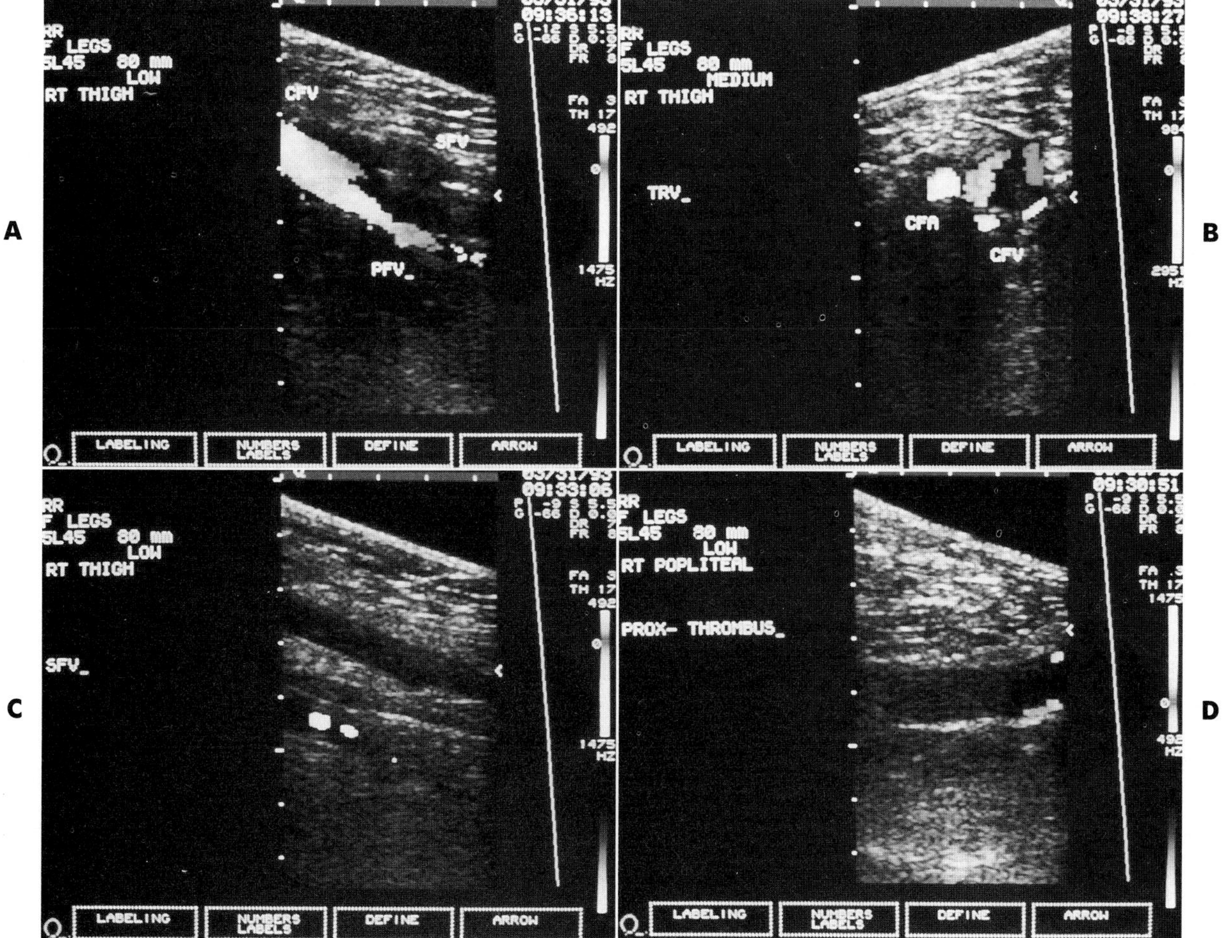

FIG. 21-50 A, Partial distal common femoral vein thrombosis, superficial femoral vein thrombosis—longitudinal view (see text). **B,** Partial distal common femoral vein thrombosis—transverse view (see text). **C,** Thrombosed superficial femoral vein, midthigh. **D,** Thrombosed proximal popliteal vein. **E,** Thrombosed distal popliteal vein with some flow around the periphery of the thrombus (see text). **F,** Thrombosis of the peroneal-tibial venous junction with some recanalization or collateralization present (see text).

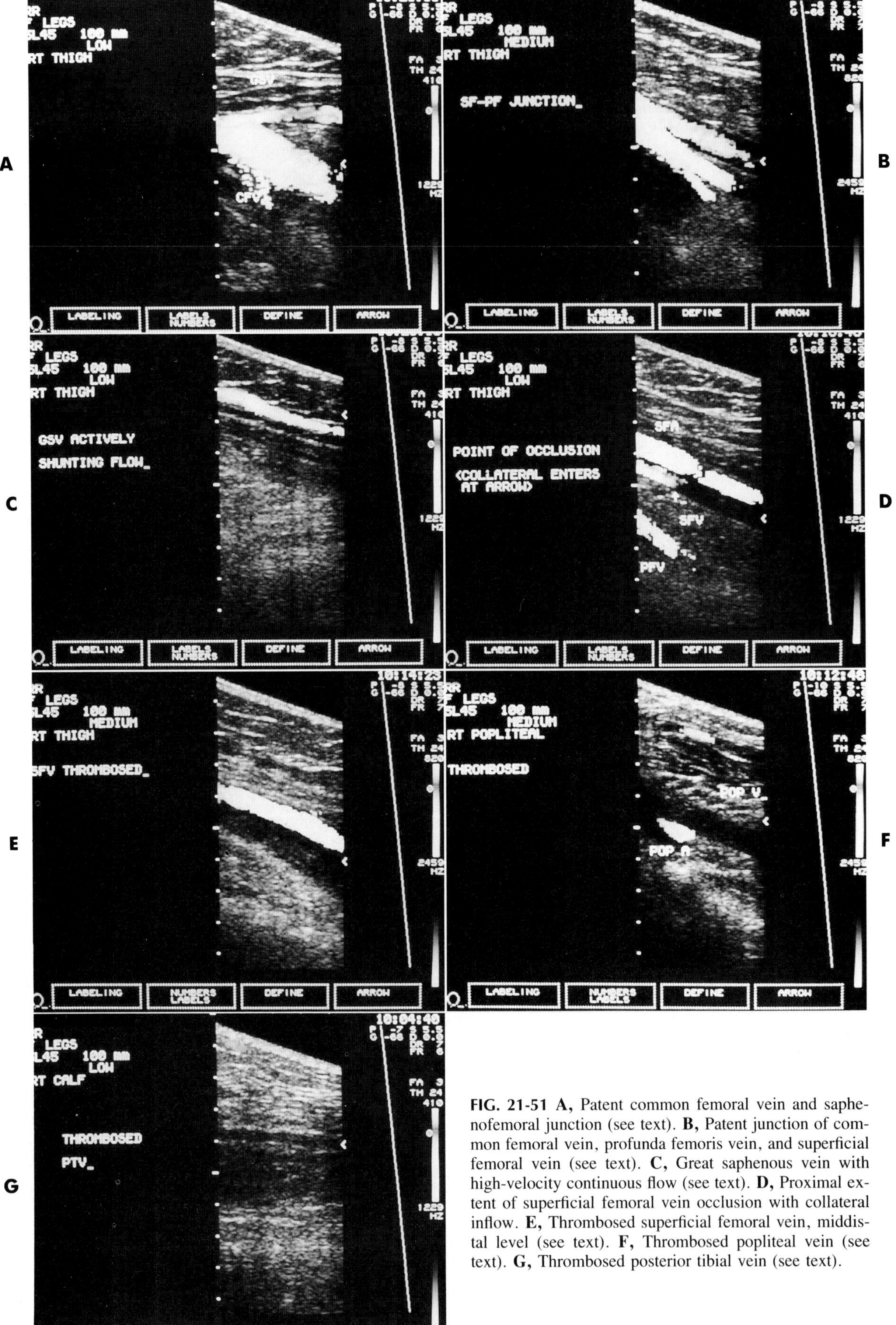

FIG. 21-51 **A,** Patent common femoral vein and saphenofemoral junction (see text). **B,** Patent junction of common femoral vein, profunda femoris vein, and superficial femoral vein (see text). **C,** Great saphenous vein with high-velocity continuous flow (see text). **D,** Proximal extent of superficial femoral vein occlusion with collateral inflow. **E,** Thrombosed superficial femoral vein, middistal level (see text). **F,** Thrombosed popliteal vein (see text). **G,** Thrombosed posterior tibial vein (see text).

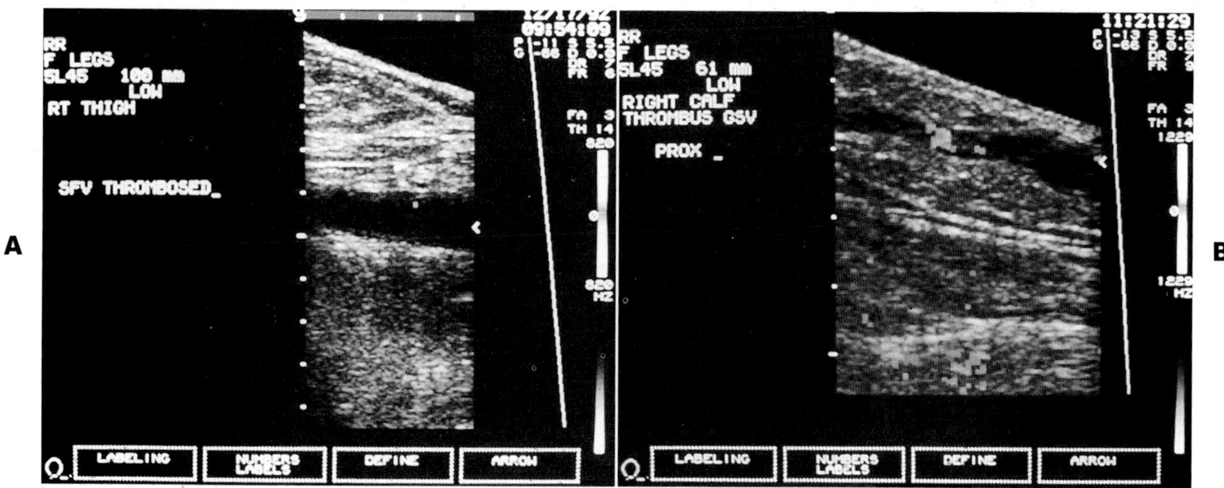

FIG. 21-52 A, Superficial vein thrombosis. **B,** Thrombus in the great saphenous vein just below the knee.

with some recanalized patent areas (Fig. 21-52, *B*; see color image).

The patient underwent heparinization, with subsequent lysis of the thrombi in the deep system and with some restored patency to the superficial system.

Case 6 (Fig. 21-53): focal thrombosis of the posterior tibial vein

This 69-year-old patient was referred with a 10-day history of focal calf tenderness and pain, as well as calf swelling that had diminished substantially during that period.

Evaluation of the posterior tibial veins at the ankle showed patent but nonspontaneous flow, which responded well to distal augmentation (Fig. 21-53, *A*; see color image). At the midcalf level, however, the posterior tibial vein was noted to be thrombosed (Fig. 21-53, *B*; see color image). Note the clearly defined arteries and the fully patent peroneal system deep to the posterior tibial. The patent distal posterior tibial veins were shunting flow to the distal great saphenous via an incompetent perforating vein just below the thrombus (not shown). The thrombosis was slightly echogenic proximal to the site in *B* and occupied both veins (Fig. 21-53, *C*; see color image); the veins were incompressible under the transducer in transverse (Fig. 21-53, *D*; see color image). The thrombosis ended at the peroneal-tibial trunk and did not propagate into the patent popliteal vein (Fig. 21-53, *E*; see color image). The anterior tibial vein was patent also (Fig. 21-53, *F*; see color image).

Above the knee, the rest of the deep and superficial systems were patent with normal flow and no evidence of thrombus or reflux.

UPPER EXTREMITY VENOUS EVALUATION

Although the major incidence of venous disease occurs in the lower extremities, the upper extremities are the site of venous thromboses that can be just as serious as those found in the legs. Since the introduction of intravenous solution administration, monitoring catheters, and dialysis operations for the patient in renal failure, the incidence of upper-extremity phlebitis has increased.[10] Like the leg veins, the upper-extremity veins may thrombose and give off potential pulmonary emboli.[10,20] The contrast method of venography may not be suitable, especially in the dialysis patient with a surgically produced arteriovenous fistula. Determining the patency of veins often becomes a factor in decisions on whether to proceed with venography, to intervene surgically, or to attempt anticoagulant therapy to resolve the problem. Use of Doppler and duplex sonography again provides an easily available and accurate method of examination.

Venous Anatomy of the Upper Extremities

Both deep and superficial systems exist in the upper extremities.

The deep venous system is of somewhat small caliber and may be difficult to evaluate in the forearm. Adequate signals and visualization can be obtained from the radial and ulnar veins, which arise from venous plexuses in the venous palmar arches. These veins run superiorly along with their respective radial and ulnar arteries and anastomose at the antecubital fossa to form the brachial vein.

The brachial vein runs superiorly along either side of the brachial artery and anastomoses with the axillary vein at the junction of the basilic (superficial) vein at the shoulder (Fig. 21-54).

The axillary vein continues superiorly into the thorax, where it becomes the subclavian vein at approximately the lateral border of the first rib. The subclavian vein then anastomoses with the internal jugular vein to form the brachiocephalic vein. The right and left brachiocephalic veins join the superior vena cava, which then empties into the right atrium of the heart (Fig. 21-55).

The superficial venous system of the upper extremity consists of two major veins, the basilic and cephalic veins.

The basilic vein begins on the ulnar side of the arm. It runs proximally on the posterior surface of the ulnar side of the arm and continues superiorly along the medial aspect of the arm to the axilla, where it joins the axillary vein. The median antebrachial vein lies between the radial and ulnar arteries and anastomoses with the basilic vein approximately 2 cm below the antecubital fossa.

The cephalic vein begins in the radial part of the dorsal

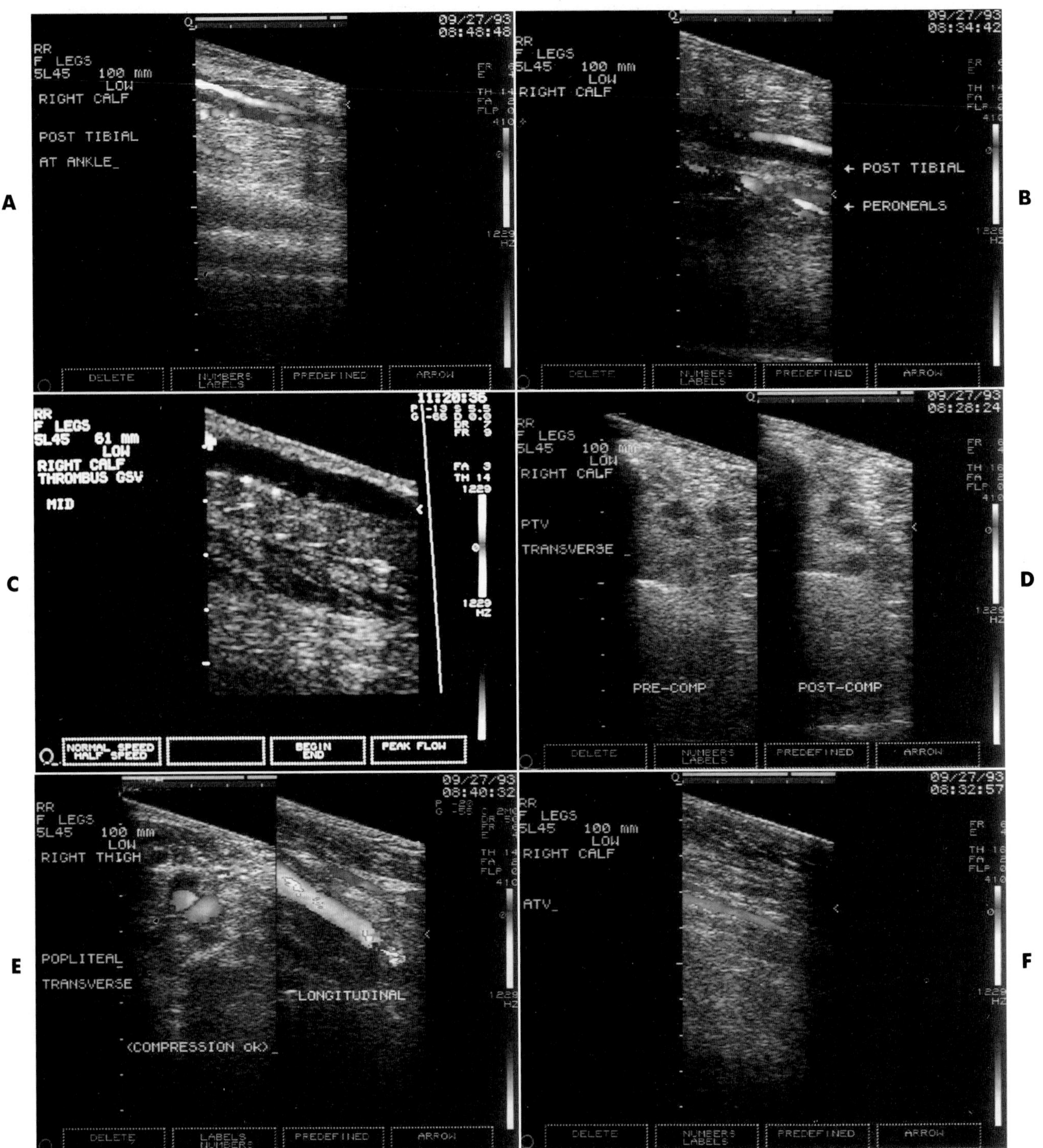

FIG. 21-53 A, Patent distal posterior tibial veins (see text). **B,** Thrombosed posterior tibial veins, patent peroneal veins. **C,** Thrombus in the great saphenous vein along the midcalf segment. **D,** Thrombosed posterior tibial vein, midcalf level, transverse plane, with and without transducer compression (see text). **E,** Patent popliteal vein (longitudinal and transverse planes). **F,** Patent anterior tibial vein.

venous network of the hand. It extends proximally around the radial border of the forearm to the antecubital fossa, where it anastomoses with the median cubital vein. It then continues up the lateral side of the arm superiorly and enters the shoulder to anastomose with the subclavian vein (Fig. 21-56).

Continuous-Wave Doppler Upper-Extremity Venous Evaluation

The patient's history is once again obtained, with emphasis on pain, discoloration, swelling, and history of recent intravenous infusions; and differentiation is made between arterial and venous disease as in the lower extremity examination.

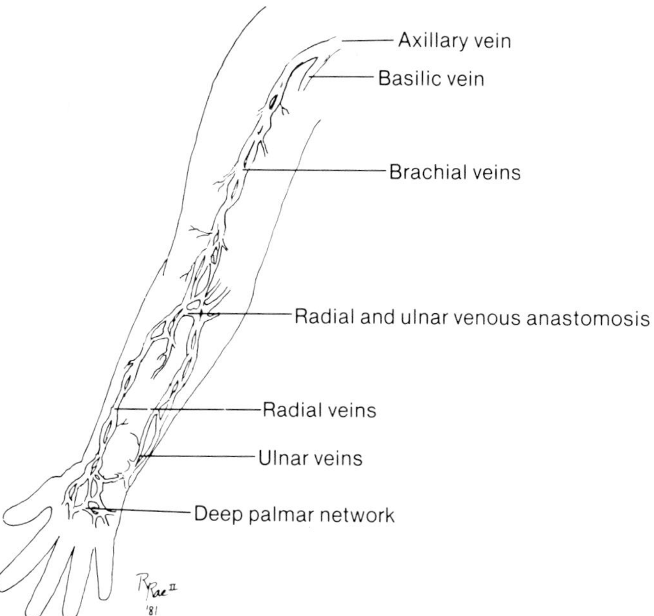

FIG. 21-54 Deep venous system of the upper extremity to the axilla.

The patient lies supine in a room with the same environmental conditions as for the lower-extremity examination.

First, the deep veins are examined when practicable. The deep veins in the forearm are not as easily assessed because of the complexity of the superficial system in the forearm. General guidelines, however, can be given. The radial and ulnar veins are located at the wrist by locating their companion arteries. The probe is then angled caudally, and the venous signal is distinguished and evaluated by the standard characteristic qualities of the normal venous signal. Note that expansion of the superior vena cava as a result of negative intrathoracic pressure may increase venous flow in the upper extremity with inspiration rather than expiration.

When the flow signal is evaluated, the forearm is compressed and released after several seconds for proximal augmentation. Distal augmentation may be performed by compression of the fleshy part of the hand. Both the radial and the ulnar veins are evaluated in this manner.

Next, the brachial vein is examined. It is monitored at its site on the medial side of the arm at the intramuscular septum. Locating the artery first may, once again, aid the examiner. The standard signal qualities are used to evaluate the venous flow signal. Distal compression is performed by compression of the forearm (Fig. 21-57), and the Valsalva maneuver is used for proximal compression. Responses should be the same as in the lower-extremity venous examination.

The axillary vein is then located by angling caudally in the axilla, medial to the axillary artery. The axillary signal may be pulsatile and is one of the few exceptions to the rule of nonpulsatility. (All pulsatile signals from this site proximally should be interpreted as normal.) Distal compression of the upper arm and forearm should be performed. Proximal compression consists of the Valsalva maneuver.

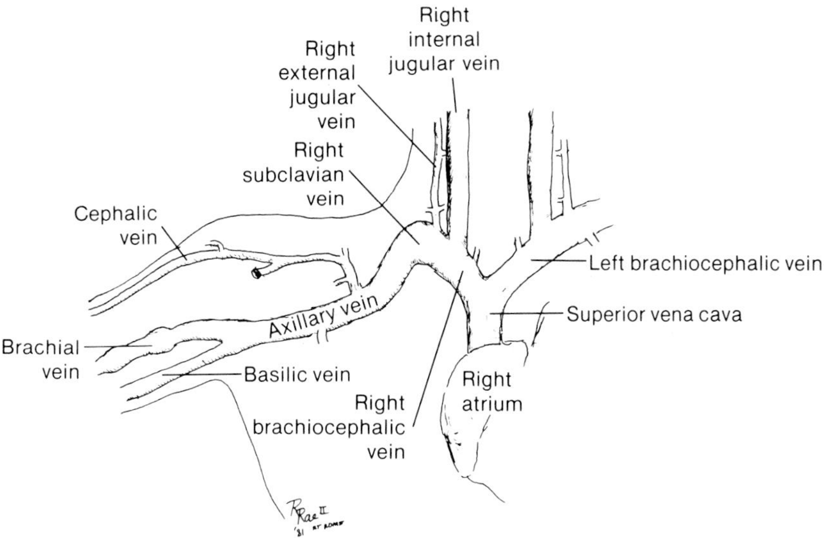

FIG. 21-55 Deep venous system in the thorax to the right atrium.

The subclavian vein is located by placing the probe either beneath the clavicle and angling superiorly and laterally or in the supraclavicular fossa and angling laterally and inferiorly (Fig. 21-58). This signal is also pulsatile and must be carefully distinguished from the subclavian artery signal. Examination is performed as for the axillary vein.

If axillary or subclavian thrombosis is indicated, the internal jugular vein should be evaluated to determine the extent of the thrombus.

The internal jugular is located by angling the probe inferiorly and laterally to either the inferior or the superior border of the sternocleidomastoid muscle. The internal jugular signal can be phasic, continuous, or pulsatile and usually is heard as a high-velocity variable hissing sound. The only maneuver performed is a Valsalva. Diminished augmentation on release implies a proximal brachiocephalic venous thrombus.[2]

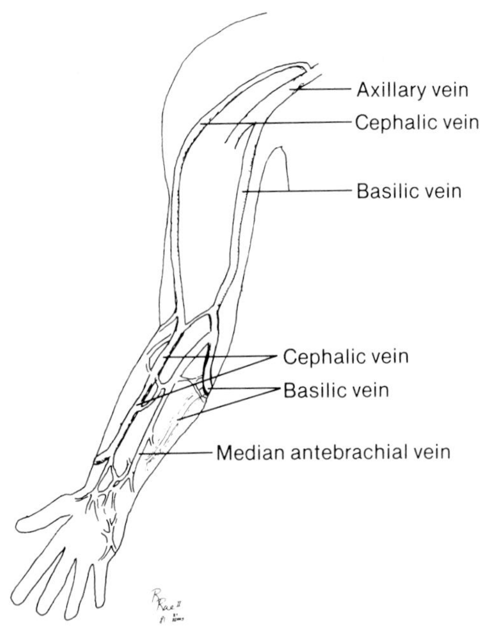

FIG. 21-56 Superficial venous system in the upper extremity.

The superficial veins are examined in a manner similar to that for the veins of the lower extremity. They can, again, be monitored anywhere along their course; they also require light probe pressure. Usually a slightly phasic or continuous signal is heard, and augmentation is performed by percussion or light compression. Reduced or absent flow may imply a thrombus near the axillobrachial junction in the cephalic vein and in the subclavian vein with diminished basilic vein flow.

In summary, these are the steps in the venous continuous-wave Doppler examination of the upper extremity:

1. Obtain the history.
2. Examine the radial and ulnar veins. Distal compression of the hand and proximal compression of the forearm may be performed for augmentation.
3. Examine the brachial vein. Distal compression of the forearm may be performed, and a Valsalva maneuver for proximal compression.
4. Examine the axillary vein, with distal compression of the forearm and Valsalva maneuver.
5. Examine the subclavian vein in the supraclavicular fossa, or underneath the clavicle in the same way as for the axillary vein.
6. Examine the internal jugular vein if there is a question of thrombus extending into the brachiocephalic vein. A Valsalva maneuver also may be performed.
7. Evaluate the basilic and cephalic veins.

See Fig. 21-59 for upper extremity venous probe site locations.

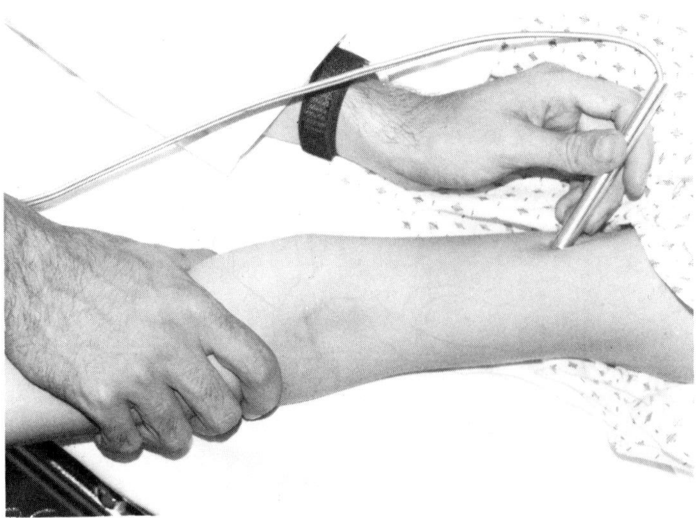

FIG. 21-57 Examination of the brachial vein with distal forearm compression. The transducer is angled against the flow.

Interpretation of the Continuous-Wave Doppler Upper-Extremity Venous Examination

In brachial vein thrombosis there is usually a continuous signal in the radial and ulnar veins. One or both may be continuous, depending on the level of the thrombus. There are poor augmentation responses with release of upper-arm compression or Valsalva.

The brachial venous signal is either absent or continuous, with a markedly reduced flow rate.

The axillary and subclavian signals are normal with normal responses to Valsalva but poor distal augmentation responses with arm compression.

The superficial veins show changes reflecting the extent of the thrombus, especially if it extends into the axillary.

In both axillary and subclavian venous thrombosis the radial and ulnar vein signals are continuous. Poor proximal augmentation can be expected.[2]

The axillary signal may be absent or continuous, depending on the location of the thrombus and collateral circulation. Both distal compression and Valsalva maneuver responses are poor.

The subclavian vein reflects the same conditions as the axillary, but if thrombosis is suspected in the proximal brachiocephalic vein, the jugular signal should be evaluated.

In the internal jugular vein a reduced Valsalva response implies a brachiocephalic venous occlusion. Flow may be reduced, depending on the extent of the thrombus.

The use of intravenous infusions tends to be the greatest cause of superficial phlebitis in the upper extremities.[2] In cases of superficial thrombus in the basilic and cephalic veins, flow is usually completely absent with poor or limited response to augmentation maneuvers. Evaluation must be based on augmentation and patency, as in the lower-extremity veins.

Venous Upper-Extremity Doppler Cases

Case 1 (Fig. 21-60): normal upper-extremity venous flow—postoperative examination

This 68-year-old woman was admitted for a mass felt in the right supraclavicular fossa, which was suspected to be a thrombosed subclavian artery aneurysm. The patient went to surgery, but the mass was found to be a subclavian vein aneurysm involving the external jugular and three adjacent veins. It was thrombosed but fortunately was off one wall of the subclavian vein and did not involve the entire circumference of the vein. It was resected, and the four involved branches were ligated. Flow was determined postoperatively.

Normal waveforms with normal phasicity, pulsatility, and augmentation maneuvers are shown. The internal jugular was checked to ensure that proximal flow was normal. There was a normal response to the Valsalva maneuver.

Venous Duplex and Color-Flow Examination of the Upper Extremity

Upper-extremity evaluation with the duplex real time scanner uses many of the same criteria as in the lower-extremity duplex venous examination, but the flow patterns are different, as mentioned above, because of the intrathoracic pressure difference, and a "phasic pulsatility" of the vein is encountered. Thrombosis retains the same appearances as those mentioned earlier, as do flow augmentation responses. The main differences are in the examination technique.

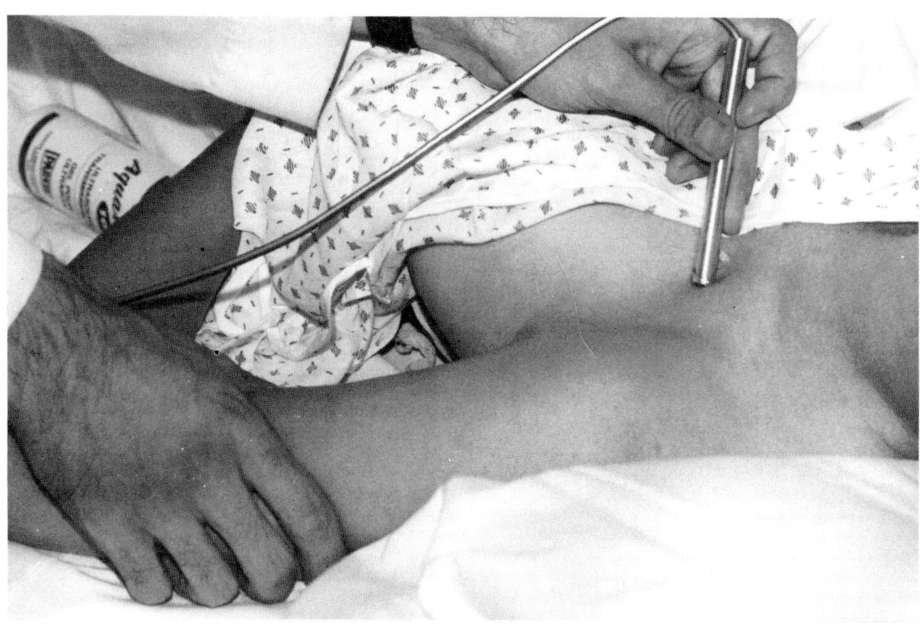

FIG. 21-58 Obtaining the subclavian venous signal.

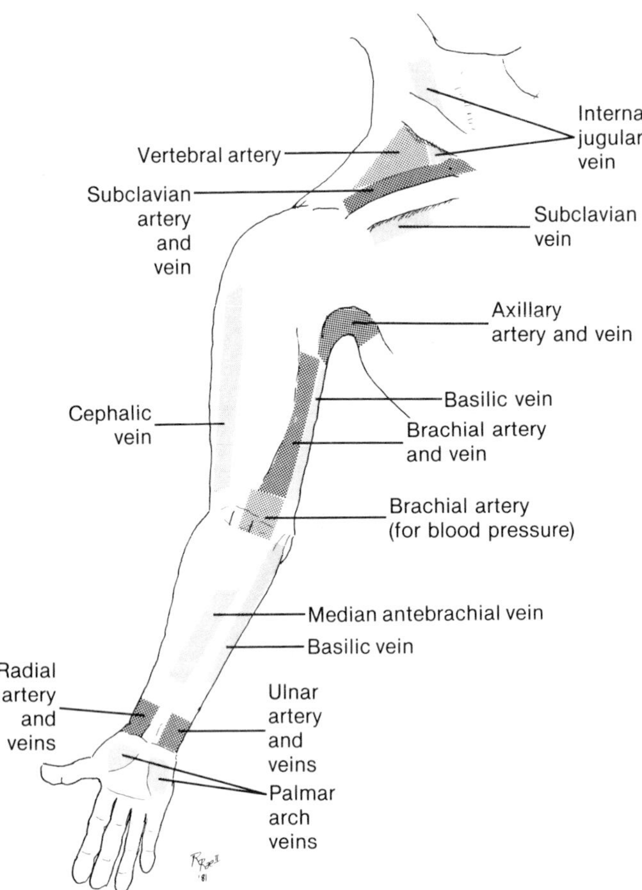

FIG. 21-59 Sites for both arterial and venous examinations of the upper extremity.

Venous Landmarks. As in the lower extremity, the examiner can use adjacent bony structures to help locate the deep veins in the arm. The radial and ulnar veins lie very superficially to the bright echo of the radius and ulna, and adjacent to the arteries. The brachial vein runs medial to the humerus and is again adjacent to the brachial artery. The axillary vein is easily located in the axilla and anteromedial to the artery. The subclavian vein is also located posterior to the clavicle and may be visualized either from above or below the clavicle. The internal jugular vein is easily found lateral to the common carotid artery in the neck.

The course of the superficial veins can vary, as discussed in the previous anatomy section. Some confusion can result near the basilobrachial junction, since both veins can be of similar dimension. Almost always, the basilic vein can be seen to run posterior and medial to the brachial vein when traced. The cephalic vein is easier to trace, since it is on the superficial and lateral aspect of the arm.

Preparation. Preliminary procedures are as with the upper-extremity Doppler venous examination, but the patient should be placed in a position that allows the easiest access to the arm being evaluated (see Positioning).

Equipment. When evaluating the upper extremity and especially the superficial veins, 7.5 or even 10-MHz linear transducers work best because of the veins' proximity to the skin surface; standoff wedges or gel pads might be beneficial in the forearm. The examiner may wish to change to a 5-MHz scanhead when evaluating the supraclavicular and axillary areas unless a frequency-agile transducer is being used. A 4-cm field depth is adequate when beginning in the forearm, but the depth may be increased if needed, especially in the shoulder areas.

Positioning. The patient is best examined in a supine position with the arm being examined nearest the examiner; very slight elevation of the thorax may help with venous filling, but the primary requirement is that the examiner be able to gain easy access to the upper arm, axilla, and supraclavicular areas. Keeping the patient supine also prevents venous collapse.[19]

Scanning Procedure. For each vein being visualized, look for the following criteria:

1. Compressibility. The vein walls should meet when compressed with the probe. Firm pressure may be required. This is best seen when done in transverse.
2. Valves should coapt (when seen) and should have thin leaflets.
3. Flow should be spontaneous and phasic (augmentation may still be necessary).
4. Color-flow patterns should be uniform and phasic, with color extending to the walls with no filling defects.

Remember that veins may be paired. Take Doppler readings frequently to ensure that veins and arteries are discriminated. Blood echoes can usually be seen moving through the vein, and phasicity can be assessed visually at times with color-flow imaging and using audible pulsed spectral Doppler.

If the patient feels discomfort in the forearm or hand, examine the radial and ulnar veins (Fig. 21-61) on the ventral aspect of the forearm. Bear in mind that they may not be as easily seen as the arm veins. Scan in longitudinal and transverse planes when practical. Compress the vein area and use the Doppler to evaluate flow characteristics.

Examine the veins in the antecubital fossa, and look for any thrombotic areas that may be present. The antecubital fossa has numerous junctures with the superficial system present, so use of the Doppler and color flow to discriminate between veins and arteries and to identify the vessels is vital.

Follow the brachial vein proximally from the antecubital fossa (Fig. 21-62; see color image) and do forearm augmentation compression maneuvers (distal augmentation) and Valsalva maneuvers (equivalent of proximal augmentation) to assess the flow characteristics and the valve functions as completely as possible. Compress the vein sequentially with the transducer (in transverse preferably) to rule out the presence of thrombus and use color-flow imaging and Doppler spectral waveforms to further evaluate the flow characteristics.

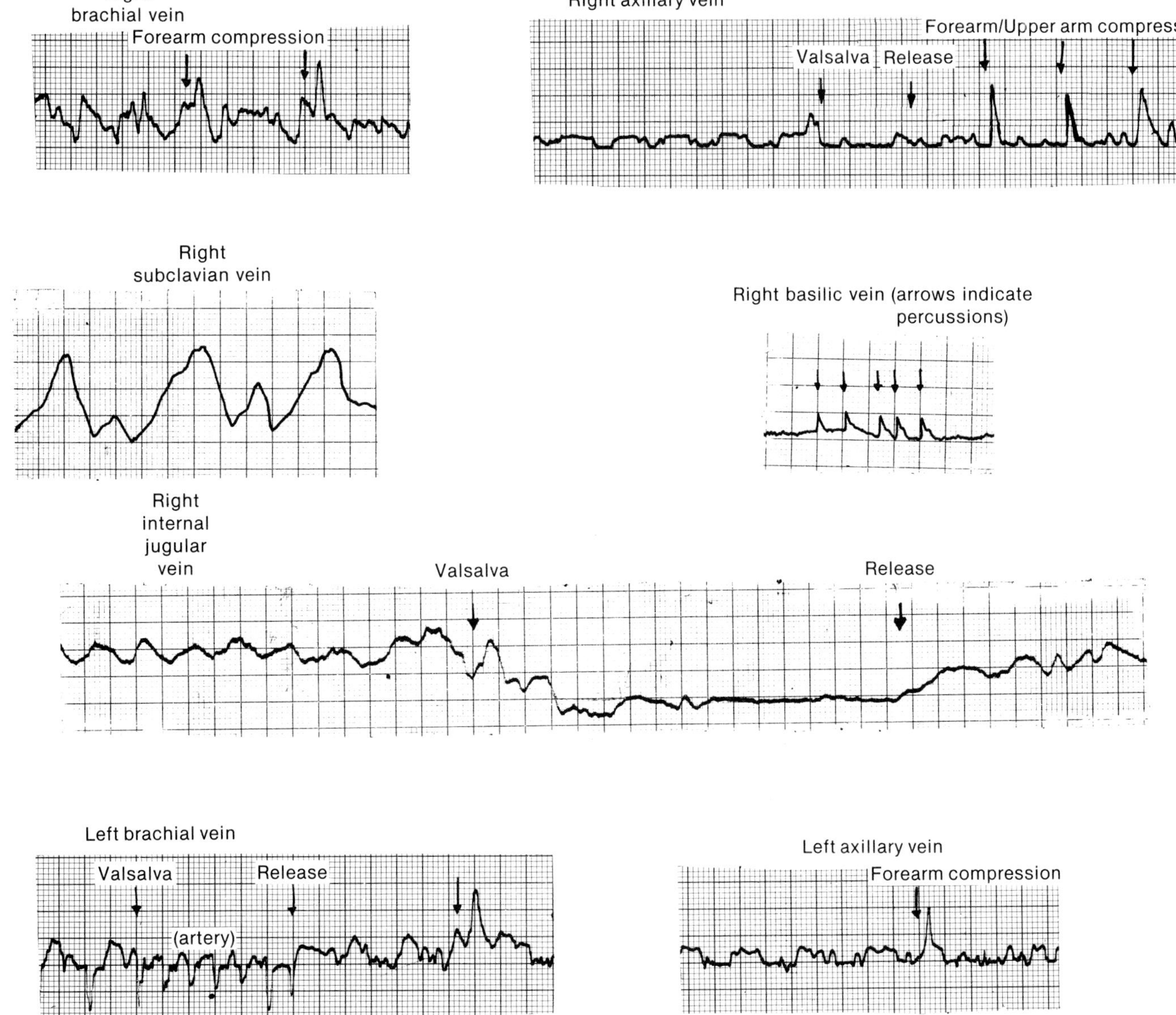

FIG. 21-60 Normal upper-extremity venous flow—postoperative examination.

Continue following the brachial vein proximally into the axilla, examining the axillary vein (Fig. 21-63; see color image) and evaluating the junction of the brachial and basilic veins (Fig. 21-64; see color image). Relocating the transducer to scan across the inferior shoulder aspect can often allow better visualization of the axillary vein and distal subclavian vein. The veins should be evaluated in both longitudinal and transverse planes when practicable; again, compress the vein area with the transducer if practicable and use color flow and Doppler spectral waveforms with proximal and distal augmentation maneuvers to evaluate the flow characteristics.

Examine the supraclavicular area (Fig. 21-65; see color images) to evaluate as much of the subclavian vein as possible from the shoulder medially until it disappears beneath the proximal clavicle. Compressing the vein with the transducer is virtually impossible at this level, so assessment of this region primarily centers on visual recognition of thrombus, use of color-flow imaging to determine patency, and use of proximal and distal augmentation maneuvers with Doppler spectral waveform analysis.[19] The cephalic vein insertion should also be evaluated at this stage of the examination, since it usually enters the subclavian vein proximal to the shoulder; this can vary in location, however.

Have the patient turn his or her head slightly away from the side being examined, then evaluate the internal jugular vein by placing the transducer on the neck just medial to the sternocleidomastoid muscle, aiming straight down (Fig. 21-66). Angling caudally into the supraclavicular area shows the proximal portion of the jugular vein; in most cases, its insertion into the brachiocephalic vein can also be visualized. Evaluate both the cervical and proximal seg-

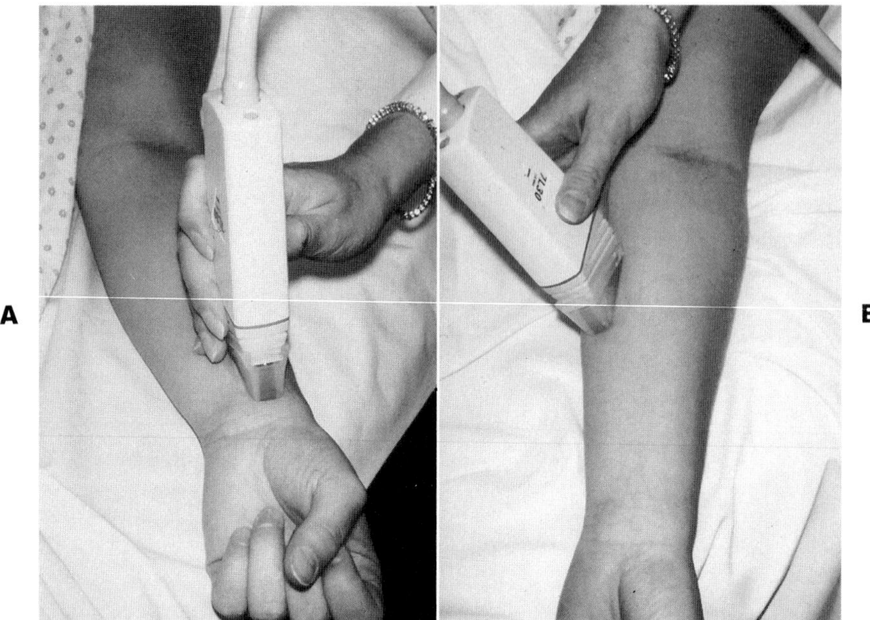

FIG. 21-61 A, Longitudinal duplex scanning position for the radial vein. **B,** Longitudinal duplex scanning position for the ulnar vein.

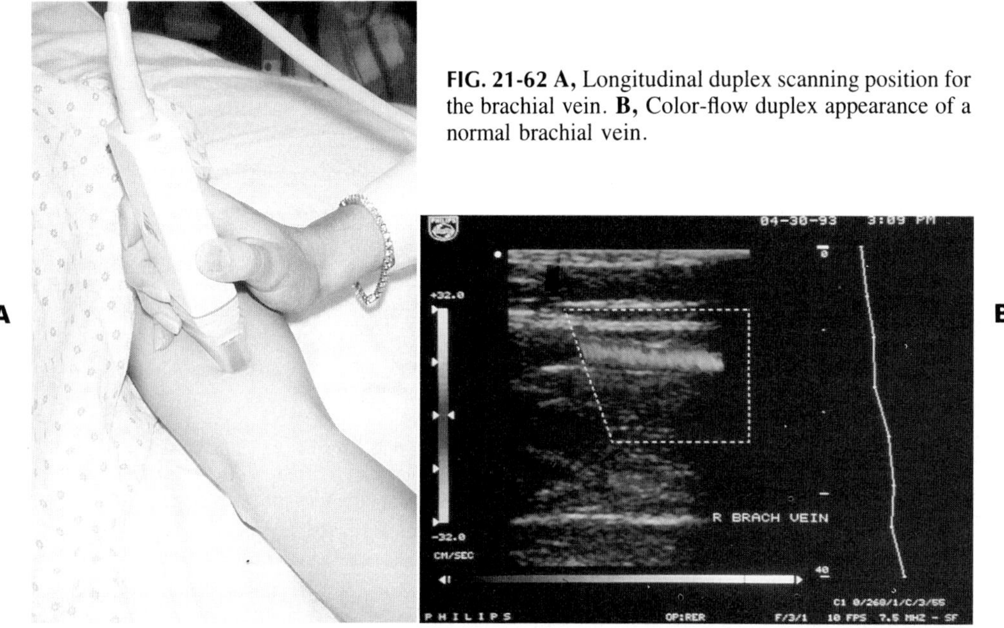

FIG. 21-62 A, Longitudinal duplex scanning position for the brachial vein. **B,** Color-flow duplex appearance of a normal brachial vein.

ments of the vein, compressing lightly in both longitudinal and transverse planes (Fig. 21-67; see color images). Color-flow and Doppler spectral waveforms again should be used to evaluate the flow characteristics, although thrombosis in this area is usually quite striking when it is present (see Case 3, Fig. 21-70). A proximal augmentation maneuver (Valsalva) can be performed and may provide additional flow information, especially if the vein does not dilate with flow decrease (the normal response) during the Valsalva maneuver.

The superficial veins can be either imaged separately at this point or included during the deep imaging of the arm veins. The cephalic vein is best evaluated by starting at its insertion into the axillary vein and progressing distally along the lateral arm. The basilic vein can be followed from its insertion at the basilobrachial junction distally and me-

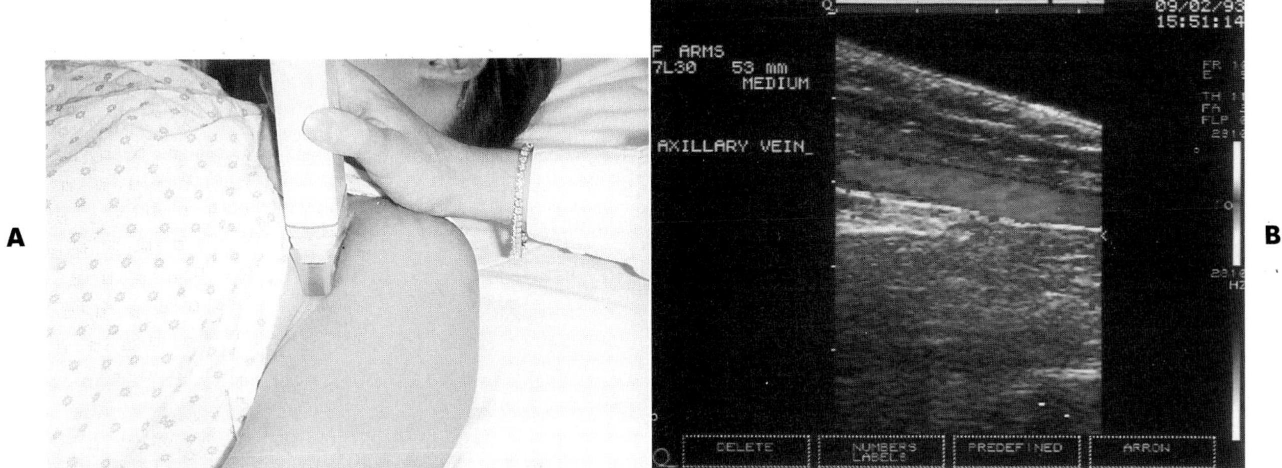

FIG. 21-63 A, Longitudinal duplex scanning position for the axillary vein. **B,** Color-flow duplex appearance of a normal axillary vein.

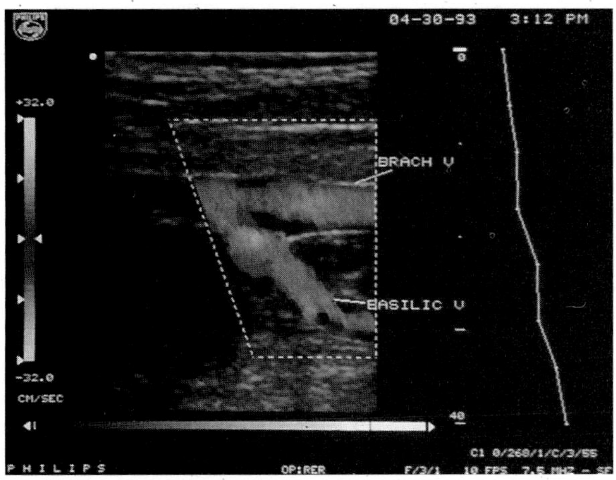

FIG. 21-64 Color-flow duplex appearance of the brachial–basilic vein junction with the normal axillary vein.

dially. These veins are extremely superficial, so a very light touch and ample coupling gel are required. Scan in longitudinal and transverse planes, compressing as you go, evaluating patency with color flow and obtaining Doppler spectral signals when necessary.

Interpretation of the Upper-Extremity Venous Duplex Examination

Normal upper-extremity venous findings

The criteria for determining the appearance of normal upper-extremity veins are virtually identical to those for lower-extremity veins, except there are fewer valves and no perforating veins. To summarize and review:

1. Normal veins are widely patent, and the walls readily coapt if compressed with the transducer.
2. Valves, when seen, are competent and thin. No reflux is apparent during augmentation maneuvers.
3. Doppler and color-flow patterns are spontaneous with normal phasic flow changes; some pulsatility is considered normal.
4. Color-flow patterns fill the visible lumen, with no filling defects or evidence of focal acceleration.

ABNORMAL UPPER-EXTREMITY VENOUS FINDINGS

The criteria for determining whether thrombus is present in upper-extremity veins are virtually identical to those for lower-extremity veins:

1. Veins with walls that do not meet under transducer compression may have thrombus of either a partially or totally obstructive nature. Thrombus appears as echogenic material within the lumen. The echogenicity increases proportionally to the age of the thrombus, the vein is dilated distal to the thrombus (usually in acute cases), and Doppler flow patterns may be continuous or of elevated velocity.
2. Color-flow patterns may be absent in occluded segments, appear in patent segments distal to an obstruction only during augmentation compression, or indicate recanalized channels through thrombus.

Technical Factor Comments. Carefully adjust the time-gain compensation and slope as well as the near and far gain and contrast controls to give the best image possible, free of artifact and reverberation. This is important, since inadequate gain settings prevent visualization of acute thrombus, and overcompensated gain creates artifacts that may be misinterpreted as thrombus, especially if a vein proves difficult to compress because of improper technique. Remember, the ideal setting allows the intimal linings to be distinctly seen, and there are some faint specular echoes of moving blood in the veins. When color flow is used, low flow-velocity thresholds and baseline shifting should be used to best show the range of velocities in the veins

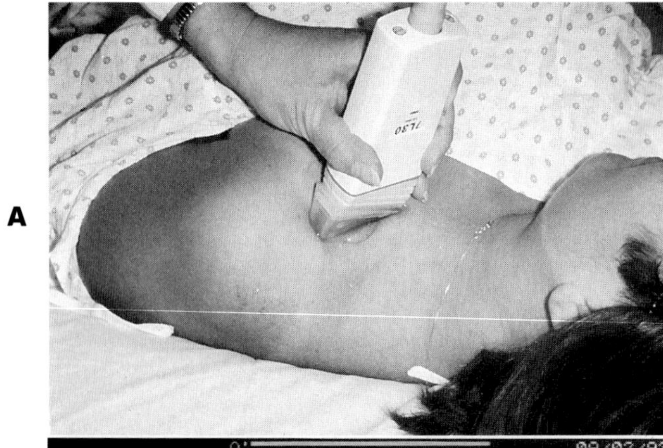

FIG. 21-65 A, Longitudinal duplex scanning position for the subclavian vein. **B,** Color-flow duplex appearance of a normal subclavian vein in the longitudinal plane. **C,** Color-flow duplex appearance of a normal subclavian vein in the transverse plane.

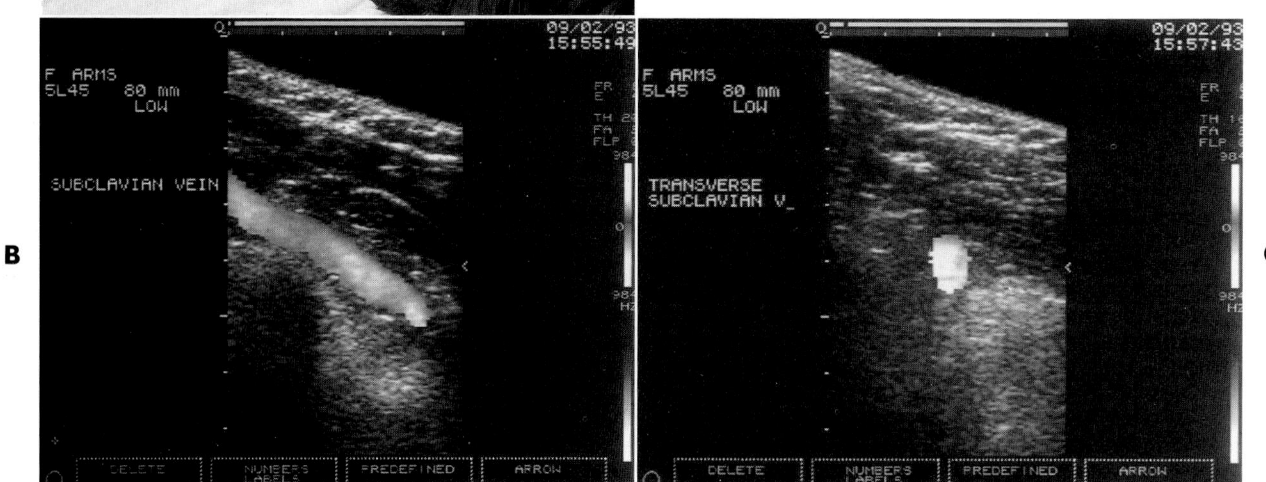

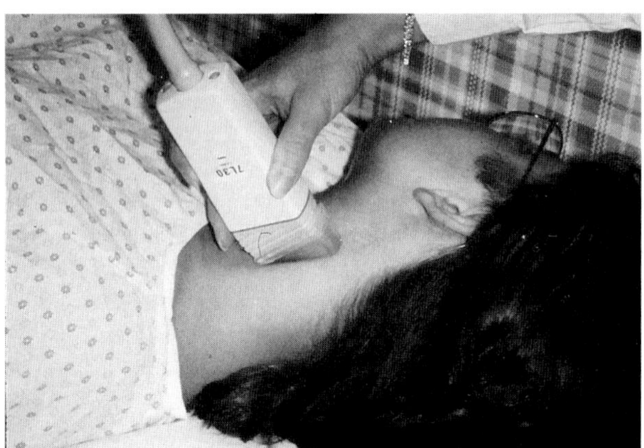

FIG. 21-66 Longitudinal duplex scanning position for the internal jugular vein.

without oversaturation or "bleeding" of the color outside of the true lumen. If velocities are increased along different segments, the color thresholds should be adjusted as needed.

Again, thrombus is classified as acute or chronic as previously discussed on page 907. Some recent evaluations of upper-extremity veins have shown relative accuracies of 85% with specificities of 90%.[19]

Upper-Extremity Venous Duplex Sonography Cases

Case 1 (Fig. 21-68): subclavian, axillary, proximal brachial vein thrombosis—chronic

This 49-year-old patient had a venographically documented venous stricture of the right subclavian vein, which was causing swelling and discoloration of the right arm and which was subsequently dilated by an intravenous balloon angioplasty procedure. There was initial relief, but 4 hours after the percutaneous transluminal angioplasty (PTA), the patient's symptoms returned with more pain and increased swelling. The patient was examined 1 week after the PTA.

Evaluation of the right distal brachial vein showed a patent vein with spontaneous but continuous flow and poor augmentation response to proximal and distal compression (Fig. 21-68, *A*; see color image). The proximal brachial vein was thrombosed with evidence of collateral flow (Fig. 21-68, *B*; see color image), and the thrombus extended into the axillary (Fig. 21-68, *C*; see color image) and subclavian (Fig. 21-68, *D*; see color image) veins, which were occupied with chronic-appearing incompressible thrombus. Evaluation of the internal jugular vein showed a patent, easily compressible vein with no evidence of thrombus within it nor was there extension of the subclavian thrombus into its origin (Fig. 21-68, *E*; see color image).

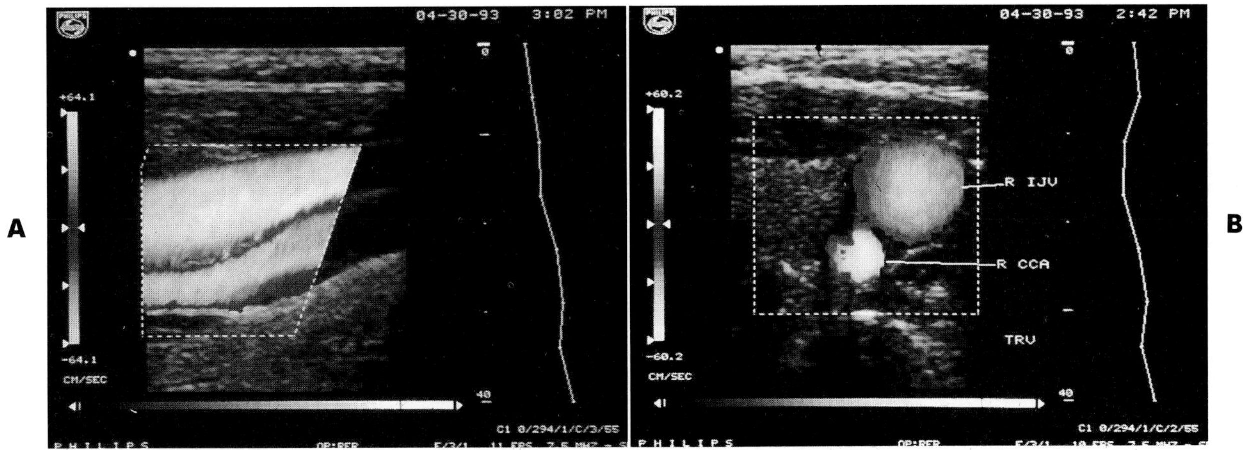

FIG. 21-67 A, Color-flow duplex appearance of a normal internal jugular vein with the internal carotid artery and carotid bulb seen deep to it in the longitudinal plane. **B,** Transverse view of the same internal jugular vein, taken somewhat more proximally with the common carotid deep and medial to it.

Case 2 (Fig. 21-69): subclavian, axillary, brachial thrombosis—chronic with collateral reconstitution

This 62-year-old patient had a history of lymphedema and a subacute segmental occlusion of the subclavian and axillary veins and was evaluated to determine whether her arm swelling was lymphedemic or venous in etiology.

The patient had diminished flow in the patent distal brachial vein (Fig. 21-69, *A*; see color image) with chronic thrombosis of the proximal brachial, axillary (Fig. 21-69, *B*), and subclavian (Fig. 21-69, *C*; see color image) veins. Despite this, a very active network of parallel collaterals with decreased phasicity drained the arm and shoulder (Fig. 21-69, *D*; see color image), with flow emptying into the subclavian vein (Fig. 21-69, *E*; see color image) proximal to the thrombus.

The flow patterns within the secondary collateral system could be considered normal (Fig. 21-69, *F*), pointing out the need for duplex examination; a continuous-wave Doppler examination without imaging would probably have missed the presence of the chronic thrombosis.

Case 3 (Fig. 21-70): brachial, axillary, subclavian, and internal jugular vein thrombosis—acute

This 63-year-old patient had a supraclavicular intravenous line in place during a recent hospital stay, developing swelling over the entire left shoulder and neck within 3 days after its removal. The patient was examined to rule out a subclavian vein thrombosis.

The distal brachial vein was patent (Fig. 21-70, *A*) but had low-velocity continuous flow (Fig. 21-70, *B*); the proximal brachial (Fig. 21-70, *C*), axillary (Fig. 21-70, *D*), and subclavian (Fig. 21-70, *E*) veins were seen to be completely filled with acute-appearing thrombus. Some accompanying early collaterals could be seen that had continuous flow. Examination of the internal jugular vein showed thrombus in the proximal (Fig. 21-70, *F*; see color image) and middle segments (Fig. 21-70, *G*; see color image) of the vessel with a patent segment distally and flow being shunted to superficial collaterals in the neck.

The patient was readmitted to the hospital for heparinization.

Case 4 (Fig. 21-71): partial residual subclavian and basilic vein thrombosis after anticoagulation

This 18-year-old patient was a baseball pitcher who had developed a subclavian, axillary, and basilic vein thrombosis; these images were from a follow-up examination about 1 month after treatment. The patient had some residual discomfort in the arm.

The right upper-extremity veins all appeared patent; there was some residual thrombus seen along the superficial wall of the basilic vein (Fig. 21-71, *A*; see color image), which was confirmed in transverse imaging because it did not allow the walls to meet on compression (Fig. 21-71, *B*; see color image).

Some residual thrombus was seen along the wall of the subclavian vein (Fig. 21-71, *C*; see color image), which appeared to be asymmetric in the transverse plane (Fig. 21-71, *D*; see color image).

The patient had no further subsequent complaints.

Case 5 (Fig. 21-72): patent deep system, superficial phlebitis, and thrombosis of cephalic vein

This 26-year-old patient was 3 weeks postpartum and had been on extensive intravenous medications through the left arm because of problems with the fetus. About 4 days before being evaluated, she developed progressive pain along the entire lateral surface of the arm up into the shoulder. A prominent red streak was present on the skin along the lateral forearm and arm from the wrist to the axilla. The lateral surface of the arm was very tender and a palpable cord was present beneath the red streak. The patient had difficulty moving the arm and there was concern of superficial

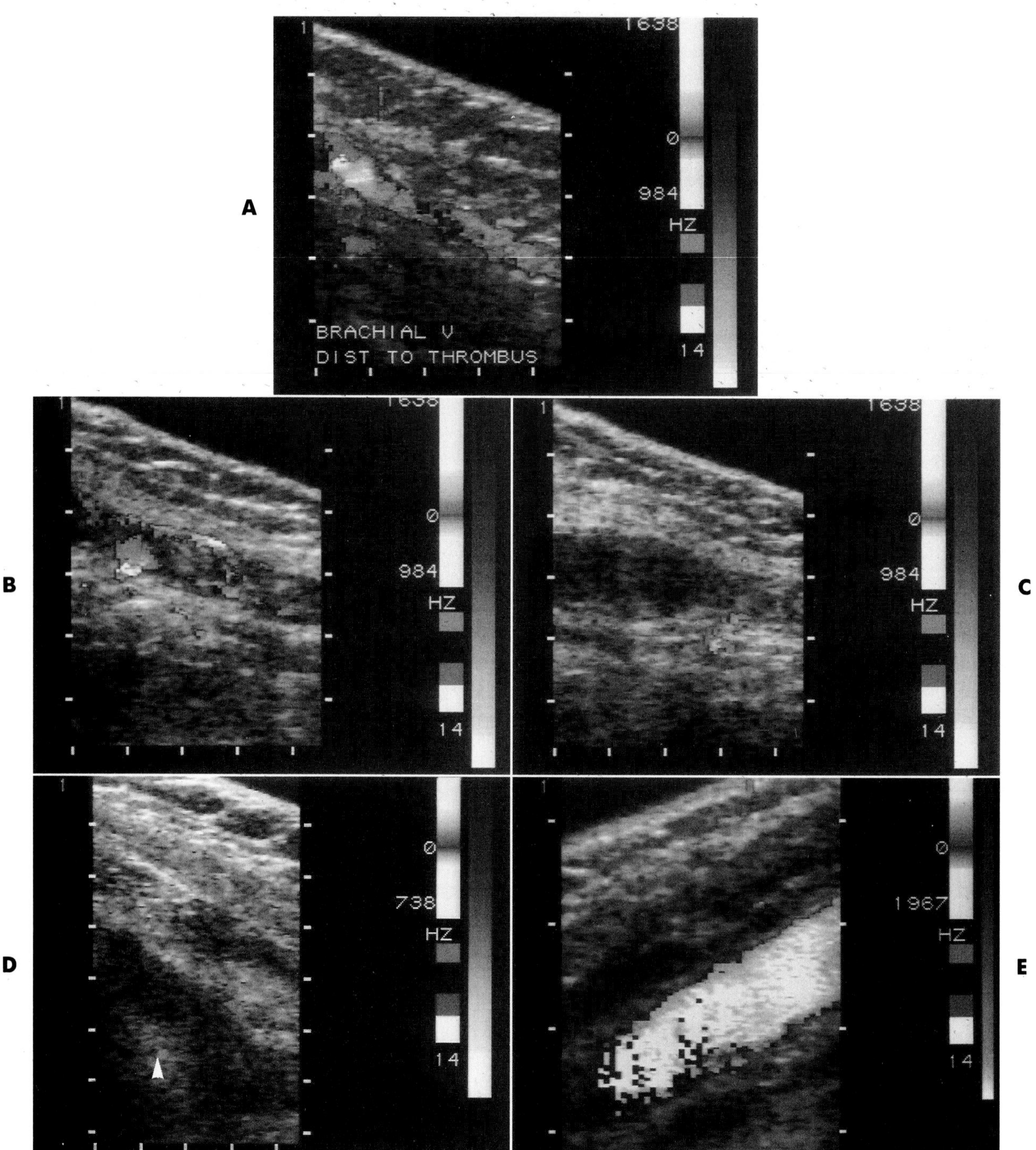

FIG. 21-68 A, Poorly augmenting patent distal brachial vein. Note edge of thrombus to left (see text). **B,** Thrombosed proximal brachial vein with collaterals (see text). **C,** Thrombosed axillary vein. **D,** Thrombosed subclavian vein (see text). **E,** Patent internal jugular vein.

phlebitis, which might have propagated into the deep veins.

Duplex examination of the brachial (Fig. 21-72, *A*; see color image), axillary (Fig. 21-72, *B*; see color image), and subclavian (Fig. 21-72, *C*; see color image) veins showed normal veins, which had normal color-flow patterns, normal compressibility, and no evidence of thrombus. The internal jugular vein was normal (Fig. 21-72, *D*; see color image). The basilic vein along the medial upper arm was also normal to its junction with the axillary vein.

The cephalic vein was completely thrombosed from the wrist level to the antecubital fossa in the forearm (Fig. 21-72, *E*; see color image); just above the antecubital fossa, the cephalic vein had a long segmental partial

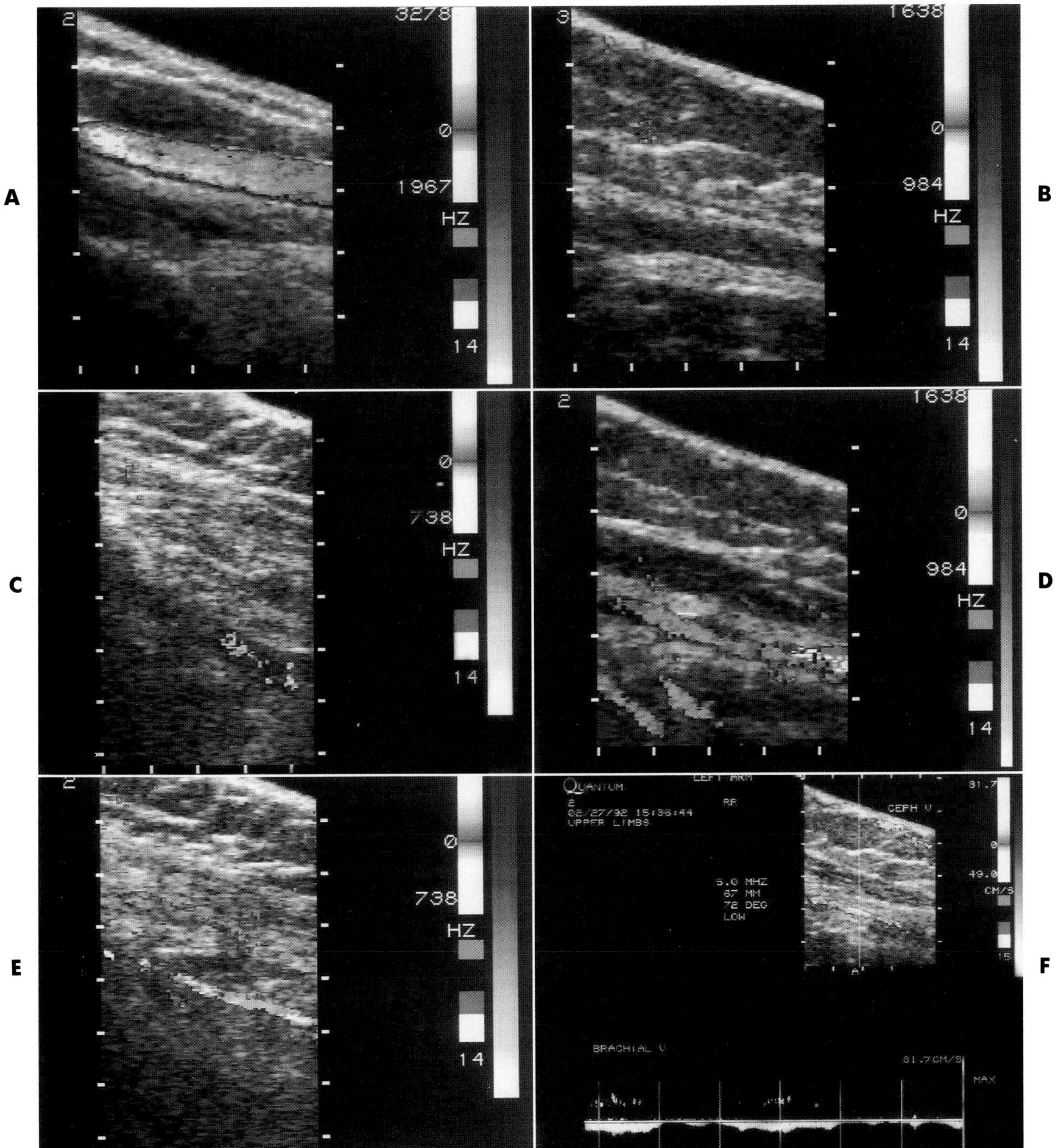

FIG. 21-69 A, Patent distal brachial vein. **B,** Thrombosed axillary vein. **C,** Thrombosed and partly recanalized subclavian vein. **D,** Active collaterals in axilla (note thrombosed axillary vein above collaterals). **E,** Patent active collateral paralleling subclavian vein. **F,** Doppler spectral signal from a collateral paralleling the brachial vein—note phasicity.

thrombosis, which allowed only partial compression of the cephalic vein (Fig. 21-72, *F*; see color image). The cephalic vein was otherwise patent and normally compressible from the midpoint of the upper arm to the cephaloaxillary junction.

The patient was treated with oral anticoagulation and antibiotics.

OTHER NONINVASIVE VENOUS TESTING

Although venous duplex sonography is considered the most important diagnostic modality in the noninvasive vascular laboratory, other methods are used to supplement duplex imaging and the use of Doppler. As stated and as specified by the Intersocietal Commission for the Accreditation

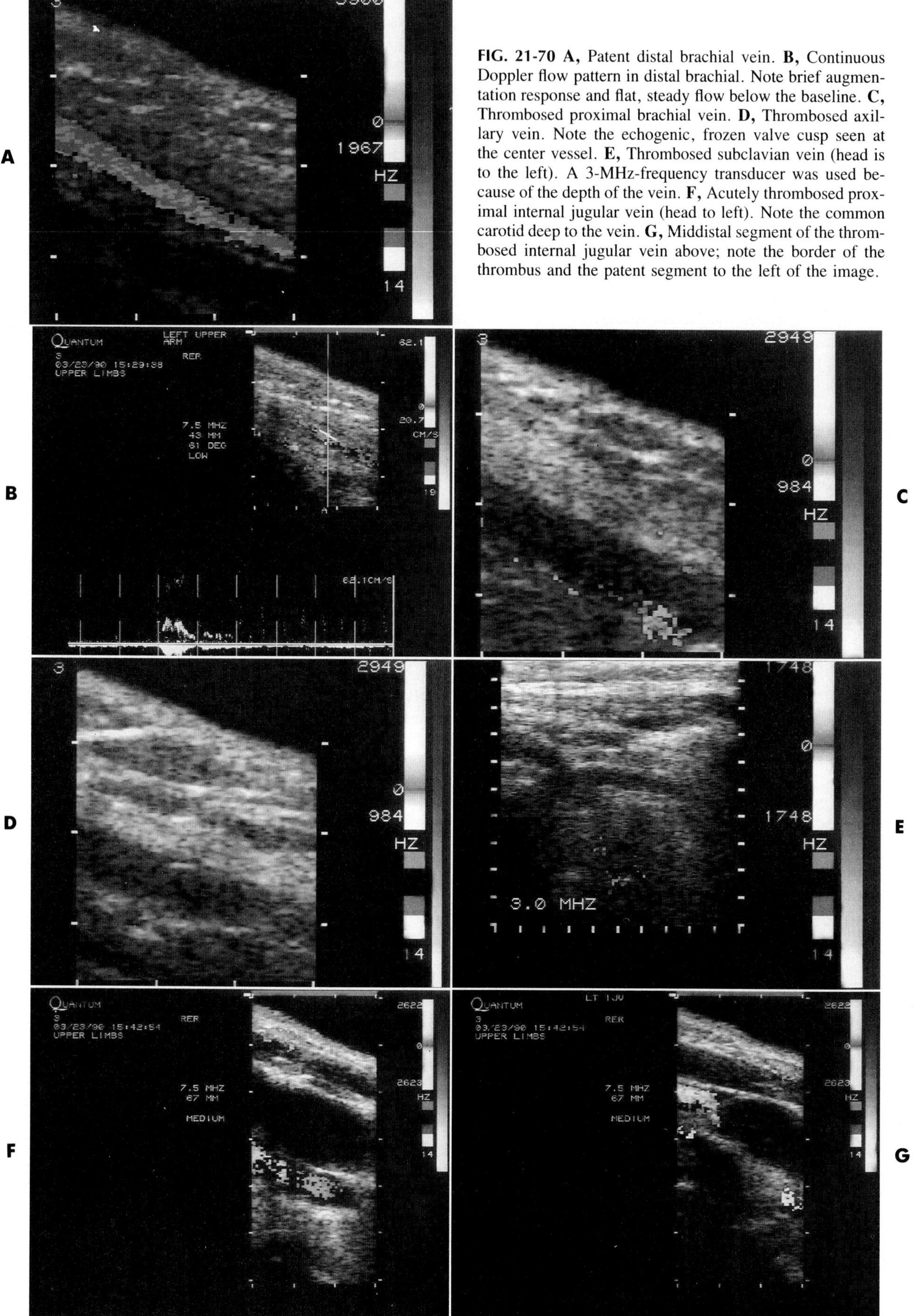

FIG. 21-70 A, Patent distal brachial vein. **B,** Continuous Doppler flow pattern in distal brachial. Note brief augmentation response and flat, steady flow below the baseline. **C,** Thrombosed proximal brachial vein. **D,** Thrombosed axillary vein. Note the echogenic, frozen valve cusp seen at the center vessel. **E,** Thrombosed subclavian vein (head is to the left). A 3-MHz-frequency transducer was used because of the depth of the vein. **F,** Acutely thrombosed proximal internal jugular vein (head to left). Note the common carotid deep to the vein. **G,** Middistal segment of the thrombosed internal jugular vein above; note the border of the thrombus and the patent segment to the left of the image.

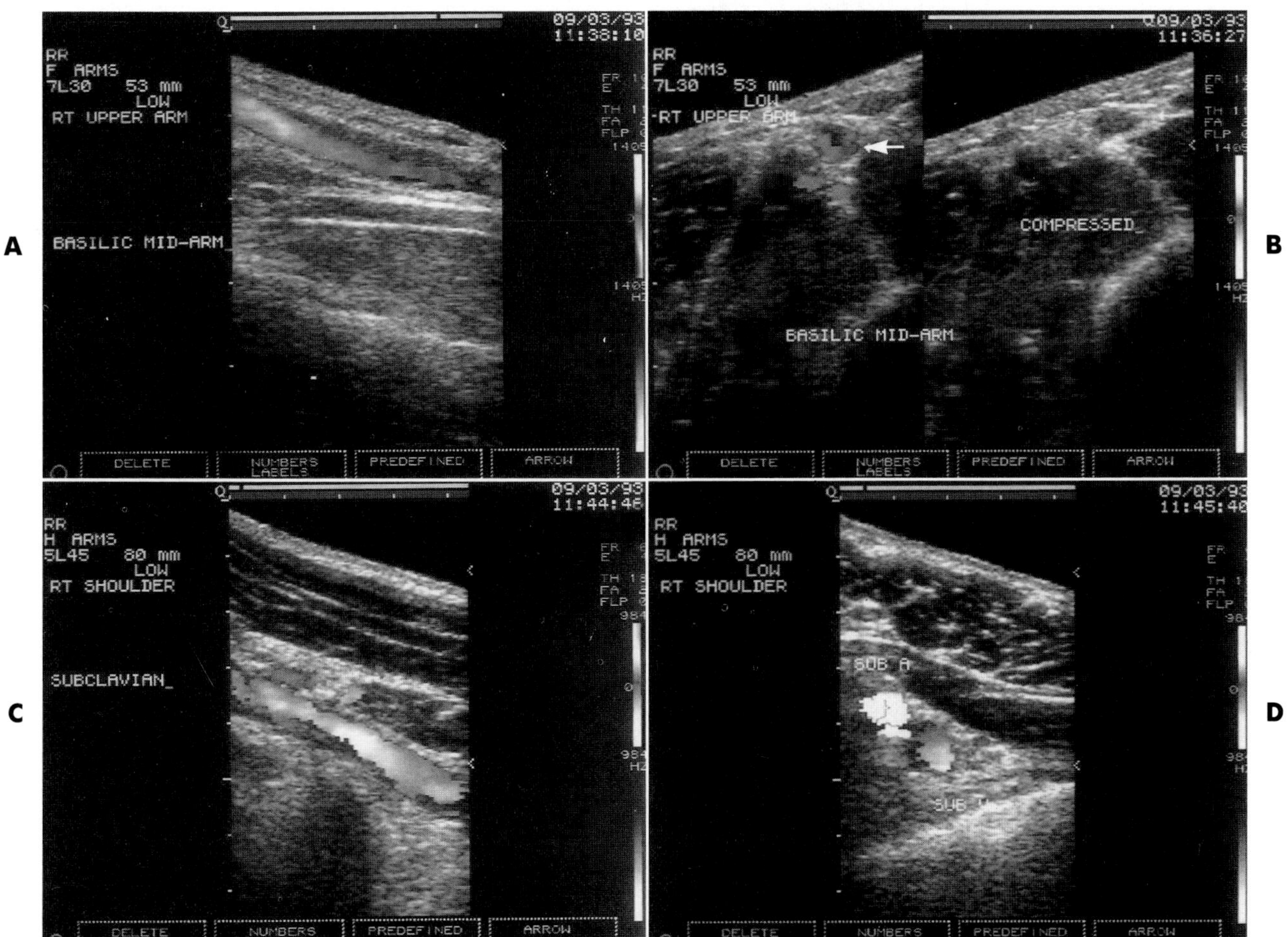

FIG. 21-71 A, Longitudinal view of basilic vein with nonobstructive partial thrombus on superficial wall. **B,** Transverse views of the above partially thrombosed basilic vein *(arrow),* before *(left),* and after *(right)* transducer compression. Note that the vein does not flatten because of the presence of the thrombus. **C,** Subclavian vein with nonobstructive partial thrombus on deep wall. **D,** Transverse view of the subclavian vein in **C.** Note the relationship of the subclavian artery (head is to left of image).

of Vascular Laboratories (ICAVL), these methods should not be used alone to diagnose deep-vein thrombosis.

VENOUS PLETHYSMOGRAPHY

Plethysmographic techniques can be used to measure limb volume changes that reflect venous filling and emptying rates in response to cuff occlusion. Several venous plethysmographic techniques and their applications are discussed in the following sections.

Phleborheography[12]

Phleborheography was initially developed by Cranley and was an outgrowth of a research polygraph; its basic principles involve comparisons of volume changes in the legs being examined with respiratory changes recorded by a pneumatic cuff placed around the chest. Respiratory waves (which correspond to phasic flow changes in the Doppler examination) are reduced or eliminated in extremities with deep-vein thrombosis (this corresponds to the continuous flow or reduced phasicity also detected with Doppler). Compression is applied through cuffs at the foot and calf to determine whether volume increases occur that are consistent with an outflow obstruction.

The test is performed with a patient lying supine and at rest in a bed with the thorax elevated 10 degrees. One cuff is placed around the chest, another at midthigh, three cuffs are closely spaced on the upper, mid, and distal calf, and a sixth cuff is on the foot. Three runs, or recordings, are made, each in a different mode.

In the A run, all cuffs are inflated to a sensing pressure of 10 mm Hg, the device recorder is calibrated, and respiratory waves are observed. The operator then activates the compress control and the device gives three bursts of 100 mm Hg pressure at half-second intervals. Baselines in normal extremities remain level, but in outflow obstruction the

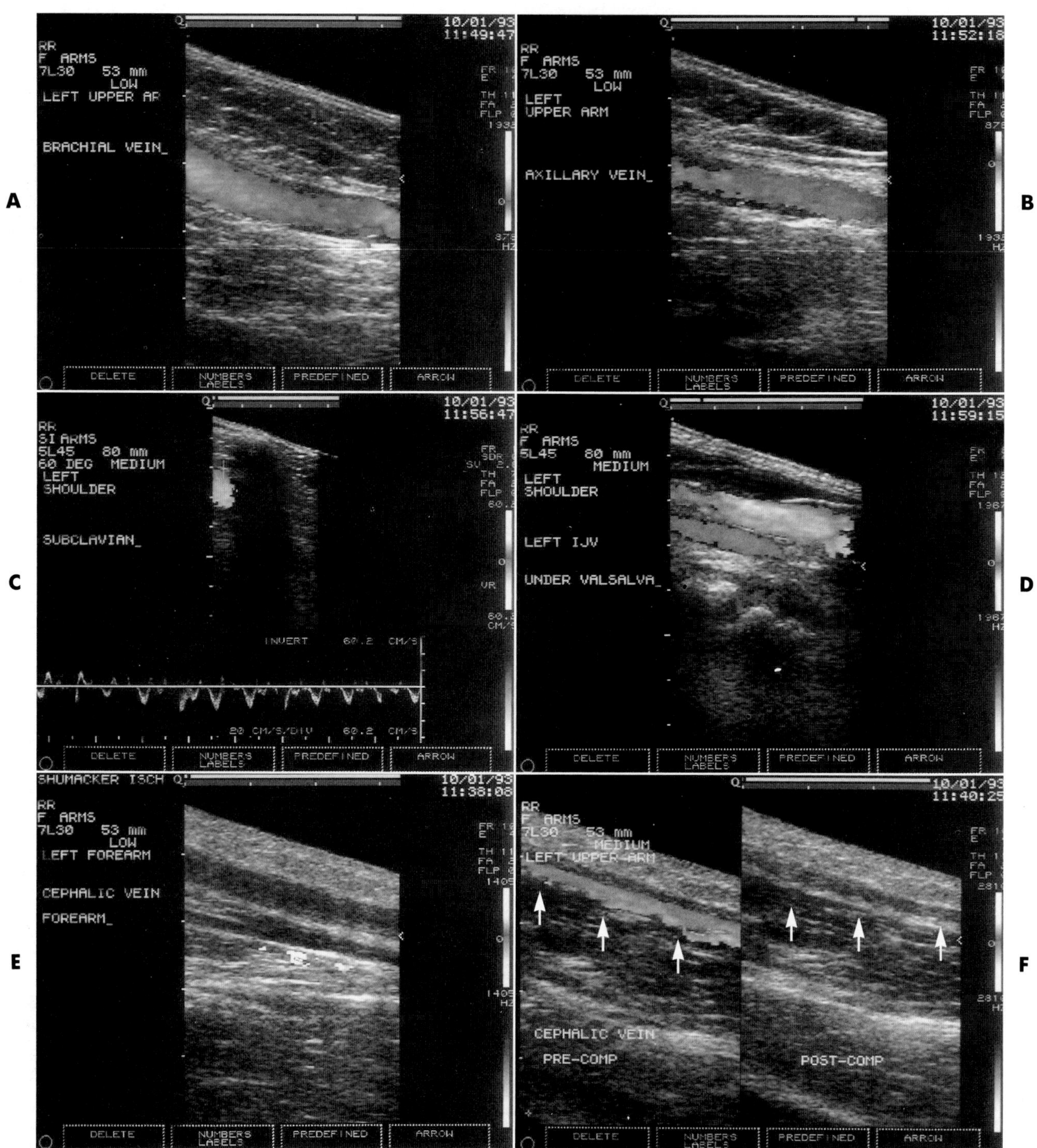

FIG. 21-72 A, Normal, patent brachial vein. **B,** Normal, patent axillary vein. **C,** Normal, patent subclavian vein (partly obscured by clavicle), showing a normal slightly pulsatile subclavian venous signal. **D,** Normal, patent internal jugular vein. **E,** Thrombosed cephalic vein in forearm. **F,** Partially thrombosed cephalic vein in upper arm, showing incomplete compressibility.

baseline rises with each compression as the volume increases. The procedure is usually repeated three times with 20 seconds between cycles allowed for venous refill.

In the B_1 run the foot cuff is placed back in a recording mode and the distal calf cuff compresses three times at 50 mm Hg. Again, the test is repeated three times, with foot emptying monitored. A rise in the baseline with each compression will be seen if outflow obstruction is present.

In the B_2 run the distal calf cuff is moved to the ankle level and compressed three times at 50 mm Hg. The run is repeated three times with foot emptying monitored. A rise in the baseline with each compression is seen if outflow ob-

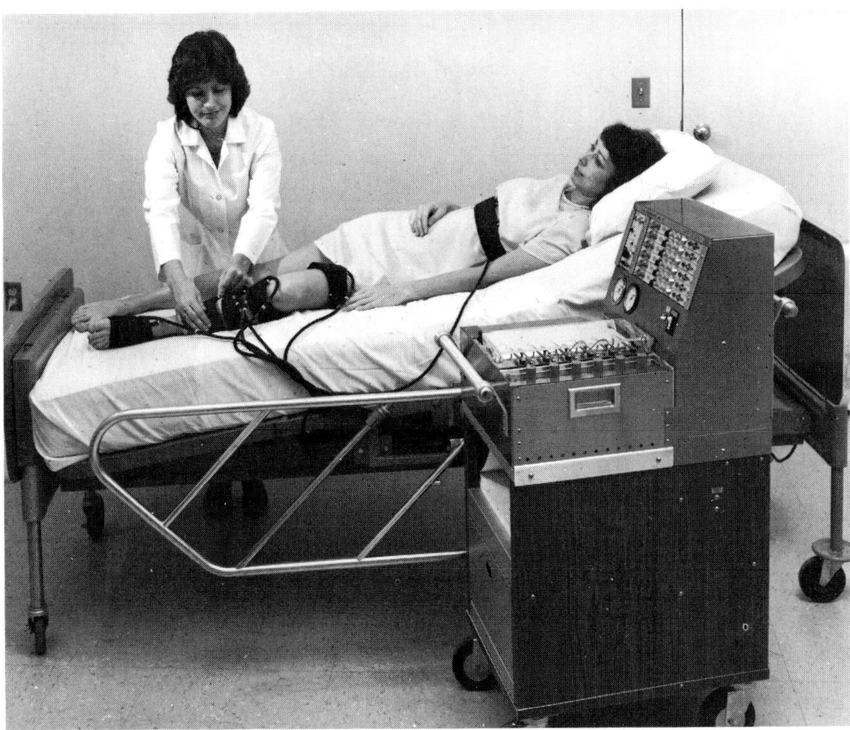

FIG. 21-73 In preparation for phleborheography of the lower extremities the patient lies quietly with the legs below heart level and six cuffs applied. (From Bernstein EB: Vascular diagnosis, ed 4. St. Louis, 1993, Mosby.)

struction is present, and foot emptying may be reduced or absent.

To summarize, a total of three runs and nine compressions (three each in runs A, B_1, and B_2) are required. The following are criteria for a normal study:

1. Normal respiratory wave amplitude averaging 50% or more of the amplitude of waves in the opposite extremity;
2. No absolute baseline rise; and
3. No dynamic baseline rise during compression.

A phleborheograph and proper positioning are illustrated in Fig. 21-73 and normal and abnormal runs are illustrated respectively in Figs. 21-74 and 21-75.

Discussion

Phleborheography equipment is no longer available and the procedure has been supplanted in many modern laboratories by venous duplex sonographic techniques. It has been quoted as having overall accuracies ranging from 59% to 96%, with the most believable statistics (from the largest series) coming in at about 92%.[12] It is mentioned here primarily as a historic note but also because it is mentioned as a secondary test in the ICAVL Essentials and Standards and because the technique still might be encountered in some laboratories.

Venous Outflow and Venous Capacitance[11,24]

Venous outflow and venous capacitance (VO/VC) can be performed using numerous plethysmographic methods; impedance plethysmography (IPG) using electrodes, strain gauges (SPG), or air-filled sensing cuffs (VPR) on the calf.

This test compares the rate of venous outflow as a volume change (i.e., calf emptying) against the maximum venous capacitance (i.e., the maximum amount of venous blood the leg veins can hold); outflow rates decrease if the proximal veins are thrombosed or obstructed.

This test is very operator-dependent and requires following the techniques to the letter to avoid errors.

The patient first lies supine for 15 minutes, then the leg being examined is elevated using foam positioning blocks or supports to a level about 27 cm above the patient's back. The leg is bent and rotated slightly laterally. A large tapered cuff is placed snugly around the patient's thigh and the capacitance electrodes, strain gauge (2 to 3 cm smaller than the circumference of the patient's calf), or VPR venous sensing cuff is placed around the widest part of the calf (Fig. 21-76). (If a sensing cuff is used, it should be inflated to 20 mm Hg for pressure-wave measurement). The plethysmograph is set to the DC mode, and the chart recorder scale is balanced so that the tracing is near the bottom of the graph and calibrated so that 10 mm on the chart is equal to 1% capacitance (if a strain gauge is used).

The thigh cuff is connected to a cuff inflator, and then the cuff is inflated to 50 mm Hg, held for 45 seconds, and released. Then 2 minutes is allowed for a resting period and the procedure is repeated. This is to increase venous tone before actually performing a measurement.

The chart is then started at a slow speed (1 mm/sec), and

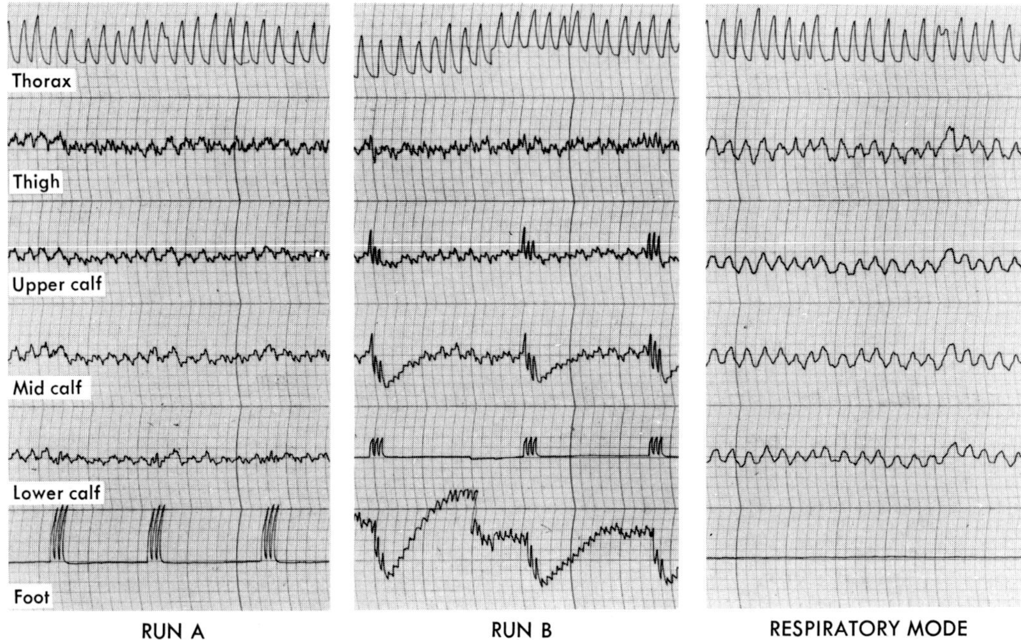

FIG. 21-74 Normal tracing. There are good respiratory waves throughout run A (foot cuff used as a compression cuff) and run B (lower calf cuff used as a compression cuff). Note the absence of a baseline shift when either the foot or lower cuff is compressed. Note also the good foot emptying in run B. The respiratory mode shows good respiratory waves after the arterial pulses have been filtered. (From Bernstein EB: Vascular diagnosis, ed 4. St. Louis, 1993, Mosby.)

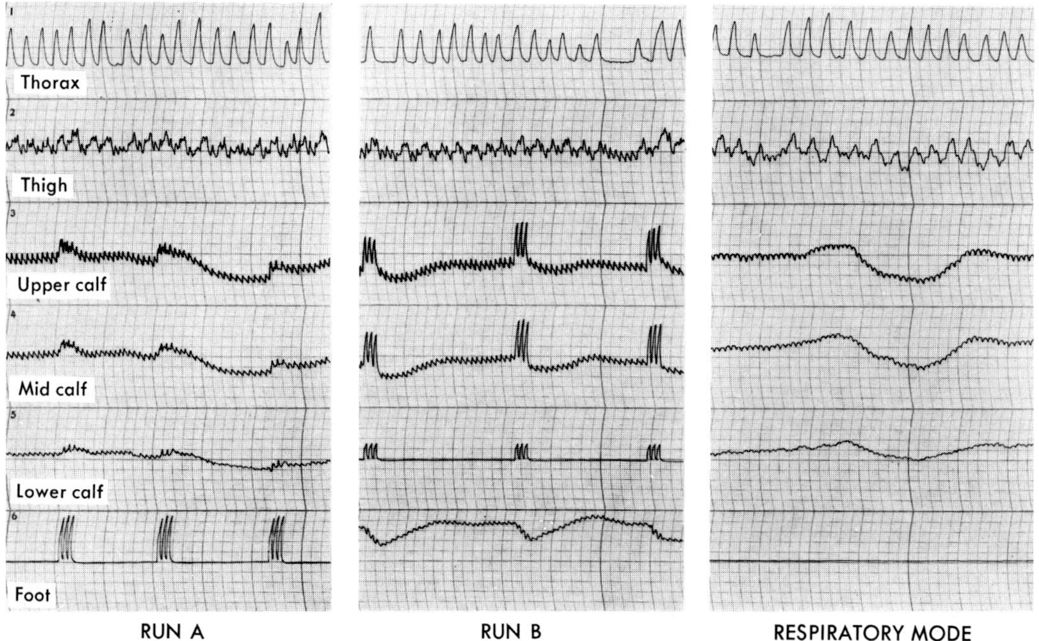

FIG. 21-75 Acute popliteal thrombosis. Note the normal respiratory waves and the absence of any baseline rise in the thigh; however, there is obliteration of the respiratory waves in the calf and baseline evaluation secondary to the foot (run A) and calf (run B) compression, indicating deep venous obstruction. Note the total absence of respiratory waves distal to the thigh on the respiratory mode trace, indicating deep venous obstruction at the popliteal level. (From Bernstein EB: Vascular diagnosis, ed 4. St. Louis, 1993, Mosby.)

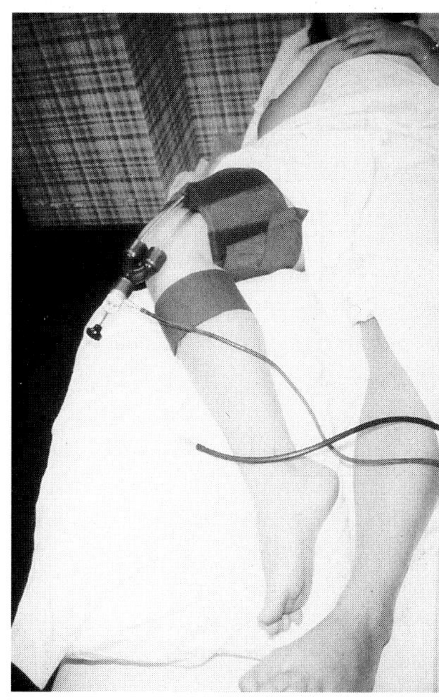

FIG. 21-76 Cuff placement and leg positioning for VC/VO examination using the VPR method.

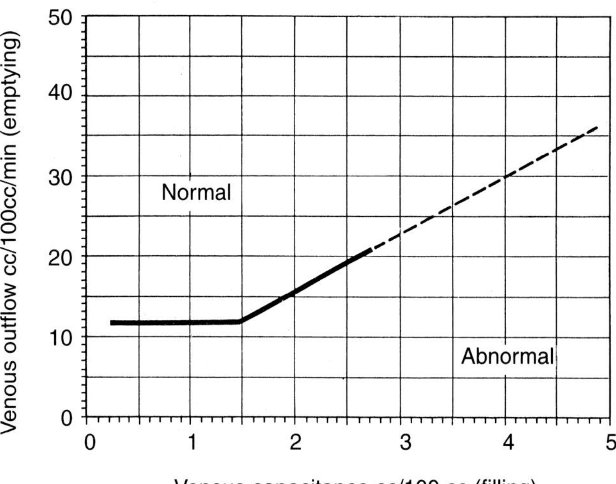

FIG. 21-77 Discriminant line chart for plotting VC/VO values from the strain-gauge plethysmography method. (Modified from Cramer M, Beach KW, and Strandness DE, Bruit 7:17, Dec. 1983; Courtesy DE Hokanson.)

the thigh cuff is again inflated to 50 mm Hg, occluding venous outflow. The tracing rises as the calf volume fills and plateaus (flattens) after about 2 minutes; this marks the point of maximum venous capacitance.

The chart speed is then set to 25 mm/sec and the thigh cuff pressure is rapidly released. The chart tracing drops, curving downward. This curve represents the venous outflow.

Interpretation

Interpreting VO/VC studies requires calculating the percentage of volume change using calipers and the millimeter divisions on the strip chart recording. Interpretive techniques are similar but the resulting calculations are often different for the VPR, strain-gauge, and impedance methods. In general the rise (capacitance) is measured in millimeters from the baseline to the highest sustained level (the plateau); outflow is measured in millimeters from the point of cuff pressure release to a point 2 or 3 seconds (depending on the criteria used) after release.

For air plethysmography (VPR), the venous outflow in millimeters (VO) is divided by the venous capacity in millimeters (VC) from the baseline, taken at 2 seconds. The result is the maximum venous outflow at 2 seconds (MVO2);

$$\text{MVO2} = \text{VO/VC}$$

Normal studies have a value of 0.80 or more at 2 seconds. If the results are equivocal, the same calculations can be performed at 3 seconds.

For IPG, the impedance change related to volume change is indicated as a baseline shift on the chart tracing but is interpreted in a similar fashion as for VPR.

For strain-gauge plethysmography, outflow is calculated in milliliters per minute by dividing the outflow in millimeters at 1 second by 60. This outflow value is then divided by the height in millimeters of the calibration marker (generally 10 mm = 1% volume), which then equals milliliters outflow per milliliter tissue per minute. Outflow exceeding 20 milliliters per 100 ml/min is considered normal. A discriminant line chart can also be used, where the percentage volume change and outflow can be calculated via a preprinted transparent overlay placed over the chart tracings and the capacitance and outflow plotted on the chart; points above the line are considered normal and points below the line are considered abnormal (Fig. 21-77). Whenever values are equivocal or abnormal, the test should be repeated at least twice.[11,24]

This study, besides being time-consuming, is also very dependent on precise patient positioning, gauge or electrode positioning, absence of chronic reflux, and the absence of collateral flow. Problems with any of the above can result in an inaccurate examination. Because of these sensitivities it has been better at detecting acute thrombosis but has little effectiveness in cases of chronic obstruction or insufficiency. It has been replaced in many laboratories by duplex imaging and Doppler. If it is performed at all, it is best done in conjunction with a duplex examination, since chronic venous problems that can affect the VO/VC results are detected by imaging. An example of a normal VO/VC study (three repetitions) is shown in Fig. 21-78.

Air Plethysmography (APG)[7,16]

In 1987, Christopoulos and Nicolaides developed a new technique of air plethysmography that uses a 5-liter-

MVO-SVC (VPR)

A

	Right #1	Right #2	Right #3	Left #1	Left #2	Left #3
SVC (mm):	25	28	26			
1 Sec Outflow (mm):	17	23	22			
2 Sec Outflow (mm):	20	26	25			
3 Sec Outflow (mm):	20	27	26			
50% Drop Time (sec):	>0.4	0.34	0.33			
80% Drop Time (sec):	>0.9	0.95	0.77			
Drop 1 Sec (%):	68	82	85			
Drop 2 Sec (%):	80	93	96			
Drop 3 Sec (%):	80	96	100			

B

MVO-SVC (VPR)

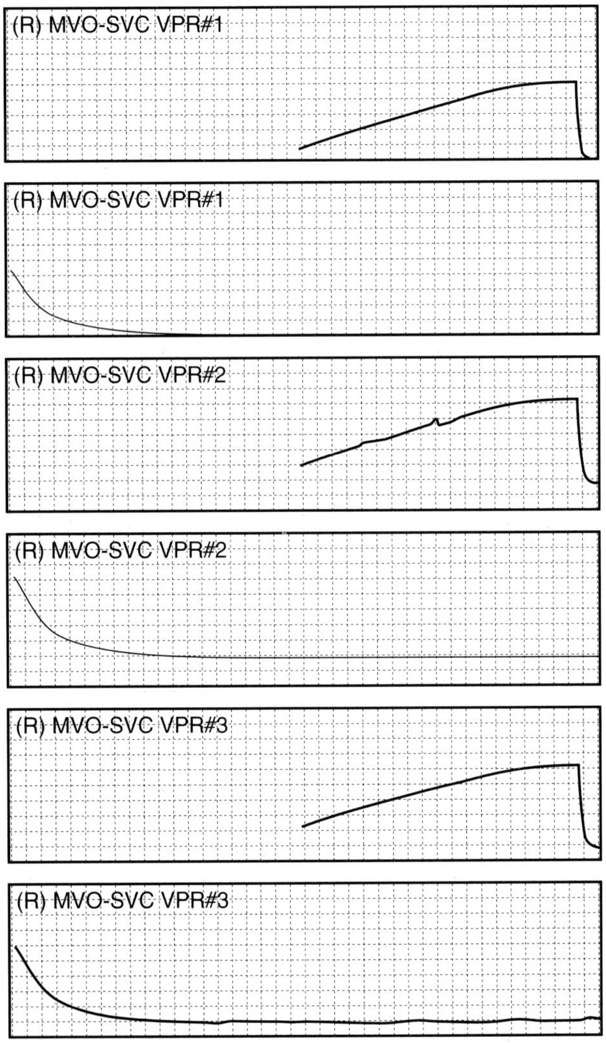

(R) MVO-SVC VPR#1

(R) MVO-SVC VPR#1

(R) MVO-SVC VPR#2

(R) MVO-SVC VPR#2

(R) MVO-SVC VPR#3

(R) MVO-SVC VPR#3

FIG. 21-78 A, VC/VO study, normal numeric values. There are three sets of data from three repetitions of the test. **B,** VC/VO study, capacitance (rising slope) and outflow (descending slope) chart recordings from the three test repetitions shown in **(A).** See text for diagnostic criteria.

capacity cuff that encloses the entire lower leg from knee to ankle. It is connected to a pressure transducer, amplifier, and chart recorder or computer interface. Before examining the patient, the cuff is placed around the limb with the patient in a supine position and is inflated to a pressure of 6 mm Hg (which secures it and enables contact with the leg surfaces). It is then calibrated by infusing 100 ml of air from a calibration syringe. The 0- and 100-ml volume values are stored in the plethysmograph and are used as a calibration reference corresponding to pen deflection ranges on the chart recorder, which run at 6 mm/sec.

The examination begins by having the supine patient rotate the leg being examined laterally with a slight knee flexion, with the heel raised or supported to keep the cuff raised off the surface of the exam table. After a 5-minute rest period to stabilize all temperature and patient factors, the cuff and APG unit are calibrated as described. The leg is next raised to empty the veins until a plateau is reached on the chart tracing (zero functional venous volume), and a zero baseline is established on the tracing.

The patient then is guided off the table (avoiding cuff contact with table surfaces) and stands up. The patient stands with the weight off the leg being examined and may hold onto a walker or some such support. The leg veins fill in the dependent position and the tracing rises, indicating volume increase. This difference between the supine and standing venous volumes is measured and equals the functional venous volume (VV).

The patient then stands on both feet and does one toe-up maneuver (standing on the balls of the feet and raising up on tiptoes, then back down), then returns to the position where the weight is back off the examined leg. A decrease in the volume (in milliliters) is noted during this maneuver, indicating blood ejected by the contraction of the calf muscle, or the ejection volume. Two to three repetitions of this maneuver are performed for comparison.

The last part of the test involves having the patient perform 10 toe-ups in sequence, one after the other, then returning to the weight-off position. The diminishing calf volume in milliliters is recorded during the toe-ups, and the calf veins refill and plateau during the standing phase following. The patient then lies back down and the leg is raised and emptied to drain the veins and record another zero-volume point. The difference between the original zero baseline and the new zero baseline after exercise equals the residual volume (RV).

Interpretation Criteria[7,16]

Air plethysmography has been considered quantitative and many of the maneuvers and criteria are noninvasive equivalents of ambulatory venous pressure, venous reflux, and calf-muscle pump function studies. These criteria are based on measurements calculated in the following ways:

1. A venous filling index (VFI) is calculated by dividing 90% of the venous volume (VV) by the length of time it takes from the onset of the standing position to fill 90% of the venous volume (VFT90);

$$VFI = 90\%\ VV/VFT90$$

Dividing the volume by the time gives the rate of refill in milliliters per second. Normal extremity veins fill slowly by arterial inflow, whereas insufficient veins fill rapidly because of retrograde flow from valvular incompetence. The VFI measures the degree of valvular insufficiency.

2. An ejection fraction (EF) is calculated by dividing the volume of blood ejected during one toe-up maneuver (EV) by the VV, then multiplying by 100 to produce a percentage:

$$EF = EV/VV \times 100$$

Normal patients generally eject more than 60% of the calf volume with each toe-up. The EF drops with valvular incompetence or venous obstruction. The EF gives the percentage of the calf volume ejected by the calf muscle pump.

3. A residual volume fraction (RVF) is calculated by measuring the residual volume (RV) after the 10 toe-ups divided by the VV, then multiplied by 100 to obtain a percentage:

$$RVF = RV/VV \times 100$$

Normal patients eject most of the blood from the extremities during exercise and thus the RVF should be low (less than 35%). Patients with chronic venous insufficiency have poor calf muscle pumps and venous reflux, and thus have a high RVF (more than 35%). RVF has correlated closely with ambulatory venous pressure measurements.[16]

An example of an APG study that illustrates these methods and indices is shown in Fig. 21-79.

Discussion

Although the current procedure and implementation are relatively new, APG is based on old technology that includes some components of water plethysmographic measurement. Despite this, the technique has shown a potential for quantifying calf muscle pump function and insufficiency levels, and in addition, it can be performed over venous compression stockings to help determine whether the stocking's compression level is adequate.[7] It also has been suggested as a method to help pinpoint patients who may develop venous ulcers.[8]

The test can only be performed on those who can stand up well and who can do toe-ups effectively. Those who are very elderly or unable to cooperate cannot be examined with APG.

If APG is performed, it should be as an adjunct to venous duplex sonographic imaging, since it does not pinpoint disease levels and areas of reflux nor is it effective above the knee.

Photoplethysmography (PPG)

A photocell can be used to determine the amount of reflux in the leg with venous valvular insufficiency. The principle here is to empty the veins of the lower leg by either exercising the calf muscle with dorsiflexion and plantarflexion of the foot or by manually compressing the calf, then measuring the time for venous refill. In this test the patient should sit comfortably on the end of an examination table or bed, with the legs hanging down and the back of the knee away from the table edge. The plethysmograph is set to acquire PPG waveforms and switched to the DC mode, and the photocell is taped with double-sided tape to an area about 3 to 6 cms anterior to and above the medial malleolus (Fig. 21-80). The location should be free of varicosities and should not be over a major vein.

Once the photocell has been attached, the examiner should balance the chart recorder pen about one half to one third of the distance from the top of the chart area, then calibrate the size and position to allow a full display of the examination output. The chart is run at a 5 mm/sec speed, so each major division on the chart paper equals 1 second.

Once a stable baseline is established, the patient is instructed to fully dorsiflex and plantarflex the foot five times, then relax. The chart normally shows five negative peaks (reflecting the flexion maneuvers) with a steadily decreasing volume, which "bottoms out" after the last flexion maneuver. The trace then slowly rises to the level of the original baseline as the veins refill and the volume in the calf veins increases. If a patient is unable to adequately flex the foot, the examiner may manually compress the calf muscle five times to empty the veins.

If the test is abnormal (see the criteria below), the examiner may repeat the test twice more, once after applying a tourniquet to the leg below the knee at midcalf (see Fig. 21-80) and again after applying a tourniquet to the leg above the knee at the thigh (after removing the calf tourni quet). As an alternative to a tourniquet, a narrow tourniquet pressure cuff can be used with enough pressure (around 40 mm Hg) to occlude the superficial veins but not the deep system. Tourniquet use is designed to help isolate reflux to the lesser saphenous, greater saphenous, or deep systems.

Interpretation Criteria

The examiner should evaluate the tracing and obtain the refilling time by measuring from the end of the last flexion maneuver to the point where the tracing reaches the original baseline. Longer refilling times are normal, whereas short refilling times imply severe reflux. Depending on whose criteria are used, refilling times greater than 23 seconds are generally considered normal, between 17 and 23 equivocal, and those less than 17 seconds are considered abnormal and suggestive of reflux.[1,6,14,18]

A more rational classification system defines the following four categories of insufficiency:[3,6]

- Refill times of greater than 25 seconds are considered normal;
- Grade I insufficiency has refill times of 20 to 25 seconds;
- Grade II insufficiency has refill times from 10 to 20 seconds; and
- Grade III insufficiency has refill times less than 10 seconds.

A

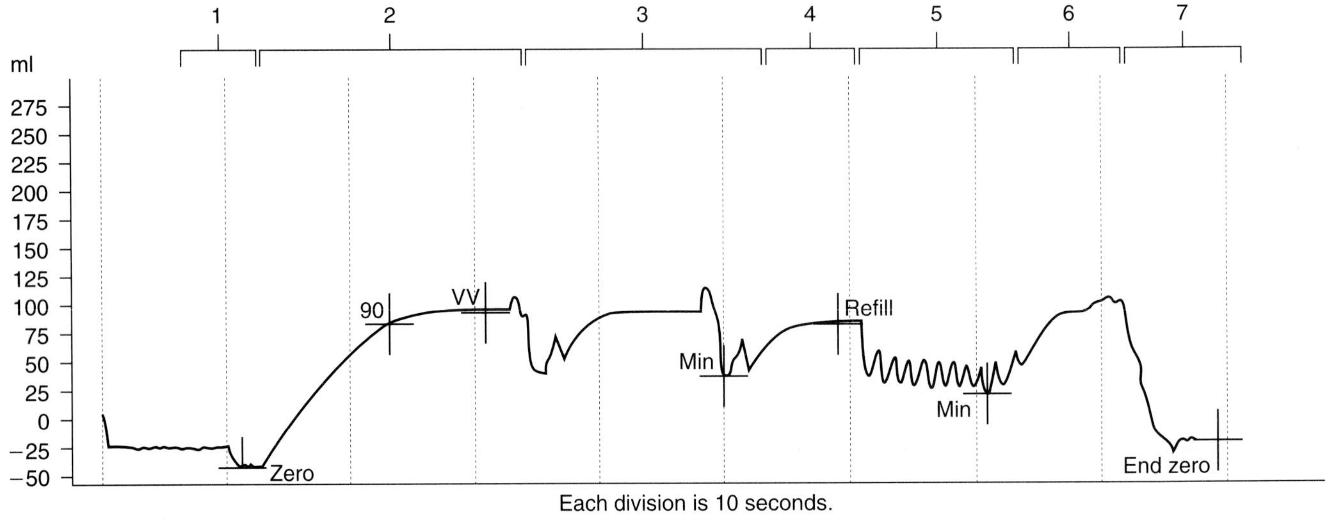

Each division is 10 seconds.

The total venous volume is .... 130.8 ml
The venous filling index (VFI) is .... 10.0 ml/sec
The ejection fraction is 34.3%
The residual volume fraction is 30.0%

Name :
SSN :
Date : 02/18/92
Test : TEST SUMMARY
Leg : Right leg with stocking.

B

Social Sec #	Name: Date: 02/18/92	RIGHT LEG	stocking	LEFT LEG	stocking	Normal Values
Obstruction	Ouflow Fraction (OF) %					>40% and
	With Superficial Occ. %					<10%
Reflux	Venous Volume (VV) ml	145.9	130.8	148.2		
ml/sec	Venous Filling Index (VFI)	10.34	10.02	9.329		<2 ml/sec
ml/sec	VFI with Superficial Occ.					<3.5 ml/s
Calf muscle pump	Ejection Volume (EV) ml	46.93	44.85	51.76		
	Ejection Fraction (EF) %	32.16	34.28	34.92		>60%
RVF	RVF % = AVP mmHg	39.86	30.00	51.58		<35%
Arterial inflow	Leg Status	Resting	Post Exc	Resting	Post Exc	
	Arterial Inflow ml/min					

NOTES:

FIG. 21-79 A, APG study. This printout illustrates the waveform changes corresponding to each part of the test; *1,* Supine, initial raising of leg to empty veins and zero the tracing. *2,* Standing, refilling veins for obtaining venous volume (VV). The 90% filling (VFT90) point also is shown. *3,* Two separate toe-ups to obtain the calf ejection volume (EV). *4,* Standing, interval refill time. *5,* Ten toe-ups in succession to calculate residual volume (RV). *6,* Standing, interval refill time. *7,* Supine, raising draining leg for second zero point. **B,** APG study. Sample data summary, with comparative values of the right leg both with and without a compression stocking. See text for a detailed description of the various indices and volume items shown here.

If tourniquets are applied, the refill times may improve or even reach normal ranges. In general:

1. If the refill times normalize with calf tourniquets, the lesser saphenous system is suspected to be incompetent.
2. If the times improve with a thigh tourniquet, then the great saphenous distribution is suspected to be incompetent.
3. If neither tourniquet improves the refill times, then the deep system is suspected to be incompetent.

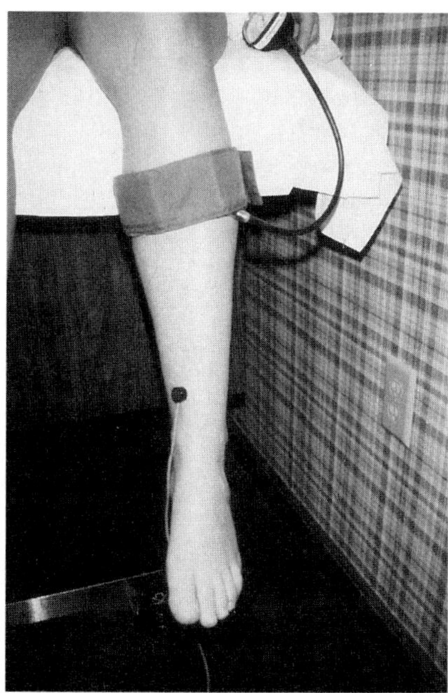

FIG. 21-80 Venous photoplethysmography. This shows proper placement of the photocell and of the calf tourniquet.

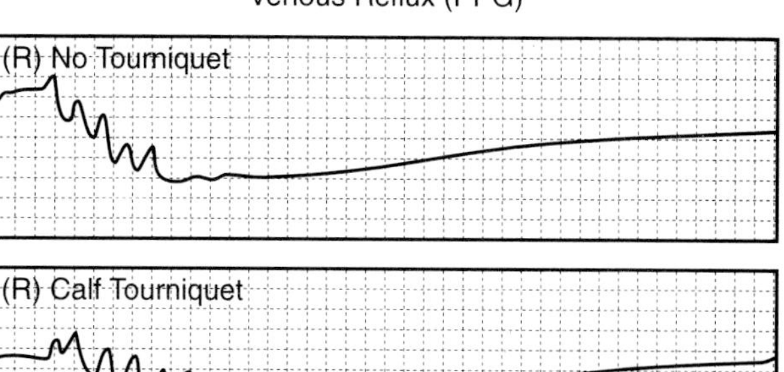

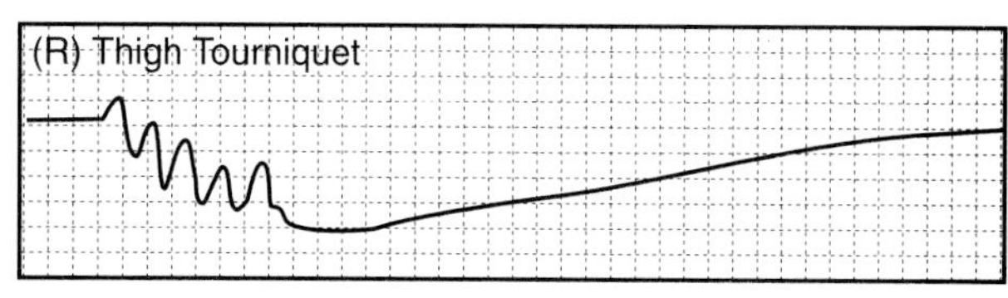

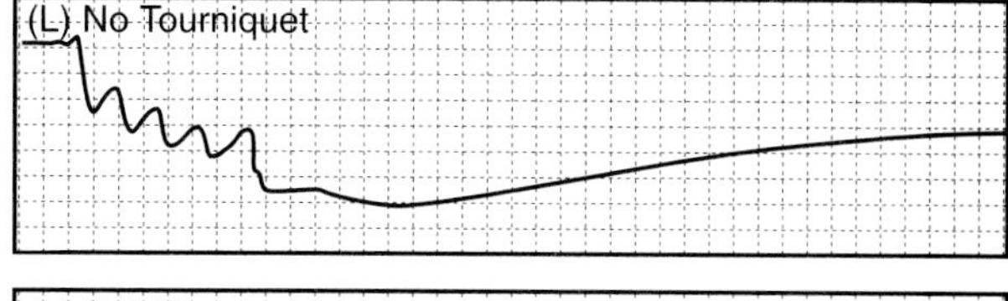

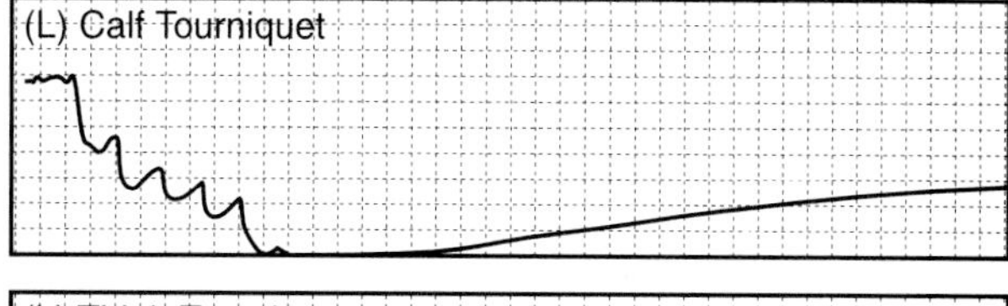

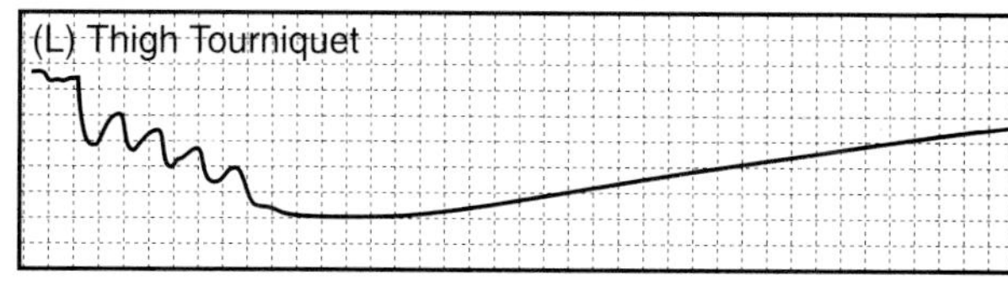

FIG. 21-81 Normal venous photoplethysmography study (see text for description).

EXAMPLES OF NORMAL AND ABNORMAL PPG STUDIES ARE SHOWN IN THE NEXT TWO CASES

Case 1 (Fig. 21-81): normal PPG

This 43-year-old patient had mild varicosities on the right with gradual swelling of both legs after standing long periods. He had no prior history of deep or superficial vein thrombosis.

The study shows normal refill times of 28 seconds in both legs, with no changes occurring after tourniquets were used at the thigh and calf.

Case 2 (Fig. 21-82): abnormal PPG

This 38-year-old patient had markedly dilated varicose veins in the right leg. He had no prior history of deep or superficial vein thrombosis.

The study shows abnormal refill times of 10 seconds in the right leg, which were not improved with tourniquet use. The left leg has normal refill times of more than 30 seconds.

A venous duplex examination showed normal deep veins bilaterally and a patent but severely incompetent great saphenous system in the right leg. The left great saphenous vein was patent and competent at all levels.

Discussion

Venous photoplethysmographic techniques can give some quantification of reflux and can screen some patients with insufficiency; but in general, it has varying effectiveness because of the variability of photocell placement, tourniquet placement, and ability of the patient to adequately perform the foot flexion maneuvers. Tourniquets do not, in practice, always isolate the superficial systems. The technique of evaluating reflux using duplex at the venous junctions with the patient standing and with uniform compression augmentation is far more effective and accurate.

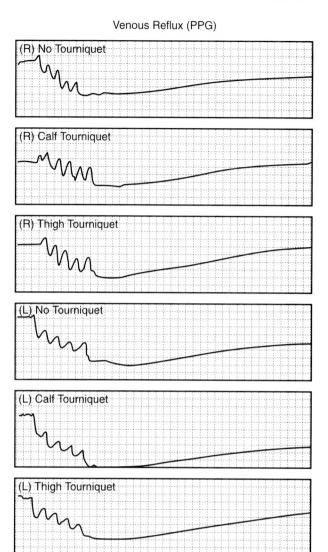

SUMMARY

Venous evaluations are among the most difficult examinations a technologist can perform, in that a great deal of subjective decision-making is required of the examiner. The technologist or sonographer must use careful technique and have a thorough knowledge of venous hemodynamics, disease processes, and the anatomy. When performing any venous study, ultrasonic or otherwise, it is important to be familiar not only with normal and abnormal findings but with the artifacts and other idiosyncrasies in the examination modalities that can cause problems and prevent one from obtaining an accurate and diagnostic examination.

In venous duplex and continuous-wave Doppler, one of the most difficult tasks for a beginner is to avoid applying

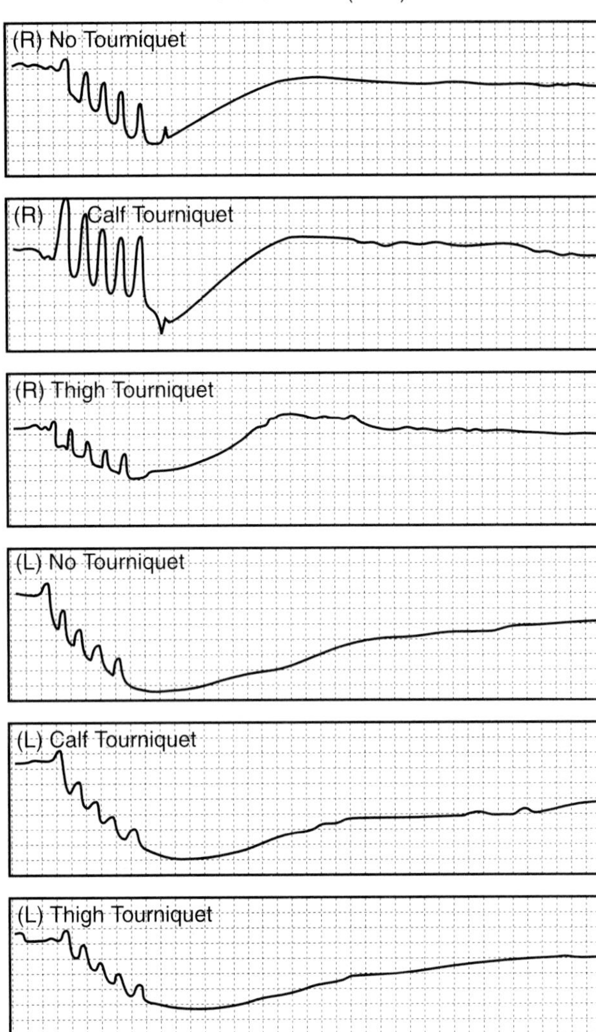

FIG. 21-82 Abnormal venous photoplethysmography study (see text for description).

undue transducer pressure. A "heavy hand" is not always catastrophic in abdominal or arterial sonography, but it can result in a completely unacceptable test result in venous studies. Not only can too much pressure occlude a superficial or deep vein, but it can alter the venous hemodynamics and even cause confusion and misinterpretation on the part of the examiner and interpreting physician alike.

Few sonographers or vascular technologists rate venous studies among their "top ten" favorite examinations; if an examination method does not hold a sonographer or vascular technologists' interest, there is a high probability that the study results will be suboptimal. It cannot be overstressed that practice and patience are the keys to succeeding when performing venous studies (or any examination, for that matter). The reader should take the time to read texts on venous disease and hemodynamics and should, above all, take venous evaluation seriously. If this is done, proficiency will follow. It also follows that with experience and success come increased interest and improved quality. Physicians often rely heavily on the sonographer or vascular technologist's findings and judgments in determining the best treatment method for venous patients, so the sonographer or vascular technologist should recognize the importance of these examinations and the need to be able to perform them well.

REVIEW QUESTIONS

1. What is a pulmonary embolus? Where can it come from?
2. What is thrombophlebitis? What usually causes it?
3. Name four different noninvasive methods used to evaluate the veins.
4. Name and describe the six characteristics of venous flow used when evaluating veins with Doppler methods.
5. Describe the deep veins of the lower extremity. Where are they located in the leg?
6. What are perforating veins? What do they communicate with? Name three areas where perforating veins can be found in the leg.
7. Name the venous sites in the leg that are evaluated with continuous-wave Doppler.
8. What is reflux and how is it checked for with Doppler, color-flow, and gray-scale imaging? What findings would you expect to see?
9. What findings would you expect to see when examining a vein segment if a thrombus is present? What do you see with gray-scale? Color-flow imaging?
10. Describe the technique used to evaluate saphenous veins for bypass use.
11. What is recanalization? Would you see it in an acute or a chronic thrombus?
12. What are differences between acute and chronic thrombus?
13. Compare the symptoms of venous disease with those of arterial disease.
14. Does venous flow move by cardiac or respiratory changes? Is pulsatility in a vein normal? Why or why not?
15. Name three surgical or nonsurgical methods of treating varicose veins.
16. Name the deep veins of the upper extremity. Name the superficial veins.
17. Name three nonultrasonic noninvasive methods of evaluating the venous systems in the extremities.
18. What are three methods used to obtain VO/VC studies?
19. What is venous capacitance? What is venous outflow?
20. Which of the nonultrasonic methods is best for obtaining quantifiable calf muscle pump information? Which is (or are) best for evaluating reflux? Which can detect venous obstruction?
21. *Venous insufficiency* is another term for what condition?

REFERENCES

1. Barnes RW, Garrett WV, et al: Photoplethysmographic assessment of altered cutaneous circulation in the post-phlebitic syndrome. Technology in diagnosis and therapy, Proc Assoc Adv Med Instrum 13:25, 1978.
2. Barnes RW, Russell HE, and Wilson MR: Doppler ultrasonic evaluation of venous disease; A programmed audiovisual instruction. Iowa City, 1975, University of Iowa Press.
3. Bergan JJ: Common anatomic patterns of varicose veins. In Bergan JJ and Goldman MP, editors: Varicose veins and telangiectasias: diagnosis and treatment. St. Louis, 1993, Quality Medical Publishing.
4. Bergan JJ: Cross-pubic bypass for iliac venous occlusion. In Bergan JJ and Kistner RL, editor: Atlas of venous surgery. Philadelphia, 1992, WB Saunders.
5. Bergan JJ: Surgical procedures for varicose veins: axial stripping and stab avulsion. In Bergan JJ and Kistner RL, editors: Atlas of venous surgery. Philadelphia, 1992, WB Saunders.
6. Blazek V, May R, Stemmer R, and Wienert V: Die Standardisiersung der LRR-Untersuchung. In May R and Stemmer R, editors: Die Licht-Reflexions-Rheographie (LRR), pp. 151-55. Erlangen, Germany, 1984, Perimed.
7. Christopoulos DG, Nicolaides AN, Szendro G, et al: Air-plethysmography and the effect of elastic compression on venous hemodynamics of the leg, J Vasc Surg 5(1):148-59, 1987.
8. Christopoulos DG, Nicolaides AN, Cook A, et al: Pathogenesis of venous ulceration in relation to the calf muscle pump function, Surgery 106:829, 1989.
9. Cornu-Thenard A and Boivin P: Treatment of varicose veins by sclerotherapy: an overview. In Bergan JJ and Goldman MP, editors: Varicose veins and telangiectasias: diagnosis and treatment. St. Louis, 1993, Quality Medical Publishing.
10. Couch NP: Axioms on venous thrombosis, Hosp Med 13:68, 1977.
11. Cramer M, Beach KW, and Strandness DE: The detection of proximal deep venous thrombosis by strain gauge plethysmography through the use of an outflow/capacitance discriminant line, Bruit 7:17, Dec 1983.
12. Cranley JJ: Diagnosis of deep vein thrombosis by phleborheography. In Bernstein EF, editor: Noninvasive diagnostic techniques in vascular disease, ed 3. St. Louis, 1985, Mosby.
13. Essentials and standards for noninvasive vascular testing. Vascular Laboratory Operations, Part II (Peripheral Venous Testing). Rockville, Md, 1993, Intersocietal Commission for the Accreditation of Vascular Laboratories.
14. Fronek A: Noninvasive diagnostics in vascular disease. New York, 1989, McGraw-Hill.
15. Goss CM, editor: Gray's anatomy. Philadelphia, Lea & Febiger.
16. Katz ML, Comerota AJ, and Kerr R: Air plethysmography (APG): a new technique to evaluate patients with chronic venous insufficiency, J Vasc Tech 15:23, 1991.
17. Kistner RL: Transposition techniques. In Bergan JJ and Kistner RL, editor: Atlas of venous surgery. Philadelphia, 1992, WB Saunders.
18. Li JM, Anderson FA, and Wheeler HB: Non-invasive testing for venous reflux using photoplethysmography: standardization of technique and evaluation of interpretation criteria, Bruit 7:25, 1983.

18b. Markel A, Manzo RA, Bergelin RO, Strandness DE: Pattern and distribution of thrombi in acute venous thrombosis, Arch Surg 127(3): 305-309, 1992.

19. Nack TL and Needleman L: Comparison of duplex ultrasound and contrast venography for evaluation of upper extremity venous disease, J Vasc Tech 16:69, 1992.
20. Netter FH and Divertie MB, editors: CIBA collection of medical illustrations, vol 7, Respiratory System. Summit, NJ, 1979, Medical Education Division, CIBA Pharmaceutical.
21. Raymond-Martimbeau P: Role of sclerotherapy in greater saphenous vein incompetence. In Bergan JJ and Goldman MP, editors: Varicose veins and telangiectasias: diagnosis and treatment. St. Louis, 1993, Quality Medical Publishing.
22. Rollins DL, Ryan TJ, et al: Diagnosis of deep venous thrombosis using real time ultrasound imaging. In Negus D and Jantet G, editors: Phlebology '85. 1986, John Libbey & Co.
23. Semrow C, Friedell M, et al: Characterization of lower extremity venous disease using real-time B-mode imaging, J Vasc Tech 11:187, 1987.
24. Sumner DS: Strain-gauge plethysmography. In Bernstein EF, editor: Noninvasive diagnostic techniques in vascular disease, ed 3. St. Louis, 1985, Mosby.
25. Talbot SR: B-Mode evaluation of peripheral arteries and veins. In Zwiebel WJ, editor: Introduction to vascular ultrasonography, ed 2. Orlando, Fla, 1986, Grune & Stratton.

CHAPTER

22

Cerebrovascular Sonography, Doppler, and Noninvasive Examinations

Richard E. Rae II

Cerebral ischemia to the brain secondary to arterial occlusion or rupture, known as stroke, is one of the leading causes of death in the world. Cerebral ischemia may manifest itself with any or all of the following symptoms:

- Vision changes, including amaurosis fugax, a monocular blindness typically described as "a shade being lowered over my eye" that may obstruct all or part of the patient's sight, blurry vision, or frank blindness
- Dizziness, with or without nausea and vomiting
- Syncopal or near-syncopal episodes, which may be described as "blacking out" by the patient
- Headache
- Transient confusion
- Hemiparesis, a unilateral weakness that may affect one or both extremities on one side of the body and may affect the face and tongue as well
- Numbness, occurring either by itself or in combination with hemiparesis, affecting limbs, face, and tongue
- Speech changes, including slurred speech (dysphasia) or complete loss of functional speech (aphasia). (The patient may know what he or she wants to say but be unable to say it.)

When the episode resolves in less than 12 hours, it is classed as a transient ischemic attack (TIA). If the attack lasts longer than 12 hours but resolves within 24 hours, it may be classed as a resolving ischemic neurologic deficit (RIND). Any debilitating ischemic attack that lasts longer than 24 hours and that may show evidence of profound cerebral damage is classed as a cerebrovascular accident (CVA). A CVA may or may not resolve with time or therapy, and if symptoms seem to increase in type and severity gradually during the episode, the stroke may be progressing as a result of an intracerebral bleed.

Causes of these ischemic episodes include the following:

1. Atherosclerotic plaque in the carotid arteries.[21] Atherosclerosis initially manifests itself as a collection of lipids in the intima, resulting in an intimal thickening process known as the *fatty streak*. Fatty streaks are smooth-surfaced, do not disrupt the intimal lining, and therefore do not obstruct blood flow. This lesion may regress or develop into the fibrous plaque. A fibrous plaque is a progression of fatty cells, collagen, and fibrous material that, as it develops, elevates the intimal lining into the lumen and progresses to a point where the lumen is significantly narrowed and may cause flow disturbance. This lesion also may regress, remain the same, or develop into a complex plaque. Complex plaques have the most potential for cerebral and arterial damage, since the fibrous and fatty lesions may have calcific changes and internal hemorrhage into the plaque, which can increase the size of the lesion. Subintimal necrosis of the lesion can occur and the smooth intimal continuity can be disrupted, resulting in an ulceration of the intima. Ulcerations can collect platelet aggregates, which cause a thrombosis to develop over the ulcer (parts or all of which may detach), or the material within the plaque can be discharged into the bloodstream. Both conditions result in embolic phenomena that can travel distally and occlude intracerebral branches and cause cerebral ischemic changes.
2. Arterial aneurysm. An aneurysm of a cerebral artery can eventually rupture and cause an intracerebral hemorrhage. Aneurysms of the internal carotid artery can develop thrombus (as in abdominal or extremity arteries), dissect, or rupture. Thrombotic aneurysms can also embolize distally.
3. Cardiac emboli. Emboli of cardiac origin can travel distally through the carotid system to the brain. Some sources for these emboli include valve vegetations, intracardiac thrombi, and myxoma.
4. Diseases of the intima, including Takayasu's and giant cell arteritis, can cause the intima to swell and occlude the lumen.
5. External compression or vascular anomaly, such as carotid body tumor, tortuosity, or kinking can severely reduce blood flow and at times even promote thrombus or plaque formation.

Many syndromes that affect the carotid arteries can remain asymptomatic or clinically silent for years; often the seemingly insignificant dizzy spell or episode of numbness is passed off by the patient until an episode occurs that does not resolve, which may lead to permanent debilitation or death.

Fortunately, many techniques have been developed to help diagnose carotid and cerebral arterial conditions, often enabling surgeons to intercede before plaques progress to the point of occlusion or imminent stroke. Cerebral and selective carotid arteriography and digital subtraction imaging remain the gold standard for diagnosing these conditions, but research and studies in recent years are beginning to challenge this view. The true gold standard is the findings at surgery, and carotid duplex sonography coupled with spectrum analysis and color-flow imaging of carotid blood flow have proven in some cases to be more accurate than arteriography.[47] Arteriography is open to radiologist variance in interpretation, and many of the fine details of plaque morphology, such as intraplaque hemorrhage, intimal ulceration, and soft plaque are impossible to assess with arteriography. Arteriograms depend on localizing filling defects, and when a smooth plaque with little encroachment on the lumen is present, or when it is on a wall obscured by contrast, false interpretations are likely (see Fig. 19-1). Sonography also allows a transverse view of the plaque and lumen unavailable with arteriography. Many vascular surgeons throughout the world are now operating on the basis of duplex sonography findings rather than arteriograms, something unthinkable a few years ago.[13] In addition, carotid duplex sonography and Doppler flow assessment are ideal for screening patients with suspected carotid problems or following up on evolving plaques because they are noninvasive and present virtually no risk to patients. Long-term follow-up of postendarterectomy patients is also practical with sonographic methods. Most patients would be reluctant to consent to arteriography every 6 months.

ANATOMY OF THE CEREBROVASCULAR CIRCULATION[21,37]

The first major vessels involved in the Doppler examination are the common carotid arteries. The right common carotid artery arises from the brachiocephalic (innominate) artery, and the left common carotid artery arises directly from the aortic arch. Both travel superiorly in the neck to just above the thyroid cartilage. Here the carotids widen into the carotid bulbs and bifurcate into the internal and external carotid arteries.

The internal carotid artery normally has no branches within the neck. It continues superiorly to enter the skull through the carotid canal. It makes several short twists, turns anteriorly and posteriorly, and then gives off its first branch intracranially, the ophthalmic artery (Fig. 22-1).

Several rare internal carotid branches can persist from fetal circulation. These are the ascending pharyngeal artery (which comes off distally to the bifurcation and often is a branch of the external carotid), the proatlantal artery, the hypoglossal artery, and the trigeminal artery (the last three come off high in the neck between the C-1 and C-3 vertebrae). The ascending pharyngeal may be seen by duplex scanning, and its presence may cause misidentification of the vessels at the bifurcation; it may be mistaken for the superior thyroid artery, which takes off the proximal external carotid at the bulb (Fig. 22-2; see color images). If there is a question, the examiner should obtain pulsed Doppler spectra from each major bifurcation vessel, using temporal artery percussion if necessary to identify the external carotid.

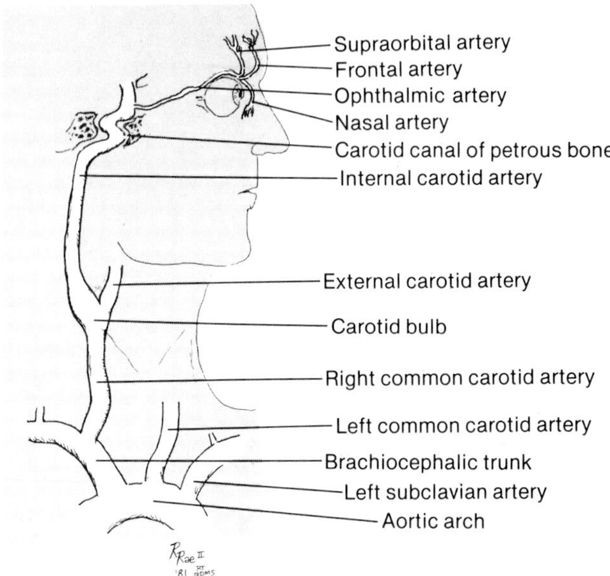

FIG. 22-1 Aortic branches and the internal carotid arterial system. (Courtesy Richard E. Rae, Indianapolis.)

The ophthalmic artery continues anteriorly into the orbit, where several branches arise and pass superiorly over the globe and exit the orbit onto the face near the orbital margin. The peripheral branches are the supraorbital, frontal (supratrochlear), and nasal (dorsal nasal) arteries. These three arteries are the most easily accessible vessels that reflect the hemodynamics of the distal internal carotid.

The supraorbital artery passes through the supraorbital notch or foramen and branches onto the forehead. The frontal artery exits the orbit at the upper medial angle and also branches onto the forehead. The nasal artery passes out of the orbit at the inferomedial angle and runs alongside the nose to anastomose with the angular artery from the external carotid (Fig. 22-3).

The external carotid primarily supplies the extracranial structures. It gives off several branches in the neck, beginning with the superior thyroid artery at the bulb and progressing up to the occipital artery, which passes posterosuperiorly toward the ear.

The next branch given off is the facial artery, at about the same level. It passes anteriorly around the inferior border of the mandible and continues superiorly to the medial corner of the orbit. It becomes the angular artery at about the corner of the mouth.

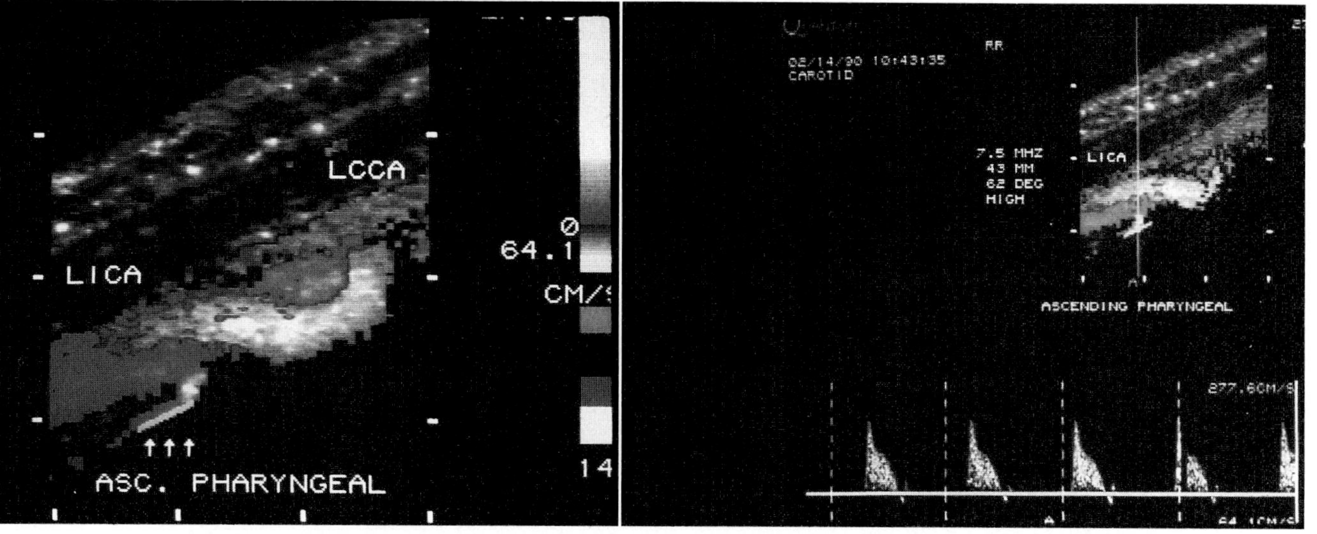

FIG. 22-2 Ascending pharyngeal artery. **A,** This color-flow duplex image clearly shows a vessel arising from a normal internal carotid origin. The external carotid artery (not shown) also had several branches in its proximal segment. **B,** A Doppler waveform from the ascending pharyngeal shows it to have a high-resistance flow pattern typical of a branch.

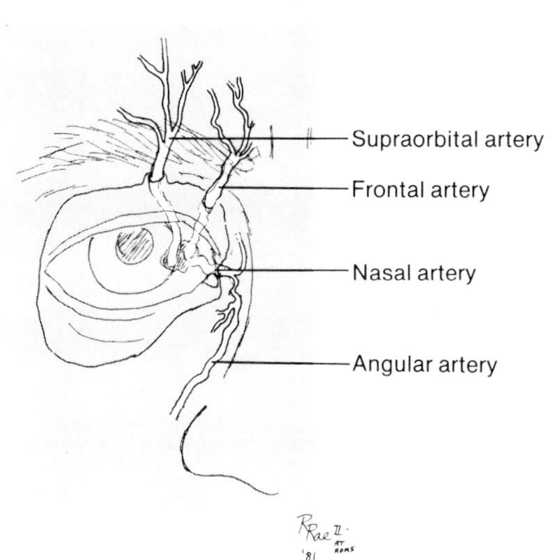

FIG. 22-3 Terminal branches of the ophthalmic artery. (Courtesy Richard E. Rae, Indianapolis.)

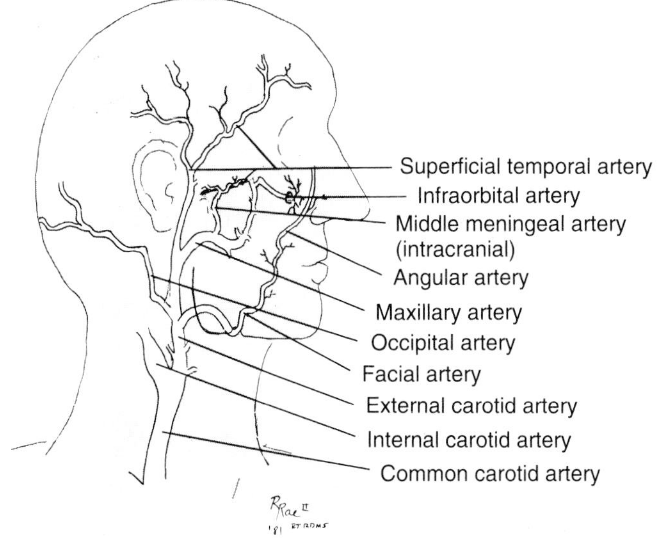

FIG. 22-4 Branches of the external carotid artery. (Courtesy Richard E. Rae, Indianapolis.)

The external carotid then continues superiorly and bifurcates into the superficial temporal and the internal maxillary arteries just below the ear.

The superficial temporal artery continues upward just in front of the ear and gives off several branches, the anterior of which branches onto the forehead.

The internal maxillary artery gives off the middle meningeal artery, which supplies the dura and floor of the cranium and then gives off deep intramaxillary branches before terminating as the infraorbital artery, which exits the skull to the superficial facial muscles through the infraorbital foramen (Fig. 22-4).

The next major arteries are the vertebral arteries. Each vertebral artery arises from its respective subclavian artery and travels superiorly and posteriorly to enter the transverse foramen of the sixth cervical vertebra. The vertebral arteries travel through the transverse foramina of the next five vertebrae until they exit the first cervical vertebra, curve anteriorly and posteriorly, and enter the skull through the foramen magnum.

On entering the skull the two vertebral arteries anastomose to form the basilar artery (Fig. 22-5).

The vertebral, basilar, and internal carotids service or are serviced by the circle of Willis, an arterial circle at the base

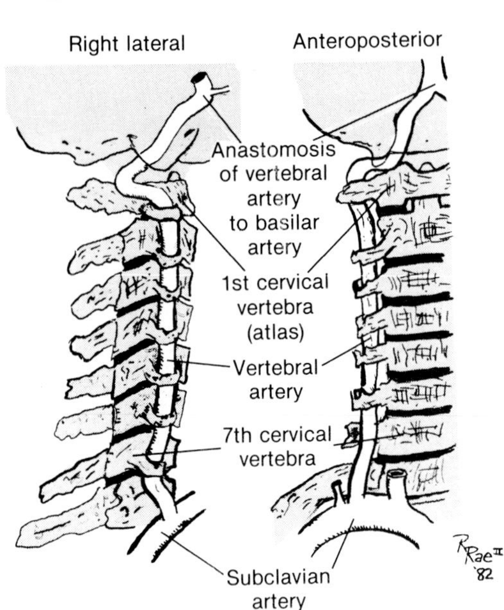

FIG. 22-5 Two anatomic views of the vertebral artery. (Courtesy Richard E. Rae, Indianapolis.)

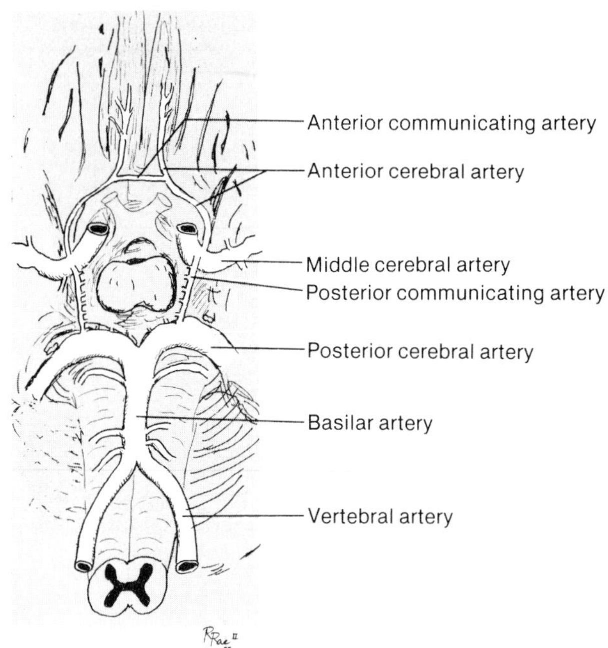

FIG. 22-6 Circle of Willis. (Courtesy Richard E. Rae, Indianapolis.)

of the brain. It is formed by the following vessels (Fig. 22-6):

1. The right and left anterior and middle cerebral arteries (which are the terminal branches of the internal carotids);
2. The posterior cerebral arteries (terminal branches of the basilar artery);
3. The anterior and posterior communicating arteries.

The cerebral arterial circle of Willis provides a common collateral pathway in cases of single or multiple arterial obstruction. For example, if one internal carotid artery is diseased or occluded, the other internal carotid artery can supply its needs by shunting flow via the circle of Willis. The basilar artery can also supply the distribution of either or both carotids in severe obstruction, as well as the vertebrals in subclavian steal syndrome (see Chapter 20).

HEMODYNAMICS AND POSSIBLE ANASTOMOSES IN CEREBRAL ARTERIAL OBSTRUCTION[8,21]

In the circle of Willis the following routes of shunting occur with obstructive disease of the internal carotid:

1. One obstructed internal carotid can be supplied by either the opposite internal carotid via the anterior cerebral and anterior communicating arteries or by the vertebrobasilar arteries via the posterior cerebral and posterior communicating arteries.
2. If both internal carotids are obstructed, they are supplied by the vertebrobasilar arteries via both posterior cerebral and both posterior communicating arteries.

Obstruction in the vertebral or carotid arteries is often masked if excellent flow is maintained in the circle of Willis. I have seen cases in which the patient with bilateral total carotid occlusion was asymptomatic and the condition was discovered during examination for a completely unrelated problem.

Obstructions can also cause anastomoses between the internal and external carotid systems. Potential anastomoses include the following:

1. Superficial temporal artery (external carotid)—supraorbital and/or frontal arteries (internal carotid)—usually on or across the forehead;
2. Facial-angular artery (external carotid)—nasal artery (internal carotid);
3. Infraorbital artery (external carotid)—nasal artery (internal carotid) via the angular artery; and
4. Middle meningeal (external carotid)—ophthalmic artery (internal carotid) with a direct intracranial connection.

When one subclavian artery is obstructed proximal to the vertebral origin, the vertebrovertebral anastomosis results in a subclavian steal. (See Chapter 20 for explanation of the hemodynamics involved and Fig. 20-102 for illustration.)

On rare occasions, vertebral artery anastomoses with the occipital artery high in the neck may draw flow from the external carotid to counteract vertebral insufficiencies.

CHARACTERISTICS OF THE DOPPLER ARTERIAL SIGNAL IN THE CEREBRAL EXAMINATION

Unlike the signal in the extremities, the normal Doppler signal in the carotid and cerebral circulation is of high velocity, and because of the low resistance of the intracranial vascular bed it does not go below the zero line (Fig. 22-7).

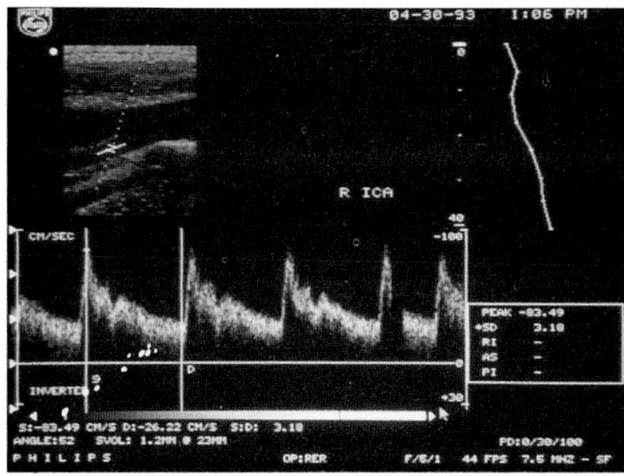

FIG. 22-7 Normal internal carotid Doppler spectral waveform, showing typical low-resistance flow pattern appearance.

The same basic components as in the extremity artery signal exist here, but there is a much shorter secondary component and a larger diastolic component. The secondary component may be absent, depending on disease or vascular resistance.

The only normal exception to low-resistance flow will be in the external carotid artery signal. This signal is still of a higher overall velocity than in an extremity artery; because of the facial branches this artery supplies, the signal is much more like that of an extremity artery and has a pattern distinct from the normal common and internal carotid signal.

In disease, blunting of systolic flow and diminishing of diastolic flow occurs proximal to a stenosis as disease increases. In cases of a complete internal carotid occlusion, diastolic flow may vanish completely and there may seem to be a reversed flow component as in the extremity artery, since there is major resistance to flow distally. Prominent bidirectional flow in the carotids may rarely be seen in cases of innominate artery occlusion and carotid steal.

CEREBROVASCULAR SONOGRAPHIC EXAMINATION TECHNIQUES

The cerebrovascular circulation and carotid arteries can be examined with one or more imaging and flow-monitoring modalities, but the Intersocietal Commission for the Accreditation of Vascular Laboratories (ICAVL) has established in their Essentials and Standards for noninvasive cerebrovascular testing that duplex ultrasonography (with or without color-flow imaging) is the primary method to be used for noninvasive evaluation.[18] Other studies, such as continuous-wave Doppler, periorbital examination, oculoplethysmography (OPG), transcranial Doppler (TCD), and transcranial duplex imaging (TCI) are considered secondary methods; they can be used in conjunction with carotid duplex, but they should not be used alone to diagnose cerebrovascular disease.

This section describes the techniques of evaluating the carotid and vertebral arteries with duplex ultrasonography and color-flow imaging, continuous-wave periorbital Doppler examination, transcranial Doppler, and transcranial duplex. Diagnostic criteria for interpretation are also presented.

The protocols and procedures here are based on numerous sources and long personal experience; the reader should note that variations on techniques and approaches may be necessary because of the architecture and idiosyncrasies of the duplex scanner in use.

The basic equipment needed for cerebrovascular examination is a stethoscope and a high-resolution duplex scanner, preferably with color-flow imaging capabilities. The 5-MHz to 10-MHz transducers allow the best imaging ranges, and pulsed Doppler frequencies should be no lower than 3 MHz. A tape recorder, multiformat camera, or color-image printer is necessary to document the examination and obtain the required images. If secondary testing is used the equipment varies according to the applications. A continuous-wave directional Doppler device, one or two pressure cuffs and inflation source, and a spectrum analyzer or strip-chart recorder are necessary for periorbital Doppler studies; a transcranial Doppler unit or duplex scanner with appropriate transcranial Doppler software and sector transducers is needed to perform transcranial Doppler or transcranial duplex imaging studies. Other devices, such as an ocular pneumoplethysmograph, may also be used (see Nonsonographic Cerebrovascular Evaluation Methods).

The first step is to obtain a history from the patient or chart. Emphasis should be placed on typical cerebrovascular symptoms, including dizziness, monocular blindness, nausea, confusion, syncope, headache, personality change, hemiparesis, numbness, and other known symptoms significant for probable carotid stenosis. If the patient has had a frank TIA or CVA, note the number of occurrences, the date of the most recent TIA or onset of CVA, the brain hemisphere affected if a CVA has occurred, whether the symptoms have resolved, and approximately how long it has taken for them to resolve, if at all.

The carotids should be auscultated with a stethoscope or carotid phonoangiograph for the presence of bruits. A bruit is heard as a low- to high-pitched squirting noise occurring with systole and may range from soft to loud. It results from intraarterial flow turbulence and is usually heard directly over the area of stenosis, although it may be detected in the distal portion of the artery as well. Bruits should be considered a significant indication of disease, especially when they occur in the asymptomatic patient, since they may indicate the presence of severe stenosis and atherosclerotic plaque.

Bruitlike sounds can be heard in patients with systolic blowing murmurs of cardiac origin that radiate through the arch to the carotids. The heart should therefore also be checked to determine whether murmurs that could be radiating are present. Bruits can, of course, be present in the subclavian or vertebral arteries if a severe stenosis exists there and can radiate distally to the carotid region. Bruits from the vertebral origin can also sound similar to carotid bruits in the cervical area. Simulated bruits caused by increased vascular dynamics can occur in young people or in individuals with low carotid bifurcations. As a rule, a bruit in the low carotid region occurring bilaterally and fading in the distal carotid and accompanied by a cardiac murmur is of cardiac origin; bruits high or midway in the neck that can be isolated by the stethoscope with no cardiac murmur are strongly indicative of carotid stenosis.

A severely stenosed external carotid artery can also cause a bruit (usually distinguished by its short duration), and many times can exist right beside a patent internal carotid. Any time a bruit or bruitlike sound is heard in the high cervical or supraclavicular area, the examiner should apply himself or herself to detecting the cause of the bruit and documenting the area of flow turbulence during the course of the examination.

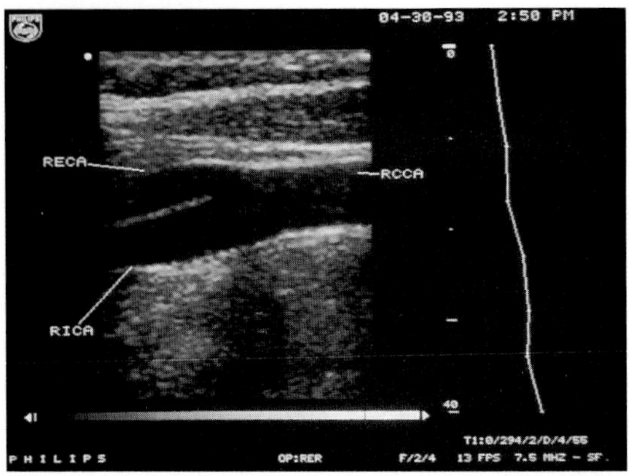

FIG. 22-8 Normal gray-scale image of the carotid bifurcation.

Carotid Duplex Sonography

Carotid duplex sonography should be the primary method used to evaluate the cerebrovascular system, with other methods used adjunctively. Although arteriography is still considered the gold standard by many, duplex correlation with surgical findings has proved quite accurate in many institutions and many surgeons perform endarterectomies based solely on the results of the carotid duplex examination.[13] Carotid duplex sonography does not eliminate arteriography, however, for evaluating structures above the mandible or intracranially, especially regarding the many small cerebral vessels inaccessible to conventional Doppler and imaging, and also since transcranial Doppler and transcranial duplex use is not widespread. Arteriography is also too risky and invasive for routine screening of patients with suspected carotid stenosis. In general, carotid imaging should never be performed without either duplex or direct carotid Doppler assessment, since imaging alone can miss a surprising number of carotid stenoses.

Description of the Carotid Duplex Real-Time Gray-Scale Image

Before performing or interpreting an examination, the technologist or sonographer must have a thorough knowledge of the appearance and anatomy of the carotid system. The reader should review the "Anatomy of the Cerebrovascular System" section in this chapter, as well as Figs. 22-1 and 22-4.

The common, internal, and external carotids appear to have sonolucent fluid-filled lumina bordered by two bright reflections, the arterial walls. The walls are lined with a low-level gray layer bordered by a fine, slightly brighter echo, thought to represent the intima of the arteries (Fig. 22-8).

Orientation of the image can vary, depending on the make of duplex scanner, but commonly cephalad is to the left and caudad to the right of the image in the longitudinal axis, with the medial side of the body to the left of the image in transverse.

The common carotid artery can be followed superiorly from the supraclavicular area and lies medial to the trachea. The even parallel echoes of the common carotid wall can be traced distally.

Usually an irregular vessel without the thicker-walled characteristics of an artery is seen either anterior to or on one side of the common carotid. This is the internal jugular vein. It can be distinguished by its lack of pulsatility, its phasic dilation and collapse with respiration, its tendency to be irregularly shaped and to widen out at the base, and the ease with which it is collapsed by light pressure from the transducer. This is much more apparent when compared with the even-diameter, thicker walls, regular pulsatility, and much more stable appearance of the common carotid.

As the transducer moves up the neck, the carotid is seen to widen out into the area of the carotid bulb. The bulb is the most common site of plaque and intimal thickening, which is usually seen to extend into the internal and/or external carotids directly above the bulb.

Contrary to what some believe, a perfect Y appearance of the carotid bifurcation is infrequently seen. The bifurcation tends to be rotated differently in certain individuals, and the appearance depends on the ability to obtain both vessels in the same view. For evaluation the internal and external carotids are best examined individually.

Longitudinally the internal carotid can be seen by moving the transducer in a posterior direction from the area of the bulb. It is a vessel generally of slightly larger diameter than the external carotid, tapering into regularly spaced walls that come off the bulb. Locating the distal common carotid and bulb, a slight counterclockwise rotation of the probe (on the right side of the neck) or clockwise rotation (on the left side of the neck) using the fingers should bring in the internal carotid origin.

The external carotid is seen by moving anteriorly and rotating the transducer central (Z) axis in a direction opposite that used to locate the internal carotid. It usually has a smaller diameter without the prominent widening frequently seen at the takeoff of the internal carotid. Branches (most commonly the superior thyroid artery near the origin or bulb and the lingual and facial branches above that) can usually be seen arising from the external carotid; finding branches confirms the visual identity of the external carotid since there are normally no branches off the internal carotid artery within the neck.

As stated in the anatomy section, several rare internal carotid branches of persistent fetal circulatory origin can occasionally be present. These are the ascending pharyngeal artery (which comes off distal to the bifurcation), the proatlantal artery, the hypoglossal artery, and the trigeminal artery (the latter three of which come off high in the neck between the C-1 and C-3 vertebrae). The ascending pharyngeal may be seen by duplex scanning in those rare cases where it occurs, and its presence may cause misidentification of the vessels at the bifurcation, since it may be mistaken for the superior thyroid artery (see Fig. 22-2). The internal and external are often transposed—the internal carotid lies medially and the external carotid laterally. The internal and external carotids also may be anterior and posterior, respectively, in one patient and inverted in another.

If there is doubt as to which artery is the internal and which is the external, several techniques can be used to assist in identification:

1. Look at the color-flow imaging pattern. The internal carotid normally has a lower intensity of color present throughout diastole; the external carotid often has more of an "on-off" appearance as flow drops to near zero in diastole because of the higher resistance in the external carotid from the branches.
2. Obtain Doppler spectra from each vessel; again, a lower-resistance pattern with flow above the baseline in diastole normally characterizes the internal carotid artery (ICA) and a higher-resistance waveform similar to that of an extremity artery waveform normally characterizes the external carotid artery (ECA) (compare the waveforms in Figs. 22-7 [ICA] and 22-9 [ECA]).
3. In cases of distal disease or vertebral insufficiency, it is possible for the external carotid to become "internalized." Flow patterns adopt a lower resistance pattern as cerebral collateral demands increase.

Occlusion of either the internal carotid or external carotid in these cases can make absolute visual identification nearly impossible by gray-scale, color-flow imaging, or Doppler. The examiner can perform temporal artery percussion to identify the external carotid. This technique is performed by first monitoring the arterial signal in the questioned bifurcation vessel using duplex and Doppler spectral waveforms; the examiner next should palpate the ipsilateral superficial temporal artery on the temple in front of the ear lobe (see Fig. 22-73 for the proper location) and feel for the pulse. Once located, the examiner should rhythmically and rapidly compress and release ("vibrate") the temporal artery and determine if there is any audible and visible effect on the signal in the artery being examined. If the artery being examined is the internal carotid, no effect on the signal occurs. If the artery is the external carotid, the rhythmic compressions cause short peaks in the signal (most visible in diastole) from brief flow reversal through the branch (see Fig. 22-9). This technique cannot be used reliably, however, if the external carotid is occluded or the temporal artery pulse cannot be palpated.

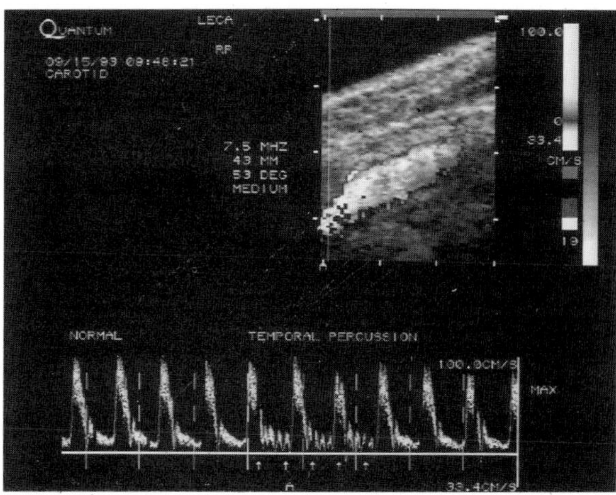

FIG. 22-9 Normal external carotid artery Doppler signal, showing the effect of superficial temporal artery percussion used to confirm Doppler identification of the external carotid. Each of the blips in diastole (marked) indicates a compression of the temporal artery.

When evaluating transversely, the common carotid appears as a rounded lumen posterior or lateral to the irregularly shaped jugular vein. The normal carotid retains its round appearance to the level of the bulb, where the diameter of the vessel becomes larger and begins to elongate as the bifurcation approaches.

The internal and external carotids are seen as two separate round lumina forming from the bulb as the transducer moves superiorly. The internal is larger than the external and positioned slightly posterior to the smaller round lumen of the external.

Disease in the carotid appears as low to moderate gray, soft, and smooth to irregularly edged deformations of the intima extending into the lumen. Calcific plaque is a bright echo with sonic dropout extending past the lesion. Calcific plaque can be incorporated into a "soft" (medium- to low-echogenic) plaque and is troublesome when the area of dropout obscures the deep wall and a superficial wall plaque is present. Ulcerated plaque can be seen as indentations or erosions in either soft-tissue plaque or the intima. For a detailed discussion of disease appearances, see *Interpretation of the Carotid Duplex Examination*.

Description of Carotid Duplex Color-Flow Characteristics

The normal color-flow pattern in the carotid artery system appears as uniform shades of red with a concentrated flow streamline (Fig. 22-10; see color images). An area of blue flow reversal or flow separation normally occurs at the carotid bulb, as described in Chapter 19, but the appear-

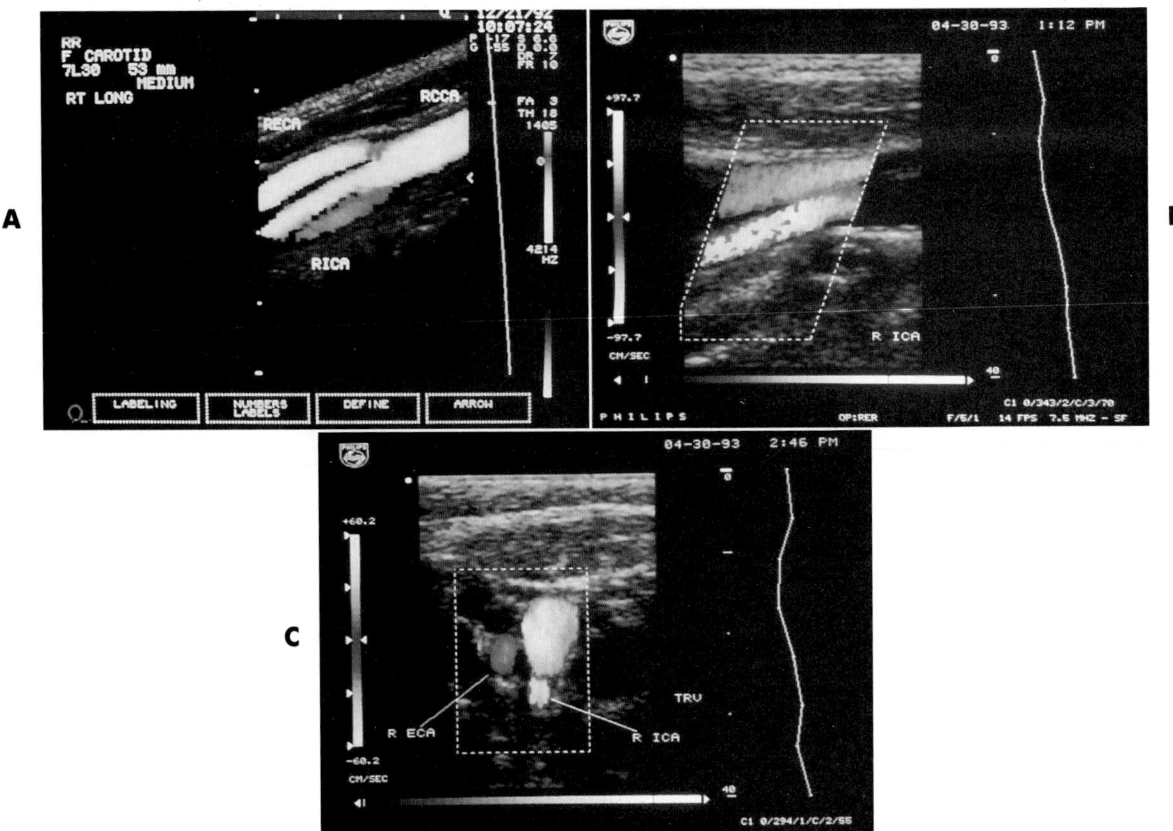

FIG. 22-10 Examples of normal color-flow imaging patterns in the carotid system. **A,** Longitudinal view of the carotid bifurcation, showing normal color-flow filling in the ICA (with an area of normal color-flow separation), ECA, and distal CCA. **B,** Longitudinal view of the internal carotid artery, with the internal jugular vein shown superficially to it, showing normal color-flow filling. **C,** Transverse image showing the relationships of the internal jugular vein, internal carotid artery, and external carotid artery (the medial side of the patient is to the left side of the image). Note the normal color-flow filling with a higher intensity of color in the ICA and a lesser, slower intensity in the ECA.

ance of shades of blue within the normal red color pattern is indicative of turbulence or flow disturbance, with the exception of some artifacts (also described in Chapter 19). Sometimes this disturbance is an expected normal variation, such as in the postendarterectomy vessel (see Fig. 22-82). In most cases, however, it implies the presence of stenosis and can occur on the downstream side of an obstruction (Fig. 22-11; see color image), within ulcerated areas, or along irregular plaque surfaces (flow eddies) (Fig. 22-12; see color image).

If color becomes regularly absent in the common or internal carotid artery at some point in the cardiac cycle (e.g., color flow is seen in systole but no color is seen in diastole—an "on-off" pattern), a distal occlusion may be implied (Fig. 22-13; see color images). Absence of color in diastole may, however, normally occur in the external carotid artery, since this finding characterizes a high-resistance vascular structure.

As mentioned in Chapter 19, the streamline can be a useful guide to the examiner, not only in determining the presence, location, and degree of stenosis, but also in size adjustment and placement of the sample volume for Doppler spectral waveform acquisition. Streamlines are also important factors in angle correction, because flow is seldom laminar through a stenosis. Axial and tangential flow jets can exist that might affect accurate alignment of the vector line (Fig. 22-14; see color image). The examiner must not, however, rely on color flow alone to determine flow velocities or patency of the vessel; color flow is most accurate and useful when combined with Doppler spectral waveforms and gray-scale evaluation with the color turned off (see below).

Examination Technique in Carotid Duplex Sonography. As discussed previously, a number of different types and configurations of duplex scanners are on the market. There are as many ways of holding and guiding the duplex transducer as there are types of transducers the vascular technologist may encounter. In spite of this the approach to imaging the carotids and vertebrals and obtaining duplex Doppler information from them is basically the same for

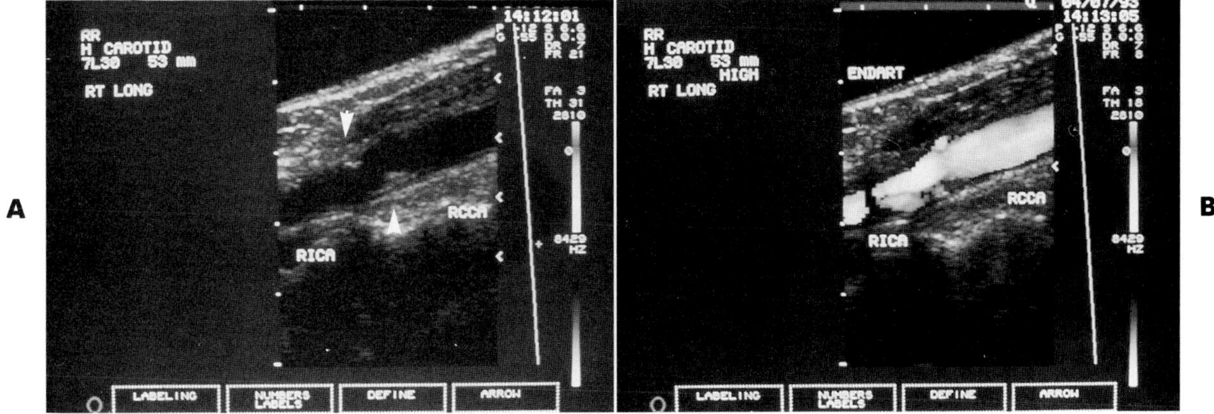

FIG. 22-11 A, Gray-scale image of an internal carotid origin with an asymmetric, ramplike recurrent stenotic plaque. **B,** Color-flow image of the same area, showing an increased streamline and blue flow separation on the distal side of the stenotic plaque.

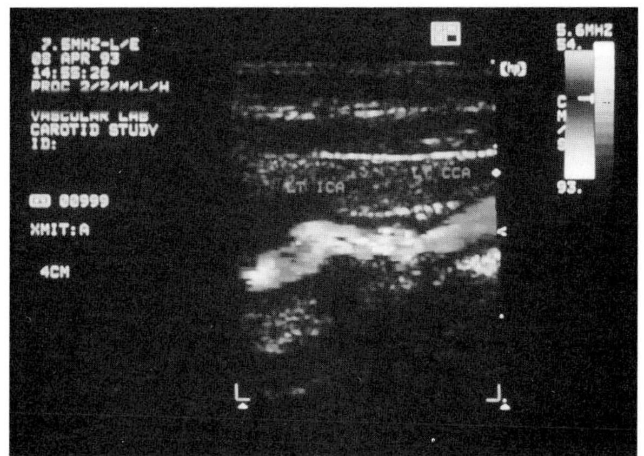

FIG. 22-12 Color-flow image of a carotid bifurcation showing blue flow eddies along the surface of an irregular plaque.

all machines. This section discusses these standard scanning techniques, all of which allow room for variation and adaptation as required.

The patient should lie supine with the head and shoulders lying on a pillow and the neck extended back to allow the examiner full access to the neck and supraclavicular area. The examiner requires the duplex scanner, a videotape recorder, a hardcopy printer or camera, and, optionally, a continuous-wave Doppler for blood-pressure measurement and periorbital examination.

On the majority of duplex scanners the image display should be oriented so that when imaging longitudinally, the head of the patient is to the left of the screen, following standard ultrasound imaging protocol. One duplex scanner (Biosound, Inc. Indianapolis, Indiana), however, orients the image sideways so that the patient's head may be at the top of the screen when the right side is being examined, and inverts the image when the left side is being examined. Some of the images accompanying the text are in this format and are so noted. When imaging transversely, the medial side of the patient should be toward the left as well. Older Biosound units place the medial side at the top of the image when examining the right side and at the bottom when examining the left side.

Initially, the carotids should be examined in the longitudinal plane. Three longitudinal approaches, or positions, afford optimal visualization of the neck vessels and allow almost the entire visible circumference of the carotids to be evaluated. Although the technologist should eventually synthesize all these positions into one smooth longitudinal examination, each of the approaches is discussed individually.

The first position used is the anterior position. The patient should turn his or her head to the left side to expose the right side of the neck, and vice versa when examining the left carotid. The sagittal plane of the head should be at about a 45-degree angle to the surface of the bed. The neck is coated with gel, and the transducer is placed on the neck, oriented for long-axis imaging. To obtain as true an anterior view as possible, the examiner should come in directly parallel with the sagittal plane of the neck (Fig. 22-15).

The examiner then examines the common carotid from the base to the bifurcation in long axis, being careful to show the artery continuously. Slight side-to-side motion of the transducer is used to pick up plaque, which may project from a lateral wall parallel with the plane of the examination (Figs. 22-16 and 22-17). It is noted, recorded on the videotape, or photographed for later reference.

On reaching the bifurcation, the examiner moves the transducer anteriorly and posteriorly to determine the takeoffs of the external and internal carotids at the bifurcation.

When the position and identification of each artery are determined, the examiner checks to see if any disease is present in the common carotid, bulb, and bifurcation areas. The transducer is moved accordingly to show the extent and degree of occlusion of the disease. Areas of disease are documented and the positioning described.

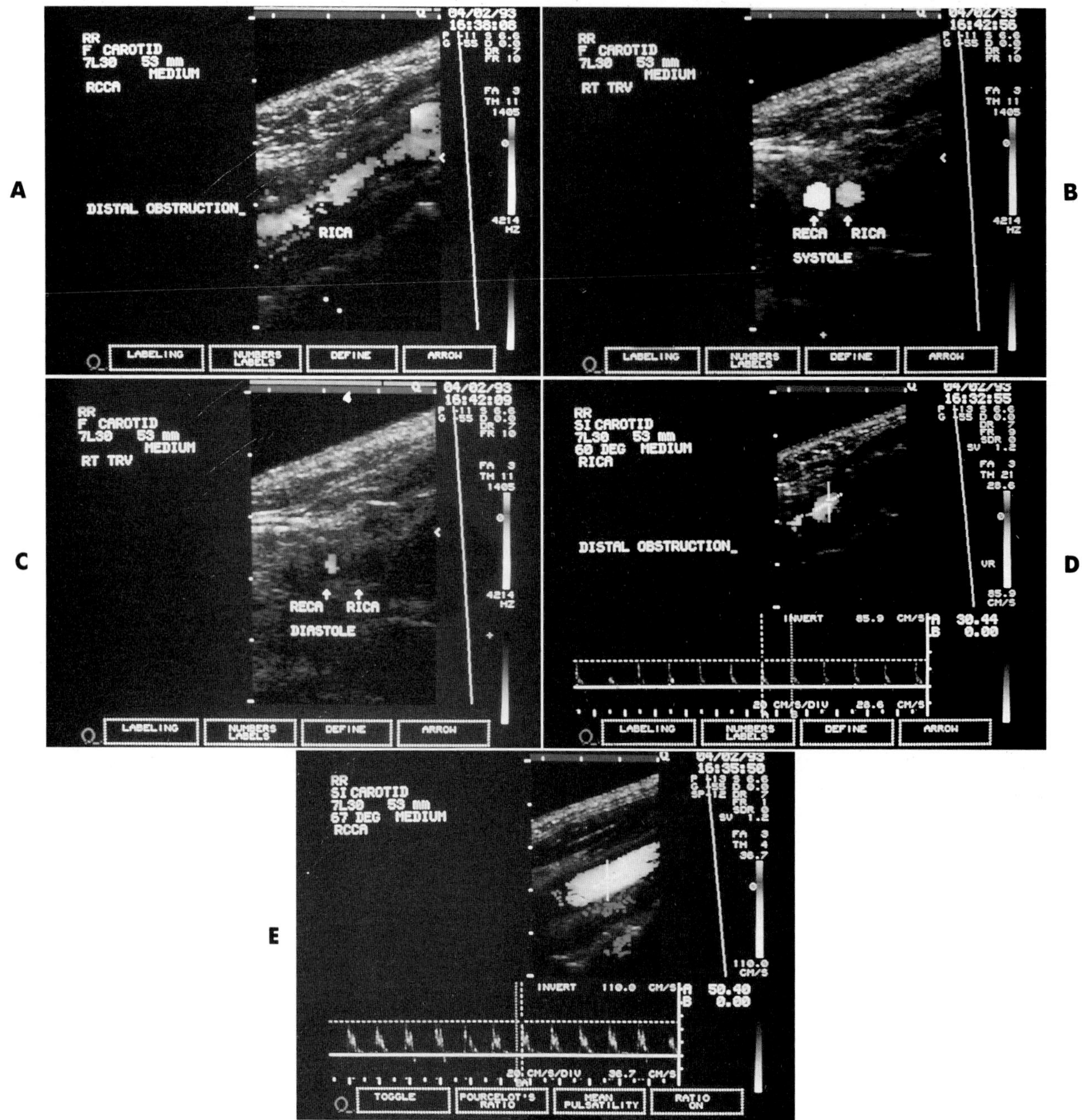

FIG. 22-13 Color-flow and Doppler spectral patterns seen in high distal ICA obstruction. **A,** Slightly stenosed but patent-appearing internal carotid artery, longitudinal view, with color flow seen in systole. **B,** Patent-appearing ICA and ECA in the transverse view, with color flow again seen in systole. **C,** Same view as in *B* but in diastole. Note absence of color flow in the ICA. **D,** Doppler spectral waveform in the ICA, showing abrupt systolic peak and absence of diastolic flow. **E,** Doppler spectral waveform in the CCA, showing the typical appearance of a preocclusion common carotid waveform with a complete absence of diastolic flow.

The examiner then determines the lie of the internal carotid and moves the transducer posteriorly toward the ear, while rotating it slightly along the plane of the long axis of the artery. The ICA is followed up as high as practicable.

The transducer next is moved anteriorly and rotated or angled to demonstrate the external carotid. As much of the artery as possible should be demonstrated.

The anterior view is not the best, since the probe comes against the mandible within the area of the bifurcation. It can, however, show disease that is not well seen in the other long-axis views.

The patient should turn his or her head a little more to facilitate the lateral position. The transducer is brought around so the beam intersects the artery perpendicular to

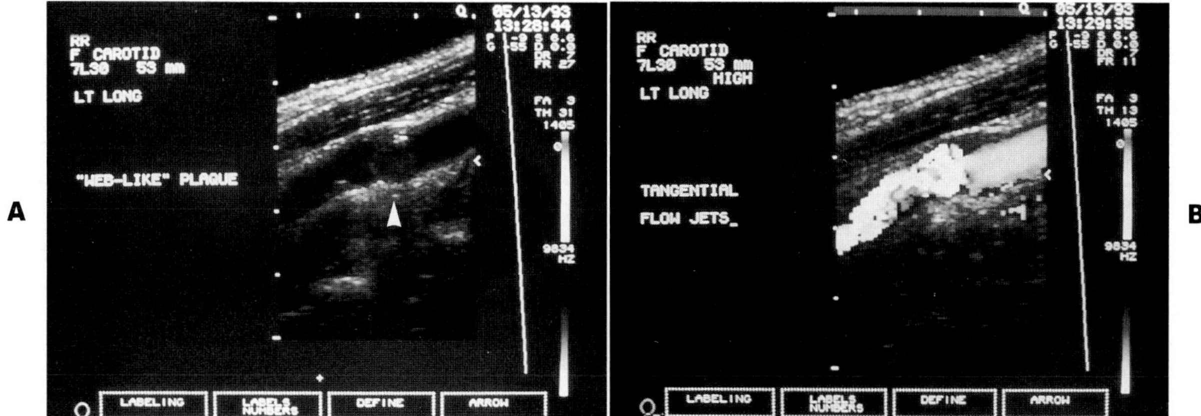

FIG. 22-14 A, Gray-scale image of a weblike soft plaque in the internal carotid artery origin. **B,** Color-flow image of the same area showing axial and tangential flow jets caused by the weblike plaque. Note the arcing appearance of the jets, which would necessitate careful alignment of the Doppler angle-correction vector line to ensure an accurate velocity calculation.

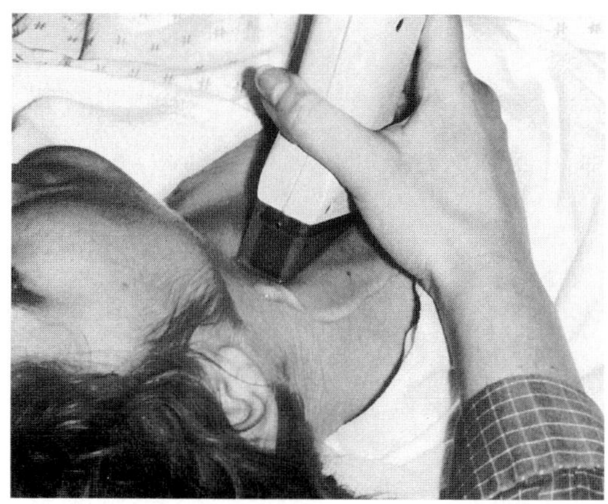

FIG. 22-15 Transducer positioning for longitudinal duplex scanning of the carotid arteries in the anterior imaging plane.

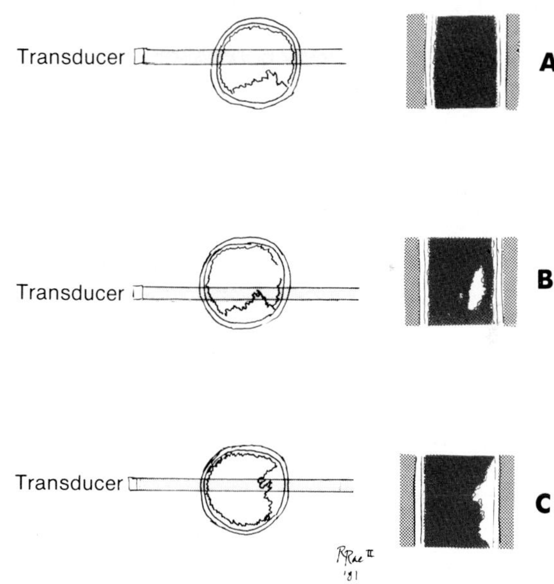

FIG. 22-16 Rocking the transducer. **A,** Plaque on the lateral walls may be missed by the parallel beam. **B,** Slight lateral motion of the transducer enables one to image the peaks of the plaque. **C,** When the transducer is moved to a different examination angle, the plaque is shown in cross section.

the sagittal plane of the head. The vessels are examined in the fashion described above (Fig. 22-18).

The patient should then turn his or her head as far as possible. In the posterior position the transducer is brought in from behind the sternocleidomastoid muscle and angled toward the anterior side of the patient. The arteries are located and examined as above. The common and bifurcation vessels may be deep in this view and not readily visualized. The Y appearance of the bifurcation tends to be seen in this position more often than in any other (Fig. 22-19).

As stated previously, these three positions can be combined into one smooth scan with the examiner compensating and instinctively turning the transducer, rocking the transducer, and shifting planes. When videotaping, the examiner should be certain to note position, where the transducer is being moved, what vessels are being imaged, the nature of the plaque and vessel walls, and the orientation of the vessel (e.g., cephalad is to the left of the image).

The carotid should appear as one continuous parallel structure (see "Description of the Carotid Duplex Real-Time Gray-Scale Image"), and it is important to show continuity (i.e., common carotid artery (CCA) to bulb, ECA connections to bulb, ICA origin, and bulb) even in cases of tortuosity, since the jugular vein is located so close to the carotid; maladjusted technical factors or a slip of the probe by an inattentive sonographer can often make the jugular seem to be part of the carotid (or even to be mistaken for it).

Some tips may help when imaging the carotids in the lon-

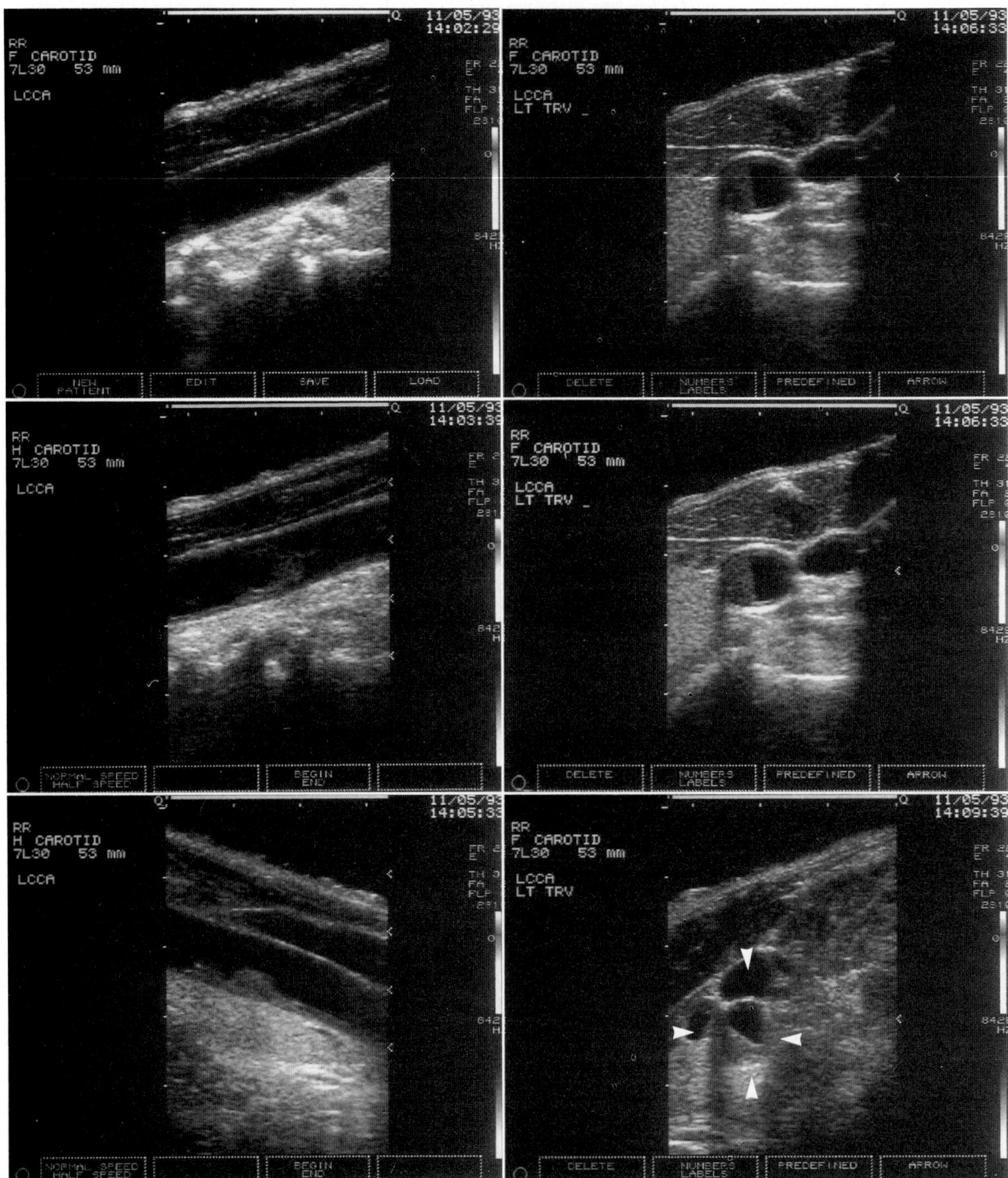

FIG. 22-17 Rocking and repositioning the transducer in longitudinal scanning. The principles are illustrated and transverse and longitudinal reference images for comparison are shown respectively. Plaque on a lateral wall is not detected by the ultrasound beam insonating through the center of a vessel (see Fig. 22-16, *A*). Slight lateral motion of the transducer reveals the peaks and surface detail of the plaque (see Fig. 22-16, *B*). Moving the transducer to a new scanning plane shows a different cross-sectional appearance of the vessel that details the plaque more clearly (see Fig. 22-16, *C*).

Continued.

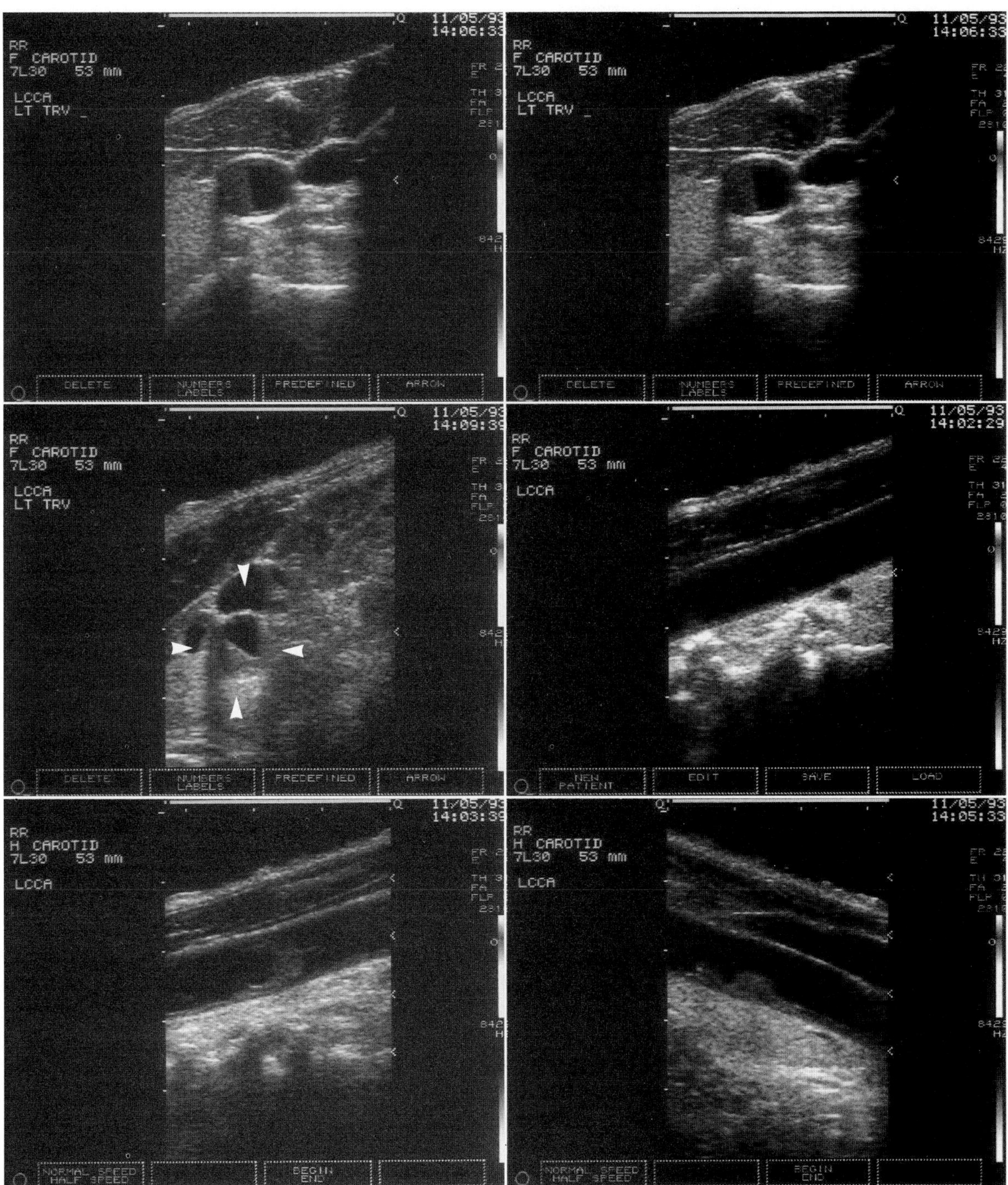

FIG. 22-17, cont'd. For legend see opposite page.

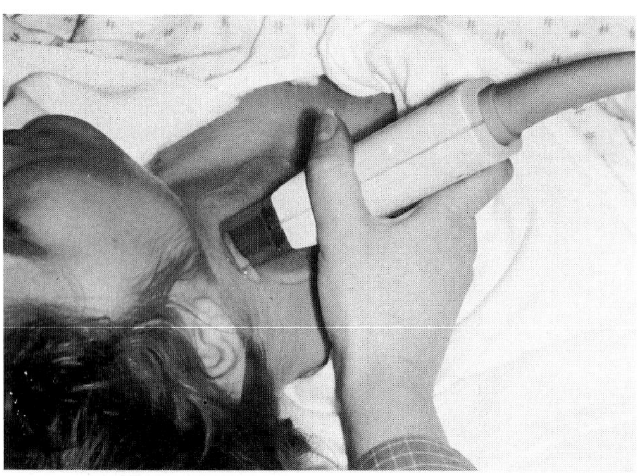

FIG. 22-18 Transducer positioning for longitudinal duplex scanning of the carotid arteries in the lateral imaging plane.

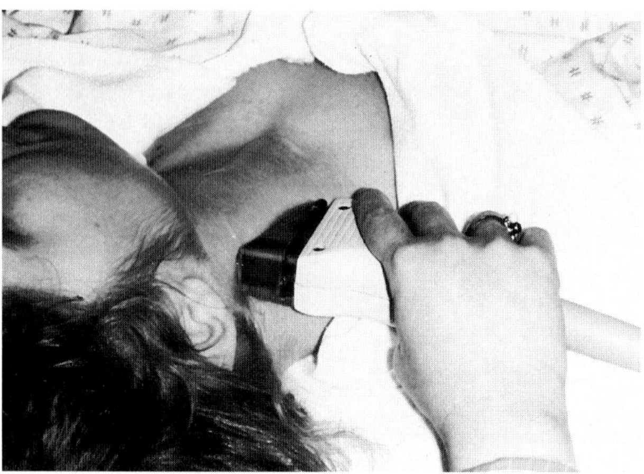

FIG. 22-19 Transducer positioning for longitudinal duplex scanning of the carotid arteries in the posterior imaging plane.

gitudinal plane. A common mistake of novice sonographers is to hold the wrist rigid when scanning, which doesn't allow him or her to follow the natural curves of the carotid. Keep the wrist loose, and use the fingers as pivot joints. Do not try to strangle the transducer. Also, novice sonographers forget to rock the transducer or change planes and positions, which often causes them to miss plaque on the lateral walls. In contrast, some move too much, sweeping past the very structures they are trying to image. Remember that distances in the carotids are very small and that you are imaging a vessel that is less than a centimeter in diameter so adjustments involve minimal motions of the transducer.

When scanning the neck, the examiner should hold the transducer around the body of the housing so that the little finger is actually in contact with the neck and in the gel, so to speak, as illustrated in the figures; this allows greater control and eliminates some of the hand and wrist fatigue that can result from holding it at the base end. This position also stabilizes the transducer better, and thus the probe is less likely to wander when the examiner is concentrating on controls or the image display. At the bifurcation, this position also helps in that the examiner can anchor the heel of the transducer (where the little finger is) at the bifurcation point and rotate the transducer along the Y axis using the thumb and fingers for more precise definition of the internal and external carotids. Remember that the common carotid is a major landmark; if you get lost while searching for the internal or external, reorient the transducer to the common carotid and begin moving cephalad again.

When using color-flow imaging, optimal color filling and saturation are obtained by setting the thresholds so that color ends at the vessel walls and does not "bleed" over into the intima or neck tissues. In longitudinal imaging the examiner may have to use a heel-toe technique along the longitudinal axis of the transducer to increase or decrease the Doppler angle and improve color-flow resolution. In transverse imaging the transducer should be angled slightly cephalad along the transverse axis to evoke a Doppler shift and ensure that flow away from the transducer appears in the proper color. In tortuous vessels the examiner may have to periodically invert the color map to accurately reflect the proper flow patterns and color assignments in the artery.

The arteries should be completely evaluated with gray scale only and color flow off if any areas of increased color-flow intensity are seen that cannot be accounted for by the joint color-flow–gray-scale image; color flow can obscure important gray-scale pathology if the flow patterns cross lateral wall lesions that would otherwise be seen (Fig. 22-20). Turning color-flow imaging off also increases the gray-scale sensitivity of the system (see the explanation in Chapter 19). It is a good idea to perform one scanning pass with the color flow off and another with color flow on to ensure that significant pathology has not been obscured; by the same token, disease that appears severe may be shown as being hemodynamically insignificant by the color-flow patterns across it.

Once the longitudinal images are obtained, the examiner should turn the probe 90 degrees to image the carotid arteries in the transverse plane. Although there is only one position here, the transducer can be directed at angles around the circumference of the neck to show the arteries and plaque surfaces optimally (Fig. 22-21).

The transducer should be placed at the clavicle level and slowly moved cephalad, following the common carotid to the bulb and bifurcation. Special attention should be given to documenting any plaque formations shown in the longitudinal views.

The area of the bifurcation should be evaluated for circumferential or partly obstructive plaques that may be at the origins but not extending into the internal or external carotids. The transducer can then be moved cephalad further to image the internal and external carotids. They should be followed cephalad as far as practicable. In cases where the internal and external carotids bifurcate at odd angles or

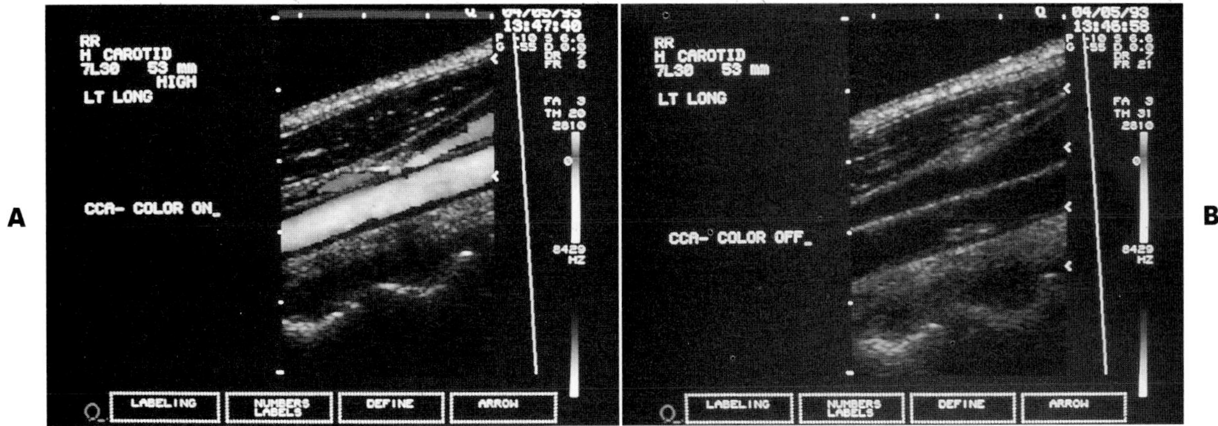

FIG. 22-20 A, Imaging of the carotid artery with color flow on shows a uniform, normal-appearing lumen with no obvious abnormalities. **B,** The color-flow information, however, obscures a lateral wall plaque that is not hemodynamically significant. This illustrates the need to examine vessels both with and without color-flow imaging on.

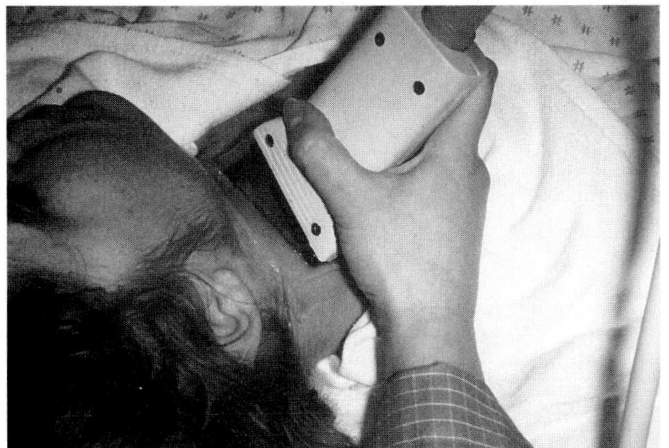

FIG. 22-21 Transducer positioning for duplex scanning of the carotid arteries in the transverse imaging plane.

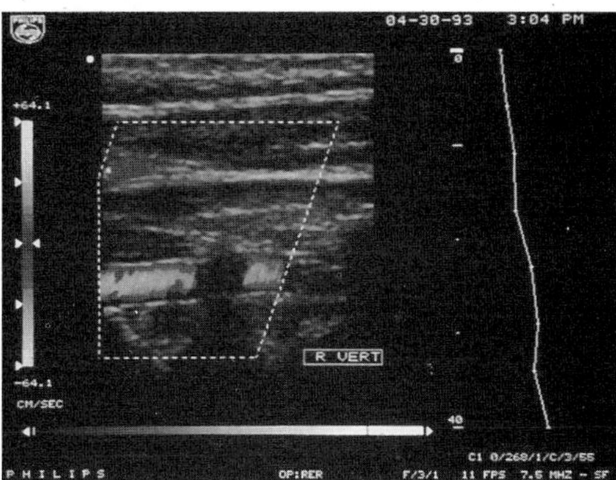

FIG. 22-22 A typical longitudinal color-flow appearance of the vertebral artery in the central cervical section of the neck, imaged between the transverse processes of the cervical vertebrae (shadow).

run deep to the transducer, accurate transverse evaluation may not be possible.

The internal carotid is generally (but not always) located posterior to the external carotid, with the external carotid positioned superficially to the deeper internal carotid on the duplex image. The examiner should bear in mind that anatomic variations frequently occur where the external carotid appears as the deeper vessel and may actually be posterior on the neck to the internal carotid. Again, the best ways to isolate and identify the bifurcation vessels are by using Doppler waveforms, color-flow pattern recognition, and temporal artery percussion in conjunction with the image appearance.

The vertebral arteries should always be included in the duplex evaluation of the carotids because they can be easily evaluated in the longitudinal plane. The origins of the vertebral arteries are often easier to evaluate using grayscale duplex to rule out disease of the origins (although some individuals do not have a satisfactory body habitus to enable easy visualization of the origins). The main trunks of the vertebral arteries can be imaged between the transverse processes of the cervical vertebrae; they are especially easy to see using color-flow imaging (Fig. 22-22; see color image).

The transducer is placed in long axis lateral to the common carotid and above the clavicle, then moved laterally and slightly cephalad (Fig. 22-23). Look for regularly spaced areas of shadowing with what appear to be vessel walls between them, then attempt to follow the vessel to its origin at the subclavian. Following the subclavian artery laterally starting at the carotid area and looking for the vertebral origin also works. The vertebral is often easier to find on the right side, since the examiner can trace the origin of the right common carotid to the innominate artery and then follow the subclavian artery laterally from the

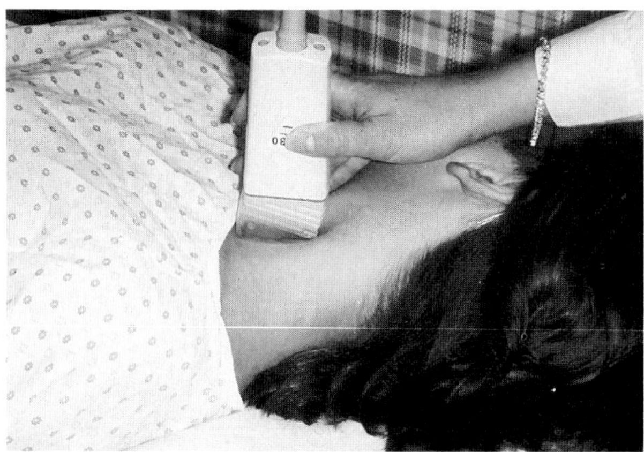

FIG. 22-23 Transducer placement for duplex scan–Doppler spectral evaluation of the vertebral artery.

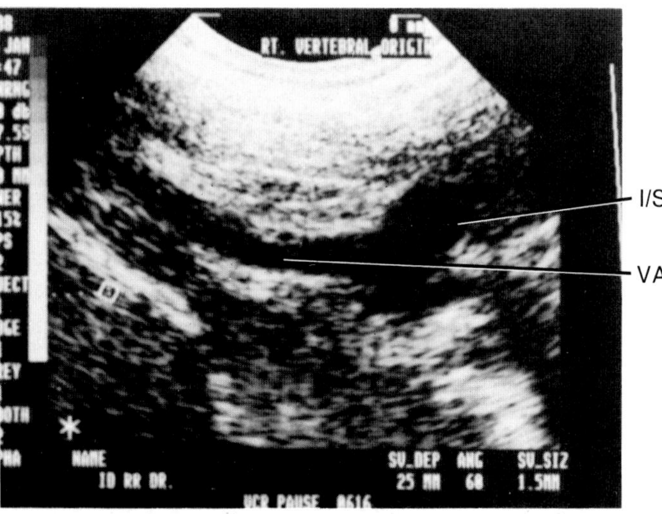

FIG. 22-24 Normal sonographic appearance of the vertebral artery origin and proximal vertebral artery.

innominate-carotid bifurcation to the vertebral origin (Fig. 22-24).

DUPLEX DOPPLER SPECTRAL WAVEFORM ACQUISITION

Gray-scale and color-flow imaging evaluation of the carotid system can demonstrate the presence of disease and allow approximate degrees of stenosis to be ascertained, but these modalities alone are insufficient to accurately grade the percentage and hemodynamic significance of the stenosis. The examiner must acquire duplex Doppler spectral waveforms from appropriate sites to document the flow states at each level of the carotid system.

During the imaging portion of the examination, the duplex Doppler should be used primarily for vessel identification and initial estimates of flow so that the examiner can concentrate on identifying the presence, location, and extent of any disease present. Once the examiner has become familiar with the location of visible plaque or stenosis, a systematic evaluation of the Doppler hemodynamics should be performed.

Duplex Doppler spectral waveforms should be routinely taken and recorded from the following:

1. The proximal common carotid artery.
2. The distal common carotid artery, just below the bulb.
3. The internal carotid artery about 1 cm distal to its origin, away from the "flared" takeoff.
4. The external carotid artery about 1 cm distal to its origin.
5. The vertebral artery, either in the proximal precervical segment or between two vertebral interspaces.

The above waveforms are sufficient in a normal carotid system. If prominent plaque is present and appears to comprise a significant stenosis either by visual estimation or with color-flow imaging, then additional waveforms should be obtained:

1. At the point of maximum stenosis, where velocities appear to be the highest.
2. Downstream to the stenosis, to document the hemodynamic effect distally.

These additional waveforms should be obtained at all stenotic sites within the common, internal, and external carotids, preferably in the longitudinal scan plane.

As each spectral waveform is obtained, the examiner should angle-correct the flow vector (see Chapter 19), using color-flow imaging to align the vector along the streamline. Electronic calipers should then be used on the spectral waveforms to measure two specific velocity factors for documentation and later interpretation. These factors are the peak systolic velocity (or frequency) and the end-diastolic velocity (or frequency). Bear in mind that Doppler velocities obtained in a transverse position cannot be angle-corrected because the precise angle of flow insonation is unknown. If some estimation of flow is required in these cases, frequency criteria should be used rather than velocity criteria.

The peak systolic velocity (PSV) or frequency is measured at the peak of the systolic component of the waveform. The end-diastolic velocity (EDV) or frequency is measured at the lowest point of diastole, usually at the end of the cardiac cycle just before the initial upslope of another systolic peak (Fig. 22-25).

More discussion on the use of these parameters in interpretation is presented next.

Carotid Duplex Examination Protocol

The following is a sample examination protocol that summarizes the technique used to evaluate the carotid system:

1. Begin in a longitudinal position and evaluate the common, internal, and external carotid arteries with gray-scale and color-flow imaging, evaluating the vessels for plaque and the presence of stenosis. Use the anterior, lateral, and posterior imaging planes as needed to opti-

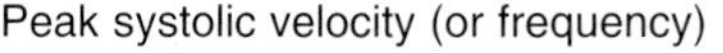

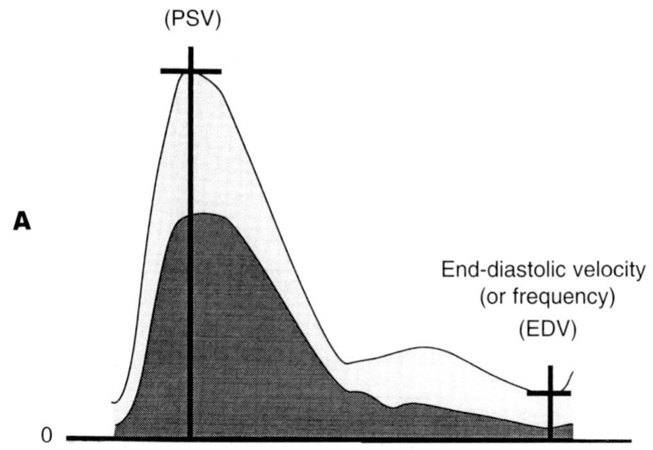

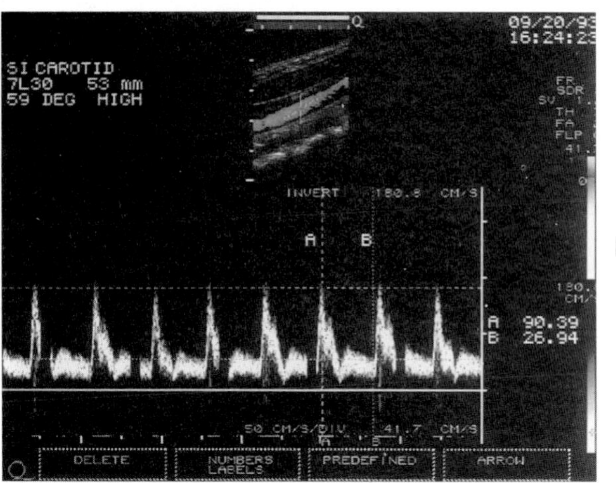

FIG. 22-25 A, Graphic showing the proper locations on the Doppler waveform to measure peak systolic velocity or frequency (PSV or PSF) and end-diastolic velocity or frequency (EDV or EDF). **B,** Doppler spectral waveform from the common carotid artery, showing these measurements being obtained (A = PSV, B = EDV).

mally visualize the vessels. If the common carotid origin and subclavian area can be seen, include these in the examination.

2. Obtain routine Doppler spectral waveforms from sample sites in the proximal and distal CCA, the proximal and distal ICA, and the ECA. Additional waveforms should be obtained at and distal to any areas of stenosis.
3. Rotate the transducer to a transverse position and evaluate the common carotid from the base of the neck, scanning cephalad to evaluate the entire cervical carotid system to above the mandible level if possible. Be certain that image orientation is consistent and demonstrate the bulb, ICA, and ECA as completely as possible.
4. Evaluate the vertebral artery from the origin and within the cervical segment, and document flow direction and appearance.
5. Repeat steps 1 to 4 for the contralateral side. (Some institutions, incidentally, prefer to switch steps 1 and 3, starting in transverse.)

TECHNICAL DIFFICULTIES IN THE CAROTID DUPLEX EXAMINATION AND THEIR RESOLUTION

Many variations in the anatomy and pathology in the carotid system can occasionally hinder the examination, mislead the examiner, or provide findings that potentially result in misdiagnosis by the interpreter. This section discusses some of these variations, the obstacles they create, and potential ways to resolve them.

Problem 1. The location of the bifurcation varies in every individual, even from side to side in some people. Occasionally the bifurcation is located partially or totally above the inferior margin of the mandible, making it unreachable by the transducer. In these cases, it is possible to miss potentially significant stenoses.

Solution. Scanning from a very posterior plane (see above), increasing image depth, and angling up underneath the mandible may improve the image and allow better visualization of the bifurcation vessels; switching to a lower-frequency transducer or from a linear to a sector or curved-linear transducer also may increase visibility.

Problem 2. Fat and prominent musculature, especially in the short-necked patient, may cause the artery to lie very deep and be out of the optimal focusing range of the transducer. Sometimes the fat and tissue have an increased acoustic impedance, which attenuates the sound beam, especially at a higher imaging frequency. Color-flow patterns may be diminished or poorly defined.

Solution. Using and optimizing focal transmit zones, if available, may help; switching to a lower-frequency transducer or boosting the transmit power (within defined practical and safe limits) may clarify the vessels and improve the color-flow image filling as well.

Problem 3. Calcified plaque, as mentioned previously, may cause prominent areas of acoustic dropout in the area of the plaque, which may obscure all or part of the bifurcation or vessel under examination if it occurs along the superficial wall. Determination of any underlying luminal reduction is thus hampered.

Solution. Changing scanning planes (e.g., from anterior to posterior), rocking the transducer across the vessel, and using color-flow imaging to search for Doppler sample placement windows and document flow patterns distal to the lesion can help minimize the effect of calcified plaque. Be aware, however, that a low percentage of calcified arteries cannot be evaluated.

Problem 4. Congenital anomalies and anatomic varia-

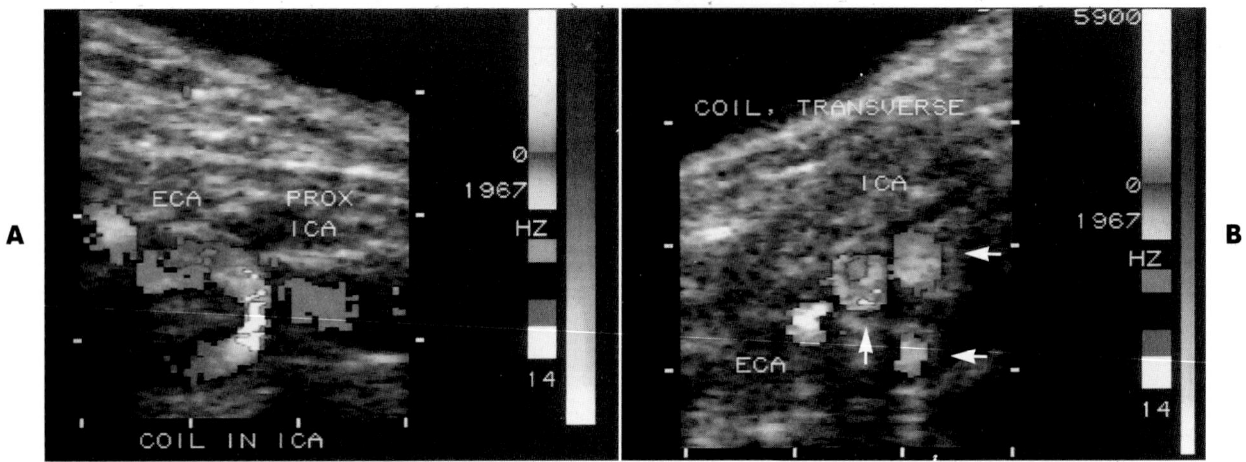

FIG. 22-26 Internal carotid artery coil. **A,** Longitudinal color-flow image partially showing loop in ICA. Note the color change to blue showing flow traveling away from the transducer face in the looped segment. **B,** Transverse image in the same patient. Note the false appearance of three lumens, all part of the same ICA *(arrows);* color-flow imaging helps delineate the flow direction in the visualized segments that make up the coil.

tions can create numerous problems for both the examiner and the interpreter.

Tortuosity of the artery makes definition of both imaging and color-flow patterns very difficult; if improperly documented, an incompletely visualized curving or twisting artery may mimic a stenosis or occlusion (especially with areas of absent or increased flow velocity from poor transducer-vessel angles). Occasionally, loops of tortuous arteries appear as more than one vessel (especially in a transverse plane) (Fig. 22-26; see color images). Tortuous vessels may appear as coils, S-shaped vessels, or bifurcations widely splayed at up to 90-degree angles from the common carotid (Fig. 22-27).

Coarctation or kinking of an artery may occur; although this may occur normally, the flow velocities may change abruptly, and a stenotic flow state may be implied if flow angles and streamlines are not carefully aligned when Doppler waveforms are obtained. Some kinks can be tight enough to actually induce a stenosis, and velocity readings confirm it; this reaffirms the need to confirm angle-streamline alignment.

Anatomic variations and anomalies can also exist, such as separate internal carotids and external carotids with no common carotid from the subclavians and low bifurcations. The variety of these anomalies precludes any set approach to evaluation, since no two may be alike.

Solution. Careful documentation of the arterial course by videotape and with color-flow imaging should be used to define the vessel or vessels very clearly so that no misinterpretation can occur. The examiner may need to rely on creativity in placing Doppler sample cursors or in finding an ideal scanning plane. It is usually possible to find one plane that allows a full visualization of the architecture of the segment.

Problem 5. The internal jugular vein may occasionally be confused with the common carotid artery (usually by the inexperienced or in cases where an abnormally high central venous pressure keeps the vein dilated).

Solution. Transverse planar imaging to compare the characteristics of the vessels seen can usually define which is the artery and which the vein. Color-flow imaging usu-

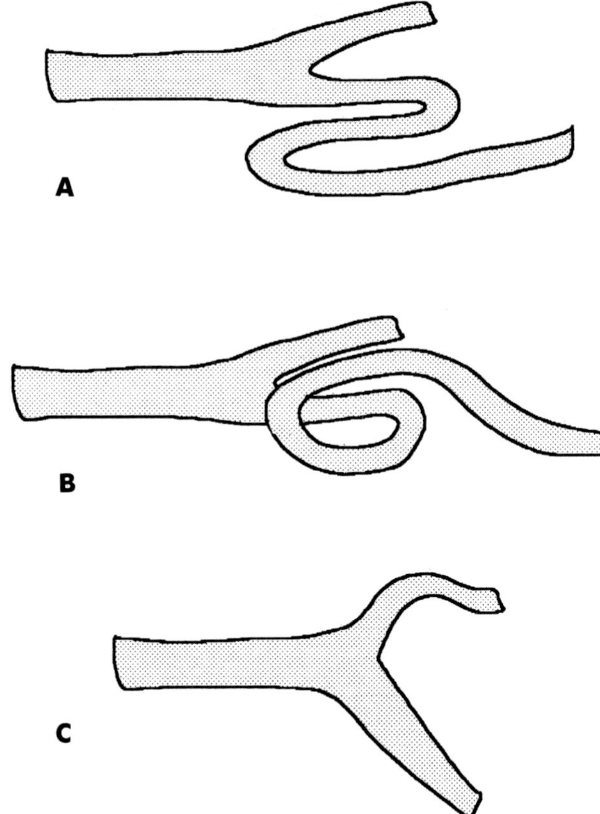

FIG. 22-27 Potential anatomic variations in the internal carotid artery and bifurcation. **A,** S-shaped tortuosity. **B,** Coil or loop. **C,** Widely splayed ICA and ECA at the bifurcation. (Courtesy Richard E. Rae, Indianapolis.)

ally provides instant recognition as well, as does spectral Doppler sampling. If in doubt, image in transverse, then have the patient perform a Valsalva maneuver; the vein should dilate markedly (if there is no proximal obstruction).

Problem 6. Transposition or inversion of the positions of the internal and external carotid arteries can cause problems for both examiner and interpreter. Misdiagnoses occur often when the external carotid is severely stenosed or occluded and the internal carotid is not, and the examiner or interpreter makes the wrong assumption regarding the flow patterns and appearances. Although the internal carotid statistically tends to harbor origin disease more often, it is indeed possible for the external carotid to be the only branch affected.

Solution. The examiner should use spectral Doppler sampling, color-flow pattern recognition, transverse imaging and size comparison, identification of any branches present off the visualized vessel, and the temporal percussion test (described previously) as needed to identify the arteries and their distinguishing features. Careful evaluation is often all that is really required.

Problem 7. Machine artifacts may mimic leading edges of plaques or specular echoes within the lumen such as are seen in homogeneous plaque.

Solution. Careful adjustment of technical factors, routine maintenance and calibration of equipment (including phantom calibration), and the use of color-flow imaging, Doppler, or both should eliminate any questionable false echoes. Color flow is especially valuable, since a significant plaque creates a filling defect in the color patterns. If a reverberation artifact or color-flow mirror-image artifact seems to be present after adjustments have been made, the examiner should simply move the transducer to see if the questioned lines or echoes move with the transducer (artifact) or stay in the same apparent location in the vessel (disease).

Finally, there is occasionally evidence of distal flow obstruction implied by resistant patterns in the Doppler waveforms and color-flow patterns in otherwise patent-appearing cervical arteries. If further information is needed, the examiner may wish to use either an indirect test (e.g., periorbital Doppler or oculoplethysmography) or a direct intracranial test (e.g., transcranial Doppler or transcranial duplex) to evaluate the distal vertebral circulation, circle of Willis, and intracranial segments of the internal carotid. These other techniques are discussed later in this chapter.

Interpretation of the Carotid Duplex Examination

On completing the examination, the study should be interpreted based on all the data collected according to guidelines established by the staff of the individual vascular laboratory or ultrasound department. These guidelines are likely to vary widely because of numerous factors and preferences, including the specialty of the interpreting physician (e.g., radiologist, vascular surgeon, cardiologist) and which published or internally generated criteria are in use.

Basic diagnostic factors should be common to every protocol, however, and these are discussed here, along with descriptions of published diagnostic criteria.

The carotid duplex examination (or for that matter, any duplex examination) should always be interpreted in conjunction with a videotape of the study. This enables the interpreting physician to appreciate the real time identification of the arteries and directly observe the changes taking place within the vessel. Since Doppler and color-flow data are dynamic, the changes with the cardiac cycle and the audible changes are more easily appreciated when videotape is used than on static hard-copy images.

Hard-copy documentation should be obtained of representative images and of Doppler spectral waveforms at the respective sites mentioned previously; in this way the extent and location of plaque, the velocity measurements, and the color-flow hemodynamics can be permanently documented for both follow-up reference and long-term storage. Some interpreters have resorted to drawing representations of plaque locations on a schematic of the carotid arteries; this older method may provide a visual estimate and record but is subject to the artistic ability of the interpreter and also does not always accurately reflect anomalous vascular changes or the precise architecture of the plaque. An actual longitudinal and transverse hard-copy image is a much better reference for both the interpreter and for technologists to use during follow-up.

Interpretation of the Carotid Duplex Image

Interpretation of the image results must take into account the Doppler spectral findings and those of color-flow imaging. Making a diagnosis based on the image alone can result in a partial and often inaccurate diagnosis, especially if color-flow imaging is not available; a patent-appearing internal carotid artery may actually be totally occluded with fresh thrombus, or a high carotid siphon or middle-cerebral artery obstruction may be present. Without accompanying hemodynamic information, the diagnostic picture is incomplete.

By the same token, direct carotid Doppler studies or periorbital examinations performed with continuous-wave probes and no imaging are only diagnostic when a stenosis is severe enough to cause significant hemodynamic alteration or turbulence. They also do not permit exact identification of the location of the stenosis and cannot generally isolate multiple stenosed segments.

Criteria for Defining and Localizing Carotid Disease

Characterizing and categorizing the visual data obtained in the cerebrovascular system can be a very involved process, one that is highly subjective and often open to variations in individual interpretation.

Although many investigators have attempted to sonographically determine what morphologic processes are taking place in a plaque (e.g., hemorrhage, calcification), atherosclerotic plaque that is visualized is generally character-

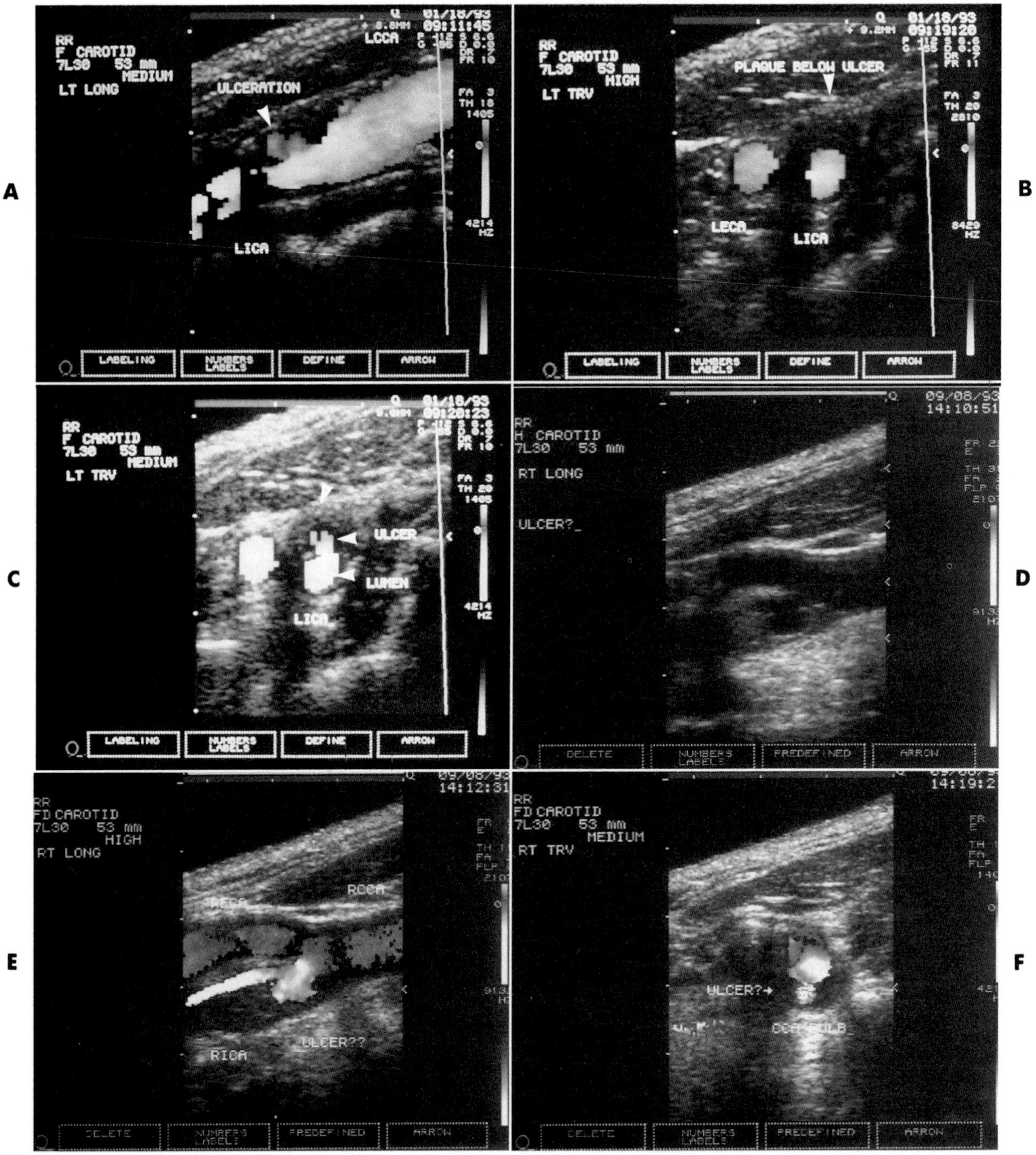

FIG. 22-28 Ulcerated plaque. **A,** Longitudinal color-flow image showing a distinct ulceration in a heterogeneous plaque on the superficial wall of the ICA origin. Note the blue color-flow reversal within the ulceration. **B,** Transverse image in the same patient, showing the proximal portion of the plaque below the ulceration. **C,** Transverse image across the ICA and plaque at the level of the ulceration. Note the distinct pocket within the plaque and the color flow reversal within it, which confirms the presence of the ulcer in two separate imaging planes. **D,** Longitudinal gray-scale image of a carotid bifurcation, showing a distinct focal ulceration in a homogeneous plaque on the posterior wall of the proximal ICA. Note the well-defined pocket. **E,** Longitudinal color-flow image showing the flow patterns into the ulceration and the jet of flow across the smooth distal taper of the plaque. **F,** Transverse image across the ECA and the ICA at the level of the ulceration. Note the well-defined borders of the plaque and the saccular appearance of the pocket. The color-flow disturbance within the ulcer again confirms its presence in two separate imaging planes.

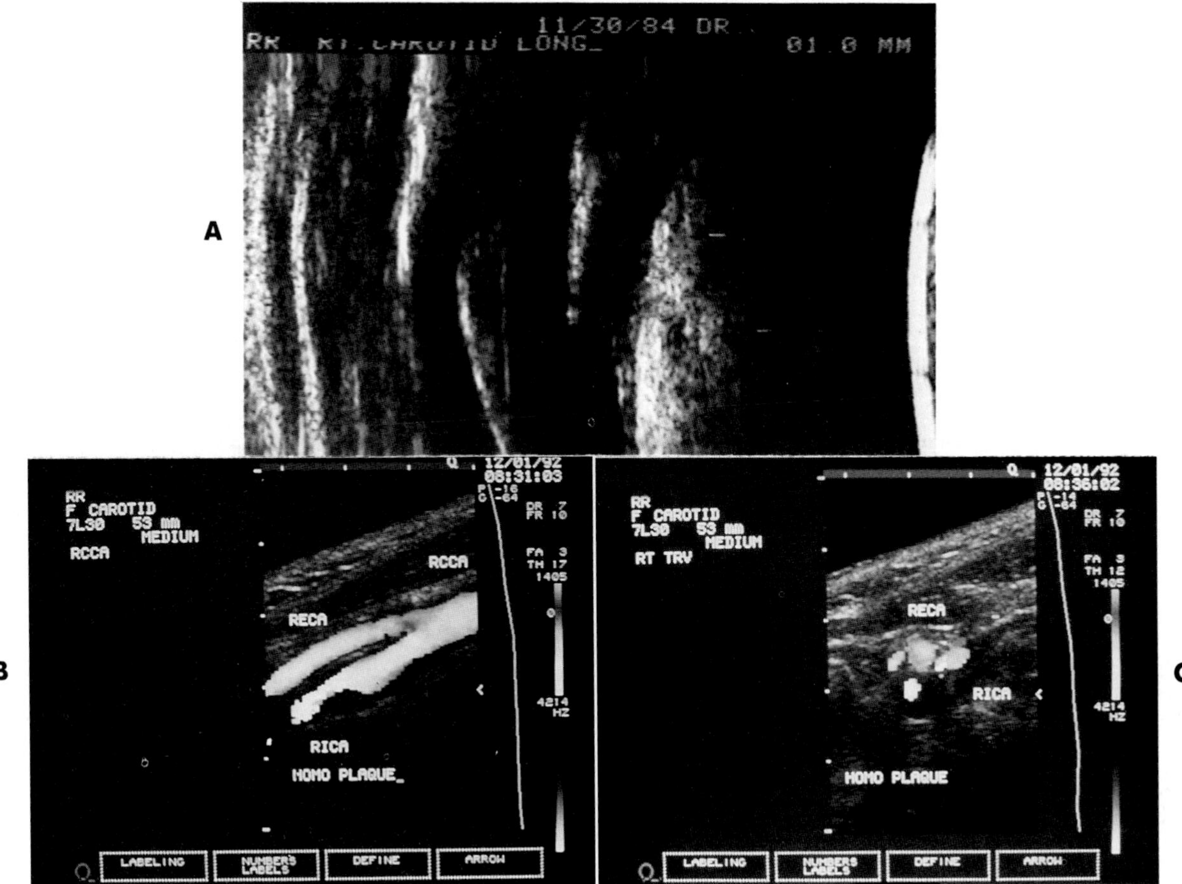

FIG. 22-29 A, Sonographic appearance of a smooth, fatty subintimal plaque. (The head of the patient is oriented toward the top in this image). **B,** Sonographic longitudinal appearance of a hemodynamically significant fatty (homogeneous) plaque in the distal ICA. **C,** Transverse view of the homogeneous plaque in the ICA shown in **B.**

ized as either homogeneous or heterogeneous in appearance.[10,46] The presence of distinct ulceration should not be diagnosed unless the ulcer is deep and can be documented in both longitudinal and transverse images (preferably with correlative color flow) (Fig. 22-28; see color images). Plaque surfaces are best classified as either smooth or irregular.[10,46]

Plaque Morphology and Sonographic Characteristics

The progressive changes in morphology and categories of plaque can be distinguished by certain patterns of appearance:

The fatty streak and fatty plaque appear as a low- to moderate-level gray homogeneous thickening or elevations of the intima, extending into the lumen from one or both walls (Fig. 22-29; see color images). The intima normally follows the vessel walls closely, making intimal thickening or plaqueing dramatically obvious when well visualized. This appearance is also typical of so-called soft plaque and thrombus.

The fibrous plaque appears as a moderate to highly echogenic luminal irregularity or focal plaque, or "mixed plaque" (Fig. 22-30). Low-level gray areas often are found alongside areas of higher echogenicity. These appear as elevations and focal enlargements into the lumen.

The calcified plaque is bright with high echogenicity and sonic dropout extending deep and parallel with the beam path (Fig. 22-31). The inability of the ultrasound beam to penetrate calcific plaque often obscures areas deep to the plaque and can obliterate the lumen, making stenosis calculation almost impossible across the plaque area. Relocation of the transducer may be necessary to look around the area of calcification. If color-flow imaging is used, flow windows can be detected more easily between shadows for Doppler sample volume placement. The color-flow streamline and presence or absence of turbulence on the distal side of a plaque shadow can also help the examiner determine whether the calcific shadow obscures a hemodynamically significant lesion (Fig. 22-32; see color images).

The complex plaque may have a speckled appearance, with areas of calcification within (Fig. 22-33). The calcium and denser-appearing areas are often the result of necrosis or intraplaque hemorrhage. The lesion also may have an extremely irregular and pock-marked appearance on the in-

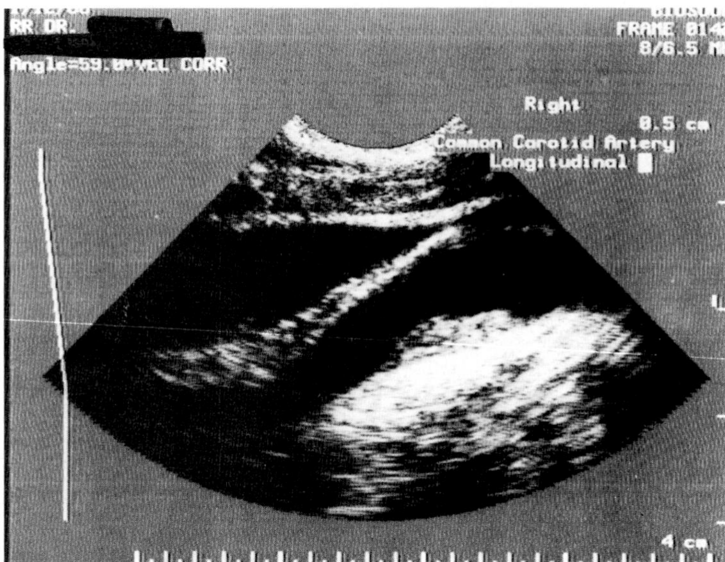

FIG. 22-30 Sonographic appearance of fibrous plaque.

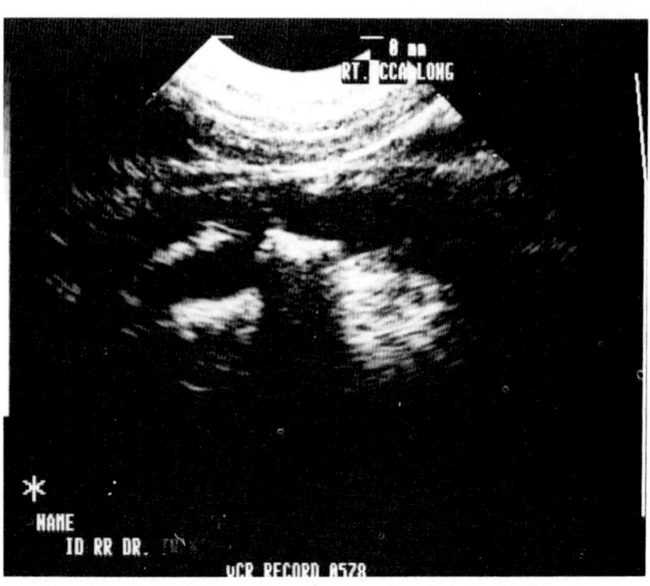

FIG. 22-31 Sonographic appearance of calcified plaque.

timal side; in some cases the fine line of the intimal lining can appear disrupted in places. Although a cratered appearance may be noted and even the occasional ulceration, ulcers should not be identified as such unless they are deep enough to be shown clearly in longitudinal and transverse planes; color-flow imaging also may confirm the presence of a flow pocket within the plaque (see Fig. 22-28).

Complete arterial occlusion usually is identified by one of the following distinctive image appearances:

1. A lumen completely filled with soft specular echoes distal to a patent vessel (Fig. 22-34).
2. A lumen completely filled with bright, heterogeneous echoes distal to a patent vessel (Fig. 22-35).
3. A chronically atrophied vessel distal to a dense echogenic plaque at the origin. The artery often tapers abruptly and may appear smaller than an accompanying vessel (e.g., the external carotid), especially in the transverse plane (Fig. 22-36; see color image).

In some cases the artery segment distal to a complete occlusion reconstitutes from collaterals or from retrograde flow through the external carotid system (Fig. 22-37; see color image).

There usually is a distinct border between the occluded and patent segments of the vessel, often at the origin of the occluded artery. Color-flow imaging demonstrates this well (Fig. 22-38; see color image).

Flow is not detectable within the occluded segment using Doppler or color flow, although a blip might be seen on the waveform, which may represent vertical motion of the vessel from proximal pulsatility rather than from an actual flow presence. With color-flow imaging, this usually manifests as a short-duration flash artifact (see Chapter 19). Doppler spectral waveforms proximal to an occlusion become characteristic of high-resistance and color-flow imaging changes and can also alert the examiner to the presence of a distal occlusion; these characteristics are discussed next.

Atypical Sonographic Abnormalities of the Carotid Artery

Carotid aneurysms

Aneurysms appear as widely dilated or ectatic areas of the common carotid, bulb, internal carotid, or external carotid but occur more frequently in the bulb or area of the internal carotid. Plaque formations, mural thrombus, calcification, and occasionally dissection of the artery may occur in combination with an aneurysm. Aneurysmal dilation usually is quite distinct compared with the normal widening of the carotid bulb area or origin of the internal

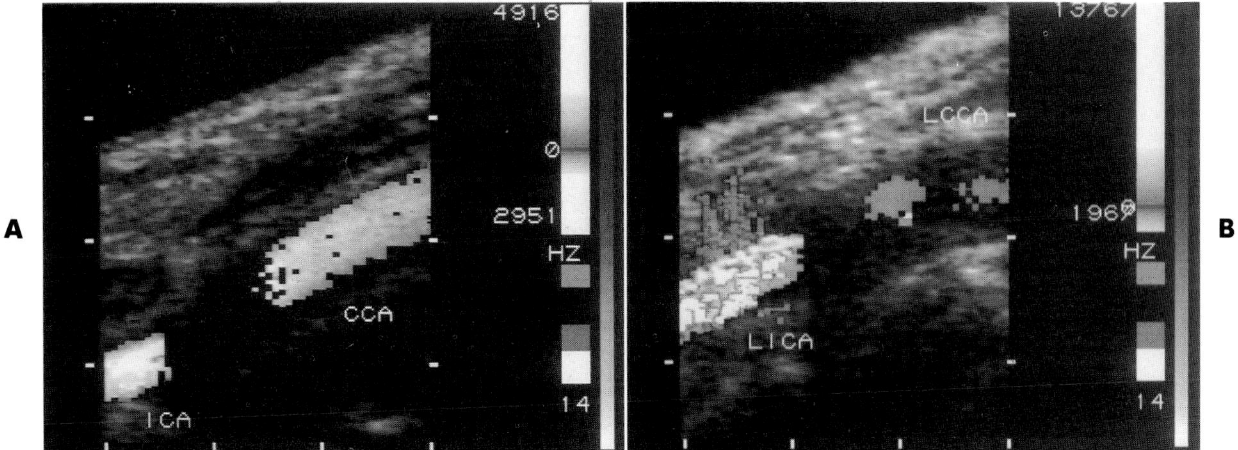

FIG. 22-32 Calcific plaque obscures the origins of the internal carotid arteries in both these examples. **A,** The color-flow patterns distal to the calcific shadow are uniform with no turbulence and a normal streamline, implying a hemodynamically insignificant stenosis. **B,** A jet streamline is seen along the superficial wall distal to the calcific shadow with marked flow separation and a visualized bruit, implying the presence of a severe stenosis hidden beneath the calcific shadow.

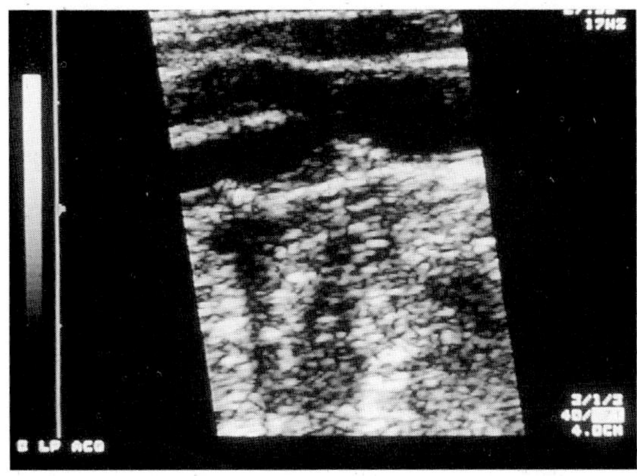

FIG. 22-33 Sonographic appearance of a complex (heterogeneous) lesion.

carotid. It is important to note that often patients are referred for suspected aneurysm in the low neck or supraclavicular region, with a prominent pulsatile mass noted. These pulsatile masses very often turn out to be prominent normal subclavian arteries or common carotid origins, which are unusually superficial and project into the supraclavicular fossa (Fig. 22-39; see color image); thus the examiner should evaluate and document any suspected aneurysm carefully.

An example of a carotid aneurysm is shown in "Carotid Duplex Sonography," case 9 (see Fig. 22-69).

Carotid dissection

Carotid dissection is not common but may manifest sonographically as a characteristic "extra lumen" within the confines of a relatively uniform-appearing carotid artery. Color-flow patterns usually make this diagnosis easier because retrograde flow may be seen in the false channel and regular antegrade flow in the true channel. Gray-scale imaging at an angle perpendicular to the dissection may help visualize the septumlike dissected inner wall. Careful evaluation with gray-scale, color-flow imaging, and Doppler spectral sampling may help reveal the inflow point. In some cases a flow entrance and a flow exit may also be detected.

An example of a carotid dissection is shown in "Carotid Duplex Sonography," case 8 (see Fig. 22-68).

Unstable lesions

The examiner should be alert to the existence of any number of unstable lesions that may occasionally be detected during the course of the carotid duplex examination. These are distinct dynamic intravascular phenomena that move or have motion within, as opposed to the typical stationary plaque. These lesions can, among other forms, manifest as loose intimal flaps, free-floating moving thrombus, pseudovalves, or partially organized liquefied thrombus within an ulcerated plaque (Fig. 22-40). The main concern is that of a potential embolic event occurring should part or all of the visualized material break free and travel cephalad. The examiner may initially see something unusual moving within the lumen or some unaccounted-for color-flow pattern; if this occurs, turn the color off and optimize the gray-scale image and focal transmit zones to allow the clearest image possible. The examiner may need to change imaging planes to catch the phenomenon at the best angle of incidence.

An example of an unstable moving thrombus is shown accompanying "Periorbital Doppler," case 2 (see Fig. 22-76).

Extracarotid lesions

Extracarotid lesions, such as carotid body tumors or chemodectomata, may be detected on a carotid duplex examination; these appear as soft-tissue homogeneous masses resembling the sonographic texture of the thyroid gland but

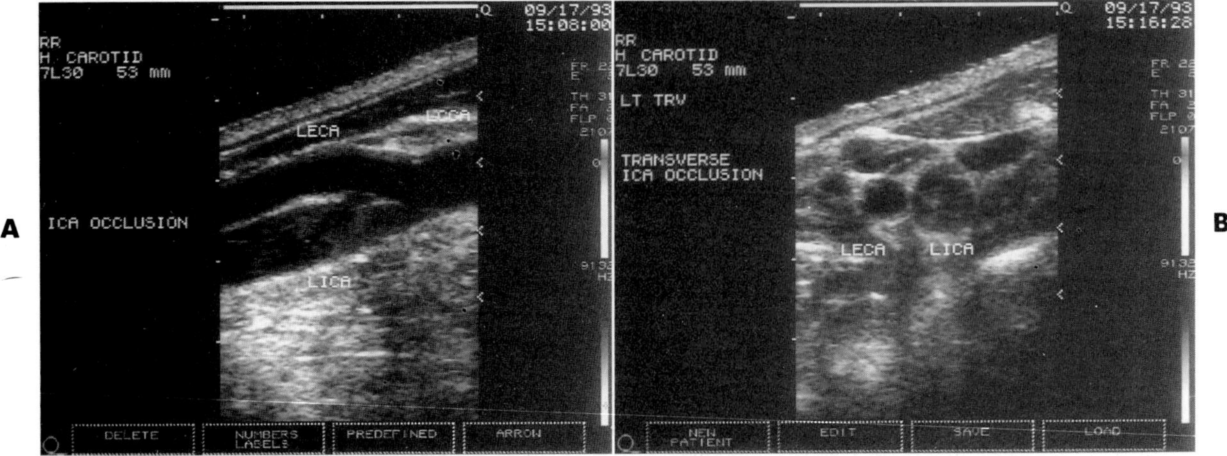

FIG. 22-34 Complete occlusion, homogeneous appearance. **A,** Longitudinal view in gray scale of an occluded internal carotid artery with homogeneous echoes filling the ICA lumen and a distinct border of occlusion at the origin of the ICA with a patent CCA and ECA. **B,** Transverse view of the occluded internal carotid artery in *A*. Note the echo-free ECA lumen to the left of the echo-filled ICA.

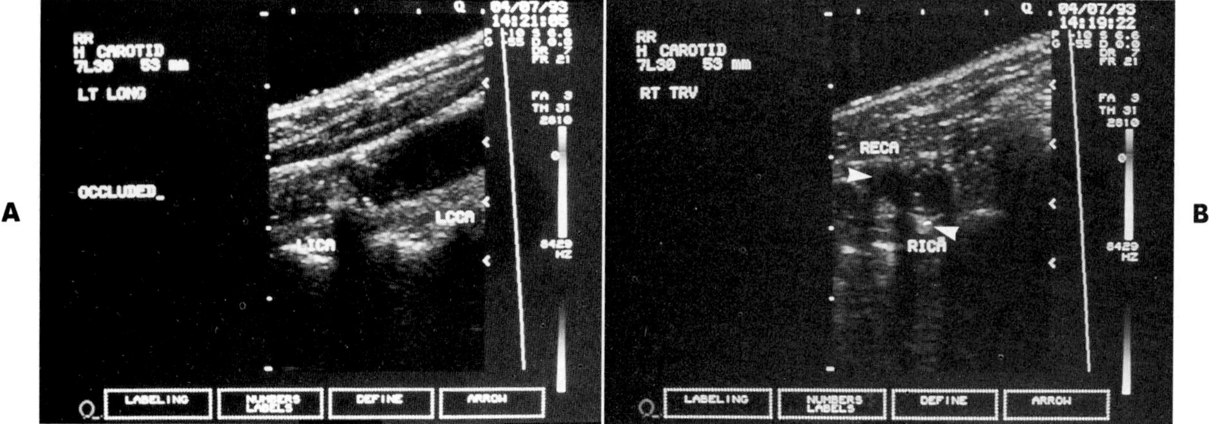

FIG. 22-35 Complete occlusion, heterogeneous appearance. **A,** Longitudinal view in gray scale of an occluded internal carotid artery with chronic heterogeneous echoes filling the ICA lumen. **B,** Transverse view of the occluded internal carotid artery in **A.** Note the mixed homogeneous and heterogeneous texture in the ICA.

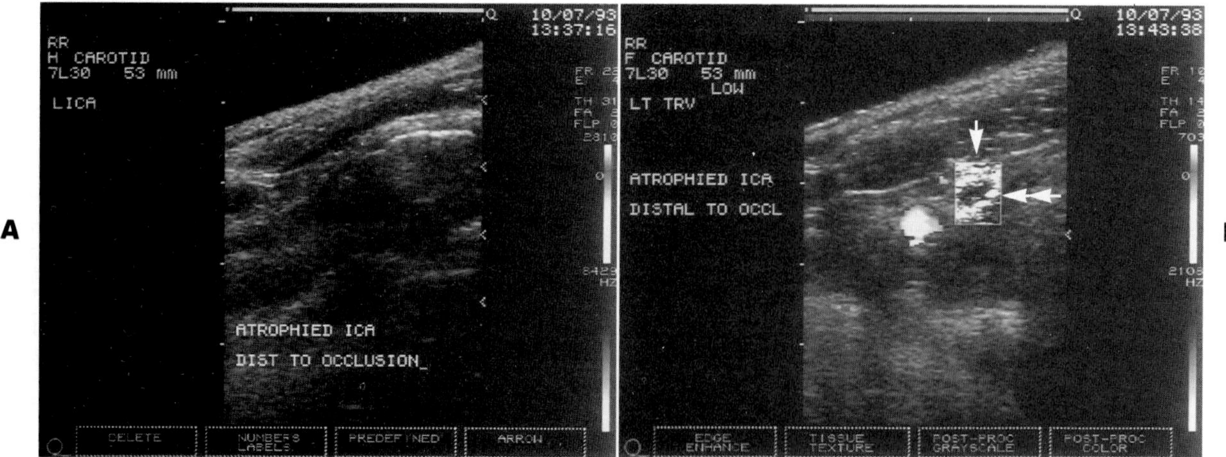

FIG. 22-36 Complete occlusion, chronic, with atrophied ICA. **A,** Longitudinal view in gray scale of an occluded internal carotid artery showing a small, tapering residual ICA distal to a large calcified origin. **B,** Transverse view of the atrophied occluded internal carotid artery in **A.** The area of the ICA has been computer-enhanced to better show the margins of the ICA against the background image. Note the small size of the ICA compared with the patent ECA (with color flow) to the left.

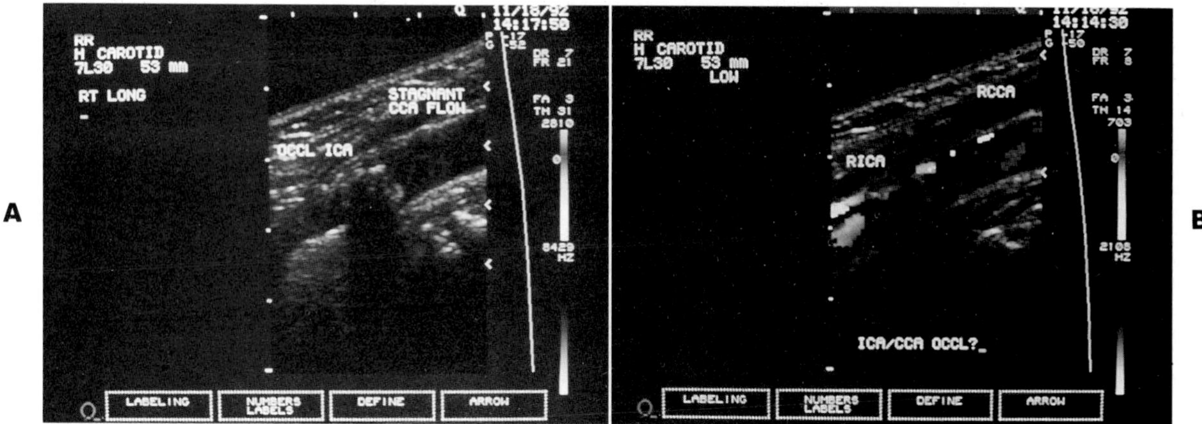

FIG. 22-37 Complete proximal occlusion with reconstituted ICA and ECA. **A,** Longitudinal view in gray scale of an occluded internal carotid artery with a dense, calcified plaque in the bifurcation and slow-moving, stagnant flow echoes in the CCA proximal to it. **B,** The same longitudinal view as in **A,** but with color flow on. Flow is seen to be present in the ECA and ICA to the left (velocity threshold is in slow-flow mode) with nonactive flow in the CCA to the right. Further evaluation showed the ECA and ICA filling slowly from a retrograde superior thyroid artery and collaterals.

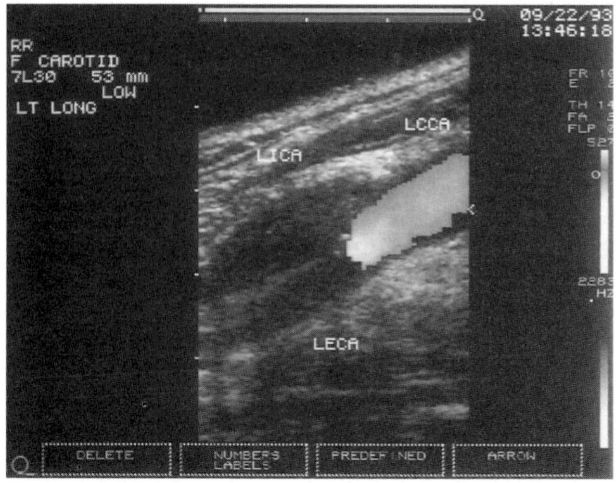

FIG. 22-38 This longitudinal color-flow image shows a completely occluded ICA and ECA with a patent CCA; note that color flow from the CCA ends abruptly at the origins of the occluded vessels and that there is homogeneous material filling both of the occluded arteries.

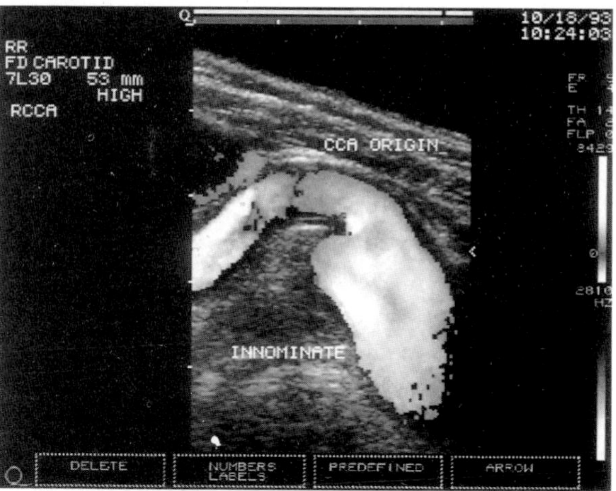

FIG. 22-39 This longitudinal color-flow image demonstrates a superficial, supraclavicularly positioned, tortuous origin of the CCA. This normal occurrence is commonly mistaken for a low-carotid aneurysm on physical examination.

with tumor neovasculature often defined within the parenchyma of the mass (Fig. 22-41). These benign or malignant masses may appear in between the internal and external carotid as outgrowths of the carotid body chemoreceptor and may expand to encompass both vessels at the bifurcation. Although the artery walls may appear to be incorporated into the mass, the lumens usually remain patent. Color-flow imaging can greatly assist the examiner in identifying a carotid body tumor, since the branching color-flow patterns of the tumor neovasculature are easily recognizable.

Methods of Calculating Luminal Reduction

Stenoses that are visualized can be measured using the scanner's integrated electronic calipers. Two types of measurements are generally obtained on carotid artery images.

Diameter calculations are performed on longitudinal images; the examiner first measures the diameter of the artery (true lumen) from superficial wall to deep wall with one set of calipers, and then measures the diameter of the residual lumen at the point of maximal stenosis (from one inner edge of the plaque to the other) (Fig. 22-42). The residual luminal diameter is divided by the vessel diameter to give an estimated percentage of diameter stenosis.

Residual lumen diameter/Vessel diameter = Percentage of diameter stenosis

This calculation is not always accurate because it depends on assuming that the plaque is symmetric in the sagittal plane being evaluated; eccentric stenoses thus cannot al-

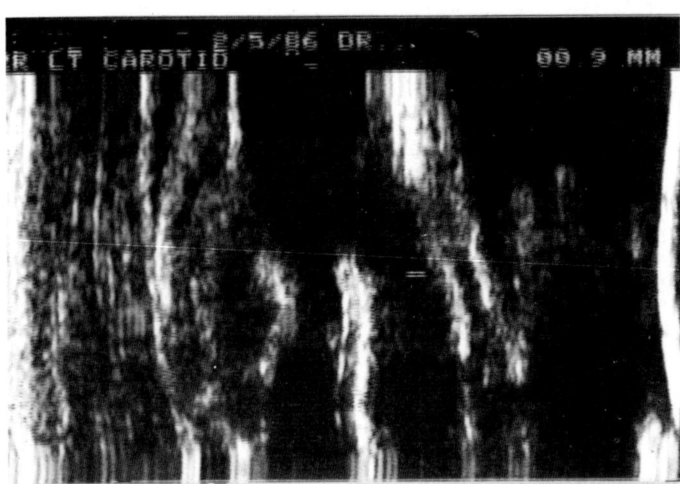

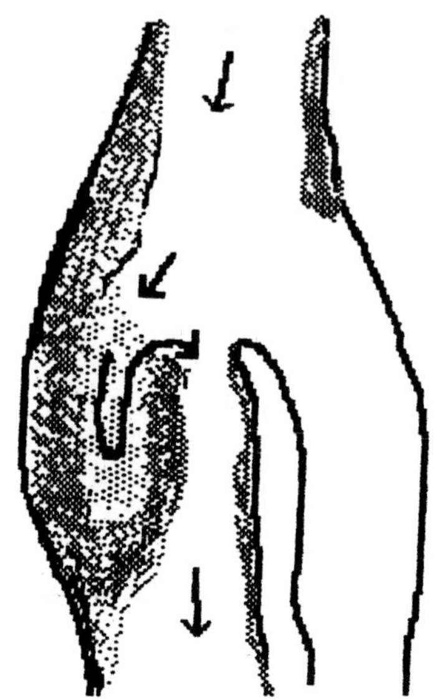

FIG. 22-40 Sonographic appearance of a turbulent unstable plaque with a diagram showing the path of blood flow into and out of the ulcer in the plaque that was visualized during duplex evaluation. (Courtesy Richard E. Rae, Indianapolis.)

ways be accurately measured.[10] Direct diameter measurements (with both true and residual lumen calculations made across the area of maximal stenosis) compare well with area stenosis measurements (see below) but, because of the technique, seldom agree with arteriographic diameter measurements. Arteriographic diameter stenosis measurements assume that the true lumen diameter is in the straight portion distal to the dilated origin of the internal carotid; the point of maximal narrowing is then measured and again calculated as above[5] (Fig. 22-43).

The potential discrepancy is that angiograms only provide a physiologic image of a filled vessel lumen and do not show soft-tissue architecture, so what may appear as a 50% or more sonographic stenosis may not calculate as a significant stenosis by arteriogram (see Chapter 19). If, ultimately, measurement correlations with arteriograms are desired, the examiner should perform diameter calculations on the ultrasound image at the same estimated locations that an arteriographer uses on an arteriographic image[36] (Fig. 22-44). The examiner should be aware, however, that interobserver and intraobserver interpretations of angiographic results vary widely and correlation may not be consistent[47] (see also Chapter 23).

Area stenosis measurements are made using electronic calipers on transverse images; the examiner first traces the outside circumference of the artery, then traces the inner circumference of the residual lumen (this measurement is made easier if color-flow imaging is used). The resulting area measurements are usually provided in square millimeters (Fig. 22-45). The residual lumen area is divided by the vessel area, then that result is subtracted from 1; the result, multiplied by 100, equals the estimated percentage of area stenosis:[10]

$$1 - (\text{Residual lumen area/Vessel area}) \times 100 = \text{Percentage of diameter stenosis}$$

Area stenosis calculations can reliably assess asymmetric stenoses and often correlate very accurately with corresponding Doppler velocity criteria.[10] One problem with area stenosis calculations, however, is that there is no similar cross-sectional arteriographic measurement; the closest arteriographic equivalent requires biplanar arteriography and summary estimation of the cross-sectional diameter.[5]

Diameter and area stenosis measurement of the plaque and the vessel can often give a better luminal reduction estimate than by visual estimation, but if they are obtained, these physical measurements should be correlated and combined with the hemodynamic criteria for estimated stenosis (see below).

IDENTIFICATION AND INTERPRETATION OF ABNORMAL CAROTID COLOR-FLOW IMAGING PATTERNS

As mentioned, color-flow imaging patterns in the carotid system correspond well to the flow patterns shown by Doppler. The normal color-flow pattern in the carotid artery system appears as uniform shades of red with a concentrated flow streamline throughout systole and diastole; no color-flow reversal (blue) is normally seen in the carotid system in diastole.

The normal common carotid has color patterns that appear as described.

The internal carotid normally has higher velocities and color intensities during systole. Some normal elevation of the diastolic intensities may occur with more intense white

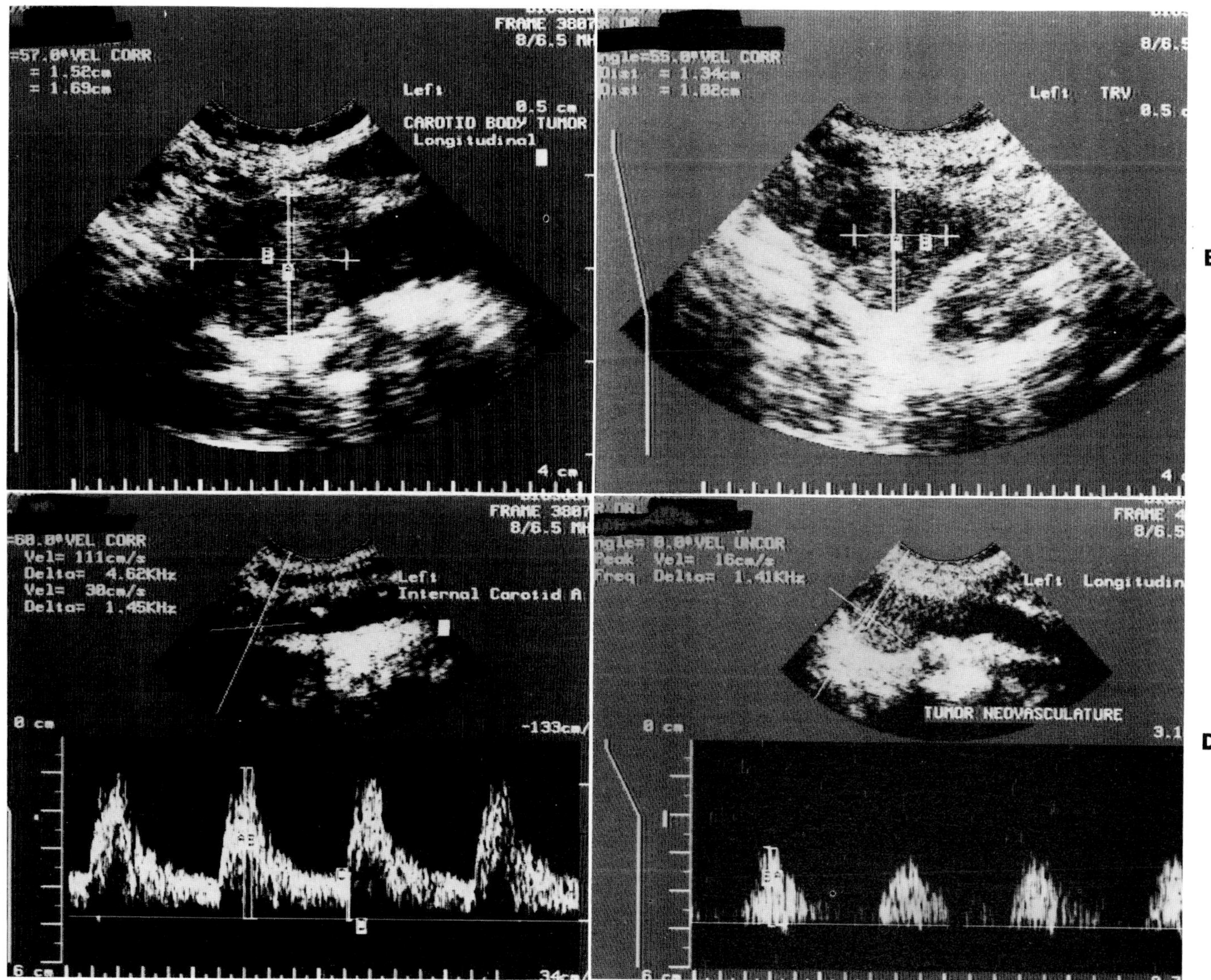

FIG. 22-41 Carotid body tumor. **A,** Longitudinal gray-scale image showing a small carotid body tumor measuring 1.52 cm by 1.69 cm by 1.02 cm; the patent CCA is to the right (the tumor is situated in the crotch of the bifurcation). **B,** Transverse view of the tumor, showing the patent lumens of the ICA (at left caliper mark) and the ECA (at right caliper mark) with the tumor between them. **C,** Internal carotid spectral waveform lateral to tumor, with normal waveform profile, PSV of 111 cm/sec, and EDV of 38 cm/sec. **D,** Examples of waveforms from tumor neovasculature.

or yellow shades than in the common carotid because of the low-resistance hemodynamics. Note that an area of blue flow reversal or flow separation may normally occur at the carotid bulb, as described in Chapter 19, but may be considered normal only if no significant plaque development is present.

The external carotid artery normally has a higher-resistance flow pattern, with a characteristic on-off pattern isolated to that vessel; absence of color in diastole normally occurs in the external carotid artery, since this finding characterizes a high-resistance hemodynamic state.

There are no criteria applicable at the time of writing to categorize the degree of stenosis by the hemodynamic changes seen in color-flow imaging. Such classification is best done using Doppler spectral waveform acquisition (see below), since velocity changes in color Doppler imaging and duplex Doppler are often related (see Chapter 19). Certain easily detectable changes in the saturation, flow streamlines, and velocity levels, however, occur at certain degrees of luminal reduction:

1. The normal streamline usually concentrates toward the center or slightly to the side distal to a flow divider. Broadening of the streamline (where instead of a bright gradient in the center, the intensities are diffusely spread

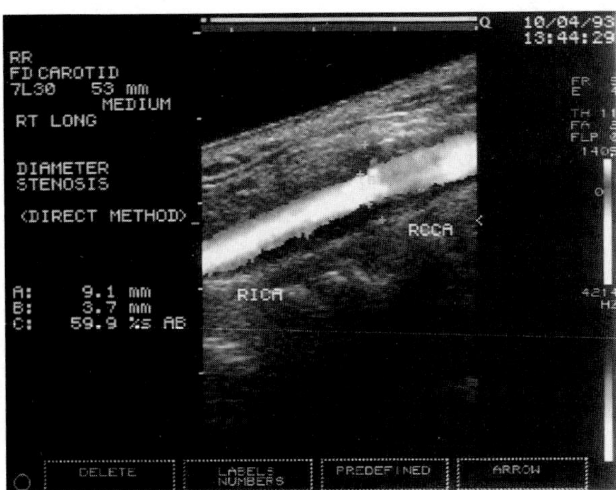

FIG. 22-42 Direct method of percentage diameter stenosis calculation measurement on a longitudinal sonographic image.

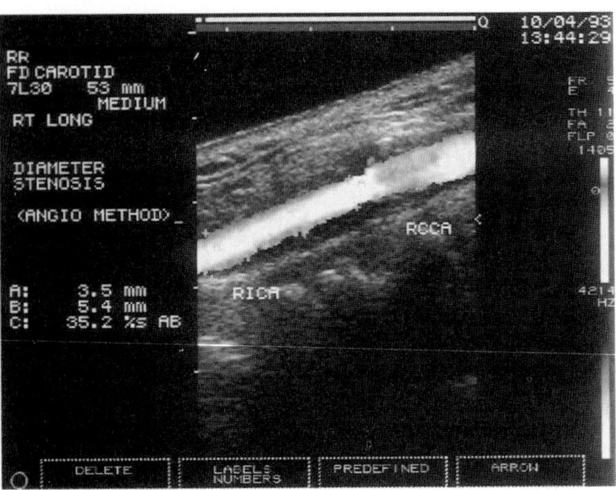

FIG. 22-44 Angiographic method of percentage diameter stenosis calculation measurement, applied to a longitudinal sonographic image.

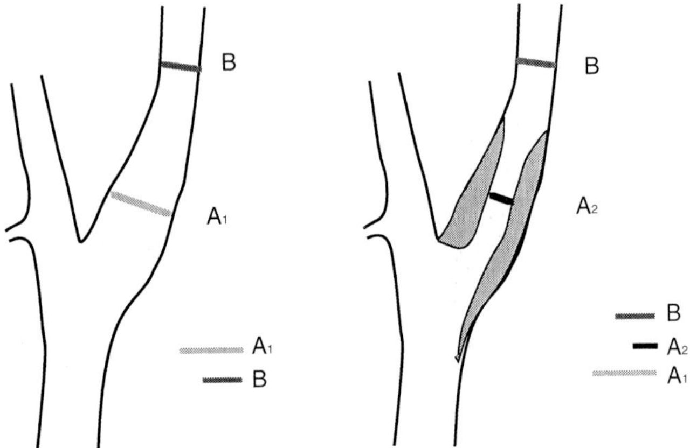

FIG. 22-43 Description of the angiographic percentage stenosis calculation method and some potential inaccuracies. **A,** The normal lumen measurement across the origin of the internal carotid (where the majority of plaque statistically forms) (A^1) is larger in diameter than the distal, straight portion of the internal carotid (B), which is normally used for angiographic comparison. **B,** In the standard method of calculating angiographic percentage of diameter stenosis the residual lumen measurement across the stenosis (A^2) is compared with the straight, nonstenosed distal ICA (B) to calculate the percentage of diameter stenosis. As is shown by the comparative line measurements, the percentage of luminal reduction is actually greater if A^2 is compared to A^1 than it is if A^2 is compared with B; unless sonographic percentage of diameter stenosis calculations follow the standard angiographic method, inaccurate correlation may occur (compare the calculations in Fig. 22-42 with those in Fig. 22-44). (Courtesy Richard E. Rae, Indianapolis.)

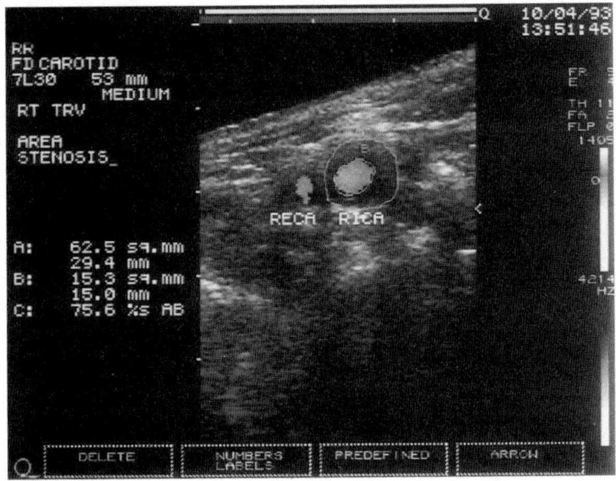

FIG. 22-45 An example of percentage area stenosis calculations on the ICA in a transverse image.

within the vessel) may suggest a proximal turbulent phenomenon, such as a proximal CCA stenosis or radiating cardiac turbulence from an aortic stenosis (Fig. 22-46). This is analogous to a disturbance of the envelope definition in a Doppler spectral waveform.

2. Highly concentrated narrow streamlines indicate a flow jet, usually appearing distal to a stenosis; there usually is a clearly defined area of blue flow separation beneath the jet directly distal to the stenotic plaque (Fig. 22-47, *A;* see color image).
3. Diastole-persistent streamlines (where a narrow streamline is almost as well defined as it is during systole) are indicative of a severe stenosis; they are analogous to the elevated and high-velocity diastolic flow seen within Doppler waveforms across high-grade stenoses (Fig. 22-47 *B;* see color image).
4. If color becomes regularly absent in diastole in the common or internal carotid artery (an on-off pattern), the existence of a distal occlusion may be implied (Fig. 22-48; see color images).
5. Mixed color-flow patterns indicate turbulence within the arterial segment, often distal to a stenosis (Fig. 22-49; see color image); this finding is very useful in cases where an extensively calcified plaque prevents

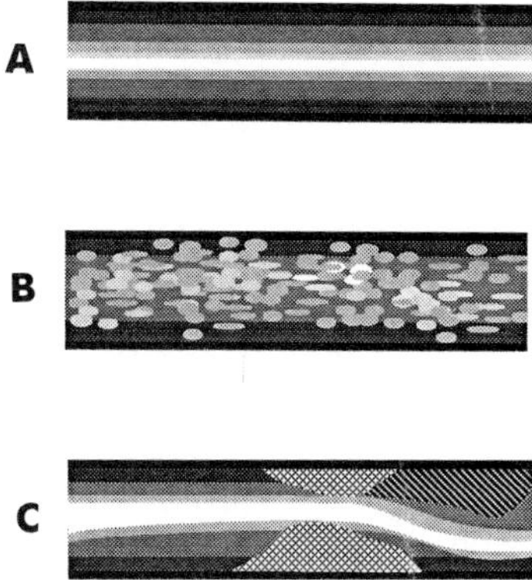

FIG. 22-46 Color-flow streamline pattern recognition. **A,** Normal laminar streamline. **B,** Diffuse, broadened streamline seen with proximal stenosis or radiating turbulence from aortic valve stenosis. **C,** Narrow jet streamline with flow separation and axial redirection, seen with severe stenosis.

determination of the underlying degree of stenosis. By evaluating the color-flow patterns distal to the calcified plaque, an examiner can determine whether the "hidden" stenosis is hemodynamically significant (see Fig. 22-32).

6. A visible bruit is an indicator of a stenosis causing a luminal reduction of greater than 60%; note that the bruit may disappear if the luminal reduction approaches the high ninetieth percentile (see Figs. 22-32 and 22-47, *A*).
7. Completely retrograde (blue) flow in the right carotid or either vertebral artery, flickering patterns (for example, the color pattern in the right internal carotid goes blank or absent during systole rather than in diastole as in number 4), or alternating blue-red patterns (with blue occurring during systole and red during diastole) are signs of pending or active subclavian steal if seen in the vertebral arteries (Fig. 22-50; see color image) and carotid

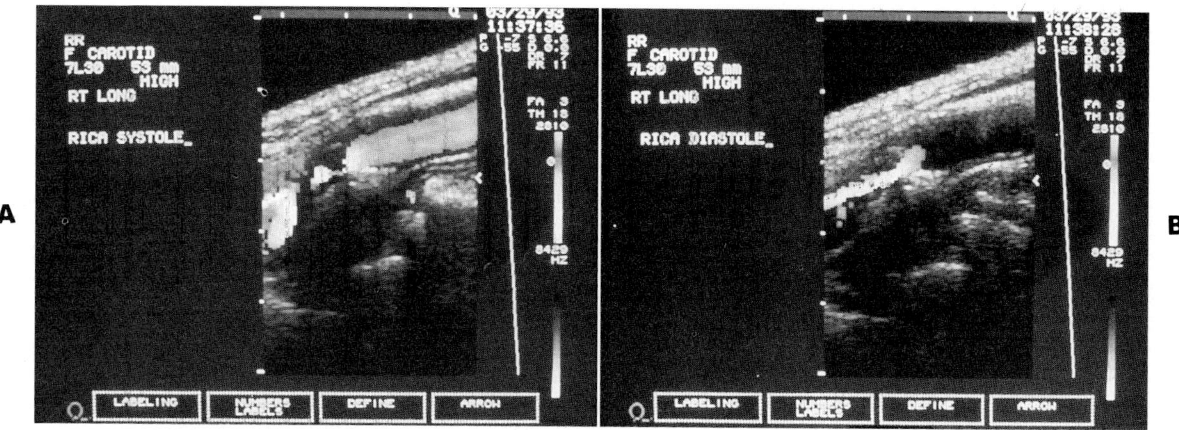

FIG. 22-47 **A,** This longitudinal color-flow image shows a severe stenosis with a tight streamline *(left)* distal to the stenosis and an area of flow separation beneath the jet in systole. Note the bruit being generated near the peak stenotic location. **B,** The same image as in **A,** taken during the diastolic portion of the cardiac cycle, shows the streamline persisting with continued elevated velocities within it.

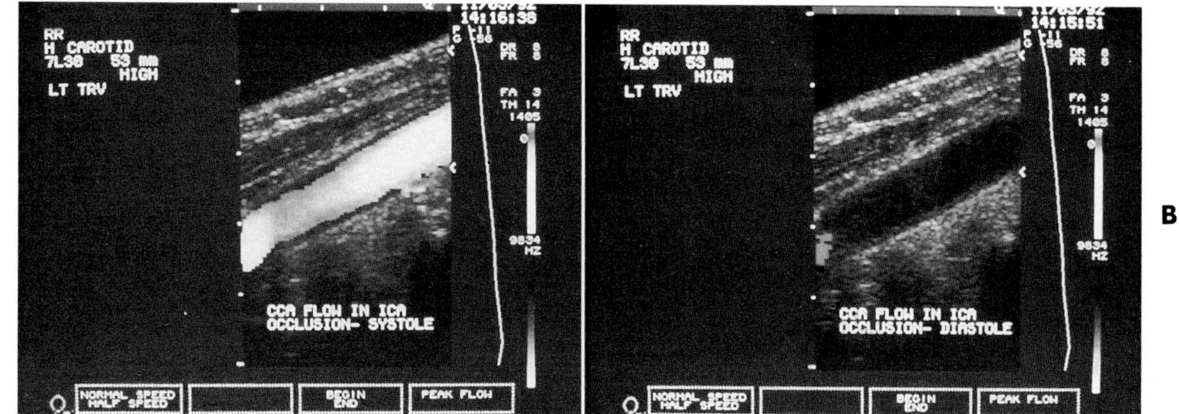

FIG. 22-48 Color-flow imaging in the common carotid in complete distal occlusion, demonstrating the on-off pattern. **A,** Color-flow image showing the common carotid pattern in systole. **B,** Color-flow image showing the common carotid pattern in diastole. Note the complete absence of color flow.

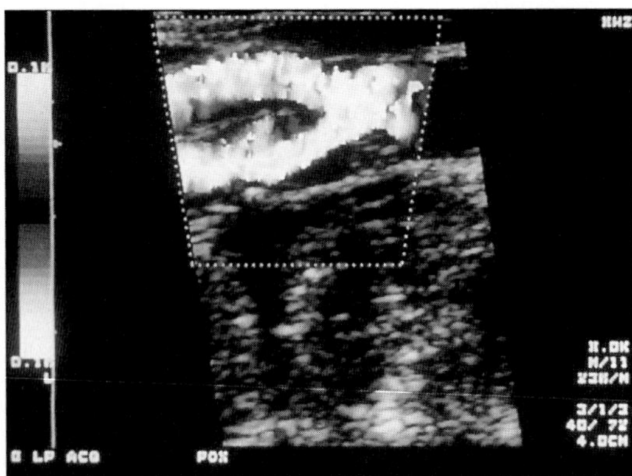

FIG. 22-49 This color-flow pattern lacks uniformity because of stenosis and luminal irregularity; numerous areas of mixed red and blue are seen from disturbed flow (some aliasing is occurring in the central streamline).

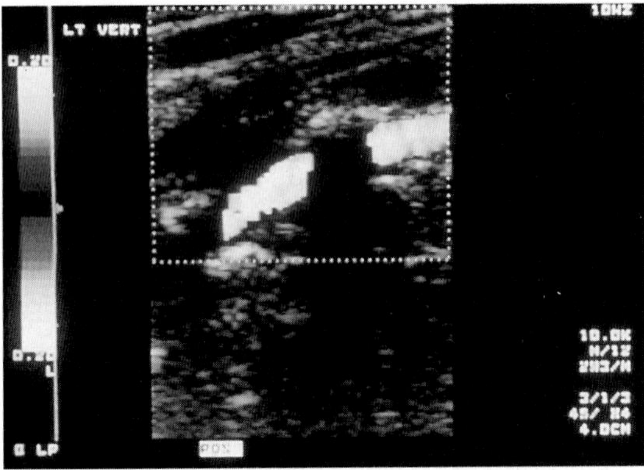

FIG. 22-50 Retrograde (blue) color-flow pattern in a vertebral artery, seen in complete subclavian steal.

steal in innominate stenosis or occlusion if seen in the right carotid artery.

The hemodynamics of subclavian steal, color-flow, and Doppler waveform appearances in the vertebral artery and the examination technique were described in Chapter 20; the hemodynamics of carotid steal are closely related, and we briefly describe the phenomenon.

If the innominate artery is severely stenosed or occluded proximal to the origin of the right common carotid artery (which arises from the innominate rather than the aortic arch; see diagram), it is possible for flow to shunt around the circle of Willis and travel in a retrograde fashion through both the vertebral and the internal carotid–common carotid to compensate the right arm (Fig. 22-51). This phenomenon is very dramatic (especially with color flow) and may manifest with flow patterns in an identical pattern to those seen in subclavian steal in the vertebral artery (see Chapter 20). The carotid retrograde or transitional flow patterns are often more pronounced if the right vertebral is occluded. Note that barring a congenital vascular developmental anomaly, retrograde flow of this type should not ever occur in the left carotid system.

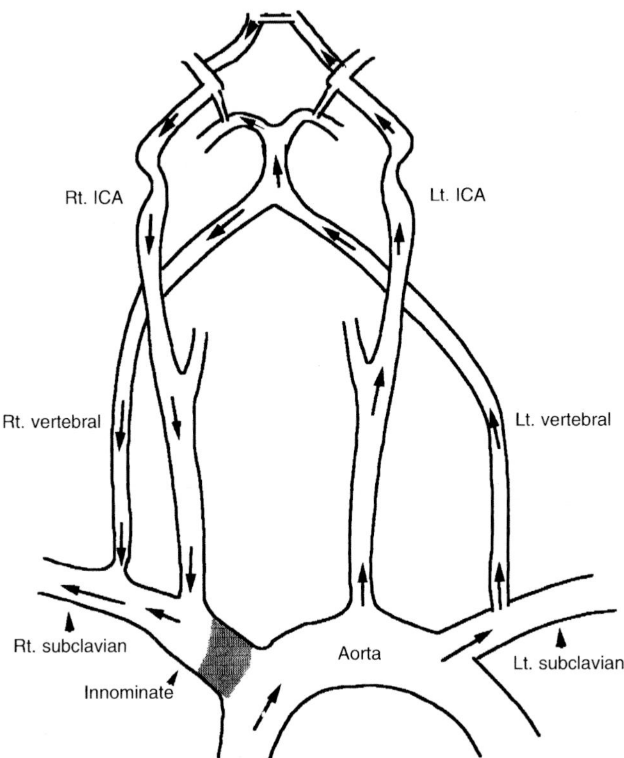

FIG. 22-51 Diagram showing the mechanism of carotid steal in innominate artery occlusion and potential collateral pathways. (Courtesy Richard E. Rae, Indianapolis.)

The degree of steal, as in the vertebral, can be determined by the following particular patterns of systolic reversal in the carotid:

1. If systolic flow goes to baseline but does not fully reverse, a flickering internal carotid color pattern may occur (which may not reflect into the common carotid if innominate pressure is still substantial). Usually a normal common carotid antegrade color pattern persists.
2. If flow reverses in systole but becomes antegrade in diastole, an alternating blue-red pattern occurs. This parallels the latent or transitional steal pattern.
3. Finally, if flow is completely retrograde throughout all of the cardiac cycle (which is rare in carotid steal), a fully blue pattern is seen.

Two examples of the carotid steal phenomenon are shown in "Carotid Duplex Sonography," cases 6 (see Fig. 22-66) and 7 (see Fig. 22-67).

Some investigators have attempted to use velocity tagging (see Chapter 19) to not only localize the point of maximum frequency and velocity shift but to attempt to quantify the velocities (Fig. 22-52; see color image); the examiner must remember that most color Doppler systems display mean velocities in color, not peak velocities (systems with time-domain color-flow processing are an exception). The examiner should not, therefore, expect the tagged velocity to correlate exactly with peak velocities obtained from the Doppler spectral waveform. Tagged veloc-

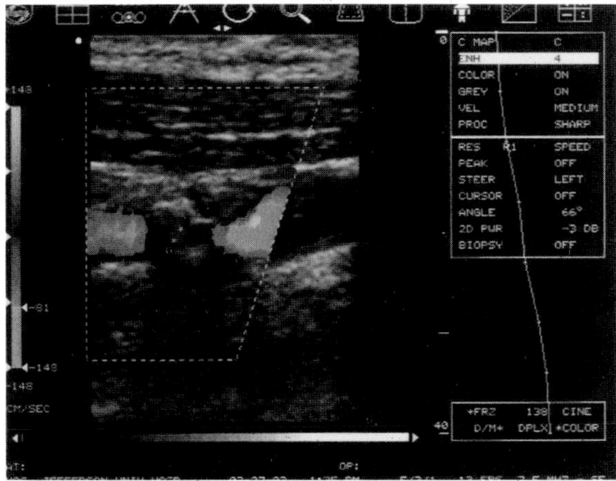

FIG. 22-52 Color-flow image of an internal carotid stenosis, showing velocity green tagging; velocities greater than 81 cm/sec (see bar at left) are colored green.

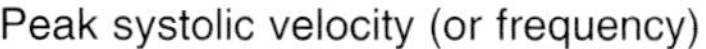

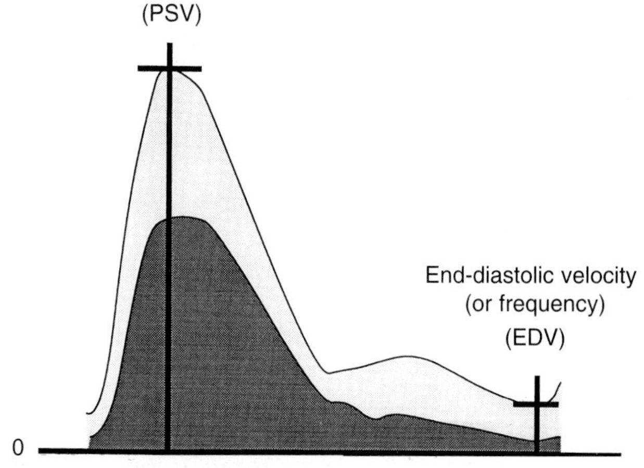

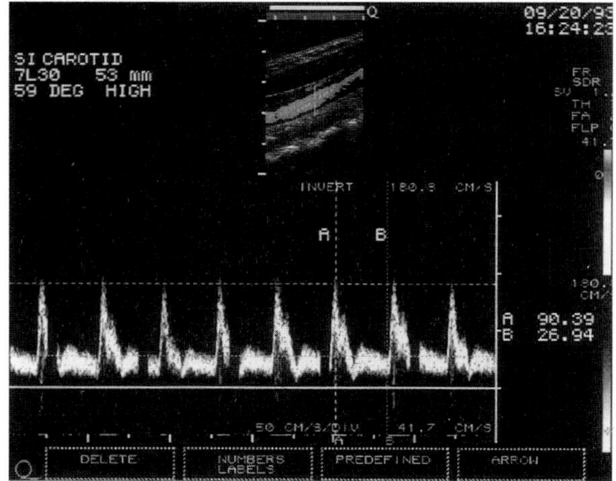

FIG. 22-53 Normal Doppler spectral waveform from the common carotid artery.

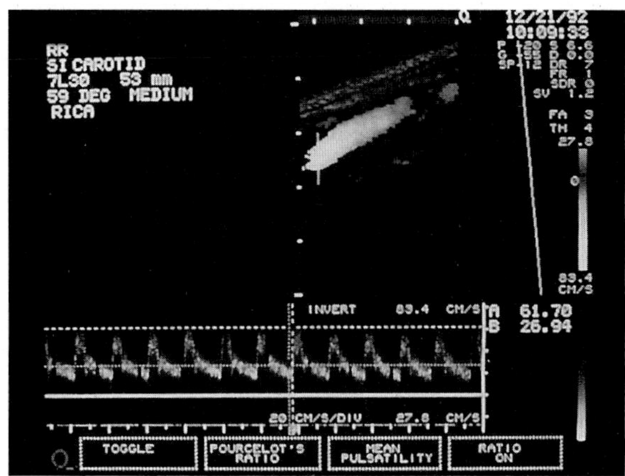

FIG. 22-54 Normal Doppler spectral waveform from the internal carotid artery.

ities can, however, serve as a guide to where the sample volume should optimally be placed for accurate Doppler spectral sampling.

Interpretation of Carotid Duplex Doppler Spectral Waveforms

Normal Carotid Waveform Patterns

Many of the criteria about interpreting the spectral display previously discussed in Chapter 19 apply to diagnosis of carotid hemodynamics and interpreting the duplex Doppler spectral waveform. A review follows:

The normal common carotid waveform has a clearly defined envelope and an uncluttered spectral window with a narrow spectral width (i.e., little if any spectral broadening) (Fig. 22-53). Peak systolic common carotid frequencies generally are under 4 KHz, and velocities are under 125 cm/sec. Some mild turbulence or flow disturbance may occur within the bulb area around the bifurcation, which is normal. Diastolic flow is clearly defined above the baseline, and there is normally no retrograde flow.

The normal internal carotid waveform is of a low-resistance quality, with most of the same characteristics as in the common carotid—a uniform envelope, little or no spectral broadening, but slightly more elevated systolic and diastolic flow (Fig. 22-54). Peak systolic common carotid frequencies also are under 4 KHz with peak velocities under 125 cm/sec.

The normal external carotid waveform, however, is of a higher-resistance quality because of the numerous branches. Again there is a uniform envelope and little or no spectral broadening. Flow generally still remains above the baseline, but systolic flow has a more rapid and sharp upstroke and flow in end-diastole generally goes close to the baseline (Fig. 22-55). A mildly prominent third diastolic component is sometimes seen. Peak frequencies and velocities vary; in general, they still are less than or equal to 4 KHz or 130 cm/sec.

Abnormal Waveform Patterns

In the presence of hemodynamically significant disease the Doppler spectral waveforms in the carotid arteries develop many qualitative changes. These waveform characteristics are directly proportional to the severity of the ste-

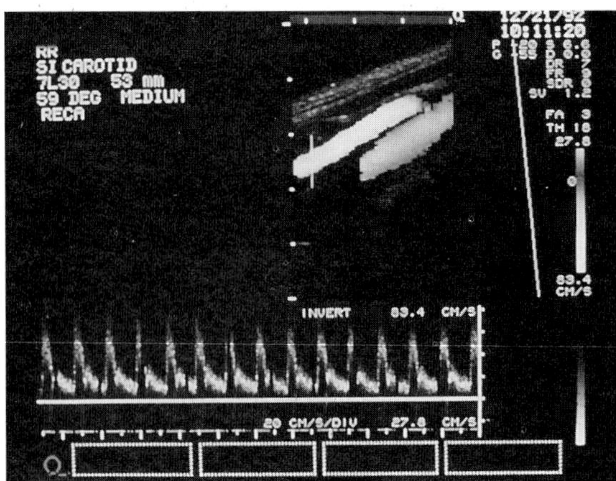

FIG. 22-55 Normal Doppler spectral waveform from the external carotid artery.

nosis (or stenoses) and not only alert the examiner to the presence of an abnormality but also aid in classifying the disease into one or more categories of severity. These characteristic flow-pattern changes have been correlated accurately with arteriographically documented luminal reduction measurements and have become reliable indicators of the approximate degree of stenosis.[50]

In general, few hemodynamic changes (except some increase in spectral broadening) are seen in the carotid waveform until a stenosis produces a luminal reduction of about 60%. At this point, several quantifiable things happen to the blood-flow waveform:

1. The spectral broadening increases proportionally with the degree of luminal reduction, approaching a spread of greater than 40 cm/sec, and the window may fill in or become absent as a stenosis increases;[10]
2. The waveform outer envelope begins to lose its definition, with significant disruption proportional to the degree of flow turbulence;
3. The peak systolic velocity (frequency) elevates above 120 to 130 cm/sec or 4 KHz; the end-diastolic velocity begins to elevate above 40 cm/sec. The more severe the stenosis and flow disruption, the higher both of these values will be.

Many of these changes are illustrated in Fig. 22-56.

Partial or complete retrograde flow in one vertebral artery suggests the presence of subclavian steal (which can be confirmed with brachial systolic pressure comparisons) (Fig. 22-57; see color images). See also the discussion of subclavian steal in Chapter 20.

If proximal innominate artery stenosis or occlusion is present, the carotid waveform on the right may become transitionally or completely retrograde as carotid steal occurs; see the discussion under number seven in the previous "Identification and Interpretation of Abnormal Carotid Color-Flow Imaging Patterns" and in "Carotid Sonography," cases 6 (see Fig. 22-66) and 7 (see Fig. 22-67) in this chapter.

Doppler spectral waveforms obtained proximal to an occlusion (or stenoses approaching the high ninetieth percentile) become characteristic of high resistance, appearing similar to an extremity artery with a loss of diastolic flow (which may drop to a velocity of zero at end-diastole) (Fig. 22-58; see color image).

Doppler Spectral Velocity Criteria for Classifying Carotid Artery Disease

As mentioned, the Doppler velocity and spectral broadening criteria measured during the examination are used by the interpreter to classify the degree of stenosis based on where the velocity and waveform criteria from the internal carotid artery fit into a specific diagnostic category. One or more of the following parameters are used in published classification tables to determine the category:

1. Peak-systolic velocity (PSV) (frequency);
2. End-diastolic velocity (EDV) (frequency);
3. Internal carotid–common carotid peak systolic velocity ratio;
4. Internal carotid–common carotid end-diastolic velocity ratio;
5. Spectral broadening in cm/sec.

The PSV or peak systolic frequency is measured at the peak of the systolic component of the waveform.[10] This is considered by some investigators to be one of the most sensitive parameters for identifying a critical stenosis (70% to 80% luminal reduction or higher), although alone it may not accurately distinguish between 60% to 80% and 80% to 99% stenosis grades.[10,31]

The EDV or end-diastolic frequency is measured at the lowest point of diastole, usually at the end of the cardiac cycle just before the initial upslope of another systolic peak (see Fig. 22-25).[10] Elevation of EDV is a very sensitive indicator for stenosis, especially when it is over 80%.[10]

The internal carotid/common carotid (IC/CC) peak systolic velocity ratio (PSVR) is calculated by dividing the peak systolic velocity number of the internal carotid by the peak systolic velocity number of the ipsilateral common carotid.

$$\text{Internal PSV/Common PSV} = \text{IC/CC PSV ratio}$$

This value normally is less than 1.8;[10] low values generally are not considered significant. This is because the internal carotid systolic velocity may occasionally be lower than average, such as in a dilated, patched vessel after endarterectomy. Elevated ratios occur at greater than 60% stenosis, and higher values are usually diagnostic for severe stenosis in combination with the other factors.[10]

The IC/CC end-diastolic velocity ratio (EDVR) is calculated by dividing the peak end-diastolic velocity number of the internal carotid by the peak end-diastolic velocity number of the ipsilateral common carotid.

$$\text{Internal EDV/Common EDV} = \text{IC/CC EDV ratio}$$

This value normally is less than 2.5.[10] The end-diastolic velocity ratio begins to elevate at a 60% stenosis; as with the PSVR, it can be a specific indicator of higher-grade stenoses (generally those over 70%)[10,36] and may help con-

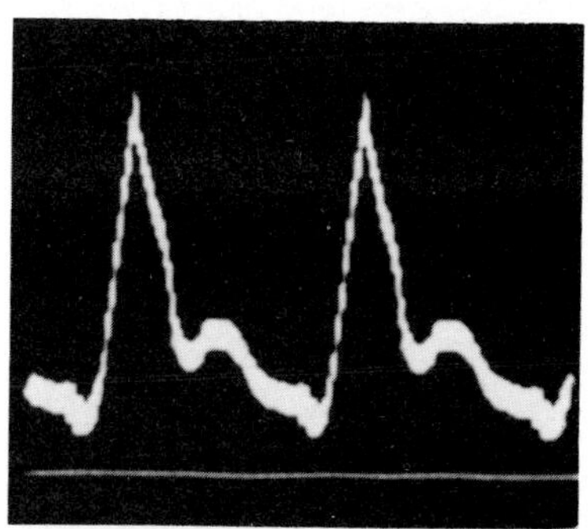

NORMAL

Narrow spectral width
Window clear using pulsed Doppler
Velocity peak does not exceed 5 kHz

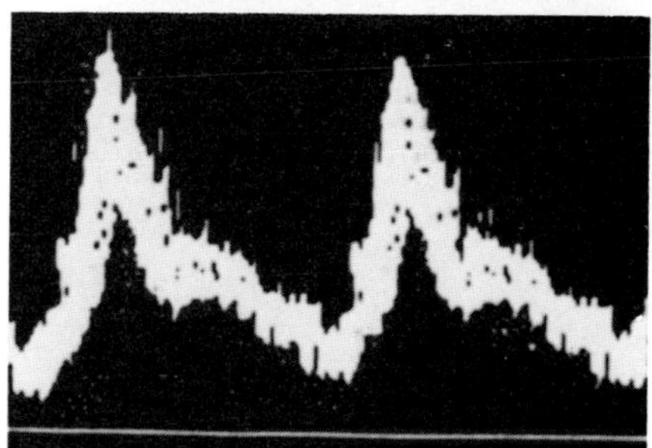

MILD (15%-50% LUMINAL REDUCTION)

Spectral width has increased
Window less clear using pulsed Doppler
Peak and velocity still within normal limits

A

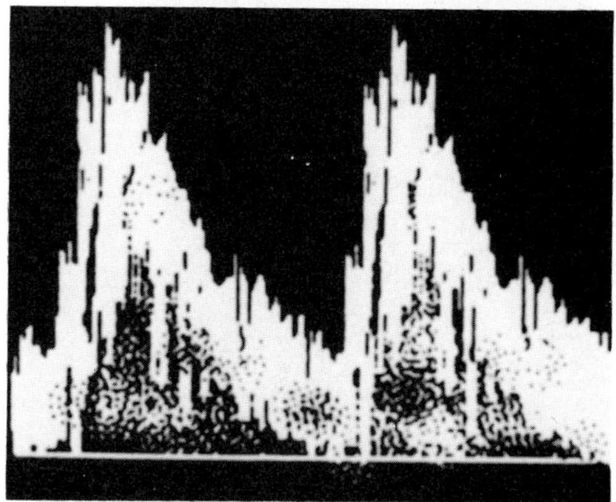

MODERATE (50%-75% LUMINAL REDUCTION)

Width is quite broad
Window fills in more
Noticeable turbulence in waveform
Systolic velocity >120 cm/s
Diastolic velocity <100 cm/s
Peak frequency is high but less than 11 kHz
Diastolic peak under 3 kHz

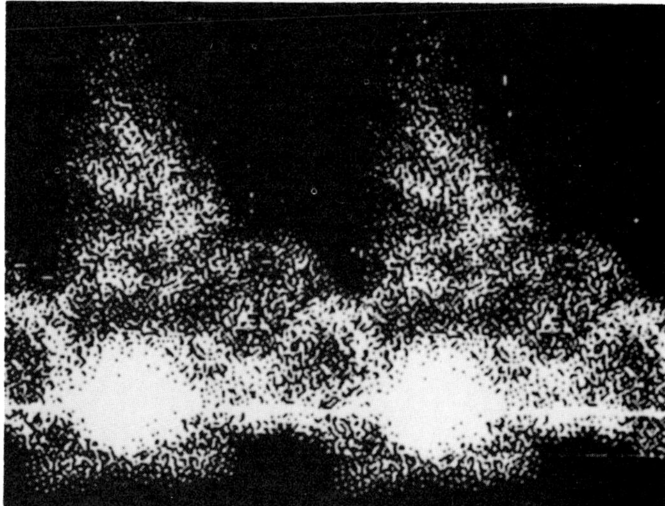

SEVERE (75%-99% LUMINAL REDUCTION)

Severe turbulence with concentration at baseline, progressing with severity
No window
Peak systolic velocities exceeding 150 cm/s
End diastolic velocities over 100 cm/s
Peak systolic >10 kHz frequency
Peak diastolic ≥3 kHz frequency
Using pulsed Doppler, peaks may be cut off or exceed 9 kHz due to aliasing

FIG. 22-56 A, Chart showing appearances in spectral signals that correspond with increases in the level of stenosis.

Continued.

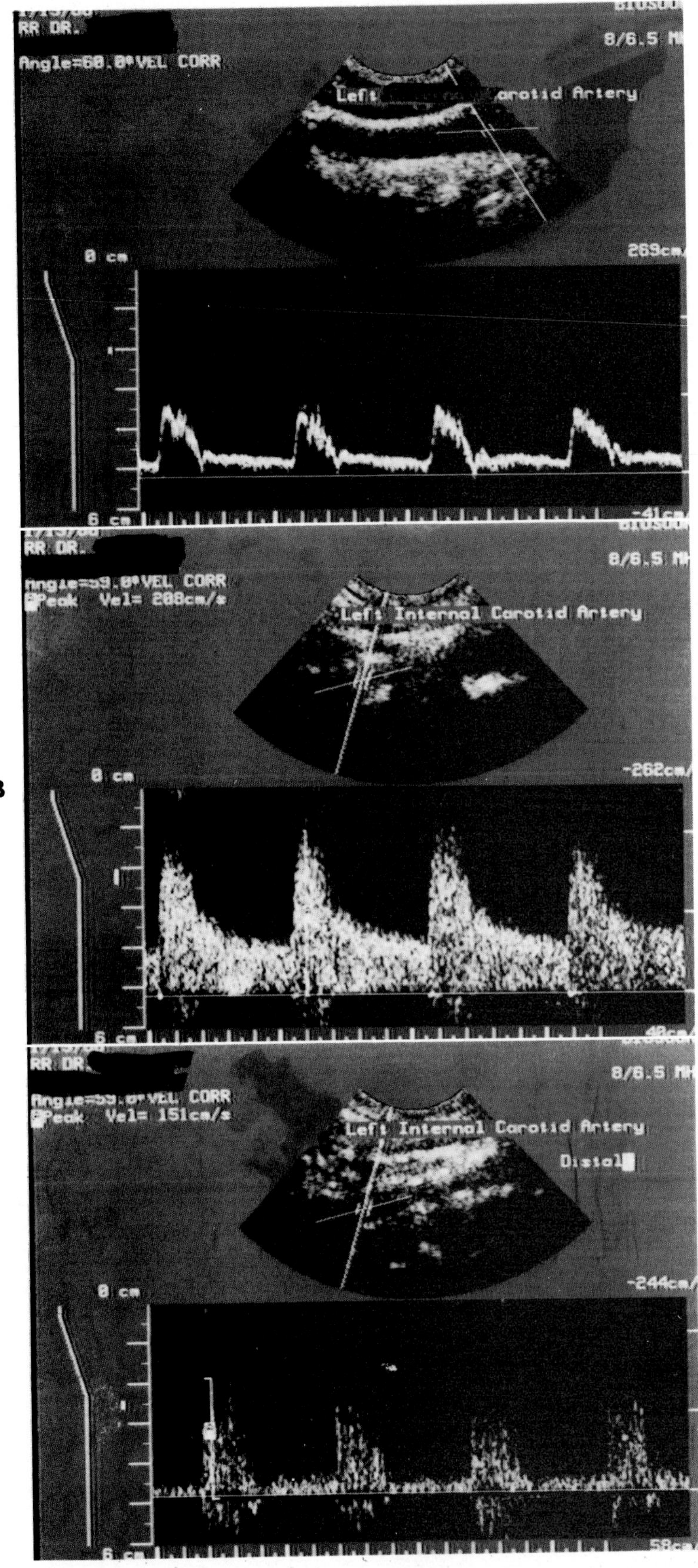

FIG. 22-56, cont'd B, Sequential example of changes below, across, and distal to a severe internal carotid stenosis. **B-1,** Prestenosis (low common carotid). **B-2,** Across stenosis. **B-3,** Distal to stenosis. *SW*, spectral width; *W*, window.

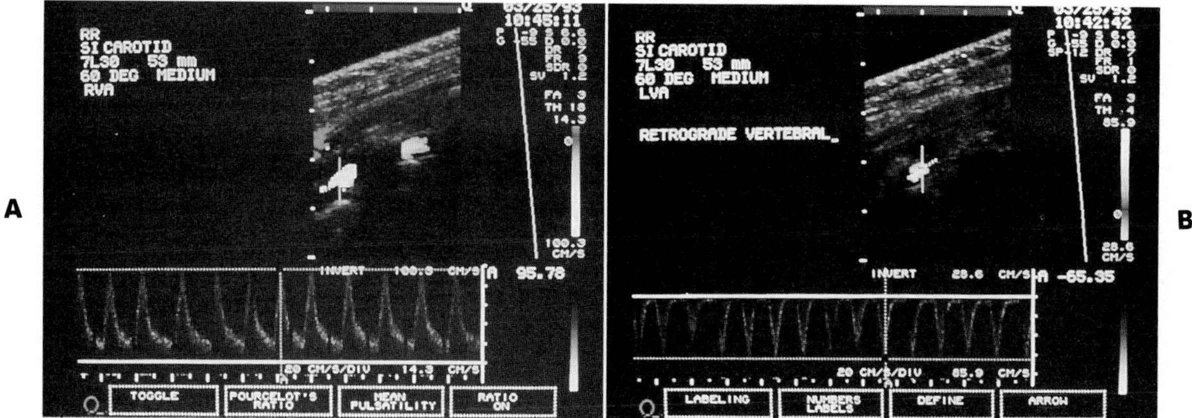

FIG. 22-57 Vertebral arteries in left subclavian steal. **A,** Antegrade Doppler flow signal in the right vertebral artery. **B,** Fully retrograde Doppler flow signal in the left vertebral artery. Note that flow is below the baseline, with a negative velocity reading (the baseline has been shifted to show the entire waveform).

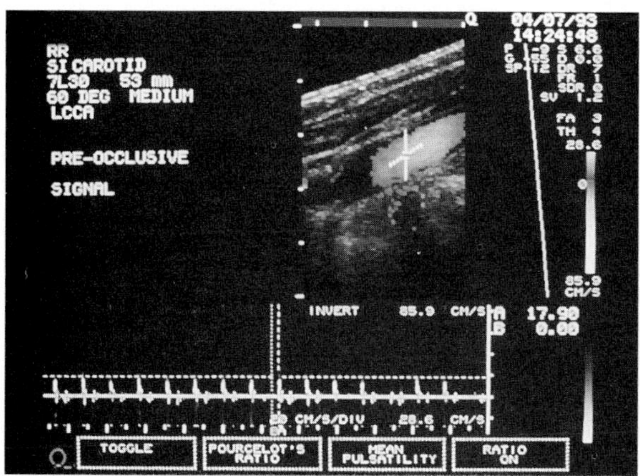

FIG. 22-58 Example of a high-resistance, low-velocity Doppler spectral waveform proximal to a complete ICA occlusion. Note that there is no diastolic flow.

firm the severity of the stenosis in combination with the other factors.[10,36] A recent study by Moneta et al. indicates that an end-diastolic velocity ratio of greater than 4.0 is significant for the presence of a 70% or greater stenosis.[36]

Quantification of spectral broadening is more often done visually than by actual caliper measurement, but the spectral bandwidth can be measured at peak systole distal to a severe stenosis using electronic calipers. One marker should be placed at the peak of the waveform and a second at the top edge of any visible window (at the baseline if a window is not present) (Fig. 22-59). Most velocity calipers measure from the baseline to the marker location, so the examiner should subtract the second measurement from the peak measurement; the result will be in centimeters per second and should represent the spectral bandwidth (SW).

$$PSV - PWV = SW$$

Peak systolic velocity (PSV) − velocity at top of window (PWV) = spectral width (SW) in cm/sec

A spectral width of 40 cm/sec or less is considered normal by some criteria. This parameter is less sensitive than the others mentioned but may be useful in supporting findings from one or more of the other four calculations.

Some specific makes of ultrasound equipment include a capability to automatically calculate a range of spectral broadening based on the range of velocities at the 50% amplitude of a spectral power histogram or to determine a percentage of window from a comparison of maximum and minimum frequency values (Fig. 22-60).[10,51] In theory the lower the percentage window number, the more spectral broadening is present; this factor, however, can sometimes be affected by improperly set Doppler gain and threshold settings. These capabilities are not present on the majority of currently manufactured systems and therefore have no universal application.

Measurement aside, the best assessment of spectral broadening is probably qualitative rather than quantitative; if the window appears to be filled in, there is probably a significant stenosis over 60%. If not, the stenosis is probably less than 60%.

Velocity Versus Frequency

Throughout this chapter references to both velocity and frequency are made; frequency values can be converted to velocity values provided the transducer frequency and angle of insonation are known. Although most ultrasound duplex scanners perform this calculation automatically, it may help the reader to know how to convert KHz to cm/sec: the frequency in KHz is multiplied by 78, then this product is divided by the cosine of the angle (cos Θ—you may need to use a scientific calculator to get this figure) times the transducer frequency in MHz, resulting in the velocity in cm/sec:

Velocity in cm/sec = 78 (frequency in KHz)/(transducer frequency in MHz)(cos Θ)

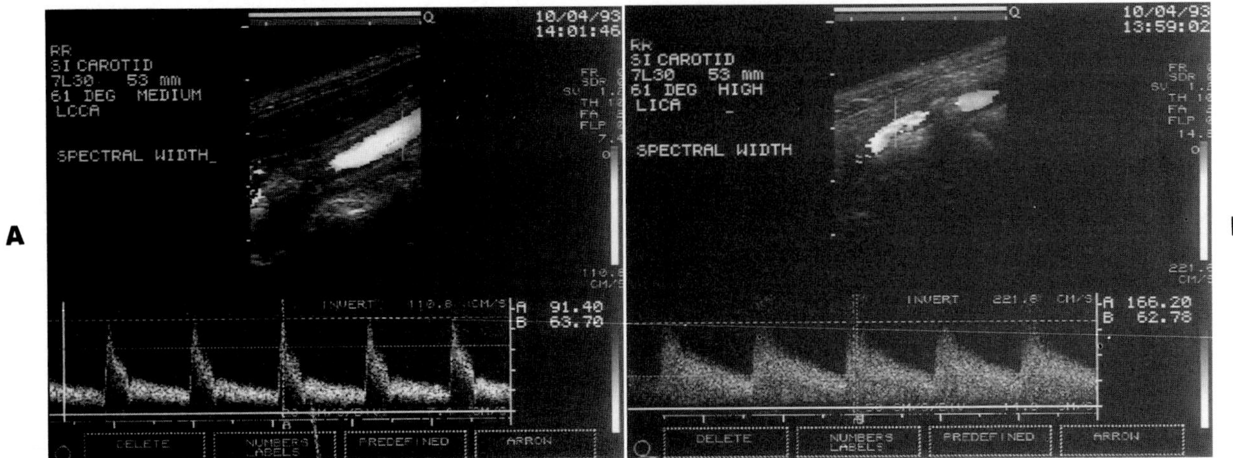

FIG. 22-59 Spectral width measurement. **A,** In this normal waveform the upper caliper *(A)* is placed at the peak of the systolic component. The lower caliper *(B)* is placed at the top of the visible window. The B reading (63.7 cm/sec) is subtracted from the A reading (91.4 cm/sec) to calculate a spectral width of 27.7 cm/sec. **B,** In this abnormal, stenotic waveform, the upper caliper *(A)* is again placed at the peak of the systolic component. The lower caliper *(B)* is subjectively placed at what appears to be the top of the window (although the window is filled in slightly and the caliper could technically be lowered). The B reading (62.8 cm/sec) is subtracted from the A reading (166.2 cm/sec) to calculate a spectral width of 103.4 cm/sec or higher.

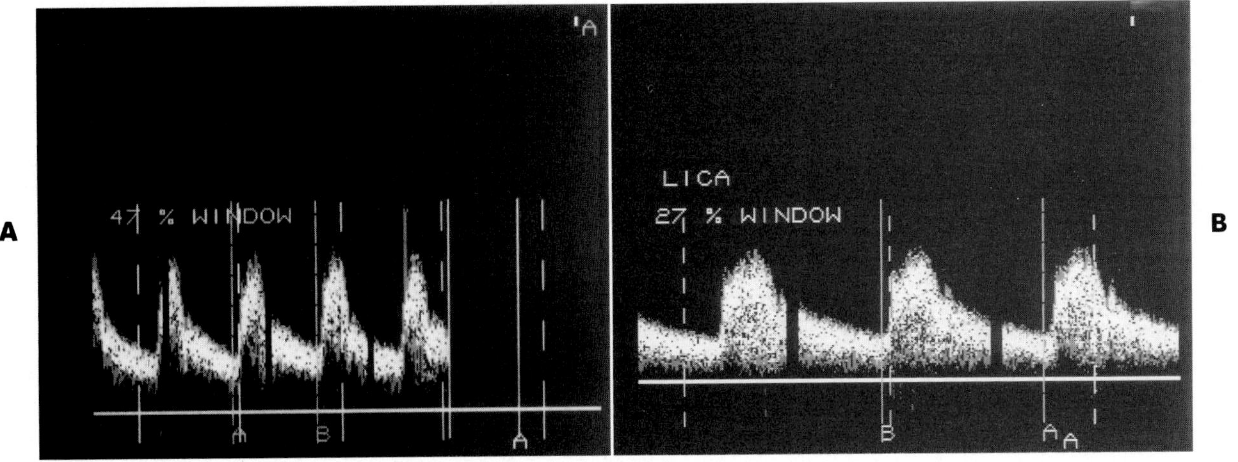

FIG. 22-60 Examples of automatic percentage window calculations. **A,** Normal waveform (47% window). **B,** Stenotic waveform (27% window).

Reporting results as velocity is currently preferred, since velocity values are universally consistent regardless of the transducer transmit frequency;[10] frequency measurements cannot be compared with other measurements (e.g., on follow-up studies) unless Doppler transducer frequency and insonation angle are identical to those used in the original study. It is important to make the distinction that this refers to Doppler transmit frequency; for example, a transducer that images at 7.5 MHz may perform pulsed Doppler at a lower frequency (such as at 5 MHz). The peak-frequency criteria limitations described here refer to the Doppler transmit frequency and not the imaging frequency.

Diagnostic Criteria Tables for Classification of Carotid Disease

Over the years many investigators have developed duplex velocity/frequency criteria for quantifying and categorizing internal carotid artery stenosis; there seem to be almost as many tables and classifications as there are published investigators. All of the criteria use peak systolic and end-diastolic velocities or frequencies; some use the IC/CC PSV ratios and EDV ratios.

Six examples of published classification criteria and tables are presented here; a vascular laboratory or ultrasound department should not blindly accept and use any of these criteria without performing some sort of internal validation study.

The following are among the reasons for internal validation:

1. Some of these criteria make assumptions that a specific Doppler frequency will be used and that all velocities or frequencies are obtained after angle correction to a specific angle of insonation.[20,25,50,51]
2. An individual laboratory's results may fail to agree with one or more categories in any one table. This is often because one or another specific make of duplex system was used exclusively by the institution that generated the criteria. It has also been demonstrated that some ultrasound systems are more accurate in their derived velocity calculations than others.[9,14]

Although the classification ranges do allow for some variability, only a self-administered periodic trial where your own system's Doppler velocity results and images are compared and correlated with arteriographic measurements can determine whether one or more of the criteria presented here will be applicable to your individual laboratory's interpretive needs.

The reader may wish to obtain and study the individual references these tables are taken from. These articles often describe the materials and methods used to derive the specific criteria, as well as details on how the criteria were validated.

Table 22-1 represents a widely used set of criteria that has been found reliable for most systems, except that it assumes the use of a 5 MHZ pulsed Doppler with a fixed 60° angle of isonation. Its simplicity of categories and disease thresholds makes it easy to remember.

A major advantage of Table 22-2 is that five different individual criteria can be cross-referenced; if two or more of the criteria agree in combination with the image characteristics, the interpreter can categorize the degree of stenosis with a fair degree of confidence. The spectral broadening measurement criteria are derived from a feature unique to one particular make of machine and are not available on devices by other manufacturers; a fair approximation, however, can be obtained using the spectral width calculation method detailed previously.

Table 22-3 uses similar diameter stenosis categories to those in Table 22-2, but provides different velocity and frequency criteria. Note the unusual angulation requirements.

The lack of velocity criteria make Table 22-4 useless for devices other than the make used to define the criteria, unless the specific Doppler transducer frequency described is used. The wide variability of angulation (from 30 to 60 degrees) also is suspect and would make repeatability and comparison of results difficult, especially between grades III and IV above. The 50% to 60% category hovers on the border of hemodynamically significant flow changes, and its value is questionable compared with other, more comprehensive data.[10]

It is interesting to note that the peak-systolic and end-diastolic criteria stated in Table 22-5 and presented in 1993 are similar to the criteria presented in 1988 by Bluth et al. (see Table 22-2).[10]

TABLE 22-1 University of Washington Criteria

Arteriographic lesion (diameter reduction)	Spectral criteria
Normal	Peak-systolic frequency < 4 KHz/peak-systolic velocity < 125 cm/sec; no spectral broadening.
1% to 15%	Peak-systolic frequency < 4 KHz/peak-systolic velocity < 125 cm/sec; spectral broadening during systolic deceleration only.
16% to 49%	Peak-systolic frequency < 4 KHz/peak-systolic velocity < 125 cm/sec; spectral broadening throughout systole.
50% to 79%	Peak-systolic frequency ≥ 4 KHz/peak-systolic velocity ≥ 125 cm/sec; end-diastolic frequency <4.5 KHz/end-diastolic velocity < 140 cm/sec.
80% to 99%	Peak-systolic frequency ≥ 4 KHz/peak-systolic velocity ≥ 125 cm/sec; end-diastolic frequency ≥ 4.5 KHz/end-diastolic velocity ≥ 140 cm/sec.
100% (occlusion)	No internal carotid flow signal, flow to zero in common carotid artery.

This long-established, very widely used table is based on criteria developed at the University of Washington[20,50].
Note that the above criteria assume a 5-MHz pulsed Doppler, a small sample volume, and a 60-degree beam-to-vessel angle of insonation.

Although not officially in Table 22-5 it should be mentioned that the NASCET data have resulted in other investigators redefining the diagnostic velocity criteria for critical stenosis at the 70% to 99% stenosis level.

A recent study by Moneta et al suggests that an end-diastolic velocity ratio of >4.0 is significant for the presence of a 70% or greater stenosis.[36] This criterium has been adopted by many institutions and can help the interpreter further categorize a grade IV stenosis above as greater or less than 70%. Also, a recent article by Hunink et al. suggests that a peak-systolic velocity of greater than 230 cm/sec may also be sensitive for detecting a greater-than-70% stenosis. Note that this threshold falls neatly between the PSV criteria presented in Table 22-2 for 60% to 79% and 80% to 99% stenoses.[31]

Table 22-6 does not present criteria for categorizing stenosis by duplex velocity data but represents the notational standard categories for cerebrovascular duplex reporting developed by the Joint Committee on Standards of the Society of Vascular Surgeons and the International Society of Cardiovascular Surgeons.[46] These standards suggest a form of shorthand for rapid reporting of plaque characteristics and the degree of stenosis. Most of the criteria that have been discussed in early sections (plaque morphology and

TABLE 22-2 Bluth, Stavros, Marich, et al. Criteria

Diameter stenosis	PSV	EDV	IC/CC PSVR	IC/CC EDVR	SB
0% (normal)	<110 cm/sec	<40 cm/sec	<1.8	<2.4	<30 cm/sec
1% to 39% (mild)	<110 cm/sec	<40 cm/sec	<1.8	<2.4	<40 cm/sec
40% to 59% (moderate)	<130 cm/sec	40 cm/sec	<1.8	<2.4	<40 cm/sec
60% to 79% (severe)	>130 cm/sec	>40 cm/sec	>1.8	>2.4	>40 cm/sec
80% to 99% (critical)	>250 cm/sec	>100 cm/sec	>3.7	>5.5	>80 cm/sec
100% (occlusion)	N/A	N/A	N/A	N/A	N/A

This table is also quite widely used. Accurate and very flexible, it was developed by a six-center task force of the Radiological Society of North America.[10]
PSV = peak-systolic velocity, EDV = end-diastolic velocity, IC/CC PSVR = internal/common carotid peak-systolic velocity ratio, IC/CC EDVR = internal/common carotid end-diastolic velocity ratio, SB = spectral broadening bandwidth measurement.

TABLE 22-3 Zwiebel Criteria

Diameter stenosis	PSV	PSF (4.5 MHz at 50 degrees)	IC/CC PSVR
0% to 40%	<80 cm/sec	<3 KHz	<1
40% to 60%	80 to 120 cm/sec	3 to 4.5 KHz	<1.5
60% to 80%	120 to 175 cm/sec	4.5 to 6.5 KHz	>1.5
80% to 99%	>175 cm/sec	>6.5 KHz	>1.8
100% (occlusion)	N/A	N/A	N/A

This table, taken from Zwiebel, categorizes data in a somewhat different manner.[51]
The table is edited somewhat to remove several atypical parameters, including those that are not available on all systems.

TABLE 22-4 Gerlach, Giyanani, Krebs Criteria

Diameter reduction	Peak-systolic frequency (4.5 MHz between 30 and 60 degrees)
Normal	
1% to 50%	<4 KHz
50% to 60%	4 to 5 KHz
60% to 80%	5 to 6 KHz
80% to >95%	>6 KHz
Occluded	

Published by Gerlach et al., this table presents a set of criteria that is arranged differently and is somewhat less comprehensive.[25]

surface characteristics) are part of this standard. Plaque morphology is classified by a "P" value:

P_1 = homogeneous
P_2 = heterogeneous

Plaque surface characteristics are notated as an "S" value:

S_1 = smooth
S_2 = minor irregularity (<2 mm deep)
S_3 = major irregularity (>2 mm deep)

For most practical purposes, the categories can be limited to S_1 (smooth) and S_2 (irregular). The hemodynamic significance (degree of stenosis) of the plaque is listed in one of five categories, notated as an H value shown in the table.

This standardized notation makes reporting of carotid disease seen on duplex much easier; for example, a heterogeneous, mildly irregular plaque that reduces the lumen by 80% could be noted as a P_2 S_2 HIV (or H_4) lesion, a normal carotid artery could be categorized as H1 (or H_1), and an occluded internal carotid could be categorized as HV (or H_5). These classifications also make data record-keeping and quality control procedures much simpler and expeditious (see Chapter 23).

DISCUSSION

Philosophies often differ among the interpreting medical staff, which can make it difficult to determine whose criteria to use or what measurements to obtain. As a general observation, radiology-based laboratories are concerned with extensively documenting image and flow data, much of which may be redundant and may not necessarily influence the patient's outcome. Vascular surgery–based laboratories often request fewer specific Doppler measurements, especially since they are more concerned with the nature of the plaque, its hemodynamic significance, and whether the stenosis is at a surgical threshold. Vascular surgeons are also often less concerned with the common carotid or external carotid arteries unless significant stenoses or irregularities are found.

Every institution has its own idiosyncrasies and departmental standards, and the image quality and velocity accuracy of every duplex system tend to differ; thus an internal validation study is ultimately the best way to evaluate all

TABLE 22-5 Faught, Mattos, van Bemmelen, et al. Criteria

Diameter reduction	PSV	EDV
0% to 29%	<110 cm/sec	<100 cm/sec
30% to 49%	≥110 cm/sec	<100 cm/sec
50% to 79%	≥130 cm/sec	<100 cm/sec
80% to 99%	≥130 cm/sec	≥100 cm/sec
Occluded		

Developed by Faught et al., the criteria in this table were established to coincide with recently defined stenosis thresholds from the North American Symptomatic Carotid Endarterectomy Trials (NASCET), European Carotid Surgery Trials, and the Veterans Affairs Cooperative Study Group asymptomatic carotid endarterectomy trials, among others.[19,30,36]

TABLE 22-6 SVS/ISCVS Notational Standard

Category	Description	Stenosis (diameter reduction)
H I	Normal to mild	0% to 20%
H II	Moderate	20% to 60%
H III	Severe	60% to 80%
H IV	Critical	80% to 99%
H V	Occluded	

Notational Standard for reporting carotid disease by the Joint Committee on Standards of the Society of Vascular Surgeons and the International Society of Cardiovascular Surgeons.

the examination parameters and diagnostic criteria to determine what classifications work best and allow an accurate and efficient interpretation of the patient's carotid disease.[9,14]

Carotid Duplex Sonography Example Cases

Although numerous examples of normal and abnormal image, color-flow, and Doppler waveforms have already been shown in previous sections, the examples presented here are intended to demonstrate specific instances of both typical and unusual carotid artery pathology and accompanying hemodynamic phenomena. Although no two cases have the same disease appearance or flow changes, these examples should familiarize the reader with a variety of abnormal occurrences in the carotid arteries.

Case 1 (Fig. 22-61): bilateral 80% to 99% ICA stenosis

The images here document a study on a 78-year-old man who presented with a TIA (left-sided transient numbness) and no carotid bruits.

On the right side a severe irregular ICA stenosis with a narrow streamline and flow separation are demonstrated in longitudinal (Fig. 22-61, *A*) and transverse (Fig. 22-61, *B*) planes. Doppler spectral waveforms at the ICA stenosis (Fig. 22-61, *C*) show significant spectral broadening, a high peak-systolic velocity (greater than 216 cm/sec, aliasing) and an elevated end-diastolic velocity (92 cm/sec). The CCA Doppler waveform is high-resistance in profile (Fig. 22-61, *D*) but has a peak-systolic velocity of 40 cm/sec and an end-diastolic velocity of 5 cm/sec. The right IC/CC PSV ratio was ≥5.40, and the right IC/CC EDV ratio was 18.40.

Using the Bluth et al. criteria (see Table 22-2), the PSV and the IC/CC PSV and EDV ratios place this right ICA stenosis well within the 80% to 99% stenosis category; the EDV itself is a shade below the 100 cm/sec breakpoint, but visual analysis of the ICA waveform (see Fig. 22-61, *C*) shows the presence of an arrhythmia that affects the diastolic height. The final interpretation reflected this diagnosis.[11]

On the left side a significant ICA stenosis is present (confirmed by color flow) but is difficult to demonstrate in long axis because of the asymmetry of the plaque (Fig. 22-61, *E*). Flow recovery is, however, seen distal to the plaque. Transverse imaging of this area is more diagnostic (Fig. 22-61, *F*) because it shows the asymmetric plaque and demonstrates the residual lumen along the medial wall. Doppler spectral waveforms at the ICA stenosis (Fig. 22-61, *G*) again show significant spectral broadening, a high peak-systolic velocity (greater than 220 cm/sec, aliasing) and a very elevated end-diastolic velocity (114 cm/sec). The relatively uniform CCA Doppler waveform (Fig. 22-61, *H*), has a peak systolic velocity of 56 cm/sec and an end-diastolic velocity of 14 cm/sec.

The left IC/CC PSV ratio was more than 3.93, and the left IC/CC EDV ratio was 8.14.

Using the Bluth et al. criteria (see Table 22-2), the PSV, EDV, and the IC/CC PSV and EDV ratios firmly place the left ICA stenosis into an 80% to 99% stenosis category. The final interpretation reflected this diagnosis.[10]

Case 2 (Fig. 22-62; see color image): greater than 95% ICA stenosis

These images (from a 66-year-old woman with left-sided TIA and no bruits) show the gray-scale appearance of what was originally diagnosed as a complete ICA occlusion by a previous arteriogram (Fig. 22-62, *A*); the internal jugular vein is the superficial vessel, with echogenic plaque seen in the proximal ICA. Color-flow imaging shows a narrow patent lumen present through the plaque in the ICA (Fig. 22-62, *B*), which was confirmed by a follow-up arteriogram taken after the duplex. The arteriogram showed a narrow string lumen that ran from the origin of the ICA to the intracranial distal ICA.

This example helps illustrate the value of color-flow imaging in detecting a small residual patent lumen.

Case 3 (Fig. 22-63; see color image): complete occlusion of the CCA/ICA/ECA

These images (from an asymptomatic 76-year-old man) demonstrate the appearance of a chronic complete occlusion of an entire unilateral carotid system.

The longitudinal view (Fig. 22-63, *A*) shows a very small common carotid and ICA area that are completely filled with echogenic material and are difficult to visually separate from the surrounding tissues. No color flow is detected. The transverse view (Fig. 22-63, *B*) shows the occluded

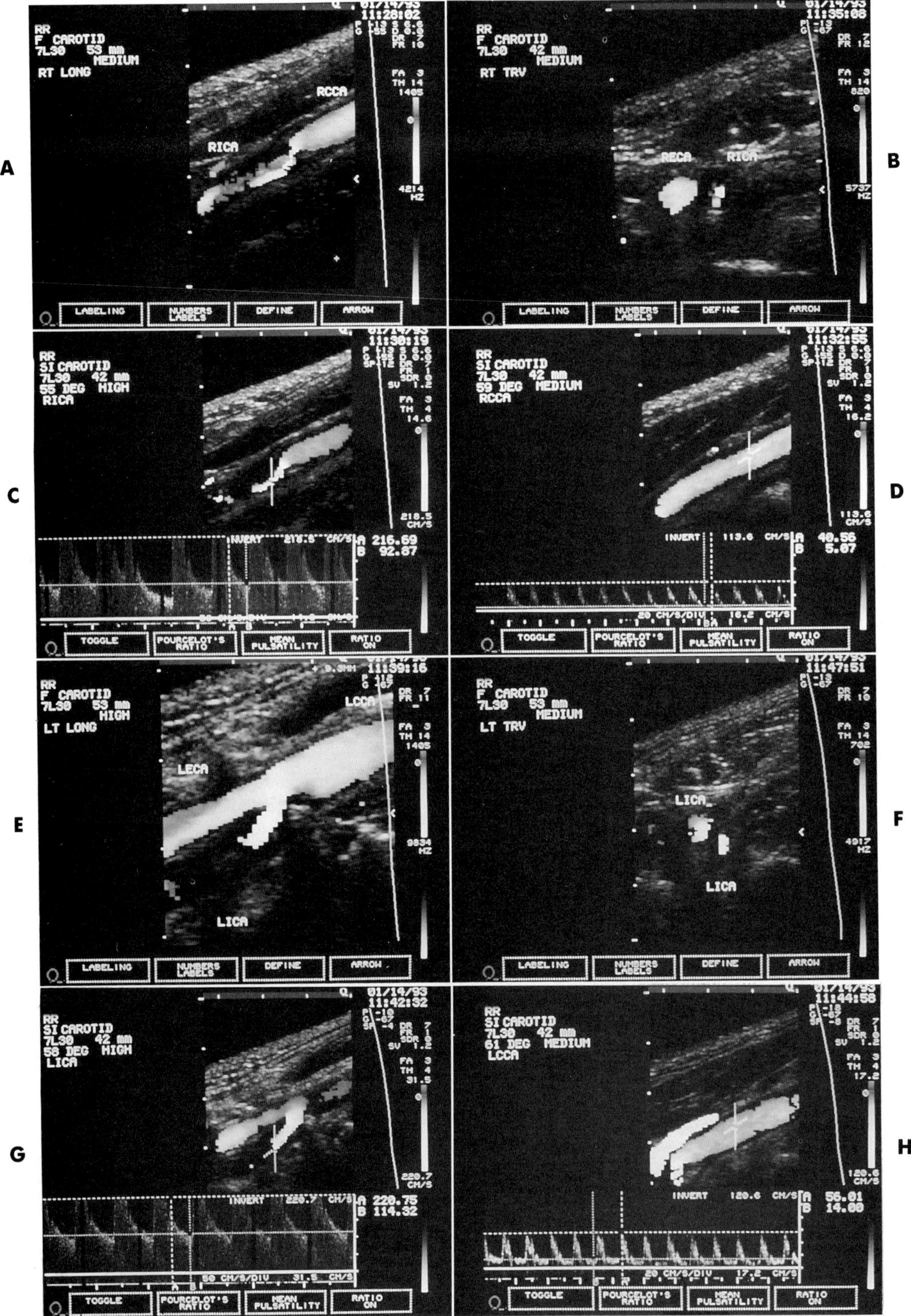

FIG. 22-61 Bilateral 80% to 99% ICA stenosis. See text for detailed description. **A,** Color-flow image, right ICA and bifurcation, longitudinal plane. **B,** Color-flow image, right ICA and ECA, transverse plane. **C,** Doppler spectral waveform, right ICA. **D,** Doppler spectral waveform, right CCA. **E,** Color-flow image, left ICA, ECA, distal CCA, longitudinal plane. **F,** Color-flow image, left ICA and ECA, transverse plane. **G,** Doppler spectral waveform, left ICA. **H,** Doppler spectral waveform, left CCA.

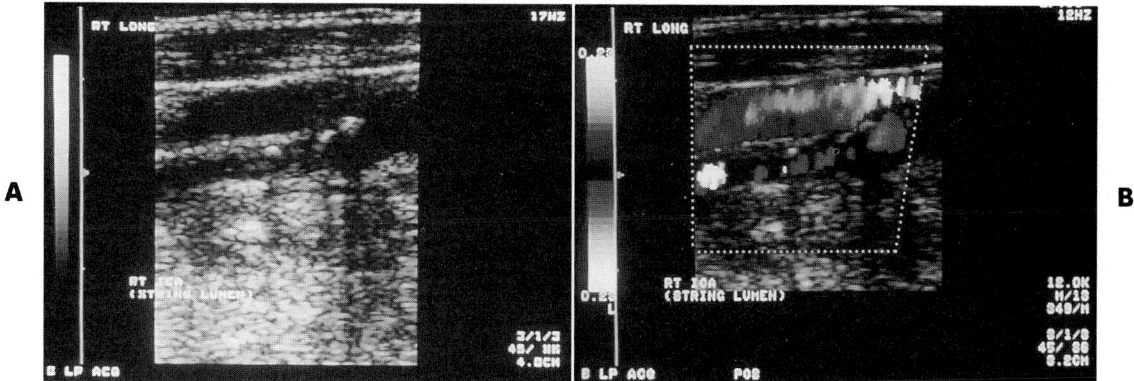

FIG. 22-62 A greater than 95% ICA stenosis. See text for description. **A,** Longitudinal gray-scale image of near-occluded ICA. **B,** Color-flow image of the same ICA, showing a narrow patent lumen.

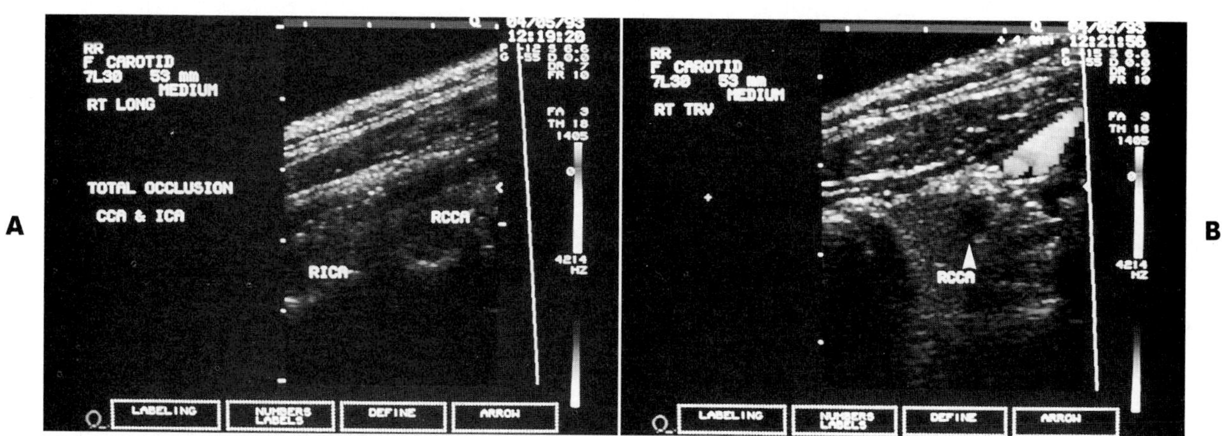

FIG. 22-63 Total occlusion of the CCA, ICA, and ECA. See text for description. **A,** Longitudinal gray-scale image showing the occluded carotid system. **B,** Color-flow transverse image of the occluded CCA, showing a patent internal jugular vein (IJV) for comparison.

CCA lumen; the color flow in the jugular vein (upper right) serves as visual confirmation of lack of patency.

Case 4 (Fig. 22-64; see color images): weblike CCA stenosis

This 66-year-old man had bilateral carotid endarterectomies in 1986. He has been asymptomatic for nearly 6 years; the unusual plaque formation demonstrated here has been serially followed since 1988 and has remained stable for that length of time.

Longitudinal color-flow imaging of the CCA and bifurcation (Fig. 22-64, *A*) shows a confusing picture; there is a flow jet along the deep wall of the distal CCA with distal turbulence that extends into the bifurcation. A small color filling defect is seen above the jet, and there is some disturbed flow separation along the wall. With color off, the architecture of the plaque becomes clearer. There is a membranous weblike lesion present in the CCA that traverses the artery (Fig. 22-64, *B*); the main flow in the lumen passes deep to it, and there is a lesser opening that allows flow in the false superficial channel to pass cephalad. The septum is best seen in the transverse plane (Fig. 22-64, *C*), as is a soft plaque at the distal superficial margin in the distal CCA (Fig. 22-64, *D*). Color-flow imaging in transverse view shows the flow patterns and openings across the lesion (Fig. 22-64, *E;* compare with *C*). Longitudinal Doppler sampling demonstrates the high-velocity jet in the lower true lumen (Fig. 22-64, *F*), which has a PSV of 203 cm/sec and an EDV of 59 cm/sec. Flow in the proximal CCA below the lesion is of normal velocity (PSV 111 cm/sec, EDV 42 cm/sec) (Fig. 22-64, *G*).

The proximal ICA (see Fig. 22-64, *A*) and ECA (not shown) are normally patent with normal velocities.

Using the Bluth et al. velocity criteria (see Table 22-2), the PSV and EDV would categorize the distal CCA stenosis into a 60% to 79% stenosis category; a distal CC/proximal CC PSV ratio of 1.8 was obtained and would be bor-

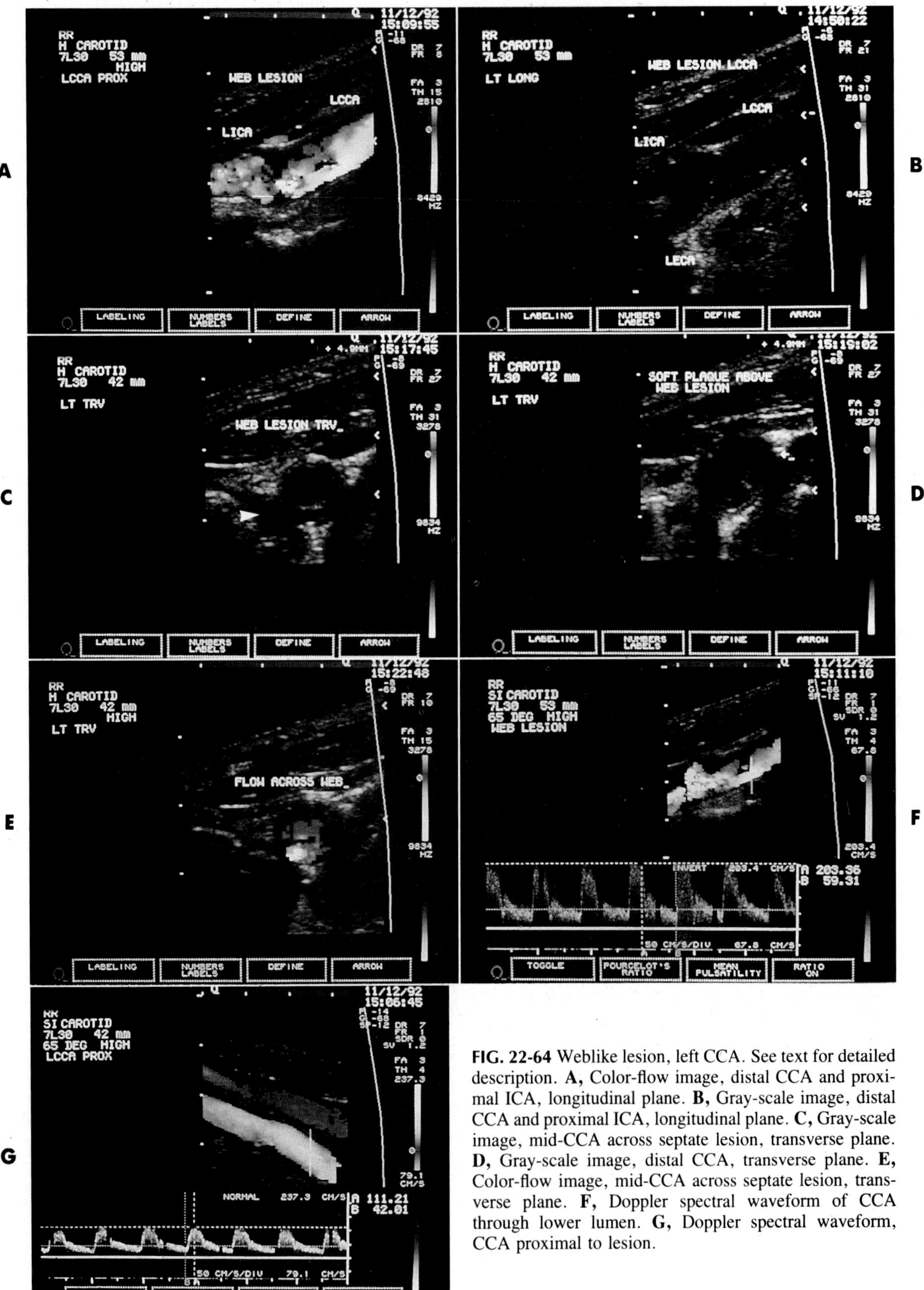

FIG. 22-64 Weblike lesion, left CCA. See text for detailed description. **A,** Color-flow image, distal CCA and proximal ICA, longitudinal plane. **B,** Gray-scale image, distal CCA and proximal ICA, longitudinal plane. **C,** Gray-scale image, mid-CCA across septate lesion, transverse plane. **D,** Gray-scale image, distal CCA, transverse plane. **E,** Color-flow image, mid-CCA across septate lesion, transverse plane. **F,** Doppler spectral waveform of CCA through lower lumen. **G,** Doppler spectral waveform, CCA proximal to lesion.

derline for the 60% to 79% category (note, however, that these criteria are intended for the internal carotid artery).[10] Serial angiographic findings on this patient have been consistent with this diagnosis.

Case 5 (Fig. 22-65; see color images): 60% to 80% distal ICA stenosis

This case (from a 68-year-old man with an asymptomatic right carotid bruit) illustrates the need to evaluate the carotids to as high a level above the bifurcation as practicable.

Longitudinal color-flow imaging of the right bifurcation shows a relatively unremarkable ICA origin (Fig. 22-65, *A*); further evaluation, however, reveals a filling defect with flow separation in the distal ICA (Fig. 22-65, *B*). Doppler spectral waveform sampling of the proximal ICA shows a borderline elevation of the PSV to 121 cm/sec (Fig. 22-65, *C*), with a substantial elevation of the PSV across the distal ICA stenosis to 257 cm/sec and an end-diastolic velocity of 72 cm/sec (Fig. 22-65, *D*).

Using the Bluth et al. criteria (see Table 22-2), the PSV and EDV categorize the distal ICA stenosis into a 60% to 80% stenosis category.[10] The final interpretation reflected this finding.

Case 6 (Fig. 22-66; see color images): carotid steal (ECA dominant)

This example, from a 64-year-old man presenting with right CVA, right amaurosis fugax, and innominate occlusion, demonstrates findings in an early carotid steal with the ECA acting as the primary collateral.

Color-flow evaluation of the right CCA shows an abnormal bidirectional pattern with retrograde flow in systole (Fig. 22-66, *A*) and antegrade flow in diastole (Fig. 22-66, *B*). This pattern was confirmed by Doppler spectral sampling (Fig. 22-66, *C*); flow is of low velocity overall.

Color-flow imaging of the right bifurcation shows very low-velocity transitional bidirectional flow in the ICA (Fig. 22-66, *D*), documented by Doppler spectral sampling (Fig. 22-66, *E*). Completely retrograde flow in the ECA is shown on color-flow imaging (Fig. 22-66, *F*) and with Doppler spectral waveform sampling (Fig. 22-66, *G*). The right vertebral artery is not a dominant contributing vessel; flow was borderline retrograde, dipping to baseline in systole but not fully reversing to a transient state (Fig. 22-66, *H*).

The image and flow data strongly suggest that the external carotid and common carotid were acting as the main

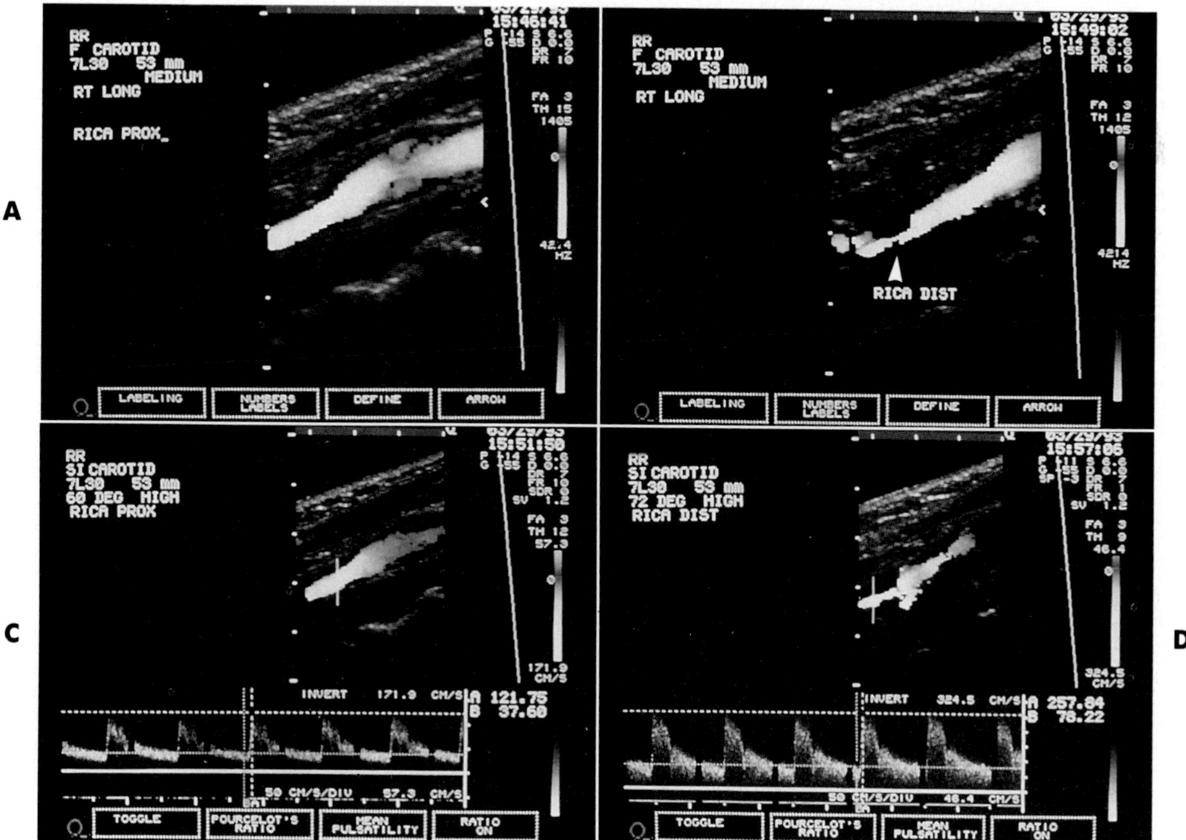

FIG. 22-65 Distal ICA stenosis. See text for detailed description. **A,** Color-flow image, proximal ICA and bifurcation, longitudinal plane. **B,** Color-flow image, distal ICA, longitudinal plane. **C,** Doppler spectral waveform of proximal ICA. **D,** Doppler spectral waveform of distal ICA, across stenosis.

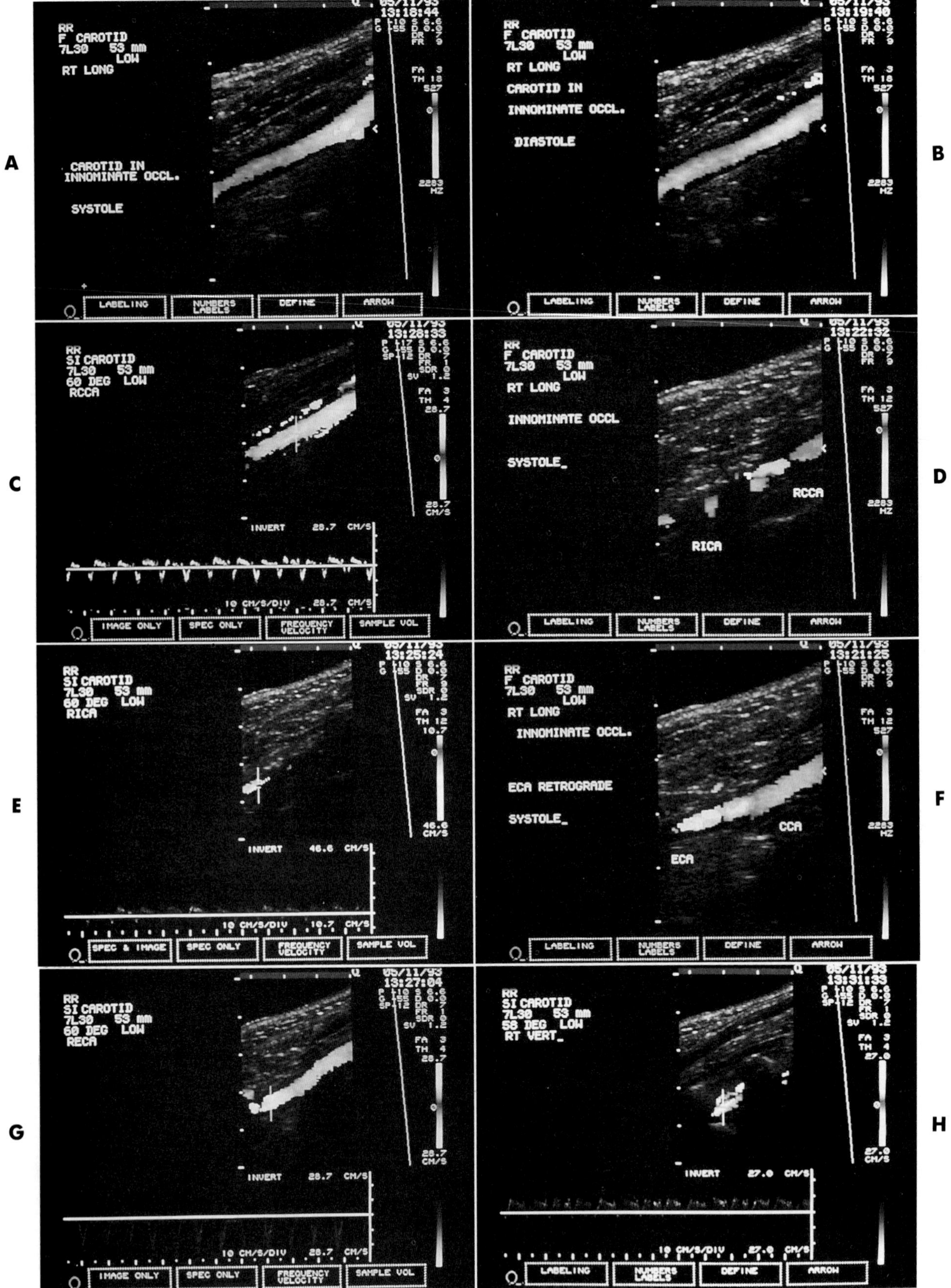

FIG. 22-66 ECA dominant early carotid steal. See text for detailed description. **A,** Color-flow image, right CCA, systole. **B,** Color-flow image, right CCA, diastole. **C,** Doppler spectral waveform with bidirectional flow, right CCA. **D,** Color-flow image of right ICA and CCA at bifurcation with transient ICA flow in systole. **E,** Doppler spectral waveform with low-velocity transient flow, right ICA. **F,** Color-flow image of right ECA and CCA at bifurcation with retrograde ECA flow in systole. **G,** Doppler spectral waveform showing retrograde flow in right ECA. **H,** Doppler spectral waveform of right vertebral artery, showing antegrade but early transitional systolic retrograde flow.

retrograde supply to compensate for the innominate stenosis. This was confirmed by an arteriogram.

The patient underwent a left subclavian PTA and a left-subclavian-to-right-CCA bypass graft, with a subsequent restoration of normal flow patterns seen on follow-up duplex examination. The patient has been asymptomatic since the procedure.

Case 7 (Fig. 22-67; see color images): carotid steal (ICA dominant)

This example, from another 64-year-old man presenting with an asymptomatic left carotid bruit, shows another example of strong carotid steal in innominate occlusion where the ICA and vertebral are dominant contributors.

Brachial systolic pressures were 84 mm Hg in the right

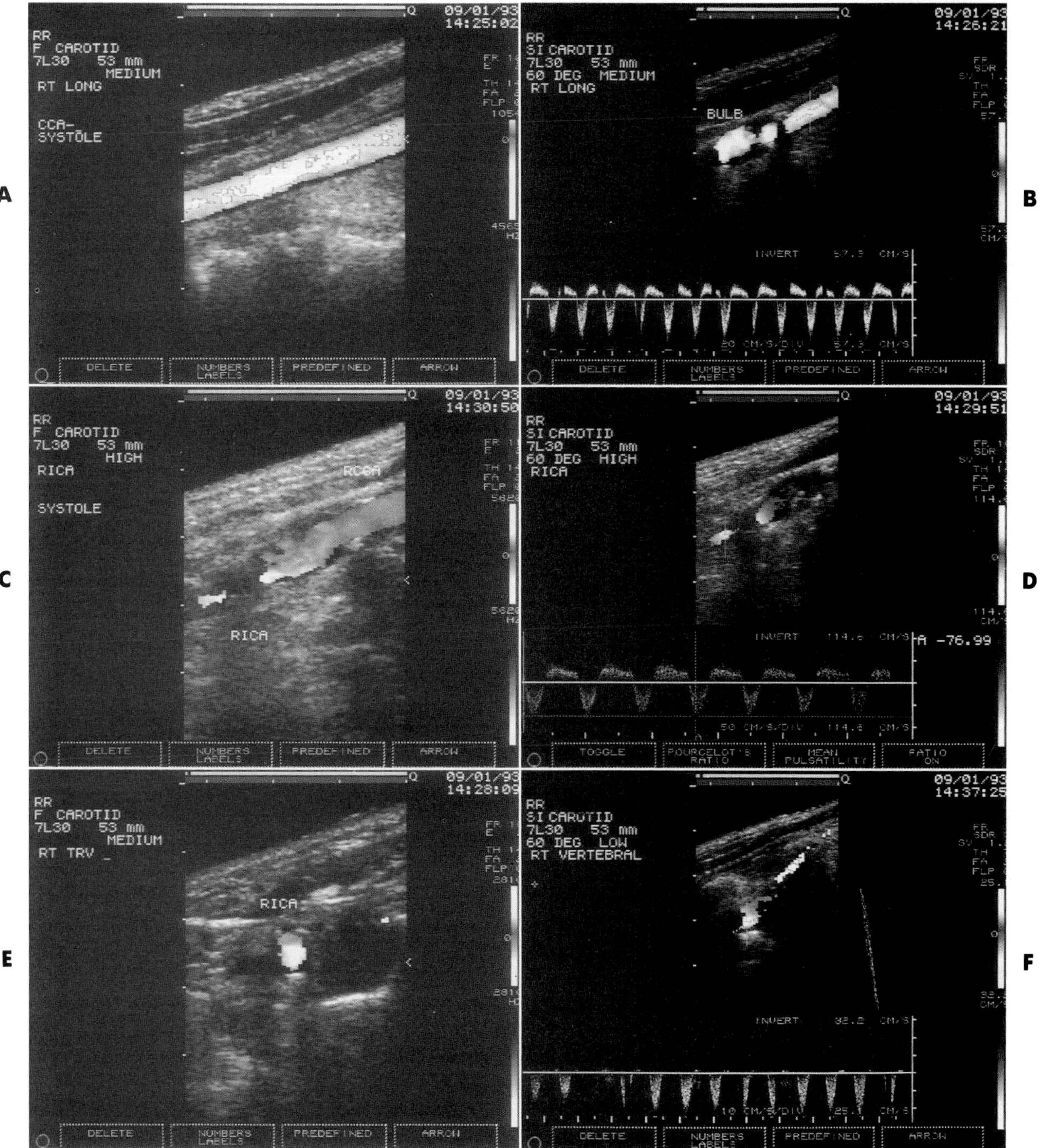

FIG. 22-67 ICA and vertebral dominant early carotid steal. See text for detailed description. **A,** Color-flow image, right CCA, systole. **B,** Doppler spectral waveform with bidirectional flow, right CCA. **C,** Color-flow image of right ICA and CCA at bifurcation in systole. **D,** Doppler spectral waveform with bidirectional flow, right ICA. **E,** Color-flow image, right ICA, transverse plane, in systole. **F,** Doppler spectral waveform with retrograde flow, right vertebral artery. *Continued.*

G H I J

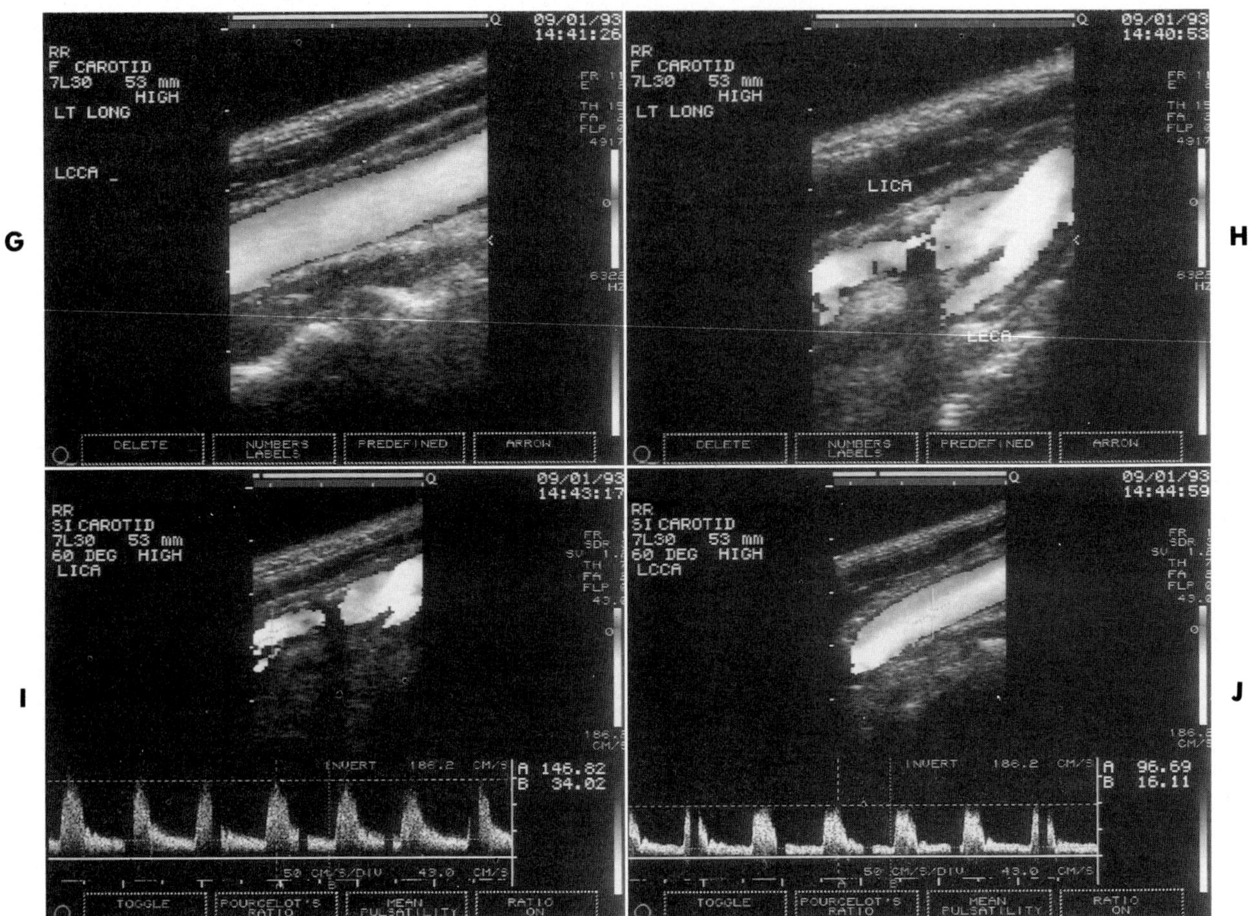

FIG. 22-67, cont'd. G, Color-flow image, left CCA, systole. **H,** Color flow image of left ICA, ECA, and CCA at bifurcation in systole. **I,** Doppler spectral waveform, left ICA. **J,** Doppler spectral waveform, left CCA.

arm and 135 mm Hg in the left arm. Color-flow evaluation of the right CCA shows an abnormal bidirectional pattern with strong retrograde flow in systole (Fig. 22-67, *A*) also demonstrated by the Doppler spectral waveform (Fig. 22-67, *B*). Color-flow imaging of the right bifurcation shows moderate-velocity transitional bidirectional flow in a moderately stenosed ICA (Fig. 22-67, *C*), again documented by Doppler spectral sampling (Fig. 22-67, *D*). This retrograde pattern is also seen in transverse images (Fig. 22-67, *E*). The right vertebral artery has completely retrograde flow (Fig. 22-67, *F*).

Compare the flow and image findings in the right carotid system with the left side. Normal antegrade color flow is demonstrated in the CCA (Fig. 22-67, *G*), a moderately stenosed ICA, and the ECA (Fig. 22-67, *H*). Doppler spectral waveforms from the ICA show moderately stenotic profiles with a PSV of 147 cm/sec and an EDV of 34 cm/sec (Fig. 22-67, *I*); the CCA has normal waveforms with a PSV of 97 cm/sec and an EDV of 16 cm/sec (Fig. 22-67, *J*). Normal directional flow was also demonstrated in the vertebral artery (not shown).

This case is a classic example of multicomponent carotid steal, with the right ICA, CCA, and vertebral all significantly supplying the innominate runoff. Arteriography confirmed the innominate occlusion and the duplex findings, additionally demonstrating that the retrograde flow was being supplied from the left side of the circle of Willis via the right posterior communicating artery and cervical collaterals.

The patient underwent an aorta-to-right-subclavian/CCA bypass performed in conjunction with coronary artery bypass grafting. This procedure restored normal flow and the patient has been asymptomatic since the procedure.

Case 8 (Fig. 22-68; see color images): common carotid dissection

This 65-year-old man had presented with a left hemispheric TIA.

Color-flow evaluation of the CCA reveals two distinct flow directions occurring side by side (Fig. 22-68, *A*); scanning in the posterior plane reveals two separate lumens divided by a septum (Fig. 22-68, *B*). The bifurcation image shows what appears to be retrograde flow in the ICA in systole (Fig. 22-68, *C*) with antegrade flow in diastole (Fig. 22-68, *D*). Transverse evaluation of the CCA (Fig. 22-68,

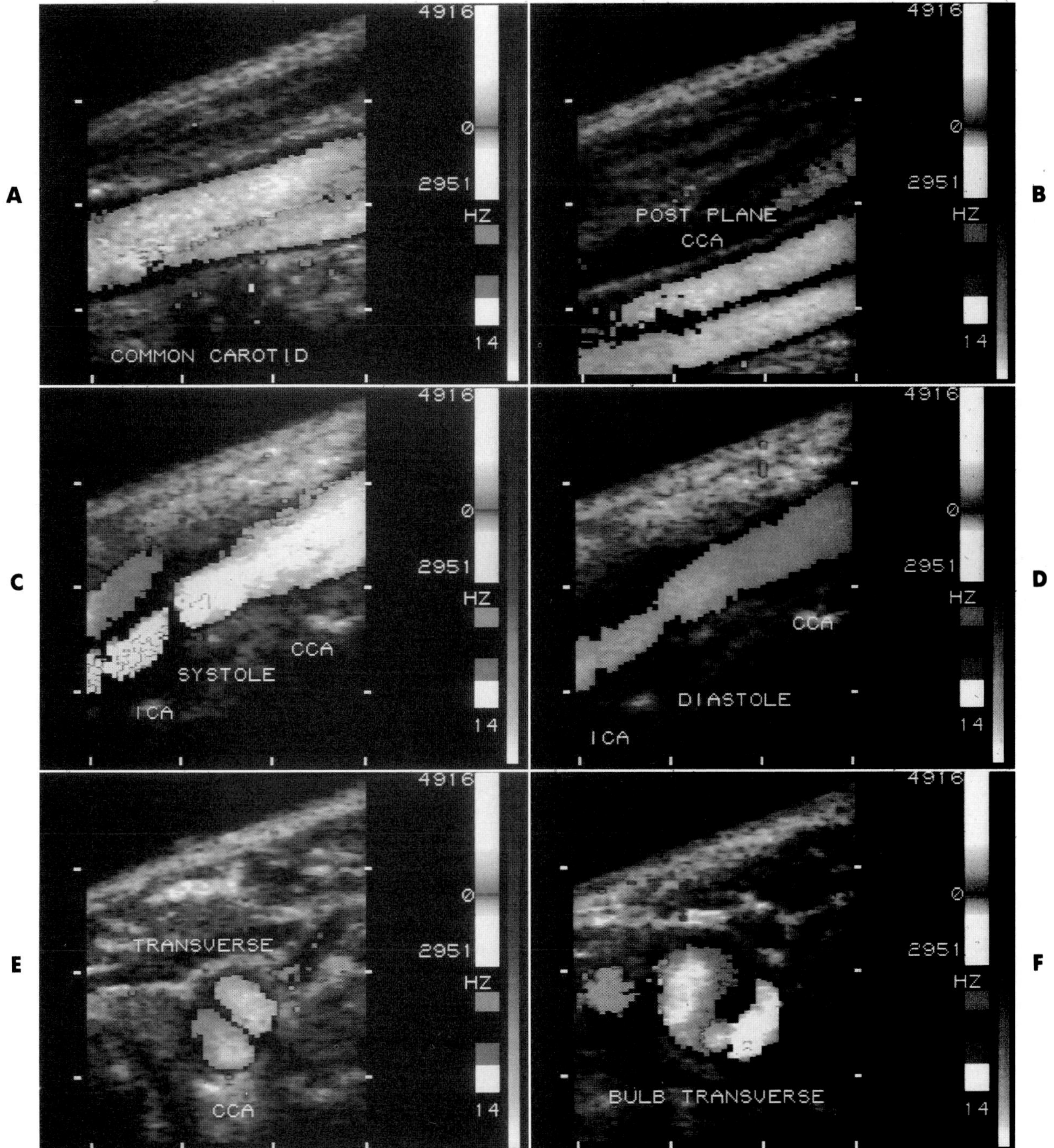

FIG. 22-68 Carotid dissection. See text for detailed description. **A,** Color-flow image, CCA, longitudinal. **B,** Color-flow image, CCA, longitudinal from posterior scanning plane, showing double lumen. **C,** Color-flow image of ICA and CCA at bifurcation in systole. **D,** Color-flow image of ICA and CCA at bifurcation in diastole. **E,** Color-flow image, CCA, transverse plane. **F,** Color-flow image, bulb area, transverse plane. *Continued.*

E) shows a double-lumen appearance, which implies a carotid dissection; the true lumen is deep (antegrade flow, red) and the false lumen is superficial (retrograde, blue). This appearance is maintained to the bulb area (Fig. 22-68, *F*), where the inflow point to the dissection is visualized. The dissection also extends into the proximal ICA (Fig. 22-68, *G*), accounting for the unusual appearance of the longitudinal images (see Fig. 22-68, *C* and *D*). Confirmation and identification of the true and false lumens is accomplished by Doppler spectral sampling; flow patterns are documented in the true lumen (Fig. 22-68, *H*) and false lumen (Fig. 22-68, *I*) in the CCA and in the true lumen (Fig. 22-68, *J*)

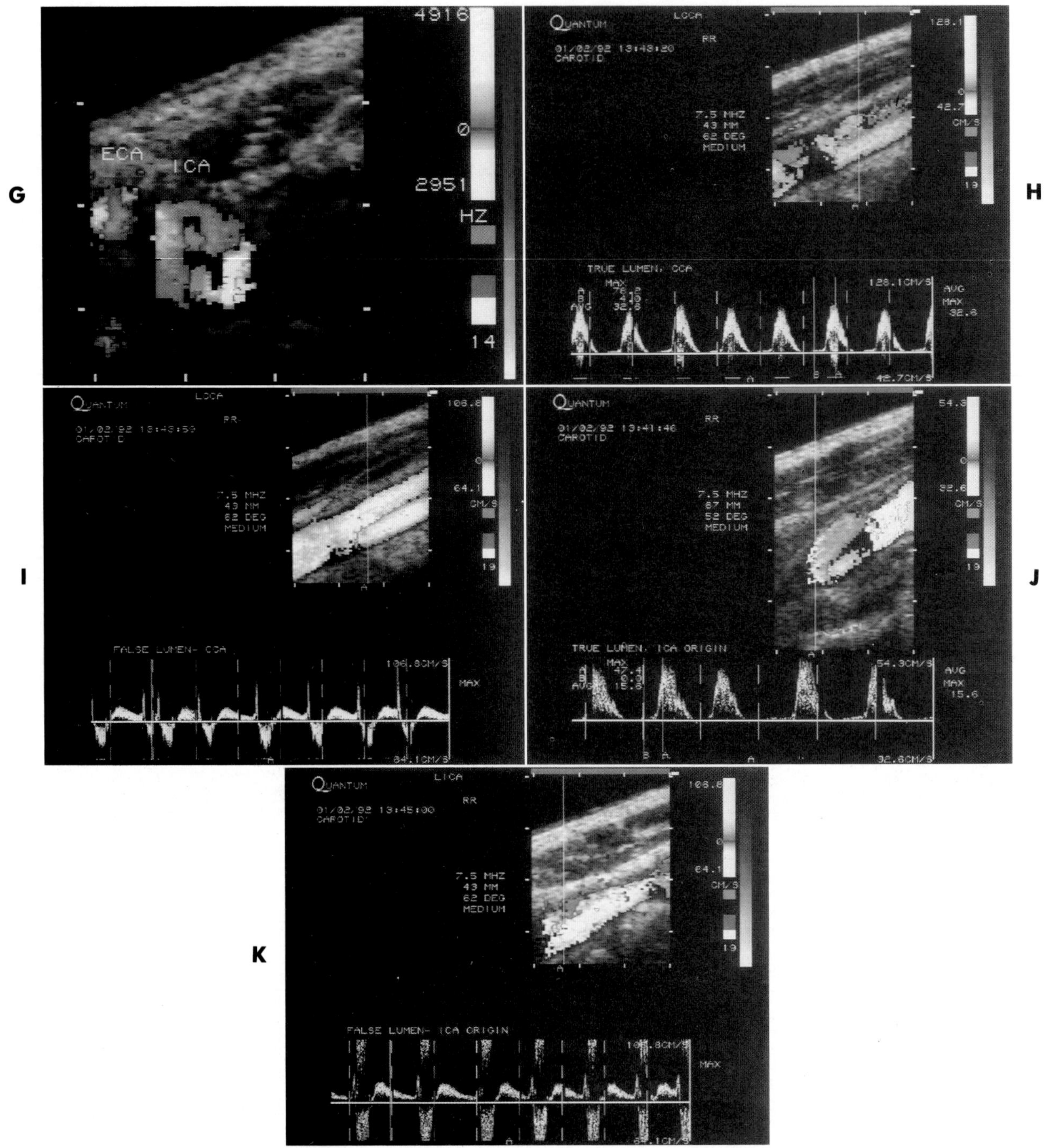

FIG. 22-68, cont'd. G, Color-flow image, ECA and ICA, transverse plane. **H,** Doppler spectral waveform in true lumen of the CCA. **I,** Doppler spectral waveform in false lumen of the CCA. **J,** Doppler spectral waveform in true lumen of the ICA. **K,** Doppler spectral waveform in false lumen of the ICA.

and false lumen (Fig. 22-68, *K*) at the ICA origin. Note the relatively normal flow waveforms in the true lumen spectra and the retrograde, abnormal transitional waveforms in the false lumen spectra.

The dissection was shown on arteriography to extend from the thoracic aorta to the origin of the CCA, then from the proximal CCA to the ICA with an inflow point in the ICA attachment and an outflow tract at the proximal CCA, as shown above by duplex. The patient underwent a left-subclavian-to-ICA Gore-Tex interposition graft procedure and has been asymptomatic since the surgery.

Case 9 (Fig. 22-69; see color images): aneurysm of right ICA origin, 20% to 59% stenosis of left ICA

This 58-year-old woman had had a right carotid endarterectomy and presented with a progressing visible pulsa-

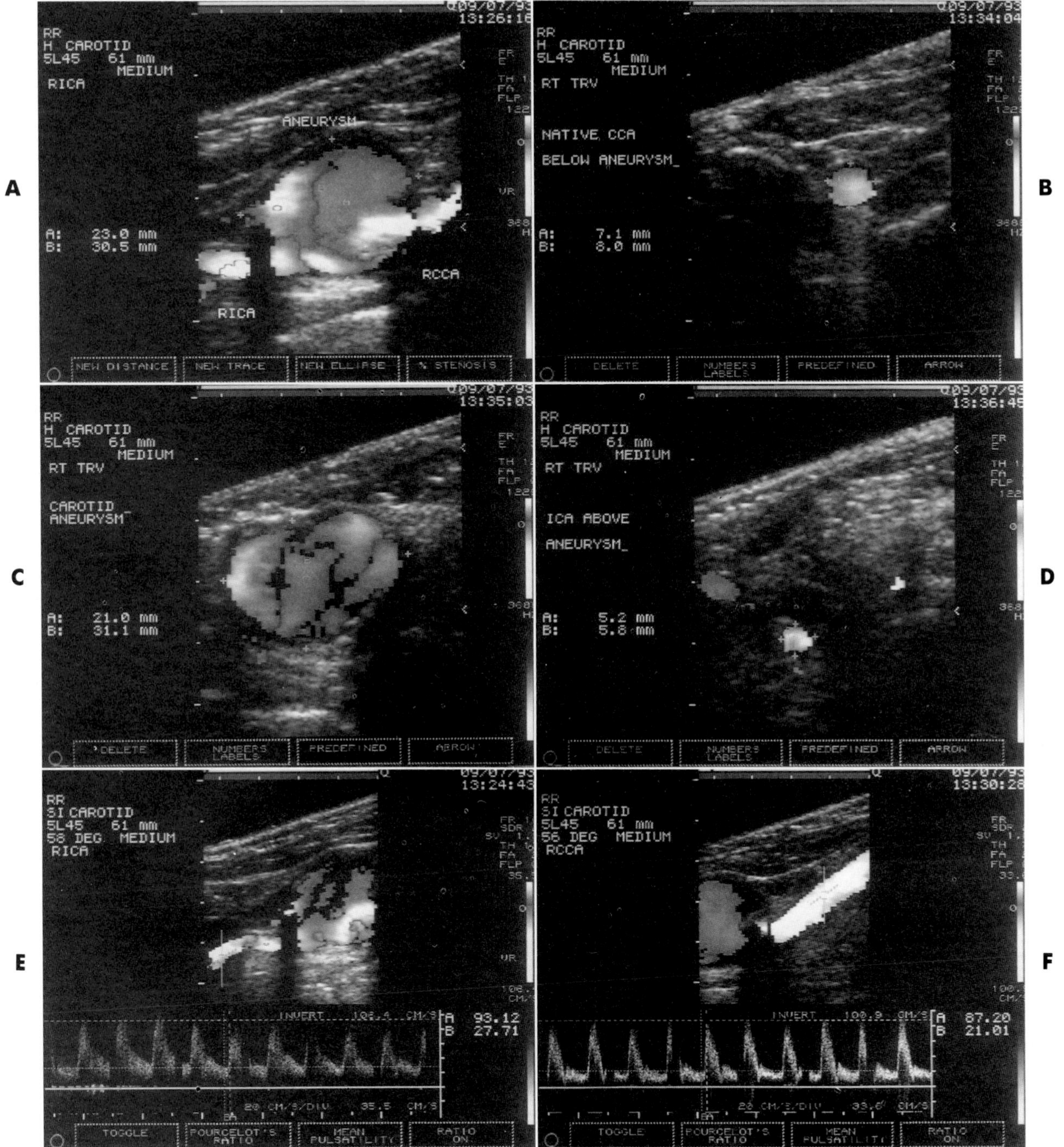

FIG. 22-69 Right carotid aneurysm and 20% to 59% left ICA stenosis. See text for detailed description. **A,** Color-flow image of right bifurcation in the longitudinal plane, showing the aneurysm and its relationship to the ICA and CCA. **B,** Transverse color-flow image of the CCA proximal to the aneurysm. **C,** Transverse color-flow image of the aneurysm. **D,** Transverse color-flow image of the right ICA distal to the aneurysm. **E,** Doppler spectral waveform in right ICA distal to the aneurysm. **F,** Doppler spectral waveform in right CCA proximal to the aneurysm.

Continued.

tile mass in the right neck, beneath the mandible area. She was otherwise asymptomatic.

Color-flow imaging of the right carotid bifurcation demonstrates a large aneurysm at the ICA origin (Fig. 22-69, *A*), measuring 2.3 cm in length and 3.05 cm in anteroposterior diameter; as can be seen, the CCA and ICA are of relatively normal caliber. This was also confirmed in transverse images of this area. The CCA below the aneurysm (Fig. 22-69, *B*) measures 7 × 8 mm, the aneurysm itself (Fig. 22-69, *C*) measures 2.1 cm × 3.11 cm, and the ICA above the aneurysm (Fig. 22-69, *D*) measures 5 × 6 mm. Proximal and distal Doppler waveforms were typically un-

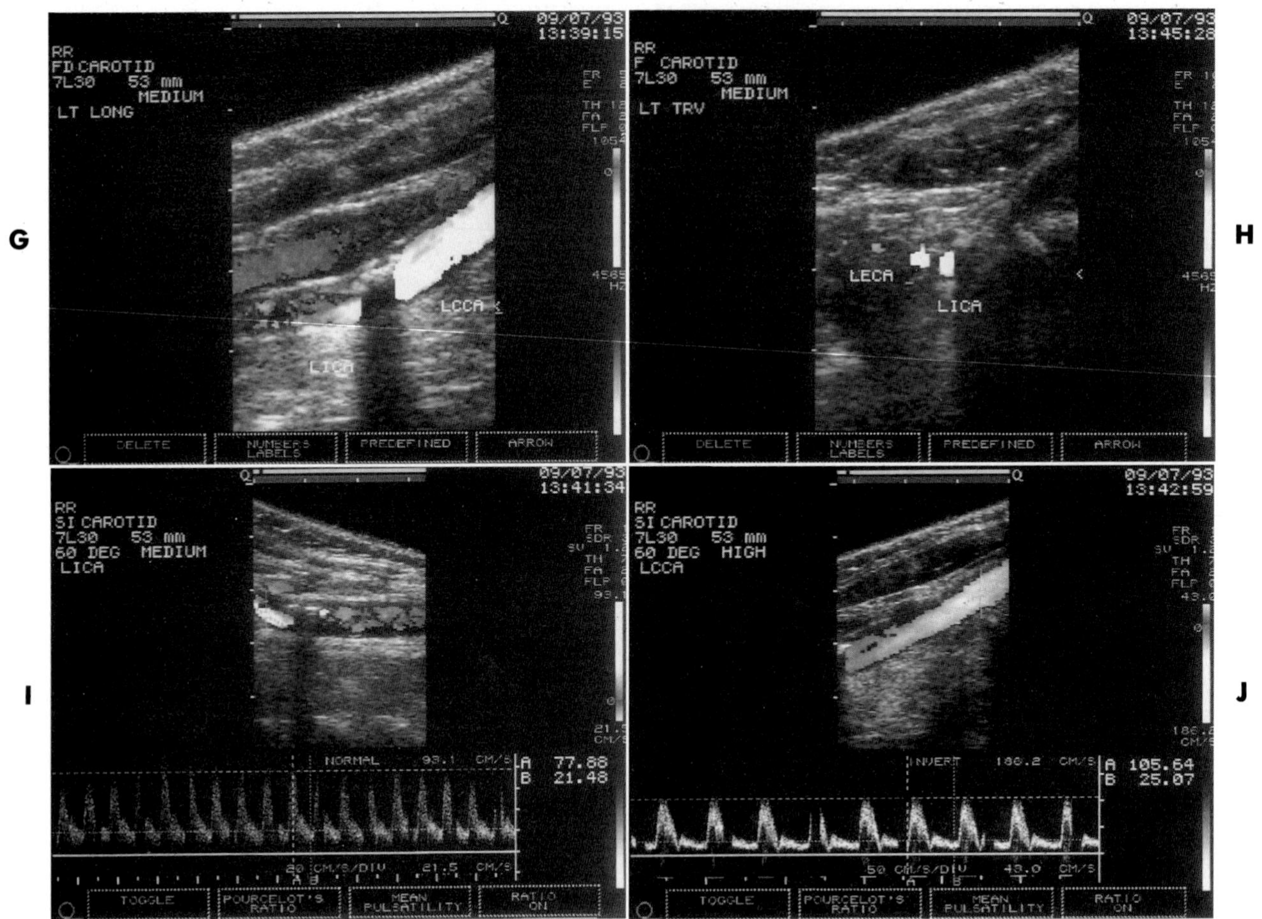

FIG. 22-69, cont'd. G, Color-flow image, left ICA and CCA at bifurcation, longitudinal plane. **H,** Color-flow image, left ICA and ECA, transverse plane. **I,** Doppler spectral waveform in the left ICA. **J,** Doppler spectral waveform in the left CCA.

affected by the aneurysm; the CCA velocities (Fig. 22-69, *E*) and ICA velocities (Fig. 22-69, *F*) are within normal limits by the Bluth et al. criteria (see Table 22-2).[10]

The left carotid was also evaluated, especially since size comparison was warranted. Imaging of the left bifurcation (Fig. 22-69, *G*) shows a complex heterogeneous plaque along the superficial wall of the ICA origin. This plaque is seen to stenose the lumen only about 50% in the transverse image (Fig. 22-69, *H*). Doppler flow waveforms from the ICA (Fig. 22-69, *I*) and the CCA (Fig. 22-69, *J*) show normal profiles with relatively normal velocities (77 cm/sec PSV, 21 cm/sec EDV in the ICA, and 105 cm/sec PSV, 25 cm/sec EDV in the CCA). The IC/CC ratio was also within normal limits, using the Bluth et al. criteria (see Table 22-2).[10]

In surgery the aneurysm was seen to involve only the proximal ICA and was distal to the bifurcation. Arteriography had implied that the ECA was involved in the aneurysm, but it was seen to be a separate vessel. The aneurysm was resected and the patient had a CCA-to-ICA Gore-Tex interposition graft placed with subsequent normal flow restoration.

Case 10: moving thrombus in CCA, occluded ICA

The carotid sonographic findings from this older but still interesting case have a bearing on the periorbital Doppler study that accompanied it. The case history and sonographic images are presented in "Periorbital Doppler" case 2 (see Fig. 22-76) at the end of the next topic.

PERIORBITAL CONTINUOUS-WAVE DOPPLER EXAMINATION

As stated in the discussion of Poiseuille's law in Chapter 20, distal to a stenosis flow pressure drops proportional to the degree of luminal reduction. In the internal carotid a lack of flow pressure causes collateral reconstitution of flow to develop from one or more external carotid branches or from circle of Willis sources to compensate for deficient flow from the obstructed vessel (see "Hemodynamics and Possible Anastomoses in Cerebral Arterial Obstructions"). This occurrence forms the diagnostic basis of the periorbital continuous-wave Doppler examination. Although this and other indirect examinations should not be used without an accompanying duplex evaluation, periorbital Doppler

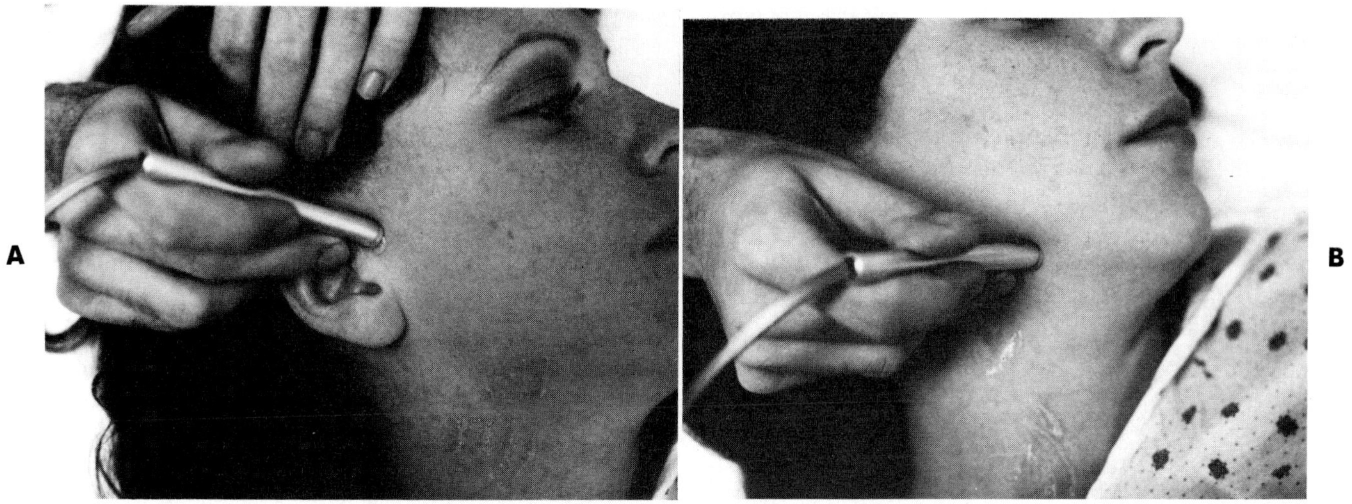

FIG. 22-70 Examination of, **A,** the temporal artery and **B,** the facial artery.

still may provide some valid information regarding the distal and intracranial circulation that would otherwise be lost or unavailable to the investigator. Periorbital studies also do not require specialized transcranial Doppler devices and take little extra time to perform.

The periorbital examination requires a bidirectional continuous-wave Doppler device with a zero-crossing strip-chart recorder or computer interface. The Doppler pencil-style probe should be used and should operate preferably at a high transmit frequency (8 MHz or 10 MHz works best).

After the carotids have been evaluated bilaterally, the examiner may wish to take continuous-wave Doppler tracings from the superficial temporal artery in front of the ear and the facial artery at the mandibular notch. These tracings may be of value in determining indirect hemodynamics; if lower-resistance flow increases strongly in either artery, collateralization may be occurring. If there is decreased or absent flow in either or both vessels, then external carotid artery occlusion may be present (Fig. 22-70).

The examiner should sit at the head of the examining table and then ask the patient to relax and close his or her eyes. The examiner should place the continuous-wave probe gently in a location just superior to the inner canthus of the eye within the orbital rim. The probe should be angled medially and cranially until the frontal artery signal is obtained (Fig. 22-71).[8,12]

When the signal is located, the chart recorder should be run at slow speed to show the direction of flow. The flow signal is normally antegrade. Retrograde flow implies a greater than 70% internal carotid obstruction.[8]

Various compression maneuvers are next performed to determine whether compression of the external carotid branches from the ipsilateral and contralateral sides causes any increase, decrease, or reversal of the frontal artery signal. The examiner steadies the probe by resting one hand

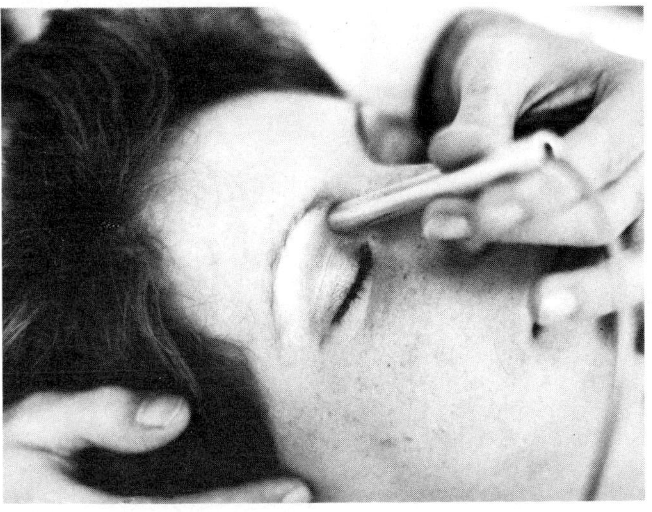

FIG. 22-71 Positioning for the frontal artery.

on the patient's chin or by steadying the examining arm in some fashion before beginning the compressions. This is to ensure that the probe does not slip off the artery during the time the compression is being attempted.

The first vessel to be compressed is the superficial temporal artery on the side being examined. Normally this either causes an increase in flow or does not affect the signal. It should be held for at least three beats and then released.

The facial artery on the same side is then compressed and held for three beats. A normal response to this compression is either an increased or an unchanged signal.

The infraorbital artery on the same side is compressed next. The normal response is an unchanged signal (Fig. 22-72).

With the probe still in place the examiner then switches hands and compresses the superficial temporal, facial, and infraorbital arteries of the opposite side of the face in turn. Compression of the contralateral arteries should not normally affect the frontal artery flow signal.

When the contralateral compressions are completed, the examination procedure is repeated for the remaining frontal artery.

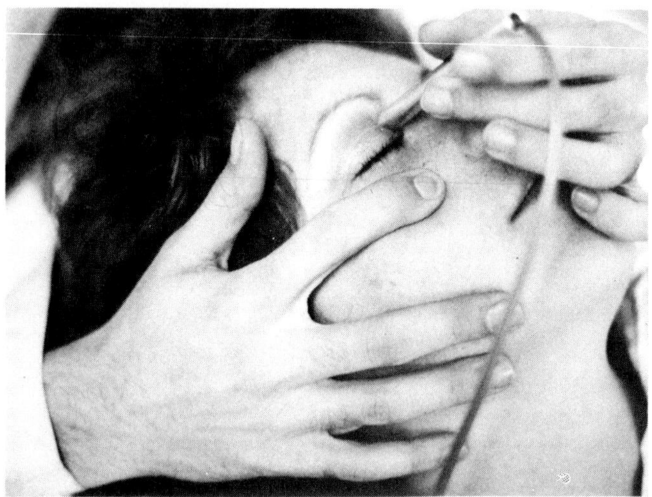

FIG. 22-72 Compression of the infraorbital artery.

The supraorbital artery should be additionally evaluated bilaterally by palpating the supraorbital notch, then monitoring the artery at that site in a similar fashion to the frontal artery. This artery should be examined in cases where frontal artery flow is absent or when determination of directional changes or collateral presence is difficult based on the frontal artery signal. Compression of the superficial temporal artery often augments the flow signal in this location. The sites for monitoring and compression are summarized and illustrated in Fig. 22-73.

Interpretation of the Periorbital Examination and Findings in Cerebrovascular Stenosis or Occlusion. The normal responses in the periorbital examination that were mentioned in the prior section are summarized here:

1. Normal flow direction in the frontal artery is antegrade.
2. Compression of ipsilateral and contralateral external branches normally either augments or does not affect the frontal artery signal.

The next section discusses what flow responses may be seen during specific obstruction thresholds and how to identify the collateralization pathways that may be present.

The frontal flow signal is an important indicator of intracerebral hemodynamics. Direction of flow is the primary diagnostic finding, but whereas stenoses generally need to exceed 75% to cause a reversal of the frontal signal, a reversal may not occur if intracranial collaterals are well de-

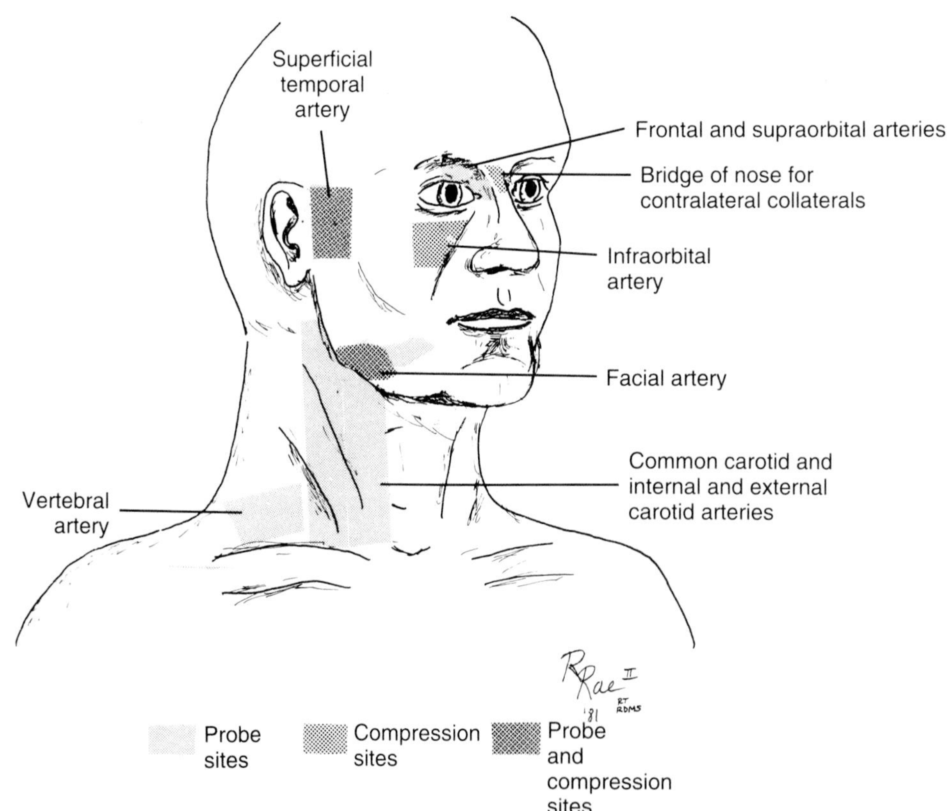

FIG. 22-73 Sites for examination and compression in the cerebrovascular and periorbital Doppler examination. (Courtesy Richard E. Rae, Indianapolis.)

veloped. The amplitude of the signal still visibly decreases in severe or subsevere internal carotid stenosis, and a bidirectional frontal signal, although not totally reversed, is an indicator that internal carotid pressure has dropped to the point where the signal is going antegrade with systole but pressure in diastole is insufficient to prevent retrograde collateral supply from dominating. It is therefore important to look not only at direction but also at amplitude when a severe stenosis is suspected of decreasing intracranial flow. The comments for interpreting the frontal signal that follow are based on clear directional changes.

In internal carotid obstruction with an ipsilateral superficial temporal artery collateral:

1. Frontal flow is retrograde, since flow travels into instead of out from the orbit.
2. Compression of the ipsilateral temporal artery either stops or reverses the flow pattern to antegrade, provided there is sufficient internal carotid pressure or another intracranial collateral supply to compensate.
3. Same-sided facial and infraorbital compression do not change the signal.
4. Contralateral compressions have no effect.

When the internal carotid is obstructed with a contralateral temporal collateral, compression of the contralateral temporal will have the same effect as in number two above. Other results will be as stated.

In obstruction with a facial collateral:

1. Frontal flow may be either antegrade or retrograde.
2. Flow is unchanged with temporal compression.
3. In retrograde flow, ipsilateral facial compression stops or reverses the signal. If a contralateral facial collateral is present, compression of the contralateral facial rather than the ipsilateral facial causes the change. Since this latter collateral can come across the bridge of the nose because of contralateral angular collateral connections, compression at the bridge should have the same effect as direct facial compression.
4. Other compressions have no effect.

When flow is antegrade, the signal still changes. The apparent antegrade signal may result from retrograde flow in the angular artery entering the nasal artery and making a U-turn to come back out the frontal artery (Fig. 22-74). The examiner should check flow in the supraorbital artery to be certain that retrograde flow in the ophthalmic artery is present.

In internal carotid obstruction with infraorbital artery collaterals:

1. Frontal artery flow usually is retrograde.
2. Temporal and facial compressions bilaterally have no effect on the signal.
3. Either ipsilateral or contralateral infraorbital compression affects the signal. The contralateral collateral network may also cross the bridge of the nose, as with the facial artery.

Intracranial or circle of Willis collaterals may also occur.[8] When the contralateral internal carotid is supplying the obstructed artery, the following occurrences will be seen:

1. The frontal artery signal is antegrade.
2. Peripheral external carotid artery branch compressions cause augmentation or no changes, as in a normal examination.

In this situation it may be necessary to compress the common carotids one at a time, for this is the only definite way to distinguish the abnormality by Doppler.

With a physician, preferably, performing the compression the carotid is located, straddled by the tips of two fingers, and compressed low in the neck for no more than two beats while the frontal signal is monitored.

The result of contralateral carotid compression should be obliteration or diminishing of the signal. Ipsilateral compression augments flow. When a vertebrobasilar collateral situation exists, contralateral common carotid compression has no effect on the frontal artery signal. Intracranial collaterals are among the hardest to diagnose with continuous-wave periorbital Doppler techniques. Proper and diligent examination can, however, limit the possibility of the existence of these collaterals going undetected.

Discussion of False-Positive and False-Negative Conditions.[8] In Doppler periorbital examinations any number of occurrences that can cause diagnostic and interpretive errors may take place. These errors are less likely when carotid duplex sonography is used as the primary adjunctive procedure. As transcranial Doppler techniques gain in use, almost all of the problems with the periorbital examination can be eliminated. Some of these errors are technical in nature; some result from inherent factors related to Doppler ultrasound measurement.

A few of the false-negative conditions are discussed first:

1. Doppler is a fairly reliable indicator of occlusion when the vessel lumen is obstructed by 70% to 80% of its transverse diameter, but this figure must be attained before pressure drops significantly in the cerebrovascular system. Diagnosis of a false-normal condition may occur when the artery is not occluded enough to reduce

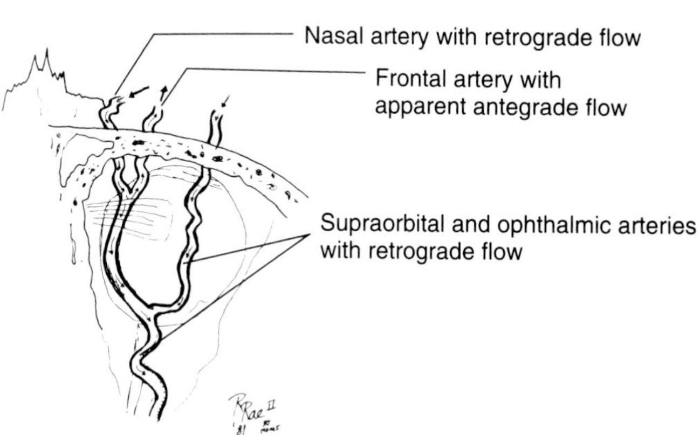

FIG. 22-74 Diagram of nasal artery flow "stolen" by the frontal artery.

flow. This factor is eliminated by the use of carotid duplex sonography and color-flow imaging (see "Carotid Duplex Sonography").
2. Many deep and nonaccessible arteries and collaterals exist that cannot be compressed or heard with the probe. These may also give a false impression of normal flow.
3. Some nonstenotic soft tissue plaques do not obstruct flow and therefore cause no audible change in the signal. With carotid duplex sonography these can be seen.
4. Sometimes both the internal and the external carotids can be stenosed or occluded simultaneously. Flow recordings of the facial and temporal arteries may imply that this obstruction is present, and these should be obtained any time a question as to the patency of the external carotid arises.
5. The frontal and supraorbital arteries can be inaccurately measured if the examiner places the probe outside the orbital rim and catches the flow signal at an incorrect angle or tries to make a reversed signal "antegrade" if unsure of the probe technique.
6. A nondirectional Doppler does not show flow direction and may lead an inexperienced examiner to believe a patient has normal flow, especially in postoperative patients.

The following are some false-positive occurrences related to the periorbital examination:

1. Excessive probe pressure may occlude the frontal or supraorbital, making flow seem reduced or absent. The probe can also slip off the artery without the examiner noticing it during compression maneuvers, occasionally giving one the idea that compression has affected the flow.
2. Flow caught leaving the forehead by an incorrectly angled probe may lead to a false diagnosis of flow reversal.
3. Monitoring the palpebral artery in the eyelid instead of the supraorbital may cause confusion, since the palpebral usually stops with temporal compression and this leads to a false diagnosis.
4. Monitoring the nasal artery can cause problems, especially if the patient fits in the category of retrograde flow (45% of normal individuals).[8] This is rarely encountered with good probe technique.
5. If the ophthalmic artery is occluded, flow is reversed. The patient usually shows signs of blindness without cerebral symptoms, however. Arteriography is indicated to specify this condition.

Common sense, care, and steady probe positioning usually produce an accurate examination.

Periorbital Doppler Cases

The following cases were done in conjunction with duplex examination and are presented as examples of the technique and its relationship to carotid disease.

Case 1 (Fig. 22-75): severe (80% to 99%) ICA stenosis

This patient presented with amaurosis fugax of the left eye. Real time sonography of the left carotid showed a large area of soft plaque occupying the proximal internal carotid but with poorly defined luminal borders (Fig. 22-75, *A*). The external carotid also appears filled with fine gray echoes at the origin (see small image in Fig. 22-75, *G*). The effect of this ICA stenosis on the hemodynamics is evident with the duplex Doppler findings. The proximal common carotid signal (Fig. 22-75, *B*) is attenuated (<45 cm/sec) and typical of a high-resistance pattern with the abnormal loss of the diastolic component. This appears with a distal obstruction that severely reduces flow. The distal common carotid signal was even more attenuated, barely reaching 20 cm/sec (Fig. 22-75, *C*). In direct contrast, there is a severe and dramatic increase in velocity in the internal carotid at the origin (Fig. 22-75, *D*), with a peak velocity of nearly 350 cm/sec with severe spectral broadening typical of the jet effect. About 2 cm distal to this, the velocity lessens a bit to 250 cm/sec, and turbulence creates strong energy concentrations at the baseline with systole and becomes more disturbed (Fig. 22-75, *E* and *F*) (compare velocities between Fig. 22-75, *D* and *F*, which are on the same scale). The PSV of more than 350 cm/sec, EDV of 100 cm/sec, and calculated IC/CC PSV ratio of 7.77 place this internal carotid artery stenosis well within the 80% to 99% reduction category of the Bluth et al. criteria (see Table 22-2).[10]

A markedly reduced and monophasic external carotid signal with none of the typical characteristics of a normal external carotid waveform is seen (Fig. 22-75, *G*). A normal left vertebral signal was obtained (Fig. 22-75, *H*). The right frontal signal was antegrade and did not change with bilateral branch compressions, (Fig. 22-75, *I*). Left frontal artery examination showed a retrograde signal (Fig. 22-75, *J*), which did not change with left-sided branch compressions. Right facial artery compression, however, caused a decrease and partial reversal of the frontal signal, showing the presence of a cross-face collateral from the contralateral facial artery. The collateral pathway across the lower bridge of the nose was confirmed with compression there.

The overall interpretation was of a severe left internal carotid stenosis of at least 90% to 95% with severe hemodynamic changes.

Case 2 (Fig. 22-76): total occlusion of distal CCA, ICA, and ECA with proximal free-floating (bouncing) thrombus

This older (but still educational) case was done before duplex was widely used; a direct continuous-wave Doppler examination was performed on the carotids to supplement the carotid sonography study. Interpreting this examination is simple; although spectrum analysis was not used, the analog waveform contour changes and elevation in relation to the zero baseline (marked with a zero) correspond closely

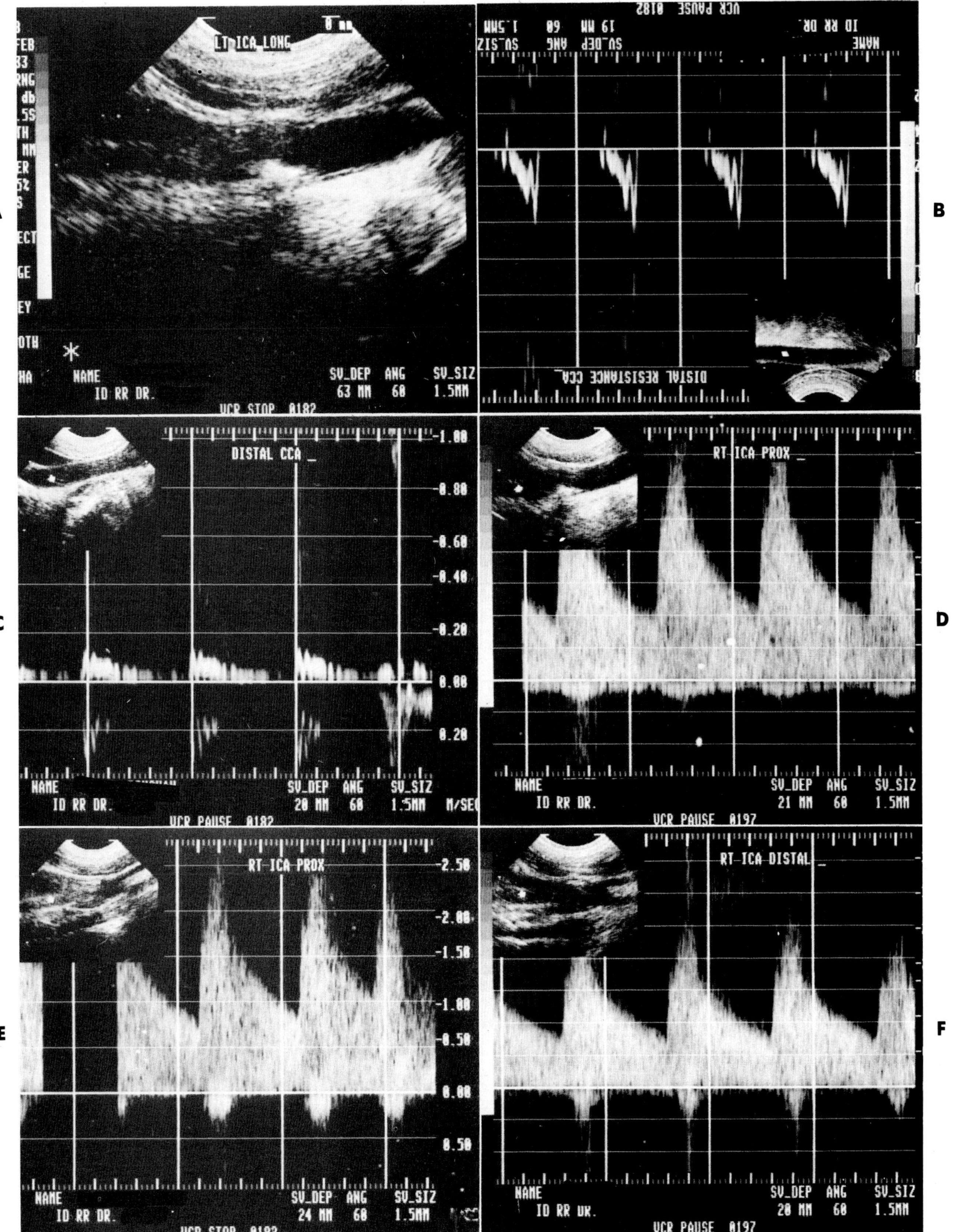

FIG. 22-75 Severe 80% to 99% ICA stenosis: Duplex and periorbital results. See text for detailed description. **A,** Gray-scale image of the distal left CCA and proximal ICA. **B,** High-resistance Doppler spectral waveform in proximal CCA. **C,** Preocclusive disturbed Doppler spectral waveform in distal CCA. **D,** High-velocity Doppler spectral waveform across ICA stenosis. **E,** High-velocity Doppler spectral waveform in proximal ICA just distal to stenosis with severe baseline turbulence. **F,** Disturbed stenotic Doppler spectral waveform in distal ICA. *Continued.*

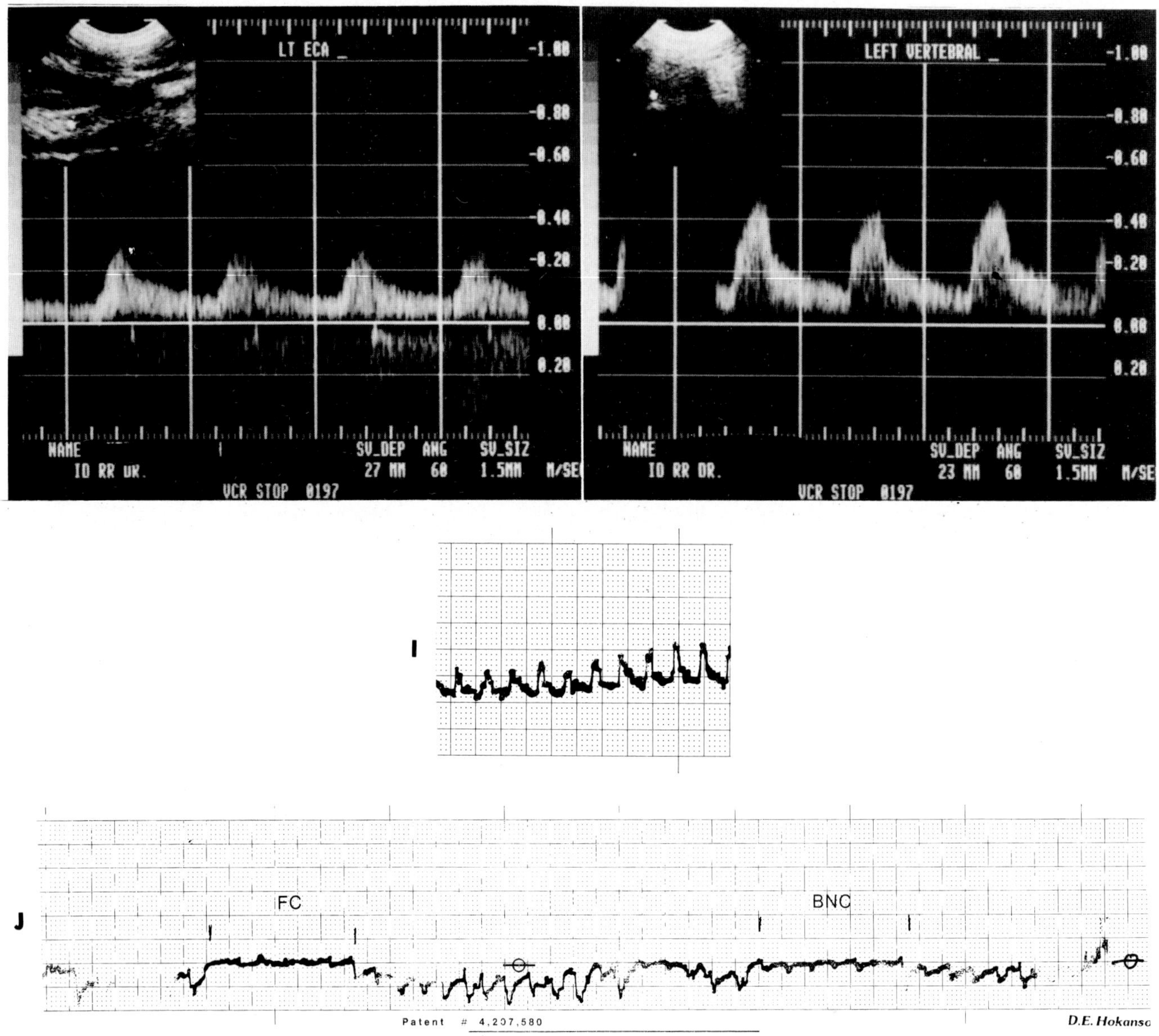

FIG. 22-75, cont'd. G, Doppler spectral waveform in the ECA. **H,** Antegrade Doppler spectral waveform in the vertebral artery. **I,** Normal antegrade right frontal artery signal with no changes during ECA branch compression. **J,** Abnormal retrograde left frontal artery signal, with changes in signal from right facial artery compression *(FC)* and compression across the bridge of the nose *(BNC)*.

and are interpreted in a similar fashion to parameters on spectral waveforms.

The real time images are interpreted sideways. In longitudinal scans the head of the patient is oriented to the top of the image; in transverse scans the medial side of the patient is oriented to the top of the image.

This 56-year-old woman was admitted for a possible coronary artery bypass operation. She had a long history of vascular disease and mitral insufficiency. She also complained of occasional dizziness and had numbness of three fingers of the right hand since an earlier cardiac catheterization. She had bilateral bruits in the carotids, and surgery was to be performed or cancelled, depending on the results of the Doppler examination and carotid sonography.

Direct carotid and periorbital findings. On the right side a normal brachial signal with a pressure of 190/100 was obtained (Fig. 22-76, *A*). The common carotid artery at the clavicle had abnormally low, practically nonexistent flow; the signal at the bifurcation was barely more than a thump. The right vertebral had normal but reduced antegrade flow. The facial artery signal was also reduced. The right temporal artery was actually reversed, implying severe collateral compensation. The ophthalmic test showed retrograde flow in the frontal artery, which was not affected by right-sided

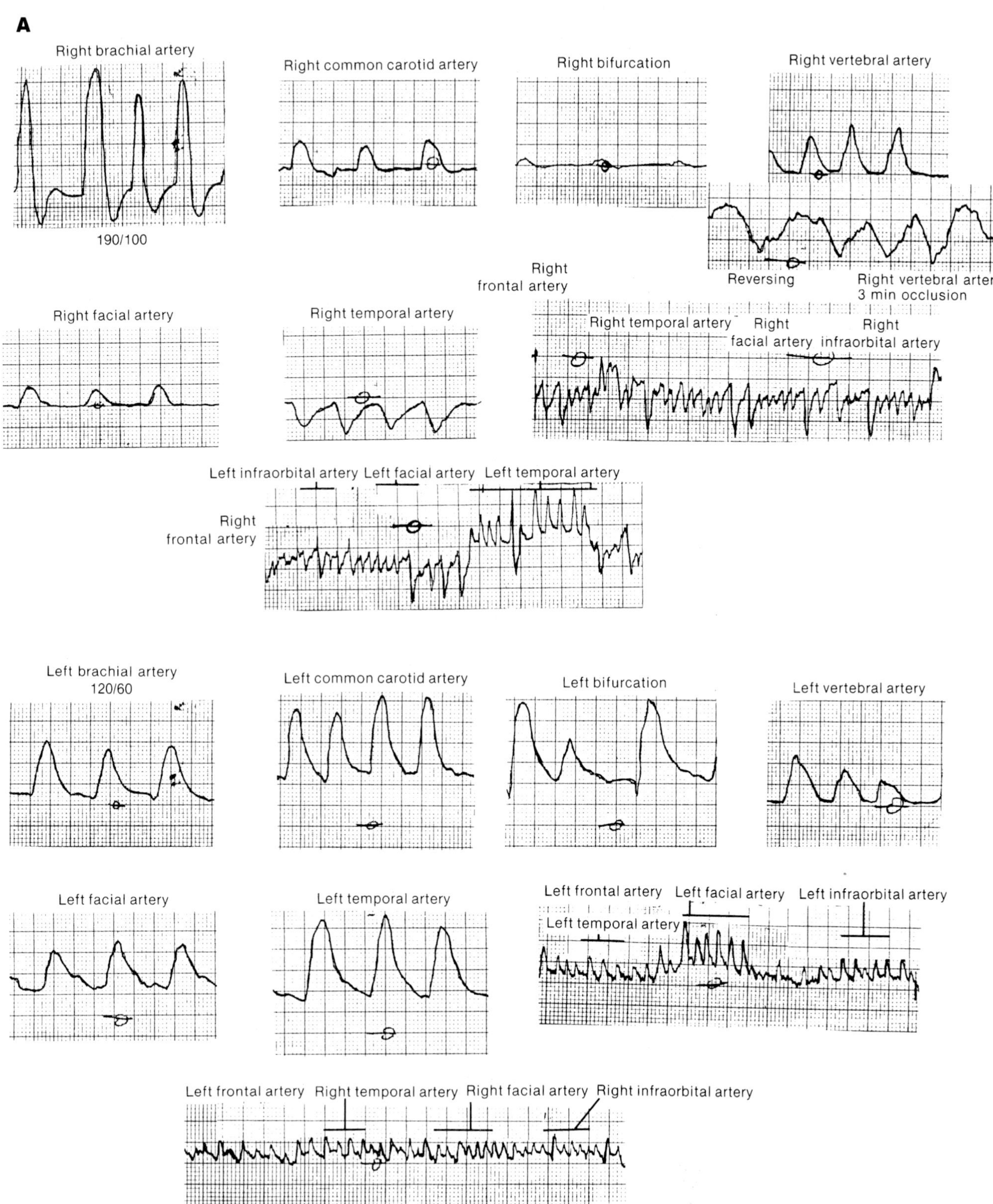

FIG. 22-76 Total occlusion of distal CCA, ICA, and ECA with proximal free-floating thrombus. See text for detailed description. **A,** Bilateral continuous-wave analog direct carotid and periorbital waveforms with findings. Real-time gray-scale carotid sonography findings. *Continued.*

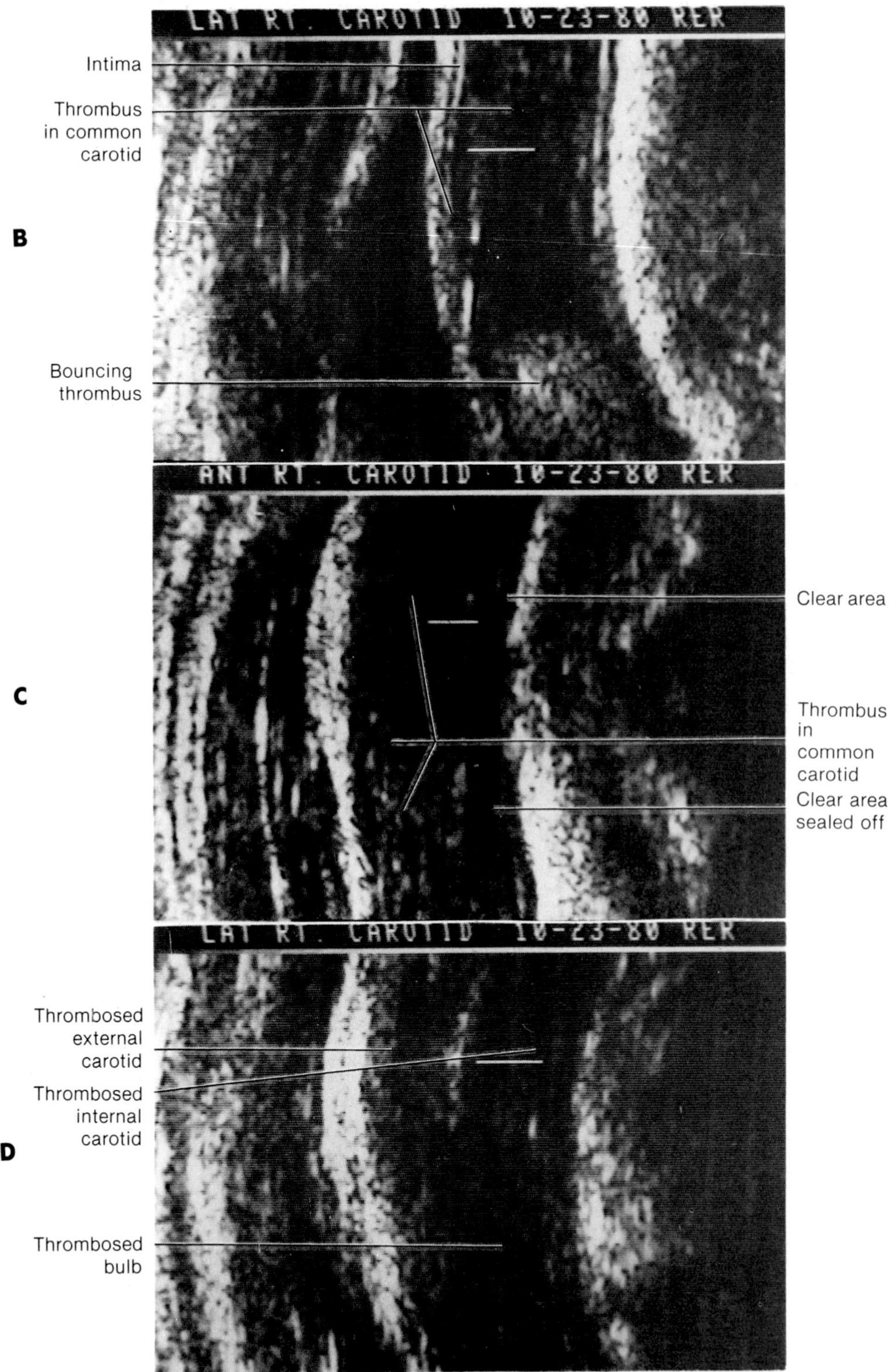

FIG. 22-76, cont'd. B, Proximal CCA with moving thrombus, longitudinal lateral scan plane. **C,** Mid-CCA with focal stationary thrombus and plaque (just distal to B), longitudinal anterior scan plane. **D,** Occluded distal CCA, ICA, and ECA, longitudinal lateral scan plane.

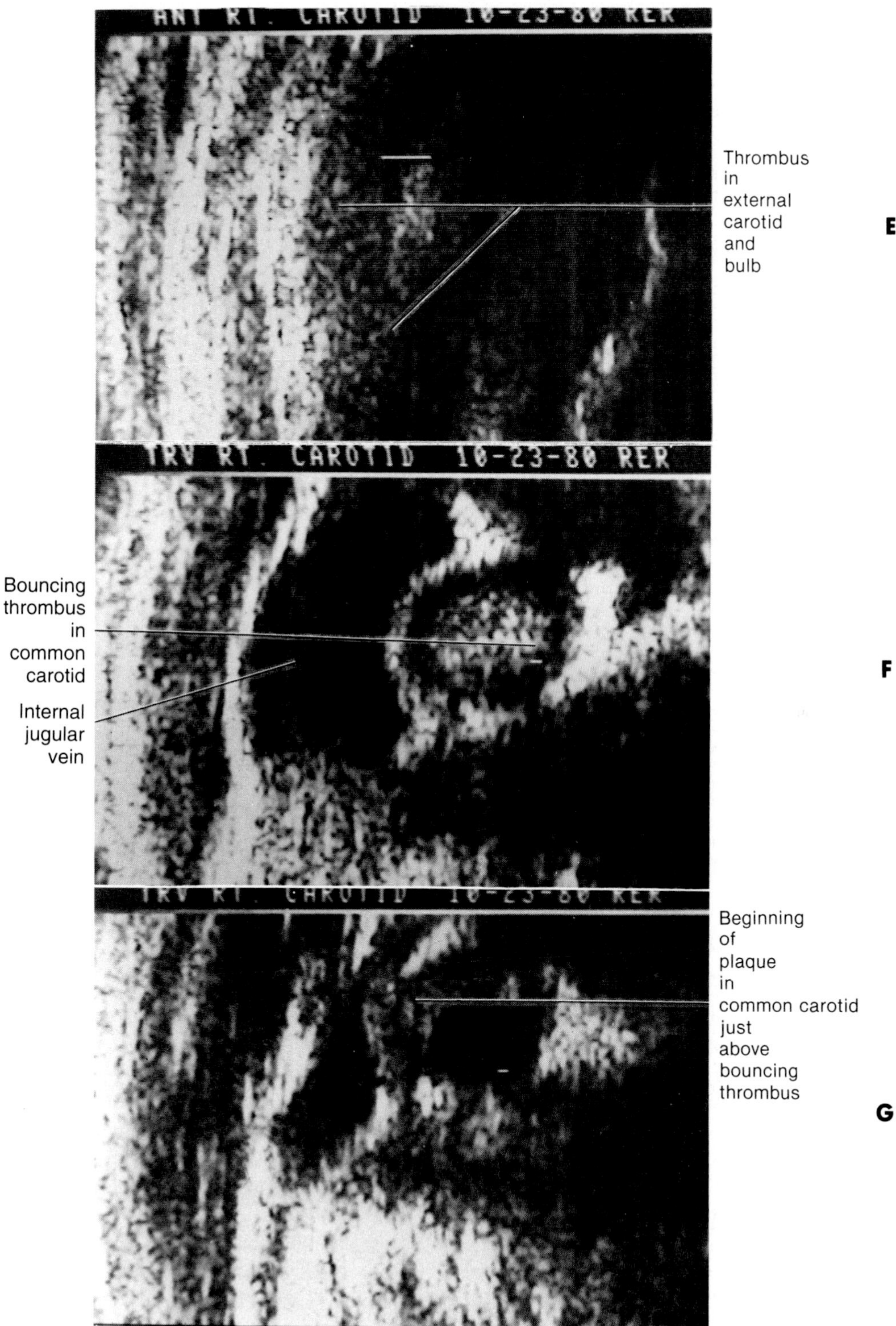

FIG. 22-76, cont'd. E, Occluded distal CCA and ECA, longitudinal anterior scan plane. **F,** Transverse view of the proximal CCA, showing the moving thrombus. **G,** Transverse view of the mid-CCA, corresponding to image *C*.

Continued.

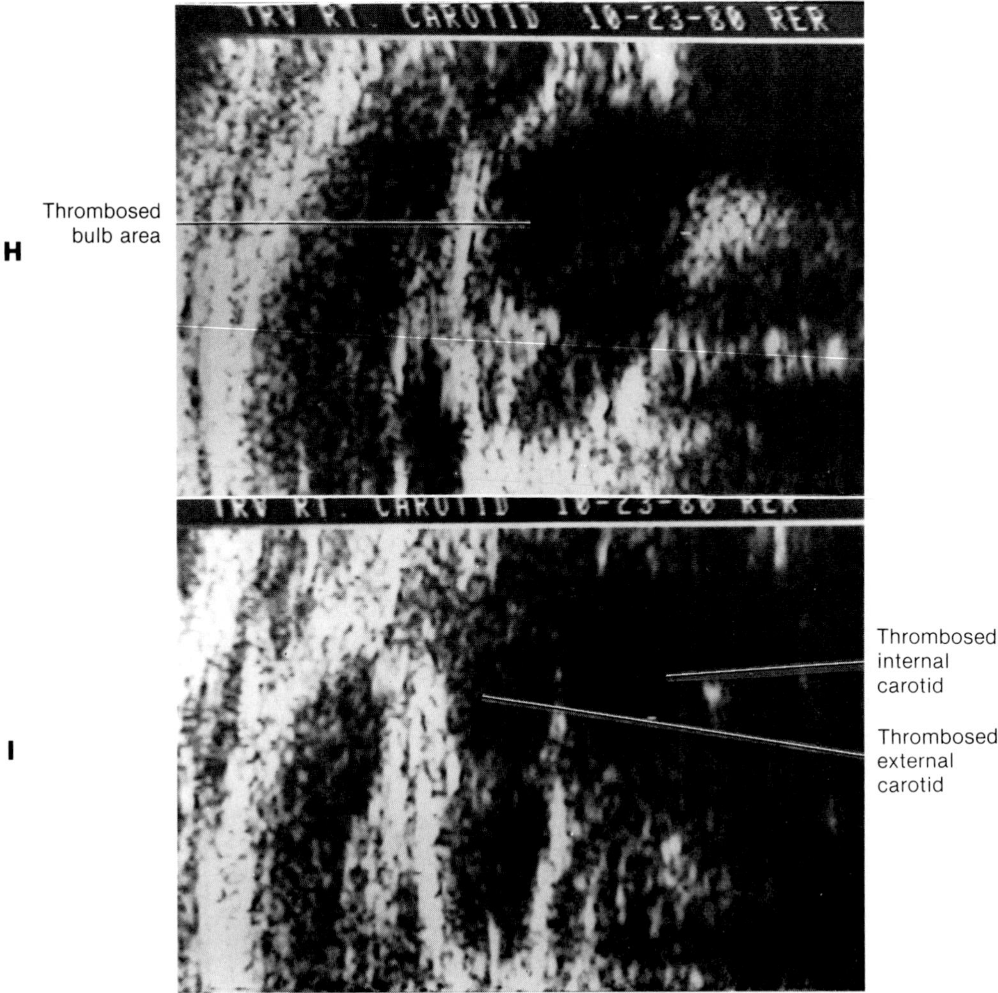

FIG. 22-76, cont'd. H, Transverse view of the occluded distal CCA and bulb area. **I,** Transverse view of the occluded ICA and ECA.

compressions. Compression of the left temporal, however, caused resumption of antegrade flow in the right frontal artery, suggesting contralateral collateralization from the left temporal artery. The other compressions had no effect. In regard to the apparent occlusion of the right common, it was thought that the frontal flow's becoming antegrade was caused by circle of Willis collateral supplies.

The left side was next examined. The left brachial artery signal was reduced and indicated subclavian stenosis and vertebral steal. A reduced antegrade vertebral signal was seen; however, postocclusive hyperemia caused a flow reversal within 10 seconds, verifying the steal. A much more normal-looking common carotid signal was noted, but throughout the carotid, there was roughening of the sound quality, implying flow problems. Bifurcation, facial, and temporal signals were of normal pattern, with some increase in flow in the temporal artery. The ophthalmic test showed an antegrade but decreased frontal signal, which increased markedly with left facial compression. All other compressions were normal. Neither right nor left supraorbital arteries were audible.

Carotid sonography findings, right side. Carotid sonography showed a thrombus occluding the right common, internal, and external carotids from the middle of the common carotid up, with a partly congealed clot floating free and moving up and down with each cardiac cycle in the low common carotid. The left side had scattered areas of plaque partly occluding the bulb and internal carotid. (See Fig. 22-76, *B* to *I* for selected examples of this case.)

A lateral view of the right common carotid artery low in the neck is shown (Fig. 22-76, *B*). The thrombus, which bounces up and down with each cardiac beat, is shown. This thrombus was completely free and unattached to the walls. Above this, the proximal portion of the congealed thrombus lining the carotid is shown. The intima is clearly seen, showing the thrombus to be separate and not a thickened part of the intima.

An anterior view was taken just above the previous image (Fig. 22-76, *C*). A much more extensive view of the thrombus is seen, as is a clear area on the deep wall that had minimal flow. This clear area was sealed off just below the bulb.

The lateral view shows the bulb and bifurcation (Fig. 22-76, *D*). The same mass of gray echoes fills the entire lumen. Doppler examination here gave an absent signal.

The anterior view gives a better perspective of the filled-in external carotid and bulb (Fig. 22-76, *E*).

In the following series of transverse views, levels have been chosen to correspond best with the longitudinal images.

A view low in the common carotid shows the transverse appearance of the moving thrombus caught in a freeze-frame image (Fig. 22-76, *F*).

A view of the area of the carotid just above the area with the moving thrombus shows the irregular edges of the thrombus and the decreased lumen (Fig. 22-76, *G*).

Another view shows an area of the bulb just below the bifurcation. The bulb is entirely filled in with echoes (Fig. 22-76, *H*). No Doppler signals could be heard.

The appearance of the internal and external carotid arteries is shown in another view (Fig. 22-76, *I*). Once again, they too are filled in, which corresponds with the findings in the long-axis images. No Doppler flow signals could be obtained.

An arteriogram was obtained and confirmed the level and extent of the occlusion in the right carotid. The right vertebral flow reduction was caused by a stenosis at the take-off of the vessel. A severe stenosis of the left internal carotid was also shown, as was a confirmation of the left subclavian obstruction and subclavian steal.

The patient was observed for 3 months until the loose bouncing clot had congealed. At that time the patient was readmitted and had another arteriogram, which showed some collateralization that filled the external carotid. The patient was taken to surgery, and a combination right carotid endarterectomy and mitral commisurotomy and repair were performed. The patient recovered and was released.

THE CAROTID DUPLEX EXAMINATION IN THE POSTOPERATIVE PATIENT

Carotid Endarterectomy

The most common procedure to alleviate stenoses of the carotid artery system is the endarterectomy. In this technique the carotid artery is exposed, then a shunt is placed in the distal common artery below the stenotic area and inserted above the stenosis into the internal carotid artery. This shunt enables the surgeon to divert the carotid flow around the area he or she intends to endarterectomize and avoid any neurologic deficits caused by lack of blood flow. An arteriotomy is made across the area of stenosis. An intimal elevator is used to dissect the intimal layer and area of plaque away from the walls, and this area is cut away. The loose ends of the residual intima are tacked down with sutures, remaining bits of plaque in the area are removed, the area is flushed with saline, and the vessel is closed. The shunt is then removed, the closure of the arteriotomy is completed, and flow is restored.

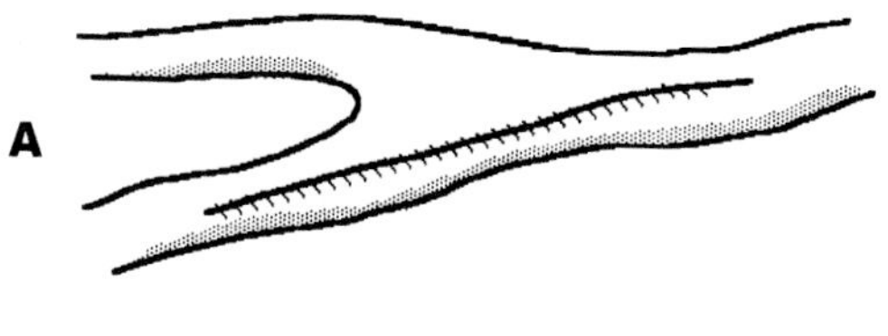

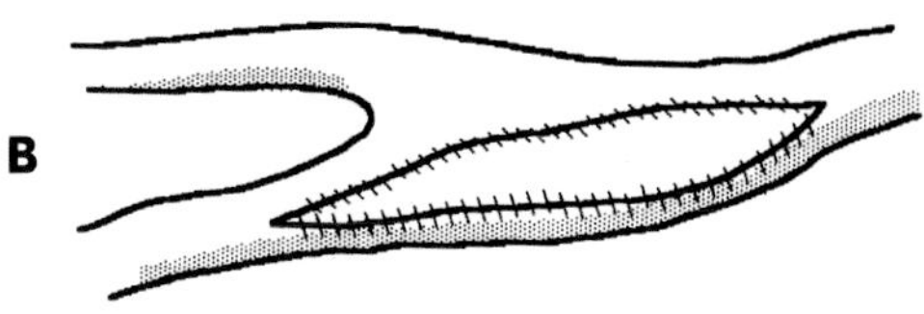

FIG. 22-77 Carotid endarterectomy closures. **A,** Standard endarterectomy. **B,** Patch angioplasty after endarterectomy. (Courtesy Richard E. Rae, Indianapolis.)

In some cases when the surgeon thinks that the artery is too small after endarterectomy, suspects probable restenosis, or is repairing a recurrent stenosis after a prior endarterectomy, a patch angioplasty may be performed as well. In this procedure the surgeon actually widens the artery by means of a patch fashioned from either synthetic material (e.g., Gore-tex or Dacron) or from a small section of autogenous saphenous or jugular vein. The edges of the arteriotomy are sutured to the outer edges of the shaped and sized patch, thus enlarging the lumen proportionally to the size of the patch (Fig. 22-77).

Complications or changes after endarterectomy may occur within the carotid artery, both of which can be easily evaluated by duplex sonography. Pseudoaneurysm formation has been associated with endarterectomy, as well as with wound infection, patching, or interposition grafts.[32] Recurrent carotid stenosis after endarterectomy can occur in 15% to 40% of cases and usually occurs in one of two categories.[32] Stenoses in the first category can develop within a year after surgery and usually result from fibrointimal hyperplasia; the other develops after 2 years and is a result of progressive atherosclerosis in the endarterectomy area. These lesions are usually treated with patch angioplasty to enlarge the vessel.[32]

The sonographic image of the carotids after endarterectomy can vary; if a straightforward endarterectomy was done, the artery generally appears very similar to a normal carotid bifurcation with perhaps a thinner wall, no defined intimal echoes in the operated area, and a step-off where the normal artery ends and the endarterectomy begins. If a patch angioplasty was performed, the repaired area will additionally appear enlarged and dilated; sometimes the suture line or patch borders can be imaged along the walls (Fig. 22-78). If the artery was patched to enlarge the vessel around a recurrent stenosis, residual stenotic material may be seen and should be monitored on subsequent follow-up examinations.

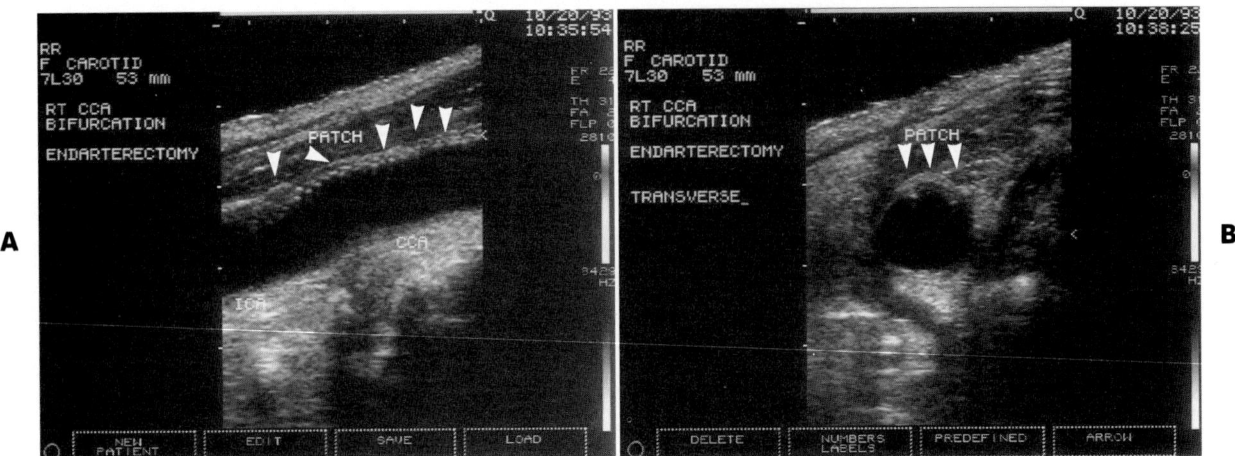

FIG. 22-78 Gray-scale duplex sonographic appearance of a carotid artery after endarterectomy with a patch angioplasty. **A,** Longitudinal image demonstrating the echoes of the patch surface *(arrows)*. **B,** Transverse image clearly showing the patch and the anastomoses on either side of it.

Fibrotic or hyperplastic stenoses often appear as narrow vessels without evidence of intraluminal stenosis, as if the vessel itself has shrunk in diameter (Fig. 22-79; see color images). Neointimal stenoses adopt the more typical appearance of stenotic plaque within the endarterectomy site (Fig. 22-80; see color images). Thrombus can also occasionally form as a reaction to wall trauma (Fig. 22-81; see color images).

Color-flow and Doppler patterns can vary in endarterectomized vessels. In nonpatched arteries the flow hemodynamics generally do not differ from those seen in normal arteries. In patched vessels a significant amount of flow disturbance and multicolor swirling or kaleidoscopic flow is seen within the endarterectomy area (Fig. 22-82; see color image). Doppler spectral flow patterns should not be obtained in these areas because of the turbulent, nondiagnostic waveform patterns that result. At the distal margin of the endarterectomy where the artery tapers and resumes a normal, unoperated caliber, some color-flow acceleration may be seen, especially if a large, dilated endarterectomy terminates into a small native artery.

Doppler patterns are often best obtained either within straight, nondisturbed segments distal to the bifurcation or in the native artery distal to the margins of the endarterectomy. Low velocities may be seen in the vessel if it is enlarged after surgery; such velocities are often normal. Elevated velocities that occur within an otherwise normal artery distal to the endarterectomy may result from the acceleration caused by diameter change (provided no distinct focal stenosis is identified). Since the margins of the endarterectomy often can be sites of recurrent stenosis, careful longitudinal and transverse evaluation of these areas should be performed to determine the significance of any flow acceleration.

If metal clips are used during an endarterectomy, these may occasionally show up as bright echoes with acoustic dropout below them, similar to calcified plaque shadows. Repositioning the transducer may help the examiner obtain an image around them.

Percutaneous Transluminal Angioplasty

Percutaneous transluminal angioplasty is periodically being used for dilation of extracranial and intracranial lesions, mostly on an investigative basis at the time of writing; the North American Cerebral Percutaneous Transluminal Angioplasty Register (NACPTAR) is part of an ongoing randomized trial determining the feasibility and utility of PTA within cerebral vessels. Angioplasty is performed frequently on subclavian and vertebral arteries, and at the common carotid origin, but has had varying success at the carotid bifurcation.[29,49] In general the best success has occurred with focal, short lesions that are not heavily calcified or rigid.

The sonographic appearance and Doppler/color-flow patterns of an internal carotid artery after angioplasty are not very different from routine imaging and flow findings; the vessel may have an apparent stretched or dilated shape and plaque may still be present, depending on the severity of the lesion (Fig. 22-83; see color image). The objective of duplex in these cases is to determine whether a hemodynamic improvement or increase in the residual luminal diameter has occurred compared with the preangioplasty state.

Carotid Bypass Grafts

Bypass grafts or reconstructive procedures are used in cases where endarterectomy will not suffice or may be inappropriate (e.g., severely stenotic carotid and vertebral origins, carotid aneurysms, recurrent stenoses with multiple repairs).

Grafts can be either of synthetic material (e.g., Gore-Tex, Dacron) or of autogenous venous origin. Bypasses

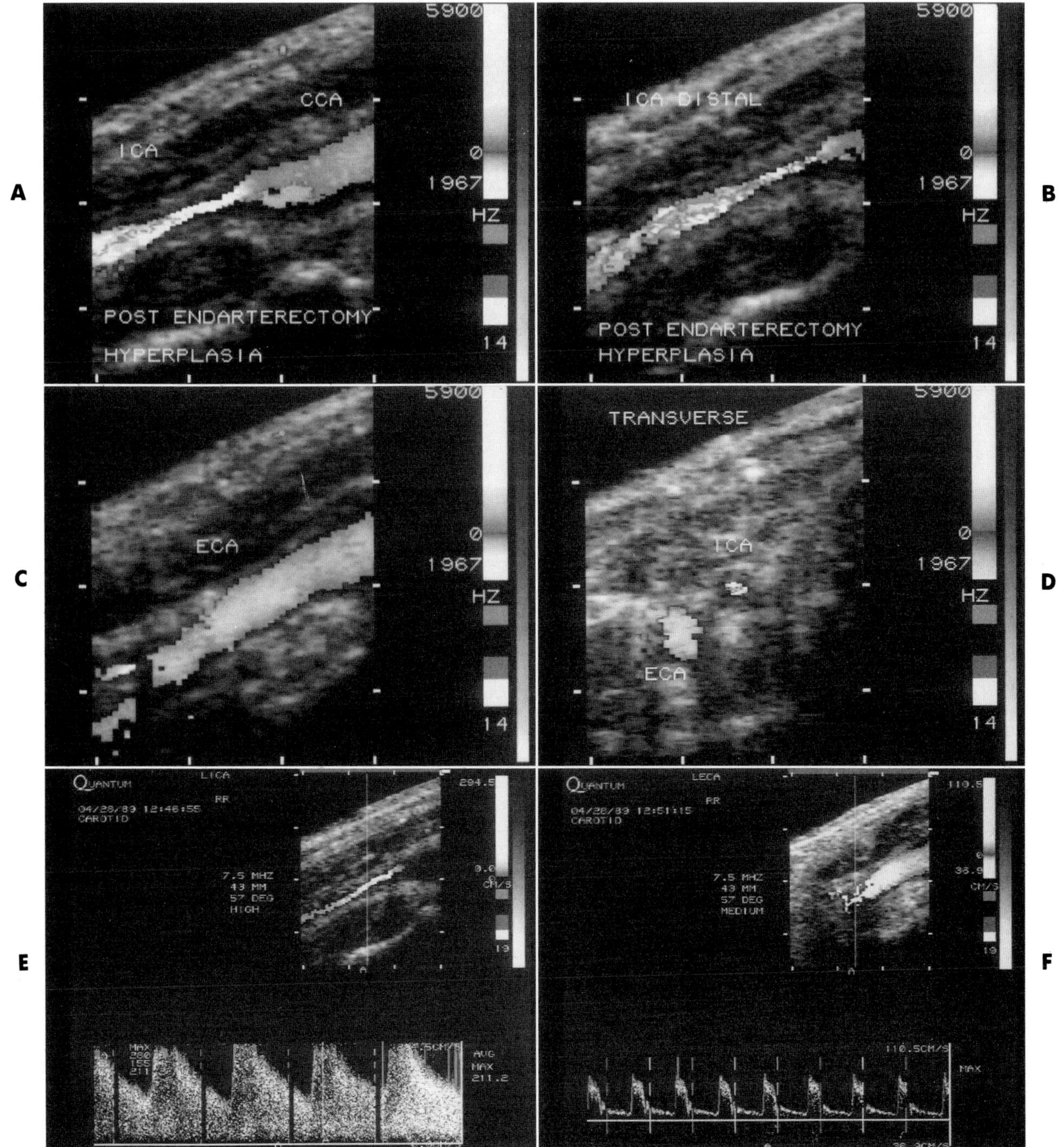

FIG. 22-79 Fibrointimal hyperplasia, after endarterectomy. **A,** Longitudinal color-flow image of the bifurcation, showing a physically narrowed proximal ICA with a high-velocity flow jet. **B,** Longitudinal color-flow image of the distal ICA, showing flow disturbance distal to the jet. **C,** Longitudinal normal color-flow image of the ECA. Compare its size with that of the hyperplastic ICA. **D,** Transverse view of the ICA and ECA. Note the small ICA lumen. **E,** High-velocity abnormal Doppler spectral waveform from the hyperplastic ICA. **F,** Normal Doppler spectral waveform from the ECA.

used to connect two separate arteries are usually synthetic, whereas saphenous vein is preferred for interposition grafts.

Some examples of bypass grafts that may be encountered by the examiner include the following:

1. *Carotosubclavian.* The carotosubclavian graft connects the subclavian artery to the ipsilateral proximal common carotid artery and is used to either restore flow to the subclavian and vertebral artery in cases of proximal subclavian stenosis, occlusion and/or subclavian steal or to restore flow to the common carotid artery in cases of

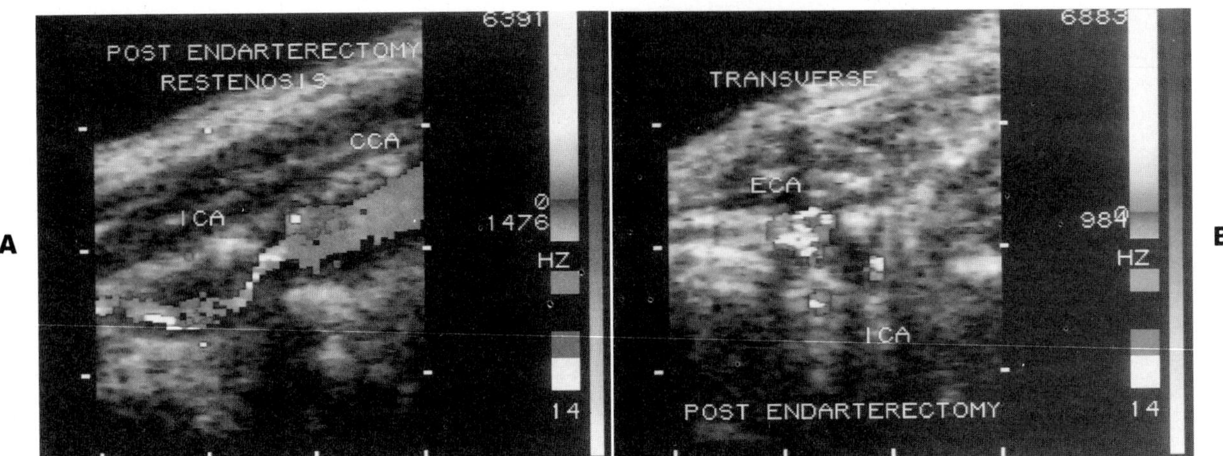

FIG. 22-80 Recurrent stenosis, after endarterectomy. **A,** Longitudinal color-flow view of an ICA after endarterectomy, showing the presence of a severe stenosis from recurrent atheroma. **B,** Transverse view of the stenosed ICA and ECA, showing the residual lumen.

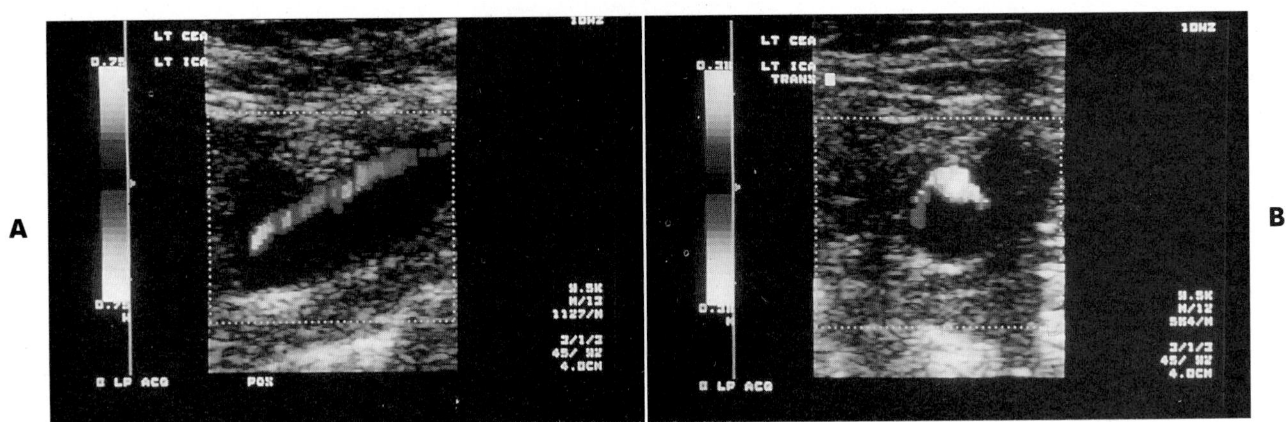

FIG. 22-81 Thrombus formation, after endarterectomy. **A,** Longitudinal color-flow view of an ICA after endarterectomy, showing the presence of homogeneous thrombus along the deep wall. **B,** Transverse view of the same ICA, showing that the thrombus is hemodynamically nonobstructive. This thrombus lysed spontaneously with no sequelae and was no longer present on subsequent follow-up studies.

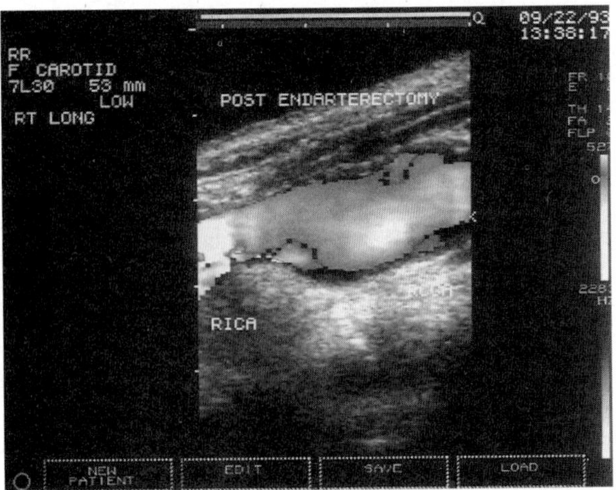

FIG. 22-82 Normal color-flow appearance in a patched carotid artery after endarterectomy.

severe origin stenosis (Fig. 22-84). The subclavian anastomosis may be difficult to see, but the carotid anastomosis is usually easily visualized. Color-flow and Doppler assessment can help the examiner determine the correct flow direction in the graft and evaluate the hemodynamics and patency of the graft.

2. *Carotocarotid.* The carotocarotid graft connects the common carotid to the contralateral common carotid across the low neck, usually inferior to the thyroid cartilage (Fig. 22-85). It shares flow from one carotid with the other. It is easily palpated and followed with duplex and color flow, and waveforms can be taken within. The anastomoses should be easily visualized. This type of bypass is infrequently performed and is seldom seen.
3. *Interposition graft.* An interposition graft is usually performed when a carotid aneurysm is present or when common carotid disease is so extensive that replace-

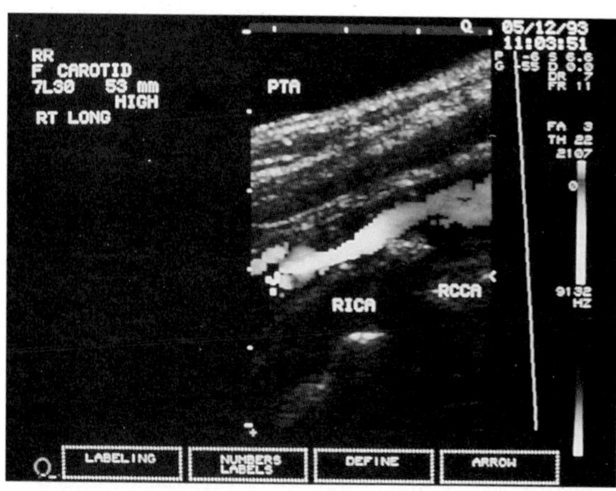

FIG. 22-83 Color-flow image of an internal carotid artery stenosis after percutaneous transluminal angioplasty. Although the residual lumen has been enlarged somewhat, residual stenotic material remains along the superficial wall.

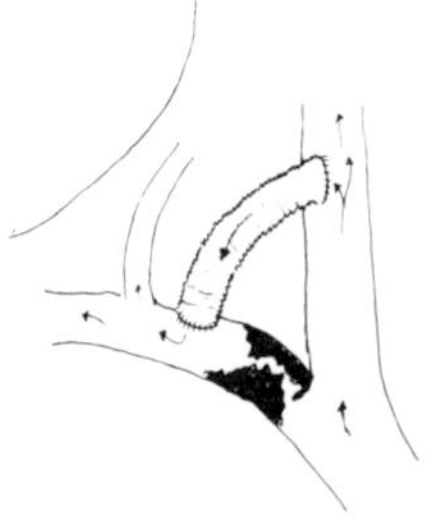

FIG. 22-84 Diagram illustrating the placement and flow mechanics of a carotosubclavian graft. If the CCA is proximally occluded instead of the subclavian (as in this example), this graft could also supply the common carotid from a patent subclavian artery. (Courtesy Richard E. Rae, Indianapolis.)

ment, excision, or exclusion, rather than endarterectomy, is indicated. Usually an end-to-end anastomosis of a vein section is performed between the native common carotid and the distal native internal carotid artery. The external carotid may be reimplanted into the graft but sometimes is excluded. The sonographic appearance is usually that of a normal carotid bifurcation or of one continuous vessel from base to mandible. The graft may be large or small, depending on the vein segment used; a shadow or diameter irregularity may mark the anastomosis points of the graft and native arteries. Color-flow and Doppler patterns are consistent as with normal vessels and generally have no distinct characteristics that the examiner need be aware of (Fig. 22-86; see color images).

Reimplantation

Reimplantation or transposition procedures may occasionally be performed to restore normal flow through the vertebral, common carotid, or subclavian arteries; some examples include the following:

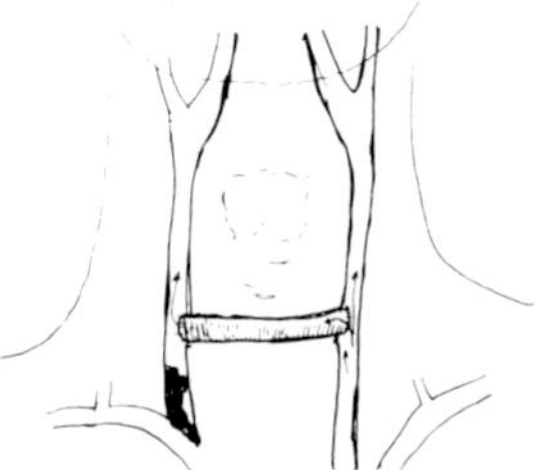

FIG. 22-85 Diagram illustrating placement and flow mechanics of one form of carotocarotid graft. (Courtesy Richard E. Rae, Indianapolis.)

1. Reimplantation of a vertebral artery into an ipsilateral proximal common carotid artery (Fig. 22-87; see color image).
2. Implantation of a subclavian artery into an ipsilateral proximal common carotid artery.
3. Transposition of a proximal common carotid artery to the ipsilateral subclavian artery (Fig. 22-88; see color image).

Many of these reconstructions lie infraclavicularly and may require a sector transducer to visualize them, although vertebrocarotid and carotosubclavian reimplantations can usually be easily seen and evaluated as illustrated in Figs. 22-87 and 22-88.

General Comments on Evaluating Patients After Surgery

The examiner needs to thoroughly evaluate any operative notes that may be available before performing a duplex examination; these notes not only describe the type of surgery performed and the date of the operation but also provide exact descriptions of the extent of the endarterectomy or type of repair procedure that was done. Patients who are referred as outpatients may not have operative notes available and do not always volunteer that they have had surgery; the examiner should look for scars on the neck and ask the patient what procedure was done. Endarterectomy scars typically appear as either fairly long scars on one side of the neck along the border of the sternocleidomastoid muscle (often in a neck fold), or sometimes as transverse scars midway up the neck. Physical signs of other procedures may appear as scars in the supraclavicular or infraclavicular areas.

There are generally no contraindications to evaluating patients after surgery with duplex either within the immediate postoperative period or in long-term follow-up (Fig. 22-89; see color image). The examiner should note, however, that duplex studies may have poor visualization of the carotid anatomy if they are routinely performed within the first 4 weeks, because of local edema and hematoma formation. Increased penetration with lower-frequency transducers may be required if emergent evaluation is necessary to rule out a postoperative restenosis or thrombosis. If an

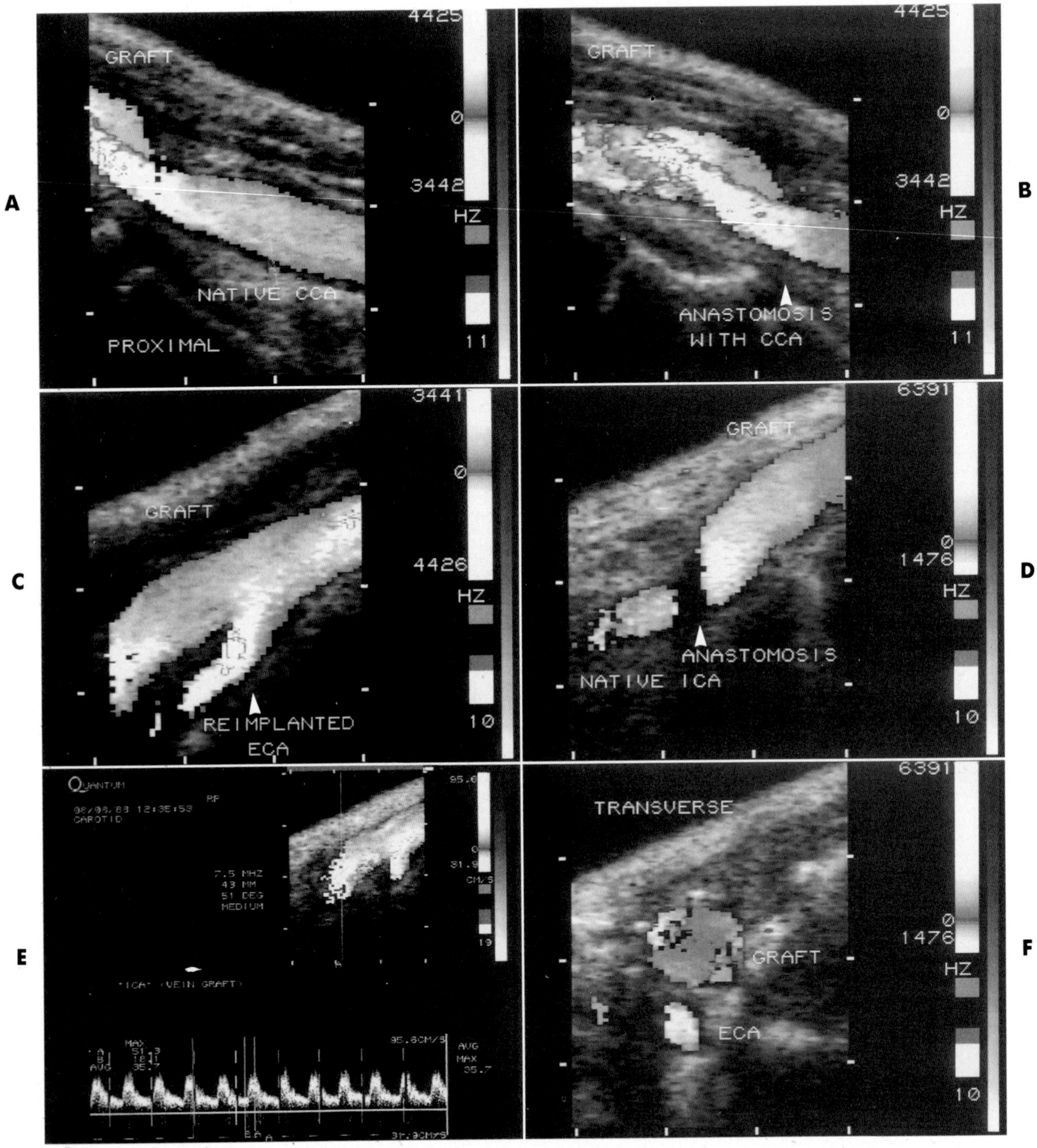

FIG. 22-86 CCA to ICA saphenous vein interposition graft. **A,** Longitudinal color-flow image of the proximal native CCA. The proximal anastomosis with the graft is to the left. **B,** Longitudinal color-flow image of the proximal graft, showing normal flow separation from diameter change. **C,** Color-flow image of the new "bifurcation" with the ECA implanted into the graft. **D,** Longitudinal color-flow image of the distal graft anastomosis with the native ICA. **E,** Normal Doppler spectral waveform in the "ICA" portion of the distal graft. **F,** Transverse view above the "bifurcation," showing the graft (which resembles an endarterectomized ICA) and the ECA.

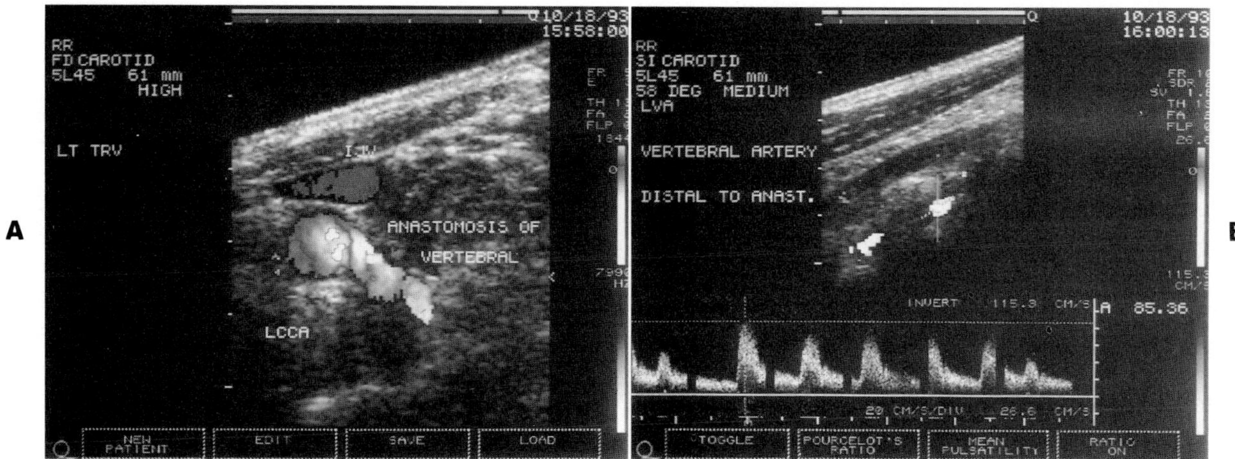

FIG. 22-87 Reimplantation, vertebral to CCA. **A,** Color-flow transverse view of a CCA with a reimplanted vertebral artery. **B,** Normal antegrade Doppler spectral waveform in the distal vertebral artery, above the anastomosis.

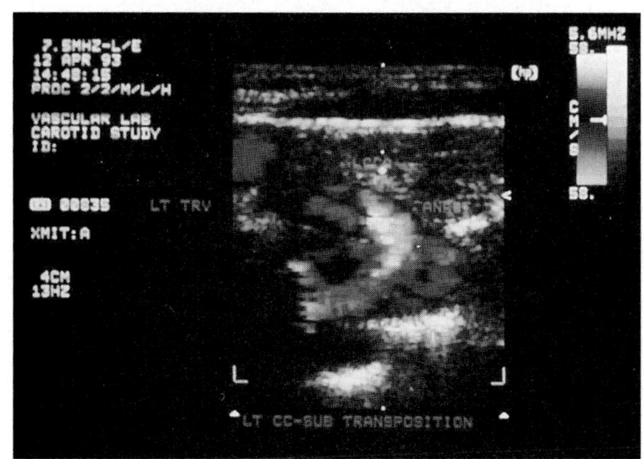

FIG. 22-88 Color-flow image of a CCA-to-subclavian-artery transposition. Although taken in the transverse plane, the view is of the long axis of the subclavian artery, with the proximal anastomosis of the transposed CCA easily identified.

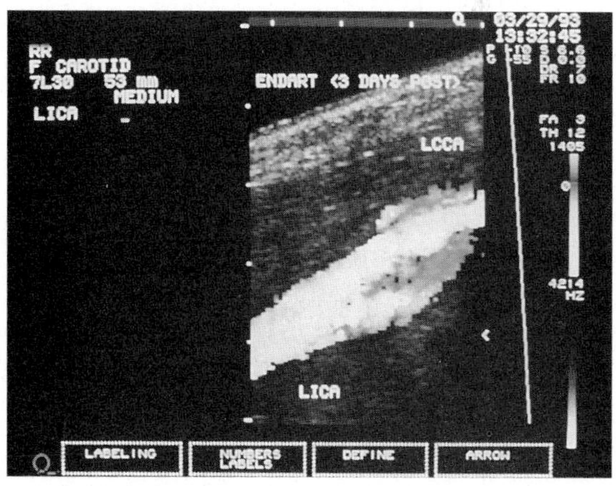

FIG. 22-89 Color-flow image of an ICA, 3 days after endarterectomy and patch angioplasty. The flow patterns are hyperemic but normal.

acute postoperative occlusion is suspected, a supplemental periorbital Doppler examination may help determine whether hemodynamically significant changes with frontal artery flow reversal have occurred.

INTRAOPERATIVE USE OF CAROTID DUPLEX SONOGRAPHY

Intraoperative duplex scanning is used by many surgeons during endarterectomy procedures; after the carotid has been exposed, this modality can help the surgeon evaluate the degree of stenosis and its precise location and extent before performing the arteriotomy, as well as allow evaluation of the hemodynamics before and after surgery within the carotid. The general technique involves placing the transducer and cable in a sterile sleeve, coupled with gel. A gel-filled cap can be placed over the sleeve where it contacts the transducer face, which helps eliminate air bubbles in the beam path. The surgical area is usually filled with saline, and the vessel is scanned through the water path. Controls and knob adjustments are made either by an attending technologist or by the surgeon through a sterile cover placed over the control panel. The appearance of the artery is similar to that described in the duplex sonography section, except that the walls and intima are always much clearer and well defined. After surgery and before the neck is closed, a second evaluation is made. Bits of plaque and remaining material are extremely easy to detect, and if they are detected, the surgeon can easily reopen and remove the material. Before intraoperative scanning was done, a deficit often was not discovered until the postoperative period, which necessitated taking the patient back to surgery and repeating the entire endarterectomy procedure.

Many surgeons find intraoperative ultrasound to be an extremely useful and cost-effective adjunctive tool to intraoperative arteriography, and its use among vascular surgeons continues to grow.

TRANSCRANIAL DOPPLER AND TRANSCRANIAL DUPLEX IMAGING

Within the last decade, new developments in Doppler and sonographic technology have enabled examiners to assess the flow and circulatory anatomy of the intracranial vault directly, using thinner areas of the skull as acoustic windows to the circle of Willis, basilar artery, terminal internal carotid, anterior cerebral, and middle cerebral and posterior cerebral arteries.

The methods used to evaluate these intracranial vessels are transcranial Doppler (TCD) and transcranial duplex imaging (often abbreviated TCI). Although the Doppler method (a nonimaging approach) may ultimately give way to the duplex imaging method, more experience and data are currently available from transcranial Doppler than from the more recent and evolving transcranial imaging modality. Knowledge and familiarity with both techniques are important, since they are complementary.

Transcranial Doppler

Transcranial Doppler was introduced by Rune Aaslid in 1982 and has developed and advanced remarkably since that time.[2] The technique is related to blind Doppler assessment (such as with direct continuous-wave Doppler), and many of the examination techniques are similar to those used in the periorbital Doppler examination, although somewhat more challenging. Even though the user has no two-dimensional image to guide sample placement, transcranial Doppler's ability to diagnose and define the intracerebral hemodynamic state has made it a very well accepted technique. It is listed as a secondary procedure in the Essentials and Standards of the ICAVL, but it also has its own TCD Essential and Standard under development (at this writing) by the ICAVL for neurology-based laboratories that do not perform noninvasive imaging or other peripheral examinations.[18]

Equipment. The device used is a bidirectional pulsed Doppler with a 2-MHz transducer, which has sufficient ability to penetrate bony structures (Fig. 22-90). The original maximum allowable power levels of 100 mW/cm^2 (SPTA) and small sample volume have recently been expanded by the FDA to allow levels of nearly 658 mW/cm^2 spatial peak/temporal average (SPTA) and a 14 by 7 mm sample volume; this allows these instruments a much greater sensitivity and diagnostic capability than was previously available.

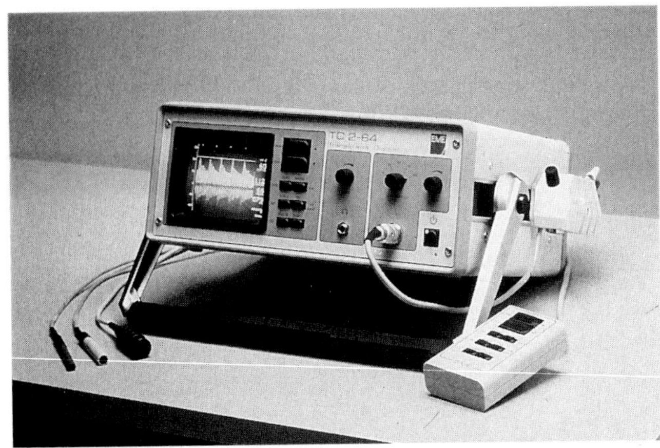

FIG. 22-90 Basic standard transcranial Doppler device. (Courtesy EME/Nicolet.)

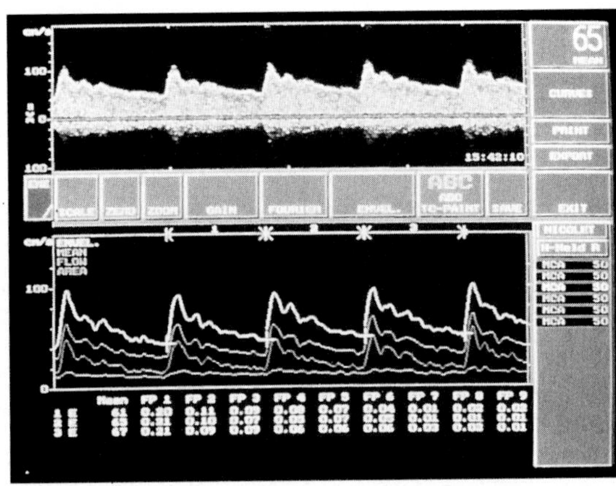

FIG. 22-91 Transcranial Doppler spectral display showing a middle cerebral artery waveform, depth, transducer, and velocity parameter indicators *(top)*, and flow profile curve analysis into peak and mean velocities, volume flow, and vessel diameter *(bottom)*. (Courtesy EME/Nicolet.)

The sample volume size can be adjusted as necessary and the sample focal depth is variable on these devices, since they by necessity must be range-gated. Depth increments range from 2 to 5 mm per step to a maximum depth of about 150 mm. The pulse-repetition rates are also adjustable, since cerebrovascular velocities are usually quite high (especially in cases of abnormality). The Doppler velocities assume an angle of 0 to 30 degrees, since the beam intercepts arterial flow at nearly that angle because of the anatomic vascular pathways. A spectrum analysis display is incorporated into these units, and external displays and computer interfaces are supported as well. The focal depth, peak and mean velocity, flow direction, pulse repetition frequency (PRF), and sample volume size are all displayed on the analysis screen, as is the spectral waveform. Some computer-based packages also allow for individual display and waveform profile analysis of the peak and mean velocities, as well as calculating a form of relative volume flow and cross-sectional vessel area (the usefulness and accuracy of volume flow in all vascular applications is still under investigation by numerous companies and institutions) (Fig. 22-91).

Transcranial Doppler devices are easily portable and can be used for bedside evaluations or can be transported to surgery for intraoperative monitoring. Many duplex scanner manufacturers are currently supplementing their transcra-

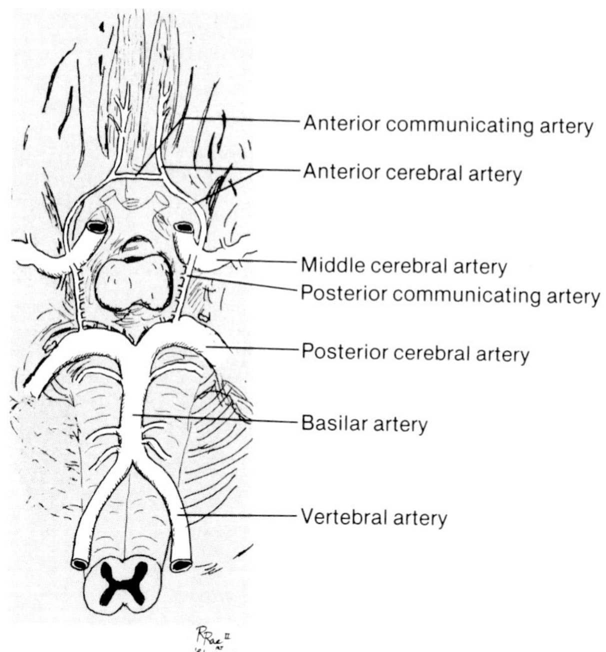

FIG. 22-92 Circle of Willis. (Courtesy Richard E. Rae, Indianapolis.)

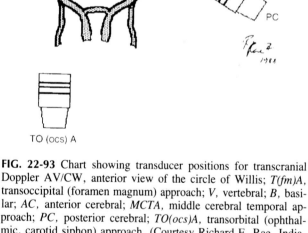

nial duplex imaging packages with the capability to perform additional blind transcranial Doppler evaluations.

Transcranial Doppler Examination Technique[24]

Before continuing, the reader may wish to review the anatomy of the intracranial cerebrovascular circulation, which is discussed toward the end of the "Anatomy of the Cerebrovascular Circulation" section at the beginning of this chapter. The arteries of the circle of Willis and posterior circulation (Fig. 22-92) that are accessible to transcranial Doppler include the following:

- Middle cerebral artery (MCA)
- Anterior cerebral artery (ACA)
- Posterior cerebral artery (PCA)
- Terminal internal carotid artery (TICA)
- Internal carotid artery (Carotid siphon)
- Ophthalmic artery (OA)
- Basilar artery (BA)
- Vertebral arteries (VA)
- Anterior communicating artery (ACoA)
- Posterior communicating artery (PCoA)

To gain access to these arteries, the ultrasound beam must penetrate the skull in some fashion. This is best accomplished through an anatomic window. In neonatal echoencephalography cranial access techniques are facilitated by the fontanelles and less-dense cranial structure, but these techniques cannot be applied to the dense, ossified adult skull. For transcranial Doppler, three standardized approaches have been established that enable the beam to enter through either natural openings (e.g., the foramen magnum, the superior orbital fissure) or through thinner, less dense parts of the skull (e.g., the anterior temporal bone).

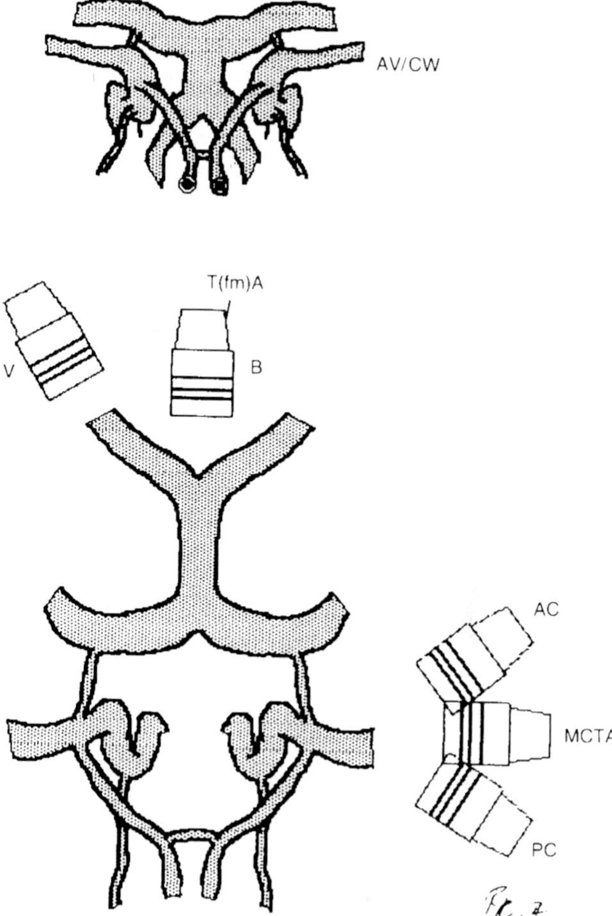

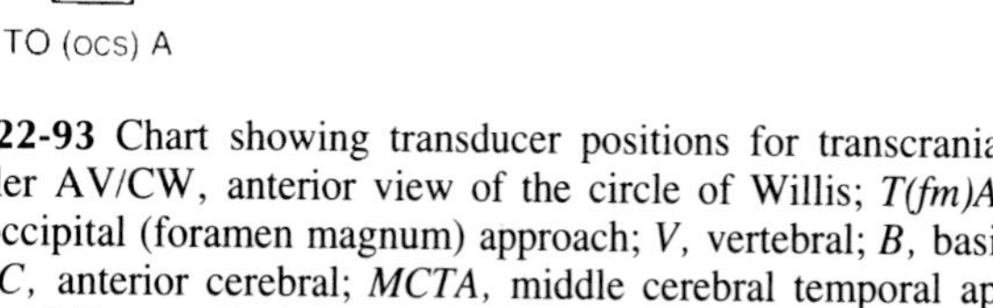

FIG. 22-93 Chart showing transducer positions for transcranial Doppler AV/CW, anterior view of the circle of Willis; *T(fm)A*, transoccipital (foramen magnum) approach; *V*, vertebral; *B*, basilar; *AC*, anterior cerebral; *MCTA*, middle cerebral temporal approach; *PC*, posterior cerebral; *TO(ocs)A*, transorbital (ophthalmic, carotid siphon) approach. (Courtesy Richard E. Rae, Indianapolis.)

The transorbital, transtemporal, and transoccipital (also called *transforamenal* or *transnuchal*) approaches (Fig. 22-93) each allow access to specific arteries; the three approaches combined allow potential evaluation of all the major cerebral arteries. The vessels accessed in each approach are identified by the following:

1. The sample volume depth;
2. The direction of blood flow in relation to the transducer (toward or away from);
3. Spatial relationships to other Doppler spectra;
4. Response to common carotid artery compressions and vertebral artery compressions.

Common carotid compression is routinely used to isolate and define collateral flow (much as in the Doppler periorbital study); its use is considered an important part of the examination despite controversies in the past. Investigative authors have stated that common carotid compression can be safely performed with no ill effects based on their experiences (among them periorbital Doppler and supraorbital photoplethysmography [PPG]) of over 10,000 patients.[6,8,17]

As stated previously, the examiner should still use caution; the CCA should be straddled between two closely placed fingertips low in the neck and still should be compressed for only about two beats (which should be sufficient time to determine the effect on the monitored Doppler signal). The vertebral artery is compressed to determine collateral effect or flow direction in the basilar artery or posterior circulation; this is accomplished along the atlantal portion by palpating the mastoid process behind the ear and compressing in the mastoid notch.

The transorbital approach is used to evaluate the ophthalmic artery and the intercranial carotid siphon segments of the internal carotid artery. Power levels should be set very low (about 10 mW/cm^2) to avoid overexposure of the lens and eye tissues to excessive acoustic power levels. The eye is closed, and the transducer is gently placed over the eyelid and coupled with gel. The beam is oriented anteroposteriorly with a slight tilt to the midline.

The OA is evaluated at a sample depth of 40 to 50 mm (Fig. 22-94). The sample depth is increased slowly as adjustments are made to keep the ophthalmic artery in the Doppler beam. At 55 to 70 mm the carotid siphon area is located and is easily discerned by the higher diastolic velocity compared with the ophthalmic signal. The different curved segments of the intracranial internal carotid where it exits the carotid canal and before it joins the circle of Willis (proximal, parasellar, curve, genu, distal and posterior, supraclinoid) are detected by flow direction. The parasellar (near the sella turcica) portion is found by angling inferiorly, and flow is toward the transducer (Fig. 22-95). The flow in the anterior curve (genu section) is bidirectional (since the beam is entering perpendicular to the flow). Locating the genu section first can help locate the other two segments. The supraclinoid segment is found by angling superiorly, and flow is away from the transducer.

The transtemporal approach is used to evaluate the middle cerebral artery, anterior cerebral artery, terminal portion of the internal carotid, posterior cerebral artery, and the anterior and posterior communicating arteries (Fig. 22-96). This approach is operator-dependent, since the examiner must locate an area in the temporal bone that is thin enough to allow an adequate acoustic window where the Doppler can penetrate the bone well. The location for transtemporal insonation is superior to the zygomatic arch, and the probe may need to be aimed anteriorly, posteriorly, or dead center, depending on which window allows the best reception of the Doppler signals from the circle of Willis arteries. The best location is found by setting the sample depth at 55 to 60 mm and then moving to obtain a clear Doppler signal from any of the arteries that lie at that depth, usually the anterior, middle, or posterior cerebral arteries and the terminal internal carotid.

The middle cerebral artery is located by reducing the sample depth by between 25 and 50 mm, which should detect it, since it is the shallowest arterial signal (Fig. 22-97). The middle cerebral flow signal is toward the transducer and diminishes with low common carotid compressions.

The internal carotid bifurcation into the middle and anterior cerebral arteries can be found at a sample depth of 55 to 65 mm and has a bidirectional signal (Fig. 22-98). The bidirectional middle and anterior cerebral bifurcation is a reference point for obtaining signals from the anterior, middle, and posterior cerebral arteries. Common carotid

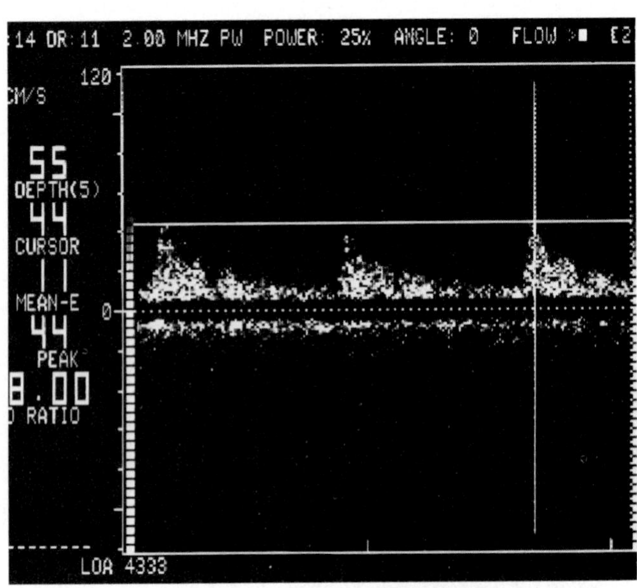

FIG. 22-94 Normal ophthalmic artery spectrum.

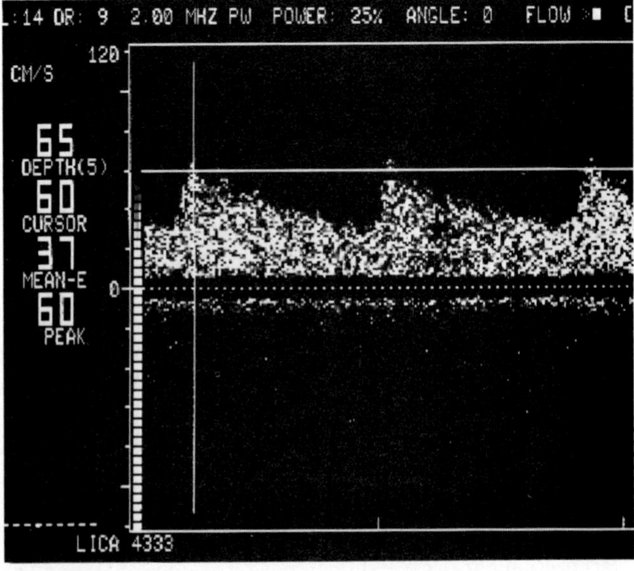

FIG. 22-95 Normal internal carotid siphon spectrum.

compressions reverse the anterior cerebral flow component if the anterior communicating artery is patent and diminish the signal if the anterior communicating artery is obstructed or absent. The middle cerebral component diminishes as mentioned previously.

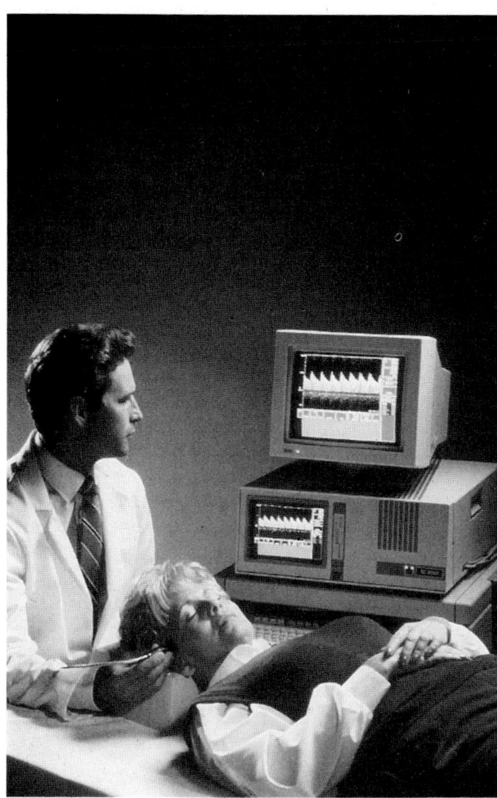

FIG. 22-96 Insonating through the transtemporal window. (Courtesy EME/Nicolet.)

The terminal internal carotid is located by angling inferior to the middle and anterior cerebral bifurcation. Flow velocities are lower than in the middle and anterior cerebral arteries, and the signal is obliterated by common carotid compression.

The middle and anterior cerebral bifurcation is relocated and the sample depth is increased to 70 to 80 mm (brain midline) while adjusting and keeping the anterior cerebral signal centered (Fig. 22-99). Flow is normally away from the transducer. Reversed signals imply cross-channel collateral flow from the opposite side, and this may occur when the ipsilateral internal carotid is severely stenosed, and the

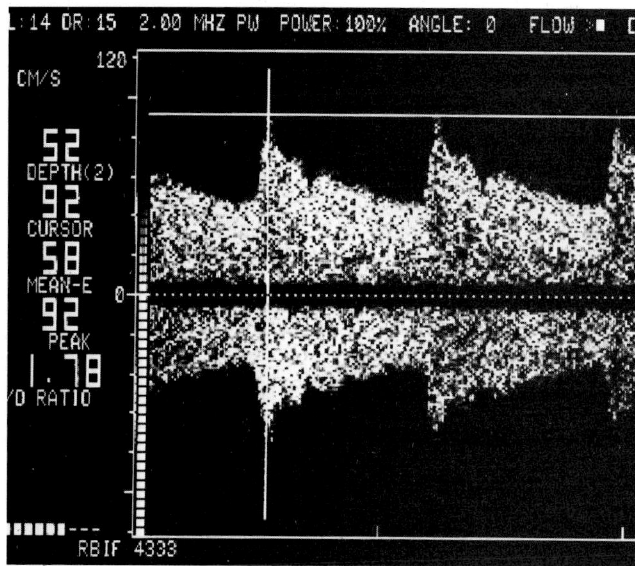

FIG. 22-98 Normal middle cerebral/anterior cerebral bifurcation spectrum.

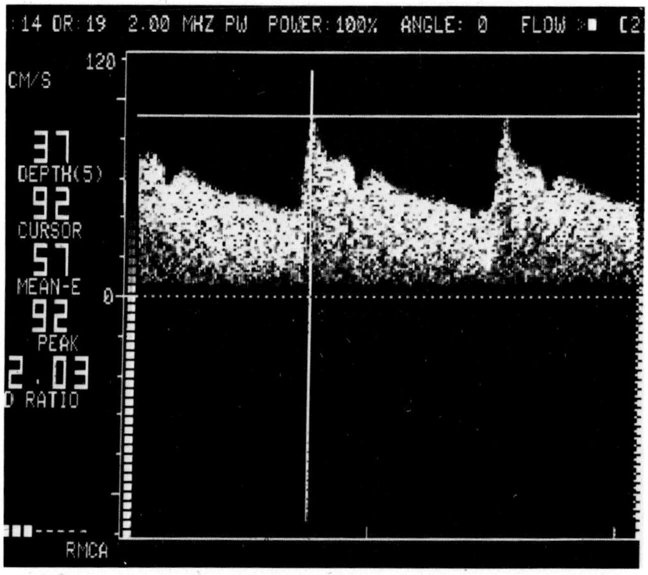

FIG. 22-97 Normal middle cerebral artery spectrum.

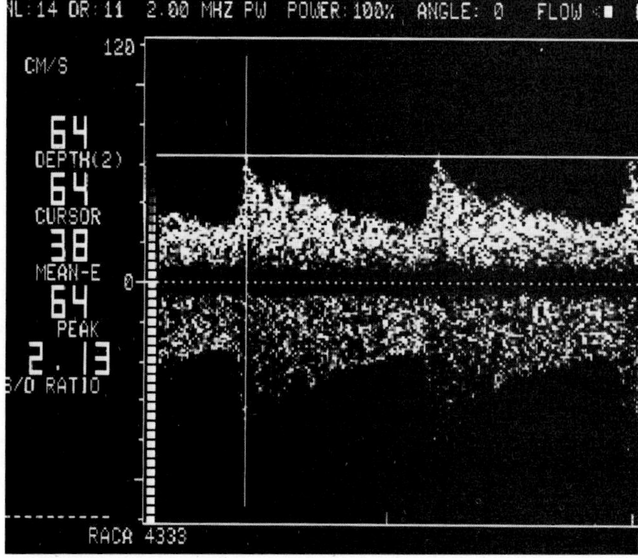

FIG. 22-99 Normal anterior cerebral artery spectrum (inverted).

contralateral anterior cerebral exhibits increased flow velocities. Common carotid compression normally reverses the anterior cerebral signal or diminishes flow in the absence of a patent anterior communicating artery. The anterior communicating artery is not normally detected unless it is acting as a collateral, when high velocities and turbulence will be noted at the 70- to 80-mm level.

The posterior cerebral artery signal is located by beginning at the middle and anterior cerebral bifurcation, increasing the sample depth by about 5 mm, then angling posteriorly and inferiorly (Fig. 22-100). Flow is toward the transducer and may occasionally be confused with the middle cerebral, but the posterior cerebral artery cannot be tracked at any depth shallower than 55 mm, whereas the middle cerebral artery can. The distal posterior cerebral artery flow signal appears to travel away from the probe or be bidirectional, since the anatomic course of the posterior cerebral changes in relation to the transducer window and the beam sweeps across the curve.

The posterior communicating artery is seldom located but appears as a turbulent, high-velocity signal when acting as a collateral and is found in a manner similar to that used for the posterior cerebral artery.

The transoccipital approach is used for the evaluation of the intracranial vertebral arteries and basilar artery. The head is slightly flexed forward and the probe is placed in the center of the suboccipital area with a sample depth of 60 to 70 mm. The probe is angled laterally right and left of midline to assess the individual vertebrals (Fig. 22-101). The sample depth is then increased until the vertebrobasilar junction is located (85 to 100 mm) and the single basilar artery signal is assessed. The probe may need to be elevated superiorly when following the arteries. The flow in the vertebrals and basilar will be away from the transducer normally. A reversed signal in one vertebral or the other with turbulence at the basilar junction is indicative of a subclavian steal, and evidence to this effect should already have been gained from earlier extracranial duplex carotid assessments.

Characteristics of Doppler Intracranial Arterial Waveforms

The normal appearance of the intracranial waveform is similar to that of the extracranial internal carotid artery, since the intracranial arterial system is also a low-resistance system. The diastolic component of the spectral waveform does not normally go below the baseline and the concentration of frequencies follows the envelope contour, as in the normal internal carotid signal (Fig. 22-102).

TRANSCRANIAL DOPPLER DIAGNOSTIC INTERPRETATION CRITERIA

The primary measurement factor used in quantifying the intracranial Doppler spectral signal is the peak systolic velocity, which is measured in the same location as on waveforms from the extracranial Doppler examination (see Fig. 22-25), or the mean velocity, which is time averaged over several waveforms. Most transcranial Doppler devices automatically calculate and display the mean velocity in real time based on the placement of the cursor along the peak (on some displays, *cursor* indicates the peak systolic frequency at placement).

Most investigators, as well the ICAVL Essentials and Standards, recommend the use of mean velocities rather than peak velocities.[18] The reason for using mean velocities is that the precise Doppler angle of insonation is not known but is assumed to be 0 degrees and no more than 30

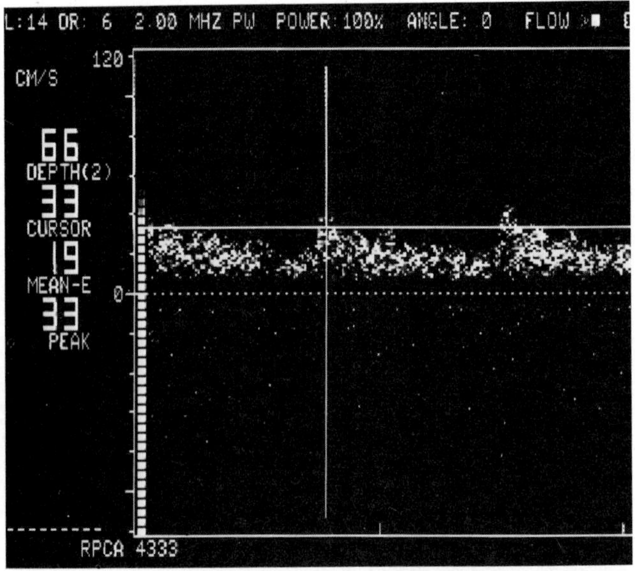

FIG. 22-100 Normal posterior cerebral artery spectrum.

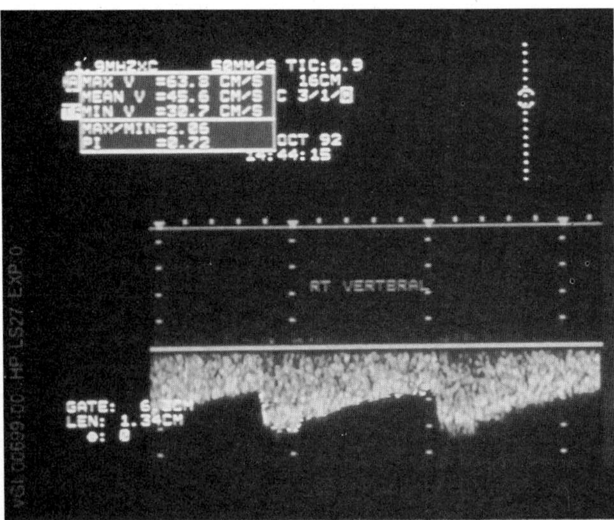

FIG. 22-101 Normal vertebral artery signal from the transoccipital approach, with flow traveling away from the transducer. (Courtesy Hewlett/Packard.)

degrees.[2] One investigator suggests reporting findings as frequencies rather than velocities for this reason.[3] Various investigators have published criteria that provide slightly different (but generally close) ranges for normal velocities in each of the vessels, and it is sometimes difficult to determine whose criteria to use. Table 22-7 shows normal PSV and mean ± standard deviation velocities compiled from Aaslid et al., DeWitt/Wechsler, and Fujioka et al. with mean frequency values from Arnolds and von Reutern.[2,3,15,24] These criteria assume an angle of 0 degrees with a 2-MHz pulsed Doppler.

ABNORMAL FLOW CRITERIA

As in the extracranial carotid duplex examination, increased flow velocities occur across a significant stenosis, in the presence of arterial spasm, or in collateral arteries. As stated previously, the increase in velocity is usually proportional to the degree of luminal reduction. Diminished waveforms and dampened pulsatility also occur distal to a severe stenosis, just as in the extracranial system or the peripheral arteries.

The direction of flow within the artery being examined is also a diagnostic factor, as are the presence and degree of flow disturbance and turbulence. Since the intracranial arteries are of small caliber, turbulent signals manifest as squeaking or whining bruit sounds with prominent harmonics; these bruits often are almost musical in nature (Fig. 22-103).

Some spectral broadening occurs naturally in intracranial arteries because of the many branches, bifurcations, and small overall calibers; spectral broadening criteria therefore do not apply, with the exception of baseline turbulence and envelope disturbance.

Certain velocity and directional findings are often consistent with specific types of intracerebral pathology; these abnormal values and findings are discussed in their appropriate subtopics.

APPLICATIONS OF TRANSCRANIAL DOPPLER AND RESPECTIVE ABNORMAL DIAGNOSTIC CRITERIA

Transcranial Doppler has been found to be useful in numerous applications, according to the American Academy of Neurology.[13] These include:

1. Detecting the presence of severe, greater than 65% stenosis in the major basal intracranial arteries;
2. Assessing the patterns and extent of collateral circulation in patients with known severe stenosis or occlusion;
3. Evaluating and following patients with vasospasm or vasoconstriction, especially after a subarachnoid hemorrhage;

TABLE 22-7 Transcranial Doppler Diagnostic Velocity Criteria Ranges

Cerebral vessel	Sample depth	PSV (cm/sec)	MV (cm/sec)	MF (KHz)
Middle cerebral artery	50-55 mm	95 ± 23	62 ± 12	2.4 ± 0.45
Anterior cerebral artery	65 mm	71 ± 18	51 ± 12	1.85 ± 0.35
Posterior cerebral artery	70 mm	56 ± 12	44 ± 11	1.53 ± 0.34
Terminal internal carotid artery	55-70 mm	89 ± 23	37 ± 6.5	—
Ophthalmic artery	40-55 mm	—	24 ± 8	—
Basilar artery	85-100 mm	56 ± 13	41 ± 10	1.63 ± 0.33
Vertebral artery	60-80 mm	45 ± 18	36 ± 9	—

PSV-Peak systolic velocity; MV-mean velocity; MF-mean frequency.

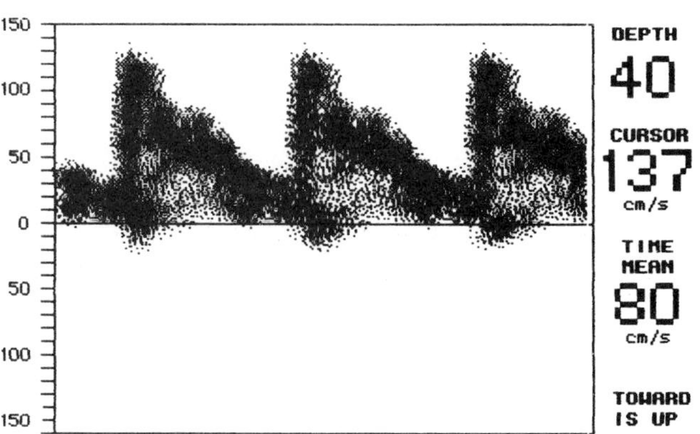

FIG. 22-102 Typical normal transcranial waveform appearance.

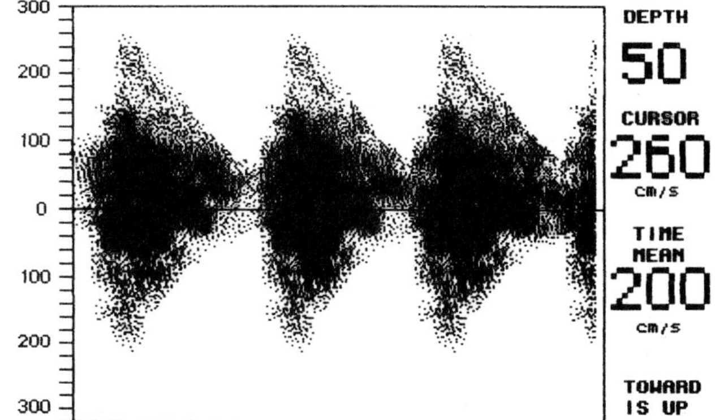

FIG. 22-103 Typical abnormal stenotic waveform appearance.

4. Detecting arteriovenous malformations (AVMs) and documenting their supply vessels and flow patterns;
5. Assessing patients with suspected brain death.

The following section addresses the utility of TCD in some of these areas and discusses diagnostic criteria used in evaluating these conditions.

Intracranial Artery Stenosis Detection

Transcranial Doppler can be used effectively to evaluate stroke patients for high-grade stenosis or occlusion in the cerebral vasculature, and to assess the success or failure of thrombolysis or cerebral percutaneous transluminal angioplasty (using protocols defined in the NACPTAR trials).

The Doppler criteria for severe stenosis in the cerebral arteries are very similar to those used for internal carotid stenosis, but no accepted universal values for categorizing degree of abnormality or grading percentages have been published. Although Mattle et al. published criteria for categorizing the diagnosis of MCA lesions, the investigative series consisted of only 61 patients, with 2 to 12 patients in each of six classification categories.[34] Detection of stenosis should therefore be subjectively based on documented velocity increases, turbulence, waveform diminution distal to the stenosis, and comparisons to the normal velocity values in Table 22-7.

Indirect Evaluation of Extracranial Disease and Collateralization

When used as an adjunct to carotid duplex sonography, transcranial Doppler can also function as an indirect study for carotid disease detection in the manner of the periorbital examination but with much more detail regarding the intracranial collateral pathways and distal effects of proximal ICA stenosis or occlusion. Flow changes in the terminal ICA may indicate the severity of the stenosis, as does reversed flow in the ophthalmic artery (the basis for the periorbital Doppler examination). Decreased velocities, diminished flow patterns, and disturbances in the middle cerebral artery often can occur as an indirect result of severe ICA stenosis, but these characteristics are not generally quantifiable. Collateral patterns through the anterior and posterior communicating arteries, however, are detectable and can be characterized by direct assessment of the anterior and posterior communicating arteries as described previously (when possible) or by using the following supporting criteria: Collateral flow through the anterior communicating artery is confirmed by reversed flow in the ipsilateral anterior cerebral artery on the side with the ICA obstruction and an increase in the contralateral anterior cerebral artery velocity that exceeds the middle cerebral artery velocity on the same side by 150%. The ipsilateral MCA also has reversed flow during ipsilateral CCA compression or decreased flow velocities during contralateral CCA compression if the anterior communicating artery is patent.[42] Collateral flow through the posterior communicating artery is confirmed by an increase in the ipsilateral proximal posterior cerebral artery velocity that exceeds the middle cerebral artery velocity on the same side by 125%. There is also an increase in the ipsilateral posterior cerebral artery during compression of the ipsilateral common carotid artery if the posterior communicating artery is patent.[42]

Transcranial Doppler also has applications in evaluating patients with subclavian steal; flow around the vertebrobasilar junction can be evaluated and directional effect established from the transoccipital window. Any cross-collateralization (including reversed flow in the basilar artery) or retrograde filling of the internal carotid artery across collaterals in innominate occlusion and/or carotid steal can also be traced and documented. Individual vertebral artery compression (accomplished by applying digital pressure at the posterior slope of the mastoid) is sometimes used to determine the flow direction in the basilar artery and enhance the degree of collateral or contributing flow from the circle of Willis to the posterior circulation.

Intracranial Vasospastic Disorders

Cerebral artery spasm often follows subarachnoid hemorrhage and is a major contributing factor to stroke deaths. Angiography is the most accurate means of assessing vasospasm but is impractical for the follow-up period required to determine a spasm's onset and resolution.

Mean-velocity interpretation criteria published by Seiler and Aaslid were developed by correlating TCD results with angiographic comparisons of the MCA diameter; velocities correspondingly increase as the vessel diameter reduces.[44]

Normal	30 to 80 cm/sec
Mild spasm	120 to 140 cm/sec
Moderate spasm	140 to 200 cm/sec
Severe spasm	≥200 cm/sec

Progression of spasm also has been followed by noting day-to-day changes in velocities; they have been observed to increase by more than 25 cm/sec per day in patients who later progress to severe vasospasm.[1]

Transcranial Doppler's clinical value in evaluating vasospasm is in its ability to detect the flow velocity changes in evolving vasospasm before the onset of ischemic neurologic deficits; this forewarning enables clinical management and prophylactic treatment to be given before severe problems occur.

Evaluation of Arteriovenous Malformations

Like techniques used to evaluate arteriovenous fistulas in extremity arteries and grafts (see Chapter 20), transcranial Doppler can help locate feeding branch vessels and occasionally the AVM itself. The flow patterns in feeding arteries are similar to those seen in arteriovenous fistulas in the extremities; there is high-velocity, turbulent flow, sometimes with decreased pulsatility. In the AVM itself the flow may be bidirectional in nature and more prominently disturbed.[33]

In a series published by Lindegaard et al. the average remote MCA mean velocity was between 44 to 94 cm/sec, tapering AVM feeder vessels had mean velocities of 75 to 124 cm/sec, and nontapering AVM feeder vessels had mean velocities of 90 to 237 cm/sec among 22 patients with cerebral AVMs.[33]

Evaluation of Brain Death

Circulatory arrest in the cerebral arterial system is not diagnosed by transcranial Doppler alone; it is made clinically and with the support of electroencephalography, radionuclide brain scan, and arteriography.

The basis of brain death determination is that flow ceases in the cerebral arteries above the circle of Willis level. As the cerebral pressure increases, the intracerebral arteries are compressed or collapse from the outer capillaries inward until the ICA in the petrous portion occludes.[28]

In the Doppler waveform, diastolic flow decreases and diminishes to the baseline as the cerebral pressure increases; ultimately a characteristic bidirectional, high-resistance waveform pattern (to-and-fro) is detected in the MCA or other cerebral vessels. With further monitoring over time, the waveform progresses to the appearance of a short spiked or blip waveform similar to that seen with vascular motion (but not flow motion) in ICA occlusion and eventually to a complete absence of detected flow.[28]

Transcranial Doppler data in brain death are not always definitive but support other findings that enable a thorough clinical determination to be made.

Other Applications of Transcranial Doppler

Transcranial Doppler is used as a monitoring tool by some investigators to evaluate changes during carotid endarterectomy, especially to determine whether to use a shunt, the continued patency of shunts during surgery, and the autoregulatory response in the MCA during cross-clamping[39] (Fig. 22-104; see color image).

Transcranial Doppler has also been used to detect gaseous microemboli during cardiopulmonary bypass so that oxygenation factors can be adjusted to reduce or eliminate neurologic events that occur as sequelae to the operation. Discontinuities and irregularities in the flow pattern can occur as the microemboli travel cephalad and result in a higher-amplitude signal. Turbulent and uniformly disturbed flow may also be seen.[40] During carotid endarterectomy, bubble emboli also may be released after removal of the clamp; these are detected by monitoring TCD as bright vertical spikes that may briefly and randomly appear in an otherwise uniform Doppler spectrum (Fig. 22-105) and that are distinct from motion artifacts.[45]

One investigator has proposed using transcranial Doppler to monitor flow in the MCA in patients with complete hemiplegia of less than 12 hours duration; preliminary findings suggested that patients with mean velocities of greater than 30 cm/sec had a good prognosis for complete recovery, whereas those with velocities of less than 30 cm/sec had a poor prognosis with less likelihood of recovery.[26]

Technical Limitations on the Performance of the Transcranial Doppler Examination

Transcranial Doppler studies cannot be performed on a small percentage of the population who have poor transtemporal windows and dense temporal bones. An insonation failure rate of about 13% is common; absent or poor temporal windows are most often found in certain racial groups, women, and older individuals.[33]

The quality of a transcranial Doppler study also depends on the technical skill of the examiner. A great deal of practice and familiarity with the operating characteristics of the device and the intracranial anatomy is necessary before reliable and diagnostic information can be obtained. The examiner also must have a "good ear" and an ability to mentally visualize where the transducer and sample volume are in relation to the signals being monitored (unless the three-dimensional device is in use). The examiner must know the proper flow directions in the

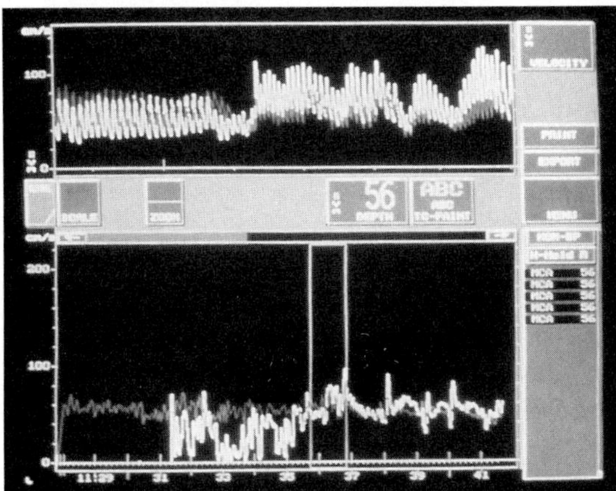

FIG. 22-104 Long-term monitoring TCD tracing during carotid surgery; the spectral envelope *(white line)* is monitored together with the blood pressure *(red line)*. The upper waveform display is an enlarged section from the lower compressed long-term display. (Courtesy EME/Nicolet.)

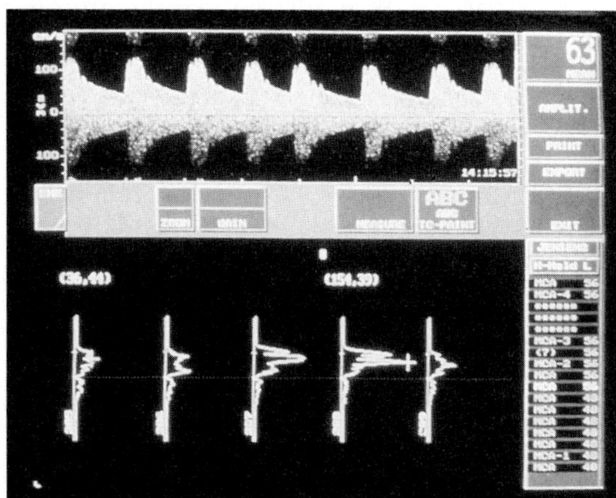

FIG. 22-105 Detection of emboli. This MCA spectrum *(top)* faintly shows an embolus passage, but an embolus spike is prominently demonstrated by the spectral amplitude display *(bottom)*; emboli are typically seen as more prominent top-to-bottom "blips" in the spectrum. (Courtesy EME/Nicolet.)

vessel being examined and be able to identify abnormalities and collaterals if detected.

Summary

Transcranial Doppler is a challenging examination technique that can be very rewarding to learn and perform; although it has been shown to have beneficial and useful diagnostic capabilities, it does not replace cerebral angiography nor should it be fully relied on unless some knowledge of the extracranial carotid and vertebral states has been acquired from a prior carotid duplex scan. By combining the two modalities a very thorough and complete picture of the extracranial and intracranial hemodynamics can be established.

THREE-DIMENSIONAL TRANSCRANIAL DOPPLER SCANNING

In addition to the standard conventional transcranial Doppler method, another supplemental technique has been developed that combines standard transcranial Doppler with a mapping method similar to that used in the older ultrasonic arteriograph. The older technique was used to map flow presence and obtain samples in carotid bifurcations by cathode ray tube (CRT) recordings of audible traces during back-and-forth sweeps of a Doppler probe over the cervical carotid arteries (Fig. 22-106).

Three-dimensional color transcranial Doppler mapping uses the same insonation techniques and protocols as conventional transcranial Doppler. Instead of a hand-held probe, however, this device uses a unique headpiece with integral 2-MHz transducers fixed to a series of position-registering X-Y-Z potentiometers (similar to B-scan arms) located on both sides of the headpiece (Fig. 22-107). The patient is examined supine and the patient's head is carefully and correctly positioned so that it is straight within the headpiece. Insonation is performed via the windows described above. The sample volume's distance from the glabella and bregma and its location relative to the transducer are tracked in space by the computer software, allowing its location to be shown in a three-dimensional representation. As the sample is advanced or relocated and waveforms and samples are stored, color-coded velocity indicators representing the flow direction and velocity at the evaluation point are manually plotted on the screen. The color map (a hue map—see Chapter 19) assigns specific shades to the sample point in 15-cm/sec steps based on the flow patterns at the sample site. Zero flow is gray. Flow toward the probe is shown (in ascending velocity order) as brown (≥15 cm/sec), orange (≥30 cm/sec), yellow (≥45 cm/sec), and red (≥60 cm/sec). Flow away from the probe is shown (in ascending velocity order) as dark blue (≥15 cm/sec), medium blue (≥30 cm/sec), light blue (≥45 cm/sec), and white (≥60 cm/sec). The Doppler waveforms and velocities at the sample site are stored at the plotted point for later recall. As the vessels are examined and the insonation sample

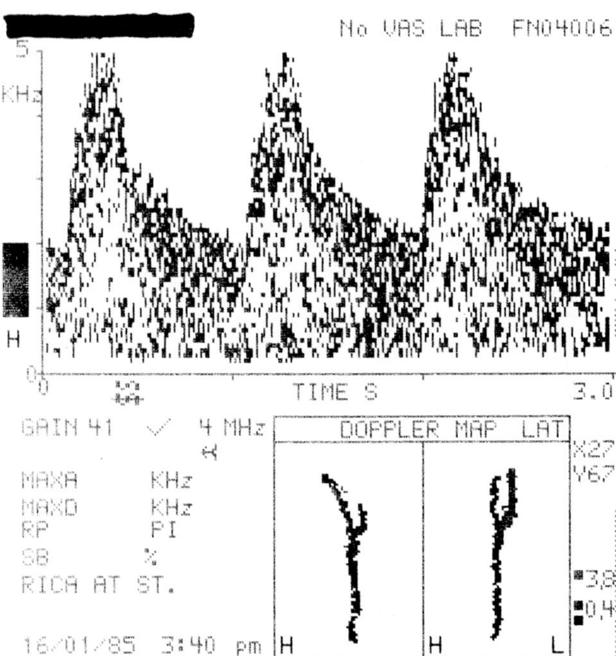

FIG. 22-106 An example of ultrasonic arteriography, showing a Doppler flow map from the carotid arteries with an ICA spectral waveform.

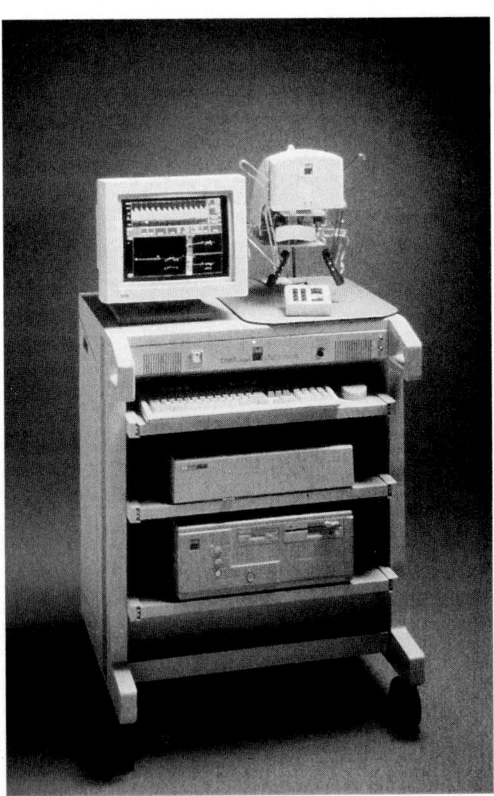

FIG. 22-107 Three-dimensional color transcranial Doppler scanner, showing the headpiece assembly sitting on the main unit to the right of the monitor. (Courtesy EME/Nicolet.)

points are plotted, an image is built up on the computer display that ultimately forms a color-coded image map of the cerebral arteries and the hemodynamic characteristics along their courses. Coronal, sagittal, and horizontal views of the resulting map can be displayed. Color-coded waveform spectra can be recalled from any point along the map and can also be displayed for hard-copy purposes[41] (Fig. 22-108; see color images).

This three-dimensional device is still widely used and has been beneficial in localizing and evaluating intracerebral artery stenoses (Fig. 22-109; see color image), AVMs, aneurysms, and potential occlusions. The mapping technique enables the abnormalities and their relations to significant portions of the circle of Willis to be compared and isolated, and the point-by-point Doppler waveform storage ability allows recall of flow dynamics and other calculations to be performed in a concise manner. This device also makes learning and performing TCD easier because of the simultaneous feedback provided by the combination of the visual spatial orientation map and the audio spectra.

Despite its utility, this device will probably ultimately be supplanted by transcranial duplex imaging as that technology improves, much as ultrasonic arteriography was made obsolete by the duplex scanner.

Transcranial Duplex Imaging

Although blind transcranial Doppler can show the intracranial hemodynamics, it does not provide a two-dimensional image of the cerebral relationships and vasculature. Transcranial duplex imaging is the next logical step and has recently become practical through technologic advances and improvements in transducer technology. The internal landmarks of the brain and intracranial vault can enable the examiner to obtain excellent images of the circle of Willis and can guide placement of the Doppler sample volume for precise measurement of the flow velocities in the arteries. An additional benefit is that angle correction can be used for (theoretically) more accurate velocity calculations.

In many ways, transcranial imaging is an evolution of real time neonatal echoencephalographic techniques applied to an adult[11] (see Chapter 16). The reader may wish to study that chapter to become familiar with the anatomy of the brain as visualized by ultrasound, since the landmarks are almost identical. Although familiarity with cerebral and intracranial landmarks benefits the examiner, identifying, visualizing, and assessing the vascular anatomy is the primary focus of the transcranial imaging examination.

Equipment. Transcranial imaging is performed with color-flow duplex instrumentation equipped with transcranial-specific annotation and waveform analysis software. Imaging is accomplished through a phased-array multielement sector transducer, usually at a 2- to 2.5-MHz image and 1.9- to 2.25-MHz Doppler transmit frequency. Most equipment displays the output power as a cranial thermal index per American Institute of Ultrasound in Medicine (AIUM) output display standards, especially given the recent approval of higher transmission power levels.

One device is a nonimaging 2-MHz pulsed Doppler transducer for additional blind TCD evaluations; the sample volume depth is graphically and numerically represented on the image in some systems for ease in tracking. Most of the

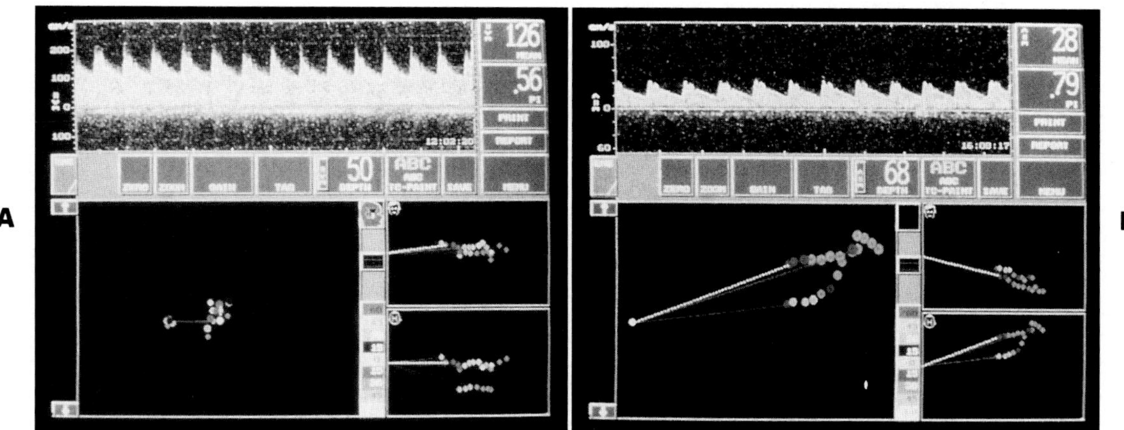

FIG. 22-108 Three-dimensional color transcranial Doppler displays. The upper third of the display shows the spectral waveform at the current sample site. The spatial maps *(bottom images)* are arranged to show a side view (lateral—*bottom left*), AP frontal view (coronal—*upper right*), and top-down view (horizontal—*lower right*) of the vessels in **A.** Flow direction toward (red hues) or away from (blue hues) the transducer in the vessels is shown by the plotted sample points. **A,** This image shows an abnormal, elevated middle cerebral artery Doppler waveform with a mean velocity of 126 cm/sec *(top),* taken from the left MCA; the top-down view clearly shows the MCAs and PCAs; the red dots localize the areas of high velocity in the insonated MCA. **B,** This image shows a normal vertebral signal *(top),* and the vertebral and basilar arteries in a top-down view (bottom—*left and lower right*) and AP frontal view (bottom—*upper right*). (Courtesy EME/Nicolet.)

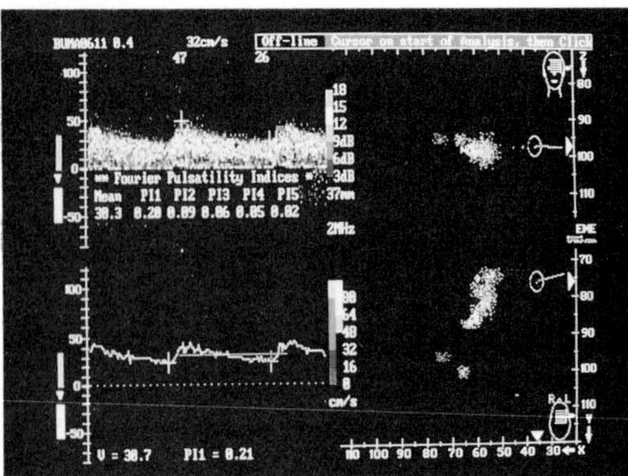

FIG. 22-109 Three-dimensional image from a patient with a traumatic ICA dissection; the left MCA has reduced pulsatility *(top left),* the left carotid siphon and ACA are not detected, and velocities and dot brightness are increased in the collateralizing left PCoA. (From F Ries. From Berstein EF, editor: Vascular Diagnosis, ed 4. St. Louis: Mosby, 1993.)

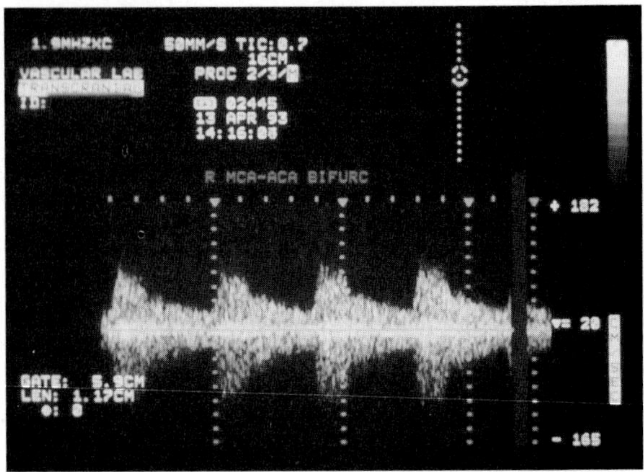

FIG. 22-110 Transcranial Doppler waveform display from "blind" examination performed on a TCD-equipped duplex scanner.

spectral display features associated with transcranial Doppler devices are duplicated on transcranial imaging systems (Fig. 22-110).

Transcranial Imaging Techniques

Transcranial imaging requires a thorough knowledge of the appearance of the intracranial vessels and the hemodynamics. Before attempting imaging, the reader should become completely familiar with the intracerebral anatomy and the transcranial Doppler examination principles described previously; transcranial imaging is an extension of almost all the principles and techniques covered.

Unlike in TCD, once the arteries have been visualized, the examiner can move the sample directly to the identified artery of interest and sample at any point along the visualized artery or circle of Willis branch. An additional advantage of transcranial imaging is that the contralateral vascular anatomy is also seen deep in the same view, so that flow reversals in cross-collateralization or areas of stenosis can be instantly identified with color-flow imaging.

Transcranial imaging is accomplished through the same access windows into the cranium as in transcranial Doppler: the transtemporal, transoccipital (transforamenal or transnuchal) and transorbital windows. The vessels that can be seen and monitored in each of the planes were described previously:

- *Transtemporal:* ACA, MCA, PCA, and ACoA and PCoA if active.
- *Transoccipital:* VA and BA and PCAs.
- *Transorbital:* OA and TICA.

When beginning the examination, the examiner should initially maximize the acoustic power (to the upper limit of 397 mW/cm^2 SPTA) until penetration is achieved and the arteries are seen, then should lower the power to the minimum levels needed to maintain good visualization and color filling. The PRF should be adjusted as low as possible to maintain sensitivity but avoiding aliasing of frequencies.

Color-flow and Doppler directional assignments should be set so that flow toward the transducer is coded as red and flow away from the transducer is coded as blue. This reflects the normal cerebral arterial flow characteristics; flow travels from the inner circle vessels outward. Vessels that are seen deep have opposite color direction shades compared with arteries in the superficial area of the image.

In the transtemporal approach (over the temporal bone above the zygomatic arch and anterior to the ear) the examiner should orient the transducer so that the scanning plane is in an axial orientation, with the transducer rotated so that the leading edge of the scan plane is slightly higher than the trailing edge to see the posterior circulation (Fig. 22-111).

Landmarks used to identify the proper insonation level and scan plane rotation include the mesencephalon, the lesser wing of the sphenoid, and the petrous pyramid of the temporal bone (Fig. 22-112). Once the proper orientation is achieved, slight angulation and rotation may be needed to visualize the arteries; the MCA usually is seen paralleling the lesser wing of the sphenoid, and the PCA is seen near the mesencephalon. The P1 segment of the PCA (the segment proximal to the PCoA insertion) usually appears red, and the P2 segment (distal to the PCoA) appears blue. Although this plane shows the circle of Willis in its entirety in certain patients, this result is not to be expected (Fig. 22-113; see color images).

Even though the contralateral vascular anatomy may periodically be seen deep in the image, the examiner should scan both sides in each temporal window to clearly and fully evaluate the vessels in an optimal fashion.

In the transoccipital approach (with the transducer in the posterior neck aiming superiorly through the foramen magnum) an angled oblique coronal orientation should be obtained by having the patient pull the chin in, placing the transducer in the nuchal area at the junction of the skull

A 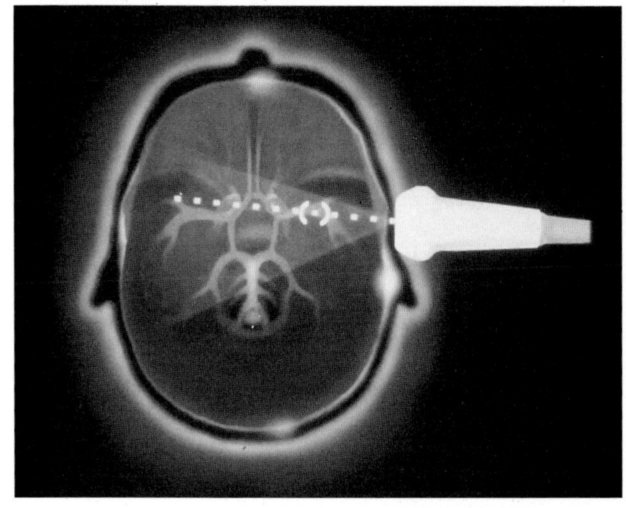

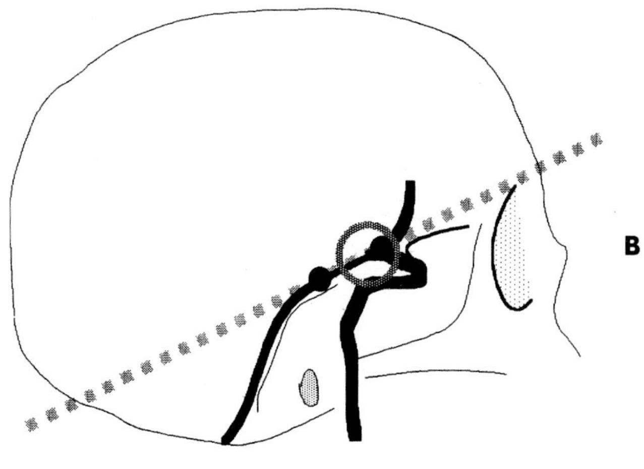 B

FIG. 22-111 A, Graphic illustrating TCI insonation of the circle of Willis, image orientation, and method of sample volume placement from a transtemporal approach and axial image plane. **B,** Lateral view of the transtemporal imaging approach, showing the proper angulation of the axial scanning plane. (**A** Courtesy Hewlett/Packard; **B** Courtesy Richard E. Rae, Indianapolis.)

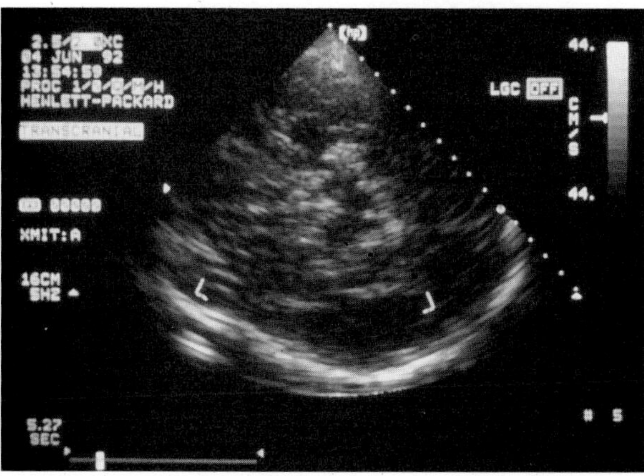

FIG. 22-112 Transtemporal axial scan showing the mesencephalon (center, heart-shaped lucency); the circle of Willis lies directly anterior to it. The lesser wing of the sphenoid bone is the bright echo to the lower left. (Courtesy Hewlett/Packard.)

and the neck, and aiming the transducer toward the nasion (the dent above the bridge of the nose) (Fig. 22-114).

The brainstem and spinal cord are the primary soft-tissue landmarks and the vertebral arteries are seen on either side wrapping anteriorly around them. The vertebrobasilar confluence and basilar artery are seen by angling upward, aiming more anteriorly, and using the posterior border of the foramen magnum (the base of the occipital bone) as a bony landmark.

Normally, image orientation shows the vertebral arteries as superficial on the image and the basilar artery as deep, with flow traveling away from the transducer (Fig. 22-115; see color image). If the duplex scanner enables horizontal flipping of the image so that the transducer "main bang" can be shown at the bottom of the display, this may help the examiner orient the vertebrobasilar junction so that the vertebrals are on the bottom and the basilar on the top, as in life. At the time of writing no display standards have been established for TCI, so this approach may work better and will be more consistent with angiographic images. The color flow in this plane may be inverted if this flipped display mode is adopted.

Because the vertebrals and basilar are seldom symmetric or textbook straight, some angulation or rotation may be required to image and evaluate them; both vertebrals and the basilar junction are not always seen in the same plane. A perfect Y vertebrobasilar image is not to be expected, just as the Y of the carotid bifurcation is seldom obtained in carotid duplex examination.

In the transorbital approach the examiner has the patient close the eye, then places the transducer over the eyelid and adjusts the output power to as low a level as possible, again to avoid overexposing the lens of the eye. By angling posteriorly and tilting and rotating the transducer, the ophthalmic artery can be seen; the carotid canal portion of the ICA, the genu, and the TICA all can be seen from this approach by angling the transducer more toward the back of the head, then pivoting inferiorly and superiorly (Fig. 22-116). The proximal ICA has a red-coded flow as it comes toward the transducer; a color transition is seen at the genu as the angle is raised anteriorly. Blue-coded flow is detected traveling away from the transducer in the TICA segment.

This examination should be repeated over each eye to ensure that both distal ICAs and TICAs are fully evaluated.

Interpretation of Transcranial Image Data and Doppler Findings

The hemodynamics of the intracranial arteries have been thoroughly described in the transcranial Doppler section. In

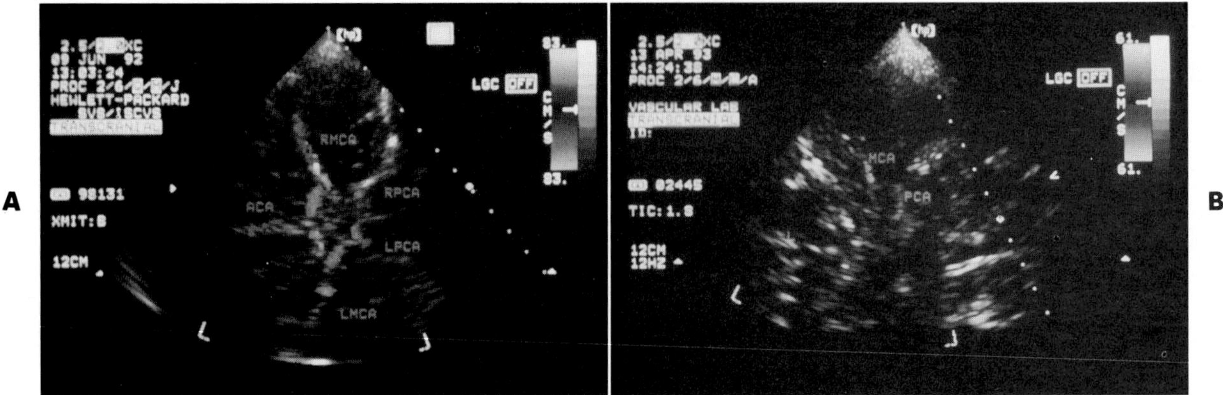

FIG. 22-113 A, Transtemporal axial color-flow scan showing an exceptional complete view of the circle of Willis. **B,** A more typical (and more likely) color-flow view of the right MCA and PCA and left ACA, seen in a 64-year-old man. (**A** Courtesy Hewlett/Packard.)

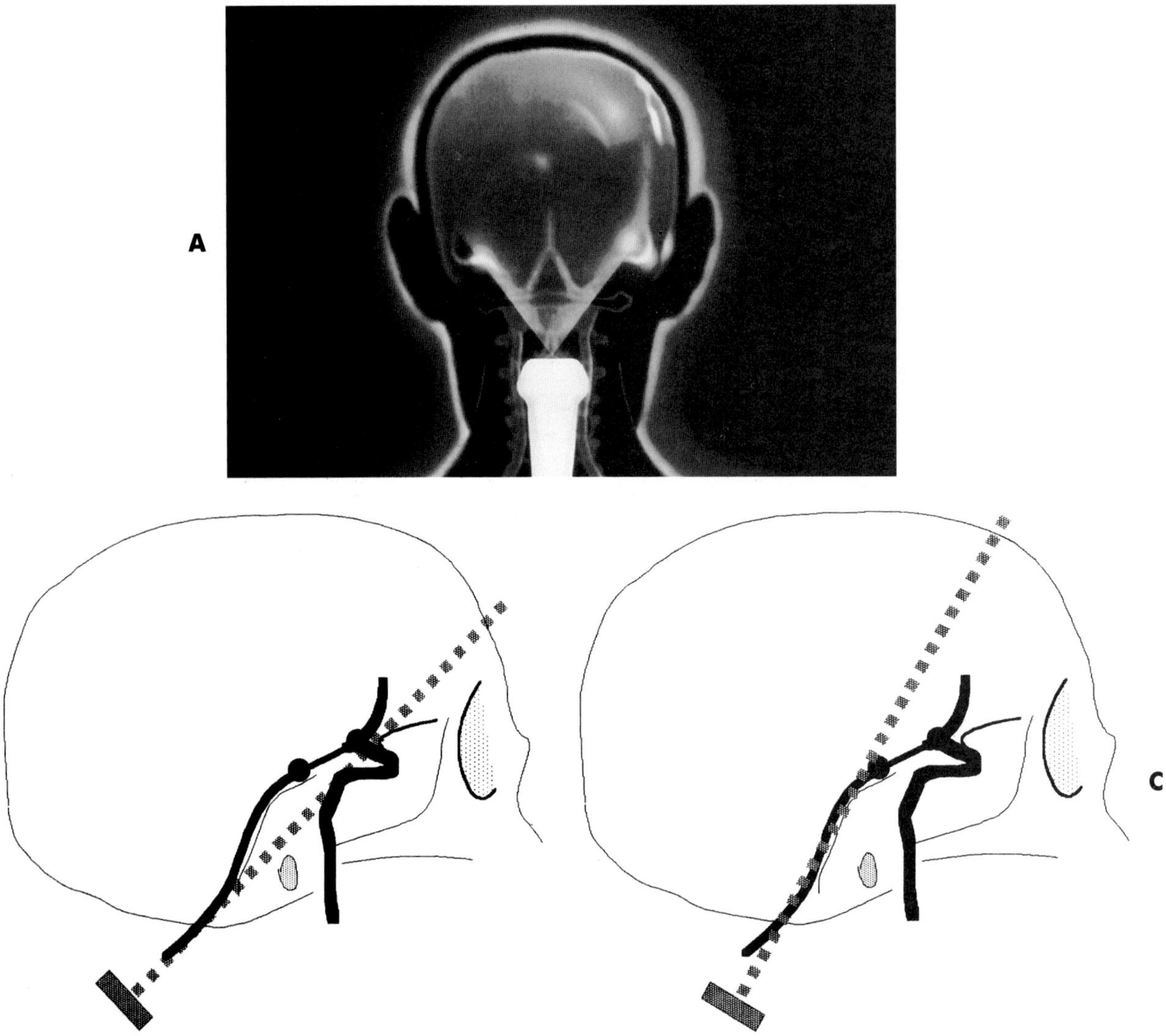

FIG. 22-114 A, Graphic illustrating TCI insonation of vertebral and basilar arteries from a transoccipital approach and oblique coronal image plane. **B,** Lateral view of the transoccipital imaging approach showing the proper angulation of the coronal scanning plane for the distal vertebral arteries. **C,** Lateral view of the transoccipital imaging approach showing the proper angulation of the axial scanning plane for the vertebrobasilar junction and the basilar artery. (**A** Courtesy Hewlett/Packard; **B** and **C** Courtesy Richard E. Rae, Indianapolis.)

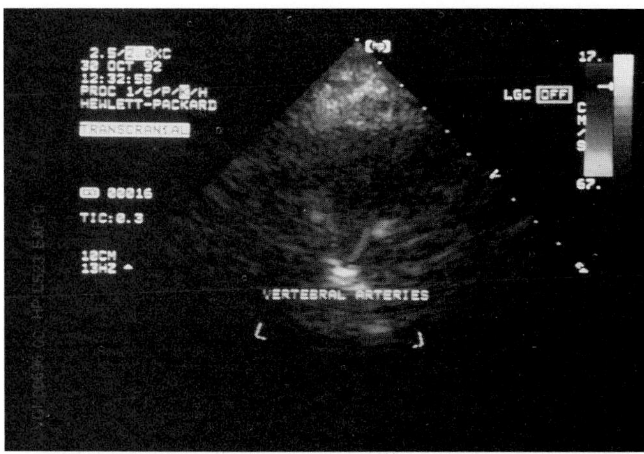

FIG. 22-115 Transoccipital color-flow scan showing both distal vertebral arteries. (Courtesy Hewlett/Packard.)

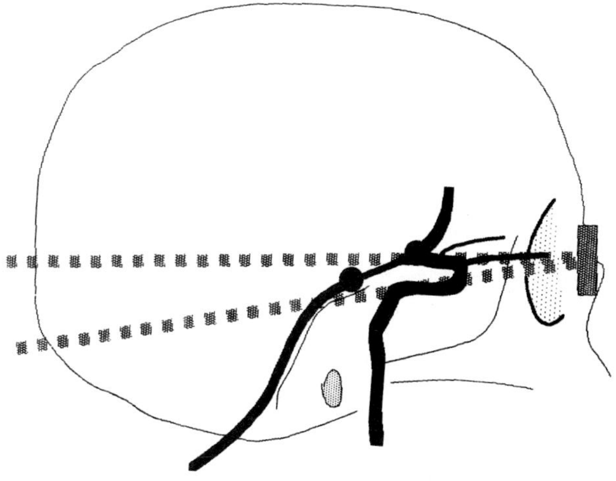

FIG. 22-116 Lateral view of the transorbital imaging approach, showing proper angulations of the scanning plane for the ophthalmic artery, carotid siphon, and terminal internal carotid artery. (Courtesy Richard E. Rae, Indianapolis.)

keeping with this, anticipated normal color-flow imaging patterns are described. Areas of stenosis or spasm should be seen as higher-velocity streamline concentrations, with visible bruits in severely stenotic regions centering at the stenosis (just as in the carotid duplex examination). Color-flow reversals should be seen with cross-collateralization following the pathways, flow patterns, and flow directions described in the transcranial Doppler section.

The appearances of normal and abnormal Doppler spectral waveforms obtained with transcranial imaging are identical to those obtained with blind transcranial Doppler (Fig. 22-117). Although common carotid compressions are freely used to enhance or isolate collateral pathways in transcranial Doppler, they are probably less important in transcranial duplex imaging, since the color-flow imaging characteristics should alert the examiner to the presence of occlusions and the existence of retrograde flow patterns. Compressions, however, may augment these pathways for on-screen confirmation and VCR recordings.

Transcranial imaging gives instant feedback on the presence and hemodynamic effect of subclavian and vertebrobasilar steal, since color-flow directional changes are dramatically seen around the vertebrobasilar junction.

Velocity Criteria and Angle Correction

It would be expected that angle-corrected velocities would be more accurate than those specified for an assumed 0- to 30-degree angle of insonation (given previously, see "Transcranial Doppler") and that new criteria would have to be developed. Interestingly enough, a study by Fujioka et al. found that angle-corrected velocities were comparable with velocities established in previously existing TCD criteria tables with little if any clinical variation; angle corrections generally resulted in Doppler vector angles of insonation of less than 30 degrees in all visualized vessels.[24] Fujioka et al. reach the conclusion that an examiner can confidently use established TCD criteria when the corrected angle is less than 30 degrees in the cerebral arteries but cautions against using corrected velocities in cases where corrected angles are greater than 30 degrees, since no established velocity criteria are available that take greater angles into account.[24]

Technical Limitations to the Performance of the Transcranial Duplex Imaging Examination

The same technical limitations of temporal bone thickness resulting from age, gender, and race apply to transcranial duplex imaging as to transcranial Doppler, but with an increased failure rate with TCI compared with TCD (47% failure for TCI as opposed to 18% failure for TCD in insonating the MCA, and 52% TCI and 28% TCD failure to insonate the PCA).[24] TCI and TCD failure rates are comparable in the vertebrobasilar segment, since there is no barrier to insonation through the foramen magnum (about 9% to 12% failure).

Although many authors have presented their initial observations or results, it should be noted that TCI is in its infancy and few if any valid data regarding its applications in abnormal cases have been published; the data in the early literature involved small series of young, normal subjects (mean ages of 30 to 48 years), whereas the study by Fujioka et al. involved a mean age of 65 years with many abnormal subjects[11,24,27,43,48]. The study by Fujioka et al. supports the existence of temporal density problems that occur with age, the insonation success rates for which are probably more applicable to the real population that this procedure will be performed on.

Summary

This section introduced the relatively new and evolving application of transcranial duplex imaging; although transcranial Doppler's applications and efficacy have been documented within the last decade, much remains to be determined regarding the usefulness and applicability of trans-

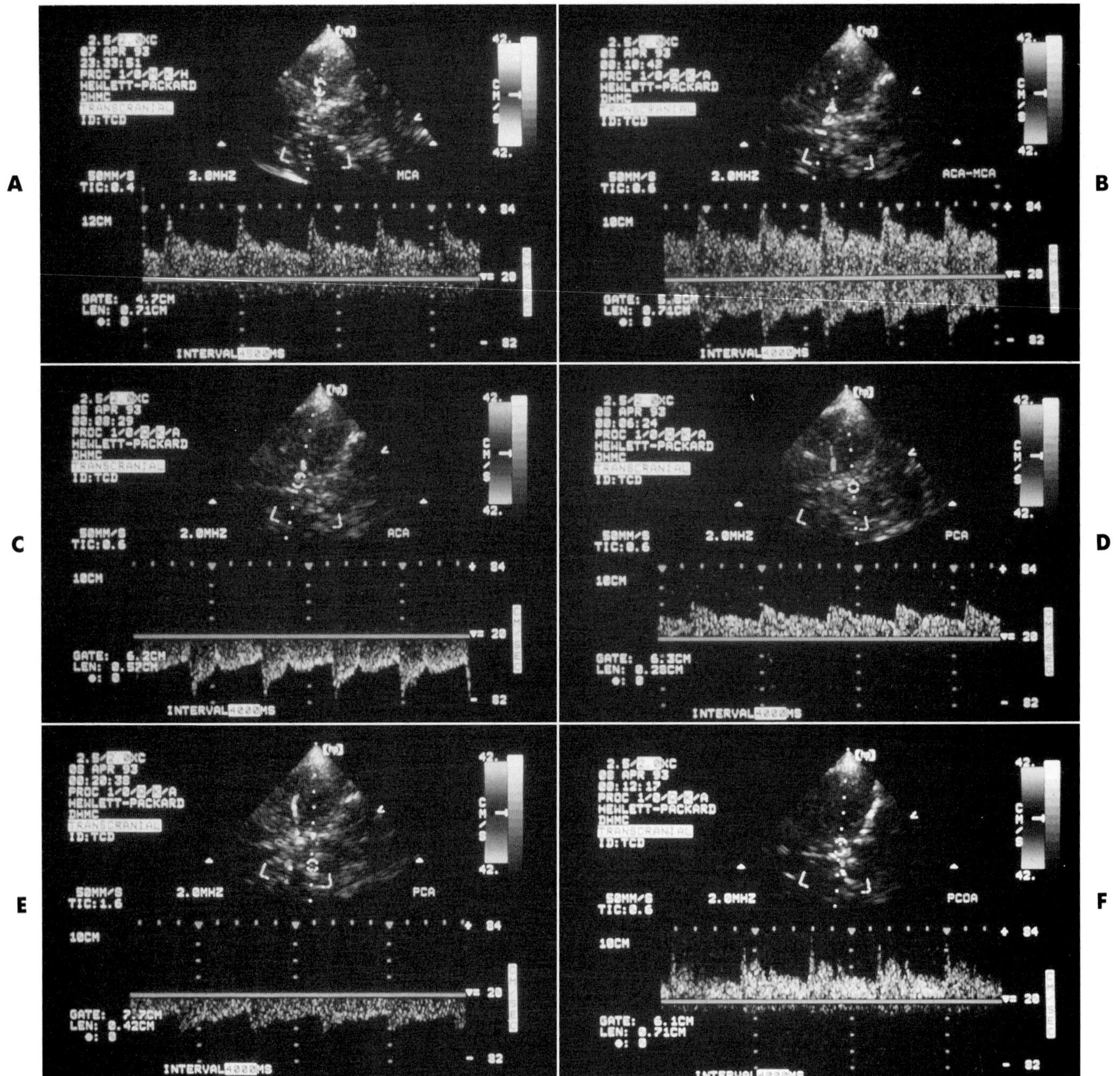

FIG. 22-117 Waveform examples obtained by transcranial duplex imaging. Transtemporal approach. **A,** Middle cerebral artery (MCA). **B,** Anterior cerebral–middle cerebral bifurcation (ACA/MCA). **C,** Anterior cerebral artery (ACA). **D,** Posterior cerebral artery, P1 segment (PCA). **E,** Posterior cerebral artery, P2 segment (PCA). **F,** Posterior communicating artery (PCoA).

Continued.

cranial imaging in the cerebrovascular system. It is recommended that TCI be used as an adjunct to standard TCD evaluation methods, especially since TCD has a statistically better chance of insonating the vessels than TCI. Since new investigative research into this modality continues, the reader is advised to review current journals to update his or her knowledge of this interesting and potentially beneficial technique.

OTHER CEREBROVASCULAR EVALUATION METHODS

A presentation of vascular techniques would be incomplete without at least a cursory mention of some other nonsonographic, noninvasive modalities, one of which is currently listed as an accepted secondary test (along with periorbital Doppler) by the Essentials and Standards of the ICAVL.[18]

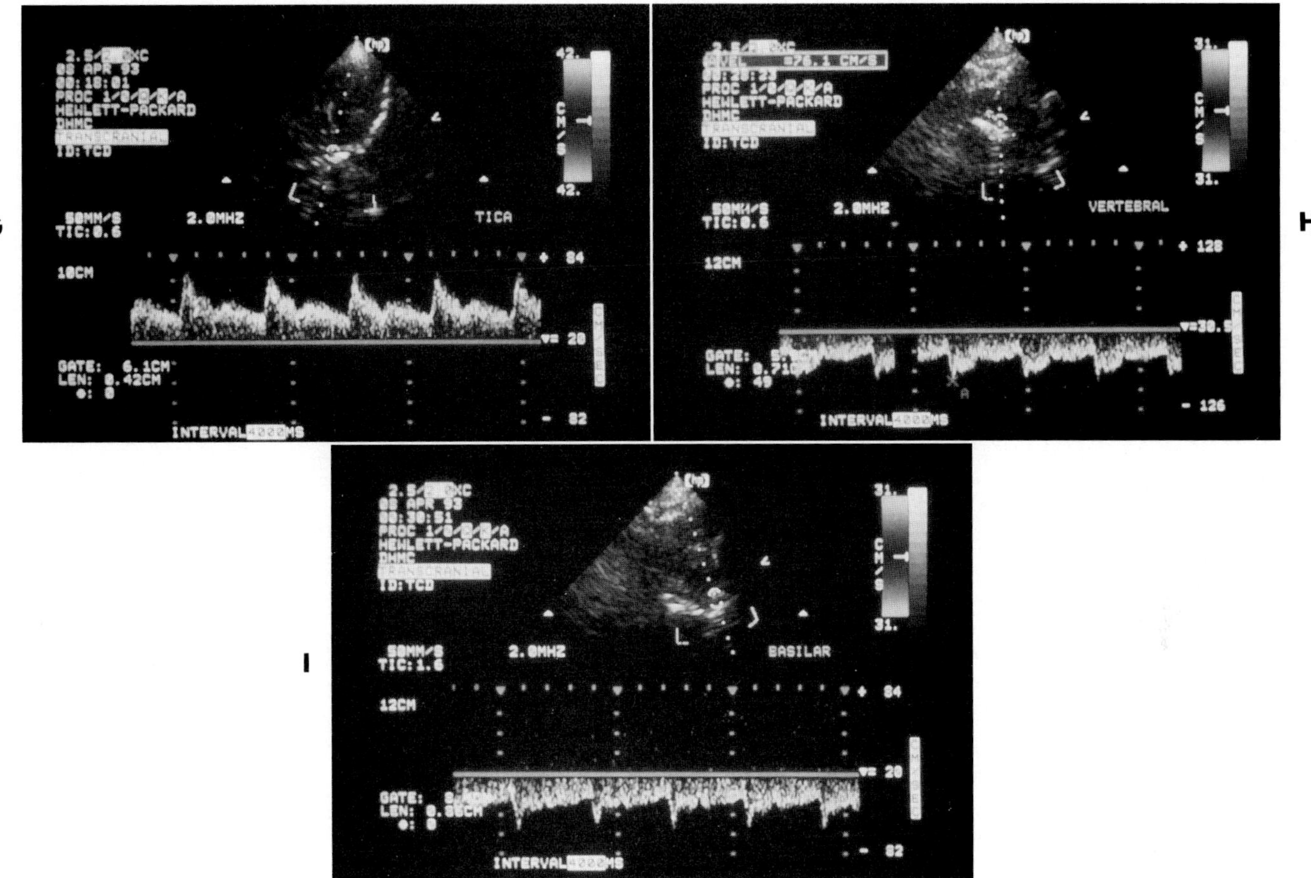

FIG. 22-117, cont'd. G, Terminal internal carotid artery (TICA). Note the prominent curved echo of the petrous bone in the reference image (right of center). Transoccipital approach. **H,** Vertebral artery (VA). **I,** Basilar artery (BA).

Duplex and Doppler assessment are standard cerebrovascular noninvasive techniques that have performed very reliably over the last two decades. They have replaced almost all indirect methods of cerebrovascular testing. Of the indirect tests mentioned here, OPG is still considered by some to be a useful adjunctive procedure and is still actively marketed by its manufacturer. Two other techniques that are less likely to be encountered in a modern laboratory include carotid phonoangiography and supraorbital PPG.

Magnetic Resonance Angiography (MRA)

Magnetic resonance angiography (MRA) is one recent development that may emerge as an alternate technique to duplex to evaluate the carotid and cerebrovascular hemodynamics.

Much of its utility and capabilities were covered in Chapter 19, as was an example of its use in the carotid system (see Figs. 19-27 and 19-28); MRA also has very useful potential in evaluating the intracerebral vasculature.

One recent investigation compared MRA image and flow data with transcranial Doppler examination and contrast angiography in nine abnormal patients and two normal volunteers. The abnormal patients had various neurologic symptoms including CVA and TIA. TCD was not performed in two of the abnormal cases, and there was one TCD technical failure because of an inability to penetrate the temporal bone. The two normal volunteers did not undergo angiography. The results of the MRA and TCD agreed in all of the six MRA-TCD-angiography comparisons, successfully detecting or ruling out collateral flow patterns. The MRA-TCD data agreed fully with the angiogram in five cases with one disparate angiogram that may have been inaccurate. TCD and MRA results agreed in both of the normal cases.[16] This investigation did not take transcranial imaging into account.

The advantages of MRA include its ability to show vascular lesions directly and its ability to show collateral pathways (e.g., fetal posterior circulation) that may not be reliably shown on TCD. Disadvantages of MRA include its lack of portability, its long acquisition time, and its expense.

Carotid Phonoangiography (CPA)

Carotid phonoangiography is basically an older technique that provides an oscilloscope method of displaying bruits, similar to phonocardiography; a microphone is placed on the neck and used like a stethoscope (the device is basically an amplified, filtered stethoscope with electronic output). The examination is usually performed at three levels within the neck (base, midneck, and high neck) and provides a visual record of bruit disturbance; audible bruit phonoangiograph patterns recorded at these levels are displayed on an oscilloscope and a Polaroid image is taken of the display. Criteria based on envelope shape and signal duration can be applied to the recorded patterns, and in theory, certain amplitudes and sound qualities correspond to specific percentages of stenosis.[23] Although both qualitative and quantitative methods have been described, the overall accuracy of this technique is poor.[23]

Comments. In practice the quality and intensity of a bruit can be subjectively evaluated by an examiner with just a stethoscope; short, abrupt bruits generally come from the external carotid, and louder, longer bruits through diastole usually are generated by the internal carotid.

Supraovbital Photoplethysmography

Supraorbital photoplethysmography is also an older, less prominent technique that uses a photoplethysmograph and chart recorder (see the discussions of photoplethysmographic technique in Chapters 19, 20, and 21). This technique is actually an alternate method of performing the periorbital Doppler examination. The use of a dual-photocell photoplethysmograph and two-channel chart recorder has been advocated,[7] but the technique can be performed with a single photocell (moved between sides) and single-channel recorder.

Two photocells are affixed with double-sided tape to the forehead, one above the medial aspect of each eyebrow, and the tracings are balanced and set to the AC amplification mode. With the recorder running, the same external branch compressions used in the periorbital Doppler examination (e.g., temporal, facial, infraorbital, and common compression) are applied individually and bilaterally. Normally, the PPG waveform is not affected by the compressions (except for the common carotid); a decrease in amplitude of greater than 33% may occur but is considered normal. A significant decrease in the pulse amplitude with a branch compression is considered evidence of a greater than 50% internal carotid artery stenosis or occlusion. If ipsilateral common carotid compression fails to eliminate or decrease the pulse waveform, then intracranial collateralization may be present, with contralateral filling through the circle of Willis implied if the pulse wave decreases with contralateral carotid compression.[7]

One study of supraorbital photoplethysmography shows it as more sensitive but less specific than periorbital Doppler. Both modalities, however, were equally unable to detect internal carotid stenoses of less than 50%.[6]

Comments. Supraorbital photoplethysmography is rarely performed in the majority of modern laboratories; if an indirect test is performed as an adjunct to carotid duplex, periorbital Doppler or ocular pneumoplethysmography tend to be the methods of choice.

Oculoplethysmography and Ocular Pneumoplethysmography

OPG was first developed in the early 1970s and achieved its main popularity through the 1980s, concurrent with the popularity of periorbital Doppler.

Two methods of oculoplethysmography have been in use, the Kartchner version (OPG-K), using a fluid displacement system, and the Gee system (OPG-G), which uses an air-vacuum technique (Fig. 22-118).

OPG-K is no longer used or available and was based on the principle that an arterial obstruction reduces pulse-arrival time; the technique involved applying fluid-filled suction cups to the sclera of the eyes and clipping photocells on the ear lobes. The eye cups measure the pulse changes from the eyes (indirectly from the internal carotid artery via the ophthalmic artery) and the photocells measure the pulsations from the ear lobe (indirectly from the external carotid artery). A normal OPG-K tracing shows the internal and external pulse waves in phase and synchronized because the pulses arrive at the same time. An internal carotid stenosis causes a delay in the pulse arrival at the eye cups; thus a phase shift between the two wave patterns occurs in an abnormal study.[17]

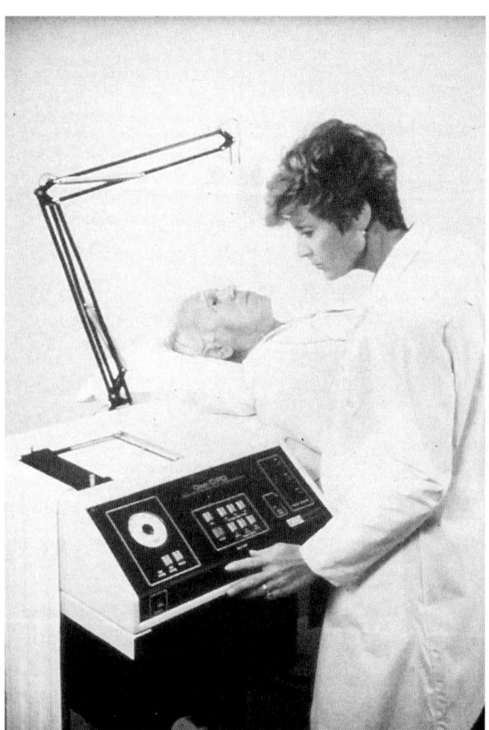

FIG. 22-118 Ocular pneumoplethysmography system (OPG-G). (Courtesy Electro-Diagnostic Instruments.)

OPG-K could detect unilateral disease very well but was poorly sensitive (70%) and specific (88%), in general because bilateral disease was difficult to accurately detect. To compensate for this weakness, OPG-K was usually done in combination with carotid phonoangiography but investigators had widely varying results. The poor sensitivity and specificity did not justify its continued use.[17]

The OPG-G technique (also referred to as *ocular pneumoplethysmography*) is different and more useful; it is based on the principle of applying vacuum pressure on the eye to increase intraocular pressure above the point where the ophthalmic pulsations are obliterated; during release of the vacuum, the point at which the pulsations return allows measurement of the ophthalmic artery pressure (OAP) (Fig. 22-119). This pressure is compared with the highest brachial systolic pressure to generate an ophthalmic pressure/systemic pressure (OP/SP) ratio in a manner that parallels the Doppler ankle-brachial ratio or forearm-brachial ratio in the extremities. Since a pressure drop occurs distal to a severe stenosis (as stated in Poiseulle's law in Chapter 20), a drop in ophthalmic artery pressure is consistent with an internal carotid artery obstruction. The pulse amplitude is also evaluated.

The procedure is performed by having the patient lie supine; the patient is asked to stare at a fixed point and to avoid blinking during the test. A topical anesthetic is applied to the eyes, and a brachial systolic blood pressure is taken from each arm with a standard sphygmomanometer and stethoscope or automated monitor. The eye cups are placed on the sclera of the eyes lateral to the cornea and gently held in place until the vacuum is activated (Fig. 22-120). A vacuum pressure of 300 mm Hg is used on normotensive individuals and 500 mm Hg on hypertensive individuals. After the vacuum is activated and the defined level is reached, the recorder is activated and the vacuum is gradually released with a corresponding decline in the tracing. A flat line usually is seen at the beginning, since the vacuum is above the occlusion pressure of the ophthalmic artery; the point at which pulse waveforms appear defines the OAP (Fig. 22-121). Alternatively, the common carotid also may be compressed during the study to determine collateral contribution, although this carries the same caveats as when it is performed in the periorbital Doppler, supraorbital PPG, or transcranial Doppler examination.

Interpretation of OPG-G Findings

The OPG-G recording and study yields three parameters used for diagnosis: the ophthalmic artery pressure, the OP/SP ratio, and the pulse amplitude. There is little agreement among investigators about what constitutes a standard diagnostic criterion. Although all the criteria commonly use a difference between the left and right ophthalmic artery pressures and the OP/SP ratio, the variability is even more widely diverse than in the carotid duplex criteria discussed above:

Gee et al.:[17]	
L-R OAP pressure differential	≥5 mm Hg
OAP	<39 mm Hg
OP/SP ratio	≤0.43
McDonald et al.:[35]	
L-R OAP pressure differential	≥5 mm Hg
OP/SP ratio	<0.66
Baker et al.[4]:	
L-R OAP pressure differential	≥5 mm Hg
OP/SP ratio	<0.66 if L-R OAP differential = 1 to 4 mm Hg <0.60 if L and R OAPs are equal
O'Hara et al.:[38]	
L-R OAP pressure differential	≥5 mm Hg
OP/SP ratio	<0.60

Pulse amplitude is usually only evaluated when extreme hypertension prevents an accurate OAP from being calculated: an amplitude difference between the two eyes of ≥2 mm on the chart tracing suggests a hemodynamically significant stenosis on the side with the lower amplitude. Eikelboom cautions against using pulse amplitude criteria when OAPs can be obtained, since this reduces the test's overall sensitivity.[19]

Contraindications and Disadvantages

This technique cannot be performed on patients who have had eye surgery, retinal detachment, implants, glaucoma, and conjunctivitis; the examination is also more difficult (and sometimes impossible) in hypertensive patients because higher vacuum levels must be used.[19,25] Sometimes the patient's hypertension is too extreme to allow accurate measurement of the ophthalmic pressure. Blinking can cause artifacts, and some institutions perform the test twice, the second time with the eyelids closed.

Patients generally find the test unpleasant and uncomfortable; the temporary blacking-out of vision disturbs many people, and sometimes ecchymoses appear on the sclera after the test, which can alarm patients. Although a careful explanation of the likelihood and lack of permanence of these occurrences before the examination may ease the patient's concerns and ensure cooperation, some patients refuse the test or are unable to tolerate it.[22]

Comments

The published diagnostic criteria for OPG-G widely disagree; indeed, this has caused many investigators to publish their results comparing each of two or more of the available criteria.[17,22] The test does not discriminate between severe stenosis and total occlusion and for this reason is

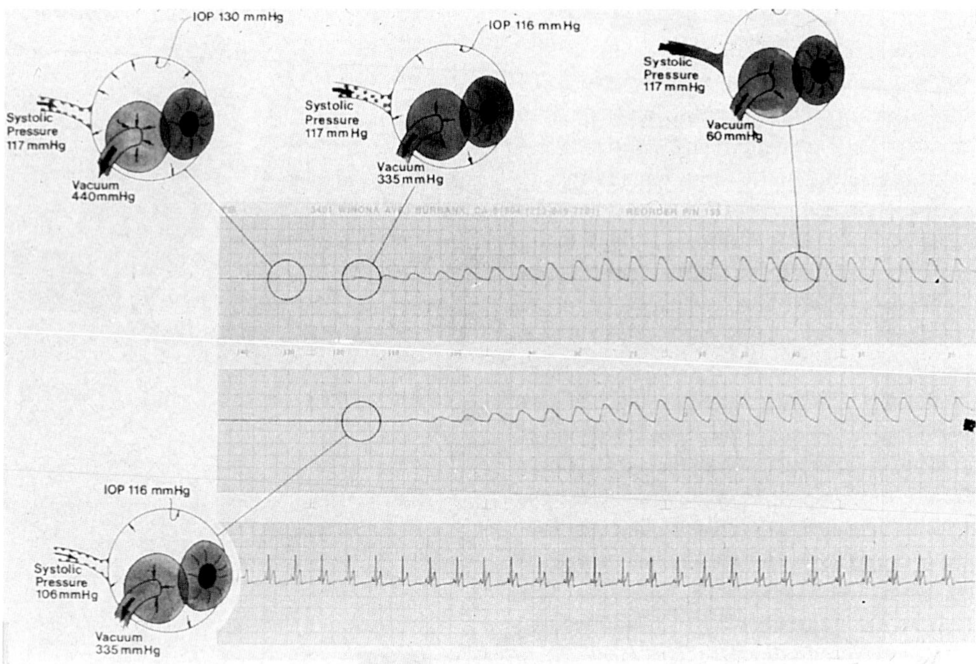

FIG. 22-119 Basic principle of ocular pneumoplethysmography and interpretation of the waveforms. This illustration shows how the pulse waveforms and ophthalmic artery flow correspond with progressive intraocular pressure decrease as the eye-cup vacuum is released. (Courtesy Electro-Diagnostic Instruments.)

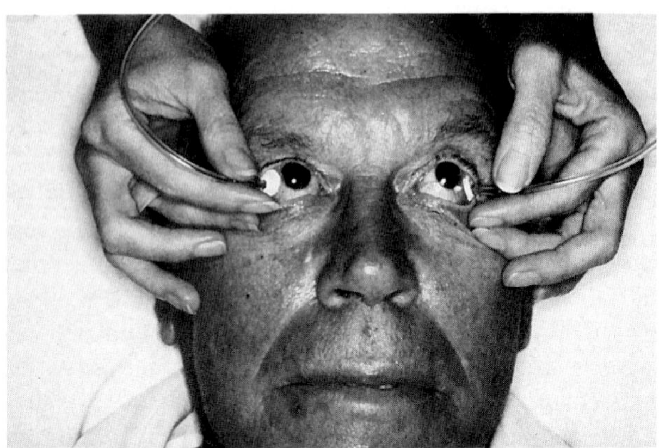

FIG. 22-120 Placement of the eyecups on the sclera for ocular pneumoplethysmography. (Courtesy Electro-Diagnostic Instruments.)

subject to the same pitfalls as the periorbital Doppler examination.

Although one recent prospective study proposes that OPG-G be used as a cost-effective screening study instead of duplex scanning for large asymptomatic populations (especially those without bruits), this is not acceptable practice and is not in line with the Essentials and Standards for ICAVL-accredited vascular laboratories.[18,22]

Although numerous clinical applications have been described for OPG, its primary application is still in the simple detection of hemodynamically significant extracranial carotid stenosis and collateralization.[17] As stated previously, OPG-G should not be used alone; if used, it should be in conjunction with a duplex evaluation.[18]

FINAL SUMMARY OF CEREBROVASCULAR TECHNIQUES

The techniques described in this chapter could be considered "venerable"; the main techniques have stood the test of time, have been beneficial, and have proved their diagnostic worth. It is unlikely that carotid duplex sonography will be an obsolete technology as a primary technique for some time, since technologic advances, such as MRA, involve expensive equipment and have yet to be made portable, inexpensive, and easily accessible to all institutions. The secondary techniques described are really supporting characters in that they may confirm or enhance a diagnosis but are seldom if ever used to initially diagnose the condition. The reader should be aware that becoming proficient in all the techniques within this chapter may not be a practical goal, but being familiar with the methods, what they show, and their benefits and limitations will enhance a technologist's or sonographer's ability to make the most of the data obtained.

Technologists or sonographers who perform one-dimensional studies seldom recognize problems other than obvi-

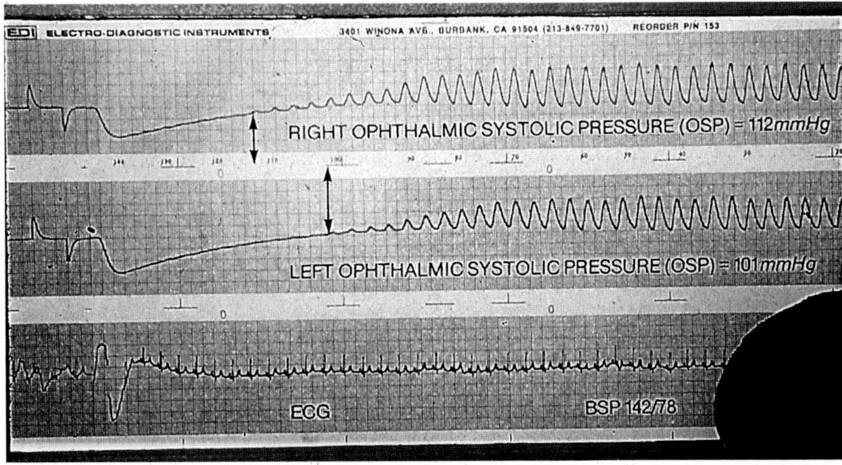

FIG. 22-121 An example of an OPG-G bilateral ocular waveform tracing. (Courtesy Electro-Diagnostic Instruments.)

ous carotid plaque. A technologist who is more well-rounded and familiar with other techniques and hemodynamic changes can confidently search for alternate findings when a duplex study of the carotids alone does not satisfactorily explain the hemodynamic or image results being obtained.

REVIEW QUESTIONS

1. List five symptoms associated with cerebral ischemia.
2. What are the differences between a transient ischemic attack, a cerebrovascular accident, and a resolving ischemic neurologic deficit?
3. Name three physical causes of cerebrovascular episodes that occur from the arterial system.
4. Which of the carotid arteries at the bifurcation supplies the brain? Which one normally has branches in the neck?
5. The vertebral arteries join what artery at the base of the skull?
6. List the arteries that make up the circle of Willis. Which one is a continuation of the internal carotid artery?
7. What is the primary hemodynamic importance of the circle of Willis?
8. Describe some potential cerebrovascular collateral pathways in unilateral internal carotid occlusion, basilar artery occlusion, and bilateral internal carotid occlusion.
9. What is a primary difference in the characteristics of the flow waveform in the cerebrovascular system compared to the extremities?
10. Describe two imaging features of the external carotid artery that distinguish it from the internal carotid artery.
11. Describe two ways to positively identify the external carotid artery by Doppler when it is otherwise indistinguishable from the internal carotid artery.
12. True or false—the presence of blue flow separation in an otherwise red-dominant color-flow image in the internal carotid origin is an abnormal finding.
13. Name the three scanning subplanes used in the longitudinal evaluation of the carotid artery.
14. True or false—the vertebral arteries cannot be identified and evaluated above the C-6 vertebra.
15. True or false—Doppler waveforms should be obtained from the common, internal, and external carotid arteries, and additional samples should be taken at and distal to any stenotic areas seen.
16. List three stages of atherosclerotic plaque morphology and how they appear with ultrasound imaging.
17. List two methods of obtaining percentage stenosis calculations. Which is more widely used? Why? Is it always accurate? Why or why not?
18. List two parameters measured on a Doppler spectral waveform that are used in diagnostic criteria. Draw a sample carotid waveform and illustrate where you would measure these parameters.
19. Why are frequency criteria less often used than velocity criteria? What range of angle correction is recommended by most of the criteria charts?
20. Convert the following frequency reading to velocity: 6 KHz with a 5-MHz Doppler transmit frequency at a 55-degree angle.
21. What three things happen to the flow-velocity waveform at a 50% to 60% degree of luminal reduction? What happens to the flow pressure in a distal arterial segment?
22. Where is the continuous-wave Doppler probe placed for the periorbital evaluation? Which artery or arteries should be monitored? What is the normal flow direction?

23. List the sites for manual compression in the periorbital examination.
24. What may happen to the artery waveform in question 22 when a severe internal carotid stenosis or occlusion is present? What happens to it when a collateral vessel is compressed?
25. Name the most common type of surgery performed on the carotid artery. Describe the sonographic, color flow, and Doppler waveform appearances in the artery after this type of surgery.
26. What is a patch angioplasty? Why is it performed?
27. Name two types of graft operation in the carotid arteries.
28. What are the mechanisms of restenosis that may occur after the surgery listed in question 25? Describe their sonographic appearance.
29. Who developed transcranial Doppler, and when was it first described?
30. Name the three different access windows to the cranium used in transcranial Doppler. List the arteries that can be accessed at each window site.
31. True or false—the anterior and posterior communicating arteries can always be detected in a normal patient.
32. Which velocity measurement is commonly used in transcranial Doppler and transcranial duplex imaging, peak systolic velocity or mean velocity? Why?
33. Name four conditions that can reliably be diagnosed or monitored with transcranial Doppler.
34. Describe the appearance of the TCD waveform in brain death.
35. List the access windows used in transcranial imaging and the arteries that can be evaluated in each.
36. What are the color-flow patterns likely to show in the circle of Willis regarding flow directions in a normal patient?
37. What are some advantages of three-dimensional transcranial Doppler scanning?
38. List the bony and soft-tissue landmarks that can be used to determine the proper insonation level in the axial and the oblique coronal planes in transcranial imaging.
39. What is a common cause of technical failure in transcranial Doppler and transcranial imaging? What factors influence this limitation? Which modality is affected most by this, TCD or TCI?
40. Name three nonsonographic methods used to indirectly evaluate carotid stenosis. Which ones are basically obsolete?
41. What is the basic principle behind ocular pneumoplethysmography? Describe the basic examination technique.
42. What parameters are used in OPG to obtain a diagnosis?
43. What are some contraindications to performing OPG?

REFERENCES

1. Aaslid R, Huber P, and Nornes H: A transcranial Doppler method in the evaluation of cerebrovascular spasm, Neuroradiology 28:11, 1986.
2. Aaslid R, Markwalder TM, and Nornes H: Noninvasive transcranial Doppler ultrasound recording of flow velocity in basal cerebral arteries, J Neurosurg 57:769, 1982.
3. Arnolds BJ and von Reutern G-M: Transcranial Dopplersonography [sic]. Examination technique and normal reference values, Ultrasound Med Biol 12:114, 1986.
4. Baker JD, Barker WF, and Machleder HI: Ocular pneumoplethysmography in the evaluation of carotid stenosis, Circulation 62(Suppl 1):11, 1980.
5. Baker WH and Hayes AC: Non-invasive laboratory evaluation: the Loyola experience. In Baker WH, editor: Diagnosis and treatment of carotid artery disease. Mount Kisco, 1979, Futura.
6. Barnes RW, Garrett WV, Slaymaker EE, Reinertson JE: Doppler ultrasound and supraorbital photoplethysmography for noninvasive screening of carotid occlusive disease, Am J Surg 134:183, 1977.
7. Barnes RW: Other noninvasive techniques in vascular disease. In Bernstein EF, editor: Noninvasive diagnostic techniques in vascular disease, ed 3. St. Louis, 1985, Mosby.
8. Barnes RW and Wilson MR: Doppler ultrasonic evaluation of cerebrovascular disease: a programmed instruction. Iowa City, 1975, University of Iowa Press.
9. Beach KW: The evaluation of velocity and frequency accuracy in ultrasound duplex scanners, J Vasc Techn 14:214, 1990.
10. Bluth EI, Stavros AT, Marich KW, et al: Carotid duplex sonography: a multicenter recommendation for standardized imaging and Doppler criteria, RadioGraphics 8:3, 1988.
11. Bogdahn U, Becker G, Winkler J, et al: Transcranial color-coded real-time sonography in adults, Stroke 21:1680, 1990.
12. Burger R, Barnes RW: Choice of ophthalmic artery branch for Doppler cerebrovascular examination: advantages of the frontal artery, Angiology 28:421, 1977.
13. Crew JR, Dean M, Johnson JM, et al: Carotid surgery without angiography, Am J Surg 148:217, 1984.
14. Daigle RJ, Stavros AT, and Lee RM: Overestimation of velocity and frequency values by multielement linear array Dopplers, J Vasc Techn 14:206, 1990.
15. DeWitt LD and Wechsler LR: Transcranial Doppler, Stroke 19:915, 1988.
16. Edelman RR, Mattle HP, O'Reilly GV, et al: Magnetic resonance imaging of flow dynamics in the circle of Willis, Stroke 21:56, 1990.
17. Eikelboom BC: Oculoplethysmography and ocular pneumoplethysmography. In Bernstein EF, editor: Vascular diagnosis, ed 4. St. Louis, 1993, Mosby.
18. Essentials and Standards for Noninvasive Vascular Testing. Vascular Laboratory Operations, Part II (Cerebrovascular Testing). Intersocietal Commission for the Accreditation of Vascular Laboratories. Rockville, Md, 1993.
19. Faught WE, Mattos MA, van Bemmelen PS, et al: Color-flow duplex scanning of carotid arteries: new velocity criteria based on ROC [receiver operator curve] analysis for threshold stenoses used in the symptomatic and asymptomatic carotid trials. Abstract from 17th Annual Meeting of the Midwestern Vascular Surgical Society. J Vasc Surg 18(3): 527-528, 1993.

20. Fell G, Phillips DJ, Chikos PM, et al: Ultrasonic duplex scanning for disease of the carotid artery, Circulation 64:1191, 1981.
21. Fields WS: Aortocranial occlusive vascular disease (stroke), Clin Symp 26:3, 1974.
22. Fisher FS, Riles TS, Oldford F, et al: Is ocular pneumoplethysmography (Gee) a cost effective screening test for asymptomatic carotid occlusive disease? J Vasc Technol 17:135, 1993.
23. Fronek A: Oculoplethysmography and carotid phonoangiography. In Bernstein EF, editor: Noninvasive diagnostic techniques in vascular disease, ed 3. St. Louis, 1985, Mosby.
24. Fujioka KA, Gates DT, and Spencer MP: A comparison of transcranial color Doppler imaging and standard static pulsed wave Doppler in the assessment of intracranial hemodynamics. Presented at the 16th Annual Conference, Society of Vascular Technologists. Washington, DC, June 2-6, 1993.
25. Gerlach AJ, Giyanani VL, and Krebs C: Applications of noninvasive vascular techniques, pp. 73-74, Philadelphia, 1988, WB Saunders.
26. Halsey JH: Prognosis of acute hemiplegia estimated by transcranial Doppler sonography, Stroke 19:648, 1988.
27. Hashimoto BE and Hattrick CW: New method of adult transcranial Doppler, J Ultrasound Med 10:349, 1991.
28. Hassler W, Steinmetz H, Pirshel J: Transcranial Doppler study of intracranial circulatory arrest, J Neurosurg 71:195, 1989.
29. Higashida RT, Tsai FY, Halbach VV, et al: Percutaneous transluminal angioplasty of the subclavian, vertebral, and basilar arteries: technical considerations, Neuroradiology 33 (Suppl):394, 1991.
30. Hobson RW, Weiss DG, et al: Efficacy of carotid endarterectomy for asymptomatic carotid stenosis, N Engl J Med 328:221, 1993.
31. Hunink MGM, Polak JF, Barlan MM, O'Leary DH: Detection and quantification of carotid artery stenosis: efficacy of various Doppler velocity parameters, Am J Roentgenol 160:619, 1993.
32. Liebman PR and Barnes RW: Complications of vascular surgery and trauma. In Greenfield LJ, editor: Complications in surgery and trauma, pp. 353-369. Philadelphia; 1984, JB Lippincott.
33. Lindegaard K-F, Grolimund P, Aaslid R, Nornes H: Evaluation of cerebral AVM's using transcranial Doppler ultrasound, J Neurosurg 65:335, 1986.
34. Mattle H, Grolimund P, et al: Transcranial Doppler sonographic findings in middle cerebral artery disease, Arch Neurol 45:289, 1988.
35. McDonald PT, Rich NM, Collins GJ Jr, et al: Ocular pneumoplethysmography: detection of carotid occlusive disease, Ann Surg 189:44, 1979.
36. Moneta GL, Edwards JM, Chitwood RW, et al: Correlation of North American Symptomatic Endarterectomy Trial angiographic definition of 70 to 99% internal carotid artery stenosis with duplex scanning, J Vasc Surg 17:152, 1993.
37. Netter FH: Ciba collection of medical illustrations, Vol 1, Nervous System. Summit, NJ, 1953 Medical Education Division, Ciba Pharmaceutical.
38. O'Hara PJ, Brewster DC, Darling RC, Hallett JW Jr: Oculopneumoplethysmography—its relationship to intraoperative cerebrovascular hemodynamics, Arch Surg 115:1156, 1980.
39. Padayachee TS, Gosling RG, Bishop CC, et al: Monitoring middle cerebral artery blood velocity during carotid endarterectomy, Br J Surg 73:98, 1986.
40. Padayachee TS, Parsons S, Theobold R, et al: The detection of microemboli in the middle cerebral artery during cardiopulmonary bypass: a transcranial Doppler ultrasound investigation using membrane and bubble oxygenators, Ann Thorac Surg 44:298, 1987.
41. Ries F: Three-dimensional transcranial Doppler scanning. In Bernstein EF, editor: Vascular diagnosis, ed 4. St. Louis, 1993, Mosby.
42. Schneider PA, Ringelstein EB, Rossman ME, et al: Importance of cerebral collateral pathways during carotid endarterectomy, Stroke 19:1328, 1988.
43. Schöning M and Walter J: Evaluation of the vertebrobasilar-posterior system by transcranial color duplex sonography in adults, Stroke 23:1280, 1992.
44. Seiler RW and Aaslid R: Transcranial Doppler for evaluation of cerebral vasospasm. In Aaslid R, editor: Transcranial Doppler sonography, pp. 118-131. Vienna; 1986, Springer-Verlag.
45. Spencer MP, Thomas GI, Nicholls SC, Sauvage LR: Detection of middle cerebral artery emboli during carotid endarterectomy using transcranial Doppler ultrasound, Stroke 21:415, 1990.
46. Thiele BL: Standards in non-invasive cerebrovascular testing. In Bernstein EF, editor: Recent advances in non-invasive diagnostic techniques in vascular disease. St Louis, 1990, Mosby.
47. Thiele BL and Strandness DE: Accuracy of angiographic quantification of peripheral atherosclerosis, Prog Cardiovasc Dis 26:223, 1983.
48. Trattnig S, Schwaighofer B, Hubsch P, et al: Color-coded Doppler sonography of vertebral arteries. J Ultrasound Med 10:221, 1991.
49. Tsai FY, Higashida RT, Matovich V, et al: Seven years experience with PTA of the carotid artery. Neroradiology 33(suppl):397-398, 1991.
50. Zierler RE: Basic and practical aspects of cerebrovascular testing. In Bernstein EF, editor: Vascular diagnosis, ed 4. St. Louis, 1993, Mosby.
51. Zweibel WJ: Analysis of carotid Doppler signals. In Zweibel WJ, editor: Introduction to vascular ultrasonography, ed 2. Orlando, Fla: Grune & Stratton.

BIBLIOGRAPHY

Bishop CCR, Powell S, Rutt D, Browse NL: Transcranial Doppler assessment of middle cerebral artery blood flow: a validation study, Stroke 17:913, 1986.

Caplan L and Committee: Assessment: transcramial Doppler. Report of the Therapeutics and Technology Assessment Subcommittee, Amercian Academy of Neurology. Position statement. American Academy of Neurology, 1989.

Feinberg WM, Devine J, Ledbetter E, et al: Clinical characteristics of patients with inadequate temporal windows. Presented at the 4th International Symposium on Intracranial Hemodynamics, Orlando, Fl, February 11-14, 1990.

Fujioka KF, Kuehn K, Sola-Pierce N, Spencer MP: Transcranial pulsed Doppler for evaluation of cerebral arterial hemodynamics, J Vasc Technol 13:95, 1989.

CHAPTER

23

Organization and Quality Assurance in the Vascular Laboratory

Richard E. Rae

VASCULAR LABORATORY ACCREDITATION

The average person would be astonished at the diversity of techniques and varying levels of expertise among the thousands of vascular laboratories in North America. Although noninvasive vascular studies should preferably be performed by qualified and experienced vascular technologists, they are very often done by office secretaries, nurses, general sonographers, respiratory therapists, ECG technicians, and radiologic technologists, among others. Many have thorough experience but others have only limited exposure (e.g., a short 3-day training course). Studies should be interpreted and supervised by trained physicians with continuing education in vascular technology; in reality the final reports are often interpreted by a huge range of individuals—vascular technologists, sonographers, chiropractors, podiatrists, neurologists, vascular surgeons, cardiologists, radiologists, and general surgeons. These individuals may or may not have the qualifications and experience to accurately diagnose the conditions being described by the study. Examinations are performed not only in hospital-based laboratories but in offices, mobile units, and nursing homes.

It goes without saying that there is potential for abuse in this system. In the past, no universal regulatory standard was in effect to certify that a vascular laboratory and its personnel were duly qualified to perform these studies, and almost anyone who knew the proper Current Procedural Technology codes (CPT codes) and International Classification of Diseases (ICD) diagnosis codes could file for insurance reimbursement. The definitions of the various noninvasive tests in the CPT do not always distinguish between simple and complex evaluations, and the Health Care Finance Administration (HCFA) became acutely aware of Medicare and insurance fraud perpetrated by the unscrupulous. The threat of government regulation of vascular laboratories and more frequent insurance denials of claims for noninvasive tests loomed on the horizon.

Fortunately, the profession recognized this danger and realized that a universal standard for certifying vascular laboratories was needed, just as the American Registry of Diagnostic Medical Sonographers (ARDMS) addressed the need for setting standards for voluntary certification of sonographers and vascular technologists. In 1990 the Intersocietal Commission for the Accreditation of Vascular Laboratories (ICAVL) was formed as a nonprofit coalition representing sponsoring medical professional organizations who universally support or use noninvasive diagnostic vascular testing. As of 1994, 11 professional organizations representing the specialties of neurology, neurosurgery, cardiology, radiology, vascular surgery, vascular research, sonography, and vascular technology had two members each on the ICAVL board of directors.

The ICAVL publishes a uniform set of essentials and standards that outlines required equipment and sets standards for noninvasive vascular testing. Part I (Organization) establishes basic standards regarding physical facilities, infection and safety procedures, physician and personnel certification, and support services;[2] Part II covers equipment capabilities and requirements, appropriate indications for testing, testing protocols, diagnostic criteria, and quality assurance for cerebrovascular, arterial, venous, and visceral vascular testing[3-6] (Fig. 23-1).

In addition to establishing these essentials and standards, the ICAVL provides a mechanism by which a vascular laboratory can apply for accreditation of the laboratory and certification that it is in substantial compliance with the published essentials and standards. Laboratories interested in obtaining accreditation document their facility's compliance by completing a self-study document (Fig. 23-2). Applicants supply records documenting all aspects of their laboratory, including personnel certification, procedure volumes, equipment maintenance, technical procedures, examples of studies performed, and quality assurance statistics, among other items. If accreditation is granted by the ICAVL, it is in effect for a 3-year period. Some applicants' applications may not initially provide a complete enough picture of their laboratory's compliance, and the laboratory site may be visited by ICAVL representatives to collect additional data regarding their application. Some laboratory sites are also randomly visited to ensure that they are continuing to comply with the essentials and standards. At the time of writing, accreditation is voluntary, but the Health

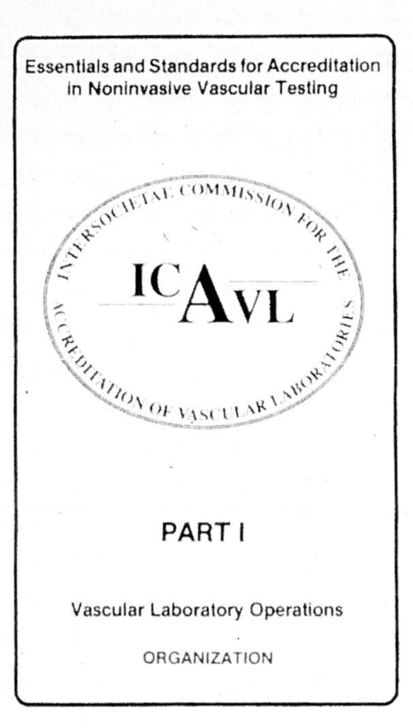

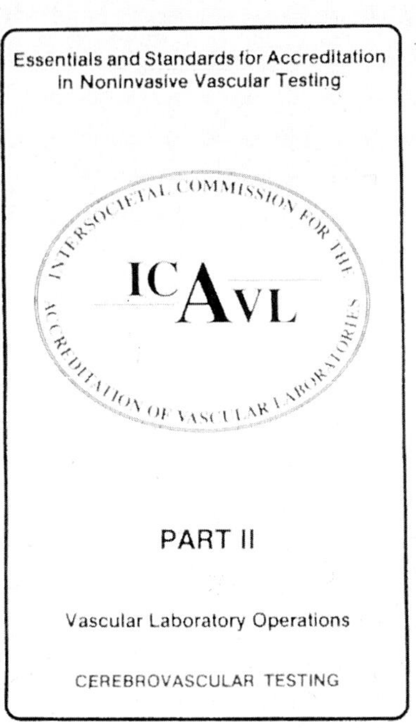

FIG. 23-1 The essentials and standards booklets as published by the Intersocietal Commission for the Accreditation of Vascular Laboratories. Part I deals with the laboratory's organization *(left)*, Part II with the essential equipment and techniques for a vascular specialty *(right)*.

Care Finance Administration (HCFA) has been monitoring the number of accredited laboratories and following the progress of the ICAVL. HCFA and insurance carrier medical directors have stated that vascular laboratory accreditation will be required for reimbursement as soon as this is practicable.

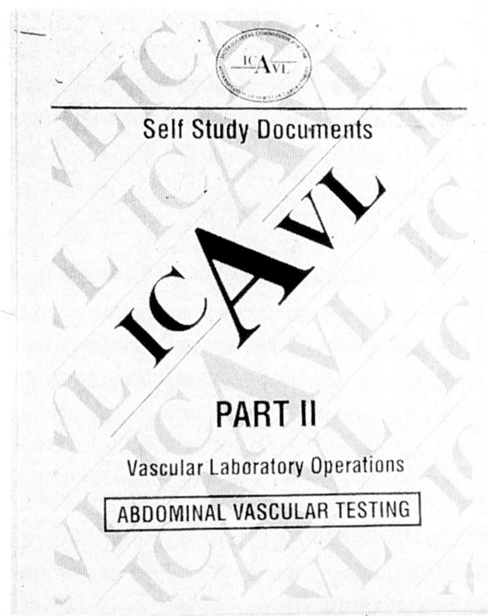

FIG. 23-2 An example of an ICAVL self-study binder with questions and space for submitting the required documentation when applying for accreditation.

VASCULAR LABORATORY ORGANIZATION

The following discussion is not intended to replace the ICAVL essentials and standards but to make the reader aware of some basic personnel and equipment requirements that a vascular laboratory needs for efficient operation.

The laboratory should have a qualified medical director, who must be a physician (MD or DO) and who should have documented experience in working with noninvasive vascular testing modalities. Over 200 physicians, noting the lack of a vascular technology certifying process specific to physicians, have taken the vascular technology certifying examination offered by the American Registry of Diagnostic Medical Sonographers, which indicates their support of the process and their recognition of the credential's high standards. Medical directors typically administer and supervise the laboratory's operations but may delegate day-by-day tasks to a designated technical director.[2]

A laboratory's technical director should preferably be a Registered Vascular Technologist, Registered Diagnostic Medical Sonographer, or Registered Diagnostic Cardiac Sonographer with significant clinical experience in vascular testing. Technical directors often deal with supervision, scheduling, and administrative tasks in addition to performing studies.[2]

Qualified medical and technical staff should have substantial documented experience or training. Staff members may have to meet minimum standards for interpreting studies that may be set by the laboratory's medical director before routinely evaluating studies. Technical staff also may be required to meet minimum proficiency standards.[2] Adequate clerical support should be provided with the goal of rapid and efficient availability of final reports on the examination, and adequate storage space should be available so that records (files, tapes, disks, and images) can be stored for the time required by law (usually 5 years or more).[2]

Equipment maintenance policies, including electrical, safety, and phantom calibration checks or manufacturer service contracts, should be in place. Patient safety, infection control, blood-borne transmission, and transducer cleaning policies that meet OSHA standards should also be implemented. Qualified nursing and CPR-certified personnel should be available, as well as emergency drugs and equipment if the situation requires them.[2] The facilities should provide enough room for efficient transport of patients in and out, and for the technologist to work comfortably; patient comfort should be a primary concern.

QUALITY ASSURANCE AND VASCULAR STATISTICS

Vascular testing procedures in a given laboratory may be based on widely published techniques. Results may be interpreted following guidelines and tables published by widely accepted authorities. It is impossible, however, for every technique or criterion to deliver foolproof results. Many radiologists do not routinely use calipers when measuring angiographic stenoses; they usually make a visual estimation, and there is often a great deal of variability between one interpreter and another.[10] The same variability can be found among physicians interpreting a noninvasive study, since both image and flow data must be used together to obtain a valid diagnostic result and one parameter may be underestimated or overestimated. What works for one laboratory may not work for another, and although many of the techniques and diagnostic methods described here can be universally applied, the only way to discern their efficacy is to perform internal validation and routine quality assurance. Quality-assurance programs are considered vital to the function of a vascular laboratory, and ICAVL essentials and standards require that they be in place in laboratories applying for vascular laboratory accreditation.[3-6]

To this end, every institution performing noninvasive vascular testing should maintain a running record of patients, using a logbook or computer data base. It is extremely important to keep track of the patients seen in the laboratory and of the tests performed on them, since valuable information can be obtained from these records regarding the laboratory's volume, physician referral patterns, utilization, technical throughput, and periodic statistics, among other items. Although logbooks are inexpensive, they can also be very difficult and tedious to work with when specific totals of patients are required, correlation data are entered or retrieved, or other numeric data is requested. A computerized data base is one of the most beneficial tools a laboratory can acquire. Although numerous vascular laboratory–specific data-base and quality-control products are available, they are all expensive and tend to be inflexible; a laboratory can easily program or create a data base itself using commonly available commercial data-base programs that can be obtained off the shelf from computer stores or mail-order houses. There are data-base creation programs for all makes and models of personal computers, and one can develop a data base easily for under $2000 (including the computer). An example of a data-base template that the reader can use as a basis for creating his or her own data base is shown in Fig. 23-3. This template also provides fields for entering correlation data.

Data should be entered into the data base either when the patient's examination is complete or during some set time at the end of the day. Before the patient's records are filed away, a designated technologist should call up the patient's data-base record and enter the results of the test (abbreviations or shorthand is helpful). As correlating angiograms or reports are received, a designated individual should look up any patients who had a noninvasive test before the angiogram, and these results should also be entered.

Information on the results of noninvasive tests should be regularly correlated or compared with any or all angiographic or surgical pathology reports available. Laboratory personnel may need to establish some mechanism so that copies of these angiographic reports can be obtained. If the vascular laboratory is part of a hospital, agreements can easily be reached with radiology and pathology departments so that these copies can be forwarded. Lists can be given to medical records personnel for cross-reference and subsequent copying, or copies of all angiogram reports can be sent to the vascular laboratory and then the data base or logbook can be referenced accordingly. It cannot be overemphasized that using a computerized data base can make this task much easier and deliver results much faster than page-by-page searches of logbooks. If the laboratory is private or part of a physician's office, correlation can be obtained through agreements with referring physicians or hospitals or by analyzing and copying needed reports from office medical records.

Correlating results involves comparing the findings from the noninvasive test against the findings of an accepted "gold standard" (usually arteriography or surgical comparison). For some cases, such as Doppler-extremity results, this can simply involve comparing tests as "normal or abnormal." For others with multicategory criteria, such as cerebrovascular studies, the comparisons must be broken down into individual categories and compared accordingly. For carotid stenosis, the individual analyzing the reports can assign estimated stenoses on arteriograms to the same categories used to record carotid stenosis by the duplex study. For example, a duplex study is reported as having a "50% stenosis in the left ICA, grade HII (20% to 59%)." An arteriogram on this patient reports "approximately 40% stenosis in the left ICA." The reviewer sees that this arteriographic measurement corresponds to a grade HII stenosis using the duplex criteria and then can enter a shorthand comparison into the log or data base ("Duplex—HII; Arteriogram—HII"). This method simplifies comparison when statistics are being calculated.

PT NUMBER ••••• PT NAME •••••••••••••••••••••••••••••••• COUNTER •
AGE ••• SEX • DATE OF EXAM ••-••-••
REFERRING MD ••••••••••••••••••••••••••••••••• LAB MD •

EXAM 1 ••••• EXAM 2 ••••• EXAM 3 ••••• EXAM 4 ••••• EXAM 5 •••••

A

PLAQUE MORPHOLOGY- RIGHT	••	PLAQUE MORPHOLOGY- LEFT	••	TECHNOLOGIST •••
PLAQUE SURFACE- RIGHT	••	PLAQUE SURFACE- LEFT	••	TAPE NO. •••••
% STENOSIS-RICA-DUPLEX	•••	% STENOSIS-LICA-DUPLEX	•••	
% STENOSIS-RICA-ARTGM	•••	% STENOSIS-LICA-ARTGM	•••	POST-OP •

VENOUS: THROMBOSIS: RIGHT • LEFT • LOCATION: RIGHT ••• LEFT •••
CHRONIC: RIGHT • LEFT • ACUTE: RIGHT • LEFT •

LEA- R • LEA- L •

CAROTID ARTGM	•	POS •	NEG •	AGREES W/CVD	•
ARTERIOGRAM	•	POS •	NEG •	AGREES W/DOPPLER	•
VENOGRAM	•	POS •	NEG •	AGREES W/DUPLEX	•
SURGERY	•	POS •	NEG •	AGREES W/TEST	•

R. Rae

PT NUMBER **07231** PT NAME **DOE, JOHN D.** ••••••••••••••••••• COUNTER **1**
AGE **57** SEX **M** DATE OF EXAM **03-25-95**
REFERRING MD **CUTTER/RÖNTGEN/HERTZ**••••••••••• LAB MD **1**

EXAM 1 **CVD** EXAM 2 **LEA** EXAM 3 **LEVDS** EXAM 4 ••••• EXAM 5 •••••

B

PLAQUE MORPHOLOGY- RIGHT	**P1**	PLAQUE MORPHOLOGY- LEFT	**P2**	TECHNOLOGIST **RER**
PLAQUE SURFACE- RIGHT	**S1**	PLAQUE SURFACE- LEFT	**S2**	TAPE NO. **00231**
% STENOSIS-RICA-DUPLEX	**H1**	% STENOSIS-LICA-DUPLEX	**H4**	
% STENOSIS-RICA-ARTGM	**H1**	% STENOSIS-LICA-ARTGM	**H4**	POST-OP **1**

VENOUS: THROMBOSIS: RIGHT **1** LEFT **0** LOCATION: RIGHT **CFV** LEFT •••
CHRONIC: RIGHT **0** LEFT • ACUTE: RIGHT **1** LEFT •

LEA- R **N** LEA- L **A**

CAROTID ARTGM	**1**	POS **1**	NEG •	AGREES W/CVD	**Y**
ARTERIOGRAM	**1**	POS **1**	NEG •	AGREES W/DOPPLER	**Y**
VENOGRAM	**1**	POS •	NEG **1**	AGREES W/DUPLEX	**N**
SURGERY	•	POS •	NEG •	AGREES W/TEST	•

R. Rae

FIG. 23-3 A, An example of a data-base template for vascular laboratory quality control, which can be created or modified using any commercial data-base software program. All the fields are alphanumeric (letters and numbers only). **B,** The same template as in **A,** now filled in with example data. The data is entered using a simple format, which permits easy searching and comparison by one or more categories. Carotid duplex and arteriographic data are entered using categories that are described in detail in Chapter 22.

Two methods are commonly used to display comparative information and obtain statistics in vascular laboratories—the 2 × 2 table and the multiple-category table. Numerous examples using these methods can be found in scientific papers and articles.

THE 2 × 2 TABLE

One method is to enter the data in a 2 × 2 table, which is acceptable if a normal-abnormal comparison is to be made between one standard and one test. The reviewer should first obtain a listing of all laboratory patients who have had a correlating angiogram during the period being evaluated. The reviewer should next sort through these patients, finding and totalling all the positive (abnormal) studies where both the noninvasive test and the angiogram agreed, then finding and totaling all the negative (normal) studies where both the noninvasive test and the angiogram agreed. These figures indicate the numbers of true-positive and true-negative studies, respectively. It is, of course, up to the laboratory medical and technical staff to determine the breakpoint for what constitutes "normal" and "abnormal" (e.g., ample indices of >.85, hemodynamically significant lesions >60%, etc.).

Next, the reviewer should sort out and total the cases where the noninvasive test was positive and the angiogram was negative, then find and total the cases where the noninvasive test was negative and the angiogram was positive. These two totals represent the numbers of false-positive and false-negative studies, respectively.

Once these four totals have been obtained (true- and false-positive, true- and false-negative), they can be entered into the table. There are many different ways of arranging the data in a 2 × 2 table; the method described here is one of the most common.[7]

First, draw the table as illustrated in Fig. 23-4.

1. Label the horizontal (X) axis across the top with the name of the standard (e.g., arteriogram, venogram). Place a plus sign (+) over the left box and a minus sign (−) over the right box.
2. Label the vertical (Y) axis along the left side with the name of the test you are comparing (e.g., lower-extremity Doppler, venous duplex). Place a plus sign (+) next to the top left box and a minus sign (−) next to the lower-left box.

To enter the data,

1. Place the number of true-positive studies in the upper-left box.
2. Place the number of true-negative studies in the lower-right box.
3. Place the number of false-positive studies in the upper-right box.
4. Place the number of false-negative studies in the lower-left box.
5. Total the left column from top to bottom (along the Y axis). Write this number beneath it. This is the total number of tests that were positive by the standard.
6. Total the right column from top to bottom (along the Y axis). Write this number beneath it. This is the total number of tests that were negative by the standard.
7. Total the top row from left to right (along the X axis). Write this number on the right upper side of the matrix. This is the total number of tests that were positive by the noninvasive test.
8. Total the bottom row from left to right (along the X axis). Write this number on the right lower side of the matrix. This is the total number of tests that were negative by the noninvasive test.
9. Add the numbers across the bottom (along the X axis) of the matrix. This is the total number of studies evaluated by the standard.
10. Add the numbers along the right side (along the Y axis) of the matrix. This is the total number of studies evaluated by the noninvasive test.
11. These two totals (9 and 10 above) should be identical. Write this number in the lower right corner outside of the matrix. This is the total number of tests evaluated for the statistical period chosen. Fig. 23-5 is an example of a completed table.

Now that the table has been created and filled in, the reviewer is ready to calculate some standard vascular percentage values that enable the following accuracy calculations to be made:[7,8]

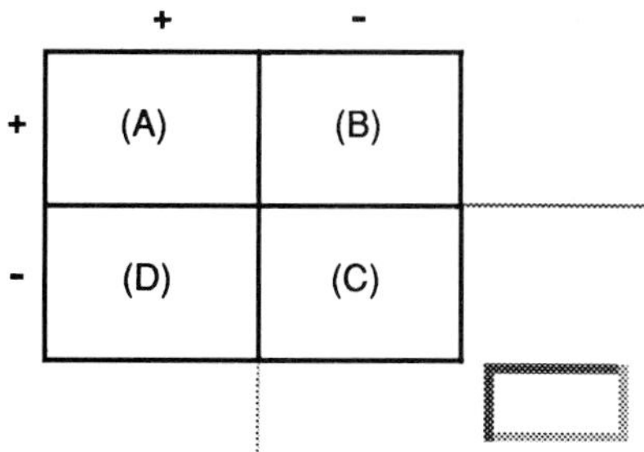

FIG. 23-4 Initial layout of the 2 × 2 table. A, B, C, and D correspond to true-positives, false-positives, true-negatives, and false-negatives.

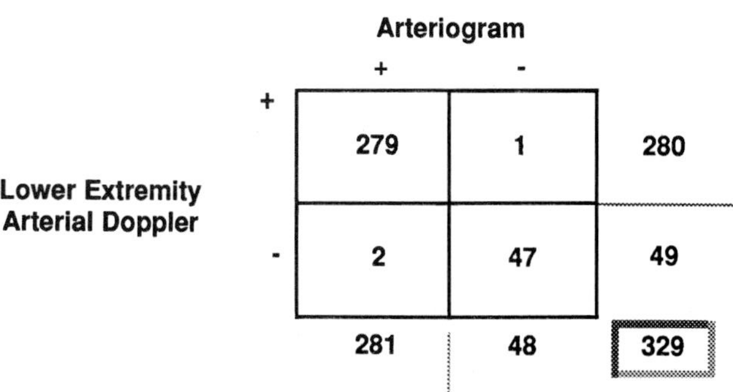

FIG. 23-5 A completed 2 × 2 table with all true and false positive and negative data entered and totaled.

Sensitivity—this is the ability of the test to actually detect a disease process—in other words, how well it can show an abnormality.

Specificity—this is the ability of the test to declare a vessel to be normal, or without disease—in other words, how well it can detect normal vessels.

Note that since vessels can only be in one group and not the other (either sensitivity or specificity), there is no mathematical relation between them. A high degree of sensitivity can be associated with any value of specificity and vice versa.[7]

Positive predictive value—this is the percentage of studies in the group that are abnormal by both the noninvasive test and the standard.

Negative predictive value—this is the percentage of studies in the group that are normal by both the noninvasive test and the standard.

Overall accuracy—this is the percentage of all the studies in the group that were correctly predicted by the test compared with the standard.

These values are calculated by the following fairly simple formulas:[8]

In these examples,

A = True-positives, B = False-positives, C = False-negatives, D = True-negatives

$$\text{Sensitivity} = \frac{A}{A + C}$$

$$\text{Specificity} = \frac{D}{B + D}$$

$$\text{Positive predictive value (PPV)} = \frac{A}{A + B}$$

$$\text{Negative predictive value (NPV)} = \frac{D}{C + D}$$

$$\text{Overall accuracy} = \frac{A + D}{A + B + C + D}$$

Fig. 23-7, p. 712, is an example of a 2 × 2 table with these statistical calculations performed. As an exercise the reader might recalculate the statistical indices in this figure using the data in the table example and the formulas above and see if the same results are obtained.

MULTIPLE-CATEGORY TABLES

Statistical analysis often requires a specific categorization of data, especially when there are many "degrees of abnormality," such as in cerebrovascular duplex examinations. A matrix table should then be used that reflects the number of diagnostic classification categories for both the test and the standard.

Since there are often many accepted criteria for carotid interpretation (see Chapter 22), the number of categories in the table may vary widely from institution to institution. The following examples are based on a 5 × 5 table, but the theory and methods can be used regardless of the number of categories.

A laboratory using a modified version of the Bluth, Wetzner Marich, et al. criteria[1] will have five categories, here also designated by the notational standard for reporting cerebrovascular noninvasive procedures recommended by the Society of Vascular Surgeons/International Society of Cardiovascular Surgeons Joint Commission:[9]

HI 0% to 19%
HII 20% to 59%
HIII 60% to 79%
HIV 80% to 99%
HV 100% (Occluded)

The procedure for creating this form of table is somewhat more complex than that for the 2 × 2 format. Please refer to the example in Fig. 23-6 for clarification of the following descriptions:

1. Draw a matrix table with five categories across and five categories down; there should be 25 boxes for data.
2. Label each column with one category from HI to HV (or with the numeric ranges) along the X axis horizontally. Label this axis with the name of the standard.
3. Label each row with one category from HI to HV (or with the numeric ranges) down the Y axis vertically. Label this axis with the name of the test.

   The reviewer analyzes the correlation results in the data base or logbook and then determines totals for each intersection of the matrix; for example, a reviewer finds eight vessels that were HI by both test and standard, five vessels that were HIV by the test but that were classed as HIII by the standard, two vessels that were HII by the test but HIII by the standard, and so on. Note that these numbers usually apply to one side or one vessel, and bilateral studies should not be averaged together. The test's accuracy at detecting disease is being evaluated and one can expect a total of twice as many in a sample group as there were examinations (unless there were some unilateral studies).
4. Once the totals for each cross-referenced category are

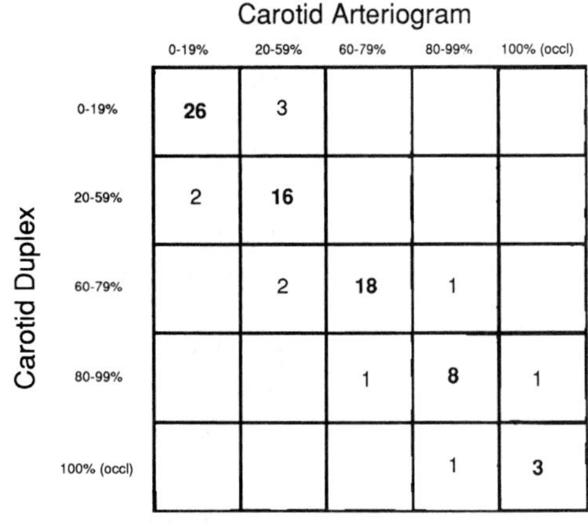

FIG. 23-6 An example of a complete 5 × 5 format table. True agreement is indicated by the diagonal axis, and examination totals and percentage agreement calculations are displayed.

obtained, the reviewer should plot these totals in the appropriate boxes on the matrix.

Once these figures are plotted, the reviewer can perform the statistical calculations.

In this format, there are the following three statistics to obtain:

Exact Correlation—this is the total number of studies in the group where the test and the standard completely agreed.

Total Examinations—this is the total number of all examinations in the study group.

Percentage Agreement—this corresponds to the overall accuracy statistic and indicates the percentage of the test study group that exactly agreed with the standard.

The following list describes how to obtain these figures:

1. Add the numbers on the main diagonal of the matrix (upper left to lower right corner). The total of these numbers gives the exact correlation figure (EC).
2. Add all the numbers in all the boxes in the matrix. This gives the total number of examinations in the study group (TE).
3. Obtain the percentage agreement by dividing the exact correlation figure by the total examination:

$$\text{Percentage agreement} = \frac{\text{EC}}{\text{TE}}$$

The total number of examinations in each category can optionally be obtained by totaling the boxes in each row and again in each column, placing the totals below the column as in the 2 × 2 table. A completed example of a 5 × 5 table with calculated statistics is shown in Fig. 23-6.

Although this method does not yield a measurement of sensitivity and specificity, the percentage-agreement statistic and the matrix data give the reviewer a very good estimate of how well the test predicted the findings compared with the standard.

INTERPRETATION OF STATISTICS

The statistics described are obtained as part of a quality-assurance program to satisfy the following needs:

1. Technologists and other laboratory staff are interested in knowing how well they are performing the tests and how accurate they are in detecting different levels of disease.
2. Physicians need to know if indeed their patient has a significant condition when the test indicates a positive result.

Although it is possible for a test to have 100% overall accuracy or 100% sensitivity and specificity, this is very rare in reality. When it occurs, it is often because a series of tests being analyzed has very low numbers or some bias has crept into the classification. By the same token, a test cannot be necessarily considered invalid if its accuracy or sensitivity appear low by a laboratory's analysis.

Once the data have been obtained and the results and statistics calculated, the reviewer should go back and analyze the specific cases that were classed as false-positive or false-negative. The reviewer needs to retrieve the reports and images from those tests and then obtain the results and films of the correlating standards that were the basis of the comparison. By doing this, it is possible to determine where errors in technique or interpretation occurred, and solutions can be proposed to help avoid similar future occurrences. On review, irregularities may also be found that caused an otherwise accurate study to have been incorrectly correlated as a false-positive or false-negative study. These irregularities can be as simple as typographic errors or as complex as misinterpretation of either the test findings or the arteriographic measurements. It is important to recognize that a "gold standard" is often only as accurate as the physician who has interpreted it. The reviewer also should never assume that the test or technique is always faulty and that the standard is always right. Arteriograms and Digital Subtraction Angiograms studies are periodically mislabeled or inverted, resulting in inaccurate or transposed interpretations. Physicians sometimes misinterpret the results; occasionally the wrong set of films has been read; problems often can be traced to unclear or garbled dictation or problems with the transcriptionist. All of these errors can potentially affect the outcome of the quality-assurance report and how it is perceived by laboratory personnel and administration. These potential sources of error emphasize the need for an intensive review of all aspects of discrepant studies. The following are some items a reviewer should keep in mind when evaluating false-positive or false-negative studies:

1. All aspects of the test should be reviewed; the final report, worksheets, images, videotapes, and waveforms. Proofread the final report to rule out typographic errors or misquoted numeric data. Check for any irregularities in technique, such as in angle correction, mistakenly identified vessels, inverted color-flow assignments, and equipment settings. Check to see if the physician departed from the diagnostic criteria used in the laboratory, or if overestimation or underestimation of stenoses or disease occurred.
2. All aspects of the arteriogram or standard should be examined. The films should be examined for any misleading shadows or views where the disease might not be clearly identified. Possible mislabeling should be checked. Calipers should be used to accurately measure diameter stenosis rather than by relying on an "eyeball estimation." Filling problems resulting from errors in technique should be identified if possible. Reports should be proofread and checked for accuracy.

IMPLEMENTING A QUALITY ASSURANCE PROGRAM

Quality assurance reports using the above methods should be compiled regularly. Statistical reviews should be performed quarterly, with an additional annual review; the latter review tends to pick up those studies that escaped initial correlation because of late or delayed reports.

Once the tabulated and calculated statistical report is ready, copies should be distributed to all vascular laboratory personnel. A meeting should be held to discuss the results with all those involved, including the medical director, technical director, laboratory staff physicians, and all staff technologists. If feasible, a round-table discussion and review of all discrepancies and discrepant studies can be performed as well. A sample quality-assurance report combining features of all the described topics is shown in Fig. 23-7.

In summary, a basic quality assurance program can be initially developed using the following guidelines:

1. Establish a computerized data base or logbook to keep track of all patients seen and all tests performed.
2. Enter abbreviated or shorthand results of the patient's tests into the data base or logbook before filing the laboratory chart.
3. Obtain any arteriographic or angiographic reports applicable to any patients in the data base whenever possible. Enter abbreviated or shorthand results of these studies into the data base or logbook and file the report with the patient's chart. Note that these results should be correlated only if done within 3 months of the test, and only if no surgical intervention occurred between the noninvasive test and the performance of the angiogram.
4. Every quarter, search through the data base or logbook and sort out all the patients who have had correlating angiographic studies within the last 3-month period. (Depending on the laboratory's volume, this may be done less frequently, perhaps every 6 months.)
5. Decide on the statistical format to use, then sort the findings into either correlating diagnostic categories or into groups of true-positives, false-positives, true-negatives, and false-negatives.
6. Enter the data into the table chosen and then calculate

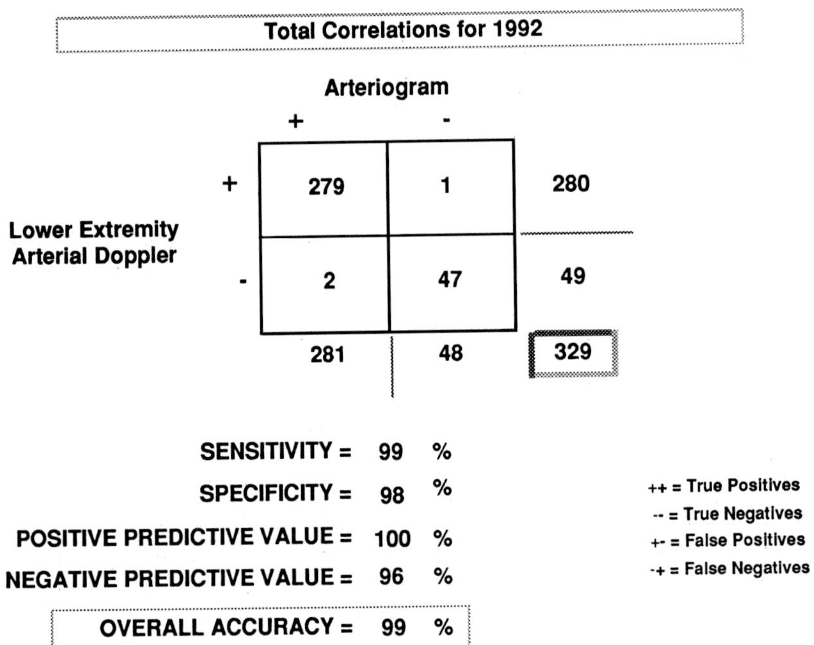

Total Correlations for 1992
Arteriogram
+
-
Lower Extremity
Arterial Doppler
+
279
1
280
-
2
47
49
281
48
329
SENSITIVITY = 99 %
SPECIFICITY = 98 %
POSITIVE PREDICTIVE VALUE = 100 %
NEGATIVE PREDICTIVE VALUE = 96 %
OVERALL ACCURACY = 99 %
++ = True Positives
-- = True Negatives
+- = False Positives
-+ = False Negatives

FALSE POSITIVES

Study done because of change in graft implied on duplex during Doppler. Arteriogram showed patent graft. Turned out to be technical error- native vessel was examined and not graft, which was laterally placed. (**)

FALSE NEGATIVES

1. Doppler- "Normal Rt. Leg" (index .96, waveforms biphasic) (***)
   A-gram- "60-70% Rt. iliac stenosis" (***)

2. Lt. leg read as normal. (***)
   Arteriogram showed significant disease but apparently not enough to cause hemodynamic changes detectable by the Doppler. (***)

FIG. 23-7 An example of a complete and detailed quality-assurance report combining a 2 × 2 table with correlation statistics and comments reflecting a review of discrepant cases. (Printout provided courtesy of Raecreations Software.)

totals, sensitivity, specificity, positive predictive value, negative predictive value, and overall accuracy or percentage agreement.

7. Identify and flag examinations that had false-positive or false-negative results. Review the data base or logbook reports for the names and obtain the laboratory files on any studies that were discrepant. Review the examinations for any irregularities.
8. Obtain, if possible, the angiogram films and reports on these patients, then review the angiograms for any irregularities.
9. If any examinations were misidentified as false-positive or false-negative after review, recalculate the statistics.
10. Summarize any or all reasons for the discrepancies and attach to the statistical report.
11. Hold a meeting of vascular laboratory staff to present the statistics and analyses and openly discuss the results. Distribute copies to all pertinent staff and administration members.

A technologist can spend a significant amount of time in quality control; patient information is best entered on a daily basis or as it is received. Spending about 15 minutes every day to maintain a data base or quality-control record eliminates the headaches of doing it all in batches or at the last minute. The effort spent pays off when the time comes to prepare a quarterly summary and statistic report. When a well-implemented quality control program is in place, a laboratory and its personnel can take pride in the knowledge that they are able to document and monitor their ability to do an effective and reliable job performing examinations.

CONTINUING EDUCATION

Vascular technologists, sonographers, and radiographers are required to submit evidence of ongoing education in their field to their credentialing organizations (e.g., the American Registry of Diagnostic Medical Sonographers [ARDMS]) and the American Registry of Radiologic Technologists [ARRT] to maintain their active status. This is done in the form of continuing education units (CEUs), which represent the number of hours spent in an educational activity, such as a meeting or seminar. CEUs are available in many forms (e.g., AMA Category I, Vascular Technology Credits [VTCs], Society of Diagnostic Medical Sonographers [SDMS] credits) and are submitted to the credentialing organization over a 3-year period (called a *triennium*). The ARDMS requires 30 credits to be acquired in each triennium. Although one would think that obtaining these CEUs would be a simple matter, budget cuts and reimbursement issues have affected travel allowances in many hospitals and private laboratories. Many technologists must either travel on their own time, attend local seminars, or fill out self-tests from journals or video presentations to obtain enough CEUs to fulfill the triennium requirements.

The ICAVL requires that continuing education opportunities of some sort be provided for the personnel of laboratories applying for accreditation.[2] With this in mind, a vascular laboratory should establish some sort of policy providing their personnel with opportunities for continuing education and allowing them time to periodically attend national or local symposia to keep abreast of nationwide issues affecting technologists. A laboratory can only remain state-of-the-art when its personnel and equipment can keep up with changes and new developments.

SUMMARY

Vascular laboratories and related administrative issues often make different demands of a technologist than does a traditional radiology or ultrasound department. Most radiology and ultrasound services incorporate most of the essential services stated in the ICAVL Essentials and Standards for Vascular Testing. Sonographers, however, are not faced routinely with statistics, nor are they exposed to the detailed research and emphasis on scientific method that rank-and-file vascular technologists are oriented toward. Because of this, there is a marked tendency in general ultrasound-based vascular laboratories to skimp or ignore quality-control and statistics issues. The ICAVL has reported that quality-control deficiencies are the single most common problem with institutions that have applied for vascular laboratory accreditation. Many commercial products are provided as aids to quality control, but these are often expensive and inflexible and cannot universally be applied to all laboratory situations. A laboratory's staff should be able to construct a low-cost database to their specifications as an alternative to expensive commercial packages. Quality assurance demands a serious commitment by all members of the medical staff and personnel in the vascular laboratory. By staffing the vascular laboratory with qualified personnel, adhering substantially to a national standard, and regularly reviewing and comparing the results of noninvasive tests performed, any vascular laboratory can be confident that the quality of service they are providing to the patient is exceptional.

REVIEW QUESTIONS

1. Name some of the potential benefits of vascular laboratory accreditation.
2. Could a podiatrist or a chiropractor be an acceptable laboratory medical director according to the ICAVL Standards? Why or why not?
3. An uncertified technologist with 3 months training and no prior vascular background is designated as the technical director in a laboratory. Why might this be unacceptable?
4. What are some basic requirements for policies in a vascular laboratory?
5. What are the advantages of a computer data base over a logbook? How long do you think it would take to

search through 100 logbook entries versus 100 computer records?

6. Why should noninvasive examinations be correlated with invasive tests? What benefits could a laboratory realize from regular correlation?
7. In statistical analysis, when should a 2 × 2 table be used, and when should a 5 × 5 or 6 × 6 table be used?
8. Name the five commonly used vascular statistical indices.
9. Define sensitivity, specificity, and overall accuracy. How are they different?
10. What is a false-positive? What is a false-negative?
11. Create a 2 × 2 table and calculate the totals and statistical indices using the following raw data:
    200 True-positives
    123 True-negatives
    2 False-positives
    1 False-negative
12. In the previous example, change the false-positive and false-negative numbers at random and recalculate the statistical indices. What happens?
13. Create a 5 × 5 table using the categories described in the chapter, plot the table, then calculate examination totals, correlation totals, and the percentage agreement using this data:
    Test HI/Standard HI = 3
    Test HI/Standard HII = 1
    Test HII/Standard HII = 6
    Test HII/Standard HI = 3
    Test HIII/Standard HIII = 7
    Test HIII/Standard HII = 2
    Test HIII/Standard HIV = 1
    Test HIV/Standard HIV = 3
    Test HIV/Standard HV = 1
    Test HV/Standard HV = 3
    Test HV/Standard HIII = 1
14. If there is a discrepancy between a noninvasive test and an arteriogram, is the test always at fault? Why or why not?

REFERENCES

1. Bluth EI, Stavros AT, Marich KW, et al: Carotid duplex sonography: a multicenter recommendation for standardized imaging and Doppler criteria, Radiographics 8:3, 1988.
2. Essentials and standards for noninvasive vascular testing. Vascular laboratory operations, Part I (Organization). Rockville, Md., 1993, Intersocietal Commission for the Accreditation of Vascular Laboratories.
3. Essentials and standards for noninvasive vascular testing. Vascular laboratory operations, Part II (Peripheral arterial testing). Rockville, Md., 1993, Intersocietal Commission for the Accreditation of Vascular Laboratories.
4. Essentials and standards for noninvasive vascular testing. Vascular laboratory operations, Part II (Peripheral venous testing). Rockville, Md., 1993, Intersocietal Commission for the Accreditation of Vascular Laboratories.
5. Essentials and standards for noninvasive vascular testing. Vascular laboratory operations, Part II (Cerebrovascular testing). Rockville, Md., 1993, Intersocietal Commission for the Accreditation of Vascular Laboratories.
6. Essentials and standards for noninvasive vascular testing. Vascular laboratory operations, Part II (Visceral vascular testing). Rockville, Md., 1993, Intersocietal Commission for the Accreditation of Vascular Laboratories.
7. Hayes A: Calculation and implication of accuracy measurements, Bruit 9:1780, 1985.
8. Lambeth A: Statistics in the vascular laboratory, Bruit 6:47, 1982.
9. Thiele BL: Standards in non-invasive cerebrovascular testing. In Bernstein EF, editor: Recent advances in non-invasive diagnostic techniques in vascular disease. St. Louis, 1990, Mosby.
10. Thiele BL, Strandness DE: Accuracy of angiographic quantification of peripheral atherosclerosis, Prog Cardiovasc Dis 26:223-226, 1983.

Glossary

ABDOMINAL AND RETROPERITONEAL CAVITIES

A

acute tubular necrosis (ATN) a common cause of acute transplant failure.

Addison's disease disease resulting from hypofunction of the adrenal cortex that is usually fatal. Signs and symptoms include hypotension, general weakness, loss of appetite and weight, and characteristic bronzing of the skin.

adrenal glands small secretory organs lying along the superomedial border of both kidneys, each composed of two endocrine glands: the cortex, which secretes a range of steroid hormones, and the medulla, which secretes epinephrine and norepinephrine.

adrenal medulla the core of the adrenal gland in which groups of irregular cells are located amidst veins that collect blood from the sinusoids; it produces epinephrine and norepinephrine.

adrenal neuroblastoma the most common malignancy of the adrenal glands in childhood and the most common tumor of infancy. It generally arises within the adrenal medulla.

adrenocorticotropic hormone (ACTH) hormone that controls the adrenal cortex.

adrenogenital syndrome hyperfunction of the adrenal cortex that results in precocious puberty in boys and masculinization of the external genitalia in girls.

adult polycystic disease a disease in which a cyst may arise from any portion of a collecting system.

agenesis of the spleen see **asplenia.**

amonium a toxic product of nitrogen metabolism.

amylase an enzyme of the pancreatic juice that causes hydrolysis of starch.

anatomic position a position of standing erect, the arms by the side with palms facing forward, the face and eyes directed forward, and the heels together with feet pointed forward.

angiomyolipoma a benign tumor that occurs most often in the kidneys.

anterior (ventral) toward the front of the body.

aorta the largest artery of the body. It distributes blood to the lower part of the body as the thoracic aorta and abdominal aorta and sends branches to the upper extremities from the ascending aorta.

aortic arch a continuation of the ascending aorta. It has three branches: the innominate or brachiocephalic trunk, the left common carotid artery, and the left subclavian artery.

aponeuroses thin, tendinous sheets attached to flat muscles.

arteriole a tiny arterial branch.

asplenia complete absence of the spleen.

B

bare area the portion of the liver that rests directly on the diaphragm.

blood urea nitrogen (BUN) the level of urea in the blood.

Bowman's capsule see **capsula glomeruli.**

C

calculi see **gallstones.**

capsula glomeruli two layers of flat epithelial cells with a space between them contained in each nephron of the kidney.

caudal toward the feet.

celiac trunk branch of the abdominal aorta that distributes to structures of the gastrointestinal tract. It gives rise to the left gastric, hepatic, and splenic arteries.

cholecystitis inflammation of the gallbladder punctuated by intermittent acute episodes, which occur when the cystic duct is obstructed by a calculus.

cholelithiasis the presence of gallstones in the gallbladder.

colic artery a left, middle, or right branch from either the inferior mesenteric or the superior mesenteric artery that distributes to the colon.

common bile duct formed by the common hepatic duct and the cystic duct.

common duct the duct formed by the junction of the cystic duct with the hepatic duct.

common hepatic duct the united right and left hepatic ducts, approximately 4 mm in diameter, which descends within the edge of the lesser omentum.

congenital renal agenesis absence of one kidney and one ureter at birth.

Conn's syndrome caused by excessive secretion of aldosterone, usually resulting from a cortical adenoma.

coronal plane any vertical plane at right angles to the median plane.

Courvoisier's sign (law) when a gallstone blocks the common bile duct, the gallbladder is smaller than usual; when the duct is obstructed in some other way, the gallbladder is dilated.

cranial toward the head.

culling inspection and destruction of abnormal or senescent erythrocytes as they pass through the spleen.

Cushing's syndrome one type of oversecretion disease of the adrenal cortex. This is produced by excessive secretion of glucocorticoids resulting from hyperplasia, a benign tumor, or carcinoma. Symptoms include increased sodium retention, muscle and bone weakness, and secretion of androgens.

cystic artery right branch of the proper hepatic artery that distributes to the gallbladder and undersurface of the liver.

D

diaphragm a dome-shaped muscular and tendinous septum that separates the thorax from the abdominal cavity.

distal away from the point of origin or away from the body.

duct of Santorini a secondary duct that drains the upper anterior head of the pancreas.

duct of Wirsung (ductus pancreaticus) the primary excretory duct of the pancreas extending the entire length of the gland.

E

enzymes protein catalysts used throughout the body in all metabolic processes.

epigastric artery a branch of the external iliac artery (inferior epigastric), the femoral artery (superficial epigastric), or the internal mammary artery (superior epigastric) that distributes to the abdominal muscles and peritoneum, the abdomen and su-

perficial fascia, or the abdominal muscles and diaphragm, respectively.
epiploic foramen the opening of the lesser sac.
external outside.

F
false pelvis see **major pelvis.**
fasciae thin sheets of tissue that cover muscles and hold them in their place.
floating gallstone some gallstones are seen to float when contrast material from an oral cholecystogram is present. This is because of the higher specific gravity of the contrast material than of the bile.
foramen of Winslow see **epiploic foramen.**

G
gallbladder a pear-shaped sac, with a capacity of 50 ml, in the anterior aspect of the right upper quadrant closely related to the visceral surface of the liver. Its function includes storage of bile for intermittent release in conjunction with eating.
gallbladder sludge thick, inspissated bile found in the gallbladder.
gallstones the small crystals of bile salts that precipitate from the bile and vary from pinhead size to the size of the gallbladder itself.
gastric artery a right, left, or short branch of the celiac, hepatic, or splenic artery that distributes to the esophagus and curvatures of the stomach.
gastroduodenal artery a branch of the hepatic artery that distributes to the stomach, duodenum, and pancreas.
gastroepiploic artery a left or right branch of either the splenic or gastroduodenal artery that distributes to the stomach and greater omentum.
Gerota's fascia see **renal fascia.**
glomerulus a cluster of nonanastomosing capillaries.
glucocorticoids steroids that play a principal role in carbohydrate metabolism. Cortisone and hydrocortisone are the primary glucocorticoids. They diminish allergic response, especially the more serious inflammatory types (rheumatoid arthritis and rheumatic fever).
glucose tolerance test a test performed to discover whether there is a disorder of glucose metabolism.

H
Hartmann's pouch created when the gallbladder folds back on itself at the neck.
hemolytic anemia the general term applied to anemia referable to decreased life of the erythrocytes.
hepatic artery (common) branch of the celiac artery that distributes to the stomach, pancreas, duodenum, liver, gallbladder, and greater omentum.
hepatic artery (proper) branch of the common hepatic artery that distributes to the liver and gallbladder.
hepatorenal recess the lowest point in the peritoneal cavity when the patient is lying supine. It is in the greatest sac just to the right of the epiploic foramen.
horseshoe kidney a defect that occurs during fetal development with fusion of the upper or lower poles, where the kidney does not ascend to its normal position in the retroperitoneal cavity.
hydronephrosis distention of the pelvis and calices of the kidney by urine resulting from an obstruction in a ureter.
hyperglycemia an effect of severe liver disease causing an uncontrolled increase in blood glucose.
hypoalbuminemia a significant lowering of the serum albumin.
hypoglycemia an effect of severe liver disease where the body becomes glucose deficient.

I
iliac artery the common iliac artery is a branch of the abdominal aorta and distributes to the pelvis, abdominal wall, and lower limbs. The external iliac artery is a branch of the common iliac artery and distributes to the abdominal wall, external genitalia, and lower limbs. The internal iliac artery is another branch of the common iliac artery and distributes to the visceral walls of the pelvis, buttocks, reproductive organs, and mid-thigh.
infantile polycystic disease a disease that causes the tubules in the distal collecting systems to dilate and form small cystic structures.
inferior below.
insulin a hormone secreted by the beta cells of the islets of Langerhans in the pancreas. It is secreted into the blood where it regulates carbohydrate, lipid, and amino acid metabolism.
internal inside.
intestinal artery branch of the superior mesenteric artery that distributes to the jejunum and ileum.
intravenous pyelogram (IVP) a roentgenogram of the kidney and ureter after the injection of a radiopaque dye.

J
jaundice the disease characterized by the presence of bile in the tissues with the resulting yellow-green color of the skin, sclerae, and body secretions.

L
labeling an orderly procedure that should be used to identify the anatomic position where the transverse and longitudinal scans have been taken.
lateral farther from the midline or to the side of the body.
left hepatic duct emerges from the left lobe of the liver in the porta hepatis and unites with the right hepatic duct to form the common hepatic duct.
lesser sac an enclosed portion of the peritoneal space posterior to the liver and the stomach.
linea alba a fibrous band that stretches from the xyphoid to the symphysis pubis and forms a central anterior attachment for the muscle layers of the abdomen. It is formed by the interlacing of fibers of the aponeuroses of the right and left oblique and transversus abdominis muscles.
lipase an enzyme secreted by the pancreas and small intestine that is capable of hydrolyzing some fats to monoglycerides and some to glycerol and fatty acids.
lithogenic bile a form of bile supersaturated with cholesterol that is found in some individuals.
lumbar artery a branch of the abdominal aorta that distributes to the abdominal walls, the vertebrae, the lumbar muscles, and the renal capsule.

M
major pelvis the portion of the pelvis found above the brim of the pelvis; its cavity is that portion of the abdominal cavity cradled by the iliac fossae.
malpighian body see **renal corpuscle.**
medial nearer to or toward the midline.
median plane a vertical plane that bisects the body into right and left halves.
mesenteric artery inferior or superior branch of the abdominal aorta that distributes to either the lower half of the colon and rectum (inferior) or the small intestine and proximal half of the colon (superior).
mesentery a double fold of peritoneum connecting an organ to the abdominal wall.
mesothelium a single layer of cells that forms the peritoneum.

metabolism the physical and chemical process whereby food is synthesized into complex elements, complex substances are transformed into simple ones, and energy is made available for use by the organism.

Mickey Mouse sign appearance of the common duct, hepatic artery, and portal vein on a transverse scan. The portal vein serves as Mickey's face, with the right ear the common duct and the left ear the hepatic artery.

mineralocorticoids steroids that regulate the electrolyte metabolism. Aldosterone is the principal mineralocorticoid; it has a regulatory effect on the relative concentrations of mineral ions in the body fluids and therefore on the water content of tissues.

minor pelvis the portion of the pelvis found below the brim of the pelvis. The cavity of the minor pelvis is continuous at the pelvic brim with the cavity of the major pelvis.

multicystic dysplastic kidney a nonfunctioning kidney whose contour and shape are very irregular and which usually contains multiple cysts of varying sizes.

multipennate muscle a muscle that contains a tendon in the center, and the muscle fibers pass to it from two sides.

N

neoplasm any new growth or development, either malignant or benign, of an abnormal tissue.

nephron a tubular excretory unit of the kidney.

O

omentum a double layer of peritoneum running to the stomach.

ovarian artery branch of the abdominal aorta that distributes to the ovary, uterus, uterine tubes, and ureter.

P

pancreatic juice the pancreas' exocrine function is to produce this juice, which enters the duodenum together with bile.

pancreaticoduodenal artery the inferior pancreaticoduodenal artery is a branch of the superior mesenteric artery, and the superior pancreaticoduodenal artery is a branch of the gastroduodenal artery. Both distribute to the pancreas and duodenum.

parietal peritoneum the portion of the peritoneum that lines the abdominal wall but does not cover a viscus.

patient position the position of the patient described in relation to the scanning table (e.g., right decubitus would mean the right side down).

pennate muscles muscles that have fibers running oblique to the line of pull, resembling a feather.

peristalsis the action of smooth muscles propelling material through vessels or the gastrointestinal tract.

peritoneal cavity the potential space between the parietal and visceral peritoneum.

peritoneal gutters passageways that conduct fluid material from one point of the peritoneal cavity to another.

peritoneal recess small, isolated, slitlike parts of the peritoneal cavity without intestine.

pheochromocytoma a tumor that secretes epinephrine and norepinephrine in excessive quantities. They may be large, bulky tumors with a variety of sonographic patterns, including cystic, solid, and calcified components.

phrenic artery the inferior phrenic artery is a branch of the abdominal aorta and distributes to the diaphragm and adrenals. The superior phrenic arteries are branches of the thoracic aorta and distribute to the upper surface of the vertebral portion of the diaphragm.

phrygian cap folding of the fundus of the gallbladder.

pitting a process by which the spleen removes granular inclusions without destroying the erythrocytes.

portal triad the common collagenous sheath that encases the liver parenchyma, the portal venous and hepatic arterial branches.

posterior (dorsal) the back of the body, or in back of another structure.

pouch of Morrison see **hepatorenal recess.**

prone lying face down.

proximal closer to the point of origin or closer to the body.

R

real time the dynamic "real-time" presentation of sequential images at varying frame rates (depending on frequency and depth).

rectus sheath a sheath formed by the aponeuroses of the muscles of the lateral group.

renal artery branch of the abdominal aorta that distributes to the kidney.

renal corpuscle Bowman's capsule and the glomerulus.

renal fascia the tissue that surrounds the true capsule and perinephric fat.

renal parenchyma the area from the renal sinus to the outer renal surface in which are found the arcuate and interlobar vessels.

renal pyramids the portion of the kidney that is composed of medullary substance, which consists of a series of striated conical masses.

renal sinus fibrolipomatosis sinus fat and fibrous tissue.

retroperitoneal fibrosis a disease of unknown etiology characterized by thick sheets of fibrous tissue in the retroperitoneal space.

retroperitoneal space the area between the posterior portion of the parietal peritoneum and the posterior abdominal wall muscles.

right hepatic duct emerges from the right lobe of the liver in the porta hepatis and unites with the left hepatic duct to form the common hepatic duct.

S

sagittal plane any plane parallel to the median plane.

septation, complete double gallbladder.

skeletal muscle muscle, composed of striated muscle fibers and having two or more attachments, that produces movements of the skeleton.

smooth muscle muscle composed of long, spindle-shaped cells closely arranged in bundles or sheets.

spermatic artery, internal branch of the abdominal aorta that distributes to the scrotum and testis.

sphincter of Oddi the circular muscle fibers that surround the end part of the common bile duct, the main pancreatic duct, and the ampulla; located at the junction of the common bile duct and the duodenum.

splenic artery branch of the celiac artery that distributes to the spleen, stomach, pancreas, and greater omentum.

superficial inguinal ring a triangular opening in the external oblique aponeuroses that lies superior and medial to the pubic tubercle.

superior above.

supernumerary kidney a rare defect where there is a complete duplicate of the renal system.

supine lying face up.

T

tendons the cords of tough, fibrous tissue that attach the ends of muscles to bones, cartilage, or ligaments.

thyroid artery, lowest branch of the aortic arch as well as the innominate and right carotid arteries that distributes to the thyroid gland.

thyroid artery, superior branch of the external carotid artery that distributes to the hyoid muscles, larynx, thyroid gland, and pharynx.
transverse plane any plane at right angles to both the median and coronal planes.
true capsule the fibrous capsule surrounding the kidney.
true pelvis see **minor pelvis.**
trypsin a pancreatic enzyme that may hydrolyze protein molecules to peptides.
tubular secretion the process in which acids and other substances the body does not need are secreted into the distal renal tubules from the bloodstream.

U
unipennate muscle a muscle in which the tendon lies along one side of the muscle and the muscle fibers pass oblique to it.
urinoma a walled-off collection of extravasated urine that develops spontaneously after trauma, surgery, or a subacute or chronic urinary obstruction.
uterine artery branch of the internal iliac artery that distributes to the uterus.

V
veins
azygos front and right side of the lumbar vertebrae.
colic right, medial, and left veins of intestines.
common iliac union of external veins draining the sacroiliac and lower lumbar region and emptying into the inferior vena cava.
cystic gallbladder.
dorsalis penis vein lying in the midline of the penis between the dorsal arteries.
ductus venosus a fetal vein that connects the umbilical vein with the inferior vena cava.
duodenal duodenum.
epigastric homonymous with epigastric artery; inferior, superficial, and superior.
gastric short, right, and left veins of the stomach and surrounding area.
gastroepiploic right and left veins of the stomach and omentum.
hepatic liver region.
hypogastric lower and middle abdomen, extending from the greater sciatic notch to the brim of the pelvis, where it joins the external iliac to form the common iliac vein.
ileocolic ileum and colon.
intercostal ribs and chest region.
interlobular renal and hepatic veins of the kidney and liver.
mammary internal vein of the breast.
mesenteric superior and inferior vein of the intestines.
ovarian ovary and broad ligament.
pancreatic pancreas.
pancreaticoduodenal pancreas and duodenum.
phlebo combining form referring to vein.
phrenic anterior and superior veins of the diaphragm.
plexus network of veins (may also refer to nerves and lymphatics).
portal liver, eventually forming sinusoids of liver.
pudendal internal and external genitalia.
pyloric pylorus and area.
renal kidney.
sacral lateral and median veins of the sacral and coccygeal areas.
spermatic spermatic cord and surrounding areas.
splenic spleen.
superior and inferior vena cava large veins that return blood to the heart. The superior vena cava returns blood from the upper extremities, and the inferior vena cava returns it from the lower extremities.
suprarenals adrenals.
thyroid inferior and superior veins of the thyroid gland and adjacent structures.
uterine uterus.
venae vasorum small veins that return blood from the walls of blood vessels themselves.
veno term referring to vein.
venules small veins.
vesical bladder.
visceral peritoneum that portion of the peritoneum that covers an organ.
voluntary muscle the movements of the skeleton produced by the skeletal muscles.

W
Waterhouse-Friderichsen syndrome malignant form of epidemic cerebrospinal meningitis characterized by the sudden onset of fever, cyanosis, petechiae, and collapse from massive bilateral adrenal hemorrhage.

SUPERFICIAL STRUCTURES

A
adenosis hyperplasia and proliferation of the epithelial component of ducts in the breast characterizing the second stage of fibrocystic disease.
aneurysm dilation of the venous wall because of high venous pressure or repeated dialysis traumas.

B
breast a differentiated apocrine sweat gland with a functional purpose of secreting milk during lactation.

C
carcinoma of the breast breast tumors that arise from the epithelium, in the ductal and glandular tissue, usually having tentacles.
infiltrating infiltration of the breast tissue beyond the basement membrane and into adjacent tissue.
noninfiltrating carcinoma of the lactiferous ducts that has not infiltrated the basement membrane but is proliferating within the confines of the ducts and its branches.
chronic hypocalcemia a disease caused by renal failure, ricketts, or malabsorption syndromes and which induces PTH secretion.
comedomastitis the dilation of the ducts in the breast filled with a secretion produced by desquamated cells from the duct wall.
Cooper's ligaments the supporting structures of the breast that provide the shape and consistency of the breast structure.
cretinism congenital hypothyroidism.
cystic disease the third stage of fibrocystic disease characterized by the involution of lobules and hyperplasia of the surrounding stroma, leading to the formation of cysts.
cystic masses lumps in the breast much like a balloon of water, well delineated but not as mobile as fibroadenomas.
cystosarcoma phyllodes an uncommon breast neoplasia and the most frequent sarcoma of the breast.

E
epididymis the first portion of the duct of the testis and its excretory system.
epididymitis the most common intrascrotal inflammation, appearing sonographically as uniform enlargement of the epididymis and most evident in the globus major.

F

fibroadenoma one of the most common benign breast tumors, the most common in childhood, and occurring primarily in young adult women.

fibrocystic disease breast syndrome with histologic changes occurring on the terminal ducts and lobules of the breast in both the epithelial and connective tissue. General symptoms are pain, nodularity, a dominant mass, cysts, and occasional nipple discharge.

G

goiter enlargement of the thyroid gland as a result of hyperplasia or neoplasia, inflammatory processes, or colloid distention of the follicles.

Graves' disease hyperthyroidism associated with diffuse goiter.

H

hydrocele of the cord the encasement of fluid in a sac of peritoneum within the spermatic cord. It can also present as a cystic mass cephalad to the testis.

hydrocele a fluid collection surrounding the testis that can be associated with infectious processes or tumors.

hyperparathyroidism

primary a state of increased function of the parathyroid glands characterized by hypercalcemia, hypercalciuria, and low serum levels of phosphate. It occurs when increased amounts of PTH are produced by an adenoma, primary hyperplasia, or rarely, carcinoma.

secondary results from chronic hypocalcemia that induces PTH secretion.

hyperthyroidism a hypermetabolic state in which increased amounts of thyroid hormones are produced as a result of pituitary-thyroid regulatory system failure. Manifestations of this condition are weight loss, nervousness, and increased heart rate.

hypothyroidism a hypometabolic state resulting from inadequate secretion of thyroid hormones. It is usually caused by an abnormality of the gland that restricts production of the hormone. Lethargy, sluggish reactions, and a deep husky voice are manifestations.

I

in situ a condition in which a carcinoma is contained and has not invaded the basal membrane structure.

iodine metabolism the mechanism for production of thyroid hormones.

M

mammary one of the three well-defined layers of the breast found between the superficial and the deep connective tissue layers.

mammography the most accurate, noninvasive method for the detection of breast lesions, especially in tissue that is predominantly fatty.

mastodynia see **mazoplasia.**

mazoplasia the first stage of fibrocystic disease characterized by an increased proliferation of the stroma and by the small number of lobules or acini.

P

Paget's disease a relatively rare tumor occurring in older women, characterized by changes in the nipple and areola.

parathyroid glands the calcium-sensing organs in the body that produce parathormone (PTH) and monitor the serum calcium feedback mechanism.

polytetrafluoroethylene a material that has become popular for use in vascular access.

precancerous mastopathy apocrine metaplasia with atypia, which carries a similar but slightly decreased risk factor compared to fibrocystic disease.

R

retromammary one of the three well-defined layers of the breast consisting of fat lobules separated anteriorly from the mammary layer by the deep connective tissue plane and posteriorly by the fascia over the pectoralis major.

S

sarcoma breast tumors that arise from the supportive or connective tissues.

scrotum a pendant sac divided by a septum into two compartments, each containing a testis, an epididymis, and a portion of spermatic cord and ductus deferens.

spermatocele a cystic dilation of the spermatic cord.

subcutaneous one of the three layers of the breast bounded superficially by the dermis and deeply by the superficial connective tissue plane.

T

testes the male organ of reproduction, found in the scrotum, that produces spermatozoa and male sex hormones.

thyroglossal duct cysts congenital anomalies presenting in the midline of the neck, anterior to the trachea, that are fusiform or spherical masses of no more than 2 or 3 cm.

thyroid an endocrine gland that maintains normal body metabolism, growth, and development.

V

varicocele cystic varicose enlargement of the veins of the spermatic cord, usually of a tortuous nature resembling a bag of worms.

NEONATAL ECHOENCEPHALOGRAPHY

A

Arnold-Chiari malformation malformation characterized by displacement of the fourth ventricle, upper medulla, and the inferior part of the cerebellum and defects in the calvarium and spinal column frequently associated with myelomeningocele, hydrocephalus, dilation of the third ventricle, and absence of the septum pellucidum.

C

caudate nuclei the inferior and lateral walls of the ventricles at the bodies and posterior part of the frontal horns.

choroid plexus an intraventricular structure lying in the floor of the lateral ventricles and extending from the temporal horns into the atria and the bodies of the lateral ventricles.

communicating hydrocephalus a type of hydrocephalus where the CSF pathways are open within the ventricular system and there is a decreased absorption of CSF.

D

Dandy-Walker malformation a malformation characterized by absence of the cerebellar vermis, cystic changes in the fourth ventricle, with the development of a large cyst in the posterior fossa and hydrocephalus.

dorsal induction changes occurring in the dorsal aspect of the embryo by which the brain and spinal cord are formed.

E

echoencephalography (ECHO) the technique of choice to visualize the neonatal brain; pulses of ultrasonic waves are beamed through the head from both sides, and echoes from the midline structures of the brain are recorded as graphic tracings.

F

focal brain necrosis necrotic lesions occurring within the distribution of large arteries mainly in term and preterm infants (infrequent under 30 weeks' gestational age).

G

germinal matrix the tissue where neurons and glial cells develop before migrating from the subventricular region to the cortex.

H

holoprosencephaly brain malformation caused by disturbances in the process of ventral induction very early in life; neuropathologic features include a single cerebrum with single ventricular activity, absence of the corpus callosum, and frontal horns and a thin membrane arising from the roof of the third ventricle, which may extend posteriorly, forming a supratentorial cyst.

hydraencephaly a large, single cavity with entire disappearance of the cerebral hemispheres.

hydrocephalus any condition in which enlargement of the ventricular system is caused by an imbalance between production and reabsorption of cerebrospinal fluid.

I

intraparenchymal hemorrhages a severe complication to SEHs/IVHs, which indicate that the brain parenchyma has been destroyed.

ischemic-hypoxic lesions generally associated with abnormal neurologic outcome, these lesions are a frequent complication of sick newborn infants.

M

multicystic encephalomalacia term used to describe multiple cavities in the cerebral tissues.

multifocal white matter necrosis (WMN) the most frequent ischemic lesion in the immature brain.

O

obstructive hydrocephalus a type of hydrocephalus characterized by interference in the circulation of the CSF within the ventricular system itself, causing subsequent enlargement of the ventricular cavities proximal to the obstruction.

P

periventricular leukomalacia see **multifocal white matter necrosis.**

porencephaly single cavity in the cerebral tissues.

S

subarachnoid hemorrhages hemorrhages that may be isolated or secondary to IVHs/SEHs, with birth trauma and hypoxia/asphyxia being the most probable causes.

subependymal hemorrhages capillary bleeding at the germinal matrix, frequently located at the thalamic-caudate groove.

subependymal-intraventricular hemorrhages (SEH/IVH) a developmental disease that is the most common hemorrhagic lesion in preterm newborn infants.

V

ventral induction changes occurring in the rostral portion of the embryo at 5 to 6 weeks' gestation, resulting in the formation of the face and forebrain.

ventriculitis a common complication of purulent meningitis in newborn infants.

OBSTETRICS AND GYNECOLOGY

A

abdominal circumference (AC) measurement of circumference of fetal abdomen at level of left portal vein. AC values are used in the determination of fetal weight.

achondrogenesis lethal autosomal recessive short-limbed dwarfism marked by long bone and trunk shortening, decreased echogenicity of the bones and spine, and "flipper-like" appendages.

achondroplasia a defect in the development of cartilage at the epiphyseal centers of the long bones producing short, square bones.

acrania condition associated with anencephaly in which there is complete or partial absence of the cranial bones.

acrocephalopolysyndactyly autosomal-dominant congenital syndrome marked by premature closure of cranial sutures resulting in a peaked head shape. Condition is associated with finger and toe anomalies (webbing or fusion). Types include Apert's syndrome, Apert-Crouzon syndrome, Chotzen's syndrome, and Pfeiffer's syndrome.

adenomyosis the inclusion of endometrial cells deep within the myometrium, which causes diffuse uterine enlargement and heavy, painful menses.

alobar holoprosencephaly most severe form of holoprosencephaly characterized by a single common ventricle and malformed brain. Orbital anomalies range from fused orbits to hypotelorism with frequent nasal anomalies and clefting of the lip and palate.

alpha-fetoprotein protein manufactured by the fetus, which can be studied in amniotic fluid and maternal serum. Elevations of alpha-fetoprotein may indicate fetal anomalies (neural tube, abdominal wall, gastrointestinal), multiple gestations, or incorrect patient dates. Decreased levels may be associated with chromosomal abnormalities.

amniocentesis transabdominal removal of amniotic fluid from the amniotic cavity using ultrasound. Amniotic fluid studies are performed to determine fetal karyotype, lung maturity, and Rh condition.

anencephaly neural tube defect characterized by the lack of development of the cerebral and cerebellar hemispheres and cranial vault. This abnormality is incompatible with life.

anomaly structural abnormality that deviates from the norm. A congenital anomaly is one present at birth.

antenatal period of time before birth.

arcuate vessels hormone-sensitive arteries running superficially in the myometrium parallel to the uterine surface that control blood delivery to the endometrium.

arhinencephaly term used to describe holoprosencephaly named after the associated absent olfactory system and corpus callosum.

asymmetric intrauterine growth retardation (IUGR) this form of IUGR usually begins in late second or early third trimester with relative sparing of head size.

B

binocular distance (BD)/outer orbital distance (OOD) measurement across both orbits, which is useful in predicting gestational age and in the detection of orbital distance abnormalities.

biometric the statistical interpretation of biologic information. In ultrasound, biometric data is analyzed in determining fetal age and growth (analysis of fetal measurements).

biophysical profile prenatal test to monitor fetal well-being using ultrasound (breathing, movements, tone, amniotic fluid) and the nonstress test (fetal heart reactivity).

biparietal diameter (BPD) the most widely accepted means of measuring the fetal head and estimating gestational age in the second trimester. The BPD is measured at the level of the thalamus and the cavum septi pellucidi.

blastocyst vesicle containing the zygote, trophoblast, and inner cell mass.

blighted ovum pregnancy that develops abnormally without an embryo (anembryonic).

blood vessels thin-walled, sonolucent, pulsatile, sinuous structures that range from 1 mm to over 1 cm in diameter.

brachycephaly fetal head shape that is widened in the anteroposterior plane and shortened in the frontal-occipital plane. Brachycephaly is determined by the cephalic index. When present, the biparietal diameter is erroneous in predicting fetal age.

breech presentation fetal pelvis is the presenting part. Various forms of a breech lie may occur. In a frank breech the legs are extended over the fetal body. In complete breech the legs are tucked in front of the body. In a footling breech the feet are the presenting parts. A single foot may also present.

C

cebocephaly form of holoprosencephaly characterized by a common ventricle, hypotelorism, and a single-nostriled nose.

cephalic index (CI) the biparietal diameter divided by the occipitofrontal diameter multiplied by 100.

cephalic (vertex) presentation fetal head is the presenting part. The fontanel, brow, or face may be the presenting structure.

cephalocele abnormal protrusion of brain tissue, meninges, and occasionally cerebral ventricles, through an opening in the skull.

cephalosyndactyly craniosynostosis and fusion of the fingers or toes.

chorion frondosum portion of chorion containing villi representing the fetal component of the placenta. Sampling site for chorionic villus procedures.

chorion laeve smooth portion of the chorion that regresses during pregnancy.

chorionic villus sampling transvaginal or transabdominal biopsy of chorionic villi during early pregnancy for the detection of chromosomal and biochemical fetal disorders.

complete abortion total evacuation of the products of conception of less than 22 weeks' gestation.

conceptus term describing the embryo and supporting membranes.

corpus luteum the remaining estrogen and progesterone cells in the follicle after ovulation.

craniosynostosis early ossification of the calvarium with destruction of the sutures. Hypertelorism frequently found in association. Sonographically, the fetal cranium may appear brachycephalic.

crown-rump length (CRL) the most accurate sonographic technique that can be used to establish gestational age in the first trimester. Measurement is taken from the top of the fetal head to the outer rump, excluding the limbs or yolk sac.

cumulus oophorus the ovum surrounded by granulosa cells.

cyclopia severe form of holoprosencephaly characterized by a common ventricle, fusion of the orbits with one or two eyes present, and a proboscis (maldeveloped cylindrical nose).

cystic hygroma dilation of jugular lymph sacs (may occur in axilla or groin) because of improper drainage of the lymphatic system into the venous system. Large septated hygromas are frequently associated with Turner's syndrome, congestive heart failure, and death of the fetus in utero. Isolated hygromas may occur as solitary lesions at birth.

D

decidua the mucous lining of the uterus thrown off after parturition.

decidua basalis decidua layer that forms the maternal aspect of the placenta found between the placenta and myometrium.

decidua capsularis endometrial membrane covering the gestational sac.

decidua parietalis membrane that lines the endometrial cavity during pregnancy.

dermoid cyst one of the more common ovarian tumors with mixed components.

dolichocephaly fetal head shape that is flattened in the anteroposterior plane and elongated in the frontal-occipital plane. Dolichocephaly is determined by the cephalic index. When present, the biparietal diameter is erroneous for predicting fetal age.

double set-up examination examination performed at delivery in a patient with vaginal bleeding and suspected placenta previa, whereby a digital examination is performed in the operating room. When previa is confirmed, a cesarean delivery is immediately performed.

dyzygotic twinning twinning resulting from fertilization of two separate ova (fraternal twins). Each fetus has a separate placenta and chorionic and amniotic sacs.

E

endometriosis a common condition in which ectopic endometrium can occur throughout the body. It is usually found on the ovaries, external uterus, and scattered over peritoneal surfaces, especially in the dependent regions.

epignathus teratoma arising from the oral cavity and pharynx.

estimated date of confinement (EDC) the estimated day of delivery as determined by the last missed menstrual period.

ethmocephaly form of holoprosencephaly in which a rudimentary proboscis-like nose is located between two closely spaced orbits with partial or complete absence of the ethmoid structures.

eventration abnormal thinning of the diaphragm because of elevation of portions of the diaphragm. May resemble a diaphragmatic hernia sonographically.

F

femur length (FL) measurement of diaphysis of femur used to determine fetal age and limb growth.

fetal acrania abnormal brain development with an associated cranial defect in the skull.

fetal microcephalus a condition marked by an abnormally small fetal calvarium.

fetoscopy ultrasound-guided fetal surgical procedure performed using a fiberoptic fetoscope to aspirate fetal blood from umbilical cord vessels, for examination of minute anatomic structures, or to biopsy fetal tissue. Certain blood and biochemical disorders can be detected.

fibroids the most common gynecologic tumor; also termed *leiomyomas* or *myoma*.

fundus the domelike top of the uterus.

G

Gartner's duct cysts large, broad ligament cysts that are continuous with the lateral walls of the vagina.

gastroschisis paraumbilical abdominal wall defect in which uncontained abdominal organs protrude into the amniotic cavity. Frequent association with intrauterine growth retardation and gastrointestinal complications.

genetic scan see **level II scan.**

gestational sac the first structure to be identified on early obstetrical ultrasound examination, it is a cystic ring like structure that occupies the fundus or mid-portion of the uterus.

growth adjusted sonar age the growth interval compared with average growth using two measurements of the fetus, one between 20 and 26 weeks, the next between 31 and 33 weeks.

H

head circumference (HC) measurement of cranial circumference obtained at level of thalamus. Measurement used to assess fetal age and cranial growth.

hemolysis breakdown of red blood cells in response to an Rh antibody, resulting in fetal anemia.

hemoperitoneum blood within the peritoneal cavity.

heterozygous achondroplasia short-limbed dysplasia that manifests in the second trimester of pregnancy. Conversion abnormality of cartilage to bone affecting the epiphyseal growth centers. Extremities are markedly shortened at birth with a normal trunk and frequent enlargement of the head.

holoprosencephaly cranial abnormality in which the forebrain (prosencephalon) fails to divide or partially divides into cerebral hemispheres or lobes. Alobar, semi-lobar, and lobar forms may occur. Varying facial anomalies may affect orbital spacing (varying degrees of hypotelorism) and formation of the nose, lips, and palate.

homozygous achondroplasia short-limbed dwarfism affecting fetuses of achondroplastic parents.

human chorionic gonadotropin (HCG) hormone manufactured by the trophoblastic cells that supply estrogen and progesterone for the pregnancy. HCG is detected in the urine of pregnant women.

hydranencephaly congenital absence of the cerebral hemispheres because of an occlusion of the carotid arteries. Midbrain structures are present, and fluid replaces cerebral tissue.

hydrocele congenital collection of serous fluid within the scrotal sac.

hydrocephalus ventriculomegaly in the neonate. Abnormal accumulation of cerebrospinal fluid within the cerebral ventricles, resulting in compression and frequent destruction of brain tissue.

hydrometrocolpos abnormality of female genital tract in which there is an abnormal collection of fluid within the uterus and vagina. Frequent association with malformations of the genital tract.

hydrops condition marked by excessive accumulation of fluid (serous) in the fetal tissues (characterized according to location: ascites, edema, anasarca). Associated with fetuses with severe immune sensitization (RH isoimmunization) or from nonimmune conditions.

hyperstimulation syndrome a condition that occurs when the ovaries continue to enlarge after ovulation.

hypertelorism abnormally wide-spaced orbits usually found in conjunction with congenital anomalies and mental retardation.

hypophosphatasia congenital condition characterized by decreased mineralization of the bones resulting in "ribbon-like" and bowed limbs, underossified cranium, and compression of the chest. Early death often occurs.

hypotelorism abnormally closely spaced orbits. Association with holoprosencephaly, chromosomal and central nervous system disorders, and cleft palate.

I

immune resistance to a disease or condition.

implantation bleed bleeding as a result of implantation of the gestational sac.

incomplete abortion incomplete expulsion of the products of conception from the uterus.

inevitable abortion abortion destined to occur because of rupture of the membranes and dilation of the cervix.

insulin-dependent diabetic diabetic pregnancy that requires insulin control in patients who have diabetes mellitus before conception.

intrapartum period of time during labor and delivery.

intrauterine growth retardation (IUGR) a decreased rate of fetal growth, usually a fetal weight below the tenth percentile for a given gestational age.

isoimmunization blood group incompatibility that occurs when fetal red blood cells enter the maternal blood. Maternal antibodies cross the placenta and destroy fetal red blood cells.

L

level II scan comprehensive sonographic examination of the fetus for exclusion, confirmation, or follow-up of a congenital anomaly. Systematic study of fetal organ systems.

leiomyomata see **fibroids.**

M

macrocephaly enlargement of the fetal cranium as a result of ventriculomegaly.

macrosomia abnormally large fetus above the ninetieth percentile for weight at any given gestational age. Macrosomia results from maternal diabetes mellitus and nonendocrine syndromes.

macrosomia index chest diameter—biparietal diameter.

mean a statistical description of the average value of a given parameter.

Meigs syndrome a benign condition consisting of massive ascites and pleural effusion.

meningocele open spinal defect characterized by the protrusion of the spinal meninges.

meningomyelocele open spinal defect characterized by the protrusion of meninges and spinal cord through the defect, usually within a meningeal sac.

menometrorrhagia irregular menstrual bleeding.

menorrhagia heavy menstrual bleeding.

microcephalus abnormally small fetal cranium with frequent association with mental retardation.

micrognathia abnormally small chin. Commonly associated with other fetal anomalies.

missed abortion pregnancy in which there is death of the fetus. In missed abortion, the products of conception remain within the uterus for at least 8 weeks.

monozygotic twinning twinning that occurs when a single fertilized egg divides (identical twins).

myomata see **fibroids.**

N

nabothian cysts cysts consisting of inspissated secretions along the canal and margin of the portio vaginalis.

neonatal period of time, in terms of the infant, immediately after birth and to the twenty-eighth day of life.

nonimmune hydrops condition in which fetal hydrops occurs, which is unassociated with fetomaternal blood group compatibility.

non–insulin-dependent diabetic diabetes that presents during pregnancy in patients without a history of diabetes (gestational diabetes). These pregnancies are most often regulated by diet, although insulin may be required to maintain blood glucose levels.

non-stress test (NST) electronic fetal heart rate monitoring that studies the ability of the fetal heart to accelerate with fetal movements. The NST is used to screen for fetal distress. Abnormal NST tests are typically followed by an oxytocin challenge test (OCT).

O

oculodentodigital dysplasia disorder marked by craniosynostosis, hypertelorism, dental abnormalities and fusion of the digits.

oligohydramnios reduction in amniotic fluid within the uterine cavity that is commonly associated with severe renal disease, intrauterine growth retardation, premature rupture of the membranes, and post-term gestation.

omphalocele anterior abdominal wall defect in which abdominal organs (liver, bowel, stomach) are atypically located within the umbilical cord. Highly associated with cardiac, central nervous system, renal, and chromosomal anomalies.

osteogenesis imperfecta metabolic disorder affecting the fetal collagen system leading to varying forms of bone disease. Intrauterine bone fractures, shortened long bones, poorly mineralized calvaria and compression of the chest may be found in type II forms.

oxytocin challenge test (OCT) electronic fetal heart rate monitoring that evaluates the fetal heart rate during uterine contractions (induced by administration of oxytocin or using nipple-stimulation method).

P

placenta previa implantation of the placenta close to or over the internal cervical os. Types include complete or total, partial, marginal, or low-lying.

- **complete or total previa** placenta completely covers the cervical os.
- **low-lying placenta** placenta implants in the lower uterine segment but does not approach the os.
- **marginal previa** placental edge is at the margin of the os.
- **partial previa** placenta partially covers the cervical os.

placental abruption the placenta separates from its site of implantation in the uterus before delivery of the fetus.

polydactyly anomalies of the hands or feet in which there is an addition of a digit. May be found in association with certain skeletal dysplasias.

polyhydramnios excessive amount of amniotic fluid, which may be associated with fetal anomalies, diabetic pregnancies, and Rh incompatibility.

prolapsed cord occurs after the rupture of amniotic membranes. The umbilical cord falls down into the vagina through the cervix. The cord is then susceptible to complete occlusion.

pseudogestational sac (decidual cast) accumulation of fluid within the endometrial cavity in ectopic gestations.

pubic symphysis a palpable midline landmark immediately anterior to the bladder, which is anterior to the uterine corpus.

pyosalpinx a pus-filled tube, resulting from an infection in the tubes most commonly from vaginal contamination and cervical ascent of bacteria.

R

renal agenesis congenital absence of one or both kidneys. Bilateral renal agenesis results in Potter's malformations and death of the newborn.

S

septic abortion an infected abortion.

serous cystadenomas simple cystic tumors usually occurring in cycling women.

shoulder dystocia delivery complication that can occur when a macrosomic fetus is delivered vaginally. There is difficulty in delivering the large shoulders after the head has passed through the vagina. Brachial plexus nerve injuries can occur.

spina bifida neural tube defect of the spine in which the dorsal vertebra (vertebral arches) fail to fuse together, allowing the protrusion of meninges and/or spinal cord through the defect. Two types exist: spina bifida occulta (skin-covered defect of the spine without protrusion of meninges or cord) and spina bifida cystica (open spinal defect marked by sac containing protruding meninges and/or cord).

spina bifida occulta closed defect of the spine without protrusion of meninges or spinal cord. Alpha-fetoprotein analysis will not detect these lesions.

standard deviation (SD) degree to which a given value deviates from the mean. Measures the variability of a distribution of parameters. In ultrasound, two standard deviations above or below the mean are considered outside of the normal range of error.

struma ovarii a teratoma composed of thyroid tissue.

symmetrical IUGR an infant small in all parameters caused by low genetic growth potential, intrauterine infection, severe maternal malnutrition, chromosomal aberration, and severe congenital anomalies.

T

tachyarrhythmia rapid beating of the heart, with rates in excess of 150, usually in the 200 to 240 range.

thanatophoric dysplasia lethal short-limbed dwarfism characterized by a marked reduction in the length of the long bones, pear-shaped chest, soft-tissue redundancy, and frequent cloverleaf skull deformity and ventriculomegaly.

threatened abortion pregnancy of less than 20 weeks complicated by bleeding or cramping. Expulsion of the products of conception may or may not occur.

tocolysis regimen using medications to stop premature labor.

transverse presentation fetus assumes a transverse orientation within the uterus.

tubo-ovarian abscess the loculation of pus resulting from the adhesive, edematous, inflamed serosa becoming further adhered to the ovary.

twin-to-twin transfusion the arterial blood of one twin is pumped into the venous system of the other twin because of an arteriovenous shunt within the placenta.

U

urethral atresia absence of the normal opening of the urethra resulting in massive enlargement of the urinary bladder.

V

ventriculomegaly abnormal accumulation of cerebrospinal fluid within the cerebral ventricles resulting in dilation of the ventricles. Compression of developing brain tissue and brain damage may result. Commonly associated with additional fetal anomalies.

version manual attempt to convert a breech fetus to a cephalic presentation to allow vaginal delivery. External cephalic version is performed through the abdomen wall using ultrasound as a guide. Version is also used to convert the second twin (Breech) during the delivery of twin fetuses.

Y

yolk sac (Vittleline duct) sac-like structure of early pregnancy, which provides nutrition for the embryo.

CARDIOLOGY

A

accessory veins intercepting veins.

aneurysm a sac formed by the dilation of the walls of an artery or a vein and filled with blood. Aneurysms may occur in any major blood vessel and include the following varieties: berry, a small saccular aneurysm of a cerebral artery, which may rupture and cause a subdural hemorrhage; cardiac, which may follow coronary occlusion; dissecting, in which blood is in between the coats of an artery; endogenous, which is due to disease of the coats of a vessel; exogenous, which is due to a wound; false, in which all the coats of the vessel are ruptured and blood is retained in the surrounding tissues; intramural, in which the blood is within the wall of the vessel; mycotic, which is produced by the growth of microorganisms in a blood vessel wall; true, in which the sac is formed by the arterial walls, one of which is unbroken (also called *circumscribed*); valvular, which is an aneurysm between the layers of a heart valve; and ventricular, which is dilation of a ventricle of the heart.

angialgia pain in a vessel; also known as *angiodynia*.

angina pectoris paroxysmal thoracic pain characterized by a feeling of suffocation and radiation of pain down the arm.

anonyma one of two large veins (right and left) that unite to form the superior vena cava. (The innominate artery is sometimes referred to as the anonyma.)

aorta the largest artery in the body. It distributes blood to the lower part of the body as the thoracic aorta and abdominal aorta and sends branches to the upper extremities from the ascending aorta.

aortic arch a continuation of the ascending aorta. It has three branches: the innominate or brachiocephalic trunk, the left common carotid artery, and the left subclavian artery.

aortic arch, hypoplasia underdevelopment of the aortic arch.

aortic arch, persistent, right aorta develops from the fourth right embryonic aortic arch; may be associated with dextroposition of the aorta as in tetralogy of Fallot.

aortic insufficiency impairment of the aorta with insufficient circulation of the blood.

aortitis inflammation of the aorta.

apex the rounded extremity of the heart pointing forward and downward and to the left. The plural form is apices.

arrhythmia variation from normal rhythm of heartbeat. This may be sinus arrhythmia; extrasystole; gallop rhythm; heart block; atrial or ventricular fibrillation and flutter; or paroxysmal tachycardia.

arterial valves semilunar valves of the aorta and pulmonary trunk.

arteriole a tiny arterial branch.

arteritis inflammation of an artery.

atrial appendage a continuation of a part of the left and right upper part of the atria (older literature refers to these appendages as auricular appendages.)

atrio a term referring to the atrium.

atrioventricular node a node at the base of the interatrial septum. It is made up of a mass of Purkinje's fibers and forms the beginning of the bundle of His. This node is also called *Aschoff's* and *Tawara's*.

atrioventricular valve valve between the atrium and ventricle of the heart. The left valve is called the *bicuspid* or *mitral valve,* and the right valve is called the *tricuspid valve*.

atrium the upper chamber on either side of the heart. The right atrium receives blood from the inferior and superior vena cava; the left receives arterial blood from the pulmonary veins. The plural form is atria.

axillary artery branch of the subclavian artery that distributes to the axilla, chest, shoulder, and upper extremity.

axillary vein continuation of the basilic vein in the upper extremity.

azygos front and right side of the lumbar vertebrae.

B

bacteremia bacteria in the blood.

bacterial endocarditis bacterial infection of the endocardium.

bicuspid valve a valve made up of two cusps, the anterior (aortic) and posterior (mural). Actually there are four cusps, including the two small commissural cusps, which are never complete in that they do not reach the anulus, or fibrous ring, around the valve and are incompletely separated from each other. This valve is also known as the *mitral valve*. It is located between the left atrium and left ventricle.

block this may be atrioventricular, sinoatrial, bundle-branch, or interventricular. In all cases, there is a blockage or obstruction to circulation.

brachial artery branch of the axillary artery that distributes to the arm. The deep brachial distributes to the inner arm structures.

bradycardia slow pulse or heartbeat.

bronchial artery a branch of either the aorta or the intercostal artery that distributes to the lungs.

bundle of His a muscular band containing nerve fibers. It arises from the atrioventricular node and connects the atria with the ventricles. It conveys stimuli from the atria to the ventricle and is sometimes called the *atrioventricular bundle* or the *AV bundle*.

C

card- and cardio- terms referring to the heart.

cardiac arrest stoppage of the heartbeat.

cardiac hypertrophy enlargement of the heart.

cardiac murmurs any adventitious sound heard over the region of the heart; may be blowing, cardiorespiratory, diastolic, harsh, presystolic, rough, or systolic.

cardiac sounds these may be diminished, intensified, or reduplicated.

cardiac veins referred to as *small, great, middle,* and *anterior veins* of the heart; also known as *venae cordis, magna, media, minimae,* and *parva*.

cardialgia heart pain; another name is *cardiodynia*.

cardiectasis dilation of the heart.

carditis inflammation of the heart.

carotid artery branch of the innominate artery (right common carotid) or the aortic arch (left common carotid) that distributes to the right or left side of the head. The common carotid further divides into the internal, distributing to the inner structures of the head, and the external, distributing to the external structures of the head.

chordae tendineae tendinous strings resembling cords that act like the shrouds of a parachute to keep the cusps in position when closed. They extend from the cusps of valves to the papillary muscles of the heart.

coarctation of aorta diffuse involvement of the aortic isthmus with narrowing and constriction of the aorta.

congestive heart failure sudden fatal cessation of the heart's action.

conus arteriosus upper and anterior angle of the right ventricle from which the pulmonary trunk arises superiorly and passes backward and slightly upward.

cor Latin term for heart.

cor pulmonale heart disease produced by disease of the lungs or of their blood vessels; pulmonary heart disease.

coronary arteries and veins blood vessels of the heart.

coronary artery a left or right artery that arises from a coronary sinus in the heart and distributes to either the left ventricle and atrium or the right ventricle and atrium.

coronary heart disease disease of the heart with involvement of the coronary vessels.

coronary vein great cardiac vein of the heart and its branches.

cusp a triangular segment of the cardiac valve; also called *leaflet*. *Cusp* means point.

D

dextrocardia the heart is displaced to the right side of the thoracic cavity.

dextroposition, aorta the aorta is displaced to the right.

diastole dilation or stage of dilation of the heart, especially that of the ventricles.

ductus arteriosus a channel in the fetus for circulation from the pulmonary artery to the aorta. This should close after birth, but if it does not, it creates a patent ductus arteriosus, a congenital anomaly.

ductus venosus a fetal vein that connects the umbilical vein with the inferior vena cava.

E

Eisenmenger's complex defects of the interventricular septum with dilation of the pulmonary artery, hypertrophy of the right ventricle, and dextroposition or dextrolocation of the aorta.

electrocardiogram a graphic tracing of the electric current produced by conduction through the heart muscle.

embolism the sudden blocking of an artery or vein by a clot or obstruction that has been brought to its place by the bloodstream. The embolus can also be air.

endarteritis inflammation of the tunica intima of an artery.

endarteritis deformans chronic endarteritis characterized by fatty degeneration of the arterial tissues, with the formation of deposits of lime salts.

endarteritis obliterans endarteritis followed by collapse and closure of smaller branches.

endocarditis infection or inflammation of the endocardium. It may be acute bacterial, subacute bacterial, mycotic (caused by a fungus), verrucous, rheumatic, or septic (malignant).

endocardium inner lining of the heart.

epicardium external covering of the heart; it is a portion of the pericardium.

F

fibroma a tumor made up of fibrous connective tissue.

foramen ovale opening between the atria in fetal life. It is normally closed after birth.

H

hemangioma a blood vessel tumor.

hematemesis vomiting blood.

hematopericardium or hemopericardium effusion of blood within the pericardium.

hematoperitoneum effusion of blood within the peritoneum.

hemothorax collection of blood in the thoracic cavity.

hypertensive heart disease high blood pressure.

I

infarction the formation of an infarct (i.e., an area of coagulation necrosis in a tissue caused by local anemia resulting from the obstruction of circulation to the area); may be embolic or thrombotic.

innominate artery branch of the aortic arch that distributes to the right side of the head, neck, and upper limbs; also called *brachiocephalic trunk.*

innominate vein a vein corresponding to the innominate artery; also called *anonyma.*

intercostal ribs and chest region.

interventricular between ventricles.

interventricular artery a branch of the left or right coronary artery that distributes to the heart ventricles or their septa.

M

mammary artery an internal artery that is a branch of the subclavian artery and distributes to the anterior abdominal wall and mediastinal structures

mammary vein internal vein of the breast.

mediastinal mediastinum.

mitral insufficiency impairment of mitral valve with malfunctioning.

mitral valve see **bicuspid valve.**

myocarditis inflammation of heart muscle.

myocardium middle muscular layer of the heart.

N

nodes see **sinoatrial** and **atrioventricular nodes.**

O

oblique, left atrium atrium.

occlusion obstruction of a blood vessel; may be caused by a thrombus or an embolus.

P

pacemaker sinoatrial node that initiates the heartbeat and regulates the rate of contraction.

palpitation rapid action of the heart felt by the patient.

panarteritis inflammation of several arteries.

patent ductus arteriosus an open duct between the great vessels, which in fetal life was a channel from the pulmonary artery to the aorta and should have closed at birth.

periarteritis nodosa inflammation of the coats of small- and medium-sized arteries with changes around the vessels and symptoms of systemic infection.

pericardiac heart.

pericarditis inflammation or infection of a membrane containing the heart.

pericardium membrane surrounding to the heart.

phlebitis inflammation of a vein.

phlebo- combining form referring to vein.

phrenic arteries the inferior phrenic artery is a branch of the abdominal aorta and distributes to the diaphragm and adrenals. The superior phrenic arteries are branches of the thoracic aorta and distribute to the upper surface of the vertebral portion of the diaphragm.

phrenic veins anterior and superior veins of the diaphragm.

plexus network of veins (may also refer to nerves and lymphatics.)

polyarteritis inflammation of several arteries.

polyserositis inflammation of the serous membranes with the serous effusion.

portal liver, eventually forming sinusoids of liver.

pulmonary arteries that originate in the conus arteriosus and distribute to the lungs.

pulmonary, right and left vessels that return blood to the heart from the lungs.

pulmonary stenosis narrowing of the opening between the pulmonary artery and the right ventricle. The stenosis may be at the site of the valve, just prevalvular, or postvalvular (arterial); also called *pulmonic stenosis.*

pulmonary valve valve at the base of the pulmonary artery; also called *semilunar valve.*

pulse variation may be alternating (pulsus alternans); bigeminal (occurring in two's); bounding; bradycardic, irregular; plateau (a pulse that slowly rises and is sustained); running; tachycardic; thready; trembling, undulating; and vibrating (jerky).

R

rhabdomyoma a malignant tumor composed of myoma and sarcoma combined.

S

semi-lunar valve pulmonary or aortic valve.

septal defects, atrial or ventricular these may be interatrial, with defects located between the atria, or interventricular, with defects located between the ventricles.

septicemia presence of pathogenic bacteria or toxins in the blood.

sinoatrial node a well-defined collection of cells at the junction of the superior vena cava with the terminal band of the right atrium. It is called the *pacemaker of the heart.*

subclavian arteries branch of the innominate artery (right subclavian) or the aortic arch (left subclavian) that distributes to the neck, upper limbs, thoracic wall, spinal cord, brain, and meninges.

subclavian veins right and left veins of the arms and upper extremity.
subcostal branch of the thoracic aorta that distributes to the region below the twelfth rib in the abdominal wall.
superior and inferior vena cava large veins that return blood to the heart. The superior vena cava returns blood from the upper extremities, and the inferior vena cava returns it from the lower extremities.
systole a period of heart contraction, especially of the ventricles. Atrial systole precedes the true, or ventricular, systole.

T

tachycardia characterized by a fast pulse or heartbeat.
teratoma a tumor composed of disorderly arrangement of tissue, the result of an embryonic defect. Teratomas also occur in the ovary.
tetralogy of Fallot this includes four anomalies as follows: pulmonic stenosis; dextroposition of the aorta; a large interventricular septal defect; and marked hypertrophy of the right ventricle; also called *Fallot's tetrad.*
thromboangiitis inflammation of the intima of a blood vessel with thrombi or clots. When obliterans is added, it means inflammatory and obliterative disease of the blood vessels.
thrombophlebitis inflammation or infection of a vein with clot formation.
transposition of the aorta and pulmonary artery aorta arising from the right ventricle and the pulmonary artery from the left ventricle; also called *transposition of the great vessels.*
tricuspid incompetency impairment of the tricuspid valve, with incompetent functioning.
tricuspid valve a valve between the right atrium and the right ventricle, consisting of an anterior, a medial (septal), and one or two posterior cusps. The depth of the commissures between cusps is variable, never reaching the anulus (Fibrous ring). Cusps are only incompletely separated from each other.

V

valves structures in a canal or passage that prevent the reflux of contents. The valves in the heart are the aortic (semi-lunar); the atrioventricular (mitral and tricuspid); and pulmonic (semilunar). Valves also occur in veins.
varicose veins swollen veins.
venae vasorum small veins that return blood from the walls of blood vessels themselves.
veno term referring to vein.
venules small veins.

PERIPHERAL VASCULAR AND VASCULAR SONOGRAPHY

A

angle correction a method of electronically compensating for the curvature of a vessel when using a steerable pulsed Doppler to obtain an accurate angle and accurate blood flow velocity.
antegrade flow flow toward the Doppler transducer face.

D

Doppler (equipment) a sonographic device that allows the measurement of moving media, such as blood, by measuring the Doppler shift of the reflected ultrasound beam.

Q

quadrature interface a Doppler feature that electronically isolates antegrade and retrograde signals and that allows displaying directional signals simultaneously in their respective directions and respective strengths.

R

retrograde flow flow away from the Doppler transducer face.

S

sample depth the variable depth at which a pulsed Doppler sample can be taken.
sample volume a Doppler gate on a pulsed Doppler that allows a specific area of the flow in a blood vessel to be sampled. The sample volume can be varied by the user from a small size to a large size.
spectral analysis a method of analyzing and displaying the frequency and flow components of a Doppler signal.
spectral broadening a change in the spectral width, which increases with flow disturbance. It can be fairly narrow with a prominent spectral window in a normal waveform, or it can be spread out and widened with filling or in absence of the window when flow is turbulent or disturbed.
spectral width during peak systole, the distance between the outer border at the peak of the waveform and the upper border of the spectral window.
spectral window a relatively clear area within the Doppler spectral waveform indicating a lack of slow-moving blood cells.

V

vector line an adjustable line seen at the sample volume, which is adjusted to obtain a Doppler vessel angle correction with a pulsed Doppler.

W

window see **spectral window.**

Z

zero-crossing circuit a Doppler circuit that averages antegrade and retrograde flow signals into a net flow readout on a chart recorder.

Index

O

P